MW01260074

Clinical Scenarios in Vascular Surgery

SECOND EDITION

Clinical Scenarios in Vascular Surgery

SECOND EDITION

Editors

Gilbert R. Upchurch Jr, MD
Chief of Vascular and Endovascular Surgery
William H. Muller Jr Professor of Surgery
Professor of Molecular Physiology and Biological Physics
University of Virginia
Charlottesville, Virginia

Peter K. Henke, MD
Leland Ira Doan Professor of Surgery
Chief, Vascular Surgery AAVA
University of Michigan
Ann Arbor, Michigan

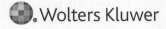

Wolters Kluwer

Philadelphia • Baltimore • New York • London
Buenos Aires • Hong Kong • Sydney • Tokyo

Acquisitions Editor: Keith Donnellan
Product Development Editor: Brendan Huffman
Production Project Manager: Bridgett Dougherty
Design Coordinator: Holly McLaughlin
Senior Manufacturing Coordinator: Beth Welsh
Strategic Marketing Manager: Daniel Dressler
Production Service: SPi Global

Second Edition

Library of Congress Cataloging-in-Publication Data
Clinical scenarios in vascular surgery / [edited by] Gilbert R. Upchurch, Peter K. Henke. — Second edition.
    p. ; cm.
  Includes bibliographical references and index.
  ISBN 978-1-4511-9213-1 (alk. paper)
 I. Upchurch, Gilbert R., editor. II. Henke, Peter K., editor.
  [DNLM: 1. Vascular Surgical Procedures—methods—Case Reports. 2. Diagnostic Techniques, Surgical—Case Reports. 3. Vascular Diseases—diagnosis—Case Reports. WG 170]
  RD598.5
  617.4'13—dc23
                                                                        2014046110

As the world continues to be more complex and chaotic,
I can always count on my wife Nancy for her calm and support;
I am thankful for her as she has never even once made me feel guilty
for all the extra time it requires to write and edit books.

— Gilbert R Upchurch, Jr., MD

To my parents, for all their loving support.

— Peter K. Henke, MD

Contributing Authors

Matthew R. Abate, MD
Resident
Section of Vascular Surgery
University of Arkansas
Little Rock, Arkansas

Joshua D. Adams, MD
Vascular Surgery Fellow
Department of Surgery
University of Virginia Health System
Charlottesville, Virginia

Gorav Ailawadi, MD
Associate Professor
Cardiac Surgery and Biomedical Engineering
Director
Minimally Invasive Cardiac Surgery
Surgical Director
Advanced Cardiac Valve Center
Chair
VCSQI Research & Writing Committee
University of Virginia Health System
Charlottesville, Virginia

Ahsan T. Ali, MD
Associate Professor
Department of Surgery
University of Arkansas for Medical Sciences
Little Rock, Arizona

Elizabeth Andraska, BA
Section of Vascular Surgery
Department of Surgery
University of Michigan
Ann Arbor, Michigan

Julie Armatas, NP
Nurse Practioner
Division of Vascular and Endovascular Surgery
University of Virginia
Charlottesville, Virginia

Shipra Arya, MD, SM
Assistant Professor
Division of Vascular Surgery and Endovascular Therapy
Department of Surgery
Emory University School of Medicine
Atlanta, Georgia

Olufunmi Onaopemipo Awonuga, MD
Resident
Division of General Surgery
Department of Surgery
University of Alabama at Birmingham School of
    Medicine
Birmingham, Alabama

Amir Azarbal, MD
Assistant Professor of Vascular and Endovascular
    Surgery
Oregon Health and Science University
Portland, Oregon

Ali Azizzadeh, MD
Associate Professor
Director
Endovascular Surgery
Memorial Hermann Heart and Vascular Institute—
    Texas Medical Center
Department of Cardiothoracic and Vascular Surgery
University of Texas Medical School at Houston
Houston, Texas

Atif Baqai, MD
Vascular Surgery Fellow
Vascular and Endovascular Surgery
University of Miami Hospital
Miami, Florida

B. Timothy Baxter, MD
Professor
Department of Surgery
Division of General Surgery
University of Nebraska Medical Center
Omaha, Nebraska

Rodney P. Bensley Jr, MD
General Surgery Resident
Beth Israel Deaconess Medical Center
Boston, Massachusetts

Scott A. Berceli, MD, PhD
Professor of Surgery and Biomedical Engineering
Chief
Vascular Surgery
Malcom Randall VA Medical Center
UF Health School of Medicine
Gainesville, Florida

Guido H. W. van Bogerijen, MD
Department of Cardiac Surgery
Samuel and Jean Frankel Cardiovascular Center
University of Michigan Health System
Ann Arbor, Michigan

Arash Bornak, MD
Assistant Professor of Surgery
Vascular and Endovascular Surgery
University of Miami Hospital
Miami, Florida

Thomas C. Bower, MD
Professor of Surgery
Department of Surgery
Division of Vascular and Endovascular
    Surgery
Mayo Clinic College of Medicine
Rochester, Minnesota

Michael B. Brewer, MD
Associate Professor of Cardiovascular
    Medicine
Division of Cardiovascular Medicine
University of Michigan Health System
Ann Arbor, Michigan

Robert D. Brook, MD
Assistant Professor of Medicine
Department of Internal Medicine
University of Michigan
Department of Internal Medicine
University of Michigan Hospital
Ann Arbor, Michigan

Stephanie M. Carvalho, BA
Clinical Research Coordinator
Massachusetts General Hospital
Boston, Massachusetts

Rabih A. Chaer, MD
Department of Surgery
University of Pittsburgh
Pittsburgh, Pennsylvania

Kristofer M. Charlton-Ouw, MD
Assistant Professor
Department of Cardiothoracic and Vascular
    Surgery
Memorial Hermann Heart and Vascular Institute—
    Texas Medical Center
University of Texas Medical School at
    Houston
Houston, Texas

Kenneth J. Cherry, MD
Professor of Surgery
Vascular and Endovascular Surgery
University of Virginia Health System
Charlottesville, Virginia

Giye Choe, MD
General Surgery Resident
Oregon Health and Science University
Portland, Oregon

W. Darrin Clouse, MD, RPVI
Mass General Hospital
Boston, Massachusetts

Dawn M. Coleman, MD
Assistant Professor of Vascular Surgery
Cardiovascular Center
University of Michigan
Ann Arbor, Michigan

Mark Conrad, MS, MD
Assistant Professor of Surgery
Division of Vascular Surgery
Massachusetts General Hospital
Harvard University
Boston, Massachusetts

Mark F. Conrad, MD, MMSc
Director
Clinical Research
Assistant Professor of Surgery
Harvard Medical School
Division of Vascular and Endovascular Surgery
Massachusetts General Hospital
Boston, Massachusetts

Michael S. Conte, MD
Professor of Surgery
Chief
Division of Vascular and Endovascular Surgery
University of California, San Francisco School of
    Medicine
San Francisco, California

Robert S. Crawford, MD
Assistant Professor of Surgery
Division of Vascular Surgery
University of Maryland School of Medicine
Co-director
Center for Aortic Diseases
University of Maryland Medical Center
Baltimore, Maryland

Jason Crowner, MD
University of North Carolina School of Medicine
Chapel Hill, North Carolina

Alan Dardik, MD, PhD
Department of Surgery
Yale University School of Medicine
New Haven, Connecticut
VA Connecticut Healthcare System
West Haven, Connecticut

R. Clement Darling III, MD
Professor of Surgery
Chief, Division of Vascular Surgery
Director, The Institute for Vascular Health and Disease
President, The Vascular Group
University of Albany
Albany, New York

Narasimham L. Dasika, MD
Associate Professor
Vascular and Interventional Radiology
University of Michigan Health System
Ann Arbor, Michigan

Mark G. Davies, MD, PhD, MBA
Houston Methodist DeBakey Heart & Vascular Center
Department of Cardiovascular Surgery
Houston Methodist Hospital
Houston, Texas

John P. Davis, MD
Resident in General Surgery
University of Virginia
Charlottesville, Virginia

Calogero Dimaggio, DO
Section of Vascular and Endovascular Surgery
Geisinger Medical Center
Danville, Pennsylvania

Paul D. DiMusto, MD
Fellow in Vascular Surgery
University of Michigan
Ann Arbor, Michigan

Salvatore Docimo Jr, DO, MS
Lutheran Medical Center
Brooklyn, New York

Audra A. Duncan, MD
Professor of Surgery
Mayo Clinic
Rochester, Minnesota

Matthew S. Edwards, MD, MS
Associate Professor, Vascular and Endovascular Surgery
Chair Vascular and Endovascular Surgery
Wake Forest University
Winston-Salem, North Carolina

Charles M. Eichler, MD
Professor of Surgery
Division of Vascular & Endovascular Surgery
Director
General Surgery Residency Program
Department of Surgery
University of California, San Francisco School of Medicine
San Francisco, California

Jonathan L. Eliason, MD
Associate Professor of Surgery
Division of Vascular Surgery
University of Michigan
Ann Arbor, Michigan

Anna Eliassen, MD
Section of Vascular Surgery
Department of Surgery
School of Medicine
University of Michigan
Ann Arbor, Michigan

James R. Elmore, MD
Section of Vascular and Endovascular Surgery
Geisinger Medical Center
Danville, Pennsylvania

Travis L. Engelbert, MD
Department of Vascular Surgery
Saint Joseph Hospital
Denver, Colorado

Guillermo A. Escobar, MD
Assistant Professor of Surgery
Vascular Surgery Division
University of Arkansas for Medical Sciences
Little Rock, Arkansas

Mark K. Eskandari, MD
Chief
Division of Vascular Surgery
Northwestern University Feinberg School of Medicine
Chicago, Illinois

Mohammad H. Eslami, MD
Associate Professor of Surgery
Division of Vascular and Endovascular Surgery
Boston University School of Medicine
Boston, Massachusetts

Zachariah K. Eslami, MD
Department of Physics
Colby College
Waterville, Maine

James M. Estes, MD
Assistant Professor of Surgery
Tufts University School of Medicine
Attending Surgeon
Division of Vascular Surgery
New England Medical Center
Boston, Massachusetts

Avery J. Evans, MD
Professor of Radiology
Neurology and Neurological Surgery
University of Virginia Health System
Charlottesville, Virginia

Peter L. Faries, MD
The Franz W. Sichel Professor of Surgery
Professor of Radiology
Chief
Division of Vascular Surgery
Icahn School of Medicine at Mount Sinai
New York, New York

Daniel Fremed, MD
Division of Vascular Surgery
Icahn School of Medicine at Mt Sinai
New York, New York

Katherine Gallagher, MD
Assistant Professor of Surgery
Division of Vascular Surgery
University of Michigan
Ann Arbor, Michigan

Antonios P. Gasparis, MD, RPVI
Associate Professor of Surgery
Division of Vascular Surgery
Stony Brook University Medical Center
Stony Brook, New York

Jonathan D. Gates, MD
Associate Professor of Surgery
Division of Vascular Surgery
Brigham and Women's Hospital
Harvard University
Boston, Massachusetts

Andrew G. Georgiadis, MD
Chief Resident
Department of Orthopaedic Surgery
Henry Ford Hospital
Detroit, Michigan

Patrick J. Geraghty, MD
Associate Professor of Surgery and Radiology
Washington University
St Louis, Missouri

David L. Gillespie, MD, RVT
Chief, Department of Vascular and Endovascular
    Surgery
Cardiovascular Care Center
Southcoast Health System
Dartmouth, Massachusetts

Peter Gloviczki, MD
Professor of Surgery
Division of Vascular and Endovascular Surgery
Mayo Clinic
Rochester, Minnesota

Prateek K. Gupta, MD
Vascular Surgery Fellow
Department of Vascular and Endovascular Surgery
University of Wisconsin Hospital and Clinics
Madison, Wisconsin

Raul J. Guzman, MD
Associate Professor of Surgery
Harvard Medical School
Beth Israel Deaconess Medical Center
Boston, Massachusetts

Pantelis Hadjizacheria, MD
Division of Vascular Surgery
Department of Surgery
University of Maryland
Baltimore, Maryland

Sukgu M. Han, MD
Clinical Fellow
Division of Vascular and Endovascular Surgery
University of California, San Francisco School of
    Medicine
San Francisco, California

Donald G. Harris, MD
General Surgery Resident
Department of Surgery
University of Maryland School of Medicine
Baltimore, Maryland

Surovi Hazarika, MD
Fellow
Division of Cardiovascular Medicine
Department of Internal Medicine
University of Virginia School of Medicine
Charlottesville, Virginia

Mark R. Hemmila, MD
Associate Professor of Surgery
Department of Surgery
University of Michigan Health System
Ann Arbor, Michigan

Peter K. Henke, MD
Professor of Surgery
Section of Vascular Surgery
University of Michigan
Ann Arbor, Michigan

Anil Hingorani, MD
Lutheran Medical Center
Brooklyn, New York

Liangge Hsu, MD
Division of Neuroradiology
Department of Radiology
Brigham and Women's Hospital
Assistant Professor
Harvard Medical School
Boston, Massachusetts

Thomas S. Huber, MD, PhD
Professor
Department of Surgery
Chief
Division of Vascular Surgery and Endovascular
    Therapy
University of Florida College of Medicine
Gainesville, Florida

Justin Hurie, MD
Assistant Professor
Department of Vascular and Endovascular
    Surgery
Wake Forest Baptist Medical Center
Winston-Salem, North Carolina

Arsalla Islam, MD
Wake Forest University
Winston-Salem, North Carolina

Elizabeth A. Jackson, MD, MPH
Associate Professor of Cardiovascular
    Medicine
University of Michigan Health System
Ann Arbor, Michigan

Benjamin Jacobs, MD
Department of Surgery
University of Michigan
Ann Arbor, Michigan

Kamran A. Jafree, MBBS
Fellow
University of Albany
Albany, New York

Amit Jain, MBBS, MS
Fellow in Vascular and Endovascular Surgery
Department of Surgery
University of Virginia Health System
Charlottesville, Virginia

Arjun Jayaraj, MBBS
Vascular Surgery Fellow
Division of Vascular and Endovascular Surgery
Department of Surgery
Mayo Clinic
Rochester, Minnesota

Mary E. Jensen, MD
Professor of Radiology
Neurology and Neurological Surgery
Department of Radiology and Medical Imaging
Director
Interventional Neuroradiology
University of Virginia Health System
Charlottesville, Virginia

William Forrest Johnston, MD
Division of Vascular and Endovascular Surgery
University of Virginia
Charlottesville, Virginia

Randolph Todd C. Jones, MD
Division of Vascular Surgery
New York University Langone Medical Center
New York, New York

William D. Jordan Jr, MD
Department of Surgery
Professor
Director
Division of Vascular Surgery and Endovascular Therapy
Program director of Vascular Surgery Residency and
    Fellowship
University of Alabama at Birmingham School of
    Medicine
Birmingham, Alabama

Jason P. Jundt, MD
Fellow
Vascular and Endovascular Surgery
Oregon Health & Science University
Portland, Oregon

Enjae Jung, MD
Division of Vascular Surgery
Department of Surgery
Washington University
St Louis, Missouri

Loay S. Kabbani, MD
Assistant Professor of Surgery
Henry Ford Hospital
Detroit, Michigan

Lowell S. Kabnick, MD, RPhS
Associate Professor
Department of Surgery
Division of Vascular Surgery
Director of Vein Center
New York University Langone Medical Center
New York, New York

Andrew S. Kaufman, MD
Uniformed Health Services
Bethesda, Maryland

Andrew Kimball, MD
Department of Surgery
University of Michigan
Ann Arbor, Michigan

Martyn Knowles, MD
Division of Vascular Surgery
Department of Surgery
University of Texas-Southwestern
Dallas, Texas

Venkataramu N. Krishnamurthy, MD
Clinical Associate Professor, Radiology and Vascular
    Surgery
Chief, Radiology Services
University of Michigan Hospital
Ann Arbor, Michigan

Hari R. Kumar, MD
Vascular Surgery Fellow
Division of Vascular Surgery
Northwestern University Feinberg School of
    Medicine
Chicago, Illinois

Christopher J. Kwolek, MD
Chief, Vascular and Endovascular Surgery
Newton-Wellesley Hospital
Training Program Director
Vascular and Endovascular Surgery
Massachusetts General Hospital
Associate Professor of Surgery
Harvard Medical School
Boston, Massachusetts

James Laredo, MD, PhD
Vascular Surgery
The GW Medical Faculty Associates
George Washington University
Reston, Virginia

Andrew Leake, MD
Department of Surgery
University of Pittsburgh
Pittsburgh, Pennsylvania

Andy Lee, MD
Department of Surgery
Beth Israel Deaconess Medical Center
Boston, Massachusetts

Byung Boong Lee, MD, PhD
Clinical Professor of Surgery
Division of Vascular Surgery
Department of Surgery
George Washington University Medical
    Center
Washington, District of Columbia

Cheong J. Lee, MD
Assistant Professor of Surgery
Vascular Surgery Division
Medical College of Wisconsin
Milwaukee, Wisconsin

Timothy K. Liem, MD
Associate Professor of Surgery
Vice-Chair, Department of Surgery
Oregon Health & Science University
Portland, Oregon

Kira N. Long, MD
Uniformed Services University
Bethesda, Maryland

G. Matthew Longo, MD
Associate Professor
Chief
Vascular Surgery
University of Nebraska Medical Center
Omaha, Nebraska

John B. Luke, MD
Division of Vascular Surgery and Endovascular
    Therapy
University of Alabama at Birmingham
Birmingham, Alabama

Fedor Lurie, MD, PhD
Associate Director
Research, Education, and Vascular Laboratory
Jobst Vascular Institute
Toledo, Ohio

Jennifer J. Majersik, MD, MS
Associate Professor
University of Utah
Salt Lake City, Utah

Rafael D. Malgor, MD, RPVI
Chief Resident
Vascular Surgery Integrated Residency
Division of Vascular Surgery
Stony Brook University Medical Center
Stony Brook, New York

Michael J. Malinowski, MD
Assistant Professor
Department of Surgery
Vascular Surgery Division
Medical College of Wisconsin
Milwaukee, Wisconsin

M. Ashraf Mansour, MD
Chair
Department of Surgery
Academic Chair
Department of Surgical Specialties
Spectrum Health Medical Group
Michigan State University College of Human
    Medicine
Grand Rapids, Michigan

Jesse Manunga, MD
Division of Vascular & Endovascular Surgery
Abbott Northwestern Hospital
Minneapolis, Minnesota

William Marston, MD
Professor
Department of Surgery
Chief
Division of Vascular Surgery
University of North Carolina School of
    Medicine
Chapel Hill, North Carolina

Elna Masuda, MD
Associate Professor of Surgery
University of Hawaii Surgical Residency
    Program
Honolulu, Hawaii

Jeff Mathew, MD
Division of Vascular Surgery
Department of Surgery
Henry Ford Hospital
Detroit, Michigan

Katharine L. McGinigle, MD, MPH
Fellow, Vascular Surgery
Duke University
Durham, North Carolina

James T. McPhee, MD
Division of Vascular Surgery
VA Boston Healthcare Systems
West Roxbury, Massachusetts
Assistant Professor of Surgery
Boston University School of Medicine
Boston, Massachusetts

Manish Mehta, MD, MPH
Professor of Surgery
Division of Vascular Surgery
The Institute for Vascular Health and Disease
University of Albany
Albany, New York

George H. Meier, MD
Chief, Vascular Surgery
University of Cincinnati
Cincinnati, Ohio

Matthew T. Menard, MD
Assistant Professor of Surgery
Brigham and Women's Hospital
Harvard University
Boston, Massachusetts

Tetsuro Miyata, MD, PhD
Department of Surgery
Division of Vascular Surgery
Graduate School of Medicine
The University of Tokyo, Japan
Tokyo, Japan

J. Gregory Modrall, MD
Professor of Surgery
Division of Vascular Surgery
UT- Southwestern
Dallas, Texas

Carla C. Moreira, MD
Vascular Surgery Fellow
Boston University Medical Center
Boston, Massachusetts

Mohammed M. Moursi, MD
Professor
Division of Vascular Surgery
University of Arkansas
Little Rock, Arkansas

Michelle Mueller, MD
Associate Professor
Vascular Surgery
University of Utah
Salt Lake City, Utah

Vijaiganesh Nagarajan, MD, MRCP
Fellow
Division of Cardiovascular Medicine
University of Virginia
Charlottesville, Virginia

Mark Nehler, MD
The Michael W. Dunaway Chair in Vascular Surgery
Vice Chair of Education for Surgery
Chief
Section of Vascular Surgery and Endovascular
    Therapy and Podiatry
University of Colorado
Aurora, Colorado

Timothy E. Newhook, MD
Resident in General Surgery
Department of Surgery
University of Virginia Health System
Charlottesville, Virginia

Louis L. Nguyen, MD, MBA, MPH
Associate Professor of Surgery
Division of Vascular & Endovascular Surgery
Brigham & Women's Hospital
Harvard Medical School
Boston, Massachusetts

Paula M. Novelli, MD
Clinical Assistant Professor
University of Michigan Health System
Ann Arbor, Michigan

Andrea T. Obi, MD
Resident in General Surgery
University of Michigan
Ann Arbor, Michigan

Marlene O'Brien, MD
Department of Surgery
University of Rochester
Rochester, New York

Gustavo S. Oderich, MD
Professor of Surgery
Director of Endovascular Therapy
Director of Clinical Research Edward Rogers
    Fellowship
Division of Vascular and Endovascular Surgery
Mayo Clinic Medical College
Rochester, Minnesota

Nicholas Osborne, MD
Assistant Professor of Surgery
University of Michigan
Ann Arbor, Michigan

Mohamed F. Osman, MD
Brigham and Women's Hospital
Boston, Massachusetts

Christopher D. Owens, MD
Associate Professor of Surgery
Division of Vascular and Endovascular Surgery
University of California, San Francisco
San Francisco, California

C. Keith Ozaki, MD
Division of Vascular and Endovascular
    Surgery
Department of Surgery
Brigham and Women's Hospital
Harvard Medical School
Boston, Massachusetts

Marc A. Passman, MD
Professor of Surgery
Division of Vascular Surgery & Endovascular
    Therapy
University of Alabama at Birmingham School of
    Medicine
Birmingham, Alabama

Himanshu J. Patel, MD
Associate Professor of Surgery
Department of Cardiac Surgery
University of Michigan Health System
Ann Arbor, Michigan

Philip K. Paty, MD
Professor of Surgery
Division of Vascular Surgery
The Institute for Vascular Health and Disease
University of Albany
Albany, New York

Philip S.K. Paty, MD
Associate Professor of Surgery
Albany Medical Center
Albany, New York

Amani D. Politano, MD, MS
Resident in General Surgery
Department of Surgery
University of Virginia
Charlottesville, Virginia

Nicolas H. Pope, MD
Resident in General Surgery
Cardiovascular Research Fellow
University of Virginia Health System
Charlottesville, Virginia

Joseph D. Raffetto, MD
Associate Professor of Surgery
Harvard Medical School
Chief of Vascular Surgery
VA Boston Healthcare System
Boston, Massachusetts

T. Konrad Rajab, MD
Clinical Fellow in Surgery
Department of Surgery
Brigham and Women's Hospital
Boston, Massachusetts

Sanjay Rajagopalan, MD
Professor of Internal Medicine
Chief, Division of Cardiology
Division of Cardiovascular Medicine
University of Maryland School of Medicine
Baltimore, Maryland

Todd E. Rasmussen, MD
Colonel USAD MC
Director
US Combat Casualty Care Research Program
Fort Detrick, Maryland
Harris B. Shumacker, Jr. Professor of Surgery
Uniformed Services University
Bethesda, Maryland

Reid A. Ravin, MD
Division of Vascular Surgery
Icahn School of Medicine at Mt Sinai
New York, New York

John Rectenwald, MD
Associate Professor of Surgery
Section of Vascular Surgery
Department of Surgery
University of Michigan
Ann Arbor, Michigan

Amy B. Reed, MD
Professor of Surgery
Division of Vascular Surgery
Penn State University
Hershey, Pennsylvania

Jorge Rey, MD
Assistant Professor of Surgery
Vascular and Endovascular Surgery
University of Miami Hospital
Miami, Florida

Yevgeniy Rits, MD
Detroit Medical Center
Wayne State University School of Medicine
Detroit, Michigan

Christopher Roark, MD
Clinical Lecturer
Department of Neurosurgery
University of Michigan Health System
Ann Arbor, Michigan

Sean P. Roddy, MD
Professor of Surgery
Division of Vascular Surgery
University of Albany
Albany, New York

Heron E. Rodriguez, MD
Associate Professor in Surgery
Division of Vascular Surgery
Northwestern University
Chicago, Illinois

Jeffrey R. Rubin, MD
Detroit Medical Center
Professor
Department of Surgery
Wayne State University School of Medicine
Detroit, Michigan

Evan J. Ryer, MD
Section of Vascular and Endovascular Surgery
Geisinger Medical Center
Danville, Pennsylvania

Wael E. Saad, MBBCh
Professor of Radiology
Division Director, Vascular & Interventional
    Radiology
Department of Radiology
University of Michigan Health System
Ann Arbor, Michigan

Julia Saraidaridis, MD
Resident in General Surgery
Massachusetts General Hospital
Harvard University
Boston, Massachusetts

Rajabrata Sarkar, MD
Professor of Surgery
Division of Vascular Surgery
University of Maryland
Baltimore, Maryland

Anna Sattah, MD
Resident in General Surgery
University of Virginia
Charlottesville, Virginia

Worthington Schenk III, MD
Professor of Surgery
University of Virginia
Charlottesville, Virginia

Marc L. Schermerhorn, MD
Chief
Division of Vascular and Endovascular
    Surgery
Beth Israel Deaconess Medical Center
Boston, Massachusetts

Marcus E. Semel, MD, MPH
Division of Vascular and Endovascular Surgery
Department of Surgery
Brigham and Women's Hospital
Boston, Massachusetts

Parthy Shah, MD
Division of Cardiovascular Medicine
University of Maryland School of Medicine
Baltimore, Maryland

Aditya M. Sharma, MBBS, RPVI
Assistant Professor
Department of Cardiovascular Medicine
University of Virginia
Charlottesville, Virginia

Alexander D. Shepard, MD
Head, Division of Vascular Surgery
Department of Surgery
Henry Ford Hospital
Detroit, Michigan

Cynthia K. Shortell, MD
Professor
Chief
Vascular Surgery
Duke University
Durham, North Carolina

Amelia J. Simpson, MD
General Surgery Resident
Department of Surgery
UW Medicine
Seattle, Washington

Matthew R. Smeds, MD
Assistant Professor of Surgery
University of Arkansas for Medical Sciences
Little Rock, Arkansas

Andrew M. Southerland, MD, MSc
Assistant Professor
Department of Neurology
University of Virginia
Charlottesville, Virginia

William M. Stone, MD
Professor of Surgery
Department of Vascular and Endovascular Surgery
Mayo Clinic College of Medicine
Phoenix, Arizona

Randall Sung, MD
Associate Professor
Department of Surgery
Surgical Director
University of Michigan Health System
Ann Arbor, Michigan

Girma Tefera, MD
Professor of Surgery
Vice Chairman, Division of Vascular Surgery
UW Health, School of Medicine and Public
    Health
Madison, Wisconsin

Mehdi J. Teymouri, MD
Division of Vascular Surgery
The Institute for Vascular Health and Disease
University of Albany
Albany, New York

B. Gregory Thompson, MD
J.E. McGillicuddy Professor and Program
    Director
Department of Neurosurgery
University of Michigan
Ann Arbor, Michigan

Robert W. Thompson, MD
Professor of Surgery
Vascular, Radiology, and Cell Biology and
    Physiology
Director
Thoracic Outlet Syndrome Center
Washington University School of Medicine in
    St. Louis
St. Louis, Missouri

Carlos H. Timaran, MD
Associate Professor of Surgery
Division of Vascular Surgery
UT Southwestern
Dallas, Texas

Jip L. Tolenaar, MD
Post-doctoral Fellow
Department of Surgery
University of Virginia
Charlottesville, Virginia

Margaret Clarke Tracci, MD
Assistant Professor
Division of Vascular and Endovascular
    Surgery
University of Virginia
Charlottesville, Virginia

Nam T. Tran, MD
Associate Professor of Surgery
Harborview Medical Center
University of Washington
Seattle, Washington

Santi Trimarchi, MD, PhD
Department of Cardiovascular Surgery
Policlinico San Donato IRCCS
Director of Thoracic Aortic Research Center
University of Milano
San Donato Milanese Milan, Italy

Gianbattista Tshiombo, MD
Department of Cardiovascular Surgery
Policinico San Donato IRCCS
Director of Thoracic Aortuc Research Center
University of Milano
San Donato Milanese Milan, Italy

William D. Turnipseed, MD
Professor of Surgery
University of Wisconsin
Madison, Wisconsin

Gilbert R. Upchurch Jr, MD
Chief of Vascular and Endovascular Surgery
William H. Muller Jr Professor of Surgery
Professor of Molecular Physiology and Biological
    Physics
University of Virginia
Charlottesville, Virginia

Omaida C. Velazquez, MD
Professor of Surgery
Division Chief of Vascular and Endovascular
    Surgery
University of Miami Hospital
Miami, Florida

Chandu Vemuri, MD
Assistant Professor of Vascular Surgery
Washington University School of Medicine in St. Louis
St. Louis, Missouri

Seth Waits, MD
Resident in General Surgery
Department of Surgery
University of Michigan Health System
Ann Arbor, Michigan

Thomas W. Wakefield, MD
JC Stanley Professor of Surgery
Section of Vascular Surgery
University of Michigan
Ann Arbor, Michigan

Bo Wang, MD
Surgical Resident
Vascular and Endovascular Surgery
University of Miami Hospital
Miami, Florida

Linda Wang, MD
Resident
Harvard Medical School
Massachusetts General Hospital
Boston, Massachusetts

Luke R. Wilkins, MD
Assistant Professor of Radiology and Medical Imaging
Section of Vascular and Interventional Radiology
University of Virginia
Charlottesville, Virginia

David M. Williams, MD
Professor of Radiology
University of Michigan Health System
Ann Arbor, Michigan

Timothy K. Williams, MD
Assistant Clinic Professor
UC-Davis
Sacramento, California

Karen Woo, MD
Assistant Professor of Surgery
Keck School of Medicine USC
Los Angeles, California

Bradford B. Worrall, MD, MSc
Professor of Neurology
University of Virginia
Charlottesville, Virginia

Kota Yamamoto, MD, PhD
Department of Surgery
Yale University School of Medicine
New Haven, Connecticut
Department of Surgery
VA Connecticut Healthcare System
West Haven, Connecticut
Division of Vascular Surgery
Department of Surgery
Graduate School of Medicine
The University of Tokyo, Japan
Tokyo, Japan

Dustin Y. Yoon, MD
Division of Vascular Surgery
Northwestern University Feinberg School
    of Medicine
Chicago, Illinois

Foreword

*C*linical Scenarios in Vascular Surgery, Second Edition, belongs on the desk of every trainee and physician caring for patients with vascular disease. This book has been markedly expanded to include the entirety of common open surgical and endovascular interventions for both arterial and venous diseases. During the more than a half decade since the first edition, the care of patients with vascular disease has undergone dramatic changes. Improvements in the diagnosis and treatment have generated many new words, new tests, and new procedures, which must be part of the lexicon of contemporary practitioners.

The most notable additions to this book are the inclusion of nearly twice as many chapters and the presence of multiple choice questions following each that will reinforce the salient information in practical terms. In addition, given the clear departure from classic lectures in a quiet auditorium or reading page after page of encyclopedic textbooks, this work is much more pragmatic and will instill common sense to patient care by rapidly assessing relevant information on the screen of one's computer, iPad, or cell phone. It is not something of the future. It is here today. Drs. Upchurch and Henke have included in the chapter authorship many individuals who are on the cutting edge of clinical vascular surgery. The knowledge gleaned from the pages they have written will enhance the reader's everyday practice and be a major benefit to those they care for.

James C. Stanley, MD
Handleman Professor of Surgery
University of Michigan

Preface

The first edition of *Clinical Scenarios in Vascular Surgery* was published in 2005. As time has passed, multiple readers constantly asked when we were going to update the book. Given the fact that no specialty has changed more than vascular surgery, we persisted in our discussions with Wolters Kluwer Health on the importance of this book to our trainees. Over the years, vascular surgery fellows in particular have used this book for oral board preparation (hopefully with some success). Now with the addition of the vascular surgery residency, this book will hopefully be even more useful. The tenet of the first edition was to provide readers with concise, focused, and data-driven clinical scenarios that could be read in a single setting. Each scenario was intended to provide the reader with an "acceptable" and safe way to manage a vascular problem.

Because vascular surgery has evolved so rapidly, in order to generate a meaningful second edition, the book needed to be greatly expanded. Thus, this edition has almost twice the number of chapters that the previous edition had. We have also done a better job of making the chapters more uniform in style. In addition, at the end of each chapter, you will find multiple choice questions, which allows the book to serve as preparation for written as well as oral exams.

In the original *Clinical Scenarios in Vascular Surgery*, we intentionally sought out younger vascular surgeons to write chapters. The idea was that they would bring new energy to the book with fresh insights. Those authors, like the editors, have aged over the last 10 years. Therefore, we used many of those same authors but asked them to update their chapters with emphasis on including new and colorful images. As we almost doubled the number of chapters, there is also greatly expanded new material specifically focused on endovascular management of vascular problems. We also have expanded the sections on venous disease and dialysis access, a large part of many vascular surgeons' practices.

We are indebted to all of the authors for their outstanding work. With exploding social media, it has become obvious that most don't buy hard cover books like they used to. However, the layout of this book translates well to the eBook format (included with the purchase of the physical copy), and each chapter can be purchased and downloaded individually similar to the way one does a song.

Anyone who edits a textbook knows that it is a labor of love. You end up harassing your friends who are, like you, often overcommitted and overworked. Once the chapters are received, they are edited on weekends and late at night, or at meetings when the subject matter allows. Our wives, Nancy and Barbara, continue to show us the love and support we need to pull off such a project. We are also indebted to Keith Donnellan, acquisitions editor, and Brendan Huffman, product developmental editor from Wolters Kluwer Health. They were so easy to work with, and this book really was almost easy to redo.

This will be the first second edition in the Clinical Scenarios series. Over the last 10 years, many people came up to us and asked for an updated version in vascular surgery. We hope that the people who asked for it, go out and buy it, and use it to improve the care of patients with vascular disease.

Gilbert R. Upchurch Jr, MD
Peter K. Henke, MD

Contents

1 Workup of Patient with Atherosclerotic Arterial Vascular Disease: Focus on Risk Factor Modification

SUROVI HAZARIKA and ADITYA M. SHARMA

Presentation

A 72-year-old woman with past medical history of hypertension and diabetes mellitus type II presents with a 3-month history of right great toe nonhealing wound. She also complains of pain in her right calf while walking more than approximately 100 feet. Pain is relieved within 3 minutes when she stops walking. She also has a 40-pack-year smoking history. She currently takes the following medications: hydrochlorothiazide 25 mg daily and metformin 500 mg twice daily. Her vital signs are normal. Physical examination is unremarkable except for nonpalpable pulses in the dorsalis pedis and the posterior tibial arteries bilaterally, with dopplerable signals.

Differential Diagnosis

Most common differentials for ulcers in the foot include venous stasis ulcers, neurotrophic ulcers, and arterial (ischemic) ulcers. Usually, venous stasis ulcers are seen on the inner aspect of the legs, above the ankles, and may affect one or both legs. They are commonly seen in patients who have venous stasis, varicose veins, or prior history of deep venous thrombosis. Neurotrophic ulcers are usually seen in patients with diabetes or other peripheral neuropathies and arise at points of increased pressure and weight bearing. Arterial ulcers are most often seen on the heels, on the tips of the toes, or between pressure points, associated with other signs and symptoms of poor arterial circulation in the affected leg such as claudication or poor pulses in the lower extremities.

Workup

The ankle-brachial index (ABI) is the most common noninvasive screening tool used for diagnosis of peripheral arterial disease (PAD). ABI is calculated as the ratio of the highest brachial systolic pressure to the highest systolic pressure in either the dorsalis pedis or the posterior tibial artery, measured in each lower extremity using a handheld Doppler. A normal resting ABI does not preclude a diagnosis of PAD, and where clinical suspicion exists, postexercise ABI should be done. A normal ABI ranges from 1.00 to 1.40, and abnormal values are defined as those ≤0.90. ABI values of 0.91 to 0.99 are considered "borderline," and values greater than 1.40 indicate noncompressible arteries. In patients with long-standing diabetes and advanced age, ABI can be nondiagnostic due to noncompressible vessels. In such cases, toe-brachial index should be used to establish the diagnosis of lower extremity PAD. Other modalities that are also helpful for diagnosis of PAD include pulse volume recording, continuous wave Doppler ultrasound, duplex ultrasound, magnetic resonance angiography, CT angiography, as well as contrast angiography.

Case Continued

The patient underwent ABI testing. Her resting ABI was 0.64 in the right and 0.76 in the left, indicating moderate arterial occlusive disease. Subsequently, she underwent a CT aortogram with runoff to the lower extremities, which showed severe long segment right superficial femoral artery severe stenosis and occluded proximal right popliteal artery.

Discussion

Lower extremity PAD is estimated to affect up to 8 to 12 million Americans. Up to 40% of these patients suffer from poor quality of life due to impaired walking ability, nonhealing wounds, and need for amputation. However, all of these patients have high risk for cardiovascular mortality and morbidity. PAD is a polyvascular disease. Sixty to ninety percent of patients with PAD also have coronary artery disease (CAD), and up to 25% have significant carotid artery stenosis. Over a 5-year period, only 1% to 2% of claudicants and asymptomatic patients develop critical limb ischemia (CLI). However, the overall 5-year mortality rate among patients all with PAD is 15% to 30% (75% of which is cardiovascular), and risk of nonfatal myocardial infarction (MI) or stroke is 20% at 5 years. Patients with CLI such as our patient have much worse cardiovascular outcomes with an annual CV mortality of 25% and annual amputation rate of 25%. This cardiovascular morbidity and mortality can be reduced significantly with use of appropriate cardiovascular medications as well as aggressive risk factor modification.

Focus on Cardiovascular Prevention Medications

Antiplatelet Therapy

The main benefits of antiplatelet therapy in patients with arterial vascular disease are from secondary cardiovascular prevention as supported by a 20% to 30% risk reduction of nonfatal MI, nonfatal stroke, or vascular death as shown by a meta-analysis of the Antithrombotic Trialists' Collaboration. In addition, in a subgroup analysis of the CAPRIE trial, clopidogrel was found to have a modest advantage over aspirin in reducing the incidence of stroke, MI, or vascular death in patients with symptomatic PAD. All the current PAD guidelines (national as well as international guidelines) recommend use of antiplatelets in patients with PAD. The ACC/AHA guidelines strongly recommend antiplatelet therapy (aspirin in daily doses of 75 to 325 mg or clopidogrel 75 mg) to reduce the risk of MI, stroke, and vascular death in individuals with symptomatic lower extremity PAD, including those with intermittent claudication or critical limb ischemia, prior lower extremity revascularization (endovascular or surgical), or prior amputation for lower extremity ischemia (class Ia). Antiplatelet therapy (aspirin in daily doses of 75 to 325 mg or clopidogrel 75 mg) is also recommended to reduce the risk of MI, stroke, and vascular death even in individuals with asymptomatic lower extremity PAD (class IIa). However, the benefit of antiplatelet therapy is not as well proven in asymptomatic patients as it is in those with symptomatic PAD such as claudication or those requiring vascular procedures or with CLI.

Statin Therapy

Several studies have focused on the outcome of PAD with treatment with HMG-CoA reductase inhibitors (statins). A subgroup analysis of PAD patients within the Heart Protection Study demonstrated a 22% relative risk reduction in the rate of first major vascular event regardless of the initial baseline low-density lipoprotein (LDL) levels. More recent studies have not only shown reduction in cardiovascular events but also reduction in amputation rates in patients with CLI and improvement in walking distance in patients with intermittent claudication. High-intensity statins are more effective in cardiovascular risk reduction compared with low-intensity statins. The current ACC/AHA guidelines recommend that all patients younger than 75 years with atherosclerotic PAD should be on a high-intensity statin (lowering LDL cholesterol [LDL-C] by ≥50%). Patients older than 75 years of age should be on at least a moderate-intensity statin (lowering LDL-C by approximately 30% to 50%) (Tables 1 and 2).

Antihypertensive Therapy

Hypertension is yet another significant modifiable risk factor for development of PAD. In the Framingham risk study, there was twofold and fourfold increase in claudication in men and women, respectively, with

TABLE 1. Medical Management of Arterial Vascular Disease

Key Steps

1. All the current PAD guidelines (national as well as international guidelines) recommend use of antiplatelets in patients with PAD.
2. More recent studies have not only shown reduction in cardiovascular events but also reduction in amputation rates in patients with CLI and improvement in walking distance in patients with intermittent claudication.
3. High-intensity statins are recommended for patients with atherosclerotic peripheral arterial disease who are younger than 75 years of age and high or moderate intensity statins are recommended for patients with atherosclerotic peripheral arterial disease. High intensity statins are more effective in cardiovascular risk reduction as compared to low intensity statins.
4. Treatment of hypertension is indicated in PAD to reduce the risk of cardiovascular complications such as stroke, MI, heart failure, and death.
5. Smoking is a powerful risk factor for development of PAD, and smokers are more likely to develop symptomatic PAD rather than symptomatic CAD.
6. Current clinical guidelines supported by multiple vascular societies, including Society of Vascular Surgery, recommend that at every visit, physicians should ask patients about their current smoking status.

Potential Pitfalls

- The overall 5-year mortality rate among patients all with PAD is 15%–30% (75% of which is cardiovascular), and risk of nonfatal MI or stroke is 20% at 5 years.
- Patients with CLI have much worse cardiovascular outcomes with an annual CV mortality of 25% and annual amputation rate of 25%.
- Patients with diabetes mellitus (DM) are at high risk for presenting with PAD complications including nonhealing ulcers with high amputation rates.

High-Intensity Statin Therapy	Moderate-Intensity Statin Therapy	Low-Intensity Statin Therapy
Daily dose lowers LDL cholesterol on average, by approximately ≥50%	Daily dose lowers LDL cholesterol on average, by approximately 30% to <50%	Daily dose lowers LDL cholesterol on average, by <30%
Atorvastatin (40) –80 mg	Atorvastatin 10 (20) mg	Simvastatin 10 mg
Rosuvastatin 20 (40) mg	Rosuvastatin (5) 10 mg	Pravastatin 10–20 mg
	Simvastatin 20–40 mg	Lovastatin 20 mg
	Pravastatin 40 (80) mg	Fluvastatin 20–40 mg
	Lovastatin 40 mg	Pitavastatin 1 mg
	Fluvastatin XL 80 mg	
	Fluvastatin 40 mg bid	
	Pitavastatin 2–4 mg	

TABLE 2. Differentiation of Various Statins with Doses Characterizing Them as Low-, Moderate-, or High-Intensity Statins

hypertension. Treatment of hypertension is indicated in PAD to reduce the risk of cardiovascular complications such as stroke, MI, heart failure, and death. In the HOPE study, in patients with PAD, ramipril reduced the risk of MI, stroke, or vascular death significantly compared to placebo. In addition, ramipril has been shown to improve claudication symptoms in randomized clinical trials. It is therefore recommended that angiotensin-converting enzyme (ACE) inhibitors such as ramipril be considered as first-line agents for treatment of hypertension in patients with PAD unless contraindicated (e.g., presence of bilateral renal artery stenosis). Although there was a theoretical concern of worsening PAD with use of beta-blocker, a meta-analysis of placebo-controlled trials using beta-blockers in patients with PAD did not show any adverse effect on walking capacity or symptoms of intermittent claudication. As such, beta-blockers can be safely used in patients with PAD if there are other ACC/AHA-supported indications for beta-blocker use.

Smoking Cessation

Smoking is a powerful risk factor for development of PAD, and smokers are more likely to develop symptomatic PAD rather than symptomatic CAD. Individuals who smoke have a twofold to sixfold increased risk of developing PAD compared to nonsmokers, and smokers with PAD have worse outcomes, with higher incidences of critical limb ischemia, amputation rates, and higher procedural

complications, including increased bypass graft failure, compared to nonsmokers. Tobacco cessation interventions are also particularly critical in individuals with thromboangiitis obliterans, as components of tobacco may be causative in the pathogenesis of this syndrome and cessation may lead to immediate relief in benefits.

Current clinical guidelines supported by multiple vascular societies, including Society of Vascular Surgery, recommend that at every visit, physicians should ask patients about their current smoking status. In addition, smokers should be assisted with counseling and developing a plan for quitting that may include pharmacotherapy and/or referral to a smoking cessation program. In the absence of contraindications, pharmacologic therapies are strongly recommended. Pharmacotherapies for smoking cessation include the following:

1. **Varenicline (Chantix)**: It is a nicotinic acetylcholine receptor partial agonist and has thus far demonstrated higher efficacy of smoking cessation compared to available alternatives. In a randomized placebo-controlled trial comparing varenicline with bupropion, varenicline produced the highest rates of abstinence at 1 year after treatment.
2. **Bupropion**: It is an aminoketone antidepressant agent that has a weak inhibitory effect on norepinephrine and dopamine reuptake. In randomized placebo-controlled trials, sustained release of bupropion at doses of 150 and 300 mg daily resulted in significant abstinence rates compared to placebo.
3. **Nicotine replacement therapy (NRT):** NRT aids in smoking cessation by reducing the urge to smoke and other withdrawal symptoms. Currently, there are multiple methods of NRT, which includes transdermal patches, gums, inhalers, sublingual tablets, and lozenges. There is currently no scientific evidence favoring one form of NRT over others, and it is possible that one form of NRT may be more effective in an individual than another form. In fact, combining two different forms of NRT such as nicotine patches with a fast-acting form such as nicotine gum or inhalers has shown to be more effective than nicotine patches alone.

Treatment of Diabetes Mellitus

DM is another strong risk factor for the development of PAD. Epidemiologic studies also show graded association between hemoglobin A1c (HgbA1c) and PAD risk in diabetic adults. Patients with DM are at high risk for presenting with PAD complications including nonhealing ulcers with high amputation rates. It is recommended that in patients with diabetes and PAD, glucose control therapies should be administered to lower HgbA1c below 7% to effectively reduce the rate of microvascular complications. In addition, the American Diabetes Association also recommends an annual evaluation for the presence of PAD in all patients with diabetes and that all patients with diabetes and PAD should be evaluated regularly for the presence of peripheral neuropathy and should receive preventive foot care to help minimize the risk of ischemic complications and limb loss. The same sentiments are echoed by the multidisciplinary guidelines by medical and surgical vascular societies.

Other Risk Factors

Although the aforementioned risk factors confer the majority of risk for PAD, other less well-established risk factors are associated with PAD. Most notably, elevated homocysteine levels have been shown associated with increased risk in vascular disease. However, there is no convincing evidence that lowering homocysteine levels in PAD results in improved outcomes. Other proinflammatory markers, such as high-sensitivity C-reactive protein and IL-6, have been associated with progression of PAD. However, the cause-effect relationship of these markers is not well understood, and their use in clinical practice is limited.

Case Conclusion

The patient was started on aspirin 81 mg daily, ramipril 2.5 mg twice daily, and rosuvastatin 20 mg daily. She was counseled on smoking cessation and started on nicotine patches as well as bupropion 100 mg twice daily. She was seen by a vascular surgeon who performed atherectomy of the right superficial femoral and popliteal artery with good angiographic outcomes. She did well with no complications. One month after surgery, she presented to the clinic with a completely healed ulcer. She had also quit smoking. Nicotine patch dose was titrated down to 7-mg patches daily. She also continued to take metformin 500 mg twice daily with better blood glucose control. Aspirin 81 mg daily, ramipril 2.5 mg daily, and rosuvastatin 20 mg daily were also continued indefinitely.

TAKE HOME POINTS

- Patients with arterial vascular disease have a significantly elevated cardiovascular morbidity and mortality, which includes increased risk of vascular-related death, MI, stroke, and high amputation rates. All of this can be significantly reduced with use of appropriate cardiovascular medications, such as statins and antiplatelet agents, as well as aggressive management of risk factors such as diabetes, hypertension, and smoking.

- Indefinite therapy with antiplatelet agents is strongly recommended in patients with PAD to reduce cardiovascular morbidity and mortality.
- All patients with PAD should be on a moderate- or high-intensity statin even if their baseline LDL-C levels are reported as "normal."
- ACE inhibitors or angiotensin receptor blockers such as ramipril should be used in patients with PAD who have either hypertension or claudication.
- Patients with past medical history or ongoing history of smoking should be assisted with counseling and developing a plan for quitting that may include pharmacotherapy and/or referral to a smoking cessation program.
- In patients with PAD and diabetes, glucose-lowering treatment should aim at reducing HgbA1c levels to below 7%.

SUGGESTED READINGS

Anderson JL, Halperin JL, Albert NM, et al. Management of patients with peripheral artery disease (compilation of 2005 and 2011 ACCF/AHA guideline recommendations): a report of the American College of Cardiology Foundation/American Heart Association Task Force on Practice Guidelines. *Circulation.* 2013;127(13):1425-1443.

Sharma AM, Aronow HD. Lower extremity peripheral arterial disease In: Gaxiola E, ed. *Traditional and Novel Risk Factors in Atherothrombosis*; 2012. ISBN: 978-953-51-0561-9, InTech, DOI: 10.5772/34227. Available from: http://www.intechopen.com/books/traditional-and-novel-risk-factors-in-atherothrombosis/lower-extremity-peripheral-arterial-disease

Stone NJ, Robinson JG, Lichtenstein AH, et al. 2013 ACC/AHA Cholesterol Guideline Panel. Treatment of blood cholesterol to reduce atherosclerotic cardiovascular disease risk in adults: synopsis of the 2013 ACC/AHA cholesterol guideline. *Ann Intern Med.* 2014;160:339-343.

CLINICAL SCENARIO CASE QUESTIONS

1. The best method for stopping cigarette smoking is:

   a. Counseling alone
   b. Varenicline (Chantix)
   c. Bupropion
   d. Nicotine replacement therapy (NRT)
   e. Pharmacotherapy along with counseling

2. Aspirin as antiplatelet therapy is indicated for how long in a patient with significant arterial vascular disease?

   a. 1 month
   b. 1 year
   c. 10 years
   d. Until they are asymptomatic
   e. Lifetime

2 Asymptomatic Internal Carotid Artery Stenosis

AMIT JAIN and GILBERT R. UPCHURCH Jr

Presentation

A 73-year-old man with a past medical history significant for hypertension, well-controlled diabetes, and hypercholesterolemia presents to your office after his family physician hears a right-sided neck bruit on routine physical examination. Social history is positive for tobacco use. His medications include a statin, a beta-blocker, an oral hypoglycemic agent, and an aspirin. On review of systems, the patient denies evidence of amaurosis fugax, motor or sensory deficits, difficulty with speech, or any previous history of a transient ischemic attack or stroke. On physical examination, the patient has a right-sided carotid bruit. His peripheral upper extremity pulses are all palpable. A duplex of the carotid arteries is recommended (Fig. 1).

■ Carotid Duplex Scan

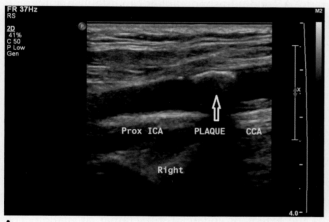

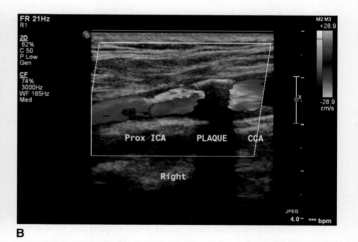

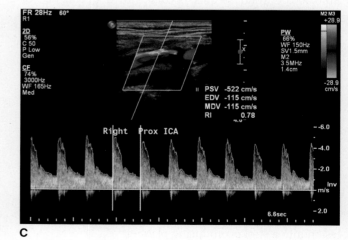

FIGURE 1 • Carotid Doppler ultrasound showing carotid bulb and proximal ICA plaque on the gray-scale image (*arrow* in **A**) and color flow image (**B**). Note the high peak systolic and end-diastolic velocities suggestive of high-grade stenosis of the proximal ICA (**C**).

■ **Carotid Duplex Scan Report**

RIGHT CAROTID SCAN: The report suggests that the carotid bulb and internal carotid artery (ICA) show evidence of heterogeneous plaque by both gray-scale and color flow imaging (Fig. 1A and B, arrow denotes extent of plaque on Fig. A).

RIGHT CAROTID DOPPLER:

CCA velocity: 110 cm/s, normal

ICA systolic velocity/end-diastolic velocity: 522/115 cm/s, 80% to 99% diameter stenosis (Fig. 1C)

ICA/CCA ratio: 4.74

ECA: normal, vertebral: antegrade

RIGHT CAROTID IMPRESSION: The right carotid study reveals an 80% to 99% diameter stenosis in the BULB/ proximal ICA. The distal end of the plaque was seen.

LEFT CAROTID IMPRESSION: The left carotid study reveals no significant disease by image. Velocities are suggestive of a less than 39% diameter stenosis in the BULB/ICA.

Differential Diagnosis

This patient has an asymptomatic high-grade right ICA stenosis. Other pathology may be noted on duplex including a carotid body tumor, a carotid artery dissection or aneurysm, or reversal of flow in the vertebral artery (secondary to "subclavian steal"). However, given the patient's smoking history, physical examination, and duplex results, the diagnosis is an asymptomatic high-grade right ICA stenosis.

Discussion

Stroke is the third leading cause of death in the United States with more than 700,000 strokes and 160,000 deaths annually. It was estimated that in 2007, nationwide stroke expenditure reached $62.7 billion with mean lifetime healthcare expenditure for each stroke patient of about $140,000. Carotid stenois occurs with a prevalence of about 2% to 9% in the general population, 5% to 9% in patients older than 65 years of age, 11% to 26% in those with coronary artery disease and as high as 25% to 49% of those with peripheral arterial disease. At present, approximately 2 million Americans are harboring asymptomatic carotid artery occlusive disease of at least 50% stenosis. About 87% of the strokes are ischemic and remaining 13% hemorrhagic in etiology. Arteriosclerosis of the brachiocephalic trunk, including the carotid arteries, causes greater than 50% of ischemic strokes. Initial plaque size, degree of stenosis, and the composition of the plaque along with some poorly understood events, including timing of plaque rupture, all play an important role in initiating the transformation of a benign carotid bifurcation lesion into a stroke-producing plaque.

The workup for a patient who presents with an asymptomatic or incidental carotid artery stenosis should be systematic. History should be directed at identifying risk factors and prior ischemic events. Physical examination should note signs of cardiac and systemic vascular disease, including assessment of peripheral pulses, examination for bruits, and careful assessment for signs of prior clinical stroke on neurologic examination. It should be noted that neither will all patients with a clinically significant lesion have a carotid bruit, nor will all the patients with a bruit have a hemodynamically significant carotid stenosis. A clinically important stenosis is present in only approximately a third of all patients with a carotid bruit. Also, every effort should also be made when taking a history to review any studies done to assess the carotid arteries in the past.

Carotid duplex ultrasonography is the recommended first screening study in patients who are suspected of having carotid artery stenosis. Duplex is widely available, is rapidly performed, is cost-effective, and carries minimal to no risk. The severity of the ICA lesion can be reliably measured based on the peak systolic flow velocity, the end-diastolic flow velocity, and the internal carotid to common carotid artery (CCA) flow velocity ratio. A good ultrasonographer can establish antegrade flow in the vertebral arteries and can also suggest diseased subclavian arteries if present. Both CT angiography (CTA) and 3D-magnetic resonance angiography (3D-MRA) with 2D-time-of-flight (2D-TOF) are useful in cases where duplex yields contradictory results or in the elucidation of concomitant proximal brachiocephalic or distal intracranial lesions. Other benefits of cross-sectional imaging include that it identifies the extent of the disease, the relationship of the carotid bifurcation to the angle of the mandible, and the tortuous course of the arteries. It is also helpful in assessing the atherosclerotic plaque burden of the aortic arch along with any ostial disease of the innominate or the left CCA, as well as the extent of collateral intracranial circulation. The traditional "gold standard" diagnostic study for carotid artery stenosis has been angiography, but it is rarely used now. Carotid angiography, however, was used in most of the randomized studies examining surgery versus medical therapy, justifying the use of carotid endarterectomy (CEA), and therefore serves as the reference standard against which other modalities are compared. In the ACAS study, confirmatory carotid angiography performed in patients with high-grade carotid stenosis on duplex criteria was associated with a 1.2% risk of stroke. It is useful in its ability to identify coexisting lesions of the great vessels and intracerebral arteries. Following a duplex scan, indications for a CTA, MRA, or carotid angiography include cases where symptoms do not correlate with the extent of carotid disease, the top of the plaque is not visualized, the vessel is extremely tortuous, the ipsilateral carotid artery is occluded, or if there is a high carotid bifurcation.

Recommendations

A right CEA is recommended given the patient's age (less than 80 years) and gender (male). A combined 3% risk of ipsilateral stroke, myocardial infarction, and death is quoted. A 5% to 10%, usually transient, cranial nerve injury risk is described. Given the patient's age (less than 80 years), lack of EKG abnormalities, no history of heart failure, and a good overall activity status (he is able to walk up a flight of stairs without shortness of breath), no further preoperative cardiac testing is performed. The patient is continued on his statin, beta-blocker, and aspirin preoperatively.

Surgical Approach

The patient undergoes appropriate monitoring including a radial arterial line and continuous percutaneous cerebral oximetry. General anesthesia is used (some surgeons prefer using cervical plexus block). The patient is placed supine in a beach chair position with neck extended and a shoulder roll underneath the scapulae. The neck is prepped including the ipsilateral ear lobe, the lower border of mandible and the sternal notch. An incision is made parallel to the anterior border of the sternocleidomastoid muscle, trying to incorporate skin lines. The platysma is divided, and the sternocleidomastoid muscle is retracted posteriorly. The carotid sheath is entered, and from this point on in the operation, sharp dissection is utilized. The facial vein is identified, ligated, and divided. Carotid artery dissection is performed with as little manipulation of the artery as possible. The vagus and the hypoglossal nerves are identified and protected. The CCA and the external carotid artery (ECA) are encircled. The patient is systemically heparinized (100 units/kg), and the ICA is encircled distal to the bulb plaque. The blood pressure

is kept at around a systolic of 150s to 160s during the time of carotid artery cross clamping. After 3 minutes of heparinization, the ICA, ECA, and the CCA are clamped. An anterior longitudinal arteriotomy is made in the CCA below the bulb and extended up the ICA until the top of the plaque is reached. A drop of >20% in the cerebral oxygen saturation from the baseline is used as an indicator to use inline shunt. (In an awake patient with cervical block, a test clamp is placed on the ICA and ECA first, and if there is no change in the neurologic exam, the CCA is then clamped). Back bleeding from the ICA is also assessed. Others use EEG monitoring or back pressure measurements of the ICA. Still others just shunt everyone. While the literature is full of multiple large case series about how to manage clamping the carotid, most would acknowledge that this is operator dependent and that most of the techniques are acceptable. The endarterectomy is begun in the CCA where the plaque is cut flush. An eversion endarterectomy of the ECA is then performed with good back bleeding. A nicely feathering plaque is removed from the distal ICA. All debris is removed. A synthetic patch is sewn in with fine monofilament suture. A bovine pericardial patch or autologous saphenous vein patch is also a viable option. Prior to completing the patch, the ECA and ICA are back bled and the CCA is bled forward. The patch is completed. Following patch closure, an intraoperative duplex scan shows normal velocities (Fig. 2A and B) with no evidence of debris. The incision is closed over a drain, and the drapes are removed. The patient is neurologically intact and is transferred to the postanesthesia care unit where he received an aspirin. The patient is discharged to home the next morning on antiplatelet and antihypertensive medications with a follow-up appointment in 4 weeks.

■ Intraoperative Carotid Duplex Scan

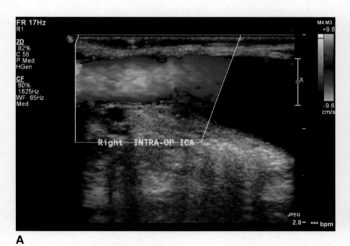

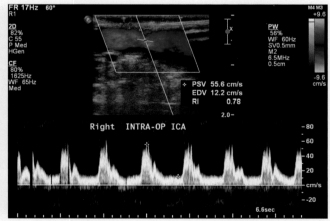

A

B

FIGURE 2 • Intraoperative carotid Doppler after patch repair showing resolution of the stenosis of the carotid bulb and proximal ICA (**A**) and return of flow velocities within normal range (**B**).

■ Duplex Scan Report (postoperatively)

Bulb: Within normal limits
ICA: Shows evidence of minimal heterogeneous plaque
ECA: Within normal limits
RIGHT CAROTID DOPPLER:
CCA velocity: 128 cm/s, normal
ICA systolic velocity/end-diastolic velocity: 56/12 cm/s, normal
ICA/CCA ratio: 0.43
ECA: normal vertebral: not imaged
RIGHT CAROTID IMPRESSION: The right carotid study reveals no significant disease (Table 1).

Discussion

Multiple large randomized controlled trials (RCTs), enrolling patients between 1980 and 2000, have established the efficacy of CEA in the setting of asymptomatic high-grade carotid artery disease. The Veterans Affairs Cooperative Study Group (VA trial) randomized 444 men with 50% to 99% to CEA and aspirin versus only aspirin and found a significantly lower incidence of primary end point of stroke and TIA in the surgery group (8% vs. 20.6%), a relative risk reduction (RRR) of 0.38 (95% CI 0.22 to 0.67) and an absolute risk reduction (ARR) of 1% over a mean follow-up of 4 years. The Asymptomatic Carotid Atherosclerosis Study (ACAS trial) randomized 1662 patients with documented carotid artery stenosis of greater than 60% to 99% by

---

TABLE 1. Carotid Endarterectomy

Key Technical Steps

1. Turn the neck to the opposite side of the incision and extend with a shoulder roll.
2. Stay a fingerbreadth posterior to the angle of the mandible to avoid marginal mandibular nerve.
3. Mobilize the sternocleidomastoid muscle and internal jugular vein laterally.
4. Dissect the common carotid first in the lower aspect of the incision and then proceed cephalad.
5. Ligate and divide the facial vein.
6. Follow the ansa cervicalis nerve cephalad to identify the hypoglossal nerve.
7. Divide the ansa and sling vessels to mobilize the hypoglossal nerve.
8. Divide the posterior digastric muscle for a more distal ICA exposure if needed.
9. Heparinize before dissecting the carotid bulb and distal ICA.
10. Shunt if poor back bleeding, >20% drop in cerebral oxygen saturation or distal ICA stump mean arterial pressure (MAP) <50 mm Hg.
11. Patch the arteriotomy for closure with Dacron, bovine pericardium, or vein.

Potential Pitfalls

- Hypoglossal and vagus nerve injury—use sharp dissection and know your anatomy.
- Chasing a thick posterior plaque in distal ICA—end the endarterectomy and tack the distal plaque with interrupted sutures.

---

ultrasound and arteriogram, to "best medical therapy" (aspirin) or to aspirin plus CEA. A 2.7-year follow-up revealed a significantly lower incidence of ipsilateral stroke and any perioperative stroke or death in the surgery group (5% vs. 11%), an RRR of 0.53 (95% CI 0.22 to 0.72) and an ARR of 3.0%. Subgroup analysis suggested men were benefited more than were women (ARR of 8% vs. 1.4%). This gender difference is often attributed to a higher presurgical stroke rate in women following arteriography. The Asymptomatic Carotid Surgery Trial (ACST) randomly assigned 3120 patients, with greater than or equal to 60% stenosis by duplex ultrasound, to immediate surgery versus deferral group. A 3.4-year follow up suggested a net 5-year risk reduction of all stroke or perioperative death in immediate CEA group versus deferral group (6.4% vs. 11.8%), an ARR of 3.1%. The risk reduction was again greater for men than women (ARR of 8.2% in men vs. 4.1% in women). A meta-analysis of these RCTs demonstrates an average of 1% stoke reduction per year with CEA in high-grade asymptomatic carotid stenosis. Hence, prophylactic CEA is likely beneficial only in the hands of surgeons with a combined perioperative morbidity and mortality of less than 3% and in patients with prolonged life expectancy.

It is important to understand that in most of these aforementioned randomized trials documenting the role of CEA in asymptomatic patients, carotid artery stenosis was defined by a greater than 60% narrowing by arteriography. These arteriographic measurements relate the size of the lumen within the bulb at the site of disease to the nondiseased distal ICA. Therefore, arteriographic results should not be confused with duplex ultrasound studies, which measure the actual amount of atherosclerotic material from the outside of the bulb compared to the remaining lumen. The described difference in technique results in inexact correlation between duplex and angiography. This is important when trying to extrapolate study data from randomized trials to clinical practice today since duplex ultrasound is often the only preoperative test performed in most patients prior to CEA.

Moreover, these trials comparing CEA to best medical therapy enrolled patients greater than 15 to 20 years ago. The standard of best medical therapy has significantly changed since then. The standard use of statins and better antihypertensive medications and availability of more potent antiplatelet drugs have led many experts to question the benefit of CEA in asymptomatic patients altogether in the present day.

Based on these randomized clinical trials and published guidelines by various societies, at present, CEA is indicated in asymptomatic patients with a carotid artery stenosis of at least 60% by arteriography or approximately 80% by carotid duplex. The majority of patients with asymptomatic carotid stenosis can be evaluated by duplex alone and do not need to undergo cerebral angiography. Surgeons who perform CEA for asymptomatic carotid disease should perform this operation with a less than 3% perioperative morbidity and mortality risk. All the patients should be treated with aspirin (81 to 325 mg) daily preoperatively and continued in the postoperative period for at least 1 to 3 months.

Carotid artery angioplasty and stenting (CAS) has been recently proposed as an alternative to CEA in both symptomatic and asymptomatic patients. The Carotid Revascularization Endarterectomy versus Stenting Trial (CREST) randomly assigned 2502 patients with greater than 50% stenosis on angiography and 70% or more on ultrasonography or CTA (47% asymptomatic and 53% symptomatic) to CEA or CAS. There was no significant difference between CEA and CAS group in the primary endpoint (a composite of any stroke, MI, or death within 30 days of the procedure) and any ipsilateral stroke during long-term follow-up of a median 2.5 years, (7.2% vs. 6.8% hazard ratio [HR] 1.1, 95% CI 0.8 to 1.5). The CEA group had a higher incidence of periprocedural MI (2.3% vs. 1.1%) and the CAS group had a higher incidence of periprocedural stroke (4.1% vs. 2.3%). Many more trials have compared CAS to CEA. Although data are suggesting similar outcomes in long-term follow-up, there is a higher incidence of periprocedural stroke with CAS particularly in older patients.

Treatment of asymptomatic carotid stenosis remains controversial, as there is a lack of level I evidence comparing either CEA or CAS versus current best medical therapy. It is still unclear whether it is beneficial to treat asymptomatic women with high-grade carotid stenosis with either CEA or CAS. The CREST-2 trial to be conducted in the near future proposes to compare, in two separate arms with CEA and CAS compared with current best medical treatment. There are other ongoing trials comparing CEA and CAS in standard-risk asymptomatic carotid stenosis patients. The US ACT 1 study of 1700 patients randomizing between CEA and CAS is near completion. The UK based ACST-2 study aims to randomize 5000 patients between CEA and CAS. Finally, the SPACE-2 study is evaluating CEA versus CAS in Germany. When these randomized trials are completed and reported, there should be enough data in the near future to further guide evidence-based treatment of asymptomatic high-grade carotid stenosis.

Case Conclusion

The patient is seen 4 weeks postoperatively and is doing well. He is encouraged to stop smoking. A follow-up visit is planned at 3 months with a repeat carotid duplex to assess the rate of ipsilateral carotid artery restenosis. It is imperative to follow the moderate contralateral left ICA stenosis as many of these patients will progress over time to develop a severe ICA stenosis requiring intervention. Following this, yearly carotid duplex scanning is recommended.

TAKE HOME POINTS

- Management of high-grade asymptomatic carotid stenosis is somewhat controversial and is evolving.
- Prophylactic CEA should be offered to patients with high-grade stenosis (greater than 80%) with low surgical risk and good life expectancy (greater than 5 years).
- Operating surgeons should have a less than 3% combined morbidity and mortality risk for CEA.
- CAS for asymptomatic disease should be limited to clinical trials until more evidence is available.

SUGGESTED READINGS

Ailawadi G, Stanley JC, Rajagopalan S, et al. Carotid stenosis: medical and surgical aspects. *Cardiol Clin.* 2002;20:599-609.

Brott TG, Hobson RW II, Howard G, et al.; CREST Investigators. Stenting versus endarterectomy for treatment of carotid-artery stenosis. *N Engl J Med.* 2010;363:11-23.

Constantinou J, Jayia P, Hamilton G. Best evidence for medical therapy for carotid artery stenosis. *J Vasc Surg.* 2013;58:1129-1139.

Executive Committee for the Asymptomatic Carotid Atherosclerosis Study. Endarterectomy for asymptomatic carotid artery stenosis. *JAMA.* 1995;273:1421-1428.

Hobson RW, Weiss DG, Fields WS, et al. Efficacy of carotid endarterectomy for asymptomatic carotid stenosis. *N Engl J Med.* 1993;328:221-227.

Huston J III, James EM, Brown RD Jr, et al. Redefined duplex ultrasonographic criteria for diagnosis of carotid artery stenosis. *Mayo Clin Proc.* 2000;75:1133-1140.

Naylor AR. The Asymptomatic Carotid Surgery Trial: bigger study, better evidence. *Br J Surg.* 2004;91:787-789.

Ovbiagele B, Goldstein LB, Higashida RT, et al. Forecasting the future of stroke in the United States: a policy statement from the American Heart Association and American Stroke Association. *Stroke.* 2013;44:2361-2375.

Roger VL, Go AS, Lloyd-Jones DM. Heart disease and stroke statistics—2011 update: a report from the American Heart Association. *Circulation.* 2011;123:e18-e209.

Usman AA, Tang GL, Eskandari MK. Metaanalysis of procedural stroke and death among octogenarians: carotid stenting versus carotid endarterectomy. *J Am Coll Surg.* 2009;208:1124-1131.

CLINICAL SCENARIO CASE QUESTIONS

1. Which of the following patients with asymptomatic carotid stenosis by duplex exam is the most appropriate candidate for carotid endarterectomy?

   a. A patient with less than 5 years of life expectancy with less than 60% carotid stenosis

   b. A patient with more than 5 years of life expectancy with less than 60% carotid stenosis

   c. A patient with less than 5 years of life expectancy with more than 60% carotid stenosis

   d. A patient with more than 5 years of life expectancy with more than 80% carotid stenosis

2. Which of the following is a key step in the exposure of the distal internal carotid artery during carotid endarterectomy for a high carotid lesion?

   a. Lateral mobilization of the sternocleidomastoid muscle
   b. Division of the facial vein
   c. Division of the posterior belly of digastric muscle and sling vessels around the hypoglossal nerve
   d. Division of the hypoglossal nerve

3 Best Medical Therapy in Asymptomatic Carotid Stenosis

VIJAIGANESH NAGARAJAN and ADITYA M. SHARMA

Presentation

A 78-year-old female with a history of diabetes mellitus and hypertension visited her primary physician for regular 6-month follow-up visit. She denied history of stroke or any symptoms suggestive of transient ischemic attacks (TIA). Her heart rate was 68 beats per minute and blood pressure was 142/92 mm Hg. Her clinical examination showed normal cardiovascular examination apart from left carotid bruit. Her HbA1c was 5.8%. Her lipid profile showed low-density lipoprotein (LDL) of 110 mg/dL and high-density lipoprotein of 42 mg/dL. She was taking metformin and metoprolol regularly.

Differential Diagnosis

Bruits are abnormal vascular sounds associated with turbulent, nonlaminar blood flow secondary to a stenotic lesion in an artery. The site of maximal intensity of the bruit gives us information regarding the possible vessel involved. Bruits heard close to the angle of the jaw are more specific for carotid artery stenosis as the bifurcation usually occurs at the level of thyroid cartilage. Other possibilities include cardiac murmurs radiating to carotids, cervical venous hum from neck veins and bruits secondary to intracranial arteriovenous malformations, and fibromuscular dysplasia. Supraclavicular bruits sometimes indicate subclavian stenosis.

Although screening for carotid artery disease is not usually advised in asymptomatic patients, carotid bruits identified on physical examination will often be evaluated for carotid stenosis. Sauve et al. investigated about carotid bruits in 1994 (NASCET trial data) and noted that the sensitivity and specificity of focal ipsilateral carotid bruit were 63% and 61%, respectively, to detect a high-grade carotid stenosis. Absence of a bruit was not a reliable marker to exclude significant carotid artery disease. In a recent meta-analysis including all studies published from 1966 to 2009, risk of TIA and stroke was significantly increased in patients with carotid bruit.

Stroke is the fourth leading cause of death and the leading cause of disability in the United States. Atherosclerosis in cervical arteries likely contributes to 15% to 20% of ischemic strokes. Hence in our patient, the next best step would be duplex ultrasonography of carotid vessels (Class IIa recommendation).

Workup of Patient

Ultrasonography in this patient showed >70% stenosis of the left carotid artery with peak systolic velocity of 280 cm/s, end diastolic velocity of 88 cm/s, and ratio of internal carotid (IC) to common carotid artery peak systolic velocity was 3.4 (Figs. 1 and 2). After being counseled about the risks and benefits of carotid intervention, the patient preferred not to undergo any revascularization. She was referred to a vascular medicine physician for optimal medical management for her carotid disease.

Recommendations for Carotid Revascularization

Current guidelines recommend revascularization only in asymptomatic patients with carotid stenosis of greater than 70% based on noninvasive imaging or more than 60% as documented by catheter angiography.

Medical Management and Risk Factor Modification

Medical optimization is a major component of management of carotid artery stenosis. Most of the trials evaluating surgical treatment options included optimal medical management in surgical arm as well. Modern medical therapy includes antiplatelet agents and statins, and aggressive risk factor modification (hypertension, cigarette smoking, diabetes, and hyperlipidemia) has dramatically reduced incidence of stroke and other cardiovascular morbidities, such as myocardial infarction (MI) and vascular deaths (Table 1).

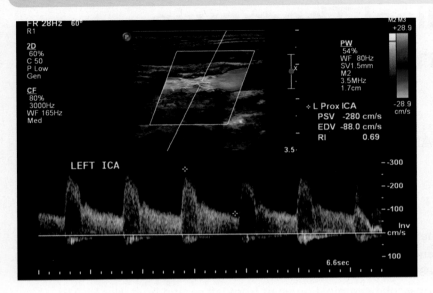

FIGURE 1 • Proximal left internal carotid artery shows elevated peak systolic velocities.

Antiplatelet Agents

The current multisocietal vascular guidelines recommend antiplatelet agents for patients with nonobstructive, as well as obstructive atherosclerotic extracranial carotid artery stenosis. Patients with carotid atherosclerosis are at increased risk of having atherosclerosis in other vascular beds, such as the coronaries. Antiplatelet agents are recommended for prevention of MI and other ischemic cardiovascular events.

The recommended drug therapy is either aspirin alone or clopidogrel alone or the combination of aspirin and extended-release dipyridamole. The dose of aspirin varied widely between trials, and hence a dose range of 75 mg daily to 325 mg daily has been recommended. There is no evidence to recommend using combination of aspirin and clopidogrel over using a single antiplatelet agent. In fact, current guidelines recommend *against* use of dual antiplatelet agents, such as aspirin and clopidogrel together, for asymptomatic carotid stenosis as it does not provide any additional benefit in reducing ischemic events but increases risk of bleeding. Dual antiplatelet therapy is only reserved for patients with other reasons to be on them, such as recently placed coronary stents, who also additionally have asymptomatic carotid stenosis.

Anticoagulant therapy with warfarin or the novel anticoagulants is not generally recommended for patients

FIGURE 2 • Gray-scale image of the proximal left internal carotid revealing echogenic calcified plaque.

TABLE 1. Differentiation of Various Statins with Doses Characterizing Them as Low-, Moderate-, or High-Intensity Statins

High-Intensity Statin Therapy	Moderate-Intensity Statin Therapy	Low-Intensity Statin Therapy
Daily dose lowers LDL cholesterol on average, by approximately ≥50%	Daily dose lowers LDL cholesterol on average, by approximately 30% to <50%	Daily dose lowers LDL cholesterol on average, by <30%
Atorvastatin (40) –80 mg	Atorvastatin 10 (20) mg	Simvastatin 10 mg
Rosuvastatin 20 (40) mg	Rosuvastatin (5) 10 mg	Pravastatin 10–20 mg
	Simvastatin 20–40 mg	Lovastatin 20 mg
	Pravastatin 40 (80) mg	Fluvastatin 20–40 mg
	Lovastatin 40 mg	Pitavastatin 1 mg
	Fluvastatin XL 80 mg	
	Fluvastatin 40 mg bid	
	Pitavastatin 2–4 mg	

with carotid artery disease with or without symptoms. The Warfarin-aspirin recurrent stroke study (WARSS) investigators performed a subgroup analysis on patients with stroke and large artery stenosis/occlusion and found no beneficial effect seen with warfarin over antiplatelet agents. But if patients have other indications for anticoagulation, like high-risk atrial fibrillation, cardioembolic stroke, or prosthetic heart valve, then anticoagulation may be recommended in such patients.

Statins

Statins have shown been to reduce ischemic stroke and overall cardiovascular risk in patients with carotid atherosclerosis. This beneficial effect is seen even if the baseline lipid levels are "normal." The SPARCL trial showed the benefit of atorvastatin in decreasing the incidence of ischemic stroke even with baseline normal LDL levels (100 to 190 mg/dL) by 22%. Two separate meta-analysis showed a 20% to 22% ischemic stroke risk reduction with use of statin therapy. This benefit is more prominent in diabetic patients with carotid atherosclerosis with the CARDS trial showing a 37% reduction in cardiovascular ischemic events and a 48% reduction in ischemic stroke by treatment with atorvastatin. Statins therapy has been shown to reduce carotid plaque progression especially as high-intensity statins are more likely to do so compared to low-intensity statins. For patients with atherosclerotic vascular disease, current guidelines recommend use of high-intensity statins, if the patients are 75 years or younger and at least moderate-intensity statins if they are older regardless of baseline lipid levels. Table 1 shows examples of low-, moderate-, and high-intensity statins with dosages.

Angiotensin Convertase Enzyme Inhibitor (ACEI) and Angiotensin Receptor Blocker (ARB)

Several trials have shown the potential for ACEI and ARBs in primary stroke reduction irrespective of their blood pressure–lowering effect. In the HOPE trial, ramipril significantly lowered ischemic stroke, cardiovascular events, and death in high-risk cardiovascular patients. The LIFE trial showed that Losartan (ARB) significantly reduced cardiovascular events beyond its role in blood pressure lowering. The SCOPE trial again showed that Candesartan (ARB) significantly reduced nonfatal strokes beyond effects of blood pressure lowering in the elderly population with isolated systolic hypertension. In the MOSES trial when ARBs were compared to calcium channel blockers, there was significant reduction in cardiovascular events especially ischemic stroke although both drugs equally lowered blood pressure. The hypothesis is that AT2 receptor stimulation by these agents cause stroke reduction as these agents provide protection against cardiovascular damage and tissue regeneration. Head-to-head trials comparing ARB and ACEI, such as the ONTARGET trial, showed a 9% greater reduction in primary stroke in patients on ARBs compared to those on ACEIs. A meta-analysis comparing ACEIs and ARBs from six randomized control trials showed that ARBs are even superior to ACEIs in stroke reduction. Patients with asymptomatic carotid stenosis should take either an ACEI or an ARB, especially if they have hypertension.

Management of Important Risk Factors
Hypertension

Hypertension is one of the most important risk factors for stroke. Multiple studies have shown linear relationship between increasing blood pressures and risk of stroke. Studies have shown decreasing blood pressure by 10 mm Hg can decrease stroke incidence up to 33%. A meta-analysis of seven randomized controlled trials showed a 24% reduction in stroke with use of an antihypertensive. Also studies like systolic hypertension in elderly program (SHEP) and Framingham heart study (FHS) showed that blood pressure is directly related to the progression of carotid stenosis as well. Controlling blood pressure is a crucial component of medical management of carotid stenosis. Guidelines recommend a target blood pressure of 140/90 mm Hg. This may not apply to patients during the acute phase of TIA or stroke who need higher pressures. Although the primary goal is to reduce blood pressure, ACEI/ARB with or without diuretics should be considered as first line agents, if possible. In the PROGRESS trial, patients with ischemic stroke who received a combination of perindopril (ACEI) and indapamide (diuretic) showed a 28% risk reduction in recurrent ischemic events.

Diabetes

The risk of ischemic stroke is increased two- to fivefold among patients with diabetes compared to those without diabetes. Carotid intima-media thickness (CIMT) was also noted to progress quicker in patients with diabetes. Current guidelines recommend treating diabetes with a hemoglobin A1c (HbA1c) target less than 7%. All patients with diabetes should receive education on exercise, diet, and glucose-lowering medications. All patients with diabetes and carotid atherosclerosis should be treated with a statin regardless of baseline lipid levels as the CARDS trial has shown to reduce overall cardiovascular risk by 37% and stroke risk by 48% by using atorvastatin in these patients even with normal lipid levels.

Hyperlipidemia

Increased risk of stroke is only mildly associated with hyperlipidemia in various clinical trials. However, reduction in LDL level with statin therapy regardless of baseline LDL levels has shown to significantly decrease the incidence of stroke. Details of the benefits of statin therapy have been discussed more in detail above under the section of medications. In patients who do not tolerate statins, other options like bile acid sequestrants or ezetimibe could be considered, but with caution and only in consultation with a preventive vascular medicine specialist as benefits from nonstatin antihyperlipidemic agents is not well established. Previous guidelines recommended treating target LDL levels; however, this is no longer recommended, and statins are recommended for all patients with clinical atherosclerotic vascular disease with far majority being treated with moderate-to-high intensity statins.

Smoking

Smoking has been well recognized as a risk factor for ischemic stroke. Smoking increases the risk of ischemic stroke by 25% to 50%. Quitting smoking decreases risk of ischemic stroke significantly within 5 years of quitting compared to those who continue smoking. Heavy smokers are noted to have a higher stroke rate compared to light smokers. Increased duration and amount of smoking also has been directly related to high-grade carotid stenosis. Hence, smoking cessation is strongly recommended to all patients with carotid artery disease.

Current clinical guidelines recommend that at every visit, the vascular physicians should ask his or her patients about history of smoking and their current smoking status. In addition, smokers should be assisted with counseling and developing a plan for quitting that may include pharmacotherapy and/or referral to a smoking cessation program. In the absence of contraindications, pharmacologic therapies are strongly recommended.

Pharmacotherapies for smoking cessation include the following:

1. **Varenicline (Chantix):** It is a nicotinic acetylcholine receptor partial agonist and has thus far demonstrated higher efficacy of smoking cessation compared to available alternatives. In a randomized, placebo-controlled trial comparing varenicline with bupropion, varenicline produced the highest rates of abstinence at 1 year after treatment.
2. **Bupropion:** It is an aminoketone antidepressant agent that has a weak inhibitory effect on norepinephrine and dopamine reuptake. In randomized placebo-controlled trials, sustained release bupropion at doses of 150 and 300 mg daily resulted in significant abstinence rates compared to placebo.
3. **Nicotine Replacement Therapy (NRT):** NRTs aid in smoking cessation by reducing the urge to smoke and other withdrawal symptoms. Currently, there are multiple routes of NRT administration, which includes transdermal patches, gums, inhalers, sublingual tablets, and lozenges. There is currently no scientific evidence favoring one form of NRT over other, and it is possible that one form of NRT may be more effective in an individual than another form. In fact, combining two different forms of NRT, such as nicotine patches with a fast-acting form such as nicotine gum or inhalers, has shown to be more effective than nicotine patches alone.

Obesity

Although we individually discussed the components of metabolic syndrome above, the impact of obesity on risk of stroke cannot be ignored. Multiple studies have shown that abdominal adiposity is associated with increased risk of stroke/TIA. Physical inactivity is another modifiable risk factor, which is linked to increased risk of stroke. So we recommend at least 150 minutes of brisk physical activity per week. Patients with morbid obesity should be considered for bariatric surgery and/or pharmacotherapy, such as phentermine/topiramate ER, orlistat, and lorcaserin.

Future Directions

The concept of personalizing care is possibly the future of atherosclerotic carotid disease, where antiplatelet therapy may be intensified based on presence of microemboli, while statin therapy is intensified based on plaque progression and morphology. However, further randomized clinical trials are needed to validate these data.

Case Conclusion

This patient was started on aspirin 81 mg PO daily and rosuvastatin 40 mg daily. She was started on losartan (ARB) for better blood pressure control. Her blood pressure during follow-up was 118/76 mm Hg. Her LDL was 68 mg/dL. She was swimming at least five times every week. She was noted to do well over the next 5 years and remains stroke free with no progression of her plaque by yearly carotid duplex (Table 2).

TABLE 2. Medical Management of Atherosclerotic Carotid Artery Stenosis

Key Considerations

1. Medical therapy for patients with carotid artery atherosclerosis should include antithrombotic agents, statins, and angiotensin-converting enzyme inhibitors.
2. Carotid artery atherosclerosis is a marker for atherosclerosis in other beds, including the coronaries.
3. Statins therapy has been shown to reduce carotid plaque progression especially as high-intensity statins are more likely to do so compared to low-intensity statins.
4. Controlling blood pressure is a crucial component of medical management of carotid stenosis. Guidelines recommend a target blood pressure of 140/90 mm Hg.
5. Quitting smoking decreases the risk of ischemic stroke significantly within 5 years of quitting compared to those who continue smoking.

Potential Pitfalls

- Dual platelet agents are known to have an increased risk of bleeding.
- Statin therapy has multiple known side effects, and therefore, patients need to be well informed of these effects prior to starting these medications.

TAKE HOME POINTS

- It is reasonable to consider screening for carotid stenosis in patients with carotid bruit. The recommended modality would be duplex ultrasonography.
- Carotid endarterectomy or carotid artery stenting may be recommended in patients with asymptomatic patients with carotid stenosis depending upon degree of stenosis. This will be discussed in a separate scenario.
- Antiplatelet therapy with either aspirin alone or clopidogrel alone or the combination of aspirin and extended release dipyridamole is recommended in asymptomatic carotid stenosis. Anticoagulant therapy with warfarin or novel anticoagulants is not recommended unless there is another indication to use them.
- Risk factor modification, especially hypertension and smoking, play a major role in decreasing the risk of stroke in patients with carotid stenosis. Consider using ACEI/ARB as first-line agents in the treatment of hypertension.
- Use of high-to-moderate intensity statins is strongly recommended in patients with asymptomatic atherosclerotic carotid disease.

SUGGESTED READINGS

Beckman JA. Management of asymptomatic internal carotid artery stenosis. *JAMA.* 2013;310(15):1612-1618.

Raman G, Moorthy D, Hadar N, et al. Management strategies for asymptomatic carotid stenosis: a systematic review and meta-analysis. *Ann Intern Med.* 2013;158(9):676-685.

2011 ASA/ACCF/AHA/AANN/AANS/ACR/ASNR/CNS/SAIP/SCAI/SIR/SNIS/SVM/SVS guideline on the management of patients with extracranial carotid and vertebral artery disease: executive summary. *J Am Coll Cardiol.* 2011;57(8):1002-1044.

CLINICAL SCENARIO CASE QUESTIONS

1. Optimal medical therapy in a patient with carotid artery stenosis would include:
   a. Smoking cessation
   b. Antiplatelet agent
   c. ARB
   d. Statin
   e. All of the above

2. A high-dose statin used to bring about a greater than 50% lowering of LDL cholesterol on average would be:
   a. Atorvastatin 80 mg
   b. Atorvastatin 20 mg
   c. Lovastatin 40 mg
   d. Fluvastatin XL 80 mg
   e. Pitavastatin 2 to 4 mg

4 Symptomatic Carotid Artery Stenosis

MOHAMMAD H. ESLAMI and ZACHARIAH K. ESLAMI

Presentation

A 65-year-old woman presented to the emergency room with right-sided paralysis and expressive aphasia. Her husband told the emergency room physician that the patient has a history of hypertension, smoking, and myocardial infarction that was treated with coronary artery angioplasty and stenting. Her husband recalls that she had an episode of slurred speech and difficulty seeing from her left eye while visiting relatives in Ireland 3 weeks ago. This quickly resolved, and she did not seek medical attention. On physical examination, she is in normal sinus rhythm and has a loud left-sided carotid bruit. Neurologically, initially, she has decreased strength (2/5) on the right side that has gradually improved to almost normal. Her facial drooping and expressive aphasia have resolved, and she is now able to communicate.

Differential Diagnosis

The most common cause of transient cerebral ischemia is embolization from atherosclerotic disease of the extracranial carotid artery and specifically from stenotic internal carotid artery (ICA). Embolization can also originate from cardiac sources (atrial thrombus, valvular vegetative disease, atrial fibrillation), fibromuscular dysplasia (FMD), stenosis of the carotid artery, carotid dissection, carotid kink or coils, aneurysms of extracranial carotid arteries, or paroxysmal arterial emboli. Neurologic symptoms may also be caused by migraine headaches and even giant cell arteritis. Considering this patient's age and cardiovascular risk factors (h/o of MI, hypertension, and tobacco abuse) and the presence of loud carotid bruit, ICA stenosis should be considered the primary source of cerebral ischemia.

Discussion

Carotid artery stenosis can cause neurologic symptoms ranging from transient cerebral ischemia to dense permanent cerebral stroke. Transient cerebral ischemia is self-limiting with neurologic deficit that lasts for less than 24 hours that completely resolves. The term encompasses different presentations, such as transient monocular blindness (TMB), also known as amaurosis fugax and lateralizing transient ischemic attacks (TIA). TMB is classically described as having a "curtain over the eye" or "a shade pulled over the eye" that clears in seconds to a few minutes. Lateralizing TIAs commonly manifest as weakness or paresthesia that affect the contralateral body. By definition, the duration of a TIA is less than 24 hours; however, they frequently last only several minutes to

an hour before resolving without a residual neurologic deficit. Physicians rarely see patients during transient attacks, and the patient's history remains the primary factor in establishing a diagnosis.

In the spectrum of presentation of carotid artery stenosis from transient to complete cerebral ischemia (stroke), there are two conditions known as crescendo TIA or stroke in evolution that need special attention. Crescendo TIA describes the situation when a patient experiences frequent repetitive neurologic attacks without complete resolution of the deficit between the episodes, producing the same deficit but no progressive deterioration in neurologic function. If a progressive deterioration in neurologic function is seen, the patient is diagnosed as experiencing a stroke in evolution. If there is a surgically correctable lesion that is identified as the primary source of cerebral embolization, these two conditions are the only time that an emergent operation is indicated.

Flow-related ischemic events are unusual due to an extremely efficient collateral blood supply to the brain, primarily through the circle of Willis. When they do occur, flow-related ischemic events are usually associated with carotid dissections often after a hypertensive crisis or traumatic injury to the carotid artery. Most commonly, cerebral ischemic attacks are caused by thromboembolic events from an arterial nidus. The arterial nidus for emboli is usually an atheromatous plaque, but emboli can also originate from lesions caused by FMD, radiation therapy, or aneurysms of the carotid vessels. A less common source is cardiac emboli, originating from an intracardiac thrombus associated with atrial fibrillation or myocardial infarction. Paroxysmal emboli, which

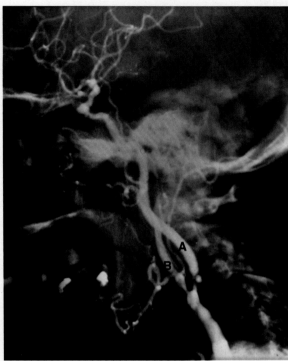

FIGURE 1 • Cerebral angiography showing severe ICA stenosis (**A**) and stenosis of ECA (**B**).

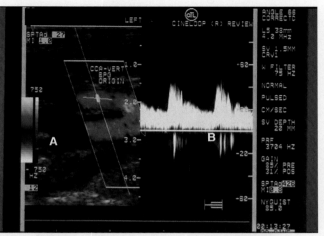

FIGURE 2 • Carotid duplex typically has two components, an image (**A**) and a waveform that shows the velocity in the ICS (**B**).

Extracranial Duplex Report

On the left side, the peak systolic velocity of 450 cm/s and end-diastolic velocity of 150 cm/s were noted at the proximal ICA. Here, significant spectral broadening of the waveform (Fig. 2B) and duplex real-time B mode (Fig. 2A) show a significant (>80% to 99%) stenosis of the proximal left ICA.

Head CT Report

No evidence of acute cerebral ischemic infarct noted. On the left cerebral cortex, multiple small punctate lesions noted suggestive of old cerebral infarcts. Clinical correlation is indicated.

Diagnosis and Recommendations

This patient has a severely stenotic and symptomatic ICA lesion. Given her neurologic symptoms that have occurred in the past and this most recent episode, urgent carotid endarterectomy (CEA) and lifelong antiplatelet therapy (e.g., aspirin) are recommended. The patient inquires about the benefits of surgery, and she is advised of a 17% absolute risk reduction of stroke and a 71% relative risk reduction of at 18 months for surgery and antiplatelet therapy compared to antiplatelet therapy alone. She asks about the use of stents and is advised that the carotid stenting is currently approved only for octogenarian and patients with prohibitive operative risks. She is informed of the operative risks of death (0.6%), stroke (1%), cranial nerve injuries (less than 1%), wound complications (less than 0.01%), bleeding (less than 0.01%), and carotid restenosis (5%). The patient and her family were assured that the risks are significantly less than not operating.

Surgical Approach

The patient is given general anesthesia, perioperative antibiotics are given, and the patient is placed in a "lawn chair" position. An incision is made anterior to

originate from a deep venous thrombus that crosses from the venous to arterial systems via a septal defect in the heart, are a rare cause of cerebral ischemic attacks that should be considered in the very young.

Although angiography has historically been considered the gold standard (Fig. 1), the initial diagnostic test is duplex ultrasonography to evaluate the extracranial carotid and vertebral arteries for occlusive lesions. The basic principle of this study is to assess anatomy, using real-time B-mode imaging, and flow dynamics, using quantitative pulsed wave Doppler, to determine the location and severity of disease. The grade of the lesion is characterized by increased velocity spectra recorded proximal to, and at, the point of maximum stenosis. Several studies have compared the accuracy of duplex ultrasound with arteriography and have determined a close correlation in stenotic estimations. Angiograms should be obtained where duplex cannot accurately determine the severity of the lesion. These situations include proximal common carotid or aortic arch lesions, contralateral carotid occlusion, high bifurcation of the carotid, and discrepancy in symptoms compared to the duplex findings. As technology advances, computed tomographic (CT) angiography and magnetic resonance arteriography (MRA) have become more useful diagnostic tools when these issues are encountered.

Recommendation

Extracranial Duplex ultrasonography was recommended as well as head CT given the lateralizing TIA.

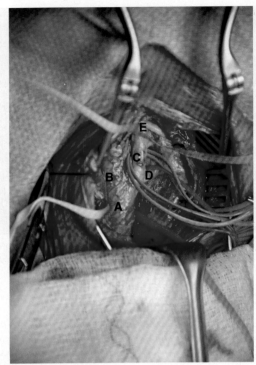

FIGURE 3 • Carotid artery exposure. **A**: Common carotid artery. **B**: Internal carotid artery. **C**: External carotid artery. **D**: Superior thyroid artery. **E**: Hypoglossal nerve.

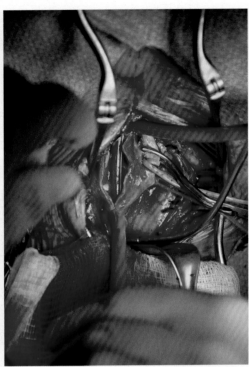

FIGURE 4 • Shunt is secured, and endarterectomy was performed. The artery is often closed with a patch.

the sternocleidomastoid muscle and carried through the platysma. The internal jugular vein is identified and retracted laterally. The dissection is carefully continued around the common carotid artery (CCA) and control obtained with a vessel loop. The vagus nerve is identified posterior to the carotid artery. The dissection is continued superiorly to the superior thyroid artery and the external carotid artery (ECA). Control of these vessels is also established with vessel loops. Care is taken to avoid direct dissection of the carotid bifurcation. The ICA is further dissected superiorly, well above the distal aspect of the atherosclerotic plaque. The hypoglossal nerve is identified superior to the bifurcation (Fig. 3). Further exposure can be obtained superiorly with division of the digastric muscle tendon. However, care must be taken not to injure the glossopharyngeal nerve. The ICA is controlled with a vessel loop. Once all the vessels are controlled, the patient is systemically heparinized, and clamps are placed on the distal ICA, proximal CCA, proximal ECA, and superior thyroid artery. An arteriotomy is made on the anterior aspect of CCA extending on the anterior aspect of ICA. A shunt is inserted, secured by Rommel tourniquets, and the integrity of the shunt is evaluated with a handheld Doppler. The endarterectomy plane is then created, and the plaque is removed (Fig. 4). If intimal flaps are present, they are secured with tacking sutures. The arteriotomy is typically closed with a patch; however, an unusually large artery may require primary

closure. Prior to completion of arteriotomy closure, shunt is removed. Back bleeding of the ICA is performed to remove any embolic potential (e.g., debris or air) before placing the last few sutures. Arterial flow is restored first to the ECA and then to the ICA. Duplex ultrasound scan is performed intraoperatively to identify any surgically correctable issues. With troublesome surface bleeding, sometimes a drain is inserted (Table 1).

Case Conclusion

The patient is awakened from anesthesia with baseline neurologic examination and intact cranial nerves. She is observed overnight and discharged home on postoperative day number 1 on aspirin. She returns to the clinic 3 weeks after surgery and will receive a duplex study every 6 months for routine post-CEA surveillance.

Discussion

The recommended therapy for symptomatic ICA stenosis is to perform CEA and in selected cases carotid stenting. As noted, the most common cause of cerebral ischemia is from embolization of an ICA stenosis. The initial mortality of an ischemic stroke is approximately 15% to 30%. Survivors have a high risk for recurrent stroke, estimated between 5% and 15% per year, implying that

TABLE 1. Symptomatic Carotid Artery Stenosis

Key Technical Steps

1. Incision is made anterior to the sternocleidomastoid muscle and carried through the platysma.
2. The internal jugular vein is identified and retracted laterally.
3. The dissection is carefully continued around the CCA and control obtained with a vessel loop.
4. The vagus nerve is identified posterior to the carotid artery.
5. The dissection is continued superiorly to the superior thyroid artery and the ECA. Control of these vessels is also established with vessel loops.
6. The ICA is further dissected superiorly, well above the distal aspect of the atherosclerotic plaque.
7. The hypoglossal nerve is identified superior to the bifurcation.
8. Further exposure can be obtained superiorly with division of the digastric muscle tendon.
9. The ICA is controlled with a vessel loop.
10. Once all the vessels are controlled, the patient is systemically heparinized, and clamps are placed on the distal ICA, proximal CCA, proximal ECA, and superior thyroid arteries.
11. An arteriotomy is made on the anterior aspect of CCA extending on the anterior aspect of ICA.
12. A shunt is inserted, secured by Rommel tourniquets, and the integrity of the shunt is evaluated with a handheld Doppler.
13. The endarterectomy plane is then created, and the plaque is removed (Fig. 4).
14. If intimal flaps are present, they are secured with tacking sutures. The arteriotomy is typically closed with a patch; however, an unusually large artery may require primary closure.
15. Prior to completion of arteriotomy closure, shunt is removed.
16. Back bleeding of the ICA is performed to remove any embolic potential (e.g., debris or air) before placing the last few sutures.
17. Arterial flow is restored first to the ECA and then to the ICA.
18. Duplex ultrasound scan is performed intraoperatively to identify any surgically correctable issues.

Potential Pitfalls

- Care is taken to avoid direct dissection of the carotid bifurcation to avoid bleeding and manipulation of the bulb.
- However, care must be taken not to injure the glossopharyngeal nerve when dissecting the distal ICA.

approximately 50% will suffer a second ischemic incident within 5 years. Carotid revascularization (CEA) leads to removal of the atherogenic ICA lesion and is therefore recommended to prevent permanent or more devastating stroke. This recommendation is based on very strong, level 1 data.

The North American Symptomatic Carotid Endarterectomy Trial (NASCET) is a large prospective study that determined a clear benefit with combined CEA and medical therapy to treat a symptomatic carotid stenosis, when compared to medical therapy alone. This study reported a 30-day operative morbidity and mortality for patients managed with CEA of 5%. At 18 months, a 7% incidence of major stroke occurred in the surgical arm of the trial, compared to a 24% incidence of major stroke in the medical arm of the trial. This difference proved highly significant. Although the previously stated data provided a general standard, many surgical centers now report lower stroke and fatality rates associated with symptomatic carotid endarterectomies. It is, therefore, important for surgeons to monitor their operative outcomes to appropriately counsel their patients preoperatively.

There is significant debate about the role of CAS in carotid revascularization that is beyond the scope of this chapter. Current evidence suggests that results from CAS are inferior to those from CEA in symptomatic patients. In a large randomized trial comparing CEA to CAS, CREST, investigators showed more devastating strokes in CAS patients than in CEA patients. Prior to CREST publications, other publications showed similar results and the current Center for Medicare and Medicaid Services in 2008 recommended CAS for patients who may not tolerate operative repair. Many studies point that the CEA results are quite acceptable even in "high-risk patients." Given that most vascular surgeons perform CAS, they may be the best specialty to counsel their patients for the appropriate intervention for their individual cases.

Treatment for patients who present with recent permanent stroke is different from patients with waxing and waning neurological symptoms. This special group of patients with recent stoke due to ICA stenosis require significant input from neurologists about the timing of CEA. In the past, these procedures were delayed for weeks. Although the exact timing is debatable, the current studies have shown that in a patient whose neurologic deficit has stabilized, surgery is advocated as soon as possible—usually within the first week after stroke. In this group of patients, CEA decreases cerebral ischemia and may improve rehabilitation and return to an improved neurologic status.

SUGGESTED READINGS

Brott TG, Hobson RW II, Roubin HG, et al. Stenting versus carotid endarterectomy for treatment of carotid artery stenosis. *N Engl J Med.* 2010;363:11-23.

Bui H, deVirgilio C. Cerebral ischemia. In: White RA, Hollier LH, eds. *Vascular Surgery: Basic Science and Clinical Correlations.* 2nd ed. Malden, MA: Blackwell; 2004:251-257.

Edwards JM, Moneta GL, Papanicolaou TG, et al. Prospective validation of new duplex ultrasound criteria for 70-99% internal carotid artery stenosis. *J Engl Med U.* 1995;16:3-7.

Eslami MH, McPhee JT, Simons JP, et al. National trends in utilization and post-procedure outcomes for carotid revascularization 2005-2007. *J Vasc Surg.* 2011;53:307-315.

Farber A, Cronenwett JL. Symptomatic carotid artery stenosis. In: Cronenwett JL, Rutherford RB, eds. *Decision Making in Vascular Surgery.* 1st ed. Philadelphia, PA: WB Saunders; 2001.

Hobson RW. Carotid artery occlusive disease. In: Dean RH, Yao JS, Brewster DC, eds. *Current Diagnosis and Treatment in Vascular Surgery*. Norwalk, CT: Appleton & Lange; 1995:28-34;88-104.

Hood DB, Mattos MA, Mansour A, et al. Prospective evaluation of new duplex criteria to identify a 70% internal carotid artery stenosis. *J Vasc Surg*. 1996;23:254-261.

Moneta GL, Edwards JM, Chitwood RW, et al. Correlation of North American Symptomatic Carotid Endarterectomy Trial (NASCET) angiographic definition of 70% to 99% internal carotid artery stenosis with duplex scanning. *J Vasc Surg*. 1993;17:152-159.

Moore WS. Extracranial cerebrovascular disease: the carotid artery. In: Moore WS, ed. *Vascular Surgery: A Comprehensive Review*. 7th ed. Philadelphia, PA: WB Saunders; 2006:617-659.

North American Symptomatic Carotid Endarterectomy Trial Collaborators. Beneficial effect of carotid endarterectomy in symptomatic patients with high-grade carotid stenosis. *N Engl J Med*. 1991;325:445-453.

Rerkasem K, Rothwell PM. Systematic review of operative risks of carotid endarterectomy for recently symptomatic stenosis in relation to timing of surgery. *Stroke*. 2009;e564-e572.

Sacco RL, Wolf PA, Kannel WB, et al. Survival and recurrence following stroke: the Framingham Study. *Stroke*. 1982;13:290-295.

CLINICAL SCENARIO CASE QUESTIONS

1. Cerebral angiograms are performed:
   a. Prior to every CEA
   b. When there is a discrepancy in symptoms compared to the duplex findings
   c. In redo CEA
   d. When radiation is suspected
   e. When FMD is suspected

2. The initial mortality from a stroke is:
   a. 5% to 15%
   b. 0% to 10%
   c. 15% to 30%
   d. 30% to 60%
   e. 90%

5 Acute Stroke after CEA

MATTHEW R. ABATE and MOHAMMED M. MOURSI

Presentation

A 65-year-old Caucasian man is 45 minutes following a right carotid endarterectomy (CEA) and is now in the recovery room. The patient underwent a CEA for a symptomatic right internal carotid stenosis measuring 86% on preoperative cerebral angiography, with the contralateral side measured as a 35% stenosis. The patient was receiving aspirin preoperatively. The operation was performed under regional anesthesia without the use of a shunt, and the carotid artery was closed with the use of a bovine pericardial patch. Initial intraoperative duplex ultrasound scan at the completion of the endarterectomy showed an intimal flap at the distal extent of the endarterectomy site requiring reopening of the artery and placement of several tacking stitches. Completion duplex ultrasound scan after this repair showed no apparent defects. The patient had no hemodynamic instability during the perioperative period and has demonstrated a normal neurologic exam until this point. Now, 45 minutes after arrival in the recovery room, the patient develops a left-sided hemiparesis involving his upper and lower extremities. In addition, he is now unable to respond to verbal commands.

Differential Diagnosis

The diagnosis with this clinical scenario is clear. This patient has signs and symptoms consistent with an acute stroke after CEA. The diagnostic dilemma involves the etiology for this stroke. The differential for the cause of an ipsilateral acute stroke after CEA includes (1) intracerebral hemorrhage, (2) watershed infarction, (3) hypoperfusion intraoperatively or postoperatively, (4) hyperperfusion, (5) embolization of atheromatous plaque or thrombus occurring intraoperatively, (6) embolization occurring postoperatively with or without a technical defect at the endarterectomy site (embolic material could be atheromatous plaque, thrombus, or platelet aggregation), (7) thrombosis of the endarterectomy site with or without a technical defect, (8) heparin-induced thrombocytopenia, (9) kink in the artery resulting in low flow, and (10) embolization from a site other than the carotid bifurcation.

Diagnostic Tests

Given that he had a lucent period in the immediate postoperative period and had a completion duplex ultrasound scan that showed no defect, this patient would be best served by simultaneously preparing the operating room for reexploration and obtaining a duplex scan of the carotid artery to determine patency.

Duplex Ultrasound Scan

Duplex Ultrasound Scan Report

Duplex ultrasound scan shows an acutely thrombosed internal carotid artery (ICA) (Fig. 1A) with Doppler waveform signal indicating no flow (Fig. 1B).

Diagnosis and Recommendation

The patient has an acute stroke secondary to a thrombosed ICA endarterectomy site, most likely due to fibrin and platelet adhesion to the endarterectomized surface. Given the thrombosed artery and the short period of time (less than 2 hours) since the CEA, the patient needs emergent reexploration of the carotid artery. Although the addition of a duplex scan in this situation is somewhat controversial, one of the cornerstones of diagnosis and treatment for an acute stroke after CEA is to determine patency of the artery. With a normal intraoperative duplex scan and a lucent period postoperatively, a duplex scan is recommended. In most hospital settings, this will not delay the required reexploration, given the portability of the duplex machine and the time required to prepare an operating room. In this situation, the ICA was thrombosed, and reexploration is indicated. However, had the duplex showed a patent artery with no defects, exploration could prove to be harmful. In that circumstance, rather than an operation, the patient would require a computed tomographic (CT) scan of the head and possible cerebral arteriography (see Discussion).

Case Continued

By the time the duplex is completed, the operating room is ready, and the patient is taken for reexploration.

Discussion

Once the carotid artery is found to be thrombosed, the patient is given systemic heparin at 100 U/kg IV bolus. In the operating room, the patient can be reexplored

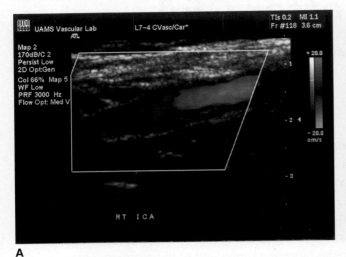
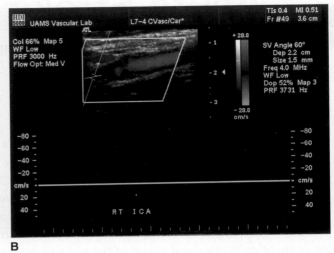

A

B

FIGURE 1 • **A:** Duplex ultrasound with thrombosed right internal carotid artery. **B:** Doppler waveform demonstrating no detectable flow within the right internal carotid artery.

under the original regional anesthetic block if the time interval between cervical block and reexploration is short and if the patient is cooperative. Otherwise, a general anesthetic is administered. The neck incision is opened, and the carotid artery is exposed, and the thrombosed artery is confirmed by visual inspection and/or handheld Doppler. In addition, any kinks or other abnormalities are identified and inspected. The common carotid and external carotid arteries are controlled with vascular clamps, and the arteriotomy is opened; note that no attempt is made to clamp the distal ICA at this time. Upon opening the artery, the thrombus is removed, and the internal carotid is allowed to back bleed into the field; if no back bleeding is observed and there appears to be thrombus extending distally, an embolectomy catheter can be used to gently remove distal clot. Care must be taken to avoid creating a cavernous sinus fistula. Once the thrombus is removed, the endarterectomized surface is inspected for defects. If any defects are identified, they are repaired by either removal of residual plaque or tacking of any intimal flaps. Alternatively, upon opening the artery, platelet aggregation may be identified. Rather than frank thrombus, a defect site may be noted. This should be removed and the defect repaired.

Surgical Approach

The patient undergoes general endotracheal anesthesia, and at exploration, the carotid artery is found to be thrombosed. The clot is removed from the distal internal carotid as well as at the endarterectomy site. No obvious defect can be identified. Therefore, an interposition saphenous vein graft is used to replace the proximal ICA. Low molecular weight dextran is started as a continuous drip. Intraoperative duplex ultrasound scan shows a widely patent interposition graft with no defects.

Case Continued

The patient awakes from anesthesia with a mild left upper extremity weakness as his only neurologic defect. The patient is placed on an additional antiplatelet agent along with aspirin. Physical and occupational therapy are initiated, and the patient is eventually sent home to continue his rehabilitation.

Case Conclusion

In this particular case, since no technical defect was observed, the presumed etiology of the thrombosis is fibrin and platelet aggregation and adhesion to the endarterectomized surface. If this is not replaced, the chance of rethrombosis is high. Therefore, a portion of greater saphenous vein was harvested from the thigh and used as an interposition graft. It is important to initiate pharmacologic antiplatelet therapy both intraoperatively with dextran as well as postoperatively, with another oral antiplatelet agent in addition to aspirin. The neck is then closed; the patient is awakened from the general anesthetic and is continued on dextran for 24 hours and antiplatelet agents. Care is taken to avoid hypotension in the postoperative period (Table 1).

Discussion

CEA has proven to be a beneficial and safe treatment for the prevention of strokes in patients with symptomatic and asymptomatic extracranial carotid artery

Key Technical Steps

1. With a normal intraoperative duplex scan and a lucent period postoperatively, a duplex scan is recommended. In most hospital settings, this will not delay the required reexploration, given the portability of the duplex machine and the time required to prepare an operating room. In this situation, the ICA was thrombosed and reexploration is indicated. However, had the duplex showed a patent artery with no defects, then exploration could prove to be harmful. In that circumstance, rather than an operation, the patient would require a CT scan of the head and possible cerebral arteriography (see Discussion).

2. Once the carotid artery is found to be thrombosed, the patient is given systemic heparin at 100 U/kg IV bolus.

3. The patient can be reexplored under the original regional anesthetic block if the time interval between cervical block and reexploration is short and if the patient is cooperative. Otherwise, a general anesthetic is administered.

4. The neck incision is opened and the carotid artery is exposed, and the thrombosed artery is confirmed by visual inspection and/or handheld Doppler. In addition, any kinks or other abnormalities are identified and inspected. The common carotid and external carotid arteries are controlled with vascular clamps, and the arteriotomy is opened; note that no attempt is made to clamp the distal ICA at this time. Upon opening the artery, the thrombus is removed, and the internal carotid is allowed to back bleed into the field.

5. If no back bleeding is observed and there appears to be thrombus extending distally, an embolectomy catheter can be used to gently remove distal clot.

6. If any defects are identified, they are repaired by either removal of residual plaque or tacking of any intimal flaps.

7. Alternatively, an interposition saphenous vein graft may used to replace the proximal ICA.

8. Intraoperative duplex ultrasound scan shows a widely patent interposition graft with no defects.

Potential Pitfalls

- Care must be taken to avoid creating a cavernous sinus fistula with passage of the embolectomy catheter too high.
- Alternatively, upon opening the artery, platelet aggregation may be identified. Rather than frank thrombus, a defect site may be noted. This should be removed and the defect repaired.
- The patient may need additional antiplatelet therapy such as Plavix in addition to aspirin. Low molecular weight dextran may be started intraoperatively and discontinued after 24 hours.

atherosclerotic occlusive disease. However, acute stroke in the immediate postoperative period remains a recognized complication with centers of excellence reporting a stroke rate in the 1% to 2% range. The management of postoperative stroke after CEA is an area where controversies still exist. Disagreement remains regarding the severity of the deficit that requires reoperation. Areas of disagreement include the role of noninvasive testing and angiography and the window of opportunity when

reoperation should be accomplished. With the advent of new helical CT scanners that can give information about the patency of the ICA in the neck and cerebral vessels in a matter of minutes, and the ability to perform perfusion sequences simultaneously, some authors would argue to perform CT angiography and perfusion CT for patients experiencing stroke in the postoperative period. Perfusional sequences can add valuable diagnostic data about the presence of hypoperfusion and areas of potentially salvageable ischemic penumbra. Theoretically, patients who will benefit most from reexploration of the operative site are those with no distal embolism of thrombus material into the middle cerebral artery or frontal branches. If distal embolization to the middle cerebral artery is present with no evidence of stenosis or occlusion at the operative site, an endovascular treatment is indicated, either with catheter-directed lytic therapy or retrieval of thrombotic material. To maximize the treatment benefit with this complication, it is imperative to have a clear, well-planned algorithm for a patient who sustains a stroke after CEA so that action can be undertaken in a timely fashion once the diagnosis is made. This involves a clear understanding of the potential etiologic mechanisms of this complication.

Not all strokes after CEA are the same; the timing of the stroke plays a large role in determining etiology and potential treatment options. A patient who undergoes a CEA under general anesthesia and awakens with a neurologic deficit has most likely sustained either an intraoperative hypoperfusion injury or an embolic event secondary to clamping or shunt placement. Upon awakening and identification of the deficit, an interrogation of the carotid artery with duplex to assess patency should be undertaken because the artery will most likely be found to be without thrombus. Reoperation is not recommended due to the potential of extending the ischemic area in the brain with any further clamping of the carotid artery. For the most part, these are locally uncorrectable situations with the likelihood of recovery being poor. Thus, the patient should be considered for a head CT scan and possibly cerebral arteriography with lytic salvage of any thrombosed intracerebral vessels.

In another scenario, a patient may develop a neurologic deficit 1 to 2 days after undergoing a CEA. In this situation, the probable cause is a cerebral hemorrhage and/or edema secondary to hyperperfusion. Hyperperfusion occurs in patients after repair of a high-grade carotid artery stenosis or in patients who present with severe bilateral stenosis. The symptom complex consists of hypertension, headache, and seizures. Diagnosis is accomplished by CT scan or magnetic resonance imaging (MRI) of the head. Treatment is blood pressure and seizure control.

More commonly, a patient has a lucent period of normal neurologic status after CEA, whether performed under general or regional anesthesia, followed by a stroke in the immediate postoperative period. The most common cause of such a post-CEA stroke is related to a technical error that results in postoperative thromboembolism. In a comprehensive review of 3062 consecutive CEA procedures, Riles et al. found that symptomatic carotid artery thrombosis occurred in 0.8% of patients but caused 40% of the postoperative strokes. These defects could serve as a point of platelet aggregation and/or initiate thrombus formation. Thromboembolism can occur secondary to errors or defect at the operative site such as an intimal flap, irregularities at the suture lines, a kink caused by elongation after endarterectomy, intramural hematoma, constricting suture line, clamp injury, ledges at the end of the endarterectomy, and/or a rough endarterectomy surface. The cause of the neurologic deficit is usually not due to obstruction of blood flow or ischemia by the thrombus, but rather from embolization of thrombus material as it was forming within the artery or from embolization originating at the distal extent of the thrombus. In addition, these defects can be the nidus for platelet aggregation, which can also embolize distally. These technical errors can and should be corrected; there is conclusive evidence to recommend decisive surgical management in the treatment of post-CEA thrombosis. If corrected in a timely fashion (1 to 2 hours), there is a high likelihood of significant neurologic recovery. Repair after this time, however, may convert a bland ischemic infarction into a hemorrhagic infarct. Any decision not to perform a reoperation in the presence of a delayed neurologic event should be supported by a study demonstrating a patent ICA without technical defects. If uncorrected, embolic events could continue to occur or the artery may progress to complete thrombosis and occlusion. If already thrombosed, restoration of flow to limit ischemia may prove to be beneficial. Rockman et al. showed that in 18 reexplorations performed for an early neurologic deficit, 83.3% clearly showed signs of thrombus or platelet aggregation. Nearly 70% of patients reexplored had either complete resolution of or significant improvement in the deficit that had been present. No patient's condition was worsened by reexploration.

At exploration, thrombus is removed from the endarterectomy site as well as the distal ICA, if present; at this stage, some authors suggest an intraoperative cerebral angiogram for identification of intracerebral thromboemboli. If these are identified, catheter-directed intraoperative lytic therapy could be initiated with good results. After these steps, the cause of the thrombosis must be sought. When these defects are identified, a decision must be made regarding the type of repair; if an obvious defect is detected and appears to be the cause of the thromboembolism, or

platelet aggregation, local repair with tacking sutures or removal of residual plaque is indicated. If no obvious defect is detected, and platelet fibrin deposition is the presumed etiology, consideration must be given to replacing the proximal ICA with an interposition saphenous vein graft. In either situation, postoperative antiplatelet therapy with high molecular weight dextran and/or another oral antiplatelet agent is recommended.

SUGGESTED READINGS

Comerota AJ, Eze AR. Intraoperative high-dose regional urokinase infusion for cerebrovascular occlusion after carotid endarterectomy. *J Vasc Surg.* 1996;24:1008-1016.

Giovanni P, Francecso V, et al. Early acute hemispheric stroke after carotid endarterectomy. Pathogenesis and management. *Acta Neurochir.* 2010;152:579-587.

Hertzer NR. Postoperative management and complications following carotid endarterectomy. In: Rutherford RB, ed. *Vascular Surgery.* Vol 2. 5th ed. Philadelphia, PA: WB Saunders; 2000:1881-1906.

Paty PS, Darling RC, Cordero JA, et al. Carotid artery bypass in acute postendarterectomy thrombosis. *Am J Surg.* 1996;172:181-183.

Radak D, Popovic AD, Radicevic S, et al. Immediate reoperation for perioperative stroke after 2250 carotid endarterectomies: differences between intraoperative and early postoperative stroke. *J Vasc Surg.* 1999;30:245-251.

Riles TS, Imparato AM, Jacobowitz GR, et al. The cause of perioperative stroke after carotid endarterectomy. *J Vasc Surg.* 1994;19:206-216.

Rockman CB, Jacobowitz GR, Lamparello PJ, et al. Immediate reexploration for the perioperative neurological event after carotid endarterectomy: is it worthwhile? *J Vasc Surg.* 2000;32:1062-1070.

CLINICAL SCENARIO CASE QUESTIONS

1. What percentage of patients have nearly complete or significant resolution of their deficit after reexploration following CEA?

    a. 20%
    b. 40%
    c. 50%
    d. 70%
    e. 90%

2. What is the primary cause for reexploration following CEA for an early neurologic deficit?

    a. Neointimal hyperplasia
    b. Atherosclerosis
    c. Thrombus or platelet aggregation
    d. Radiation changes to wall
    e. Patent CEA

6 Cerebral Hyperperfusion after Carotid Artery Endarterectomy

MARCUS E. SEMEL, LIANGGE HSU, and C. KEITH OZAKI

Presentation

A 67-year-old male with a history of dyslipidemia, essential hypertension, and a chronically occluded left internal carotid artery (ICA) is referred to your office after his primary care physician (PCP) detects a right carotid bruit on routine physical examination. The patient takes aspirin, a beta-blocker, an angiotensin-converting enzyme (ACE) inhibitor, and a statin. The PCP obtained a carotid duplex, which reveals a high-grade 80% to 99% stenosis of the right ICA with a peak systolic velocity of 462 cm/s, end diastolic velocity of 142 cm/s, and an occluded left ICA. A thorough history and physical examination does not identify any cardiac or neurologic symptoms/signs, and the exam is otherwise noncontributory. His blood pressure in the office is 148/66 mm Hg. Electrocardiogram is normal. The patient is offered and accepts a right carotid endarterectomy (CEA). In the meantime, he returns to his PCP for perioperative optimization, and the dose of his ACE inhibitor is increased. Several weeks later, he undergoes a right CEA. It is performed under general anesthesia with routine shunting and patch angioplasty—the operation is uncomplicated. In the postanesthesia care unit, he is neurologically intact. His initial blood pressure is 165/72 mm Hg but drifts down to 82/58 mm Hg after several hours. He is asymptomatic.

Differential Diagnosis

The differential diagnosis for hypotension after CEA includes hypovolemia, cardiac dysfunction, sepsis, anaphylaxis, and neurally mediated mechanisms. This last category includes autonomic dysfunction from stimulation of the carotid baroreceptors in the freshly endarterectomized bulb. Hypotension may also serve as an initial sign of an intracranial event.

Approach

Postoperative blood pressure instability after CEA demands a thorough bedside evaluation. The accuracy of the blood pressure reading should be verified. The therapeutic strategy depends on the etiology of the hypotension. If nonneural mechanisms (e.g., hypovolemia, cardiac dysfunction) are ruled out, and on examination the patient demonstrates no neurologic deficit suggestive of cerebral ischemia, then alpha agonists (e.g., phenylephrine) may be given via continuous infusion to maintain perfusion to vital organs.

Case Continued

Based on this patient's low intraoperative fluid resuscitation record, early postoperative oliguria, unremarkable physical examination results, and normal ECG, intravascular volume depletion is determined to be the cause of his relatively low blood pressure. He receives 1 L of lactated Ringer's solution. Immediately after receiving Ringer's solution, the patient's blood pressure returns to 140/80 mm Hg. Six hours later, his blood pressure is 184/97 mm Hg with a heart rate of 86 beats per minute (bpm), and he remains asymptomatic.

Differential Diagnosis

A common mechanism for postoperative hypertension after CEA is the endogenous hormonal response to pain or anxiety. Additionally, patients may have missed doses of chronic antihypertensive medications. Notably, other patients after CEA suffer idiopathic postoperative hypertension that stands outside of these known mechanisms.

Approach

Pain therapy is titrated to avoid oversedation, which would impair the ability to perform serial neurologic examinations. For hypertension that is not related to pain, sodium nitroprusside or nitroglycerin holds the advantage of rapid blood pressure reduction and short pharmacologic half-life (permits easy titration). When beta-adrenergic receptor blockade would also be beneficial, a short-acting beta-blocker infusion is another easily titrated medication.

Discussion

The relatively narrow risk/benefit ratio of CEA and the systemic atherosclerosis in these often high-risk patients demand close perioperative attention to minimize complications. In the situation of perioperative blood pressure instability, high vigilance is mandatory. Perioperative hypotension and hypertension have been associated with increased incidences of neurologic and cardiovascular events. Recently published data suggest an increased risk for 30-day mortality, stroke, and cardiac complications in patients with postoperative hemodynamic instability after CEA. Among patients receiving intravenous vasoactive medication after CEA, there was an increase in the 1-year risk for death or stroke.

There are no clearly defined criteria for an acceptable blood pressure range after CEA, and the clinician must consider the patient's baseline pressure. Although founded on limited data, many clinicians would consider systolic pressures over 160 mm Hg or less than 100 mm Hg to be indications for intervention in the short term. Hypotension due to autonomic dysfunction usually resolves within 24 hours of CEA. Idiopathic hypertension after CEA is seen more commonly in patients with preoperative hypertension and high-grade carotid stenosis.

Case Continued

A short course of labetalol brings the patient's blood pressure below 140 mm Hg with a pulse rate of 62 bpm. He is restarted on his ACE inhibitor and discharged to home on postoperative day 1. However, 48 hours postoperatively, he calls your office with the complaint of a throbbing frontotemporal right-sided headache. At your recommendation, he comes to the hospital's emergency department where his blood pressure is 168/93 mm Hg, he is neurologically intact, and he receives acetaminophen without relief. Four hours later, he vomits and then suffers a grand mal seizure. He is admitted to the intensive care unit.

Differential Diagnosis

The symptoms of cerebral hyperperfusion are primarily neurologic with the distribution of potential diagnoses following suit. Patients may present with altered mental status, confusion, headache, cortical symptoms (ranging from hemiparesis/hemiplegia, hemianopsia, and aphasia to obtundation), seizure, and signs/symptoms of intracerebral hemorrhage.

Beyond hyperperfusion, altered mental status and confusion may be attributable to postoperative delirium or narcotic pain medication resulting in oversedation.

The headache associated with cerebral hyperperfusion is ipsilateral with either a frontotemporal or a periorbital distribution but may be diffuse in nature. It is sometimes described as throbbing, but may be migrainous. As a result, migraine and cluster headaches appear on the differential, but even if the patient has a history of headaches, it is important to remain vigilant for post-CEA complications. Cortical symptoms raise concern for postoperative stroke and early after surgery should be considered the result of a technical complication until proven otherwise. Seizure may be due to stroke, hemorrhage, or trauma or may be medication induced. Intracerebral hemorrhage, which is the most feared complication of cerebral hyperperfusion, may also be the result of stroke, trauma, neoplasm, or uncontrolled hypertension.

Approach

An emergency duplex ultrasound scan confirms right ICA patency. Transcranial Doppler (TCD) can be used to measure cerebral blood flow velocity in the middle cerebral artery (MCA). The diameter of the MCA is not altered by autoregulation, and therefore, changes in velocity correlate well with changes in MCA perfusion. In cerebral hyperperfusion, TCD may show a 150% to 300% increase in the ipsilateral MCA velocity.

Computed tomography (CT) of the head without contrast serves as an initial screen for intracranial bleeding. Intracranial hypodensities on CT scan may be infarctions or edema. Notable CT findings include diffuse or patchy white matter edema, mass effect, petechial, or massive ipsilateral hemorrhage. Single photon emission CT (SPECT) can be useful for detecting alterations in brain perfusion and is sensitive for differentiating between ischemia and hyperperfusion. Similarly, diffusion-weighted magnetic resonance imaging (MRI) can help distinguish between infarctions or edema. Notable MRI findings include white matter edema, focal infarction, and local versus more diffuse hemorrhage (Figs. 1 and 2).

MRI and CT Angiography Results

Case Conclusion

The patient partially recovers but clinically has a dense left hemiplegia. The next day, his mental status deteriorates into a coma and his pupils are bilaterally fixed and dilated. He dies 2 hours later. At autopsy, the endarterectomy site is widely patent and without thrombus. There is a massive right hemispheric hematoma and brainstem herniation through the foramen magnum.

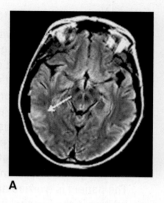 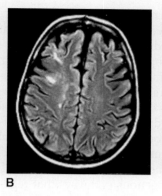 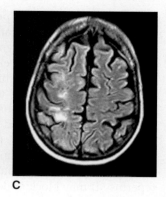

FIGURE 1 • **A–C:** Multiple FLAIR images demonstrate increased T2 signal of the subcortical white matter in the right MCA distribution (**A**, *white arrow*) without associated diffusion-weighted imaging abnormality consistent with hyperperfusion changes and not infarct.

A   B   C

Discussion

After endarterectomy for a high-grade carotid stenosis, the ipsilateral brain vasculature is exposed to perfusion pressures and blood flow substantially higher than it has seen—often in years. It is theorized that the chronically ischemic intracranial arterioles lose the ability to auto-regulate in response to sudden changes in perfusion pressure. Colloquially, these patients have "exhausted" their cerebrovascular reactivity, and the net result is increased cerebral blood flow after the carotid artery is reopened. When measured by techniques such as brain perfusion CT scan, xenon CT scan, nuclear medicine SPECT scan, or TCD, up to 9% of patients develop early postoperative cerebral blood flow well above that required for metabolic needs, with flows reaching four times baseline. Although the majority of these patients suffer no significant clinical consequences from reperfusion, about 15% to 30% of patients with a greater than 100% increase in cerebral blood flow develop cerebral hyperperfusion syndrome.

The reported incidence of clinically apparent cerebral hyperperfusion syndrome following CEA ranges from 0.04% to 1.2%, and in some series, mortality may be as high as 75%. Cerebral hyperperfusion syndrome is not limited to the post-CEA patient—it is recognized as a potential complication of any condition that results in loss of vascular autoregulation or causes that result in endothelial dysfunction with increased permeability and subsequent breakdown of the blood-brain barrier.

The pathophysiology of this syndrome probably relates to reactive hyperemia, which leads to cerebral edema and hemorrhage. It shares physiologic features with other reactive hyperemia syndromes, such as ischemia/reperfusion of an ischemic limb, heart, or bowel. The exact etiology remains unknown though it has been associated with malignant hypertension, eclampsia, immunosuppressive agents in the transplant population, and autoimmune disease.

Clinical symptoms and signs include severe ipsilateral headache, seizures, intracranial hemorrhage, and death. In post-CEA cases, symptoms usually develop within the first 2 weeks postoperatively, with a median of about 3 days. Risk factors that have been described include high-grade carotid stenosis, preoperative and postoperative hypertension, contralateral carotid occlusions, prior cerebral infarcts, use of anticoagulant and antiplatelet agents, and recent contralateral CEA. While identification of patients who will proceed to complications of cerebral hyperperfusion syndrome remains largely unpredictable, there are data to suggest that patients with a treated stenosis of greater than 90%, a contralateral stenosis of greater than 80%, and long-standing preprocedural hypertension have a 15% to 20% risk. Among patients with bilateral carotid stenosis, the interval between procedures may affect the incidence of developing cerebral hyperperfusion syndrome—a higher incidence has been observed in patients undergoing contralateral CEA less than 3 months after their first operation.

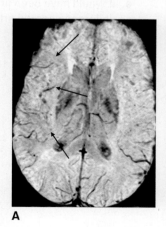 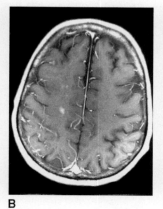 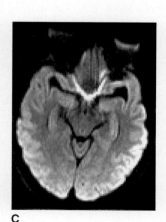

FIGURE 2 • On susceptibility-weighted imaging, (**A**) there is asymmetry with increased signal void of vessels of the right MCA (*black arrows*) with small focal areas of enhancement (**B**) and normal DWI (**C**) consistent with hyperperfusion and increased leakiness of vessels.

A   B   C

Close monitoring of perioperative blood pressure, and intervention if indicated, is advocated to prevent cerebral hyperperfusion syndrome, even though normotensive patients have developed fatal cerebral bleeding. Intraoperative surgical techniques to reduce blood pressure instability, including minimization of surgical dissection between the origins of the internal and external carotid arteries, may avoid damage to the carotid baroreceptor nerves. Similarly, routine use of lidocaine local anesthetic at the carotid sinus (to blunt autonomic stimulation as the carotid plaque is removed and the bulb reperfused) may block endogenous pathways that regulate blood pressure and heart rate in the early postoperative period. Because many patients stay in the hospital for only very limited time periods after routine CEA, discharge instructions must emphasize both blood pressure monitoring and control as an outpatient, and immediate medical attention for severe headache. In patients who exhibit early symptoms of cerebral hyperperfusion, the avoidance of antiplatelet and anticoagulant agents has also been advocated, as well as measures to avoid cerebral edema. Rarely, selected patients respond to intracranial decompressive procedures. While there have been promising data published on use of the free radical scavenger edaravone to prevent cerebral hyperperfusion syndrome, it is based on one nonrandomized study, and there have been no corroborating data or additional studies to date.

SUGGESTED READINGS

Abou-Chebl A, Yadav JS, Reginelli JP, et al. Intracranial hemorrhage and hyperperfusion syndrome following carotid artery stenting: risk factors, prevention, and treatment. *J Am Coll Cardiol.* 2004;43(9):1596-1601.

Karapanayiotides T, Meuli R, Devuyst G, et al. Postcarotid endarterectomy hyperperfusion or reperfusion syndrome. *Stroke.* 2005;36(1):21-26.

Moulakakis KG, Mylonas SN, Sfyroeras GS, et al. Hyperperfusion syndrome after carotid revascularization. *J Vasc Surg.* 2009;49(4):1060-1068.

Tan TW, Eslami MH, Kalish JA, et al. The need for treatment of hemodynamic instability following carotid endarterectomy is associated with increased perioperative and 1-year morbidity and mortality. *J Vasc Surg.* 2013;59:16-24.

van Mook WN, Rennenberg RJ, Schurink GW, et al. Cerebral hyperperfusion syndrome. *Lancet Neurol.* 2005;4(12):877-888.

CLINICAL SCENARIO CASE QUESTIONS

1. A 64-year-old female with a history of hypertension and left carotid stenosis of greater than 80% undergoes an uncomplicated right carotid endarterectomy for an asymptomatic greater than 90% stenosis. The following day, she is preparing for discharge from the hospital when the nurse makes a final check of her vital signs. The nurse calls the house officer to report that the patient's blood pressure is 194/106 mm Hg. The house officer evaluates the patient who has no complaints, is neurologically intact, and has a flat, clean neck incision. The patient is worried about holding up her son who is waiting in the hospital lobby to drive her home. The next most appropriate step in management is:

   a. Emergency neck exploration in the operating room
   b. Discharge from the hospital with blood pressure checks at home
   c. Immediate management of the patient's hypertension
   d. Noncontrast computed tomography (CT) scan to rule out intracranial hemorrhage
   e. Single-photon emission CT (SPECT) to evaluate brain perfusion

2. Two days after hospital discharge, the patient's son calls your office to say that his mother has a throbbing headache over the right side of her forehead. She returns to the hospital with a blood pressure of 178/92 mm Hg. She is alert, oriented, and remains neurologically intact. A noncontrast head CT rules out hemorrhage. Magnetic resonance imaging of the brain demonstrates white matter edema without evidence of diffusion-weighted imaging abnormality. She is started on an intravenous nitroglycerin infusion and admitted to the intensive care unit for close observation. Which of the following statements about the patient's headache is true?

   a. Combination therapy with butalbital/acetaminophen/caffeine is first-line management.
   b. It is likely the result of postoperative hypovolemia.
   c. Full anticoagulation is necessary to prevent a conversion to stroke.
   d. Risk factors include a treated stenosis greater than 90% and a contralateral stenosis greater than 80%.
   e. It would have been prevented had the patient undergone carotid artery stenting.

7 Symptomatic Carotid Endarterectomy—Carotid Artery Stenting

DUSTIN Y. YOON and MARK K. ESKANDARI

Presentation

A 65-year-old right-handed gentleman with a history of tobacco use, myocardial infarction status post coronary bypass, and left carotid endarterectomy (CEA) 5 years ago now presents with crescendo transient ischemic attacks (TIAs). The patient states that these episodes started 2 months ago and occur several times per week. Each episode lasts 20 to 30 minutes and is associated with mild right arm weakness and blurry vision on the left side. No loss of consciousness occurs. On neurologic examination, the patient is grossly intact with mild right pronator drift. Ultrasound reveals peak systolic velocities of 380 cm/s in the left proximal internal carotid artery (ICA), and magnetic resonance angiography (MRA) of the head/neck shows two focal high-grade stenoses of 90% in this same region (Fig. 1). He remains compliant with aspirin and clopidogrel since his initial CEA.

Differential Diagnosis

The incidence of recurrent carotid stenosis is variable and depends on the definition of restenosis, method of diagnosis, and interval follow-up, with an estimated range of 8% to 19%, of which only 3% are symptomatic. Identification and management of restenosis is primarily dictated by two factors: (1) length of time from index procedure to diagnosis of restenosis and (2) the presence/absence of clinical symptoms.

A stenosis identified within the immediate post-operative period is often residual disease after an incomplete CEA rather than recurrent stenosis. Restenosis within the first 36 months is often a result of neointimal hyperplasia and is generally a smooth and homogenous lesion that is less prone to embolization. Restenosis after this 36-month post-operative period is generally a result of progressive or new atherosclerotic disease and has been associated with risk factors that include age less than 60 years, female sex, smoking, diabetes, and hypertension. Surgical management of post-CEA restenosis should be individualized and generally reserved for asymptomatic patients with greater than 80% or symptomatic patients with ≥50% lesions. However, consensus guidelines have yet to be made.

Though unlikely in this patient, differential diagnoses include new-onset atrial fibrillation (or other sources of thromboembolic disease), vasculitis, fibromuscular dysplasia (FMD), carotid dissection/aneurysm, extensive intracranial carotid disease, and migraine headaches.

Workup

The most robust assessment and follow-up data for recurrent carotid stenosis are provided by the Asymptomatic Carotid Atherosclerosis Study (ACAS) and are surveyed by noninvasive duplex ultrasonography. Color duplex ultrasound remains the preferred first-line imaging modality for evaluation although the recommended frequency of surveillance remains controversial. With the advent of contrast-enhanced MRA and now multidetector computed tomographic angiography (CTA), the anatomy of the aortic arch and circle of Willis can be assessed for carotid artery stenting (CAS) suitability. Furthermore, CTA can enhance the identification of calcification, vessel tortuosity, and any cerebral abnormalities, all of which are important for preoperative planning and post-operative monitoring. Prior to surgery, appropriate preoperative risk stratification with concomitant medical optimization with aspirin, clopidogrel, and statins should be performed.

In this patient, Figure 1 shows two focal high-grade lesions of the left ICA.

Diagnosis and Treatment—Redo CEA or Stent?

Substantial controversy exists regarding the natural history, histopathologic significance, and threshold for intervention of post-CEA restenosis as well as the appropriate method of treatment. Although patient care should be individualized, most vascular surgeons would generally accept that symptomatic patients with ≥50% lesions

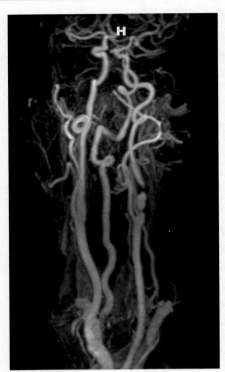

FIGURE 1 • MRA of the head/neck shows two high-grade focal lesions at the proximal left ICA and at the level of C1.

should be treated. Generally, CAS has been recommended to high-risk patients with prior neck external beam irradiation, prior neck dissections/tracheostomies, inaccessible lesions unamenable to CEA (above the C2 level), and those with limited cervical spine mobility. While many centers show high patency rates in the immediate post-CEA CAS period, the long-term durability is inconclusive. Nevertheless, CAS has been continuously justified for its minimally invasive approach, the histopathologic nature of neointimal hyperplastic lesions more amenable to dilation, and the low risk for cranial nerve injury, with some studies showing up to 18% risk of nerve injury with redo CEA.

Several meta-analyses have been performed comparing the complication rates of redo CEA versus CAS in this post-CEA population. While the results are widely variable, there are trends toward lower perioperative cardiac complications, lower rate of procedure-related stroke, and lower cranial nerve injuries with CAS. These trends, however, are difficult to tease out with respect to early versus late restenosis, and some data show the highest risk of periprocedural stroke/death with CAS within 7 days of symptoms. Most studies show no difference in mortality between the two treatment groups.

This patient, who has high preoperative risk factors and late restenosis, opted to enroll in the high-risk Stenting and Angioplasty with Protection in Patients at High Risk for Endarterectomy World Wide (SAPPHIRE WW) trial and undergo CAS.

Surgical Approach

Approximately 50% of all patients undergoing CEA have clinically relevant coronary artery disease, and myocardial death is the most common cause of mortality in these patients. While the North American Symptomatic Carotid Endarterectomy Trial (NASCET) excluded patients with recent unstable angina and myocardial infarction, they showed high cardiovascular complication rates. The initial results of the randomized SAPPHIRE trial comparing CEA with CAS in patients with high risk for open surgery showed that CAS was noninferior in comparison to CEA and had trends toward lower complication rates. Enrollment and results are still ongoing in the high-risk registry, but, in general, most vascular surgeons would agree that high-risk, symptomatic patients with contraindications or challenging redo CEA should undergo CAS.

Unless contraindicated, all patients should be on dual antiplatelet regimen of aspirin and clopidogrel preoperatively. Preprocedural imaging with MRA or CTA should be obtained to carefully evaluate aortic arch morphology and origin and abnormalities of supra-aortic vessels (i.e., tortuosity, calcification, severe angulation), and to take accurate measurements of the lesion and carotid arteries (Table 1).

Figure 2 shows the intraoperative selective angiogram of the left carotid artery and confirms the MRA findings of two high-grade focal lesions of the left ICA. Figure 3 shows successful stent deployment with no residual stenosis, and Figure 4 shows completion intracranial angiogram without any perfusion deficits.

Special Intraoperative Considerations

Intraoperative neuromonitoring is of utmost importance during the procedure. Continuous electrocardiographic and intra-arterial monitoring should be obtained throughout the procedure. The level of speech and motor function should be evaluated frequently by asking the patient simple questions or by use of a toy honking device on the contralateral side of affected lesion.

The use of embolic protection devices (EPDs) is mandatory for reimbursement in the United States, and transcranial Doppler is a useful adjunctive technique for detecting stroke, especially when crossing calcified lesions. Excessive manipulation of the 0.014-inch guidewire of the EPD should be avoided and not advanced too far as the intracranial portion of the ICA is prone to dissection.

Post-operative Management

All patients who undergo CAS should undergo frequent neuromonitor checks in the post-operative period, as strokes most often are detected within the first 6 hours post-operatively. We have all patients undergo duplex ultrasonography within the first month post-operatively and at least annually thereafter. Regardless of timing, all patients should be carefully followed with a carotid surveillance program.

TABLE 1. Symptomatic Carotid Endartectomy- Carotid Artery Stenting

Key Technical Steps

1. Obtain retrograde access via common femoral artery followed by a 5-French introducer access sheath. Brachial access can be obtained if femoral access is not possible but is more cumbersome and less desirable.
2. Obtain a diagnostic aortic arch angiogram in a 35- to 40-degree left anterior oblique projection by placing a pigtail catheter over a guidewire in the ascending aorta.
3. Selectively cannulate the common carotid artery with a preshaped guiding catheter (i.e., DAV [Cook], IMA, Vitek [Cook]) and obtain a selective angiogram of the carotid bifurcation and intracranial circulation (AP and lateral views).
4. Administer systemic intravenous anticoagulant (unfractionated heparin or Angiomax) to achieve an activated clotting time (ACT) of >250 seconds to reduce perioperative stroke risk.
5. Using a 0.014-inch guidewire, cross the stenotic lesion, deploy the embolic protection device (EPD), and ensure adequate wall apposition and brisk filling through filter element. Distal balloon and proximal occlusion with or without flow reversal are alternative options for embolic protection.
6. If necessary, predilate with a 3- or 4-mm balloon at low inflation pressures and cross the lesion with the self-expanding stent with roadmapping technique. Prior to angioplasty, systemic intravenous administration of 0.4 mg of atropine may reduce the incidence of bradycardia.
7. Size the diameter and length of the stent, typically to the largest portion of the vessel and 1 mm larger than CCA diameter and deploy.
8. Post-dilate the narrowest portion of the stent (typically 5 mm) and obtain a post-deployment angiogram.
9. Retrieve the EPD and obtain completion angiogram of carotid and intracranial circulation to rule out dissection and/or other complications (i.e., flow-limiting embolism).
10. Remove catheter, wire, sheath, and selectively close the arteriotomy with a closure device.

Potential Pitfalls

- The most devastating complication is distal embolization visible on completion angiogram. Although results can vary, catheter-directed thrombolysis, aspiration thrombectomy, and/or thrombus maceration have been suggested as neurorescue maneuvers.
- Ensure that catheter tips are not placed into the sidewall of arteries or near any lesions to avoid any jet effect or manual embolization.
- Carefully examine access sites for hemostasis and monitor for future complications (i.e., pseudoaneurysm, hematoma, arterial embolism).

Case Conclusion

The patient recovers in the post-anesthesia care unit without issues or change of neuromotor status from his preoperative baseline. He is discharged within 23 hours, and 1-month carotid duplex shows no evidence of restenosis. His TIAs have completely resolved, and he returns to work within several days of his surgery.

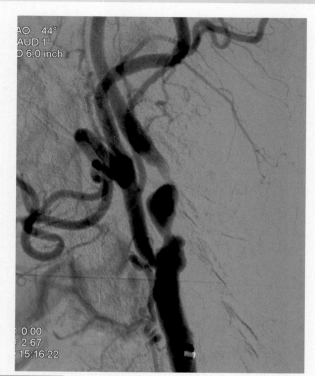

FIGURE 2 • Intraoperative angiogram showing patency of left CCA and ECA. Approximately 80% stenosis of the distal ICA at the C1-C2 level.

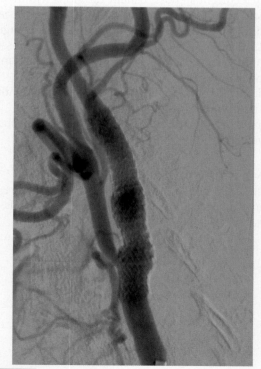

FIGURE 3 • Intraoperative angiogram post–stent deployment crossing the orifice of the ECA. Angiogram shows no flow-limiting dissection, intraluminal filling defect, or residual stenosis and preserved flow to the ECA.

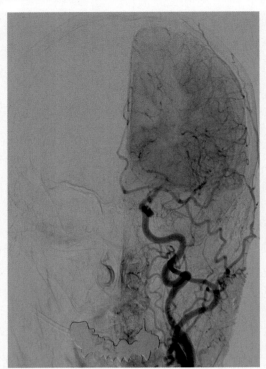

FIGURE 4 • Intraoperative cerebral angiogram showing filling of the anterior middle cerebral arteries with no cross filling to the collateral circulation.

TAKE HOME POINTS

- Early recurrent stenosis usually develops within 3 years and is secondary to neointimal hyperplasia.
- Medical optimization, accurate preoperative imaging for CAS suitability with CTA or MRA, and risk assessment of CAS versus CEA should be performed on an individual basis.
- Intraoperatively, the patient should undergo continuous neuromonitoring for embolic evaluation.
- All patients should undergo post-operative carotid surveillance.

SUGGESTED READINGS

AbuRahma AF, et al. Primary carotid artery stenting versus carotid artery stenting for post carotid endarterectomy stenosis. *J Vasc Surg.* 2009;50(5):1031-1039.

Attigah N, et al. Redo surgery or carotid stenting for restenosis after carotid endarterectomy: results of two different treatment strategies. *Ann Vasc Surg.* 2010;24(2):190-195.

Barnett HJ, et al. Benefit of carotid endarterectomy in patients with symptomatic moderate or severe stenosis. North American Symptomatic Carotid Endarterectomy Trial Collaborators. *N Engl J Med.* 1998;339(20):1415-1425.

de Borst GJ, et al. Carotid angioplasty and stenting for post-endarterectomy stenosis: long-term follow up. *J Vasc Surg.* 2007;45(1):118-123.

Keldahl ML, et al. Carotid artery stenting using proximal balloon occlusion embolic protection. *Perspect Vasc Surg Endovasc Ther.* 2010;22(3):187-193.

Lal BK. Recurrent carotid stenosis after CEA and CAS: diagnosis and management. *Semin Vasc Surg.* 2007;20(4):259-266.

Rantner B, et al. The risk of carotid artery stenting compared with carotid endarterectomy is greatest in patients treated within 7 days of symptoms. *J Vasc Surg.* 2013;57(3):619-626.

CLINICAL SCENARIO CASE QUESTIONS

1. A 61-year-old male comes into your clinic complaining of right-sided vision loss for 2 to 3 minutes. He also notes some left-sided arm paresthesias and weakness. His history is significant for 1-pack-per-day smoking and right carotid endarterectomy 3 years ago. On physical examination, no neurologic deficits are elicited, but duplex ultrasonography reveals 75% stenosis of his right ICA and 50% stenosis of his left ICA. Which of the following statements is not true?

   a. He has amaurosis fugax secondary to emboli from his right ICA plaque.
   b. Carotid artery stenting is an acceptable treatment for his right ICA.
   c. He is a candidate for CEA on the right but not the left.
   d. The patient is a candidate for either CAS or CEA bilaterally.

2. Which of the following risk factors is the strongest indication to perform a carotid artery stent versus a carotid endarterectomy in a restenotic patient after traditional endarterectomy?

   a. Prior neck lymph node dissection
   b. C2-C3 cervical spine fusion
   c. Uncontrolled diabetes with HbA1c of 12.5%
   d. Angina with three-vessel coronary disease

8 Intimal Hyperplasia after Carotid Artery Stenting

MARTYN KNOWLES and CARLOS H. TIMARAN

Presentation

A 69-year-old male with a history of peripheral arterial disease, coronary artery disease, hypertension, and carotid artery stenosis, who underwent right carotid artery stenting (CAS) 4 years prior to presentation, follows up for routine carotid duplex ultrasound surveillance. He denies any history of transient ischemic attack (TIA), stroke (CVA), or amaurosis fugax. On physical examination, he has no carotid bruits and is neurologically intact.

Workup

His previous carotid duplex from a year earlier revealed a peak systolic velocity (PSV) of 103 cm/s in the left internal carotid artery (ICA), 108 cm/s in the left common carotid artery (CCA), an end diastolic velocity (EDV) of 32 cm/s, yielding an ICA/CCA ratio of 1.1. On the right, PSV was 162 cm/s in the ICA, 79 cm/s in the CCA, with an EDV of 54 cm/s, yielding an ICA/CCA ratio of 2.1. The study was consistent with left carotid artery minimal stenosis, 1% to 39%; right carotid artery moderate stenosis was 40% to 59%.

The current duplex reveals a PSV of 97 cm/s in the left ICA, 107 cm/s in the CCA, an EDV of 23 cm/s, yielding an ICA/CCA ratio of 0.9. On the right, PSV is 388 cm/s in the ICA, 52 cm/s in the CCA, an EDV of 94 cm/s, yielding an ICA/CCA ratio of 7.4. Interpretation: left carotid artery minimal stenosis, 1% to 39% unchanged from previous study; right carotid artery severe stenosis, 70% to 99% significantly worsened from previous study (Fig. 1). A CT angiogram of the head and neck is obtained and reveals a severe, greater than 80%, stenosis with intraluminal thrombus in the right ICA (Fig. 2). The patient is immediately placed on a heparin drip and admitted for repair.

Differential Diagnosis

The patient has an asymptomatic recurrent high-grade in-stent stenosis of the right ICA after previous CAS. Other less likely disease processes that may account for the restenosis include carotid body tumor, carotid artery dissection, trauma, aneurysm, or fibromuscular dysplasia. However, given the history of CAS and high-grade in-stent restenosis, carotid artery restenosis is more likely. In symptomatic patients, the differential diagnosis for a TIA or cerebrovascular accident (CVA) following carotid intervention includes recurrent stenosis from myointimal hyperplasia or progressive atherosclerosis, embolic phenomenon (atrial fibrillation or other cardiac causes), or vasculitis.

Discussion

Restenosis is a serious complication after carotid intervention. Following carotid endarterectomy (CEA), the incidence of restenosis is between 5% and 20%, which is only symptomatic in less than 5% of patients. Within the first 3 years, recurrent stenosis is typically from intimal hyperplasia. Lesions that typically develop after this time are more often due to advancing or de novo atherosclerotic disease. Recurrent stenosis is more common in women, those who continue to smoke, and patients with diabetes, hypercholesterolemia, or hypertension.

Restenosis after carotid intervention is frequent when only balloon angioplasty is performed, as reported in the CAVATAS trial with 14% 1-year restenosis compared to 1% after CEA. In more recent studies, in which routine stenting is performed, similar rates of restenosis between CAS and CEA are reported, usually in the range of 0.6% to 18%. Patients who undergo CAS for recurrent stenosis after CEA, or have a history of neck irradiation or cancer, appear to be at higher risk.

Diagnosis of restenosis after CAS requires careful assessment. Ultrasound criteria for restenosis after CAS are different from nonstented arteries because of the inherent effects the stent has on the artery, and the type of stent. Vessel compliance is decreased and frequently alters the ultrasound flow velocities. Stent design may also affect blood flow velocities, with open cell stents more likely to remain closer to normal velocities due to less of an effect on compliance. New modified criteria have been proposed after CAS; however, no standardization has been adopted. Peak systolic velocities over 300 cm/s and ICA/CCA ratio over 4.3 have been found to be consistent with stenosis greater than 70%. Careful examination with B-mode and color Doppler can also elucidate luminal narrowing. Carotid duplex ultrasonography should be sought after 1 month postprocedure for a new baseline and then v every

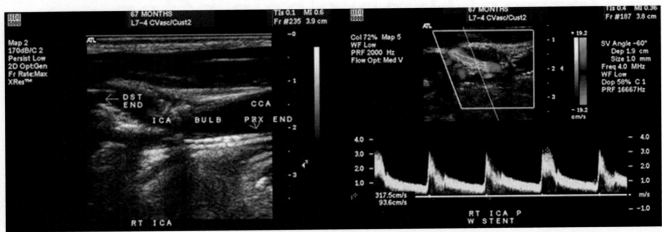

FIGURE 1 • B-mode imaging of the right carotid artery reveals a patent carotid stent with severe in-stent restenosis in the proximal ICA. Color Doppler and spectral ultrasound analysis of the right ICA revels high peak systolic velocities >300 cm/s consistent with a high-grade stenosis within the stent.

6 months for the first 2 years, when intimal hyperplasia is more likely, then yearly thereafter.

Diagnosis and Treatment

Recurrent stenosis after CEA can be treated with either redo CEA or CAS. Redo CEA is associated with a stroke risk of 3% to 5% and carries a higher risk of cranial nerve injury. Accordingly, CAS has become a popular treatment modality for recurrent stenosis after CEA avoiding the risk of cranial nerve injury and a general anesthetic. However, there are complications associated with CAS, including bradycardia and hypotension after balloon dilatation and stent placement. Because of the ability to avoid anatomic and physiologic constraints, such as history of cranial nerve injury, neck immobility, neck irradiation, tracheostomy, previous neck surgery, or high lesions, CAS is now considered first-line therapy for carotid stenosis among anatomic high-risk patients.

The decision to treat a patient with carotid restenosis is not straightforward as the majority of patients are asymptomatic. Global perfusion, contralateral carotid flow, severity of symptoms, medical comorbidities, interval since carotid intervention, and rapid progression need to be considered to define the type of treatment. Asymptomatic low- and moderate-grade stenoses are typically treated with antiplatelet agents and serial surveillance ultrasonography. Historically, symptomatic or high-grade (>80%) stenosis, especially in those with contralateral occlusion, has been treated with repeat intervention. Lesions caused by myointimal hyperplasia are thought to have a lower risk of embolism and can regress, and therefore, reintervention during the first 2 to 3 years is typically avoided in the absence of symptoms. Angiography is an important part of the evaluation of patients with restenosis and allows accurately characterization of lesions.

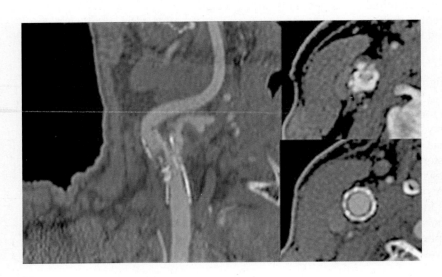

FIGURE 2 • CT angiogram revealing the right carotid stent with encroachment of the stent within the lumen in the central portion causing a high-grade stenosis with intraluminal thrombus. Cross-sectional images reveal severe intrusion of the stent in the midportion compared to the edges.

Options for Surgical Repair

The majority of in-stent restenoses are treated with balloon dilatation with regular or cutting balloons. At each treatment, reinitiating double medical therapy with aspirin and Plavix is recommended. Uncommonly, restenting is required for lesions that do not respond to angioplasty alone, or stenoses at or beyond the edges of the stent. In cases where percutaneous intervention is unsuccessful, or the patient is at high risk for embolization, open endarterectomy with explantation is recommended. Care should be given to avoid any manipulation of the carotid bifurcation to avoid embolization. According to recent observational studies, triple antiplatelet therapy with aspirin 325 mg for life, clopidogrel 75 mg for a month, and cilostazol 100 mg twice daily for 3 months may be given to decrease the likelihood of further restenosis after CAS for recurrent stenosis, especially if associated to prior irradiation, neck cancer, or previous CEA restenosis. Randomized clinical trials supporting this regimen are still missing.

Case Conclusion

The patient is admitted and placed on intravenous heparin. The likely presence of intraluminal thrombus makes endovascular management with percutaneous angioplasty a less attractive alternative of treatment. A CEA with explantation of the carotid artery stent and patch angioplasty is performed under general anesthesia with arterial monitoring via a radial arterial line. Intraoperative plain x-ray films are taken showing severe intrusion of the stent from external compression (Fig. 3). The neck is prepped and draped, and an incision is made along the anterior border of the sternocleidomastoid muscle (SCM). The platysma is divided, and the SCM is retracted laterally, allowing visualization of the internal jugular vein (IJV). The facial branch is ligated, and the IJV is retracted laterally. Because of the intraluminal thrombus, carotid manipulation is kept to a minimum, and the patient is heparinized (100 U/kg) with a goal of an activated clotting time (ACT) >250. Careful dissection allowing control of the CCA, external carotid artery (ECA), and ICA with vessel loops is performed. After raising the systolic blood pressure to >140 mm Hg, clamps are placed sequentially on the ICA, ECA, and CCA. A stump pressure is checked and found to be 35 mm Hg. Dissection of the carotid bulb and an arteriotomy are performed, which required transection of the stent from the CCA to ICA (Fig. 4). A #8 Argyle shunt is placed and flow confirmed with a handheld Doppler probe. The endarterectomy is performed starting in the CCA toward the ICA. An eversion endarterectomy of the ECA is also performed with good back bleeding. Endarterectomy allows removal of the carotid stent with thrombus noted in the lumen until a good distal end point is identified. All debris is removed. A bovine pericardial patch is sewn in with fine monofilament suture. Prior to completing the repair, the shunt is removed, and back bleeding of the ECA and ICA, as well as forward bleeding of the CCA, allows removal of any debris or air. The patch is completed, and an intraoperative duplex study is performed ensuring there are no flaps. The heparin is partially reversed, and the incision is closed. The patient is awakened, and prior to extubation, he is noted to be neurologically intact. His neurologic exam and blood pressure are monitored in the intensive care unit for 24 hours, prior to discharge. He is sent home on aspirin as antiplatelet therapy (Table 1).

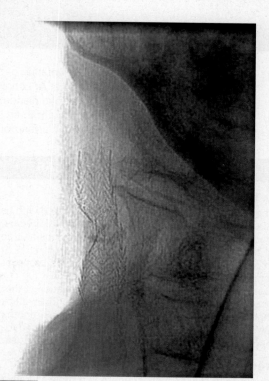

FIGURE 3 • X-ray of the carotid stent showing severe intrusion of the stent from external compression due to restenosis.

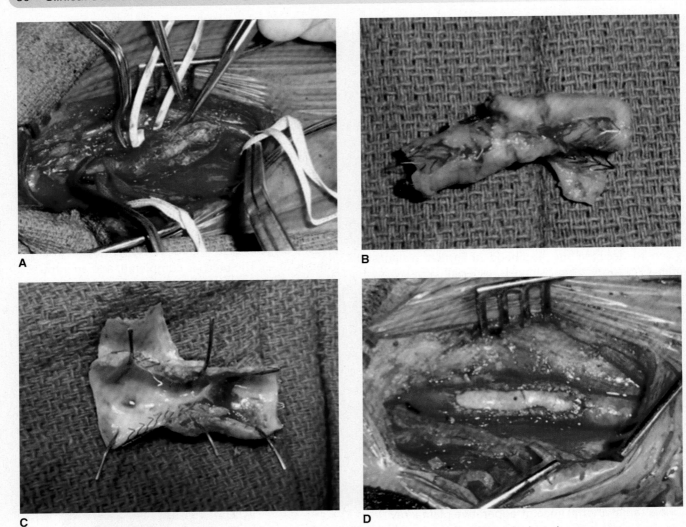

FIGURE 4 • A CEA with explantation of the carotid artery stent and patch angioplasty is performed under general anesthesia. **A:** Longitudinal arteriotomy is performed. **B:** The crushed stent is removed en bloc with the carotid plaque. **C:** The stent is transected longitudinally, and a floating thrombus is demonstrated adherent to an ulcerated plaque within the stent. **D:** A bovine pericardial patch is used to repair the carotid arteriotomy.

TABLE 1. Intimal Hyperplasia after CAS

Key Technical Steps

1. The majority of in-stent restenoses are treated with balloon dilatation with regular or cutting balloons.
2. At each treatment, reinitiating double medical therapy with aspirin and Plavix is recommended.
3. Uncommonly, restenting is required for lesions that do not respond to angioplasty alone, or stenoses at or beyond the edges of the stent.
4. In cases where percutaneous intervention is unsuccessful, or the patient is at high risk for embolization, open endarterectomy with explantation is recommended.
5. Care should be given to avoid any manipulation of the carotid bifurcation to avoid embolization.
6. According to recent observational studies, triple antiplatelet therapy with aspirin 325 mg for life, clopidogrel 75 mg for a month, and cilostazol 100 mg twice daily for 3 months may be given to decrease the likelihood of further restenosis after CAS for recurrent stenosis, especially if associated to prior irradiation, neck cancer, or previous CEA restenosis.
7. A CEA with explantation of the carotid artery stent and patch angioplasty is acceptable therapy in this setting.

Potential Pitfalls

• Randomized clinical trials supporting a triple therapy (aspirin, plavix, pletal) regimen in this scenario are lacking.
• There are data to suggest that cranial nerve injury is higher in the setting of open surgery compared with an endovascular approach.

Postoperative Management

The patient is seen after 2 weeks for a wound check. He is doing well and on daily aspirin. A 30-day carotid duplex ultrasound reveals a patent endarterectomy site without restenosis. After the 1-month scan, routine yearly follow-ups with carotid duplex imaging are recommended.

TAKE HOME POINTS

- Risk of restenosis after CAS appears to be comparable to open endarterectomy.
- Risk of restenosis seems to be increased in those treated for recurrent stenosis after a CEA or those with previous neck irradiation or cancer.
- Consideration for triple antiplatelet therapy should be entertained initially in high-risk patients, including aspirin, clopidogrel, and cilostazol. Aspirin 325 mg id maintained as a long-term mainstay therapy.
- Close serial follow-up of patients with duplex ultrasonography is imperative.
- Because of alterations in flow velocities after CAS, the 1-month postprocedural duplex ultrasound should be used as a new baseline.

SUGGESTED READINGS

Aburahma, AF, Bates, MC, Stone, PA, et al. Comparative study of operative treatment and percutaneous transluminal angioplasty/stenting for recurrent carotid disease. *J Vasc Surg.* 2001;34(5):831-838.

AbuRahma AF, Maxwell D, Eads K, et al. Carotid duplex velocity criteria revisited for the diagnosis of carotid in-stent restenosis. *Vascular.* 2007;15(3):119-125.

Brott TG, Hobson RW II, Howard G, et al. Stenting versus endarterectomy for treatment of carotid-artery stenosis. *N Engl J Med.* 2010;363(1):11-23.

Endarterectomy for asymptomatic carotid artery stenosis. Executive committee for the asymptomatic carotid atherosclerosis study. *JAMA.* 1995;273(18):1421-1428.

North American Symptomatic Carotid Endarterectomy Trial, Collaborators. Beneficial effect of carotid endarterectomy in symptomatic patients with high-grade carotid stenosis. *N Engl J Med.* 1991;325(7):445-453.

Yadav JS, Wholey MH, Kuntz RE, et al. Protected carotid-artery stenting versus endarterectomy in high-risk patients. *N Engl J Med.* 2004;351:15:1493-1501.

CLINICAL SCENARIO CLOSING QUESTIONS

1. The most common time to develop intimal hyperplasia in a carotid stent is at:

   a. 1 week
   b. 1 month
   c. 1 to 2 years
   d. 10 years
   e. 20 years

2. Reintervention of a CAS should occur when the stent is:

   a. >40% stenosed
   b. >60% stenosed
   c. >20% stenosis with posterior circulation symptoms
   d. >80% stenosed
   e. Occluded

9 Carotid Artery Stent/Neck Approach/Difficult Arch

LINDA WANG and CHRISTOPHER J. KWOLEK

Presentation

A 74-year-old female is referred by another vascular surgeon for a second opinion concerning the management of a critical right internal carotid artery (ICA) stenosis. She denies any focal motor or sensory deficits, speech difficulties, or visual changes. The patient is 14 years status post resection of a right-sided tonsillar carcinoma with chemoradiation. Her past medical history is significant for diabetes, hypertension, and hyperlipidemia. She is a nonsmoker and currently taking aspirin 81 mg/d, simvastatin 20 mg/d, and metformin 500 mg twice a day. On physical examination, the patient is a well-appearing Caucasian female who looks her stated age. Vital signs are notable for a regular pulse of 70 beats per minute, blood pressure of 152/67 mm Hg in the left arm and 168/75 mm Hg in the right arm, and a respiratory rate of 16. Her physical examination is significant for a right carotid bruit, palpable carotid pulses bilaterally, and well-healed scar tissue from previous neck surgery and radiation. Her neurologic exam is intact.

Differential Diagnosis

Any patient with a history of neck radiation is at risk for developing ipsilateral carotid artery stenosis. This patient's history of radiation 14 years prior puts her at high risk for developing radiation-induced vascular disease. She additionally has cardiovascular risk factors, such as hypertension and hyperlipidemia, which put her at increased risk for developing atherosclerotic disease.

Workup

It is important to know about cardiovascular risk factors in patients presenting with carotid artery stenosis. More specifically, a history of diabetes, hyperlipidemia, myocardial infarction, stroke, a positive family history of premature atherosclerosis, and smoking are particularly pertinent. A full neurologic and pulse examination should be performed in any patient presenting with carotid artery disease.

Carotid duplex examination should be used to evaluate for the presence of calcification and thrombus as well as for the degree of stenosis by measuring elevation in peak systolic velocity (PSV) and end diastolic velocity (EDV). In the present case, ultrasound demonstrates a severe right ICA stenosis with a PSV of 506 cm/s, EDV of 228 cm/s, and ICA to common carotid artery (CCA) ratio of 10.4 as shown in Figure 1. She had no significant left-sided stenosis.

Computed tomography angiography (CTA) can help define arch anatomy and disease, vessel tortuosity, calcification, and intracranial disease. CTA to evaluate these characteristics in patients being considered for carotid artery stenting (CAS) is routinely used. This patient's CTA is shown in Figure 2. Magnetic resonance imaging (MRI) and magnetic resonance angiography (MRA) can also be used for evaluation of arch and cerebral vessels as well as to evaluate for acute and chronic stroke.

Diagnosis and Treatment

The patient has a critical right ICA stenosis. One option for treatment would involve open surgical exploration with a carotid artery endarterectomy (CEA) or a carotid artery interposition grafting. However, there are several things to consider in a patient who has undergone prior radiation and/or dissection. Radiation induces skin changes that can compromise nutrient delivery and therefore affect wound healing. Scar tissue from previous dissections can complicate subsequent open procedures and also increases the risk of nerve injury.

Carotid angioplasty and stenting is therefore a reasonable alternative. Minimizing the risk of stroke during this procedure is of the utmost importance. Transfemoral carotid stenting has been shown to have a higher incidence of new microembolic lesions on diffusion-weighted MRI when compared to proximal carotid artery occlusion with flow reversal. However, the current commercially available proximal balloon occlusion systems require placement through a 9-French femoral sheath and can significantly increase the risk of embolic events in patients with tortuous and diseased aortic arches. Direct

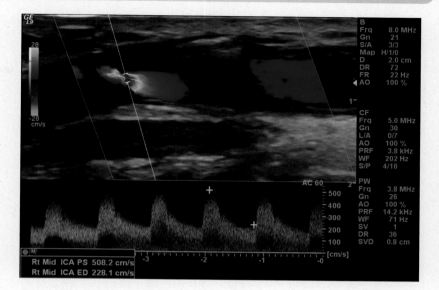

FIGURE 1 • Preoperative carotid duplex ultrasound demonstrating severe right ICA stenosis.

CCA access via a supraclavicular incision with proximal occlusion and flow reversal was thus developed to overcome these limitations.

To minimize the risk of periprocedural stroke and embolization, the patient should be started on aspirin, clopidogrel, and a statin 3 to 5 days before the intervention if the patient is not already taking those medications.

Surgical Approach

Direct cervical carotid access with flow reversal was designed to combine the advantages of both CEA and CAS by pairing direct carotid access with proximal occlusion and flow reversal to provide embolic protection during stenting. In contrast to traditional CAS, the procedure starts at the neck instead of the groin. Direct carotid access is intended to minimize the risk of microemboli and stroke associated with arch navigation.

The procedure is done under local anesthesia and minimal sedation to be able to assess intraoperative neurologic status. The patient is pretreated with glycopyrrolate to prevent procedure-induced cardiac vagal reflexes. An ultrasound is performed to confirm the length from the clavicle to the carotid bifurcation (minimum of 5 cm), to identify the depth of the CCA, and to identify a potential puncture site free from calcification and thrombus. Control of the CCA is accomplished through a small transverse incision above the clavicle with placement of a Rummel tourniquet or vessel loop.

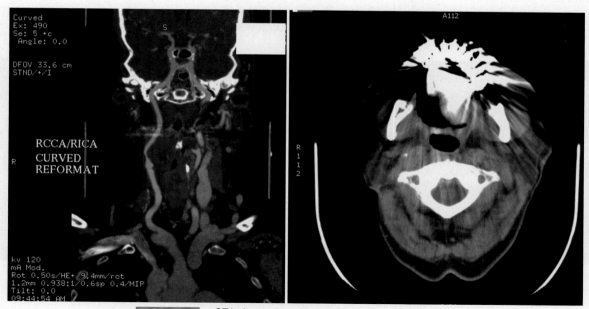

FIGURE 2 • CTA demonstrating critical right ICA stenosis.

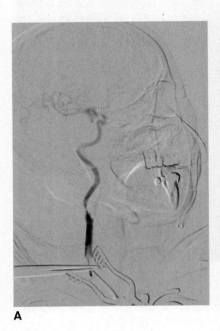

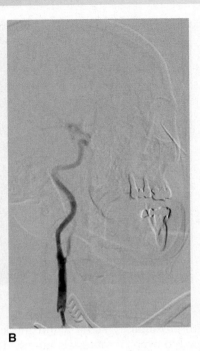

A   **B**

FIGURE 3 • Intraoperative angiography demonstrating critical right ICA stenosis (**A**) and completion angiogram after CAS (**B**).

A 5-0 prolene suture is placed as a U-stitch in the anterior wall of the CCA. The patient is systemically heparinized to maintain an activated clotting time (ACT) greater than 250 seconds, and a micropuncture needle is introduced through the U-stitch into the CCA. Angiography is then performed to confirm a greater than or equal to 80% stenosis and locate the lesion (Fig. 3A). An Amplatz Super Stiff wire with a 1-cm floppy tip is introduced into the CCA while staying below the level of the lesion. The entry site is then dilated with an 8-French dilator. The flow reversal cannula is introduced 2.5 cm into the CCA (Fig. 4A), and cervical and intracranial angiograms are performed.

After suturing the carotid sheath to the chest wall, a second access sheath is placed in the contralateral femoral vein. The two sheaths are connected via a flow controller, thereby creating an arteriovenous shunt that diverts embolic debris away from the brain (Fig. 4B). Flow reversal is established at the start of the procedure, providing embolic protection before any manipulation of the carotid lesion. The CCA is then completely occluded, and complete flow reversal is established. The stenosis is crossed with a 0.014-inch guidewire. A self-expanding carotid stent is placed and postdilated with a 4- or 5-mm balloon. A completion angiogram is performed (Fig. 3B). The cannula is removed, and the previously placed U-stitch is tied. Protamine is then given for heparin reversal. Hemostasis is confirmed, and closure is completed with placement of a closed suction drain. The femoral venous cannula is removed, and pressure is applied (Table 1).

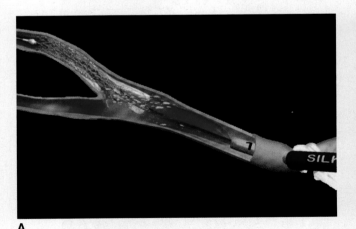

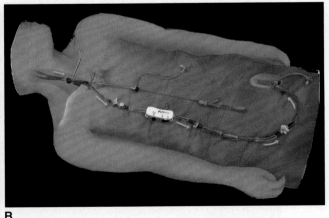

A   **B**

FIGURE 4 • **A:** Direct CCA access with placement of arterial sheath for flow reversal system. **B:** Flow reversal system with (1) arterial sheath in right CCA, (2) arteriovenous shunt with flow controller, (3) proximal inline filter, and (4) venous sheath in left common femoral vein.

TABLE 1. Carotid Artery Stent/Neck Approach/Difficult Arch

Key Technical Steps

1. Ultrasound to confirm a 5-cm minimum distance from the carotid bifurcation to the clavicle
2. Small incision above the clavicle with dissection down to the CCA
3. Micropuncture needle placement and confirmation angiogram
4. Introduction of the flow reversal cannula into the CCA
5. Placement of venous return sheath in the contralateral femoral vein
6. Connection of the flow reversal filter and tubing
7. Occlusion of the CCA with a Rummel tourniquet or vessel loop
8. Crossing of the stenosis with a guidewire and placement of a self-expanding stent
9. Completion angiography
10. Removal of arterial sheath and CCA closure

Potential Pitfalls

- Embolization to the brain if arterial sheath is placed too close to the bifurcation
- Hypotension and bradycardia at the time of stent deployment
- Creation of a dissection flap with access and placement of CCA sheath

Special Intraoperative Considerations

Extensive carotid calcification or severe intraluminal thrombus may become apparent upon either perioperative ultrasound or during direct CCA access. If these factors are significant to the point of compromising cannula introduction and orientation, then one should consider aborting the procedure.

Occasionally, significant vessel tortuosity can be encountered when mobilizing the CCA. If it is unclear which end is proximal, then preoperative imaging should be carefully reviewed. Alternatively, one side of the vessel can be temporarily clamped to determine which end is pulsating. If the tortuosity of the vessel compromises the ability to safely insert the cannula into the correct orientation, then one should consider terminating the procedure.

Postoperative Management

The postoperative period in patients undergoing this procedure is similar for other endovascular interventions. Immediately after the procedure, the patient should lie flat for a minimum of 3 hours with head elevation. An ice pack can be applied to the supraclavicular incision to minimize swelling. Frequent neurologic exams should be performed to assess for signs of stroke, and blood pressure should be closely monitored.

Complaints of a severe, unilateral headache are concerning for reperfusion injuries, and imaging should be promptly obtained. The closed suction drain output should be documented, and typically, the drain can be removed the next day. Aspirin, clopidogrel, and a statin should be continued for all patients. You can consider discontinuing clopidogrel 6 weeks following the procedure. The patient should be followed with repeat ultrasound imaging at 1 month, 6 months, 12 months, and then annually following the procedure.

Case Conclusion

The patient tolerated the procedure well and was admitted overnight. Her drain was removed the next morning. Four weeks after she was discharged, the patient returned to clinic for a follow-up visit. Her neck incision was well healed, and her neurologic status was intact. Carotid duplex ultrasound showed no evidence of stenosis (Fig. 5). She was maintained on antiplatelet therapy and a statin.

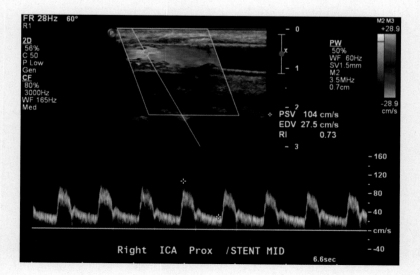

FIGURE 5 • Completion carotid duplex ultrasound demonstrating patent right ICA stent.

TAKE HOME POINTS

- When considering a CAS intervention, initial diagnostic imaging should include carotid duplex ultrasound and CTA.
- Periprocedural antiplatelet and statin therapy are critical to minimizing embolization and stroke in the peri- and postprocedural period.
- Patients with a hostile neck, secondary to radiation or prior surgery, may be at increased risk for wound complications and nerve injuries with open surgical repair.
- Direct cervical carotid access with flow reversal can provide a safe method of performing carotid angioplasty and stenting, while minimizing the risk of embolic events.

SUGGESTED READINGS

Bijuklic K, et al. The PROFI study (Prevention of Cerebral Embolization by Proximal Balloon Occlusion Compared to Filter Protection During Carotid Artery Stenting): a prospective randomized trial. *J Am Coll Cardiol.* 2012;59(15):1383-1389.

Bonati LH, et al. New ischaemic brain lesions on MRI after stenting or endarterectomy for symptomatic carotid stenosis: a substudy of the International Carotid Stenting Study (ICSS). *Lancet Neurol.* 2010;9(4):353-362.

Pinter L, et al. Safety and feasibility of a novel transcervical access neuroprotection system for carotid artery stenting in the PROOF Study. *J Vasc Surg.* 2011;54(5):1317-1323.

Sfyroeras GS, et al. Results of carotid artery stenting with transcervical access. *J Vasc Surg.* 2013;58(5):1402-1407.

CLINICAL SCENARIO CASE QUESTIONS

1. Which of the following imaging studies should be obtained when considering a carotid artery stenting intervention?

   a. CTA
   b. Carotid duplex ultrasound
   c. Diagnostic transfemoral arch angiography
   d. a and b
   e. All of the above

2. Which of the following is not a significant consideration in patients who have undergone prior neck radiation and/or dissection?

   a. Increased risk for nerve injury during CEA
   b. Compromised wound healing status
   c. Increased risk for radiation-induced vascular disease
   d. Compromised postoperative respiratory status

10 Carotid Artery Aneurysm

MICHAEL B. BREWER and KAREN WOO

Presentation

A 70-year-old female with a past medical history significant for hypertension and smoking presents with several episodes of transient left arm weakness. Each episode lasted several hours, consisted of weakness and numbness of the left arm and hand, and resolved completely. The patient also reports one instance of right eye blindness, described as a dark curtain being drawn down over her vision, which also completely resolved. She has no other medical problems, has no previous surgeries, and is on no medications. Physical examination is remarkable only for a right carotid bruit. She has no residual neurologic deficits, has no pulsatile masses, and has strong pulses throughout.

Differential Diagnosis

The patient's symptoms are consistent with transient ischemic attack (TIA) and amaurosis fugax. These symptoms have a broad differential diagnosis and have a nonvascular cause in up to 30% of cases. For this reason, a careful and thorough history should be elicited, with a focus on cerebrovascular disease and its risk factors. While atherosclerotic disease of the carotid arteries (primarily the internal) is the most likely etiology, the differential should include cardiac embolic phenomena, extracranial carotid artery aneurysm (ECAA) or dissection, arteritis (due to medications, irradiation, infection, or trauma), sympathomimetic drugs (e.g., cocaine), and fibromuscular dysplasia. Systemic illnesses, such as hypercoagulability or Marfan's syndrome, should be considered as well.

Duplex ultrasound is the initial imaging modality of choice, as it is simple, readily available, noninvasive, and well established. Its limitations include an inability to identify high lesions and overestimation of degree of stenosis in the presence of a contralateral carotid artery occlusion.

Workup

A bilateral carotid duplex is ordered. An image from the right carotid is shown in Figure 1.

Carotid Duplex Ultrasound Scan Report

The duplex ultrasound examination of the left carotid artery is normal. On the right, the duplex demonstrates an aneurysm at the bifurcation of the common carotid artery (CCA) and bulb approximately 3 cm in diameter. The aneurysm appears to involve the right internal carotid artery (ICA). There is moderate intraluminal thrombus within the ECAA.

Discussion

Traditionally, carotid arteriography has been the gold standard for evaluation of ECAAs. However, this convention is shifting with the increasing availability and diagnostic accuracy of computed tomographic angiography (CTA) and magnetic resonance angiography (MRA). CTA allows for visualization of the carotid artery, the aneurysm wall, and any associated thrombus or calcification. Additionally, it can reveal other surrounding neck pathology and allows for orientation with other anatomic landmarks with three-dimensional reconstruction. CTA provides the additional benefit of avoiding the invasiveness, access complications, and 1% stroke risk associated with carotid arteriography. Most surgeons would proceed to CTA as the next necessary preoperative step in the evaluation of ECAA. A carotid arteriogram is shown in Figure 2, with a corresponding CTA shown in Figure 3.

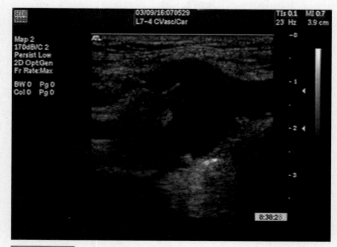

FIGURE 1 • Carotid duplex.

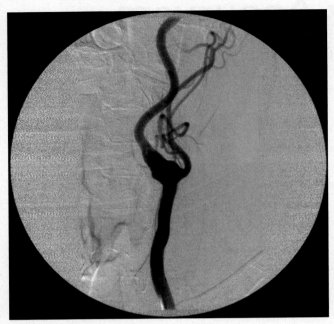

FIGURE 2 • Carotid artery angiogram.

Carotid Artery Angiogram Report

Angiography confirms the diagnosis and demonstrates a right ECAA involving the right ICA. The lesion is well removed from the petrous portion of the ICA, and there is no evidence of fibrodysplasia. Both the angiogram and CTA provide quality images with similar information.

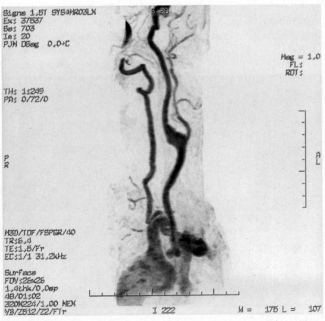

FIGURE 3 • CTA 3D reconstruction.

Diagnosis and Treatment

The patient is diagnosed with an ECAA, which, left untreated, carries a poor prognosis with stroke and death rates approaching 50%. For this reason, the presence of an ECAA is an indication for operative repair, and size >2 cm is an absolute indication. One could argue, however, that in poor operative candidates or patients with small, incidental, asymptomatic aneurysms, observation with serial duplex scans and antiplatelet therapy could be employed. In these cases, aneurysm growth or the development of symptoms would be indications to intervene.

The conventional operative approach is open surgical repair; however, more and more authors are describing good results with endovascular deployment of covered stent grafts. As these lesions are extremely rare, the approach will most likely depend on surgeon experience.

Discussion

ECAAs are rare, representing 0.4% to 4% of all peripheral aneurysms. Most tertiary centers treat fewer than 1 per year, and most reports in the literature are small case series spanning decades. Like most aneurysms, an ECAA is defined as a localized area of increased artery caliber of 50% over that of normal adjacent artery or reference values (ICA: 0.55 cm male, 0.49 cm female; carotid bulb: 0.99 cm male, 0.92 cm female). Unlike other aneurysms, ECAAs are not associated with aneurysms of other anatomical locations. There is a 15% to 20% incidence of carotid aneurysm on the contralateral side. ECCAs are 2.5 times more common in males, occur at an earlier age than carotid occlusive disease (53 to 56 years), and are frequently associated with hypertension (62%).

The most common presentation of ECAAs is related to thromboemboli, followed by mass effect, as rupture is rare. Sixty-seven percent present with TIA, 33% report amaurosis fugax, 21% have nonhemispheric symptoms (blurry vision or equilibrium disturbance), and 8% present with stroke. Presenting symptoms from mass effect include palpable pulsatile mass, dysphagia, or cranial nerve dysfunction. Many ECAAs are asymptomatic and found incidentally on CT scans done for other reasons or on routine surveillance carotid duplex.

Historically, ECAAs were most commonly due to peritonsillar infection. Currently, most series report atherosclerosis as the most common etiology. Postoperative pseudoaneurysms are also relatively common but represent a different clinical entity that is treated in much the same fashion. Less common causes of ECAAs include trauma, dissection, dysplasia, and infection. Regardless of cause, the most common location is the carotid bulb (95%) with extension into the proximal ICA. Extension into the carotid siphon can occur, highlighting the importance of preoperative imaging.

Until the 1970s, operative management of ECAAs was carotid artery ligation and was associated with a mortality of approximately 30%. More recent data suggest a lower mortality rate with ligation (11% to 12%). However, operative management has evolved significantly since that time, and preservation of internal carotid continuity is considered essential. Current operative strategies range from complete carotid reconstruction with autogenous vein graft to simple aneurysmorrhaphy. Other options include synthetic graft reconstruction, external carotid artery (ECA) to ICA transposition, aneurysmorrhaphy with patch angioplasty (using Dacron or bovine pericardium), and resection with primary end-to-end anastomosis or graft interposition. Combined major stroke and mortality rates for these procedures are generally accepted as 9% (3% to 20%).

Endovascular therapy consists of carotid angiography, followed by placement of a covered stent graft across the aneurysm. Depending on the location of the aneurysm, coil embolization of the ECA may be required to prevent type II endoleak. Endovasular repair is associated with fewer cranial nerve injuries and shorter recovery time than open surgical repair. Hybrid procedures consisting of open ECCA repair, followed by endovascular repair of a separate, more cephalad carotid aneurysm, have also been described.

Case Continued

The patient's risk factors for anesthesia and surgery are minimal. Informed consent is obtained, and she is started on antiplatelet therapy with aspirin. She is then taken for elective open repair of her carotid aneurysm.

Surgical Approach

The goal of surgical treatment is resection of the aneurysm with restoration of arterial continuity, while simultaneously avoiding neurologic complications due to thrombosis or embolism. The operative approach to ECAA repair is similar to that of elective carotid endarterectomy. General endotracheal anesthesia is recommended because these procedures may be complex and have a protracted duration. The patient is positioned on a shoulder roll with adequate neck extension and rotation. The neck, upper chest, and groin (if the saphenous vein is to be used as a conduit or patch) are prepared and draped in standard sterile fashion. A cervical incision is made along the anterior border of the sternocleidomastoid muscle at the level of the carotid bifurcation. The platysma muscle is divided using electrocautery, and the carotid sheath is entered. The internal jugular vein is reflected laterally, and the facial vein is ligated. The ECAA is then exposed with minimal manipulation to avoid causing emboli. The posterior belly of the digastric muscle and the omohyoid muscle can be mobilized and, if necessary, divided to facilitate atraumatic dissection

of the carotid. Care is taken to preserve the vagus and hypoglossal nerves, which may adhere to the aneurysm and can easily be injured. Once dissection is satisfactory, systemic heparin is administered. The CCA proximally and the ICA distally are controlled with vascular clamps. If the distal extent of the aneurysm is high and not amenable to clamping, intraluminal balloon occlusion devices may be used. The ECA is routinely ligated at this point, with the potential for reimplantation if collateral circulation is inadequate. Intraluminal shunts may be used selectively if there are signs of impaired intracranial collateral blood flow, if the patient has had a prior stroke, or universally depending on surgeon preference. The aneurysm is then resected, and an end-to-end carotid-carotid interposition graft with spatulation of the distal ICA anastomosis is created. Reversed saphenous vein is generally the preferred conduit, but synthetic graft may be used with good results if vein is limited (Table 1).

Markedly tortuous carotid arteries with limited aneurysm involvement occasionally may be treated by simple aneurysm resection and primary reanastomosis or reimplantation of the carotid artery. Simple open aneurysmorrhaphy with patch angioplasty can be performed in selected patients with saccular aneurysmal disease, although the long-term success of this operation has not been established definitively. If the ECA is sizable, it can be ligated and transposed to the distal ICA to reestablish in-line flow. Finally, ICA artery ligation is rarely necessary, but if such an approach is required, postoperative anticoagulation should be considered to prevent stroke from cephalad propagation of thrombus in the ligated distal ICA stump.

Once repair is accomplished and hemostasis achieved, the platysma should be closed with absorbable suture material according to the surgeon's preference, followed by skin. Closed suction drainage is generally not necessary but can be considered if a large potential space is left after resection of the aneurysm. If general anesthesia was used, the patient should be awakened without undue Valsalva and a thorough neurologic assessment performed to assess for any deficits. Acute neurologic events within hours of surgery should prompt emergent operative exploration to evaluate for technical failure of the repair and surgically correct any problems discovered.

Case Continued

The ECAA is resected and replaced with a saphenous vein interposition graft sewn end to end with the CCA proximally and to the ICA distally. The distal anastomosis is generously spatulated to avoid anastomotic stenosis. The ECA is not reimplanted. Postoperatively, the patient does well with no evidence of stroke, but her tongue now deviates to the right on protrusion.

TABLE 1. Carotid Artery Aneurysm Repair

Key Technical Steps

1. The operative approach to ECAA repair is similar to that of elective carotid endarterectomy. General endotracheal anesthesia is recommended because these procedures may be complex and have a protracted duration.
2. The patient is positioned on a shoulder roll with adequate neck extension and rotation. The neck, upper chest, and groin (if the saphenous vein is to be used as a conduit or patch) are prepared and draped in standard sterile fashion.
3. A cervical incision is made along the anterior border of the sternocleidomastoid muscle at the level of the carotid bifurcation. The platysma muscle is divided using electrocautery, and the carotid sheath is entered. The internal jugular vein is reflected laterally, and the facial vein is ligated. The ECAA is then exposed with minimal manipulation to avoid causing emboli.
4. Care is taken to preserve the vagus and hypoglossal nerves, which may adhere to the aneurysm and can easily be injured.
5. Once dissection is satisfactory, systemic heparin is administered.
6. The CCA proximally and the ICA distally are controlled with vascular clamps.
7. If the distal extent of the aneurysm is high and not amenable to clamping, intraluminal balloon occlusion devices may be used.
8. The ECA is routinely ligated at this point, with the potential for reimplantation if collateral circulation is inadequate.
9. Intraluminal shunts may be used selectively if there are signs of impaired intracranial collateral blood flow, if the patient has had a prior stroke, or universally depending on surgeon preference.
10. The aneurysm is then resected, and an end-to-end carotid–carotid interposition graft with spatulation of the distal ICA anastomosis is created. Reversed saphenous vein is generally the preferred conduit, but synthetic graft may be used with good results if vein is limited.
11. Markedly tortuous carotid arteries with limited aneurysm involvement occasionally may be treated by simple aneurysm resection and primary reanastomosis or reimplantation of the carotid artery.
12. If the ECA is sizable, it can be ligated and transposed to the distal ICA to reestablish in-line flow.
13. Once repair is accomplished and hemostasis achieved, the platysma should be closed with absorbable suture material according to the surgeon's preference, followed by skin closure.

Potential Pitfalls

- ICA artery ligation is rarely necessary, but if such an approach is required, postoperative anticoagulation should be considered to prevent stroke from cephalad propagation of thrombus in the ligated distal ICA stump.
- Acute neurologic events within hours of surgery should prompt emergent operative exploration to evaluate for technical failure of the repair and surgically correct any problems discovered.

Discussion

Cranial nerve injury during repair of ECAAs is common due to anatomic displacement and adherence from local inflammation. The vagus and hypoglossal nerves are the most commonly injured. Incidence varies widely between reports (0% to 66%), but most reports cite a rate between 5% and 10%. These injuries usually represent a transient cranial neuropraxia, resulting from traction injuries, and resolve within months. Complete transection leads to permanent loss of nerve function.

Case Conclusion

The patient returns 2 years later with a pulsatile mass deep to the incision on the right neck. Carotid duplex is performed, revealing a 2-cm aneurysmal degeneration at the distal anastomosis of her previous aneurysm repair. The patient is otherwise asymptomatic, and her tongue deviation has resolved.

Discussion

ECAAs in patients with previous neck surgery pose a significant problem. These most commonly arise as pseudoaneurysms after endarterectomy. Strong consideration should be given to endovascular repair rather than open surgical repair in a redo neck. Reoperation on the carotid artery increases the incidence of cranial nerve injury and other operative morbidity. Endovascular exclusion of the ECAA using a covered stent graft is the procedure of choice.

Surgical Approach

The goal of endovascular therapy is complete exclusion of the aneurysm by landing a covered stent graft from the CCA, across the aneurysm, to the ICA. The operative approach is similar to that of elective carotid artery stenting. Local anesthesia is recommended in order to continuously evaluate the patient's neurologic status. Femoral access is obtained, and a flush catheter is used to perform arch angiography. The target CCA is selectively catheterized, and a wire is advanced into the ECA for support. A sheath is then placed into the CCA, through which an embolic protection device is placed into the distal ICA. The stent graft is then introduced, positioned across the aneurysm with at least 1 cm of apposition both proximally and distally, and deployed. Balloon postdilation of the landing zones followed by completion angiography is then performed. The embolic protection device is removed. Depending on the position and the patency of the ECA, it can be coil embolized prior to graft deployment. In this case, the patient's ECA had already been ligated at the initial operation.

TAKE HOME POINTS

- ECAA can present with thromboembolic symptoms to the brain and/or compressive symptoms to the surrounding nerves, esophagus and trachea.
- The initial imaging modality of choice for ECAA is duplex ultrasound.
- Size >2 cm of an ECAA is an absolute indication for repair.
- Treatment options vary based on the nature of the aneurysm and the anatomy.
- If redundancy exists in the carotid and the aneurysm can be resected with a primary repair, this is the treatment of choice.
- If a primary repair cannot be performed, an interposition saphenous vein graft can be performed.
- Endovascular repair with a stent graft can be considered if the anatomy is favorable, with minimal tortuosity and appropriate proximal and distal landing zones.

SUGGESTED READINGS

Attigah N, Kulkens S, Zausig N, et al. Surgical therapy of extracranial carotid artery aneurysms: long term results over a 24-year period. *Eur J Vasc Endovasc Surg.* 2009;37(2):127-133.

Donas KP, Schulte S, Pitoulias GA, et al. Surgical outcome of degenerative versus postreconstructive extracranial carotid artery aneurysms. *J Vasc Surg.* 2008;49(1):93-98.

Li Z, Chang G, Yao C, et al. Endovascular stenting of extracranial carotid artery aneurysm: a systematic review. *Eur J Vasc Endovasc Surg.* 2011;42(4):419-426.

Srivastava SD, Eagleton MJ, O'Hara P, et al. Surgical repair of carotid artery aneurysms: a 10-year, single-center experience. *Ann Vasc Surg.* 2010;24(1):100-105.

Stanley JC. Extracranial carotid artery aneurysms. In: Ernst CB, Stanley JC, eds. *Current Therapy in Vascular Disease*. 4th ed. St. Louis, MO: Mosby; 2001:104-108.

Szopinski P, Ciostek P, Kielar M, et al. A series of 15 patients with extracranial carotid artery aneurysms: surgical and endovascular treatment. *Eur J Vasc Endovasc Surg.* 2005;29(3):256-261.

Zhou W, Lin PH, Bush RL, et al. Carotid artery aneurysm: evolution of management over two decades. *J Vasc Surg.* 2006;43(3):493-496.

CLINICAL SCENARIO CASE QUESTIONS

1. The most common presentation of extracranial carotid artery aneurysm is:

   a. Stroke
   b. Dysphagia
   c. Rupture
   d. Transient ischemic attack
   e. Hoarseness

2. During open repair of a fusiform aneurysm involving the carotid bulb and proximal internal carotid artery, the distal common carotid artery and internal carotid artery distal to the aneurysm are found to be tortuous. The ideal management of this aneurysm should be:

   a. Resection with vein graft interposition
   b. Resection with prosthetic graft interposition
   c. Resection with primary anastomosis
   d. Resection of the anterior wall with prosthetic patch
   e. Resection of the anterior wall with vein patch

11 Internal Carotid Artery Fibromuscular Dysplasia

MARY E. JENSEN and AVERY J. EVANS

Presentation

A 49-year-old woman presented to her primary care physician after a 5-minute episode of left amaurosis fugax, followed by a headache. She was initially seen by an ophthalmologist who noted a normal eye exam with intact visual fields, but identified a left carotid bruit. Her past medical history was important for sicca syndrome, hyperlipidemia, and mitral valve prolapse (MVP). She was taking pravastatin 40 mg qd at the time of the event; afterward, aspirin, 325 mg qd, was added to her medications. She was a nonsmoker, had no family history of cardiovascular disease, and had no personal history of hypertension. She denied any recurrent visual changes, neurologic abnormalities, or history of headaches. At physical examination, her vital signs and neurologic exam were normal. She had bilateral carotid bruits, left greater than right. A known left-sided thyroid nodule was stable.

Differential Diagnosis

The differential diagnosis of amaurosis fugax is extensive and can be divided into circulatory, ocular, and neurologic etiologies (Table 1). This patient's history of MVP, hypercholesterolemia, sicca syndrome (also known as Sjögren's syndrome) (SS), and a headache associated with the visual disturbance give rise to several potential diagnoses (Table 1).

The presence of a bruit, and the unilateral nature and duration of the visual loss, are indicative of an embolic etiology from a carotid stenosis, most likely from bifurcation disease. This patient's history of hypercholesterolemia puts her at risk for atherosclerotic disease, but she is young for advanced disease and has no other risk factors. Carotid artery dissection is a strong consideration, particularly when headache and/or neck pain is reported or Horner's syndrome symptoms (ptosis, miosis, anhidrosis, and enophthalmos) are present. Visual disturbance or loss from a carotid dissection may be from decreased retinal perfusion caused by low flow, or from thrombus forming on the dissection flap or in the false lumen, which embolizes to the retinal artery or to portions of the brain that supply the optic radiations. Intrinsic vascular diseases that result in turbulent flow or stenosis, such as fibromuscular dysplasia (FMD) or large vessel arteritides, are other possibilities.

With the patient's history of MVP, a cardiac embolic source must be excluded. SS is a chronic autoimmune disease in which the exocrine glands are damaged or destroyed. Eye dryness may result in blurry vision but not visual loss unless the cornea is injured. However, inflammatory vasculitis involving small vessels is associated with SS and can involve the brain and cranial nerves.

Lastly, visual disturbance, usually binocular, is common with migrainous disease, but this patient had no history of chronic headaches.

TABLE 1. Causes of Amaurosis Fugax

Circulatory
Embolic (cardiac, carotid, IV drug use)
Hypoperfusion (carotid or ophthalmic stenosis, cardiogenic)
Malignant hypertension
Inflammatory disorders, e.g., giant cell arteritis
Hypercoagulable states
Polycythemia
Vasospasm
Iatrogenic

Ocular
Glaucoma
Retinal or posterior vitreous detachment
Intraorbital hemorrhage
Orbital tumor
Optic disc drusen
Dry eye syndrome
Keratitis
Blepharitis
Iritis

Neurologic
Migraine syndrome
Papilledema
Pseudotumor cerebri
Optic neuritis
Multiple sclerosis
Vasculitis, e.g., SLE
Intracranial tumor
Psychogenic

Workup

Carotid Dopplers were negative for bifurcation plaque, and a transthoracic echocardiogram (TTE) did not demonstrate valve vegetations or mural thrombus. Since cardiac and carotid bifurcation disease were excluded by sonography as potential embolic sources, the next step was to evaluate those portions of the carotid artery that are difficult to see on carotid ultrasound; that is, the aortic arch and brachiocephalic origins, and the retromandibular segments.

Computed tomographic angiography (CTA) (Fig. 1A and B) showed bilateral internal carotid artery (ICA) irregularities consisting of concentric and eccentric plications with intervening saccular outpouchings ("string of beads") and a focal dissection with an expanded lumen on the left (Fig. 1A). The diseased segments extended from the C1-C2 level to the skull base. The diagnosis of bilateral ICA FMD was made based upon the noninvasive imaging findings and confirmed by cervicocerebral angiography (Fig. 2), where no flow limitation or thrombus formation was noted. Also, angiographic evaluation of the renal arteries at the same time showed mild-to-moderate FMD.

Diagnosis of Cerebrovascular FMD

This patient's radiographic studies demonstrated the classic appearance of FMD, with the focal areas of dilatation and constriction involving the distal ICAs, evidence of a dissection flap, variable caliber of the diseased segments compared to the normal ICA, and similar involvement of the renal arteries.

Prevalence

FMD is a noninflammatory, nonatherosclerotic vascular disease originally described in 1938 by Ledbetter and Bergland and labeled as "fibromuscular hyperplasia" by McCormack et al. in 1958. The prevalence of FMD in the population is unknown, but it is more common in women than in men by a ratio of 9:1. The U.S. Registry for FMD published its initial results in 447 patients and found the incidence of renal and cerebrovascular FMD in their participants to be nearly equal, contradicting previous data that found the incidence of renal FMD greater than cerebrovascular FMD by almost 2:1. The prevalence of cerebrovascular FMD has been reported as ranging from 0.3% to 3.2% based upon consecutive cerebral angiographic studies. The cause of FMD is also

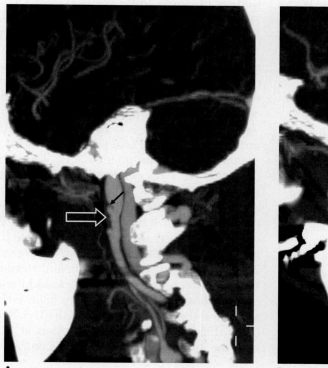
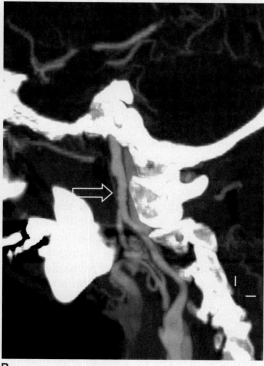

A   **B**

FIGURE 1 • Sagittal maximum intensity projection (MIP) images from computed tomographic angiography (CTA) of the neck (**A and B**) show bilateral internal carotid artery (ICA) short-segment irregularities consisting of concentric and eccentric plications with intervening saccular outpouchings ("string of beads") (*open arrows*) at the C1-C2 level. On the left, there is a focal dissection with visualization of the flap (*arrow*, **A**) and expansion of the lumen distal to the flap to the carotid canal.

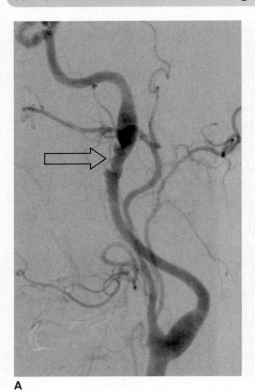

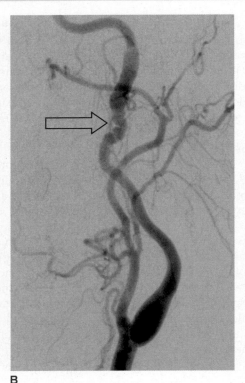

A   **B**

FIGURE 2 • Lateral images from distal subtraction angiography (DSA) of the left **(A)** and right **(B)** common carotid bifurcations confirm the abnormalities of the distal ICAs. The "string of beads" is better seen on the DSA (*open arrows*) and shows the intervening areas of stricture and dilatation, particularly on the right. Again noted is the dissection flap on the left with distal dilatation of the vessel. The right ICA also shows mild dilatation of the vessel proximal to the skull base.

unknown, and although hormonal factors have been proposed, none have been proven. Evidence supports a genetic susceptibility to FMD, and two small studies suggest a relationship between cigarette smoking and the risk of FMD.

Pathology

In 1971, Harrison and McCormack published a paper on the classification of FMD, dividing lesions into medial, intimal, and adventitial/periarterial types, according to the arterial layer most affected. The medial variant is the most common, accounting for greater than 90% of all cases. It is characterized by deposition of loose collagen in zones of degenerating elastic fibrils, resulting in fibromuscular ridges causing circumferential stenoses, with intervening areas of smooth muscle loss and subsequent arterial dilatation. The result is the "string of beads" appearance on imaging, which is found primarily in the mid-to-distal portions of the internal carotid and vertebral arteries.

Intimal FMD accounts for 1% to 2% of all cases and is caused by accumulation of fibrous tissue in the intima with preservation and reduplication of the internal elastic lamina, resulting in focal or tubular angiographic stenoses.

Adventitial FMD is seen in less than 1% of cases and shows collagen deposition in the adventitia with extension into the periarterial tissue and focal infiltration of lymphocytes. Tubular stenosis is the most common radiographic appearance.

Clinical Presentation

The clinical manifestations of cerebrovascular FMD are highly variable and often nonspecific. Data from 447 patients enrolled in the U.S. Registry for FMD show the most common symptom is headache (60%), often of the migrainous variety (50%). Pulsatile tinnitus or a "swooshing" sound was described by 27.5% of participants, followed by neck pain and dizziness/lightheadedness (20% to 26%). Cervical bruit was the presenting sign in 22% of patients; reported neurologic events included hemispheric TIA (13.4%), cervical artery dissection (12.1%), completed stroke (9.8%), and amaurosis fugax (5.2%).

FMD is associated with carotid dissection and intracranial aneurysm. It has been estimated that 15% to 20% of cervical artery dissections are FMD related. In the U.S. Registry, dissections at any location were noted in 19.7%, 20% of those patients had multiple dissections, dissections were more common in males, and the most common location was the carotid artery, followed by the renal artery and the vertebral artery. In the U.S. Registry, 17% of participants reported an aneurysm at any location, with the prevalence of asymptomatic intracranial aneurysms reaching 7.3%.

Differential Diagnosis

Standing Waves

A pattern of "ripples" may be seen in a vessel downstream from the catheter tip during contrast injection. These undulations are concentric and regularly spaced, with no intervening areas of stricture or dilatation. "Standing waves" are thought to be due to irritation or spasm of the vessel during injection and are relieved by catheter removal or intra-arterial infusion of a vasodilator. This phenomenon should not be confused with FMD.

Atherosclerosis

FMD is usually associated with young individuals without cardiovascular risk factors, making it easier to distinguish from atherosclerotic disease. Atherosclerotic disease is most likely to occur at branch points in the proximal portions of the brachiocephalic arteries and the carotid bifurcation and often show signs of calcification within the plaque or vessel wall. FMD is located in the distal portions of the ICA and vertebral arteries, or in ECA branches, and has the "string of beads" appearance, which is not associated with ASVD.

Inflammatory Arteriopathies

Large artery vasculitides, such as Takayasu's and giant cell arteritis, may mimic the tubular stenoses noted with FMD. However, these arteriopathies often consist of long, smooth tapering stenoses of the brachiocephalic origins and proximal aspects of the carotid and vertebral artery, which are not typical locations for FMD. Inflammatory markers, such as erythrocyte sedimentation rate and C-reactive protein, are often positive in inflammatory arteriopathies and not in FMD.

Spontaneous Dissection

Although FMD is implicated in spontaneous cerebrovascular dissections, other etiologies include collagen-vascular disorders, such as Marfan's and Ehlers-Danlos syndromes; atherosclerosis; hyperextension during sports or exercise; and mild blunt force trauma. Evaluation of uninvolved cervicocerebral vessels or the renal arteries may show the typical findings of FMD to make the diagnosis.

Segmental Arterial Mediolysis

This noninflammatory, nonatherosclerotic arteriopathy is caused by lysis of the outer media of the arterial wall, resulting in segmental changes including stenoses, dissections, and aneurysm formation. The imaging characteristics are often indistinguishable from FMD, and pathologic findings may also be similar. However, the clinical profile and location of involved vessels in segmental arterial mediolysis (SAM) is markedly different from FMD. SAM most commonly involves the splanchnic vessels of late middle-aged and elderly individuals who present with abdominal or flank pain, distention, falling hematocrit, and hypovolemic shock. Dissections of peripheral arteries unrelated to the aorta with pseudoaneurysm formation, often multiple, is indicative of SAM.

Imaging Evaluation

The increased detection of cerebrovascular FMD may be associated with the increased awareness of its association in the presence of renal FMD and the availability of high-quality noninvasive imaging that permits evaluation of vascular territories outside of the symptomatic one. Duplex ultrasound, CTA, and magnetic resonance angiography (MRA) are all suitable for cerebrovascular FMD diagnosis, and the latter two have the additional advantage of allowing concurrent parenchymal evaluation. However, catheter angiography remains the diagnostic gold standard, and flow and pressure measurements across stenoses can be performed at the same.

Duplex Ultrasound

This imaging modality is noninvasive, widely available, and relatively inexpensive and gives both anatomic and flow-related information. Velocity shifts indicative of stenosis with associated turbulence of color flow, beading, and tortuosity of the mid-to-distal cervical ICA are evidence of FMD. One limitation of the technique is the lack of specific velocity-based criteria for severity of stenosis that has been angiographically validated. The standards for atherosclerotic stenosis do not apply, and less-skilled vascular labs may misinterpret FMD for atherosclerotic stenosis. Duplex ultrasound can be used as surveillance imaging, with annual studies performed initially, and less frequent testing after stability has been recognized. This approach was given a class IIa recommendation by the 2011 multisocietal guidelines for extracranial carotid and vertebral disease.

CTA and MRA

There are no clinically validated studies in the comparison of CTA or MRA to catheter angiography for the diagnosis of cerebrovascular FMD. However, multidetector CTA is routinely used for the evaluation of extracranial and intracranial disease, including atherosclerosis, FMD, dissection, and cerebral aneurysms, and displays detailed anatomy in multiple planes using maximal intensity and three-dimensional projections. T1-fat saturation sequences are particularly useful in the detection of FMD-associated dissections. MRA has the advantage of not using radiation or iodinated contrast making it a useful screening tool, but its sensitivity and specificity in the detection of FMD are unknown.

Cerebral Angiography

Digital subtraction angiography (DSA) is the "gold standard" in the evaluation of FMD due to its superb spatial resolution and digital magnification capabilities that allows disease detection in the smallest vessels. The three most common angiographic patterns identified are the "string of beads" appearance, smooth tubular stenosis, and smooth tubular dilatation with an associated outpouching. Also, DSA has a higher detection rate of small intracranial aneurysms than does CTA or MRA.

However, the diagnosis of FMD is readily and reliably made with high-quality noninvasive imaging, and angiography is often reserved for symptomatic patients in whom intervention is contemplated, when the diagnosis or severity is in question, or for hemodynamic evaluation or investigation of a source of thrombus.

Treatment of Cerebrovascular FMD

Medical Therapy

The incidental finding of FMD may require nothing more but the knowledge of its presence and surveillance. The decision to treat is dependent upon the nature of the lesion, (for example, stenosis, dissection, and degree of vascular involvement); the presence of symptoms and prior events related to the disease; presence and size of intracranial aneurysms or extracranial pseudoaneurysms; and comorbidities. There are no randomized controlled trials in this patient population to provide guidance.

The 2011 multisocietal statement supported the following medical therapies in patients with FMD:

1. Use of antiplatelet therapy in asymptomatic and symptomatic patients with carotid FMD as long as there was no contraindication for its use (Class IIa evidence)
2. Management of cervical artery dissection with heparin or low molecular weight heparin followed by oral anticoagulation with warfarin for 3 to 6 months and then antiplatelet therapy (Class IIa evidence)
3. Modification of cardiovascular risk factors such as hypertension treatment, smoking cessation, and statin therapy in accordance with published consensus guidelines

Revascularization of Carotid or Vertebral Artery FMD

The 2011 multisocietal guidelines did not recommend revascularization of carotid FMD for asymptomatic patients, regardless of the stenosis severity (Class III). Revascularization is reserved for those patients who are symptomatic with cerebral or retinal ischemic events (Class IIa). Appropriate candidates are patients suffering from recurrent ischemic symptoms despite best medical therapy or where antiplatelet or anticoagulation therapy is contraindicated and in lesions with symptomatic flow-limiting dissections and/or compressive pseudoaneurysms.

In this patient, a second episode of left-sided amaurosis fugax occurred despite single-agent antiplatelet therapy, and the decision was made to treat her with mechanical dilatation of the affected segment.

Surgical Treatment

In the past, revascularization of symptomatic lesions was performed with surgical exposure of the extracranial ICA and graduated dilatation of the stenosis using a series of rigid dilators with progressively larger diameters or a balloon catheter. Proximal clamping of the vessel and back bleeding allowed associated debris to be flushed out of the artery. The major disadvantages to this approach were the need for surgical arterial exposure of the carotid artery and the inability of the operator to assess the affected segment during the procedure. Much of the technique was based upon "feel," as kinks, coils, stenotic segments, and intimal flaps were negotiated with the dilators.

Regardless of the technical difficulties, perioperative stroke rates in major series were acceptable (1.4% to 2.6%), long-term primary patency rates were high (94% in one series), and late stroke development was low (1.2% to 3.8%). Still, the development of endovascular techniques provided a minimally invasive way of dilatation with image-guided monitoring of the procedure and its results and contemporaneous detection of complications. For these reasons, treatment of symptomatic FMD is now performed primarily by endovascular means.

Endovascular Treatment

Endovascular treatment of FMD targets the "string of beads" segment caused by hypertrophic smooth muscle and fibrous elements involving the media. Most FMD lesions require only angioplasty to disrupt the fibrous rings, but stenting may be needed for recalcitrant lesions, postangioplasty flow-limiting dissections, and compressive pseudoaneurysms. Patients are started on dual antiplatelet therapy prior to treatment to minimize thrombus formation during and after the procedure.

Technical Considerations

Treatment is usually done with the patient under conscious sedation or managed anesthesia care (Table 2). A good neurologic examination is performed before the procedure to determine baseline status. Femoral access is obtained, and an appropriately sized femoral sheath is placed. The sheath can be upsized by one French to allow for arterial monitoring through its sideport. If the plan is to use a long arterial sheath such as a Shuttle sheath (Cook Medical, Bloomington, IL) for carotid treatment, then a radial arterial line is placed for monitoring. With the patient fully heparinized, a diagnostic angiographic study of the entire cerebrovascular system is done with a standard 5F tapered catheter to identify all vessels with FMD, assess the collateral circulation, and evaluate the targeted vessel. Important information includes length and location of the diseased segment; diameter of the adjacent normal vessel; identification of dissection, pseudoaneurysm or clot formation; tortuosity of the artery; presence of proximal disease; and collateral circulation to the downstream territory. The diagnostic catheter is replaced with a large-bore guide catheter or sheath, suitable for both angioplasty balloon catheters and stent systems. If the aortic arch is tortuous, the guide catheter is advanced over an exchange length guidewire with its

TABLE 2. Carotid Angioplasty/Stenting for FMD

Key Technical Steps

1. Obtain femoral access and fully heparinize the patient.
2. Perform diagnostic cervicocerebral angiography with a diagnostic catheter.
3. Determine working projection, and measure length of diseased segment and diameter of normal vessel.
4. Select appropriate microguidewire/distal protection device, balloon catheter, and stent (in case stenting is required for recalcitrant lesion or angioplasty complication).
5. Remove diagnostic catheter and place an appropriately sized guide catheter or sheath in the common carotid artery.
6. Cross lesion with microguidewire/distal protection device under roadmapping guidance.
7. Position balloon catheter across diseased segment and slowly inflate to nominal diameter of normal vessel.
8. Deflate balloon and perform control angiogram; check the patient's neurologic status; repeat if needed.
9. Remove balloon and leave microguidewire/distal protection device across the lesion; repeat neuro checks and control angiograms every 5 minutes for total of 20 minutes to evaluate for clot formation.
10. Perform control angiogram of the intracranial circulation to evaluate for any distal emboli.
11. If a stent is required for a recalcitrant lesion or dissection, place it at this time over the microguidewire/distal protection device.
12. Perform control angiogram after placement of stent as above.
13. Remove microguidewire or capture and remove distal protection device.
14. Perform final postangiogram.
15. Remove guide catheter, perform angiogram of puncture site, and use closure device to seal site if possible.

Potential Pitfalls

- Creation of a vascular dissection or occlusion requiring stenting
- Clot formation on treated segment requiring intra-arterial glycoprotein IIb/IIIa inhibitor administration
- Loss of vascular access from below that may require navigation from the contralateral side across the circle of Willis with snaring of the microguidewire
- New neurologic deficit caused by distal embolization requiring intracranial thrombolysis/clot extraction
- Significant vasospasm from vessel manipulation requiring intra-arterial infusion of a vasodilator such as verapamil
- Hemodynamically significant "in-stent" stenosis requiring angioplasty

tip placed in the external carotid artery to avoid inadvertent engagement of the ICA. The guide catheter is then advanced into the common carotid artery in anticipation of the treatment portion of the procedure.

Vascular Access

Angioplasty and stenting of a carotid artery in the setting of FMD presents some special challenges and considerations. As far as planning the technical aspects of the case,

the decision that will determine the approach is the size of the stent that will be used or available if needed. Most carotid angioplasty and stenting takes place in the setting of atherosclerotic disease, a fundamentally different lesion than FMD. Because the stent always extends into the carotid bulb and usually into the common carotid, the stent size must be 9 to 10 mm, and, at the moment, stents in this size range are only available in a 6-French device. Consequently, the stent delivery system requires a 6-French guide sheath or an 8-French guiding catheter. With FMD, the length of the diseased segment varies but rarely, if ever, involves the carotid bifurcation or common carotid artery. Consequently, the choice of stent usually need not be in the 9 to 10 size range. Stents in 5- to 8-mm sizes usually suffice, and these stents are available on 4- to 5-French delivery systems. Specifically, 5- and 6-mm stents can be found on 4-French delivery systems, and 7- and 8-mm stents on 5-French delivery systems. Once the stent size has been determined, the appropriate guiding catheter is chosen. For 4- and 5-French delivery systems a 6- or 7-French guiding catheter is advanced through a femoral sheath. If a 6-French device is necessary, a 6 long sheath exchanged directly into the common carotid artery is the best choice. Long sheathes are also appropriate for tortuous arterial systems where extra support is necessary for device delivery.

Angioplasty

Angioplasty alone should be attempted first. The vessel should be angioplastied to the nominal diameter of the normal artery with a balloon that is long enough to treat the entire length of the abnormal vessel in one inflation (Fig. 3). FMD is easily dilated, and a compliant balloon, such as a Hyperglide (Covidien, Irvine, CA) (Fig. 3A), is perfectly adequate for the angioplasty. Distal protection is not as important with FMD as it is in ASVD since stretching or disruption of the fibrous rings are unlikely to result in distal embolization. In fact, it may not be practical or safe to deploy a device if there is no safe extracranial "deployment zone" distal to diseased portion.

The vessel is fragile and easily dissected. It may have multiple webs and areas of outpouching, dissection flaps, or pseudoaneurysm formation. Crossing with a 0.014-inch guidewire and a microcatheter is prudent, and if distal protection is to be employed, an "over-the-wire" device delivered through a microcatheter, such as a Spider (Covidien, Irvine, CA), is indicated, rather than an "all-in-one" distal protection device. Forming the tip of the microguidewire into a tight "J" shape may facilitate passage through the diseased segment. Once the lesion has been crossed, access must be maintained, and if use of any "over-the-wire" devices is anticipated, then an exchange-length wire should be used.

Postangioplasty

The vessel should be evaluated with an angiogram. If the result is good, the wire should be left across the lesion and control angiograms performed every 5 minutes for

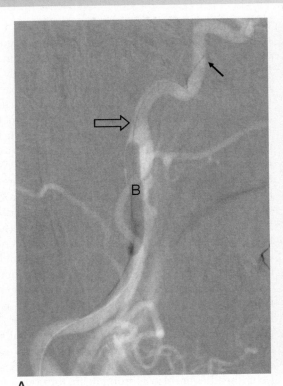

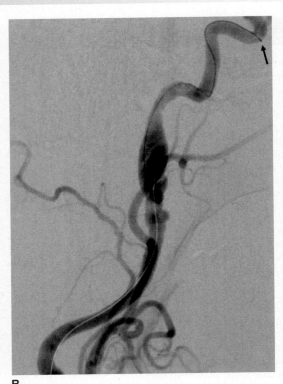

A   B

FIGURE 3 • Lateral roadmap image from DSA of the left ICA during angioplasty **(A)** and control angiogram following treatment **(B)**. The left common carotid artery was accessed with a 6-Fr Shuttle sheath, and a 4 mm × 30-mm compliant balloon (Hyperglide, Covidien, Irvine, CA) was advanced over a 300-cm exchange microwire in which the tip had been placed in the precavernous segment of the ICA **(A**, *arrow)*. The balloon *(B)* was slowly inflated to 4 mm, the diameter of the normal ICA, and then deflated. Care was taken to not angioplasty across the edge of the carotid canal **(A**, *open arrow)* to avoid creating a dissection. Control angiogram **(B)** showed no discernible change in the appearance of the vessel, although "waisting" was noted during balloon inflation. The wire tip was noted to advance during removal of the balloon catheter *(arrow)*, reminding the operator to image the tip during the procedure lest it advance intracranially.

20 minutes. If the vessel remains patent and does not begin to thrombose, the wire can be removed and the procedure ended. If the vessel develops thrombus, a bolus of a glycoprotein IIb/IIIa inhibitor should be given intra-arterially, and the vessel stented as soon as the visible thrombus in the vessel has cleared.

In the clinical scenario presented, the patient was symptom free for 4 years when she presented with word-finding difficulties and new left amaurosis fugax. A repeat DSA showed the development of a pseudoaneurysm at the level of the dissection flap (Fig. 4A and B). Since the patient had failed best medical therapy and her symptoms were escalating, the decision was made to stent the affected segment.

Stenting

Before angioplasty is performed, the carotid should be measured and an appropriate self-expanding stent chosen for bailout if it becomes necessary. A single stent should be used that can cover the whole diseased segment (Fig. 4). It should be sized for the widest part of

the vessel so that there will be good wall apposition in all parts of the vessel. Poststenting, the vessel should be observed again for approximately 20 minutes to insure that it remains patent and without platelet aggregation.

Potential Pitfalls

It is possible in these cases to dissect the artery, lose access from below, and not be able to recross the flap. Consequently, it is imperative that a complete cerebral angiogram be performed before the treatment so that the cerebral collaterals can be evaluated. If the patient is at risk for ischemia or infarct in the event of a carotid dissection and/or occlusion, the operators must be prepared to institute general anesthesia and perform a rescue procedure. In this circumstance, arterial access is acquired through the other femoral artery and a catheter placed in the contralateral carotid. A microcatheter and guidewire are maneuvered up the carotid, across the anterior communicating artery, and then retrograde down the dissected carotid. The wire is then captured with a loop snare, and the loop snare and microcatheter are pulled up the carotid through the

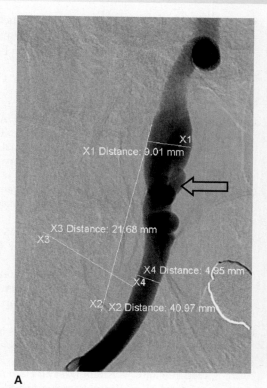
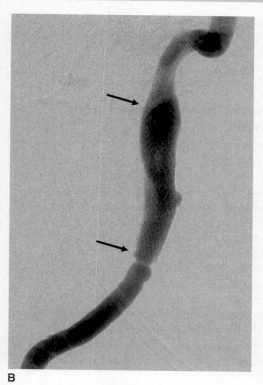

A   **B**

FIGURE 4 • Lateral images from DSA of the left ICA during planning for stent placement **(A)** and control angiogram following treatment **(B)**. Important measurements **(A)** are shown in the planning image, including the minimum and maximum diameters and the length of the vessel segment to be stented. Note that the outpouching **(A**, *open arrow*) associated with the dissection flap has enlarged and is now a pseudoaneurysm causing some mild compression of the adjacent vessel. Stenting was performed with a 10 mm × 40-mm Precise stent (Cordis Corporation, Bridgewater, NJ). After stenting, the diseased segment **(B**, *arrows*) has smoothed out with minimal filling of a single outpouching along the anterior border. There is focal concentric vasospasm at the proximal end of the stent without flow limitation.

FIGURE 5 • Sagittal MIP **(A)** and axial source image **(B)** from a CTA performed 12 months later shows mild mismatch of the stent/vessel at its proximal portion **(A**, *arrow*) but excellent wall apposition at the distal end within the dilated segment of vessel **(A**, *open arrow*; **B**). No in-stent stenosis of the carotid lumen **(C)** was noted on the study.

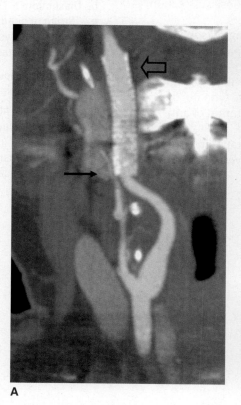
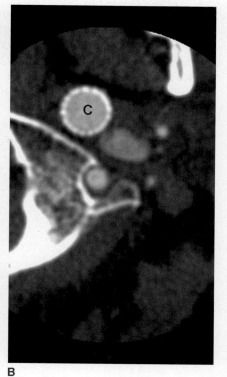

A   **B**

dissection, providing access. An exchange wire is placed through the microcatheter. Once access is obtained, the carotid is then angioplastied and stented. If the anterior communicating artery is absent, the posterior communicating artery can be accessed in the same fashion.

Postoperative Management and Surveillance

The postoperative management is the same regardless of whether the patient has undergone angioplasty or stenting. Routine postangiography neurologic and femoral checks are instituted; a poststudy carotid ultrasound is performed if the treated area is located in an accessible place. Patients who required glycoprotein IIb/IIIa inhibitors may need a short-term continuous infusion following the procedure. Dual oral antiplatelet therapy is continued for 3 to 6 months, at which time a daily single agent is given for life.

The timing of follow-up visits is at the operator's discretion. Return of a carotid bruit, TIA, or stroke should be investigated with imaging, usually CTA or ultrasound with DWI MRI for patients with neurologic symptoms. For the asymptomatic stent patient, ultrasound or CTA (Fig. 5) is performed at 6 to 12 months to evaluate for in-stent stenosis.

TAKE HOME POINTS

- FMD is a noninflammatory, nonatherosclerotic systemic vasculopathy that may present with variable and nonspecific symptoms, TIA, or stroke or may simply be an incidental finding on vascular imaging.
- The classical imaging finding of FMD is the "string of beads" appearance in addition to stenosis, dissection, and pseudoaneurysm formation.
- FMD should be considered in a young person with a carotid bruit, stroke, or TIA or any patient with a swishing sound or pulsatile tinnitus.
- The majority of patients with FMD will never experience a neurologic event, but for those who do, the first line of treatment is usually institution of antiplatelet therapy.
- For individuals who fail medical therapy, endovascular mechanical revascularization of the vessel with balloon angioplasty usually suffices.

- Patients with more complicated lesions such as dissection, compressive pseudoaneurysm formation, or hemodynamically significant stenosis can be treated with stent placement.

SUGGESTED READINGS

Brott TG, Halperin JL, Abbara S, et al. ASA/AACF/AHA/AANN/AANS/ACR/ASNR/CNS/SAIP/SCAI/SIR/SNIS/SVM/SVS guideline on the management of extracranial carotid and vertebral artery disease: executive summary. Circulation. 2011;124:489-532.

Cronenwett JL, Johnston W. Rutherford's Vascular Surgery. 7th ed., Chapter 97: Carotid artery disease: fibromuscular dysplasia. Philadelphia, PA: Elsevier; 2010.

Olin JW, Froehlich J, Gu X, et al. The United States registry for fibromuscular dysplasia: results in the first 447 patients. Circulation. 2012;125:3182-3190.

Olin JW, Gornik HL, Bacharach M, et al. Fibromuscular dysplasia: state of the science and critical unanswered questions. A scientific statement for the American Heart Association. Circulation. 2014;129:1048-1078.

Persu A, Touze E, Mousseaux E, et al. Diagnosis and management of fibromuscular dysplasia: an expert consensus. Eur J Clin Invest. 2012;42:338-347.

Touze E, Oppenheim C, Trystram D, et al. Fibromuscular dysplasia of cervical and intracranial arteries. Int J Stroke. 2010;5:296-305.

CLINICAL SCENARIO CASE QUESTIONS

1. The most common imaging finding in cerebrovascular FMD is:

   a. Tubular stenosis
   b. Dissection
   c. "String of beads" appearance
   d. Pseudoaneurysm formation
   e. Vascular dilatation

2. Which of the following does not need to be treated during angioplasty/stenting?

   a. Disruption of fibrotic rings
   b. Vascular dissection
   c. Stroke
   d. Carotid occlusion
   e. Hemodynamically significant vasospasm

12 Occluded Internal Carotid Artery with Symptoms

CHRISTOPHER ROARK and B. GREGORY THOMPSON

Presentation

A 45-year-old right-handed female mechanic is referred to your office because she has been falling at work. The patient states that these episodes began 6 months ago and have been slowly increasing in frequency, now occurring three to four times per week. She typically notices that after lying under a car in shop she will "abruptly fall down" if she gets up too fast and starts walking quickly. She recovers nearly immediately after falling to the ground. There have been no witnessed episodes of shaking, loss of consciousness, urinary incontinence, or tongue lacerations. This began in the early spring and has progressively worsened through the summer months. She initially felt it was related to dehydration, and she notes fewer "spells" on the days when her water consumption is elevated. She does not regularly go to the doctor and takes no medications. On physical examination, she is neurologically intact. She hand-carries a 24-hour EEG report that is read as normal.

Differential Diagnosis

The patient is describing "drop attacks." These are characterized by sudden falls without loss of consciousness or warning signs. Key differentials for drop attacks are seizure, cardiac, and thromboembolic causes. Seizures or cardiac events causing these symptoms would often lead to loss of consciousness and would be associated with other neurologic or physical symptoms. Seizures are often—but not always—followed by variable periods of time where the patient does not feel at his or her baseline. This patient is immediately "back to normal." Thromboembolic phenomena, although common, typically result in an isolated neurologic deficit (e.g., arm weakness only, aphasia only, visual complaints only) during a particular episode. This patient does not describe any focal neurologic deficits and has a normal neurologic exam. The association with postural changes and hydration status could certainly point to a primary cardiac cause of these events and warrants further investigation.

Workup

Holter Monitor

A Holter monitor is ordered, and the patient wears this for 1 week. During this time, she is released back to work and has another attack. There are no arrhythmias noted that would expect to be causative.

MRI/MRA

An MRI/MRA of the brain is performed to look for mass lesion, hydrocephalus, stroke, or vascular abnormality.

Report: No mass lesions, hydrocephalus, or large territory infarcts are noted. The left internal carotid artery (ICA) appears to drop out near its terminus. This could represent severe stenosis or occlusion. There are multiple dilated collaterals at the base of the brain. The right ICA is smaller in caliber at its terminus than would be expected.

Diagnostic Cerebral Angiography

A formal cerebral angiogram is the definitive test for evaluating the cerebral vasculature (both intra- and extracranial).

Report: Rapid, severe tapering of the left ICA at its terminus with some stenosis of the proximal anterior and middle cerebral arteries (Fig. 1). Moderate tapering of the distal ICA on the right is seen. Small collateral vessels are seen at the base of the brain ("puff of smoke"). External carotid artery runs demonstrate a widely patent superficial temporal artery (STA) without evidence of stenosis or vasculitis.

Xenon CT Scan

To assess the degree and limits of the patient's collateral circulation, tests that can now be performed include positron emission tomographic (PET) scan, magnetic resonance imaging (MRI) scan with perfusion/diffusion, computed tomographic (CT) scan with perfusion, or xenon CT scanning. In this case, xenon CT scan is ordered.

Report: Xenon CT scan reveals decreased baseline cerebral blood flow in the left ICA distribution (Fig. 2).

Diagnosis and Treatment

The angiogram solidifies the diagnosis of moyamoya disease and demonstrates collateral circulation to the frontal, temporal, and parietal lobes. The xenon CT scan

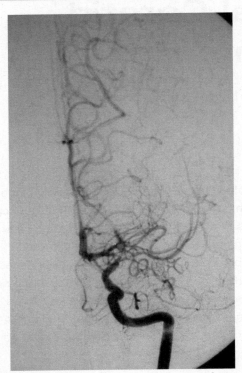

FIGURE 1 • AP angiography with left ICA injection demonstrating rapid tapering of ICA terminus with numerous dilated collateral vessels at the base of the brain.

confirms the presence of diminished perfusion in the left hemisphere. While surgery for isolated atherosclerotic carotid occlusion has fallen out of favor after the results of two randomized controlled trials (RCTs) demonstrated no benefit, surgical revascularization as a primary treatment of moyamoya disease (a cerebral proliferative angiopathy) is still understood to be of benefit.

This patient presented with symptoms of hemispheric hypoperfusion. Medical therapy relies on antiplatelet agents to minimize thromboembolic complications, of which this patient has had none. Given her young age, symptomatology, and line of work, she would be expected to derive significant benefit from cerebral revascularization.

Surgical Approach
Surgical Decision Making

The results of the EC-IC bypass trial published in 1985 resulted in a significant decrease in the number of these procedures being performed. Significant concerns were raised regarding the large number of patients operated on outside of the trial and the lack of hemodynamic evaluation in the selection of patients. The Carotid Occlusion Surgery Study (COSS) trial was designed to address the hemodynamic risk associated with stroke in the setting of ICA occlusion. The COSS trial was stopped for futility reasons after a planned interim analysis demonstrated no benefit for the surgical arm in the primary outcome ([1] all stroke and death from 30 days after surgery and [2] ipsilateral ischemic stroke within 2 years of randomization). EC-IC bypass volume has subsequently continued to decline. Today, EC-IC bypass is largely reserved for patients with moyamoya disease who have continued to have ischemic strokes despite maximal medical therapy (usually antiplatelet agents such as aspirin). Surgical treatment of moyamoya disease (via direct EC-IC bypass or indirect methods) has been shown to decrease the rate of symptomatic progression to 2.6%.

Key Technical Steps

The patient is placed in a Mayfield head-holder to provide three-point fixation. While the patient is in the supine position, the head is turned to the right. A Doppler probe is then used to demarcate the branches of the STA in the scalp. After identification of a suitable donor vessel, the head is shaved and prepped in a sterile fashion. A skin incision is made next to the donor vessel so that it can be identified clearly and dissected free from the surrounding connective tissue. The incision is lengthened so that a small craniotomy may be performed beneath the temporalis muscle. A distal branch of the middle cerebral artery (MCA) is identified on the cortical surface as the recipient vessel. The donor and recipient vessels are joined in an end-to-side anastomosis with an 9-0 monofilament suture. A handheld Doppler probe

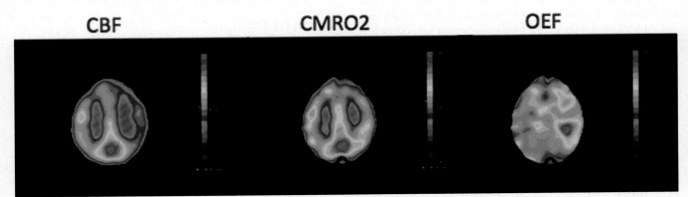

FIGURE 2 • Severe reductions in perfusion pressure below the autoregulatory limit produce a decline in regional cerebral blood flow (CBF) greater than in cerebral oxygen metabolism ($CMRO_2$), thus causing an increase in regional oxygen extraction fraction (OEF).

is used to ensure adequate flow across the anastomosis. When a suitable STA cannot be found, saphenous vein or radial artery can serve as a conduit between the EC and IC circulation.

Potential Pitfalls

EC-IC bypass is dependent on the presence of adequately sized vessels to allow for direct anastomosis. In an adult, the STA usually will have a similar caliber to a cortical MCA branch. Children may not have requisite vessel size to accept and bypass and this contributes to the preference for indirect bypass techniques often used in pediatric moyamoya cases. Occasionally, a surgeon will encounter an inadequate or damaged STA. The preoperative angiogram must be carefully studied to assess the caliber of the STA and whether use of the frontal or parietal branch is preferable. Damage to the STA during the initial opening can also preclude a direct STA-MCA bypass. In cases where an adequate STA is not present, one can use the saphenous vein or radial artery as an interposition graft.

Obstruction of STA during replacement of bone flap and closure can ruin an otherwise technically successful operation. It is imperative to evaluate, and modify if necessary, the bone flap to accommodate a traversing STA. The superficial temporalis fascia near the anastomosed STA must also not be closed tightly such that flow is impeded.

Ischemic stroke is a known risk of any EC-IC bypass procedure. These procedures should be performed at centers with an acceptably low rate of ischemic complication, given that this is the outcome surgery is designed to avoid (Table 1).

TABLE 1. Occluded Internal Carotid Artery with Symptoms

Key Technical Steps

1. Supine position with three-point Mayfield fixation of the head
2. Preop Doppler ultrasound to identify course of STA
3. Skin incision immediately adjacent to course of STA
4. Dissection of STA from surrounding connective tissue, leaving a small cuff
5. Extend incision to allow for craniotomy beneath temporalis muscle
6. Identify appropriate recipient branches of the MCA
7. End-to-side anastomosis of vessels using 9-0 monofilament suture
8. Doppler ultrasound and intraoperative fluorescence angiography to check patency of anastomosis

Potential Pitfalls

- Inadequate or damaged STA
- Stenosed or "Backwalled" anastomosis
- Intraoperative or immediate postoperative hypotension
- Obstruction of STA during replacement of bone flap and closure
- Ischemic stroke

Special Intraoperative Considerations

If there is no suitable recipient vessel in the MCA territory, one must consider indirect bypass (more proven benefit in children) or review the angiogram to determine the feasibility of a more posterior bypass utilizing the occipital artery. This presents difficulties with anastomosing in eloquent cortex. The Sylvian fissure can be split in order to find a more proximal MCA branch, but the tolerance for cross-clamping of the vessel for anastomosis in an already compromised hemisphere makes this a higher risk procedure. An alternative is using the saphenous vein or radial artery as an interposition graft, both of which have their own advantages and disadvantages. Intraoperative hypotension must be avoided and frequent communication with the anesthesia team is of paramount importance.

Case Continued

The patient was offered medical or surgical therapy. The risks and benefits of both modalities were presented, and the patient provided informed consent for STA-MCA bypass.

Postoperative Management

The patient was sent to the ICU postoperatively for close blood pressure monitoring and regulation. The single most important aspect of postoperative care is the strict avoidance of hypotension. The patient was also placed on full-strength ASA. In patients who require use of the radial artery for the interposition graft, calcium channel blockers should be started as arterial interposition grafts have a higher risk of vasospasm in the postoperative period.

An intact patient who neurologically declines with lateralizing signs should have a stat head CT performed to rule out a mass lesion (subdural or epidural hematoma) at the operative site. If the patient is stable on postoperative day (POD) 1, he or she may be transferred to the general ward and progress to discharge.

Case Conclusion

The patient underwent an uneventful STA-MCA bypass and was discharged on POD 2. She had complete resolution of her symptoms and was working full time without problem 6 weeks later. Angiography on POD 1 confirmed the patency of the bypass (Fig. 3). Angiography at 6 months demonstrated maturation of flow through the bypass (Fig. 4).

TAKE HOME POINTS

- ICA occlusion in the setting of moyamoya disease is still an accepted indication for EC-IC bypass.
- EC-IC bypass has been proven in two RCTs to be of no benefit for atherosclerotic ICA occlusion, and bypass is now reserved for rare cases of crescendo symptoms with failure of medical management and radiographic evidence of hypoperfusion.

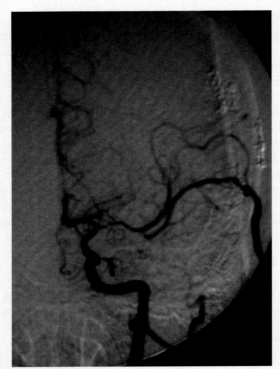

FIGURE 3 • Angiogram demonstrating patent STA-MCA bypass graft and improved perfusion of distal MCA vessels.

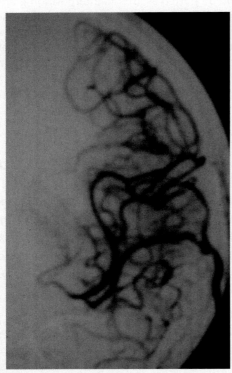

FIGURE 4 • Angiogram showing continued patency and excellent filling of MCA distribution on selective ECA injection.

- Angiography is the gold standard and should include evaluation of the external carotid arteries (ECAs) to determine the adequacy of extracranial vessels for anastomosis.
- Meticulous technique must be used during dissection of the STA.
- Bone and scalp closure must be performed in such a fashion as to not occlude the successfully constructed anastomosis.
- ICU monitoring is essential for early detection of life-threatening postoperative hypotension, bleeding, or seizure.

SUGGESTED READINGS

Amin-Hanjani S, Barker FG, Charbel FT, et al. Extracranial-intracranial bypass for stroke-is this the end of the line or a bump in the road? *Neurosurgery.* 2012;71(3):557-561. doi:10.1227/NEU.0b013e3182621488

Failure of extracranial-intracranial arterial bypass to reduce the risk of ischemic stroke. Results of an international randomized trial. The EC/IC Bypass Study Group. *N Engl J Med.* 1985;313(19):1191-1200.

Fung LW, Thompson D, Ganesan V. Revascularisation surgery for paediatric moyamoya: a review of the literature. *Childs Nerv Syst.* 2005;21:358-364.

Grubb RL, Derdyn CP, Fritsch SM, et al. Importance of hemodynamic factors in the prognosis of symptomatic carotid occlusion. *JAMA.* 1998;280:1055-1060.

Powers WJ, Clarke WR, Grubb RL Jr, et al. Extracranial-intracranial bypass surgery for stroke prevention in hemodynamic cerebral ischemia: the Carotid Occlusion Surgery Study randomized trial. *JAMA.* 2011;306(18):1983-1992.

Scott RM, Smith ER. Moyamoya disease and moyamoya syndrome. *N Engl J Med.* 2009;360:1226-1237.

Sundt TM. Was the international randomized trial of extracranial-intracranial bypass representative of the population at risk? *N Engl J Med.* 1987;316:814-816.

Yonas H, Smith HA, Durham SR, et al. Increased stroke risk predicted by compromised cerebral blood flow reactivity. *J Neurosurg.* 1993;79:483-489.

CLINICAL SCENARIO CASE QUESTIONS

1. Moyamoya disease involves which of the following?

    a. Complete occlusion of the external carotid artery at its terminus

    b. Rapid tapering of the proximal internal carotid artery

    c. Rapid tapering of the distal internal carotid artery and its bifurcation

    d. Severe stenosis of the distal middle cerebral artery

2. Among the four steps outlined below in the performance of an EC-IC bypass, which is the earliest?

    a. Identification of a suitable recipient vessel

    b. Doppler identification of the STA

    c. Performance of a small craniotomy beneath the temporalis muscle

    d. Prepping and draping the operative field

13 Recurrent Carotid Stenosis

ANDY LEE and RAUL J. GUZMAN

Presentation

A 61-year-old man with a history of hypertension and coronary artery disease previously underwent bilateral carotid endarterectomies (CEA). His most recent CEA was performed on the left side 12 months ago. The right CEA was performed 2 years ago. He presents to your office for routine follow-up. On questioning, he admits to having two episodes of left eye blindness over the last month that each resolved over 10 to 15 minutes. Physical examination is notable for a left-sided cervical bruit. A carotid duplex ultrasound is performed.

Carotid Duplex Ultrasound Scan Report

Right common and internal carotid arteries without significant stenosis.

Left common carotid artery (distal): 80% to 99% stenosis.

Left internal carotid artery: 15% to 49% stenosis.

Differential Diagnosis

Recurrent carotid stenosis has an incidence of 4% to 16% in patients evaluated by serial duplex ultrasound following CEA. As patients with recurrent stenosis are typically asymptomatic, this reported incidence varies widely depending on the measurement criteria, methods, and duration of postoperative follow-up. Restenosis identified within the immediate postoperative period likely represents an incomplete endarterectomy with residual disease or technical defect after surgery. The characteristic homogeneous neointimal lesion seen in restenosis is usually discovered in patients experiencing recurrence within the first 3 years after endarterectomy. Late recurrences are more often due to progressive atherosclerosis.

In symptomatic patients, the differential diagnosis for stroke or transient ischemia attack following CEA includes recurrent carotid stenosis, new-onset atrial fibrillation (or other cardiac sources of embolic disease), vasculitis, and lacunar infarction.

Workup

The diagnosis of recurrent carotid stenosis is most commonly made on routine postoperative surveillance using duplex ultrasound. According to the Society for Vascular Surgery (SVS) clinical guidelines, patients undergoing CEA should be followed by exam and carotid duplex ultrasound testing within 30 days after their procedure. Patients without significant hemodynamic abnormality on initial duplex will usually have the study repeated in 6 months and thereafter on a yearly basis. Studies demonstrating stenosis greater than 50% should be repeated every 6 months or sooner if symptoms occur. A new cervical bruit that develops in an asymptomatic patient after CEA should be promptly evaluated by duplex ultrasound for recurrent carotid stenosis.

Adjunctive imaging modalities, such as computed tomography, MRI, and contrast angiography, may be employed when the duplex ultrasound does not provide sufficient anatomic definition or when there is a question about the proximal or distal vasculature. Computed tomography angiography (CTA) can provide excellent anatomical detail, especially when considering an endovascular approach. Physical examination should include a careful neurologic evaluation with a focus on cranial nerves to assess for stroke or any postoperative deficits.

Up to 50% of patients undergoing reoperation for recurrent carotid stenosis have an asymptomatic, high-grade lesion that was incidentally discovered through duplex ultrasound screening. Closure by patch angioplasty at the time of primary CEA has been shown to reduce the risk of developing restenosis. Data from the Carotid Revascularization Endarterectomy versus Stent Trial (CREST) suggest that female sex, hypertension, diabetes, and dyslipidemia were risk factors for recurrent stenosis after stenting or endarterectomy. Smoking has also been shown to be an independent predictor of restenosis but only after CEA.

Case Continued

The patient is scheduled for CTA to further evaluate his cerebrovascular anatomy.

CT Angiogram Report

The right common carotid artery (CCA) and internal carotid artery (ICA) are patent with mild calcified plaque and minimal luminal narrowing.

The left distal CCA shows an 80% stenosis. The left ICA is patent with 2 cm luminal narrowing but no focal stenosis (Fig. 1).

Recurrent Carotid Stenosis, Symptomatic

Diagnosis and Treatment

Several factors are considered when selecting the most appropriate treatment for recurrent carotid stenosis. Interval since CEA, severity of stenosis, medical

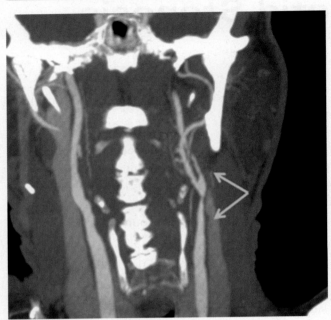

FIGURE 1 • CTA of neck, coronal view. *Yellow arrows* identify restenosis in the distal CCA.

comorbid conditions, status of the contralateral carotid, and presence or absence of symptoms are the key considerations. Asymptomatic, low-grade, or immediate-grade lesions are usually managed using antiplatelet therapy. Intervention should be considered for high-grade (greater than 80%) or symptomatic lesions, especially those associated with contralateral carotid occlusion. Preoperative imaging plays an essential role in characterizing the recurrent lesion, and these anatomic data must be considered in combination with the history and comorbid conditions of the individual patient in selecting the best method of intervention.

Redo CEA with patch angioplasty is the standard operative approach used to treat recurrent carotid stenosis. It carries a risk for cranial nerve injury in 7% to 20% of patients. Interestingly, data from regional databases with larger sample sizes have suggested that redo CEA is associated with higher rates of stroke/death/MI compared with primary CEA, but there was no difference in cranial nerve injury.

More recently, carotid angioplasty and stenting (CAS) has been employed in the treatment of postendarterectomy restenosis. In cases of early restenosis (less than 3 years), the homogenous lesion from myointimal hyperplasia is thought to be smooth and less likely to result in lesion embolization during wire traversal. The method allows for the avoidance of redo surgery in those patients with dense scar tissue. National vascular registry data show better outcomes for carotid artery stenting in restenotic compared with primary lesions. Other appealing features of carotid stenting include the use of local anesthesia making it a suitable alternative for those patients thought to be at increased risk for general anesthesia. Bradycardia during balloon inflation and femoral pseudo-

aneurysm formation are potential complications unique to angioplasty and stenting. Stenting is not associated with cranial nerve injury, and it therefore may be a more appropriate option for patients with a prior nerve injury, neck irradiation, radical neck dissection, permanent tracheostomy, limited cervical spine mobility, or other conditions that might predispose to a difficult dissection.

Although some centers have suggested that short-term morbidity and mortality events for CAS are comparable to redo CEA, the long-term durability of this procedure remains unknown. Traditionally, carotid stenting has not been employed for late carotid restenosis where recurrent atherosclerotic disease is the most common etiology, or for lesions with ulcerations, free-floating thrombus, or tortuous arterial anatomy. The use of embolic protection devices including filters or retrograde flow systems may help to reduce the stroke risk during carotid stenting, but the benefit has yet to be definitively established in randomized trials. It remains to be seen whether the emergence of carotid protection devices will expand the application of endovascular management to include these lesions with greater risk for embolic complications.

At present, data from outcome studies do not favor one particular operative approach over another as patients with postendarterectomy restenosis exhibit increased risk of adverse events regardless of which procedure is used. The general agreement has been that carotid stenting should be considered for patients with early restenosis whose risk for redo CEA or other open repair is unacceptably high. In the absence of any prospective randomized and controlled trials, the management of patients with recurrent stenosis remains difficult, and the choice of reintervention should be individualized to the patient's personal risk factors.

Case Continued

The patient is informed of the two different approaches available. Complications that are discussed for surgery include stroke, myocardial infarction, cranial nerve injury, bleeding, infection, and death. Complications related to stenting include access site issues such as bleeding, leg ischemia, and pseudoaneurysm formation. A 4% risk of stroke is balance against the lower risk of postprocedure MI and cranial nerve injury. The patient chooses carotid stenting.

Surgical Approach
Carotid Artery Stenting

Carotid stenting should be performed under local anesthesia. Intravenous sedation should be minimized because it may interfere with intraoperative neurologic assessment. Femoral access is most commonly employed. Balloon inflation during angioplasty is sometimes associated with symptomatic bradycardia that may seldom require transvenous pacemaker placement.

With carotid stent procedures, placement and passage of filters or wires across a lesion can be challenging, particularly when there is tortuosity of the internal carotid artery. The use of stiffer accompanying wires can help straighten the artery to facilitate access. Vessel manipulation may induce vasospasm complicating further instrumentation. Pre-stent dilation of a stenotic area can lead to hemodynamic instability such as bradycardia and hypotension, requiring close anesthesia monitoring and administration of atropine. It is important that a post–stent placement arteriogram is obtained to examine for appropriate placement and flow beyond the carotid bifurcation (Table 1).

Redo Carotid Endarterectomy

When chosen, redo CEA or carotid reconstruction is performed through an incision parallel to the anterior sternocleidomastoid muscle in an approach similar to that employed for primary operation. Dissection is carried directly through the plane of scar with lateral reflection of the sternocleidomastoid muscle. Patch angioplasty should be combined with redo endarterectomy whenever possible. Intraoperative shunting is commonly employed because of the increased operative time compared with primary CEA. If redo endarterectomy with patch angioplasty is not possible, common-to-internal carotid bypass with synthetic or saphenous vein graft is performed, and this has been used in up to 50% of patient undergoing reoperation in some series. Patch angioplasty alone has also been reported with good results in patients with myointimal hyperplasia where endarterectomy is not possible. Limited comparative data on the different operative approaches for carotid restenosis are available (Table 2).

Case Continued

The patient is taken to the operating room, where under minimal sedation and local anesthesia, right common femoral artery access was obtained. The left carotid artery

TABLE 2. Redo CEA

Key Technical Steps
1. Vertical incision parallel to anterior SCM
2. Dissect through plane of scar tissue to mobilize jugular vein and muscle laterally
3. Expose carotid vessels to obtain proximal and distal control
4. Place shunt as needed
5. Assess characteristics of lesion for possible endarterectomy with patch angioplasty
6. Bypass when necessary
7. Obtain hemostasis

Potential Pitfalls
- Difficulty of reoperative dissection and endarterectomy
- Cranial nerve injury
- Excessive bleeding from scar tissue

was selected, and a sheath was passed into the common carotid artery. A filter wire was then passed across the lesion and opened without difficulty. The area of stenosis was predilated using a 2-mm balloon. A stent was then positioned across the lesion, deployed, and postdilated using a 4-mm balloon. Completion angiography demonstrated good luminal improvement. The patient remained fully aware and without neurologic findings. The sheath and catheter were removed, and hemostasis was obtained using a closure device (Fig. 2).

TABLE 1. CAS

Key Technical Steps
1. Aspirin and Plavix beginning a minimum of 48 hours prior to procedure
2. Knowledge of aortic arch anatomy from preoperative imaging or arch aortogram
3. Percutaneous access and carotid cannulation
4. Selective cerebral arteriography
5. Crossing carotid stenosis
6. Placement of embolic protection devices
7. Balloon dilatation of stenosis
8. Deployment of stent and angioplasty
9. Repeat carotid arteriography

Potential Pitfalls
- Access site complications (hematoma, pseudoaneurysm)
- Atheroembolism from wire manipulation
- Hemodynamic instability

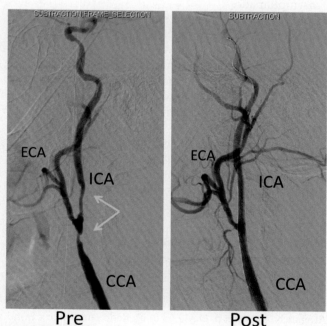

FIGURE 2 • Operative angiograms pre and post carotid stent placement. Left image pre-stent angiogram with *yellow arrows* indicating region of stenosis at distal CCA with extension into ICA. Right image, post stent placement demonstrate improved luminal diameter.

Postoperative Management

After carotid stent placement, the patient is closely monitored for neurologic changes, blood pressure maintenance, and access site problems. The following day, renal function is assessed as needed for evidence of contrast-induced nephropathy. Any changes in neurologic status should raise concerns for stent thrombosis. A dual antiplatelet regimen usually aspirin and clopidogrel is generally continued for at least 1 month then a single agent is continued indefinitely. Patients return for noninvasive imaging at 1 month, 6 months, and annually to assess patency.

Case Conclusion

The patient is discharged from the hospital on the first postoperative day on aspirin and clopidogrel. Postoperative carotid duplex performed 1 month later shows no evidence of restenosis.

TAKE HOME POINTS

- Recurrent carotid stenosis occurring within 3 years of the initial procedure is associated with neointimal hyperplasia.
- Recurrent carotid stenosis occurring after 3 years is associated with progression of atherosclerosis.
- Patients with recurrent carotid restenosis are often asymptomatic.
- Risk factors for restenosis include female sex, small artery size, hypertension, hyperlipidemia, smoking, and diabetes.
- In patients with symptomatic carotid restenosis or those with an asymptomatic lesion greater than 80%, open or endovascular revascularization is performed.
- Redo CEA and carotid stent procedures are associated with similar perioperative stroke/death/MI risks in patients with recurrent carotid stenosis.
- In patients with an asymptomatic recurrent carotid stenosis less than 80%, antiplatelet therapy is usually continued with close surveillance for lesion progression or symptoms.

SUGGESTED READINGS

AbuRahma AF, Abu-Halimah S, Bensenhaver J, et al. Primary carotid artery stenting versus carotid artery stenting for postcarotid endarterectomy stenosis. *J Vasc Surg.* 2009;50(5):1031-1039.

Attigah N, Külkens S, Deyle C, et al. Redo surgery or carotid stenting for restenosis after carotid endarterectomy: results of two different treatment strategies. *Ann Vasc Surg.* 2010; 24(2):190-195.

Bowser AN, Bandyk DF, Evans A, et al. Outcome of carotid stent-assisted angioplasty versus open surgical repair of recurrent carotid stenosis. *J Vasc Surg.* 2003;38(3):432-438.

Brott TG, Halperin JL, Abbara S, et al. 2011 ASA/ACCF/AHA/ AANN/AANS/ACR/ASNR/CNS/SAIP/SCAI/SIR/SNIS/ SVM/SVS guideline on the management of patients with extracranial carotid and vertebral artery disease: executive summary: a report of the American College of Cardiology Foundation/American Heart Association Task Force on Practice Guidelines, and the American Stroke Association, American Association of Neuroscience Nurses, American Association of Neurological Surgeons, American College of Radiology, American Society of Neuroradiology, Congress of Neurological Surgeons, Society of Atherosclerosis Imaging and Prevention, Society for Cardiovascular Angiography and Interventions, Society of Interventional Radiology, Society of NeuroInterventional Surgery, Society for Vascular Medicine, and Society for Vascular Surgery. Developed in collaboration with the American Academy of Neurology and Society of Cardiovascular Computed Tomography. *Catheter Cardiovasc Interv.* 2013; 81(1):E76-E123.

Dorigo W, Pulli R, Fargion A, et al. Comparison of open and endovascular treatments of post-carotid endarterectomy restenosis. *Eur J Vasc Endovasc Surg.* 2013;45(5):437-442.

Fokkema M, Jan de Borst G, Nolan BW, et al. Carotid stenting versus endarterectomy in patients undergoing reintervention and prior carotid endarterectomy. *J Vasc Surg.* 2014:59(1): 8-15.

Hobson RW II, Goldstein JE, Jamil Z, et al. Carotid restenosis: operative and endovascular management. *J Vasc Surg.* 1999;29(2):228-235; discussion 235-238.

Lal BK. Recurrent carotid stenosis after CEA and CAS: diagnosis and management. *Semin Vasc Surg.* 2007;20(4):259-266. Review.

O'Hara PJ, Hertzer NR, Karafa MT, et al. Reoperation for recurrent carotid stenosis: early results and late outcome in 199 patients. *J Vasc Surg.* 2001;34(1):5-12.

Ricotta JJ, O'Brien-Irr MS. Conservative management of residual and recurrent lesions after carotid endarterectomy: long-term results. *J Vasc Surg.* 1997;26(6):963-972.

CLINICAL SCENARIO CASE QUESTIONS

1. A 60-year-old woman returns to clinic for annual follow-up 4 years after undergoing an uncomplicated left CEA with patch angioplasty for a symptomatic carotid stenosis. On her most recent ultrasound carotid duplex, there is an 80% to 99% carotid stenosis. She remains clinically asymptomatic. Which of the following best characterizes this lesion?

   a. This lesion is the result of neointimal hyperplasia within the postoperative period.

   b. On gross and angiographic appearance, this lesion is generally smooth and homogenous in appearance.

   c. Ultrasound is not the preferred modality to assess restenosis.

d. Restenosis at this time is likely due to progressive atherosclerotic narrowing involving inflammatory mechanisms.

e. Because it is a result of ongoing vascular injury secondary from the initial surgery, smoking is not a risk factor for this recurrence.

2. When choosing the method of revascularization for a patient with carotid restenosis, what is an appropriate rationale for choosing endovascular management?

a. Recurrences that occur within 3 years after primary CEA are usually due to neointimal hyperplasia that likely carries a lower risk of embolization during wire traversal.

b. Clinical data suggest an absolute benefit with an endovascular approach to carotid restenosis because it is associated with no risks for perioperative neurologic events.

c. An open operation for restenosis is not possible because there is no intima.

d. Antiembolic protection devices used during carotid stenting prevent restenosis.

e. All patients with asymptomatic carotid restenosis benefit from reintervention.

14 Symptomatic External Carotid Artery Disease

SEAN P. RODDY, R. CLEMENT DARLING III, and KAMRAN A. JAFREE

Presentation

An 82-year-old right-handed man with hypertension, hypercholesterolemia, history of tobacco use, and coronary artery disease presents with multiple episodes of amaurosis fugax. He denied other focal symptoms and had no prior stroke. On physical examination, he had a right carotid bruit. Neurologic examination was unremarkable. A duplex study from 2 years ago demonstrated an occluded right internal carotid artery (ICA). He has no history of head or neck cancers and has never had any radiation treatments.

Differential Diagnosis

The differential diagnosis for amaurosis fugax focuses on atheroembolism from the heart to the area of brain involved. Atheroemboli primarily develop at the carotid bifurcation and usually involve the ICA origin, although an atherosclerotic plaque may reside in the aortic arch and great vessels. In the setting of an occluded ICA, emboli may be released from the ICA stump or from disease in the external carotid artery (ECA), which provides an important collateral pathway for cerebral blood flow in the presence of ICA occlusions or severe stenosis. Cardiac thrombus, especially in individuals with atrial fibrillation, valvular heart disease, or ascending aortic disease, has the potential for distal embolization, but this is not usually associated with retinal artery events.

Workup

The patient undergoes a duplex ultrasound examination of the carotid arteries, which reveals a normal right common carotid artery (CCA). The right ICA is occluded with a severe stenosis of the right ECA shown in Figure 1. The left carotid system has mild plaque in both the ECA and ICA. The vertebral arteries are patent, with antegrade flow. No evidence of aneurysmal disease is identified. Ultrasound is a quick, cost-effective, office-based procedure without radiation that helps identify the majority of extracranial carotid pathology. In this case, it not only confirms the prior occlusion of the ICA but also identifies the significant ECA stenosis that has developed. It cannot assess intracranial or intrathoracic pathology.

Cross-sectional imaging (either magnetic resonance or computed tomography [CT]) is usually the next step from the aortic arch to the intracranial vessels. In this patient, CT angiography identifies no aortic arch pathology, confirms the ICA occlusion and ECA stenosis, and rules out aneurysms, arteriovenous malformations, and intracranial hemorrhage. Alternatively, contrast arteriography of the aortic arch and great vessels may be performed with selective catheterization of the carotid arteries. Two cervical carotid selective angiographic images are listed in Figures 2 and 3 confirming the ICA occlusion and the ECA origin occlusive disease.

For completeness, the patient should undergo cardiac evaluation, including transesophageal echocardiography, for both perioperative risk assessment and source of atheroemboli. In this patient, the cardiac evaluation revealed a left ventricular ejection fraction of 50%, mild mitral regurgitation, normal ascending aorta, and no atrial or ventricular thrombus.

Diagnosis and Treatment

From these data, the most probable source of emboli is the stenotic ECA. The proximal ICA stump was occluded on duplex evaluation 2 years ago and is therefore less likely the etiology. If the ICA was previously patent, acute ICA occlusion and distal ICA thromboembolism could be a source for amaurosis fugax. The ascending aorta and proximal great vessels do not have a significant atherosclerotic plaque burden as an alternate etiology. Recommendation was made for ICA ligation and ECA endarterectomy with patch closure.

Surgical Approach

Open surgical reconstruction remains the gold standard for this pathology. The patient is placed supine under regional or general anesthesia based on surgeon preference. The carotid artery is exposed through a longitudinal neck incision. Systemic anticoagulation is achieved typically with intravenous heparin. The ICA is suture ligated. A CCA and ECA endarterectomy is performed. Prosthetic, vein, or endarterectomized ICA is typically used for patch closure.

A newer alternative recently described by Naylor et al. and Kouvelos et al. involves an endovascular approach

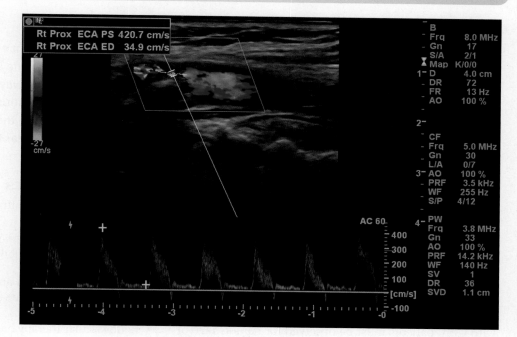

FIGURE 1 • Duplex ultrasound image of the right carotid artery bifurcation demonstrating a severe stenosis in the right external carotid artery and a right internal carotid artery occlusion.

with carotid artery stenting using bare metal stents with and without embolic protection versus ICA stump exclusion using a stentgraft that covers the ICA origin and extends into the ECA. Tapering from the CCA to the ECA is an obvious concern when using one of the current commercially available nontapered stentgrafts. Validation of this technique by others is required.

Special Intraoperative Considerations

For standard carotid endarterectomy (CEA), care should be taken to avoid the vagus and hypoglossal nerves. The surgeon must protect and separate the vagus nerve from the carotid artery so it is not caught when the vascular clamps are applied. The hypoglossal nerve traverses the superior aspect of the dissection field and can be avoided

FIGURE 2 • AP contrast arteriogram of the right common carotid artery demonstrating internal carotid artery occlusion and a stenotic, irregular external carotid artery.

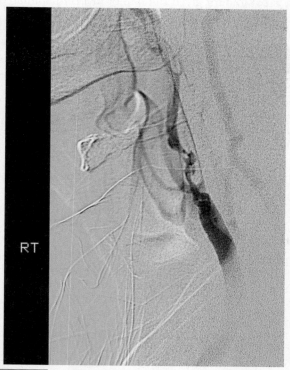

FIGURE 3 • Straight lateral contrast arteriogram of the right carotid artery demonstrating internal carotid artery occlusion and a stenotic, irregular external carotid artery.

by transection of the artery and vein to the sternoclei-domastoid muscle that tethers it. When ICA ligation and a CCA/ECA endarterectomy are performed, the ECA at the distal end point is skeletonized to a more significant degree than during standard CEA. The superior laryngeal nerve passes posterior to the ECA prior to entering the larynx. Dissection of the ECA and its branches distal to the atherosclerotic plaque should be performed as close as possible to the vessel wall to ensure that the nerve is separated from the adventitia.

Shunting may be performed routinely or on demand in the course of standard CEA. During ICA ligation and ECA/CCA endarterectomy, the same concerns apply though the incidence of shunt use in several series is minimal.

Patients receive systemic anticoagulation to prevent thromboembolic events during CEA. Hemostasis at the completion of the procedure is therefore critical.

Postoperative Management

Given an arterial anastomosis and use of anticoagulation with CEA, patients must be observed for hemorrhage or hematoma formation that may even compress the airway requiring operative exploration. Alternatively, thromboembolic events may lead to transient ischemic attack or stroke that also may require operative exploration and arterial reconstruction.

Elevated blood pressure occurs in over 20% of normotensive patients after CEA. Poor control of blood pressure in the postoperative period increases the risk of developing cerebral hyperperfusion syndrome. Cardiac monitoring is paramount given the rate of myocardial infarction that approaches 5% in some series (Table 1).

TABLE 1. External Carotid Artery Endarterectomy

Key Technical Steps

1. The patient is placed supine under regional or general anesthesia based on surgeon preference.
2. The carotid artery is exposed through a longitudinal neck incision.
3. Systemic anticoagulation is achieved typically with intravenous heparin.
4. The ICA is suture ligated.
5. A CCA and ECA endarterectomy is performed.
6. Prosthetic, vein, or endarterectomized ICA is typically used for patch closure.

Potential Pitfalls

- Avoid superior laryngeal nerve injury.
- Given an arterial anastomosis and use of anticoagulation with CEA, patients must be observed for hemorrhage or hematoma formation that may even compress the airway requiring operative exploration.
- Thromboembolic events may lead to transient ischemic attack or stroke that also may require operative exploration and arterial reconstruction.
- Elevated blood pressure occurs in over 20% of normotensive patients after CEA. Poor control of blood pressure in the postoperative period increases the risk of developing cerebral hyperperfusion syndrome.

Case Conclusion

The patient underwent endarterectomy with polytetrafluoroethylene (PTFE) patch angioplasty. An ulcerated plaque was found at the origin of the ECA with fresh thrombus. There were no neurologic sequelae, and the patient has remained asymptomatic in 5-year follow-up.

TAKE HOME POINTS

- Ultrasound helps identify the majority of extracranial carotid pathology.
- Angiography is necessary to delineate the anatomy.
- Endarterectomy with patch angioplasty is the treatment of choice.
- Dissection of the ECA and its branches should be performed close to the vessel wall to avoid superior laryngeal nerve injury.
- Endovascular therapy has been used in some case reports in selected patients with acceptable results.

SUGGESTED READINGS

Barnett HJM, Peerless SJ, Kaufman JGE. Stump of internal carotid artery a source for further cerebral embolic ischemia. *Stroke.* 1978;9:448-456.

Gertler JP, Cambria RP. The role of external carotid endarterectomy in the treatment of ipsilateral internal carotid occlusion: collective review. *J Vasc Surg.* 1987;6:158-167.

Karmody AM, Shah DM, Monaco VJ, et al. On surgical reconstruction of the external carotid artery. *Am J Surg.* 1978; 136:176-180.

Kouvelos GN, Koutsoumpelis AC, Klonaris C, et al. Endovascular repair of external carotid artery disease. *J Endovasc Ther.* 2012; 19(4):504-511.

Kumar SM, Wang JCC, Barry MC, et al. Carotid stump syndrome: outcome from surgical management. *Eur J Vasc Endovasc Surg.* 2001;21:214-219.

Naylor AR, Bell PR, Bolia A. Endovascular treatment of carotid stump syndrome. *J Vasc Surg.* 2003;38:593-595.

CLINICAL SCENARIO CASE QUESTIONS

1. What is the traditional management of the patient undergoing an external carotid endarterectomy?

   a. Operative endarterectomy with patch
   b. Anticoagulation alone
   c. Antiplatelet therapy alone
   d. Eversion internal carotid endarterectomy
   e. Carotid to subclavian artery bypass

2. The first test for a patient who presents with amaurosis fugax in the setting of an ICA occlusion is what?

   a. MRA of the head
   b. Duplex ultrasound
   c. Four-vessel cerebral angiography
   d. Computed tomography angiography
   e. CO_2 angiogram of the head

15 Carotid Artery Dissection

ANDREW M. SOUTHERLAND, JENNIFER J. MAJERSIK, and BRADFORD B. WORRALL

Presentation

A 47-year-old right-handed man presented with abrupt onset right-sided head and neck pain while shoveling snow. Six hours later, he noticed his left hand was not working as well so his wife called 911. Past medical history is significant for migraine headaches with visual aura and mild hypertension, but no other vascular risk factors. Family history is negative for stroke or other vascular disease. On physical examination, his blood pressure is 153/93 mm Hg with vital signs otherwise stable. He has no cervical bruits, normal cardiac auscultation, and regular and symmetric pulses. Cranial nerve exam reveals mild right-sided tarsal lid ptosis and anisocoria (right pupil 2 mm, left 4 mm) more pronounced in the dark. Additional neurologic exam reveals a mild left pronator drift and weakness of the left hand with slowed finger tapping and 4/5 grip strength. Neurological exam is otherwise intact.

Differential Diagnosis

Abrupt onset of focal neurologic symptoms localizing to an arterial territory is always concerning for an acute stroke. In this case, differential diagnosis includes ischemic versus hemorrhagic stroke subtypes, complicated migraine headache given the head pain and his past history, or an acute neuromuscular injury given the association with exertional activity. Other causes of stroke in the young include thromboembolism from acquired or congenital cardiac disease; transient vasculopathies, such as reversible cerebral vasoconstriction syndrome (RCVS); genetic vasculopathies, such as moyamoya; or occult hypercoagulable states; the etiology remains cryptogenic in many cases. Hemorrhagic stroke subtypes, such as aneurysmal subarachnoid hemorrhage, should present with a more profound "worst headache of life."

The key physical finding in this case is the presence of lid ptosis and miosis on the right, hallmark signs of oculosympathetic palsy or Horner's syndrome, representing injury to the carotid plexus of ascending postganglionic sympathetic fibers innervating the superior tarsal and pupillary dilator muscles (Fig. 1). The constellation of abrupt head and neck pain, Horner's syndrome, and stroke-like symptoms in a relatively young adult is consistent with cervical artery dissection and requires immediate vascular imaging of the cervicocerebral arteries.

Workup

An MRI and MRA of the head and neck are obtained. On diffusion-weighted imaging (DWI), brain MRI reveals wedge-shaped areas of restricted diffusion in the right frontal cortex, consistent with acute infarctions of likely thromboembolic origin (Fig. 2). Neck MRA demonstrates a "tapered" occlusion of the right internal carotid artery (ICA) several centimeters distal to the bifurcation (Fig. 3A). The left ICA has a "tonsillar loop" but is otherwise widely patent and regular (Fig. 3B). Intracranial MRA demonstrates delayed cross-filling of the right middle cerebral artery (MCA) from the left carotid circulation via a patent anterior communicating artery (AComm) (Fig. 3C).

Discussion

Cervical artery dissection (CeAD)—*dissection of the carotid or vertebral arteries*—is a significant cause of stroke in young and middle-aged adults, mostly occurring between the ages of 30 and 50 with women being younger than men at time of event. In contrast to other causes of ischemic stroke in older adults related to chronic vascular disease, CeAD typically occurs in young, healthy patients without known atherosclerosis or cardiovascular risk factors. A small proportion (less than 2%) can be attributed to known monogenic connective tissue disorders, such as vascular Ehlers-Danlos or Marfan's syndrome, but most patients are phenotypically normal. Another 10% to 20% of cases are associated with fibromuscular dysplasia (FMD) of the cervical arteries. The majority of cases are considered *spontaneous* and often associated with cervical neck exertion ranging from violent coughing to chiropractic manipulation. A subset results from major neck trauma involving cervical spine injuries with a majority from motor vehicle accidents (Table 1).

In the spontaneous form, the true pathology leading to dissection is unknown but is likely multifactorial

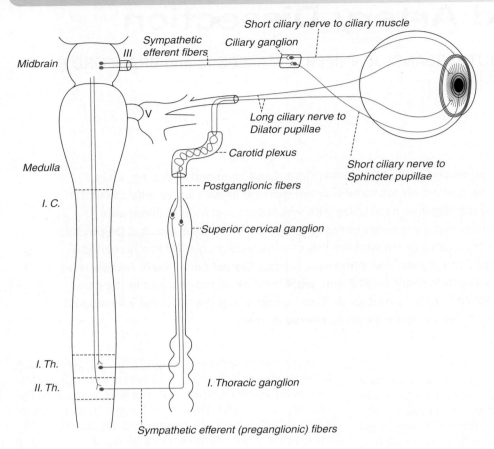

FIGURE 1 • Sympathetic trunk and carotid plexus (Gray's Anatomy—public domain).

including both environmental and genetic predisposition to weakening of the arterial wall. Shear force exertions with lateral rotation or hyperextension of the neck leads to an intimal tear and intramural hematoma dissecting the medial or adventitial layers. Strokes occur by hematoma expansion occluding the true lumen contributing to large-artery territory infarcts or thromboemboli from the site of dissection occluding downstream vascular territories.

About 70% of CeAD cases present with stroke or transient ischemic attack (TIA). Carotid dissections lead to stroke by either carotid occlusion from the intramural hematoma or thromboembolism from the site of intimal injury. Carotid dissection most often presents as a stroke or TIA in the MCA or anterior cerebral artery (ACA) territories. Vertebral artery dissection most often manifests as ischemia in the posterior circulation, presenting as an acute vestibular syndrome

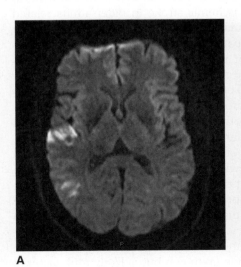
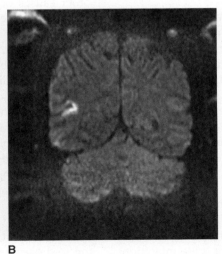

FIGURE 2 • MRI/DWI sequences. **A:** Axial. **B:** Coronal.

A

B

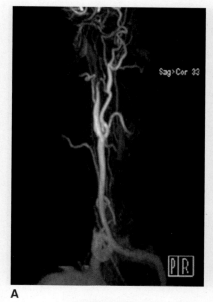
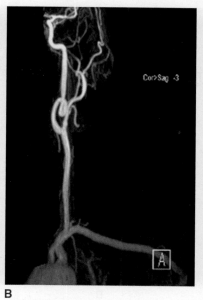
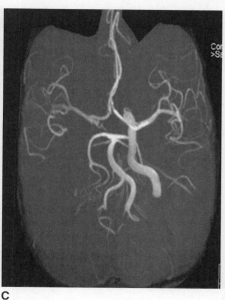

A   **B**   **C**

FIGURE 3 • MRA head and neck. **A:** Left ICA with tapered occlusion. **B:** Right ICA with tonsillar loop. **C:** Delayed cross-filling of right MCA via left carotid circulation and patent AComm.

of vertigo and ataxia or a more circumscribed lateral medullary (Wallenberg) syndrome or cerebellar stroke. The latter is of particular concern in this young patient population given the subsequent risk for cerebellar edema and posterior fossa herniation as a neurologic emergency. Thromboembolic events may occur several days or even weeks after the initial dissection event, creating a high-risk period in need of optimal stroke prevention.

A remainder of cases present with local signs only, comprising pain, Horner's syndrome, or cranial neuropathies from local arterial insufficiency to the nerve

proper. The pain of carotid dissection is typically in the face or lateral neck, while vertebral artery dissections predispose to pain in the occipital or posterior cervical region—often described as *tearing* or *cricking*. Migraine or history of migraine headaches has also been associated with CeAD.

Up to 20% of cases of CeAD occur in multiple cervical arteries *simultaneously,* so called *polyarterial clustering* that suggests an underlying arteriopathy of unclear etiology. This is further suggested by reported associations with other nonatherosclerotic vasculopathies, including intracranial and aortic aneurysms, FMD, aortic root dilatation, and nonspecific arterial tortuosity and kinking.

Diagnosis and Treatment

In the present case, the clinical presentation is confirmed by imaging as a diagnosis of acute ischemic stroke secondary to right ICA dissection with thromboembolic infarcts in the right MCA territory. The imaging diagnosis of CeAD depends on verifying the presence of intramural hematoma in the arterial wall. The gold standard is an MRI of the neck with T1 fat-saturated or fat-suppressed sequences highlighting arterial wall expansion and narrowing of the true artery lumen (Fig. 4). Additional radiologic signs of CeAD on vascular imaging include evidence of an intimal flap or extracranial dissecting aneurysm (Fig. 5). In the case of arterial stenosis or occlusion, a smooth *tapering* or *flame-shaped* appearance indicates expanding intramural hematoma, as opposed to an ulcerated plaque or abrupt occlusion more indicative of atherosclerosis or intraluminal thrombus. The layering hematoma of CeAD may also

TABLE 1. Cervical Artery Dissection

Potential Pitfalls

- Failing to obtain an accurate history, including any presence of head, face, or neck pain or the concurrence of cervical exertion, that might heighten suspicion for CeAD.
- Failing to perform a thorough neurological exam—missing key signs of stroke or Horner's syndrome.
- Failing to order appropriate imaging of the cervical arteries if CeAD is suspected (e.g., MRA/CTA head *and* neck as first-line imaging, MRI T1 in the neck with fat-saturated or fat-suppressed sequences to image intramural hematoma, or conventional cervicocephalic angiography).
- Unnecessarily treating a dissecting aneurysm or stenosis. In the case of spontaneous CeAD, the arteries may be more vulnerable to iatrogenic injury. Interventional or surgical treatment is therefore reserved for patients progressing with cerebrovascular symptoms despite optimal antithrombotic therapy.
- Delay in prescribing early antithrombotic therapy in CeAD for stroke prevention.

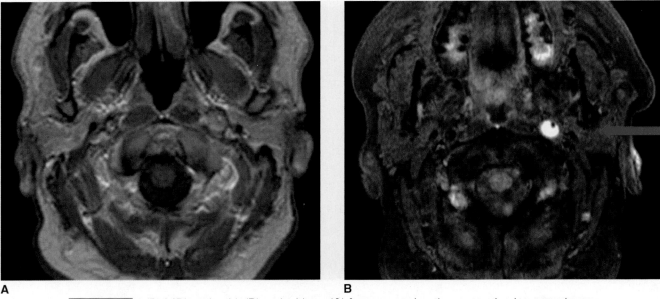

A   **B**

FIGURE 4 • T1 MRI neck with (**B**) and without (**A**) fat suppression demonstrating intramural hematoma of the left internal carotid artery (*arrow*). The *black dot* represents the true lumen.

give the view of a luminal *crescent* or *half moon* in axial sequences on MRA or CTA (Fig. 6).

The location of the lesion also typifies CeAD. Carotid dissections typically occur several centimeters distal to the bifurcation in the mid-cervical segment or just distal to entry into the petrous canal. Vertebral artery dissections most commonly occur in the V3/V4 segment where the artery exits the C2 foramen making a turn to enter the dura. In this way, vertebral artery dissections are more likely than carotid artery dissections to extend into the intradural (or intracranial) segment by which they can present with rupture and subarachnoid hemorrhage (SAH).

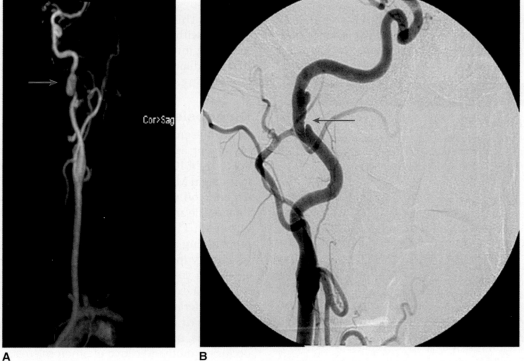

A   **B**

FIGURE 5 • **A:** Right ICA pseudoaneurysm on neck MRA (*red arrow*). **B:** Intimal flap on cervical angiography (*red arrow*).

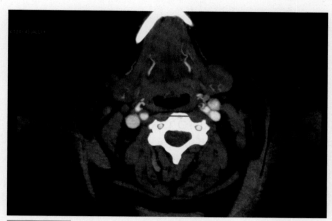

FIGURE 6 • Half-moon–narrowed lumen of the right ICA on axial CTA (*red arrow*).

The risk for ischemic stroke and recurrent dissection is highest in the first days and several weeks following the initial dissection event (approximately 25%), consistent with the likelihood of an underling arteriopathy. Diagnosing CeAD early is therefore paramount in order to initiate stroke prevention with an antithrombotic. Classically, anticoagulation with therapeutic warfarin is the recommended treatment, particularly if intraluminal thrombus is revealed on vascular imaging. However, a number of observational studies have found no difference in outcomes between patients treated with anticoagulation versus antiplatelet therapy alone. An ongoing prospective randomized trial of anticoagulation versus antiplatelet therapy in CeAD will hopefully shed light on optimal medical therapy (www.clinicaltrials.gov NCT00238667). Additional concern for hemorrhagic risk may also dissuade anticoagulation, such as hemorrhagic conversion of an infarct or extension of a vertebral artery dissection into the intradural space where it may be prone to SAH. The use of novel anticoagulants, such as direct thrombin inhibitors (dabigatran) or factor Xa inhibitors (rivaroxaban, apixaban), continues to be studied in this population.

As an additional note, CeAD is not a known contraindication to intravenous tissue plasminogen activator (IV tPA) for treatment of acute ischemic stroke. Several small observational studies have reported that use of IV tPA in this setting is relatively safe compared to use in more common stroke types.

Endovascular or surgical therapy in the treatment of CeAD is generally reserved for a small minority of cases who progress with cerebrovascular events despite optimal medical therapy. The vast majority of cases have a good prognosis with antithrombotic therapy alone, with roughly 75% achieving hemodynamically significant recanalization and 50% complete recanalization at 6 months. Moreover, the *polyarterial clustering* observed in many spontaneous cases of CeAD likely represents a transient arteriopathy, during which the arterial wall is more vulnerable to iatrogenic injury from cerebrocervical angiography or surgical manipulation.

With time for vessel healing, the risk of long-term recurrence after the first few months is low (1% to 2% per year), compared to the initial period of vulnerability surrounding the dissection event. Despite many case reports describing endovascular treatment of extracranial dissecting aneurysms as a sequela of CeAD, these are generally considered benign entities particularly when remaining asymptomatic and are often identified incidentally as chronic manifestations of an incident dissection.

While not necessarily recommended by evidence, patients are often warned against exertional activities of the neck during a convalescent period of time after the dissection. At around 3 months, a repeat vascular imaging study can confirm expected arterial recanalization and vessel wall healing, at which time further decisions about long-term antithrombotic therapy can be made. A long-term benefit of lifetime antiplatelet therapy in this population is unknown, although many practitioners recommend it nonetheless.

Case Conclusion

The patient is started on warfarin (goal INR 2 to 3) with a bridge of low molecular weight heparin. He passes a swallow evaluation and is discharged with outpatient physical and occupational therapy for his hand. He is seen again at 3 months at which time he exhibits no residual weakness or focal neurologic deficits. Repeat CTA showed partial recanalization of his right carotid artery with non–flow-limiting stenosis and minimal vessel irregularity. Decision was made to discontinue warfarin in favor of daily aspirin.

TAKE HOME POINTS

- Cervical artery dissection is a major cause in stroke in young and middle-aged adults without additional vascular risk factors.
- The clinical presentation of cervical artery dissection often includes symptoms of stroke or TIA, Horner's syndrome, and abrupt head and neck pain. Carotid dissections manifest as large artery or thromboembolic strokes in the MCA and ACA territories. Vertebral artery dissection most commonly present as lower brain stem or cerebellar stroke.
- Gold standard diagnosis includes radiologic confirmation of intramural hematoma, intimal flap, or dissecting aneurysm by T1 fat-saturated MRI, CTA, MRA, or cerebrocervical angiography.

- Antithrombotic therapy with either anticoagulation or antiplatelet therapy is the mainstay of stroke preventive treatment, particularly in the high-risk period shortly following the dissection event. Comparative trials are ongoing.
- Surgical or endovascular treatments are reserved for highly selected cases of symptom recurrence despite optimal medical therapy.
- The true etiology of spontaneous cervical artery dissection remains unknown, but polyarterial clustering and transience of risk suggest an underlying arteriopathy. Genetic and environmental studies to identify the pathology are ongoing.

SUGGESTED READINGS

Debette S, Grond-Ginsbach C, Bodenant M, et al. Differential features of carotid and vertebral artery dissections: the CADISP study. *Neurology.* 2011;77:1174-1181.

Debette S, Leys D. Cervical-artery dissections: predisposing factors, diagnosis, and outcome. *Lancet Neurol.* 2009;8:668-678.

Debette S, Metso T, Pezzini A, et al. Association of vascular risk factors with cervical artery dissection and ischemic stroke in young adults. *Circulation.* 2011;123:1537-1544.

Debette S, Metso TM, Pezzini A, et al. CADISP-genetics: an International project searching for genetic risk factors of cervical artery dissections. *Int J Stroke.* 2009;4:224-230.

Dittrich R, Nassenstein I, Bachmann R, et al. Polyarterial clustered recurrence of cervical artery dissection seems to be the rule. *Neurology.* 2007;69:180-186.

Kennedy F, Lanfranconi S, Hicks C, et al. CADISS Investigators. Antiplatelets vs anticoagulation for dissection: CADISS nonrandomized arm and meta-analysis. *Neurology.* 2012;79(7):686-689.

Nedeltchev K, Bickel S, Arnold M, et al. R2-recanalization of spontaneous carotid artery dissection. *Stroke.* 2009;40: 499-504.

Schievink WI, Debette S. Etiology of cervical artery dissections: the writing is in the wall. *Neurology.* 2011;76:1452-1453.

Southerland AM, Meschia JF, Worrall BB. Shared associations of nonatherosclerotic, large-vessel, cerebrovascular arteriopathies: considering intracranial aneurysms, cervical artery dissection, moyamoya disease and fibromuscular dysplasia. *Curr Opin Neurol.* 2013;26(1):13-28.

Tzourio C, Cohen A, Lamisse N, et al. Aortic root dilatation in patients with spontaneous cervical artery dissection. *Circulation.* 1997;95:2351-2353.

CLINICAL SCENARIO CASE QUESTIONS

Given the nature of this book, we would ask that everyone provide two multiple choice single best answer questions for their chapter. We will try to offer CME credit for this activity. Please do not include true or false questions or questions that end in an answer that involves all of the above.

1. A patient presents with abrupt-onset lateralized head and neck pain, aphasia, and right-sided weakness. On exam, the patient is noted to have anisocoria with a right pupil noted to be larger than the left. Which cervical artery would you expect to be involved in this syndrome?

    a. Right internal carotid
    b. Left internal carotid
    c. Right vertebral
    d. Left vertebral

2. A 60-year-old man with hypertension and dyslipidemia receives a CTA of the neck for workup of a left cervical bruit. He is found to have mild-to-moderate atherosclerotic stenosis in the left carotid bifurcation. Incidentally, a small non–flow-limiting pseudoaneurysm is found in his right vertebral artery. When questioned further, he recalls a motor vehicle accident many years prior sustaining no major injuries except self-limited "whiplash." What is the appropriate management of the pseudoaneurysm?

    a. Further diagnostic imaging with digital subtraction angiography (DSA).
    b. Repeat CTA in 3 months for serial monitoring.
    c. DSA with planned angioplasty and stenting.
    d. No further workup is required.

16 Carotid Body Tumors

THOMAS C. BOWER

Presentation

A 58-year-old man is referred to you by his primary care physician for evaluation of slowly enlarging bilateral neck masses. The patient has sporadic mild pain in the upper right neck. He has a 50-pack-year history of smoking and drinks occasional alcohol. He has developed moderate hypertension over the past year, controlled with two medications. He has not had palpitations or other cardiac problems. He has some occupational hearing loss, but no dysphagia, odynophagia, or visual changes. He has a morning cough but has not had fevers or a sore throat. He believes an aunt may have had some type of neck tumor. On physical examination, he has a regular heart rate of 95 beats per minute and a blood pressure of 140/86 mm Hg. The thyroid gland is mildly enlarged. There is a 3-cm immobile mass high in the right neck and a 2-cm mass in the mid left neck just below the angle of the jaw. The left neck mass can be moved laterally but not vertically. Carotid and upper extremity pulses are normal. No bruits or thrills are present in the neck. There is mild erythema in the posterior pharynx but no ulcerations or masses. There are no cardiac murmurs. There are a few coarse rhonchi on auscultation of the lungs. Neurologic examination is within normal limits, including cranial nerves.

Differential Diagnosis

The differential diagnosis for an anterior neck mass in an adult male includes benign and malignant thyroid tumors; adenopathy from metastatic head and neck cancer; tumors of the salivary gland, larynx, or parathyroid; lymphadenitis or lymphoma; and carotid body tumor or carotid aneurysm. The most likely diagnosis in this patient is carotid body tumors (CBTs). Most CBTs can be moved laterally but not in a cranial-caudal direction (Fontaine's sign). They are not expansile like an aneurysm. While the tumors are hypervascular, only 40% of patients have a bruit over the mass. Chronic hypoxemia may play a role in their development.

Evaluation

A complete blood count with differential and thyroid-stimulating hormone level are normal. A color flow duplex ultrasound scan of the neck shows a normal thyroid gland, mildly enlarged cervical lymph nodes with fatty centers, and three masses in the neck, two on the right side and one on the left. The larger upper right neck mass cannot be fully imaged, measures about 3.5 cm but looks solid. The remaining masses splay each carotid artery bifurcation, are hypervascular, and measure between 2 and 2.5 cm in maximum diameter. The common, internal, and external carotid artery velocities are normal.

These findings are suspicious for bilateral carotid body tumors. The upper right neck mass is indeterminate but could represent a vagal tumor or a paraganglioma of the cervical sympathetic chain. While CBTs in most patients are sporadic (75%), the bilateral CBTs, and a relative with a neck tumor in this patient, suggest a familial syndrome.

Approximately 20% to 25% of patients have a family history of paragangliomas, and the tumors may be multicentric. CBT carries a low risk of malignancy. Even though patients rarely present with symptoms, such as headaches, flushing, or palpitations, the presence of bilateral tumors in this man, and a possible family history, warrant additional biochemical, genetic, and radiologic tests.

Biochemical testing is done with a 24-hour urine collection for metanephrines and catecholamines. Succinyl dehydrogenase subunit mutations are common in patients with bilateral tumors and/or a family history. A Mayo Clinic study found 94% of patients with a positive family history and 71% with bilateral tumors to have a genetic mutation. These include subunits SDHB on chromosome 1p35-36 and SDHD on chromosome 11q23. Importantly, metachronous paragangliomas occur in one third of patients with a genetic mutation, which emphasizes the importance of surveillance studies in this subset.

Radiologic imaging is done with ^{123}I-metaiodobenzylguanidine scintigraphy, or CT or MRI studies of the chest and abdomen to exclude other paragangliomas. CT angiography of the head and neck provides better anatomic detail about tumor location, its superior and medial extent, size, volume, and characterization than ultrasonography. In this patient with multiple tumors, the ultrasound study did not fully image the tumors, so CTA would be very useful.

Size, volume, and anatomic location referable to the angle of the mandible and the upper cervical vertebrae

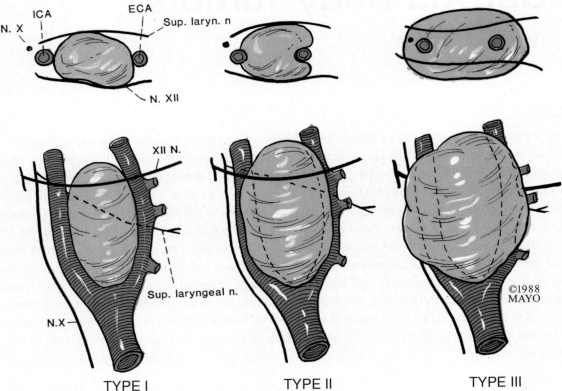

FIGURE 1 • The Shamblin classification of carotid body tumors predicts the difficulty of surgical resection. Class I tumors are localized and easily resected. Class II tumors adhere to or partially surround the carotid arteries. Class III completely surround or encase at least one of the arteries. (ECA, external carotid artery, ICA, internal carotid artery.) (Reprinted with permission from the Mayo Clinic and Hallett JW Jr et al.)

on the CTA determine risk of operation, including injury to adjacent cranial nerves. Ease of resection can be predicted by the Shamblin classification of the tumor (Fig. 1). This classification is determined by the preoperative imaging studies, the operative findings, and pathologic analysis. Class I tumors are localized to the carotid bifurcation and easily resected. Class II tumors partially surround the external and internal carotid arteries but may be adherent to them. Class III tumors completely encase at least one of the arteries and are the most difficult to resect. In general, the larger the tumor size and the more encased the internal carotid artery is, the more difficult the operative resection, the higher the risk of cranial nerve injuries, and the greater the potential need to replace or patch the artery.

Surgical Approach

This patient proved to have nonfunctioning tumors, all isolated to the neck. The SDH genetic analysis was positive, and additional family members were scheduled to be screened. CT imaging of the chest and abdomen showed no other paragangliomas. Select images of the CT of the head and neck are shown in Figure 2. The next steps are planning and executing the operation.

Surgical considerations and patient counseling include the need to embolize the tumor, the risk of cranial nerve injury, the side to treat, and operative preparations. Most tumors less than 3 to 4 cm in diameter or 20 cm³ can be resected without adjuncts, such as embolization. Patients with larger tumors may benefit from cerebral arteriography with selective embolization of feeding vessels the day prior to operation to facilitate operation and lessen blood loss. Most of the arterial feeders originate from the external carotid artery, particularly, the ascending pharyngeal branch (Fig. 2D). The goal of embolization is to decrease tumor vascularity as much as safely possible. While intuitively it might seem that the risk of cranial nerve injuries would be lower if the tumor shrinks and it is less vascular, that has not been a consistent correlation. In the Mayo Clinic report, tumor embolization was safe with no patient sustaining a transient ischemic attack, stroke, or access-site complication in 33 patients treated from a cohort of 131 who had CBT resection. Embolization allowed for a significantly higher number of simple excisions, less need for temporary carotid clamping, and lower blood loss than those not treated by preoperative embolization. However, cranial nerve injuries were no different between the two groups.

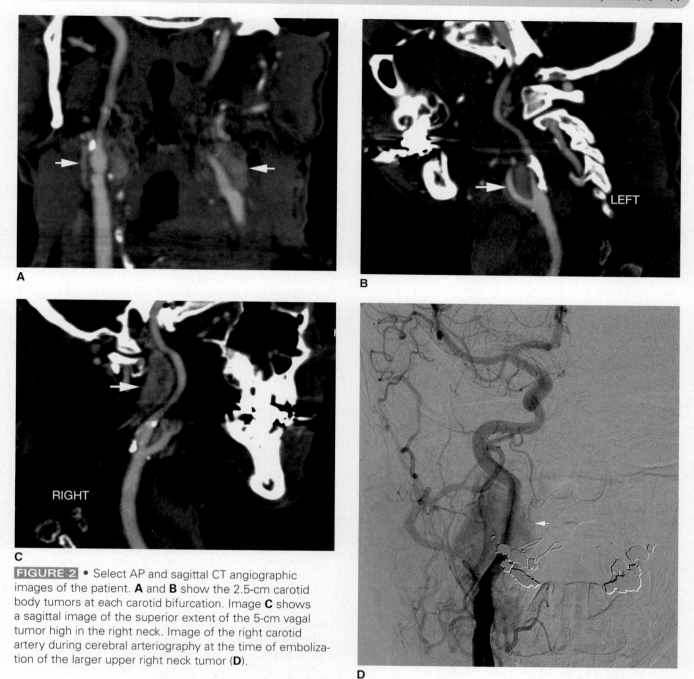

FIGURE 2 • Select AP and sagittal CT angiographic images of the patient. **A** and **B** show the 2.5-cm carotid body tumors at each carotid bifurcation. Image **C** shows a sagittal image of the superior extent of the 5-cm vagal tumor high in the right neck. Image of the right carotid artery during cerebral arteriography at the time of embolization of the larger upper right neck tumor (**D**).

The risk of stroke during tumor excision is exceedingly low in experienced hands. Nonetheless, cranial nerve injuries remain problematic for patients with large tumors (Shamblin III). For this reason, most good-risk patients are considered for surgical resection, unless a tumor has been nonfunctional and stable in size for years and the patient is old (greater than 70 to 80 years), or rarely if the tumor is large and asymptomatic but when surgical resection risks significant disability from cranial nerve injuries. Although nerve injuries occur in one third of patients or more with large tumors, the permanent

cranial nerve deficits that are clinically evident 1 year after resection was only 6% in the Mayo Clinic series. The most common temporary nerve injuries were the marginal mandibular branch of the facial nerve (13%) and the hypoglossal nerve (12%).

The primary cranial nerve injury in this patient may be to the vagus nerve, given that the upper right neck tumor could originate from that nerve.

There is some controversy regarding which tumor should be resected first. One approach is resection of the larger tumor first, as this may pose the greatest threat to the patient. Should the individual sustain a cranial nerve injury, the smaller contralateral tumor can be either observed or treated by alternative means, such as radiation therapy. Significant growth of the contralateral tumor occurs in less than 10% of patients with bilateral carotid body tumors who only have unilateral resection. Other surgeons suggest resection of the smaller tumor first, because of the lower risk of cranial nerve injuries. In this way, if a cranial nerve injury occurs after the second operation to remove the larger CBT, both sides will have been treated.

Nasotracheal intubation is used for patients with lesions that extend to the C2 vertebral body or higher. Subluxation of the mandible is rarely used, except for tumors that extend to the skull base. Tumor extension into the skull mandates input from neuro- or otorhinolaryngologic surgeons with expertise in dealing with such lesions. Surgical assistance from an experienced head and neck cancer surgeon is beneficial to free cranial nerves in patients with large tumors located high in the neck. Some CBTs that extend high into the parapharyngeal space require identification and protection of the facial and glossopharyngeal nerves and the cervical sympathetic trunk. Electroencephalography is often used. The key steps of the operation are as follows. The common carotid artery is dissected free. The vagus and hypoglossal nerves are identified early in the course of operative dissection. The distal internal and external carotid arteries are isolated after identification and mobilization of the hypoglossal nerve away from the tumor. In patients with posterior or medial extension of the tumor, it is important to identify and free away the superior laryngeal nerve. Resection is generally done in a cranial-to-caudal direction. Bipolar diathermy helps control some of the small feeding branches along the inner aspects of the internal and external carotid arteries. Larger feeders along the carotid bifurcation and the ICA and ECA are separately ligated and divided.

Temporary arterial clamping is needed in less than one fourth of patients, and only 10% will need some type of carotid artery reconstruction. However, the surgeon should always be prepared to clamp and reconstruct the carotid artery, particularly in patients with large tumors. The thighs should be prepped for possible saphenous vein harvest in these cases. Should carotid clamping be needed, intravenous heparin is administered to achieve a therapeutic activated clotting time (≥200 to 250 seconds). Carotid reconstruction is accomplished with a patch or saphenous vein interposition graft in select cases. Intraoperative duplex ultrasound imaging is done to assess technical outcome for those who require significant manipulation, clamping, or reconstruction of the carotid artery.

Pitfalls from resection occur because of poor operative preparation, inadequate exposure, dissection in a subadventitial plane along the artery, or a lack of an organized approach to removal of the tumor (Table 1).

TABLE 1. Carotid Body Tumor

Key Technical Steps

1. Patients with larger tumors may benefit from cerebral arteriography with selective embolization of feeding vessels the day prior to operation to facilitate operation and lessen blood loss.
2. Nasotracheal intubation is used for patients with lesions that extend to the C2 vertebral body or higher.
3. Subluxation of the mandible is rarely used, except for tumors that extend to the skull base.
4. Some CBTs that extend high into the parapharyngeal space require identification and protection of the facial and glossopharyngeal nerves and the cervical sympathetic trunk.
5. The common carotid artery is dissected free.
6. The vagus and hypoglossal nerves are identified early in the course of operative dissection.
7. The distal internal and external carotid arteries are isolated after identification and mobilization of the hypoglossal nerve away from the tumor.
8. In patients with posterior or medial extension of the tumor, it is important to identify and free away the superior laryngeal nerve.
9. Resection is generally done in a cranial-to-caudal direction.
10. Bipolar diathermy helps control some of the small feeding branches along the inner aspects of the internal and external carotid arteries.
11. Larger feeders along the carotid bifurcation and the ICA and ECA are separately ligated and divided.
12. The surgeon should always be prepared to clamp and reconstruct the carotid artery, particularly in patients with large tumors. The thighs should be prepped for possible saphenous vein harvest in these cases. Should carotid clamping be needed, intravenous heparin is administered to achieve a therapeutic activated clotting time (≥200 to 250 seconds). Carotid reconstruction is accomplished with a patch or saphenous vein interposition graft in select cases. Intraoperative duplex ultrasound imaging is done to assess technical outcome for those who require significant manipulation, clamping, or reconstruction of the carotid artery.

Potential Pitfalls

- Pitfalls from resection occur because of poor operative preparation, inadequate exposure, dissection in a subadventitial plane along the artery, or a lack of an organized approach to removal of the tumor.
- Hypoglossal and vagus nerve injury—use sharp dissection and know your anatomy.

Case Conclusion

The patient undergoes successful preoperative embolization of the two right neck tumors. Nasotracheal intubation is used because of the high location of the larger tumor. The hypoglossal nerve had to be retracted to accomplish the resection.

Both tumors were excised, removing a few fibers of the vagus nerve from which the higher tumor originated. Postoperatively, he has some tongue deviation to the right side, mild hoarseness in voice, and coughs when swallowing liquids. A swallowing study identifies some penetration in the posterior pharynx to thin liquids. Swallowing exercises are initiated by the speech pathologist, thicker consistency of foods is given, and the patient recovers normal swallowing 1 month after operation.

After operation, patients should have neurologic function monitored closely, including cranial nerve functions. Blood pressure can be labile in some patients, so continuous BP monitoring is useful. Patients with large tumors (Shamblin class II or III) and those with vagal tumors carry risk of cranial nerve injuries. Swallowing studies to assess risk of aspiration and engagement of a speech pathologist are helpful should patients have disabilities from cranial nerve injury.

TAKE HOME POINTS

- Carotid body tumors can be sporadic or familial. Familial tumors often are bilateral and multicentric. Patients have a succinyl dehydrogenase mutation.
- CBTs are rarely functional or malignant, but those with the familial history or bilateral tumors should undergo a 24-hour urine screening for metanephrines and catecholamines.
- CT or MR angiography of the head and neck is the most useful study to plan operative treatment.
- Tumors more than 4 cm in diameter or 20 cm³ benefit from preoperative embolization to decrease vascularity and facilitate surgical resection.
- Nasotracheal intubation, with or without mandibular subluxation, is used for individuals with large tumors located above the C2 vertebral body on sagittal imaging.
- Large tumors (Shamblin class III) carry the highest risk of cranial nerve injuries, though most injuries prove to be temporary after 1 year unless the nerve is resected.

SUGGESTED READINGS

Basal BE, Myers EN. Etiopathogenesis and clinical presentation of carotid body tumors. *Microsc Res Tech.* 2002;59:256-261.

Hallett JW, Nora JD, Hollier LH, et al. Trends in neurovascular complications of surgical management for carotid body and cervical paragangliomas: a fifty-year experience with 153 tumors. *J Vasc Surg.* 1988;7:284-291.

Kruger AJ, Walker PJ, Foster WJ, et al. Important observations made managing carotid body tumors during a 25-year experience. *J Vasc Surg.* 2010;52:1518-1522.

La Muraglia GM, Fabian RL, Brewster DC, et al. The current surgical management of carotid body paragangliomas. *J Vasc Surg.* 1992;15:1035-1045.

Moore WS, Colburn MD. Carotid body tumors. In: Fischer JE, Baker RJ, eds. *Mastery of Surgery.* 4th ed. Philadelphia, PA: Lippincott Williams & Wilkins; 2001:397-408.

Nora JD, Hallett JW, O'Brien PC, et al. Surgical resection of carotid body tumors: long-term survival, recurrence, and metastasis. *Mayo Clin Proc.* 1998;63:348-352.

Power AH, Bower TC, Kasperbauer J, et al. Impact of preoperative embolization on outcomes of carotid body tumor resections. *J Vasc Surg.* 2012;56:979-989.

Wang SJ, Wang MB, Barauskas TM, et al. Surgical management of carotid body tumors. *Otolaryngol Head Neck Surg.* 2000;123:202-206.

Westerband A, Hunter GC, Cintora I, et al. Current trends in the detection and management of carotid body tumors. *J Vasc Surg.* 1998;28:84-93.

CLINICAL SCENARIO CASE QUESTIONS

A 40-year-old man is referred with a 5-cm "vascular" mass found on ultrasound imaging, which splays the internal and external carotid arteries. He has no symptoms other than recent-onset hypertension. Two other first-degree relatives had similar neck tumors.

1. The following is pertinent to the evaluation of this patient:
   a. Electrocardiogram
   b. Chest x-ray
   c. Twenty-four-hour urine studies for metanephrines and catecholamines
   d. Genetic testing for aneurysms

2. A 37-year-old man is found to have a 6-cm right carotid body tumor that encases most of the internal and external carotid arteries (Shamblin III). He has developed mild dysphagia, has no hypertension, and is otherwise asymptomatic. His family history is unremarkable. CT angiography shows the superior extent of the tumor to be at the base of the C1 vertebral body.

   Appropriate operative preparation and execution include:
   a. Oral endotracheal intubation, resection of the tumor, and replacement of the carotid artery with a prosthetic graft
   b. Preoperative embolization, nasotracheal intubation, and EEG monitoring with plans to resect the tumor and reconstruct the carotid artery as necessary
   c. Oral endotracheal intubation, EEG monitoring, and resection of the tumor with ligation of the carotid artery
   d. Oral endotracheal intubation, subluxation of the jaw, and tumor resection to include the adjacent cranial nerves

17 Carotid Artery Trauma

MOHAMED F. OSMAN and JONATHAN D. GATES

Presentation

A 51-year-old man presents to the emergency department with a stab wound sustained 12 hours ago to the right side of the neck. He describes a tender mass around the area. He admits to mild clumsiness and numbness in his left hand and left leg, but denies difficulty with breathing or swallowing, vocal changes, hematemesis, hemoptysis, or other neurologic symptoms. Examination of the neck reveals multiple small wounds and a 2-cm stab wound to zone II (between the cricoid cartilage and the angle of the mandible) of the right neck just anterior to the sternocleidomastoid muscle (SCM) with a moderate-sized firm pulsatile hematoma (Fig. 1). There is no active bleeding, air bubbling from the wound, or crepitus in the neck. He is in no respiratory distress or stridor and has no palpable thrill or bruit on auscultation of the neck. The patient is hemodynamically stable and has no wounds in other regions of the body. Neurologic examination reveals a mild left pronator drift and a mild decrease to light touch sensation in the left arm and left leg.

Differential Diagnosis

This man has suffered a single stab wound to the neck with a moderate-sized hematoma. A focused and detailed clinical evaluation reliably identifies patients with vascular injuries who require treatment. A negative physical examination with observation has a negative predictive value of 90% to 100% for vascular injuries. In the event that there are no obvious clinical signs of vascular or aerodigestive tract injury, it is essential to determine the depth of this wound through local exploration. If the wound is small, it must be explored with the use of local anesthesia to enlarge the wound and determine whether or not it has penetrated the platysma. If the wound is large and gaping, often elevation of the tissue is sufficient to determine that the platysma has been violated. Wounds that are superficial to the platysma are treated with debridement and closure while deeper wounds classify as penetrating trauma and raise the suspicion for deeper injury to vital structures in the neck.

This patient has soft signs of vascular injury, namely a stable neck hematoma in the setting of an injury tract in the vicinity of major vessels. Other soft signs include history of bleeding at the scene, cranial nerve injury, and unequal upper extremity blood pressure measurements. Soft signs allow time for further investigation with selective operative exploration as an option. Hard signs include refractory hypotension, pulsatile bleeding, bruit or thrill, expanding hematoma, and loss of pulse with stable or evolving neurologic deficit. Hard signs mandate urgent exploration. Ninety-seven percent of patients with hard signs have a vascular injury, as opposed to only 3% of those with soft signs.

Early airway evaluation and a low threshold for airway control are paramount in the initial evaluation of these patients with significant neck wounds. There is no evidence for airway compromise in this case. Obvious signs of airway injury (respiratory distress, hemoptysis, stridor, or air bubbling from the wound) are indications for operative exploration and repair. There is no obvious sign of esophageal or pharyngeal injury as there is no air bubbling from the wound during the act of swallowing and no reported odynophagia. Clinically, he has evidence of a mild right hemispheric stroke. At the top of the differential, one must consider penetrating injury to the carotid artery with an acute mild stroke from embolic debris. Spinal cord, cranial nerves (IX, X, XI, and XII), and brachial plexus injuries are other possibilities but are inconsistent with this physical exam.

Workup

Given that the patient is hemodynamically stable, the wound has penetrated deep to the platysma, and soft signs of vascular injury are present, further workup is essential and appropriate. Preoperative CT scan of the head is essential in this stable patient to delineate the presence or absence of suspected stroke and determine whether or not there is a hemorrhagic component. Computerized tomographic angiography (CTA) has become an invaluable screening tool for arterial injuries in some locations, the neck being one of them. In the setting of penetrating cervical injuries, CTA has a 90% sensitivity and 100% specificity for vascular injuries that require treatment. This study modality, CTA, may be limited in the setting of metallic foreign bodies such as bullet or

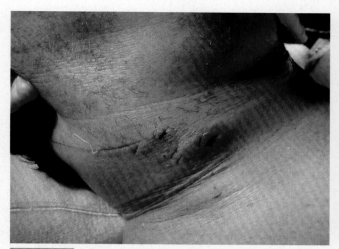

FIGURE 1 • Stab wound to zone II of the neck.

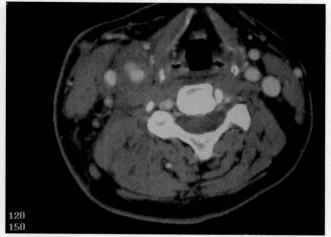

FIGURE 3 • CTA of the neck reveals a right common carotid pseudoaneurysm.

missile fragments (especially shotgun injuries) obscuring the cervical vasculature through artifact. Arteriography taken in various planes allows the radiographer to vary the relationship of the stationary fragment to the underlying vasculature without artifactual degradation of the image. Angiography supplies additional information and is perhaps more sensitive with respect to minor intimal injury. Angiography was at one point the diagnostic study of choice before the availability and speed of the current generation of CT scan machines. Arteriography has become a second-line diagnostic study in the presence of artifact but also has the distinct advantage that it offers therapeutic endovascular interventional options at the same time. CTA is much more widely employed in these scenarios due to its ease of availability and plethora of useful information.

Ultrasonography has become the standard screening tool for carotid disease in the elective evaluation of suspected atherosclerotic disease. It has been used for

penetrating neck trauma, but its utility is limited to zone II neck injuries. In addition, subcutaneous air, fragments, and hematomas make ultrasound less reliable. Magnetic resonance angiography (MRA) may aid in the diagnosis of arterial injury but requires the patient be moved to the magnetic resonance suit, rendering the patient less available for ongoing care and perhaps at risk for movement of any metallic foreign body subjected to the magnetic field.

In this case, CT scan of the head without intravenous contrast revealed a 3-cm ischemic, nonhemorrhagic stroke in the right frontal lobe anterior to the motor strip (Fig. 2). The neck CT with intravenous contrast showed an extraluminal collection of contrast at the distal common carotid artery consistent with a pseudoaneurysm with preservation of antegrade flow (Figs. 3 and 4). An angiogram was performed with an option for an endovascular solution; however, the potential contamination of the neck wound from aerodigestive content was a concern (Fig. 5).

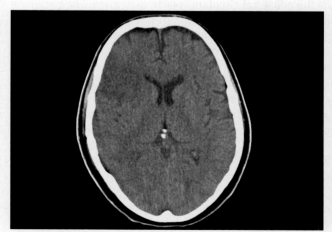

FIGURE 2 • CT scan of the head shows a bland stroke in the frontal lobe.

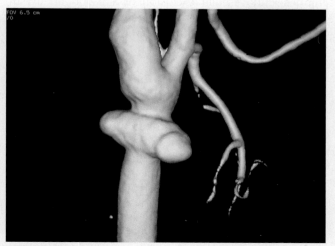

FIGURE 4 • Three-dimensional reconstruction of the CTA of the neck demonstrating the pseudoaneurysm.

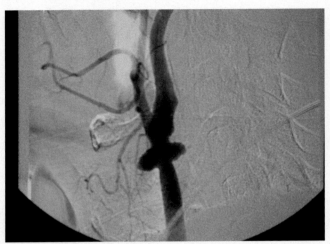

FIGURE 5 • Formal angiogram of the right carotid artery showing a similar picture to Figure 4.

Diagnosis and Treatment

This patient has penetrating trauma to the right common carotid artery with localized pseudoaneurysm formation. The arterial wall has been disrupted, and the leaking arterial blood is contained by surrounding hematoma and periarterial tissues. This resulted in a moderate-sized bland infarct of the right frontal lobe. A small thrombus or more likely a platelet plug must have formed at the site of the injury or from turbulence within the pseudoaneurysm and embolized to the brain causing an ischemic stroke. The carotid lesion also may rupture, given the tenuous nature of the wall of the pseudoaneurysm. Clinically, the stroke is relatively small. Radiologically, it is of moderate size and hemorrhagic transformation with revascularization is of concern.

Catheter-based endovascular interventions in trauma have evolved from the early embolization of end vessels, to stent placement, and currently covered stents for larger defects in the wall of arteries. For zones I and III injuries, endovascular exclusion of a pseudoaneurysm, partial transection, or arteriovenous fistula remain viable options. Self-expanding covered stents can be safely delivered to these locations with limited morbidity. The anatomically inherent difficulty of attaining good open surgical exposure and control (proximal control in zone I and distal control in zone III) in these injuries makes the endoluminal approach an attractive option. This approach may avoid the morbidity of a median sternotomy, high thoracic incision, or difficult dissection at the base of the skull. Another advantage is that endoluminal therapy can be performed with the patient under local anesthesia, allowing direct assessment of the patient's neurologic status.

Zone II vascular injuries should be treated by operative repair. Moreover, the possible need for anticoagulation and dual antiplatelet therapy during and after the procedure may represent a risk of transformation of the bland infarct into hemorrhagic infarct. The traumatic nature of the wound, late presentation, and potential aerodigestive tract injury raise the issue of foreign body and infection risk should a covered stent be deployed. If the wound were to become infected, the presence of a covered stent may complicate the situation. Surgical options include exploration and repair of the arterial injury with intraoperative intravenous heparin and secondary prophylaxis with aspirin perioperatively. The risk of intracranial bleeding would be less, and this approach would allow definitive evaluation of the airway and digestive tract as well as allow the option of definitive wound care and removal of a foreign body if present. One must continue with the evaluation of the aerodigestive tracts using bronchoscopy and either endoscopy or water-soluble contrast study.

Special consideration should be given to patients who present with coma, dense hemispheric stroke or documented carotid thrombosis. Currently, the only preoperative outcome predictive marker is the injury-to-revascularization time duration. Early revascularization in this group has consistently demonstrated improvement or stabilization of neurologic function. Late revascularization (more than 24 hours from the time of injury) exposes the patient to the risk of developing reperfusion injury, cerebral edema, uncal herniation, and death. Minor carotid injuries, intimal defects, or small pseudoaneurysm in selected neurologically stable patient can be safely managed nonoperatively.

Surgical Approach

Electroencephalography (EEG) monitors are placed on the head to monitor brain function while the patient is under general anesthesia of the case. If EEG monitoring is not available, then an intravascular shunt may be used, or back pressure may be measured once the clamp is placed on the common carotid artery. If the injury and the repair involve only the common carotid artery, then the overwhelming majority of the time there should be no ipsilateral cerebral ischemia, but it is not impossible as the collateral circulation is an unknown. The patient is kept supine and in a slight Trendelenburg position with the neck carefully positioned for maximal exposure and the head mildly rotated away from the side of injury. The patient is prepped from the chin down to the bilateral knees in anticipation of the need for a thoracic incision or saphenous vein harvest. In vascular trauma, one must anticipate the unexpected and be prepared for proximal and distal control of the common carotid and internal/external carotid arteries, respectively, so as to minimize hemorrhage and time of potential neurologic ischemia prior to addressing the pseudoaneurysm (Fig. 6).

The most common incision for exposure of the unilateral carotid artery is a vertical oblique incision over the anterior border of the SCM, from just above the angle of the mandible to the region of the sternoclavicular joint. Retraction of the SCM laterally will expose the internal

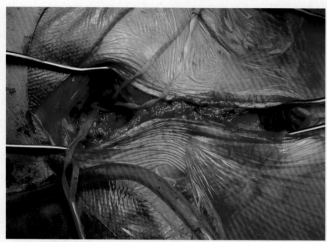

FIGURE 6 • Operative exposure starting with proximal and distal control.

jugular vein, with the carotid artery lying posteromedially to the vein. Care should be taken not to injure the vagus nerve located in the posterior carotid sheath. Ligation and division of the facial vein will expose the carotid bifurcation and allow mobilization and control of the internal and external carotid arteries. Associated injuries of the internal jugular vein or external carotid artery may be repaired, but in most cases, these vessels can be ligated rapidly if the injuries are complicated and extensive. If this was the case here, this approach would then allow attention to be directed to the pseudoaneurysm and the common carotid injury. Ideally, the surgeon should strive for proximal and distal control outside of the hematoma surrounding the site of injury. This may be difficult in that it requires careful exposure of the distal vessels in a limited field of view.

Some zone I injuries may be controlled and repaired through a cervical incision, but proximal zone I injuries may require extension inferiorly into a median sternotomy or anterolateral thoracotomy; hence, the need for skin preparation ahead of time and wide draping as to leave all options on the table. Mobilization and superior retraction of the brachiocephalic veins will expose the aortic arch, innominate artery, and proximal left common carotid artery. Zone III carotid injuries are the most difficult to obtain adequate exposure and distal control. In this case, the cervical incision can be extended superiorly into the posterior auricular area, and the digastric muscle followed by the occipital artery can be divided, with care taken to avoid injuring the hypoglossal, glossopharyngeal, and facial nerves. Maximal exposure of the distal internal carotid artery may be obtained by anterior subluxation and fixation of the mandible before the incision is made (Tables 1 and 2).

Once the arteries are exposed and controlled, heparin is given, the pertinent arteries are clamped, and the pseudoaneurysm is exposed to define the injury.

TABLE 1. Carotid Artery Trauma

Zone I Injuries
- Encompasses the area between the clavicles and the cricoid cartilage
- Includes the innominate vessels, the origin of the common carotid artery, the subclavian vessels and the vertebral arteries, the brachial plexus, the trachea, the esophagus, the apex of the lung, and the thoracic duct
- Difficult surgical exposure because of the presence of the clavicle but possible
- Carry a guarded prognosis because of critical structures involved

Zone II Injuries
- Encompasses the area between the cricoid cartilage and the angle of the mandible
- The most prevalent penetrating neck wounds
- Contains the carotid and vertebral arteries, the internal jugular vein, the trachea, and the esophagus/pharynx
- More accessible to clinical examination and surgical exploration
- Because of their accessibility, injuries in zone II carry a more favorable prognosis

Zone III Injuries
- Extends between the angle of the mandible to the base of the skull
- Includes the distal internal carotid and vertebral arteries and the pharynx
- Zone III is not amenable to easy physical examination or surgical exploration and presents unique therapeutic and diagnostic challenges because of its secluded nature and the critical structures spanning this locale

The artery is opened longitudinally from the common carotid artery into the internal carotid artery as would be done for atherosclerotic disease. If EEG were not available, one could measure stump pressures of the internal carotid artery with the common carotid clamp in place or routinely insert an endoluminal shunt. Once the back wall is repaired with 6-0 or 7-0 Prolene sutures, a saphenous vein patch is secured to the arteriotomy in usual fashion and the shunt, if used, is removed prior

TABLE 2. Hard and Soft Signs of Vascular Injury

Hard Signs	Soft signs
• Severe active or pulsatile bleeding	• Stable, small- to moderate-sized hematomas
• Large expanding or pulsatile neck hematoma	• Minor bleeding or history of bleeding
• Absent or diminished distal pulse	• Mild hypotension responding well to fluid resuscitation
• Bruit on auscultation or thrill on palpation	• Unequal upper extremity blood pressure measurements
• Unexplained refractory hypotension	

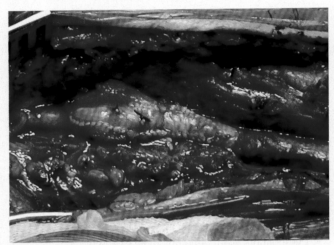

FIGURE 7 • Operative picture of the vein patch reconstruction across the common carotid artery to the internal carotid artery.

to completion of the anastomosis (Fig. 7). The wound tract must be followed throughout its entirety to ensure that no other structures in the neck have been injured. A Jackson-Pratt drain is placed through a separate incision, and the platysma and skin are closed separately. The patient neurologic exam is evaluated upon emergence from anesthesia.

In addition to patch angioplasty described here, primary repair, internal to external carotid artery transposition, and interposition grafts are other technical strategies depending on the degree of damage and disruption of the native anatomy. Carotid ligation should be reserved for the patient in whom repair is not technically possible, such as in injuries at the base of the skull or in patients with established ischemic infarction of the brain with late presentation. In hemodynamically unstable patients, placement of a temporary intraluminal carotid shunt and delayed carotid artery reconstruction may be considered. Temporary intraluminal shunting with return to the operating room for definitive repair has become an essential part of damage control surgery. The use of the shunt in the carotid circulation in this manner is limited, and certainly, shunt thrombosis could be problematic if it were associated with subsequent neurologic damage.

Postoperative Management

Upon recovering from anesthesia, the neurologic assessment is performed and repeated every hour. The patient must be monitored in a critical care setting for signs of cerebral edema and intracranial hypertension. Postoperative bleeding, hematoma with airway compromise, and hypotension are all known potential postoperative complications after carotid surgery. Hypertension is to be avoided because of the danger of acute stroke, cerebral hyperperfusion syndrome, or disruption of the arterial repair.

Case Conclusion

The patient undergoes an unremarkable postoperative course. Follow-up CT scan of the head demonstrates no further exacerbation of the previously noted frontal ischemic stroke. He is started on aspirin preoperatively, and this is continued postoperatively for secondary prophylaxis. The Jackson-Pratt drain is removed on postoperative day one. The patient is discharged home with outpatient neurorehabilitation program.

TAKE HOME POINTS

- As with all trauma care, it is critical to look at the whole patient and consider the best course of action for the individual patient in light of all injuries. It is important to consider the impact of other injuries on the ability to anticoagulate the patient.
- Penetration of the platysma defines significant penetrating neck trauma.
- Ninety percent of carotid injuries are penetrating.
- In vascular trauma, anticipate the unexpected, prep widely, and consider all potential proximal and distal control strategies in advance.
- Beware that the zones of the neck are reference points but some penetrating wounds may pass through one, two, or all three.
- Hard signs of vascular injury mandate immediate operative exploration.
- Soft signs of vascular injury mandate further investigations and allow selective exploration.
- CTA is the diagnostic test of choice in stable patients and in many cases has supplanted the use of formal arteriography. There is a more limited role for angiography in light of the availability and quality of the images obtained through current CT scanning technology.
- Catheter-based endovascular intervention is potentially a valuable tool for stable patients with injuries in zones I and III injuries.
- Evaluation of the aerodigestive tract with endoscopy, contrast studies, or direct inspection is an essential part of the evaluation and management of penetrating neck trauma.

SUGGESTED READINGS

Brywczynski JJ, Barrett TW, Lyon JA, et al. Management of penetrating neck injury in the emergency department: a structured literature review. *Emerg Med J.* 2008;25:711.

Hoyt DB, Coimbra R, Potenza BM, et al. Anatomic exposures for vascular injuries. *Surg Clin North Am.* 2001;81:1299-1330.

Kumar SR, Weaver FA, Yellen AE. Cervical vascular injuries. Carotid and jugular venous injuries. *Surg Clin North Am.* 2001;81:1331-1344.

Lane JS, Jamshidi R, Messina LM. *Management Principles for Vascular Trauma. Mastery of Vascular and Endovascular Surgery.* Lippincott Williams & Wilkins; Philadelphia, PA 2004:611-617.

Tisherman SA, Bokhari F, Collier B, et al. Clinical practice guideline: penetrating zone II neck trauma. *J Trauma.* 2008;64:1392.

CLINICAL SCENARIO CASE QUESTIONS

1. Hard signs of vascular injury in the neck include all EXCEPT:

   a. A single episode of mild hypotension
   b. Active arterial hemorrhage
   c. Large neck hematoma
   d. Bruit on auscultation or thrill on palpation

2. The surgical approach to carotid artery injury includes all EXCEPT:

   a. Wide skin preparation to include the neck, chest, abdomen, and groins bilaterally.
   b. Rule out other bodily injuries.
   c. Cerebral monitoring or other forms of assessment of adequate cerebral perfusion.
   d. Physical exam alone is adequate to manage large stable neck hematomas in neurologically intact patients.

18 Same Day Discharge after CEA

MARK G. DAVIES

Presentation

A 65-year-old female presents for her annual physical examination, and on auscultation, her physician finds a right carotid bruit. She is on both an aspirin and a statin. She has known hypertension, controlled with a beta-blocker. There is no other relevant past medical or surgical history. On auscultation, her physician finds a right carotid bruit, which had been present on her exam last year. She is normotensive. There are no other relevant cardiovascular findings. She has a normal neurologic status. A carotid duplex exam was performed last year, which had demonstrated a 60% right carotid stenosis at the bulb with a normal homogeneous, highly echogenic plaque. Her current blood workup reveals a normal hematologic and biochemical panel. A lipid profile reveals a cholesterol level of 180 mg/dL and an LDL level of 90 mg/dL. Her HDL is 50 mg/dL, and her triglycerides are 130 mg/dL. Hemoglobin A_{1c} is normal.

Differential Diagnosis

The differential diagnosis in this case for a carotid bruit is that of carotid disease or transmitted valvular disease. The presence of the carotid duplex from the previous year assists in the determination of the origin of the bruit. The absence of neurologic symptoms and signs strongly suggests that this lesion is asymptomatic. It should, however, be restudied to demonstrate stability.

Workup

A second scheduled carotid duplex exam is performed, which now demonstrates a greater than 90% right carotid stenosis at the bulb with a heterogeneous echolucent plaque (Fig. 1A and B). Due to the progression in stenosis and a change in plaque morphology, the patient is referred for evaluation by a vascular surgeon. The carotid duplex is reviewed, and it shows the bulb is in the mid-neck and accessible. A preoperative transcranial Doppler (TCD) is performed to risk stratify the plaque, and it reveals microemboli on the ipsilateral side. An echocardiogram shows no valvular disease and a normal ejection fraction with normal wall motion. EKG shows sinus rhythm. In light of the TCD findings, a noncontrast CT scan of the brain is performed and reveals no ischemic or embolic lesions.

Diagnosis and Treatment

This is a morphologically high-risk asymptomatic progressive carotid lesion in a healthy 65-year-old female with no contraindications to intervention that has received proper preventative medical therapy.

Medical Therapy

The medical therapies appropriate to consider in these patients are antiplatelet, antihypertensive, antilipid, and in diabetics, angiotensin system inhibitors. All patients with diagnosed carotid disease have systemic atherosclerosis and benefit from maximal cardiovascular risk factor modification. In a symptomatic patient, clopidogrel or an equivalent should be administered in addition to acetylsalicylic acid (ASA). Naive patients should be started on statins as even a loading dose has been shown to have systemic benefits. Current national guidelines on antilipidemic, antihypertensive, and diabetic management should be followed. There is no evidence to support stopping any antiplatelet agent preoperatively, and all other medications should be continued to prevent rebound phenomena postoperatively. One caveat is insulin, which should be reduced commensurate with the fasting period.

Timing of Surgery

Symptomatic disease should be treated within 1 month of presentation or earlier if the patient is neurologically stable. There is no good data to determine the timing of surgery for asymptomatic disease, but the 1-month rule appears appropriate to follow. Acute occlusion and crescendo Transient Ischemic Attacks (TIAs) accelerate the timing of surgery and need to be balanced against the neurologic condition of the patient.

Use of TCD

TCD is not widely available, but its ability to differentiate high-risk lesions from low-risk lesions is significant in the preoperative period, and it represents a very good tool for intraoperative monitoring.

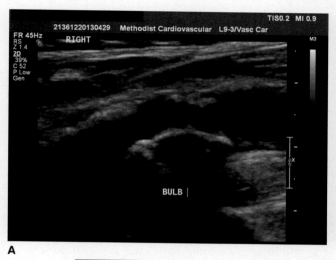
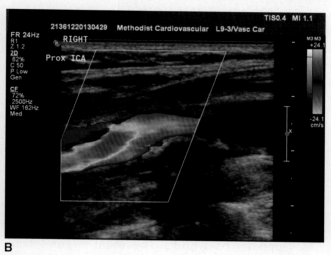

FIGURE 1 • A gray-scale image (**A**) and color flow image (**B**) from carotid duplex demonstrating a greater than 90% right ICA stenosis with a heterogeneous plaque.

Use of CT Scan

Routine CT scan for asymptomatic disease has not been validated, but its importance lies in the differentiation of presumed asymptomatic carotid stenosis and symptomatic carotid stenosis.

Use of Follow-up Carotid Duplex

There are no well-defined algorithms for carotid duplex imaging postprocedure (carotid endarterectomy [CEA] or Carotid artery Stenting [CAS]). Postoperative duplex is used to follow the contralateral side if disease has been identified and to follow the ipsilateral side for restenosis and recurrent disease. A reasonable follow-up algorithm would be 1 month, 6 months, and yearly postoperatively moving to greater intervals after the second year.

Surgical Approach

Indication

Surgery is indicated because the patient has progressive stenosis despite adequate medical management and has microemboli on TCD. This represents a high-risk category of asymptomatic carotid stenosis. The patient does not match any physiologic or anatomic criteria for carotid artery stenting, and CEA is appropriate provided the provider has a stroke and perioperative event rate less than 3%. If the provider is enrolled in the Vascular Quality Initiative, this is readily available.

Throughput Considerations

The patient should be sent to the preanesthesia assessment clinic to ensure clearance and avoid delays on the day of surgery. First case start allows for a more rapid discharge cycle for the uneventful CEA patient.

Procedure

The patient may have either a cervical block or a general anesthetic. TCD on the middle cerebral artery (MCA) is used for cerebral monitoring. The patient is placed supine in 20-degree reverse Trendelenburg with the neck hyperextended and turned to the contralateral side. An ultrasound probe is used to determine the level of the bifurcation. A transverse incision is made on the neck with its midpoint based on the border of the sternocleidomastoid muscle (SCM). The internal jugular vein is retracted posteriorly. Dissection is carried out to mobilize and control the common carotid artery (CCA) followed by the external carotid artery (ECA) and the internal carotid artery (ICA). On reaching the carotid sheath, 1 to 2 mL of 1% lidocaine is injected into perivascular sheath to reduce the risk of bradycardia. The facial vein is ligated. Care is taken to identify and avoid the vagus nerve near the CCA (it may be anterior). As the ICA is dissected free, the patient is heparinized and care taken to mobilize and protect the hypoglossal nerve. Once all vessels are controlled, a shunt is identified and prepared. On confirmation of an Activated Clotting Time (ACT) over 250 seconds, clamping of the ICA, ECA, and CCA is performed. An arteriotomy is then performed and extended proximally and distally to gain access to a good lumen. At this stage, a shunt may be placed from ICA to CCA and flow confirmed by handheld Doppler.

Intraoperative TCD of the MCA flow will permit a quantification of the flow pre- and postclamping. A 50% reduction would suggest placement of a shunt. Using a Freer elevator, a dissection plane is developed in the proximal media, and all plaque is removed. Care is taken distally and when transition from the CCA to the ECA. End points are established and any debris removed. Fronds are removed tangentially. The distal end point is tacked with 7-0 Prolene sutures and the vessel patched with Dacron, Polytetrafluoroethylene (*PTFE*), or bovine pericardial patch material. Prior to final closure, the shunt, if present, is clamped and removed, and all vessels are vented. On closure, the ICA is released. Repair sutures are performed, and then, the ICA is occluded at its origin, and flows are reestablished from CCA to ECA and 30 seconds later to ICA. Any additional repair sutures are performed if required. Intraoperative imaging (duplex) is performed and heparin reversed with protamine to return the ACT to normal. The wound is closed over a drain after ensuring no venous bleeding during a Valsalva maneuver.

The following are potential pitfalls of the operation as it is routinely conducted that can be considered general or procedure specific

General

1. *High bifurcation*: The bifurcation may be higher than anticipated and compromise the procedure. Preoperative or in room ultrasound to identify the level of the bifurcation can prevent this unexpected event.
2. *Bradycardia*: Manipulation of the bifurcation can result in significant bradycardia. This event is preventable by injection of local anesthetic into the carotid sheath prior to full exposure or by placement of an esophageal pacer.
3. *Blood Pressure control*: Unexpected hypo- and hypertension can occur generally due to anesthesia techniques, but persistent hypertension may result in postprocedure hematoma or signal an intracranial bleed.
4. *Patch or eversion*: Both patch closure and eversion techniques are acceptable and superior to primary closure. If there is a problem doing the eversion technique or the end result is suboptimal, then conversion to a patch technique should be considered.
5. *Failure to anticoagulate*: ACT should be checked after heparinization, and failure to heparinize in spite of adequate unit/kg dosing of heparin should raise the question of administration issues or antithrombin III deficiency.
6. *Abnormal coagulation*: Appearance of white clot should raise the specter of *Heparin-induced thrombocytopenia (HIT)* and a HIT protocol should be followed.

Procedure Specific

1. *Seizure*: Seizure can occur during the procedure under Monitored Anesthetic Care (MAC). This can result from underlying epilepsy, an intracranial bleed, or inadvertent injection of local anesthetic into the carotid circulation at the time of a cervical block or during the actual procedure.
2. *Distal flap*: Completion imaging may reveal a defect in up to 30% of cases, but the finding of a distal flap mandates reexploration and repair. This can result from a poor end point, injury due to a shunt, or injury due to a clamp.
3. *Distal stenosis*: Distal stenosis is most often found on completion imaging and requires re-exploration (Table 1)

Postoperative Management

The following are consideration in postoperative management:

TABLE 1. Same Day Discharge after CEA

Key Technical Steps
1. Ensure perioperative monitoring with TCD or EEG if not shunting.
2. Transverse incision with midpoint based on anterior border of SCM.
3. Mobilize SCM posteriorly.
4. Identify the CCA, ECA, and ICA, and dissect the patient off the carotid arteries.
5. Inject local anesthetic into the carotid sheath to prevent bradycardia.
6. Ligate the facial vein, identify and protect the vagus and hypoglossal nerves
7. Heparinize and ensure an adequate ACT
8. Prepare a shunt if one is to used.
9. Clamp the ICA, ECA, and CCA in that order.
10. Ensure adequate arteriotomy, place the shunt, and perform the endarterectomy.
11. Inspect and remove debris.
12. Tack the distal end points.
13. Close with a patch of your choice.
14. Postoperative imaging with Duplex or arteriography.
15. Reverse heparinization.
16. Ensure adequate hemostasis.

Potential Pitfalls
- Bradycardia during carotid dissection
- Injury to the vagus nerve or recurrent laryngeal nerve
- Inadequate distal anatomic dissection
- Inadequate anticoagulation
- Intimal flap
- Distal stenosis on closure
- Too many repair sutures compromising the lumen

---

1. *Postoperative hypertension*: Blood pressure in the immediate postoperative period should be tightly controlled to levels consistent with preoperative levels. Patients should be encouraged to take their antihypertensive medications preoperatively to help avoid this condition. Persistent or unusual hypertension may signal an intracranial bleed or hyperperfusion syndrome. CT scan and TCD should be considered if the hypertension is resistant and associated with any neurologic symptoms or signs.
2. *Postoperative hematoma*: Postoperative hematoma can occur due to a venous bleed, and doing a Valsalva prior to closure will allow determination of the security of venous ties ligatures. Arterial bleeding can occur immediately or in the early postoperative period. A drain does not prevent a symptomatic hematoma, and airway compromise is generally due to edema rather than true compression. Re-exploration is recommended.
3. *Postoperative neurologic injury*: Cranial nerve injury due to injury to the marginal mandibular nerve or recurrent laryngeal nerve is described and is avoided by careful dissection and judicious use of retraction techniques.
4. *Postoperative stroke*: Postoperative stroke can manifest as recapitulation of symptoms of prior stroke or as new symptoms. Hypertension in this setting makes

an intracranial bleed a possibility. If this is identified in the room, reexploration and imaging are mandated. If in the *post-anesthesia care unit (PACU)*, immediate imaging or return to the OR is mandated. In both cases, imaging will dictate intervention. Postoperative stroke after PACU should prompt immediate duplex and CT scan. In all cases, neuroradiologic rescue must be considered if appropriate.

5. *Hyperperfusion syndrome*: Patients who present with persistent headaches after the procedure must be considered to be at risk of either a cerebral event or hyperperfusion syndrome. Administration of propranolol can alleviate the symptoms and consideration of a CT scan to rule out a subarachnoid hemorrhage and TCD to rule out hyperperfusion syndrome should be made.

6. *Follow-up*: The patient should be followed up with duplex imaging at 1 month, 6 months, and 1 year thereafter to assess the operative side for restenosis and monitor the contralateral side for progression of disease if appropriate.

Case Conclusion

On closure, the patient is recovered from anesthesia and reassessed neurologically before moving to the PACU. A 2- to 4-hour wait in the PACU allows for the patient to stabilize and facilitate a move to a high dependency unit for monitoring. Patients should be allowed to sit at 30- to 60-degree recumbent to facilitated reduction in edema around the airway. A clear liquid diet is recommended, and oral meds resumed. If there are no issues, the patient can have the drain removed and can be discharged after 6 to 8 hours on home medications.

TAKE HOME POINTS

- The patient must receive maximal cardiovascular risk modification prior to surgery.
- Patients require surgery only if their stenosis is greater than 80% on duplex and have positive TCD.
- The stroke rate at 1 year for best medical therapy is now 1.5%; thus the surgical risk of stroke must be lower than this.
- Patients should be sent for preoperative anesthesia assessment and the expectations of discharge within 23 hours set.
- Preoperative or in room ultrasound should be used to localize the bifurcation.
- Local anesthesia in the Carotid sheath prevents bradycardia.
- Dissection technique should be considered dissection of the patient off the carotid artery.

- Check ACTs before clamping ECA-ICA-CCA.
- The distal end should be tacked.
- Patch and eversion CEA are equal in trained hands.
- Completion imaging is essential.
- Neurologic exam prior to leaving the room.
- Blood pressure management expedites a patient's course for discharge.
- Multiple studies have documented that certain patients are eligible for discharge same day following CEA.

SUGGESTED READINGS

Constantinou J, Jayia P, Hamilton G. Best evidence for medical therapy for carotid artery stenosis. *J Vasc Surg.* 2013;58(4):1129–1139.

Executive Committee for the Asymptomatic Carotid Atherosclerosis (ACAS) Study. Endarterectomy for asymptomatic carotid artery stenosis. *JAMA.* 1995;273:1421–1428.

Kakisis JD, Avgerinos ED, Antonopoulos CN, et al, The European Society for Vascular Surgery guidelines for carotid intervention: an updated independent assessment and literature review. *Eur J Vasc Endovasc Surg.* 2012;44(3):238–243.

Kuy S, Seabrook GR, Rossi PJ, et al. Management of carotid stenosis in women. *JAMA Surg.* 2013;148(8):788–790

Raman G, Moorthy D, Hadar N, et al. Management strategies for asymptomatic carotid stenosis: a systematic review and meta-analysis. *Ann Intern Med.* 2013;158(9):676–685

Ricotta JJ, Aburahma A, Ascher E, et al, . Updated Society for Vascular Surgery guidelines for management of extracranial carotid disease: executive summary. *J Vasc Surg.* 2011;54(3):832–836.

van Lammeren GW, den Hartog AG, Pasterkamp G, et al, Asymptomatic carotid artery stenosis: identification of subgroups with different underlying plaque characteristics. *Eur J Vasc Endovasc Surg.* 2012;43(6):632–636.

CLINICAL SCENARIO CASE QUESTIONS

1. What is the current stroke risk for patients with asymptomatic carotid stenosis who are placed on maximal medical therapy?

   a. 1%
   b. 1.5%
   c. 2%
   d. 2.5%
   e. 3%

2. What is the rate of defects found on completion duplex imaging after carotid endarterectomy?

   a. 5%
   b. 10%
   c. 15%
   d. 20%
   e. 25%

19 Subclavian Steal Syndrome

MICHAEL J. MALINOWSKI and CHEONG J. LEE

Presentation

A 67-year-old male presented with 3 months of increasing left upper extremity numbness and tingling with strenuous use. The patient has recently also developed gangrene to the tip of his third digit within the past 3 weeks with symptoms of vertigo. According to the patient's wife, he also has had a few episodes of unsteadiness while walking needing to support himself at points of ambulation. The patient was evaluated initially by his primary care physician and referred for evaluation. He has no evidence of prior stroke or transient ischemic attacks.

Differential Diagnosis

Although the presentation of this patient illustrates multiple symptoms pointing to subclavian artery stenosis, the differential diagnosis must be carefully reviewed. Berger's disease in young male patients with extensive tobacco use can present with upper extremity tissue loss and ulceration, but without the proximal branch symptoms of vertebrobasilar insufficiency. When considering inflammatory etiologies, both Takayasu's arteritis and giant cell arteritis can cause similar groupings of symptoms including upper extremity ischemia and vertebrobasilar symptomatology and should be strongly considered if there is evidence of elevated inflammatory markers, such as C-reactive protein and erythrocyte sedimentation rate, along with imaging studies featuring proximal branch vessel disease. In an older patient in the sixth or seventh decade of life, consideration must include native atherosclerotic disease especially in patients with renal failure and heavy tobacco use. Although primary Raynaud's must be considered, the fact that disease progression has resulted in tissue loss generally rules out primary disease. The multitude of etiologies for secondary Raynaud's disease, however, remain in the differential diagnosis.

A posterior distribution ischemic stroke must be strongly considered in this patient given the issues with coordination and balance and should be ruled out to prevent long-term morbidity of an undiagnosed cerebrovascular event. Since the patient has a subacute presentation, this scenario is unlikely embolic, although this may be considered.

In the case of subclavian stenosis, atherosclerotic disease is by far the most common etiology requiring a diameter stenosis of greater than 75%. Multivessel involvement is seen in up to 40% of patients presenting with symptomatic disease.

Workup

Full imaging of the subclavian artery by ultrasonography is limited by bony landmarks, including the clavicle. Flow dynamics, such as spectral broadening and elevated velocities, seen in the artery around the stenotic lesion should prompt further imaging, especially in concert with flow reversal in the ipsilateral vertebral artery. The gold standard of diagnostic imaging is conventional angiography provided by an arch angiogram. With the advent of advanced CT imaging and reconstruction software, computed tomography angiography (CTA) and magnetic resonance angiography (MRA) can effectively evaluate the proximal subclavian artery for stenotic lesions; however, these modalities are strictly diagnostic, as opposed to angiography that allows for assessment of translesion pressure gradients and direct endovascular therapy. Disadvantages of aortography include local arterial trauma, risk of stroke with arch manipulation, and nephrotoxicity with contrast administration. With a high percentage of these patients with proximal branch vessel disease also having concomitant coronary disease, coronary evaluation with transthoracic may be useful in assessment of cardiac function. Although the most common orientation of the transverse branch vessels involves three separate trunks of the innominate, left carotid and left subclavian arteries, aberrant arch anatomy including bovine arch orientation is present in up to 16% to 24% of patients. For evaluation of open operative revascularization, this is a less important point; however, in the context of endovascular revascularization including subclavian stenting, it is critical.

Aberrant vertebral anatomy also plays an important role not only in treatment but also in disease physiology. An aberrant left vertebral origination off the aortic arch between the left common carotid and subclavian arteries occurs in 6% of patients and an aberrant right subclavian artery origination occurs in 0.5% to 1.0% of patients.

Diagnosis and Treatment

Initial awareness of proximal subclavian stenosis may manifest itself as asymmetry in upper extremity blood pressures with a 20 mm Hg difference between upper arm brachial systolic pressure measurements. A patient presenting with vertebrobasilar insufficiency with resultant vertigo, nausea, imbalance, and diplopia, a duplex of the ipsilateral vertebral artery, will often show signs of flow reversal. Yet, this duplex finding alone is common in asymptomatic patients as well. For patients with left-sided subclavian stenosis and prior coronary bypass grafting with origination from the left internal mammary artery, subclavian-coronary steal may occur leading to myocardial ischemia, angina, and possible infarction. More proximal innominate and common carotid artery stenosis and occlusions tend to present with ipsilateral hemispheric symptoms, including aphasia and hemiparesis.

When symptoms are present a thorough physical examination, to check upper extremity pulses and associated bruits along with a comprehensive neurologic exam, should be performed followed by duplex sonography. Often angiography can be successfully used not only for diagnosis but for treatment as well. As discussed, CTA and MRA imaging is a useful adjunct to angiography, and even transesophageal echocardiography may be employed to further evaluate and characterize the level of aortic arch disease prior to intervention, but these remain diagnostic modalities only.

The main indication for treatment is the presence of symptoms, including upper extremity ischemia, vertebrobasilar symptoms, or sequelae of subclavian-coronary and subclavian-carotid steal. There are no clear guidelines of when to intervene on asymptomatic patients, if ever, but a suitable indication to consider is in a patient with high-grade left subclavian stenosis with an anticipated internal mammary artery to coronary artery bypass.

Surgical Approach

Endovascular and open techniques are both available options for treatment of symptomatic subclavian stenosis. With the advent of improved stent technology, lower

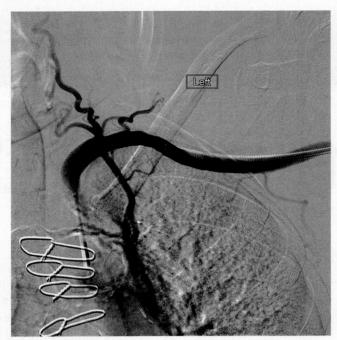

FIGURE 1 • Retrograde subclavian angiography demonstrating origin stenosis of the left subclavian artery and a patent left internal mammary artery graft in a patient with coronary-subclavian steal syndrome.

profile delivery systems and knowledge of endovascular limitations including appropriate patient selection, proximal orificial subclavian stenting is considered by most as a first-line treatment. This utilizes either femoral or brachial access with the use of wire and catheter cannulation of the lesion with thru-wire access followed by angioplasty and stent placement. Retrograde brachial access is preferred in the setting of hostile arch or aortoiliac anatomy (Fig. 1). This often requires open exposure of the vessel depending upon the device and sheath sizes required to treat the lesion. With regard to stent positioning and placement, for orificial lesions, this requires proximal stent placement into the aortic lumen to prevent inadequate treatment of the underlying spillover lesion (Fig. 2).

Carotid-Subclavian transposition

A transverse incision is made in a supraclavicular location approximately 1 fingerbreadth above the clavicle, starting medial to the clavicular head of the sternocleidomastoid muscle to obtain access to the common carotid and subclavian arteries. The omohyoid muscle is divided after retraction of the scalene fat pad laterally. The internal jugular and vagus nerves are retracted laterally. The common carotid artery is mobilized circumferentially, and proximal subclavian exposure is performed including division of the vertebral vein. The vertebral and internal mammary arteries are isolated and controlled. The subclavian is transected after appropriate heparinization (ACT > 250) and transposed with an end-to-side

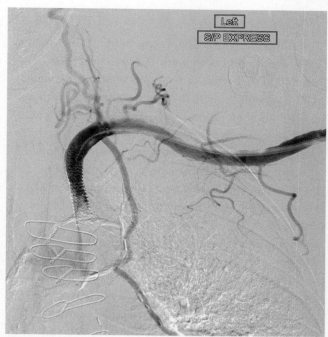

FIGURE 2 • Retrograde subclavian angioplasty and stent placement in a patient with a left internal mammary artery graft.

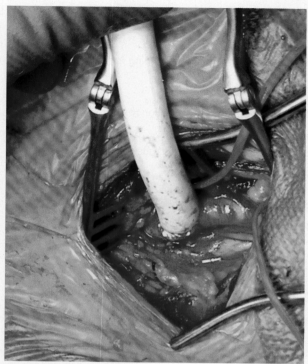

FIGURE 4 • Distal subclavian anastomosis is constructed first prior to the carotid anastomosis.

anastomosis to the common carotid artery (Fig. 3). The remaining subclavian stump is then oversewn, and layers are closed. This particular reconstruction should not be employed in the setting of coronary steal related to the internal mammary perfusion as this would require a clamp to be placed proximal to the internal mammary takeoff for the transposition.

Carotid-Subclavian Bypass

The same basic exposure of the common carotid and subclavian arteries are performed as in a transposition; however, a much more limited dissection of the subclavian artery is required since mobilization is not a requisite for this procedure. The common carotid is exposed by

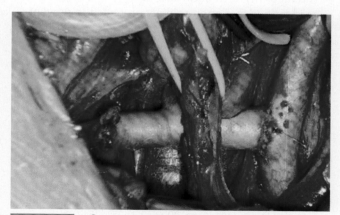

FIGURE 3 • Carotid to subclavian transposition.

retracting both sternocleidomastoid muscle and internal jugular vein laterally after division of the platysma. The distal insertion of the bypass on the subclavian artery is exposed with division of the anterior scalene after clear delineation and protection of the phrenic nerve as it courses lateral to medially inferiorly along the scalene. For left-sided procedures, the thoracic duct must be managed by either careful identification and protection or controlled ligation to prevent inadvertent injury. After adequate heparinization, the bypass is performed with proximal and distal end-to-side anastomosis from the carotid to subclavian artery with prosthetic graft in a retrojugular tunnel. Given that the subclavian artery situates in a relative "hole," we recommend performing the distal subclavian anastomosis first as the exposure becomes limited once the proximal carotid artery anastomosis is completed (Fig. 4). In this bypass, unlike most bypasses within the arena of vascular reconstructions, prosthetic conduit of Dacron or PTFE has shown superior 5-year patency results compared to vein conduit and is the preferred choice (Table 1).

Intraoperative Considerations

The key surgical pitfalls of both open revascularizations include hemorrhage control and preservation of underlying structures including the phrenic nerve, thoracic duct, and vagus nerve. The primary consideration for hemorrhage control is especially important when discussing transposition versus bypass, since meticulous control

TABLE 1. Carotid-Subclavian Bypass

Key Technical Steps

1. Supraclavicular incision extending from the medial head of SCM
2. Divide omohyoid
3. Divide anterior scalene fat pad
4. Perform retrojugular dissection to get to the common carotid artery
5. Look for the phrenic nerve on the anterior scalene muscle
6. Divide the anterior scalene muscle directly on top of the subclavian artery
7. Perform the distal subclavian anastomosis first prior to performing the proximal carotid anastomosis
8. Graft should lie retrojugular

Potential Pitfalls

- Thoracic duct leak: take time to ligate and divide the lymphatics in the anterior scalene fat pad
- Injury to the phrenic nerve—lies on top of the anterior scalene muscle
- Injury to the vagus nerve during the retrojugular approach to the carotid
- Handling of the subclavian artery—the subclavian artery is softer in comparison to other peripheral arteries; recommend performing the anastomosis using parachute technique

Case Conclusion

The patient in this scenario was sent for CRP and ESR, which were both within normal limits. On examination, his left radial pulse was nonpalpable with a greater than 20 mm Hg difference with the contralateral blood pressure. On CTA, he had a type I arch anatomy with proximal subclavian occlusion. On duplex evaluation, there was retrograde flow within the left vertebral artery and monophasic distal subclavian waveforms. His preoperative MRA showed no intracranial parenchymal brain infarct. He was treated with a left carotid-subclavian bypass and discharged on postoperative day two with initial follow-up surveillance duplex with mean peak systolic flow velocities of 56 cm/s and anastomotic velocities <250 cm/s. He required isolated partial digit amputation of the distal IP joint space and has healed the amputation site with no further vertebrobasilar symptoms.

of the proximal subclavian stump and oversewing are critical to prevent stump retraction into the thorax and uncontrolled hemorrhage.

Otherwise, meticulous dissection is required for both open revascularizations since similar exposures are required for both, including identification of the medially coursing phrenic nerve as it travels inferiorly along the anterior scalene muscle, which can be aided by a nerve stimulator as needed. The vagus nerve is generally located in a posterolateral position in the carotid sheath and must be visualized and protected from clamp injury primarily during carotid manipulation. The thoracic duct is the main concern in left-sided interventions as it joins the jugular and subclavian veins. Since retraction and manipulation around the duct can be fraught with potential tear and injury, often division may be required for adequate exposure and prevention of a chyle leak.

Postoperative Management

The stroke risk is generally considered to be less than a standard carotid endarterectomy at less than 2% to 3%. This procedure is tolerated well by most patients. Cardiac comorbidity is still a significant concern due to the coexistence of coronary disease in this patient cohort and usually requires a short postoperative acute nursing requirement for postoperative neurologic exams and telemetry. Normally, a routine antiplatelet and statin regimen is initiated with surveillance 6-month duplex evaluation for graft patency.

TAKE HOME POINTS

- Multiple modes of imaging are useful for workup of subclavian steal, including duplex ultrasonography, CTA, MRA, and traditional angiography; however, the presence of symptoms in light of appropriate anatomy is a necessary requirement for intervention.
- Angiography allows determination of extent of disease as well as enabling the surgeon to interrogate translesion pressure gradients and intervene in focal orificial stenosis with angioplasty and stenting.
- For more complex atherosclerotic lesions, open revascularization is relatively low risk in appropriate patient populations and has durable long-term patency with prosthetic graft reconstructions or transposition.
- The vagus nerve, thoracic duct, and phrenic nerve should be identified and appropriately protected to prevent significant morbidity.
- With the associated comorbid cardiac disease found in a majority (>40% of patients) with symptomatic branch vessel disease, cardiac and neurologic monitoring is a mainstay to adequate and safe postoperative monitoring.

SUGGESTED READINGS

Berguer R, Morasch MD, Kline RA, et al. Cervical reconstruction of the supra-aortic trunks: a 16-year experience. *J Vasc Surg.* 1999;29(2):239-246; discussion 246-248.

Morasch MD. Technique for subclavian to carotid transposition, tips, and tricks. *J Vasc Surg.* 2009;49(1):251-254.

Stone PA, Srivastiva M, Campbell JE, et al. Diagnosis and treatment of subclavian artery occlusive disease. *Expert Rev Cardiovasc Ther.* 2010;8(9):1275-1282.

Takach TJ, Duncan JM, Livesay JJ, et al. Contemporary relevancy of carotid-subclavian bypass defined by an experience spanning five decades. *Ann Vasc Surg.* 2011;25(7):895-901.

CLINICAL SCENARIO CASE QUESTIONS

1. A 78-year-old woman presents with progressively worsening angina pectoris 5 years following a coronary artery bypass utilizing the left internal mammary artery. A CTA demonstrates occlusion of the left subclavian artery at the origin. Which of the following is the management strategy of choice?

   a. Left carotid-subclavian transposition
   b. Left carotid-subclavian bypass with reversed saphenous vein
   c. Left carotid-subclavian bypass with PTFE
   d. Left subclavian artery stent
   e. Redo coronary artery bypass

2. A 58-year-old male metal sheet worker presents to clinic with progressively worsening symptoms of vertigo and imbalance. On physical examination, you note an absence of a left radial pulse. Which of the following would you expect to find on duplex sonography?

   a. Peak systolic velocity of 150 cm/s in the left subclavian artery
   b. Spectral broadening in the left common carotid artery
   c. Reversal of flow in the left vertebral artery
   d. Reversal of flow in the left internal carotid artery
   e. Tardus-parvus waveforms in the innominate artery

20 Aberrant Right Subclavian Artery

NICOLAS H. POPE and GILBERT R. UPCHURCH Jr

Presentation

A 35-year-old female presented to her primary care physician complaining of dysphagia to solid food. Her past medical history and physical examination were unremarkable. Noninvasive blood pressure measurements were equal in both upper extremities. A barium swallow study was ordered and demonstrated a posterior filling defect consistent with external compression of the esophagus (Fig. 1). Upper endoscopy revealed no mucosal pathology and a posterior, pulsatile, extraluminal mass in the proximal esophagus with significant narrowing of the esophageal lumen. Mannometric studies done at this time were unremarkable, and no biopsies were taken.

Differential Diagnosis

The differential diagnosis of dysphagia is broad and includes both benign and malignant esophageal tumors, mechanical esophageal pathologies such as Zenker's diverticulum, benign esophageal strictures, webs or rings, peristaltic and neuromuscular disorders, and extrinsic compression of the esophagus by other mediastinal masses or vascular structures. Given the findings of pulsatile external compression, a retroesophageal aberrant right subclavian artery (RSCA) should be highly suspected as a cause for this patient's symptoms.

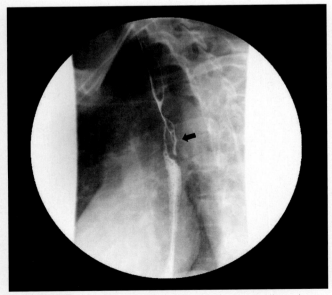

FIGURE 1 • Upper gastrointestinal barium swallow demonstrating contrast filling defect in the proximal esophagus (*arrow*).

Discussion

Aberrant right subclavian (RSCA), or Lusorian artery, is a common variant of normal aortic arch anatomy, occurring in 0.5% to 1.0% of the population. It is thought to be the result of obliteration of the right fourth aortic arch during development. The RSCA then originates at an aortic diverticulum first described by Kommeral distal to the left subclavian. From there, it takes a variable course across the mediastinum to the right upper extremity. Retroesophageal Lusorian artery may present with dysphagia, as in the case presented. Workup of dysphagia begins with a barium swallow and EGD to look for more common pathologies. When a Lusorian artery is suspected, angiography has historically been the gold-standard for diagnosis. This has largely been replaced by computed tomography angiography, as it is noninvasive and allows for visualization of the entire mediastinum. Lusorian artery aneurysms are present in up to 60% of aberrant RSCAs and should uniformly be repaired, as the incidence of rupture is high.

Case Continued

CT angiography was performed (Fig. 2).

Diagnosis and Recommendation

The diagnosis is aberrant origin RSCA with clinically significant compression of the esophagus. Traditionally, this requires open transposition through a right supraclavicular and sternotomy incisions and reanastomosis to the left carotid artery in an end-to-side manner. Advances in endovascular therapy have allowed for a less-invasive treatment option through a hybrid approach. This involves right carotid-subclavian bypass to revascularize the right upper extremity followed by occlusion of the origin of the

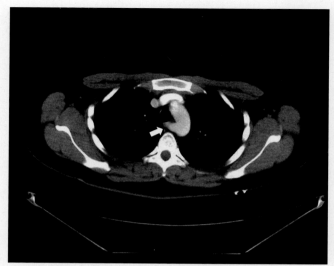

FIGURE 2 • CTA demonstrating retroesophageal course of an aberrant right subclavian (Lusorian) artery (*arrow*).

aberrant artery with Amplatz occlusion device and covering of the ostium with a covered stent graft. Relief from dysphagia symptoms is typically excellent once flow in the retroesophageal portion of the artery is eliminated by either open or endovascular approach (Table 1).

Treatment Approach
Open Surgical Repair

Open repair of a nonaneurysmal Lusorian artery involves transposition of the distal portion of the aberrant subclavian artery with reanastomosis to the right carotid artery to supply the right upper extremity. A prosthetic graft may be used to complete the carotid-subclavian bypass if there is difficulty mobilizing sufficient length of Lusorian artery to complete a tension-free anastomosis. Next, ligation of the proximal Lusorian artery proximal to its retroesophageal course is performed. This is accomplished through a left thoracotomy. The Lusorian artery is identified and mobilized both proximal to its retroesophageal course. The proximal portion of the artery to the left of the esophagus is oversewn in two layers with polypropylene suture. Care must be taken not to injure the thoracic duct, which may enter the right jugulo-subclavian commissure in these patients.

Hybrid Approach
Subclavian Revascularization

After discussion with the patient, she elects to proceed with carotid-subclavian bypass and endovascular occlusion. Preoperatively, a CTA of the head and neck is performed to ensure adequate flow to support the additional burden of the proposed bypass and avoid steal phenomenon. She is brought to the hybrid suite and positioned in the supine position. General endotracheal anesthesia is induced, and a right carotid-subclavian

TABLE 1. Aberrant Right Subclavian Artery

Key Technical Steps

1. The aberrant right subclavian (Lusorian) artery and proximal right carotid artery are exposed through a right supraclavicular incision.
2. The Lusorian artery is mobilized, and control of the artery is obtained both proximal and distal to its retroesophageal portion.
3. The patient is heparinized, and the Lusorian artery is clamped and divided to the left of the esophagus.
4. The distal Lusorian artery is freed from its retroesophageal course and brought to the proximal right carotid artery such that it is neither under tension nor redundant.
5. A small Satinsky clamp is placed on the lateral portion of the proximal right carotid artery, and the Lusorian artery is anastomosed in an end-to-side fashion.
6. Duplex exam of the exposed Lusorian artery confirms a patent anastomosis. Distal pulses in the right upper extremity are also checked to ensure adequate perfusion.
7. Alternatively, a common carotid artery to RSCA bypass may be performed.
8. The proximal Lusorian artery stump is oversewn in two layers with a running polypropylene suture through a left thoracotomy.
9. The incision is closed in several layers.

Potential Pitfalls

- The thoracic duct may enter the venous circulation on the right rather than left jugulo-subclavian junction. Injury to the thoracic duct may result in right chylothorax.
- Insufficient mobilization of the distal Lusorian artery may result in significant tension on the carotid-subclavian anastomosis, increasing the chance of pseudoaneurysm formation.
- Inadequate closure of the broad-based proximal Lusorian artery stump may result in catastrophic stump blowout or pseudoaneurysm formation.
- The thoracic aorta may need to be replaced if the artery stump is aneurysmal or associated with a dissection.

bypass is performed through a supraclavicular incision. Bypass can be accomplished either by direct transposition or with a synthetic interposition graft. The thyrocervical trunk may be ligated if necessary to allow better mobilization of the proximal RSCA prior to beginning the anastomoses. The patient is heparinized prior to placement of vascular clamps. Transposition is completed in an end-to-side fashion with running polypropylene suture. Once complete, on-table Doppler exam can confirm adequacy and direction of flow. The field is inspected for hemostasis, and a drain is left in the wound bed (Table 2).

Endovascular RSCA Exclusion

Due to the difficulty in safely ligating the proximal RSCA through a supraclavicular incision, we prefer to accomplish this by an endoluminal approach. First,

TABLE 2. Hybrid Technique

Key Technical Steps

1. Imaging confirming patent carotid arteries and antegrade vertebral flow is reviewed.
2. A right supraclavicular incision is made, and the right common carotid artery is dissected near its origin.
3. The aberrant RSCA is dissected free as proximally as can safely be achieved through the given incision.
4. The thyrocervical trunk can be ligated if additional mobilization is necessary.
5. Prior to the placement of vascular clamps, heparin is given systemically.
6. The distal RSCA is transposed to the right carotid artery in an end-to-side manor, or a Gortex interposition graft is used to complete the anastomosis.
7. Complete hemostasis is achieved, and a drain is brought out through a separate stab incision.
8. The incision is closed in several layers.
9. Angiogram documents origin of RSCA. Artery and branches are either coiled and/or plugged.
10. Endovascular stent graft is placed to cover the origin of the aberrant artery.

Potential Pitfalls

- Significant right carotid stenosis increases the chance of cerebral steal syndrome postoperatively.
- Anastomoses performed under tension increases the chance for pseudoaneurysm formation. If the right common carotid and RSCA cannot be transposed easily after complete mobilization, a synthetic interposition graft should be used.
- While less likely with a right supraclavicular approach, injury to the thoracic duct is still possible while dissecting the proximal RSCA. Care must be taken to protect this structure if encountered, and drain output should be monitored postoperatively.
- Although rare, there is a small risk of paraplegia following placement of a thoracic aortic stent graft to cover the origin of the aberrant artery.

arterial access is gained of the right femoral artery. An arterial sheath is placed, and an angled guide-wire is advanced into the proximal descending aorta. A pigtail catheter is advanced over the guide-wire and a contrast injection given to provide a road map for the remainder of the procedure. The origin of the RSCA is then selected, and additional contrast is given to confirm the absence of additional branches proximal to the planned sight of occlusion immediately proximal to the right vertebral artery. The guide-wire is then exchanged for a super stiff wire, and an appropriately sized occlusion device is deployed 2 cm beyond the origin of the RSCA. An appropriately oversized stent graft is then introduced via the right femoral sheath. The bare proximal portion of the stent graft is placed at the proximal landing zone between the left subclavian and aberrant right subclavian origins, such that the covered portion of the graft will cover the origin of the aberrant RSCA. If needed,

a second covered stent graft may be placed distally to ensure complete exclusion of the RSCA origin. The stent grafts are then ballooned to prevent graft migration and endoleak. A completion aortogram is then performed to ensure complete exclusion of the aberrant RSCA.

Case Conclusion

Postoperatively, the patient is monitored for signs of neurologic changes or right upper extremity malperfusion. At 1 month, a CT confirmed good position of the stent grafts without evidence of endoleak. Follow-up imaging is obtained at 6 months and then at 12-month intervals. These demonstrate continued occlusion of the retroesophageal aberrant RSCA and no evidence of endoleak. The patient had immediate and continued resolution of her symptoms

TAKE HOME POINTS

- Aberrant RSCA (Lusorian artery) may be diagnosed incidentally or may present with symptoms of dysphagia.
- Aneurysmal aberrant RSCAs require intervention as they have a high rate of rupture.
- Symptomatic, nonaneurysmal patients frequently have good improvement in their symptoms following open or hybrid repair.
- Open carotid-subclavian bypass or subclavian transposition followed by endovascular occlusion and covering of the origin of an aberrant RSCA is a less invasive for repair.

SUGGESTED READINGS

Attmann TBM, Muller-Hulsbeck S, Cremer J. Two-stage surgical and endovascular treatment of an aneurysmal aberrant right subclavian (lusoria) artery. *Eur J Cardiothorac Surg.* 2005;27:1125-1127.

Davidian M, Kee ST, Kato N, et al. Aneurysm of an aberrant right subclavian artery: treatment with PTFE covered stent-graft. *J Vasc Surg.* 1998;28:335-339.

Freed K, Low VH. The aberrant subclavian artery. *AJR Am J Roentgenol.* 1997;168:481-484.

Lacroix VAP, Philippe D, Goffette P, et al. Endovascular treatment of an aneurysmal aberrant right subclavian artery. *J Endovasc Ther.* 2003;10:190-194.

Shennib HDE. Novel approaches for the treatment of the aberrant right subclavian artery and its aneurysms. *J Vasc Surg.* 2008;47:1066-1070.

Simon RW, Lachat M, Pfammatter T, et al. Giant aneurysm of an aberrant right subclavian artery from the left aortic arch. *J Thorac Cardiovasc Surg.* 2006;132:1478.

CLINICAL SCENARIO CASE QUESTIONS

1. Which of the following is *not* true of an aberrant right subclavian (Lusorian) artery?

   a. Aberrant course of the artery is variable, but frequently retroesophageal.

   b. The origin is typically distal to the normal position of the origin of the left subclavian artery.

   c. Though frequently undiagnosed, they are present in 4% to 8 % of the population.

   d. Dysphagia is the most common presenting symptom.

2. Which of the following is *not* true regarding treatment of an aberrant right subclavian (Lusorian) artery?

   a. A right carotid-subclavian bypass is required prior to endovascular occlusion of an aberrant RSCA in order to perfuse the right upper extremity.

   b. Carotid-subclavian bypass may be accomplished by direct transposition or with a synthetic interposition graft.

   c. Dysphagia symptoms usually improve or resolve following open or hybrid repair of a retroesophageal Lusorian artery.

   d. Aneurysmal aberrant RSCA (Lusorian artery) can be expectantly managed and infrequently requires repair for rupture.

21 Subclavian and Axillary Artery Aneurysms

AMIT JAIN and KENNETH J. CHERRY

Presentation

A 56-year-old Caucasian female with a past medical history of Marfan's syndrome presented to clinic for evaluation of painless swelling below her left clavicle. She noticed this swelling a few months previously. She had a strong family history of Marfan's syndrome involving her father and 2 of her 13 siblings. She denied any tingling, numbness, or cold sensation in her left upper extremity. She had gastroesophageal reflux disease with hiatal hernia, controlled with medications, and was status post inguinal hernia repair and bilateral lens implants. She had an ECHO 6 months earlier that showed a normal heart and aortic root. On physical examination, she had intact radial, ulnar, and brachial pulses with equal and normal blood pressures in both arms. There was a pulsatile, expansile painless swelling in the left infraclavicular region, measuring approximately 3 × 4 cm. Motor and sensory functions of the left upper extremity were normal.

Differential Diagnosis

A supra or infraclavicular pulsatile and expansile mass raises the possibility of subclavian or axillary artery aneurysm. Thoracic outlet syndrome, especially with a cervical rib, may be an etiology. In the presence of a cervical rib, the subclavian pulse is often palpable high in the neck rather than in its usual "subclavian" position. Poststenotic dilatation of the subclavian artery beyond a mechanical thoracic outlet obstruction or chronic soft and bony tissue damage to the artery is seen in this situation.

A pseudoaneurysm may develop at access sites in the axillary artery for central line and placement of cannulas during cardiac operations. A pseudoaneurysm may also form at the proximal anastomotic site of an axillary-femoral bypass graft and may present as a pulsatile swelling in the infraclavicular area and deltopectoral groove. These pseudoaneurysms may or may not be infected. Connective tissue disorders, like Marfan's syndrome and Ehlers-Danlos syndrome, may present with true and false aneurysms of the subclavian or axillary arteries. Endovascular interventions may cause pseudoaneurysms, as may noniatrogenic blunt and penetrating trauma.

Workup

Given the history of Marfan's syndrome in this patient with a palpable, painless, pulsatile, and expansile mass in the left infraclavicular region and a high suspicion for aneurysm, a computed tomography angiogram (CTA) was obtained. CTA revealed a broad fusiform aneurysm of the left axillary artery with maximal transverse diameter of 2.4 cm over a 4.3-cm long segment (Fig. 1A and B). There was a small 1.8-cm fusiform aneurysm of the contralateral axillary artery over a 2.0-cm length. The rest of the vessels in the chest, abdomen, and pelvis were normal.

Were there acute limb ischemia secondary to macro or microembolism from this axillary aneurysm, a traditional arteriogram might have been indicated to ascertain the degree of forearm and digital ischemia. Macroembolism might also be treated with lysis simultaneously.

Diagnosis

A 2.4-cm true left axillary artery aneurysm secondary to Marfan's syndrome was diagnosed.

Discussion

Subclavian and axillary artery aneurysms are rare, accounting for only about 1% of all peripheral arterial aneurysms. Of these, more than 85% involve the subclavian artery. Aneurysms of the proximal subclavian artery are usually secondary to "atherosclerotic" degenerational disease. Aneurysms of the distal subclavian artery and axillary artery are frequently secondary to thoracic outlet syndrome. Crutch trauma is the etiology in approximately 50% of axillary artery aneurysms with atherosclerosis, infection, fibromuscular dysplasia, dissection, and connective tissue disorder, like Ehlers-Danlos syndrome, comprising the other etiologies. In addition to these entities, aneurysms of these vessels may be seen in patients with various types of inflammatory arteritis, like Takayasu's and temporal arteritis.

Most subclavian and axillary artery aneurysms are symptomatic with about 10% of cases asymptomatic at

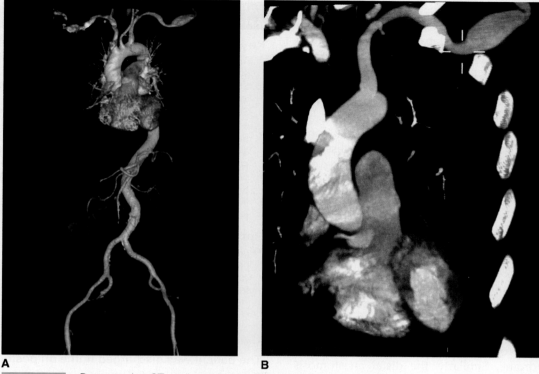

A   **B**

FIGURE 1 • Preoperative CT angiogram with 3D (**A**) and 2D MPR (**B**) reconstructions showing left axillary artery fusiform aneurysm.

presentation. Symptoms are usually secondary to compression of adjacent structures by the aneurysm or to ischemia from distal embolization. Rupture is rare but can be seen with large aneurysms of the proximal subclavian artery. About two thirds of symptomatic patients present with thrombosis of the aneurysm or a distal macro- or microembolization, causing hand or digit ischemia. Chronic ischemia may present as weakness and easy fatigability of the upper extremity with absent radial or ulnar pulses. Large proximal subclavian artery aneurysms may cause compression of the superior vena cava (facial swelling), sympathetic chain (Horner's syndrome), and/or recurrent laryngeal nerve (hoarseness). Patients may also present with shoulder, arm, or hand pain and brachial plexus palsy with upper extremity paresthesias. Dysphagia lusoria may be present in the case of an aberrant right subclavian artery. These embryonic arteries are susceptible to aneurysm degeneration. Rupture is dramatic and is one of the few causes of arterial-esophageal fistula. Rupture may occur in the presence of Ehlers-Danlos or Marfan's syndrome as well.

In patients presenting with ischemic upper extremity symptoms, histories of smoking, sensitivity to cold, and use of vibratory tools should be sought. Buerger's disease and Raynaud's syndrome need to be in the differential. Aneurysms of the ulnar artery from blunt trauma to the artery at the hook of the hamate are seen in patients who use their hands as tools of force. These often embolize and cause digital ischemia. Noninvasive vascular lab testing along with duplex examination is useful in differentiating large vessel pathology from small vessel diseases. A hypercoagulable workup, antinuclear antibody, and erythrocyte segmentation rate may be valuable additions to routine complete blood count and serum chemistries.

Bilateral synchronous symptoms are usually an indication of systemic collagen vascular or rheumatologic disease in most cases, and are seldom arterial per se in etiology. The distal subclavian artery and the entire axillary artery may be studied by a duplex ultrasound. Duplex is noninvasive and can effectively rule out the presence of a distal aneurysm and is excellent for follow-up. Ultrasound is of no benefit with proximal subclavian aneurysm. CTA or magnetic resonance angiograms (MRA) are very helpful in operative planning. Conventional angiography is indicated when ischemic digital symptoms are present, as it can assess distal vessels in detail, something CTA and MRA cannot do well. It can simultaneously serve a therapeutic purpose if there is a need for thrombolysis or if the aneurysm is amenable to endovascular treatment.

As most of these aneurysms are symptomatic at presentation, treatment is generally recommended for all cases unless a small aneurysm is detected in patients who can be treated for the underlying causal factor (e.g., thoracic outlet syndrome). Even in those cases, it is rare to leave the artery unattended. Treatment is usually open surgical resection with prosthetic graft bypass for replacement of either the subclavian or the axillary artery.

Surgical Approach

This 56-year-old female with Marfan's syndrome and a 2.4-cm asymptomatic left axillary artery aneurysm was offered open surgical repair. With the patient in supine position and under general anesthesia, the left arm was extended on an arm board and prepped circumferentially along with the left neck, chest, and shoulder. Through an infraclavicular incision, the pectoralis major muscle fibers were split and the pectoralis minor tendon was divided. The artery was carefully dissected free, proximal and distal to the aneurysm, taking care to avoid injuries to the brachial plexus. Proximal control was obtained just below the clavicle, and the small muscular branches arising directly from the aneurysm were ligated. After heparinization (100 U/kg) to keep the activated clotted time close to 300 seconds, and control of the proximal and distal artery, the aneurysm was opened. Back-bleeding posterior branches were oversewn from within the aneurysm. An 8-mm polyester graft was cut on a slight bevel and anastomosed end to end proximally to the subclavian artery with No. 4-0 Prolene monofilament running suture. A felt strip pledget was used to reinforce the anastomosis given her Marfan's syndrome. Similarly, the distal anastomosis was performed after cutting the graft to an appropriate length to avoid tension as well as redundancy. Flow was restored and hemostasis achieved after reversing anticoagulation. The wound was closed in layers. The radial and ulnar pulses were restored (Table 1).

TABLE 1. Subclavian and Axillary Artery Aneurysm Repair

Key Technical Steps

1. Always treat the underlying cause of the aneurysm if possible (thoracic outlet syndrome).
2. Sternotomy (right) or thoracotomy (left) may be needed for control of the proximal subclavian artery.
3. Supraclavicular and infraclavicular incisions may be used either alone or in combination for exposure.
4. Supraclavicular—Mobilize the scalene fat pad cephalad and laterally with ligatures to avoid injury to the lymphatic ducts and postoperative lymph leak, preserve the phrenic nerve, and divide the anterior scalene muscle to expose the subclavian artery.
5. Infraclavicular—Split the pectoralis major fibers and divide the pectoralis minor tendon for exposure of the axillary artery.

Potential Pitfalls

- Inadequate proximal exposure or control
- Injury to phrenic nerve, brachial plexus, or thoracic duct
- Using small venous conduit to replace a large subclavian artery

Case Conclusion

The patient was discharged home on postop day 2 without any complication. On follow-up in the clinic in 6 weeks, a CTA (Fig. 2A and B) was obtained, which showed a patent normal caliber left axillary artery with intact run off.

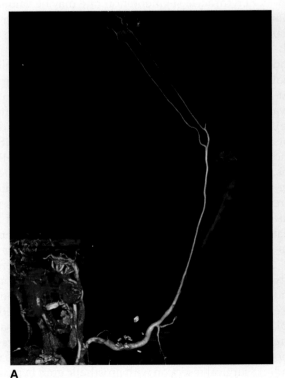
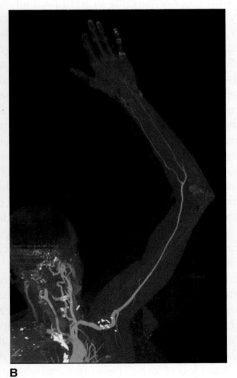

A   **B**

FIGURE 2 • Postoperative follow-up CT angiogram of left upper extremity with 3D (**A**) and 2D MPR (**B**) reconstructions showing normal left axillary artery.

Discussion

Acute upper extremity embolization, in a nonthreatened limb with intact motor and sensory function, may be treated with catheter-directed thrombolysis to reopen distal circulation before definitive open surgical or endovascular repair of the aneurysm. Rarely, ligation of the aneurysm and a long-segment bypass to a distal open arterial segment may be necessary; using a venous conduit in such cases is prudent. Poststenotic subclavian artery aneurysm secondary to thoracic outlet syndrome should be treated simultaneously with appropriate thoracic outlet decompression. A supraclavicular approach may be used for both arterial reconstruction and the first rib resection in such cases. Often an infraclavicular incision is necessary for distal control. If the graft spans the clavicle, then the first rib must be excised to allow adequate space for the graft. Experience has shown that failure to excise bone in these situation will result in an occluded graft. Aneurysms of more proximal subclavian artery require either a sternotomy (for the innominate and right subclavian arteries) or a thoracotomy (for the left subclavian or an aberrant right subclavian artery). The axillary artery, however, can be approached from an infraclavicular incision with extension or a separate incision in the axilla or the upper arm as needed.

Endovascular options are limited secondary to short-segment landing zones, tortuous course of the arteries over the rib and under the clavicle and the origins of several important branches (right carotid, vertebral and internal mammary arteries) that may be close to the aneurysmal arterial segment. However, in selected patients, the use of covered stents and stent graft exclusion of these aneurysms have been successful. With technological advancements in endovascular therapy, more subclavian and axillary artery aneurysms may become amenable to endovascular repair.

TAKE HOME POINTS

- Subclavian and axillary artery aneurysms are rare.
- Distal thromboembolism, the most common presentation, may manifest as digital ischemia in the setting of palpable radial and ulnar pulses (blue finger syndrome).
- Most of these aneurysms are symptomatic at presentation, hence the need for treating all but the very small incipient aneurysms sometimes seen with thoracic outlet syndrome.
- Doppler ultrasound is an excellent initial and follow-up study for peripheral aneurysms, with CTA and MRA being mostly used for surgical planning.

- Prosthetic replacement has good long-term patency for subclavian and proximal axillary artery. If the shoulder joint must be passed and the reconstruction taken from supra or infraclavicular area to the brachial artery, vein is preferred.
- Aneurysms secondary to thoracic outlet compression must be repaired simultaneously with surgical first rib resection for outlet decompression, unless the aneurysm is very small and has no associated thromboembolization.
- Median sternotomy and left thoracotomy may be necessary for proximal control in the repair of proximal right and left subclavian artery aneurysms, respectively.
- Endovascular options are good alternatives in appropriately selected patients with suitable aneurysm location and anatomy.

SUGGESTED READINGS

Baudier JF, Justesen P, Astrup M, et al. Endovascular treatment of subclavian artery aneurysm. *Ugeskr Laeger.* 1999;161:1774.

Bower TC, Pairolero PC, Hallett JW Jr, et al. Brachiocephalic aneurysm: the case for early recognition and repair. *Ann Vasc Surg.* 1991;5:125-132.

Cury M, Greenberg RK, Morales JP, et al. Supra-aortic vessels aneurysms: diagnosis and prompt intervention. *J Vasc Surg.* 2009;49:4-10.

Hilfiker PR, Razavi MK, Kee ST, et al. Stent-graft therapy for subclavian artery aneurysms and fistula: single-center mid-term results. *J Vasc Interv Radiol.* 2000;11:578.

Hobson RW II, Isreal MR, Lynch TO. Axillo-subclavian arterial aneurysms. In: Bergan JJ, Yao JST, eds. *Aneurysms.* New York: Grune & Stratton; 1982:435-447.

Pairolero PC, Walls JT, Payne WS, et al. Subclavian-axillary artery aneurysms. *Surgery.* 1981;90:757.

Timaran CH. Upper extremity aneurysms. In: Rutherford RB, ed. *Vascular Surgery.* 7th ed. Philadelphia, PA: WB Saunders; 2010:2128-2131.

CLINICAL SCENARIO CASE QUESTIONS

1. Which of the following is the most common presentation of subclavian and axillary artery aneurysm?

   a. Rupture
   b. Horner's syndrome
   c. Distal thromboembolism
   d. Asymptomatic presentation

2. The most appropriate exposure for proximal subclavian artery aneurysm is:

   a. Supraclavicular
   b. Infraclavicular
   c. Combined supra and infraclavicular
   d. Median sternotomy for right and thoracotomy for left subclavian artery

22 Treatment of Combined Symptomatic Carotid and Subclavian Artery Atherosclerosis

JAMES M. ESTES

Presentation

A 65-year-old woman presents with a 3-week history of intermittent right hand numbness, dizziness, and flashing colored lights in both eyes. The episodes last a few minutes and then completely subside. Her past medical history includes type 2 diabetes mellitus, hypertension, hyperlipidemia, and hypothyroidism. Physical examination reveals bilateral cervical bruits and an absent brachial pulse in the left arm.

Differential Diagnosis

This patient's neurologic symptoms are consistent with both vertebrobasilar and hemispheric ischemia. The flashing colored lights in a binocular distribution suggest involvement of the visual cortex in the posterior cerebrum, and the dizziness may be related to ischemia of other hindbrain structures. These symptoms are indicative of symptomatic subclavian steal.

Evidence of subclavian artery disease is occasionally discovered on routine physical examination in older patients with atherosclerotic risk factors. However, surgical reconstruction for this condition is unusual and represents less than 5% of arterial cases in busy academic centers, according to Evans and Shepard. The Joint Study of Extracranial Arterial Occlusion found associated subclavian or innominate disease in 17% of patients undergoing arteriography for suspected carotid disease, according to Fields and Lemak.

The true incidence of severe subclavian artery disease is largely unknown, because most patients are asymptomatic and are discovered incidentally after finding either decreased pulses or a lower blood pressure in one arm. Symptoms generally reflect vertebrobasilar insufficiency and typically include dizziness, visual symptoms, and syncope. The classic symptoms of vertebrobasilar insufficiency induced by arm exercise are uncommon, and in most cases, the symptoms are provoked by orthostatic maneuvers or excessive dosages of antihypertensives. Arm claudication may be present as well, but overt arm or hand ischemia is uncommon and usually indicates multilevel occlusive disease. The presence of hemispheric or monocular symptoms suggests coexisting carotid bifurcation disease.

A subset of patients who have had coronary bypass using the left internal mammary artery (LIMA) may present with recurrent angina due to hemodynamically limiting subclavian disease proximal to the LIMA origin. This condition is referred to as *coronary steal syndrome*.

The hand and arm numbness suggest ischemia in the distribution of the middle cerebral artery, implicating a critical carotid lesion as a cause, most likely from a hemodynamic and not embolic etiology in this case. An angiogram is ordered.

Workup
Arch Aortogram

Arch aortogram demonstrates severe proximal left subclavian artery disease, a moderately severe lesion in the proximal left common carotid artery, and severe left carotid bifurcation disease (Fig. 1).

Delayed arteriographic sequence demonstrates retrograde left vertebral flow and filling of the subclavian artery distal to the occlusive lesion (Fig. 2).

Diagnosis and Treatment

Symptomatic left subclavian steal and carotid atherosclerosis.

Left carotid endarterectomy, intraoperative retrograde angioplasty/stenting of the proximal left common carotid artery, carotid-to-subclavian bypass using 8-mm PTFE.

The initial diagnostic test of choice is duplex ultrasound imaging. Often the subclavian lesion can be identified, and the presence of retrograde vertebral flow confirms the diagnosis of subclavian steal. It is also crucial to assess the carotid bifurcations, because significant coexisting disease is common and should be considered for contemporaneous

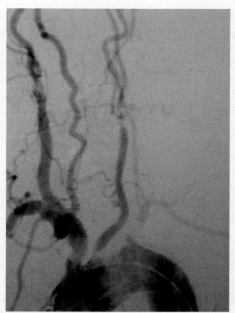

FIGURE 1 • Arch aortogram revealing stenosis at the origin of the left common carotid artery, stenosis at the left carotid bifurcation, and occlusion of the left subclavian artery.

treatment. Arteriography is the definitive test because it provides a dynamic and more detailed view of overall anatomy, particularly the origins of the great vessels, which are difficult to identify with ultrasonography.

Treatment is indicated when symptoms of cerebral or arm ischemia are present. The most common surgical procedures performed are carotid-subclavian bypass and subclavian-carotid transposition. Our preference is bypass using a short 8-mm polytetrafluoroethylene (PTFE) graft,

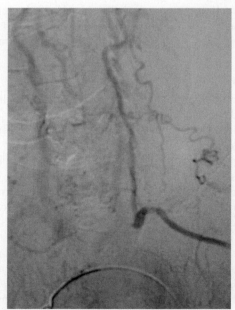

FIGURE 2 • Delayed imaging demonstrating collateral filling of the left subclavian artery via retrograde flow in the left vertebral artery. These findings are characteristic of subclavian steal syndrome.

because the transposition requires much more proximal dissection of the subclavian artery, putting the thoracic duct, phrenic nerve, and vertebral artery at greater risk of injury.

If the ipsilateral carotid artery is not suitable for inflow, extra-anatomic configurations such as axillo-axillary, subclavian-subclavian, and even femoro-subclavian bypasses can be constructed. However, direct great vessel reconstruction is preferred in these circumstances, using a graft off the ascending aorta in patients medically fit enough to tolerate median sternotomy.

Endovascular treatment of subclavian disease is also an important therapeutic option. In general, long-term patency is modestly reduced compared with surgical reconstruction. Yet, this approach may be more desirable for patients with more significant comorbidity or active myocardial ischemia from coronary steal.

Surgical Approach

This patient has both symptomatic subclavian steal and ipsilateral carotid bifurcation disease. Surgical management is complicated by the moderate focal stenosis of the left common carotid origin, which renders it disadvantageous as inflow for a carotid subclavian bypass. You elect to perform a carotid-to-subclavian bypass and carotid endarterectomy with endovascular treatment of the common carotid artery disease, because the lesion is focal and the remainder of the artery is normal. The alternatives of aortocarotid/subclavian bypass or extra-anatomic reconstruction are less desirable for this patient because of her comorbidities.

The patient is positioned for carotid endarterectomy, with the neck extended and rotated to the right. The subclavian and proximal carotid arteries are dissected out through a medial supraclavicular incision. The clavicular head and a portion of the sternal head of the sternocleidomastoid muscle are divided. The phrenic nerve is gently retracted medially and the anterior scalene muscle divided, exposing the subclavian artery. A second incision is made along the upper anterior border of the sternocleidomastoid muscle, providing the typical exposure required for carotid endarterectomy.

Via the supraclavicular incision, a tunnel is made posterior to the jugular vein for the bypass, avoiding injury to the vagus nerve. The common carotid anastomosis is performed first to an 8-mm externally supported PTFE graft, which facilitates positioning of the graft on the lateral aspect of the vessel for a favorable lie. Prior to completing the anterior wall of the anastomosis, a short 9-French sheath is advanced through the arteriotomy retrograde down the common carotid artery and then controlled with a Rummel tourniquet. Using road-mapped angiographic imaging, an 8-mm self-expanding stent is placed across the lesion, followed by an 8-mm angioplasty balloon. The stent is positioned to flare slightly into the aortic lumen. Completion angiography is performed. At this time, the sheath is removed and the anastomosis completed. The graft is tunneled behind the jugular vein, and the subclavian anastomosis is performed.

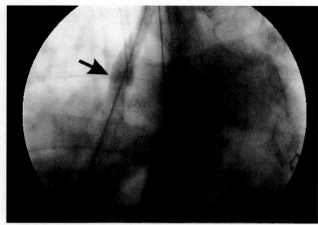

FIGURE 3 • Completion angiogram following primary stenting of the origin of the left common carotid artery (*arrow*).

After deployment of the stent, the vessel is vigorously flushed prior to completion of the bypass. Carotid endarterectomy is then performed using a Dacron patch and routine shunting as the last step to minimize the development of stasis thrombi on the fresh patch and neointima during clamping of the common carotid artery for the bypass and stent. A closed suction drain is placed in the supraclavicular incision.

Intraoperative Angiography Report

Intraoperative completion arteriogram following primary stenting and touch-up angioplasty of the proximal common carotid artery reveals no residual stenosis (Fig. 3; *arrow* indicates the treated area of the vessel).

Case Conclusion

Postoperatively, the patient's blood pressure and neurologic status are closely monitored. The drain can usually be removed by postoperative day 1 or 2. Excessive lymphatic drainage that does not abate necessitates reexploration and ligation of thoracic duct or lymphatic branches. Length of inpatient stay is typically 1 to 2 days (Table 1).

TABLE 1. Carotid Subclavian Bypass

Key Technical Steps
1. Supraclavicular incision
2. Identify and protect phrenic nerve
3. Mobilize subclavian artery
4. Mobilize common carotid artery
5. Identify and protect vagus nerve
6. Tunnel graft behind jugular vein
7. Do carotid anastomosis first to lateral side of vessel

Potential Pitfalls
• Injury to phrenic or vagus nerves
• Injury to thoracic duct

Discussion

This case illustrates the utility of combined surgical and endovascular treatment options for complex great vessel disease. Although the carotid stent could have been placed preoperatively as a separate procedure, advantage is taken of the retrograde intraoperative approach to clamp the distal common carotid artery and protect the cerebral circulation from potential atheroembolization during crossing of the lesion and stent deployment.

The precise role of surgical versus endovascular treatment for subclavian artery occlusive disease has yet to be defined. At experienced centers, carotid-subclavian bypass or transposition can be done with a very low complication rate and 5-year patency rates of 90% and is the procedure of choice in patients who are acceptable operative risks. Endovascular treatment is a good option for patients with significant comorbidity and high operative risk but confers inferior long-term patency, ranging from 59% to 68% (4-year follow-up). Data also suggest that long-term patency is better with angioplasty alone, as in-stent restenosis occurred frequently, though Henry et al. found no difference in long-term patency for stenting versus angioplasty alone. Contemporary treatment most commonly employs primary stenting, with 5-year primary patency as high as 84% (Takach et al.).

In summary, intervention for subclavian artery occlusive disease is uncommon but is indicated in those with symptoms of cerebral or arm ischemia, as well as cardiac ischemia in patients with LIMA bypass and proximal subclavian disease. Several therapeutic options are available, ranging from endovascular techniques to direct arch reconstruction. Appropriate therapy should be individualized based on anatomy and comorbidity to maximize long-term durability and minimize periprocedural risk.

TAKE HOME POINTS

• The initial diagnostic test of choice is duplex ultrasound for a subclavian lesion.
• The presence of retrograde vertebral flow confirms the diagnosis of subclavian steal.
• Treatment is indicated when symptoms of cerebral or arm ischemia are present.
• The most common surgical procedures performed are carotid-subclavian bypass and subclavian-carotid transposition.
• If the ipsilateral carotid artery is not suitable for inflow, extra-anatomic configurations such as axilloaxillary, subclavian-subclavian, and even femorosubclavian bypasses can be constructed. However, direct great vessel reconstruction is preferred in these circumstances, using a graft off the ascending aorta in patients medically fit enough to tolerate median sternotomy.
• Endovascular treatment of subclavian disease is also an important therapeutic option.

SUGGESTED READINGS

Cina CS, Safar HA, Lagana A, et al. Subclavian carotid transposition and bypass grafting: consecutive cohort study and systematic review. *J Vasc Surg.* 2002;35:422-429.

Evans JR, Shepard AD. Upper extremity occlusive disease. In: Ernst CB, Stanley JC, eds. *Current Therapy in Vascular Surgery.* 2nd ed. Philadelphia, PA: BC Decker; 1991:178-181.

Fields W, Lemak N. Joint study of extracranial arterial occlusion. *JAMA.* 1972;222:1139-1143.

Henry M, Amor M, Henry I, et al. Percutaneous transluminal angioplasty of the subclavian arteries. *J Endovasc Surg.* 1999;6:33-41.

Schillinger M, Haumer M, Schillinger S, et al. Risk stratification for subclavian artery angioplasty: is there an increased rate of restenosis after stent implantation? *J Endovasc Ther.* 2001;8:550-557.

Takach TJ, Duncan JM, Livesay JJ, et al. Brachiocephalic reconstruction II: operative and endovascular management of single-vessel disease. *J Vasc Surg.* 2005;42:55-61.

CLINICAL SCENARIO CASE QUESTIONS

1. Which structure is *most* vulnerable to injury during supraclavicular exposure of the subclavian artery?

   a. Vertebral artery
   b. Thoracic duct
   c. Phrenic nerve
   d. Vagus nerve

2. Most patients with subclavian steal syndrome have:

   a. Chronic stable angina following remote CABG
   b. Arm claudication
   c. No symptoms
   d. Drop attacks

23 Upper Extremity Embolic Disease

JUSTIN HURIE

Presentation

A 65-year-old woman, who had a cerebrovascular accident 6 weeks ago, presents to the emergency department with right upper extremity pain and numbness for 5 hours. She had been recovering well at home and had minimal residual right-sided weakness after her cerebrovascular accident. The patient notes having difficulty moving her right arm and has severe pain in her hand. Her past medical history includes tobacco use and hypertension. Her current medications included aspirin and hydrochlorothiazide. She has no prior history of a cardiac arrhythmia. On physical examination, her pulse is 120 beats per minute and irregular, and her blood pressure is 110/60 mm Hg. Her cranial nerves are intact, and she has no evidence of cerebral ischemia. Her right hand is cool, painful, and mottled. She has palpable left radial and brachial pulses. She has a strong right brachial pulse but has no arterial signal at her wrist when interrogated with a handheld Doppler. She has decreased strength and sensation in her right hand. Her abdomen is soft, and she has palpable femoral and pedal pulses in her legs.

Differential Diagnosis

The patient has evidence of upper extremity ischemia based on physical examination. Potential sources of upper extremity ischemia include the following:

1. Cardiac embolus
2. Acute on chronic upper extremity arterial disease
3. Embolus from a proximal aneurysm
4. Traumatic injury
5. Proximal dissection

Workup

The patient has evidence of a new cardiac arrhythmia, as well as acute limb ischemia (ALI). It is common for patients with ALI to have multiple acute and chronic medical problems that must be treated appropriately and contribute to a high short-term mortality rate. An electrocardiogram suggests atrial fibrillation without evidence of acute myocardial ischemia. Although the patient denies chest pain, a troponin level should be checked and may be trended in order to evaluate for underlying myocardial damage.

Approximately 80% of patients with ALI have an embolism from a cardiac source. Diagnostic tests, such as duplex, computed tomography angiography (CTA), and/or conventional arteriography, may be considered, but minimizing delay in treatment for severe ALI is essential. This patient needs prompt revascularization to keep the total ischemic time less than 6 hours in order to minimize the risk of permanent muscle and nerve damage. Arteriography with thrombolysis may be an option for patients with less advanced ischemia but may delay reperfusion that could be achieved more rapidly with surgery. Physical examination is critical to localize the site of occlusion in the setting of ALI. In the setting of normal contralateral perfusion, presence of a water-hammer pulse at the brachial artery on the affected limb suggests that she would be a good candidate for open brachial thromboembolectomy.

Diagnosis and Treatment

The patient should be started on full-dose intravenous (IV) heparin (100 U/kg bolus and 18 U/kg/h) to decrease the risk of recurrent cardiac emboli from atrial fibrillation. The patient's heart rate is controlled with an intravenous beta-blocker. She is prepped for the operating room.

When the etiology of ALI is not as clear by history and physical examination, additional information may be gathered through performance of a CTA. CTA may further delineate the extent and level of embolism and be the best imaging modality to demonstrate an aneurysm. Conventional arteriography may provide an alternative option for diagnosis with the benefit of possible intervention. Arteriography only demonstrates luminal diameter so may not clearly show a proximal aneurysm. Due to the high level of spatial resolution, arteriography may demonstrate a subtle proximal lesion (Fig. 1).

Surgical Approach

The patient is taken to the operating room emergently (Table 1). Her right arm in entirety as well as one thigh are prepped and draped in the usual sterile fashion.

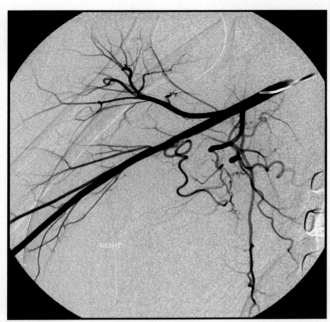

FIGURE 1 • Angiography demonstrating a subtle proximal lesion involving the brachial artery.

The thigh may be interrogated with an ultrasound prior to prepping in order to assure access to the great saphenous vein should a bypass or vein patch be required. An open thromboembolectomy under local anesthesia with IV sedation may be performed if the patient is able to cooperate; otherwise general anesthesia may be required. The brachial artery may be exposed through a transverse or longitudinal incision. Care should be taken to avoid injury to the median nerve that courses with the brachial artery. Vessel loops may be used for proximal and distal arterial control and a transverse arteriotomy performed. A catheter embolectomy may be performed with 2- to 4-French Fogarty balloons based on the size of the vessel. The balloons should only be inflated while withdrawing the balloons in order to prevent injury to the vessel. The balloons should be passed until no additional thrombus is obtained and there is evidence of good inflow and adequate back bleeding. In this case, thrombus is extracted from the brachial artery, and the artery is repaired using interrupted 6-0 Prolene suture. The hand becomes pink, and the patient has a palpable pulse.

Special Intraoperative Considerations

If there remains unsatisfactory perfusion to the hand after embolectomy, an on table angiogram may be performed through the exposed brachial vessel (Fig. 2). An angiogram may help to distinguish between residual thrombus and vasospasm, which more frequently affects vessels of the upper extremity compared to the lower extremity. There is debate regarding whether routine completion

---

TABLE 1. Upper Extremity Embolectomy

Key Technical Steps

1. The patient is taken to the operating room emergently.
2. Her right arm in entirety as well as one thigh are prepped and draped in the usual sterile fashion. The thigh may be interrogated with an ultrasound prior to prepping in order to assure access to the great saphenous vein should a bypass or vein patch be required.
3. An open thromboembolectomy under local anesthesia with IV sedation may be performed if the patient is able to cooperate; otherwise general anesthesia may be required.
4. The brachial artery may be exposed through a transverse or longitudinal incision. Care should be taken to avoid injury to the median nerve that courses with the brachial artery.
5. Vessel loops may be used for proximal and distal arterial control and a transverse arteriotomy performed.
6. A catheter embolectomy may be performed with 2- to 4-French Fogarty balloons based on the size of the vessel. The balloons should only be inflated while withdrawing the balloons in order to prevent injury to the vessel. The balloons should be passed until no additional thrombus is obtained and there is evidence of good inflow and adequate back bleeding. In this case, thrombus is extracted from the brachial artery, and the artery is repaired using interrupted 6-0 Prolene suture.
7. Examine the hand and make sure it becomes pink and has a palpable pulse.

Potential Pitfalls

- If there remains unsatisfactory perfusion to the hand after embolectomy, an on table angiogram may be performed through the exposed brachial vessel. An angiogram may help to distinguish between residual thrombus and vasospasm, which more frequently affects vessels of the upper extremity compared to the lower extremity. Adjuvant steps that may be useful to restore perfusion include repeat attempts at embolectomy or use of over the wire embolectomy catheters. Tissue plasminogen activator may also be administered intra-arterially in order to help clear residual distal thrombus. Finally, suction embolectomy catheters may also allow additional clot retrieval although may be cumbersome when used directly at the brachial artery.
- In patients with evidence of severe limb ischemia and profound neurologic impairment, a forearm fasciotomy should be performed.

---

angiography may help decrease the rate of target vessel reocclusion.

Occasionally, patients have evidence of residual thrombus that was not cleared after the initial attempt at open embolectomy. Adjuvant steps that may be useful to restore perfusion include repeat attempts at embolectomy or use of over the wire embolectomy catheters. Tissue plasminogen activator may also be administered intra-arterially in order to help clear residual distal thrombus. Finally, suction embolectomy catheters may also allow additional clot retrieval

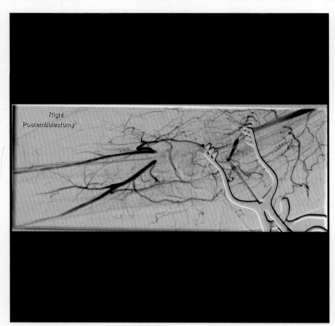

FIGURE 2 • Postembolectomy angiogram demonstrating residual occlusion of the right brachial artery.

although may be cumbersome when used directly at the brachial artery.

In patients with evidence of severe limb ischemia and profound neurologic impairment, a forearm fasciotomy should be performed.

Postoperative Management

It is important to continue the heparin throughout the case and in the postoperative setting. Patients with ALI remain at an elevated risk for recurrent embolization. Warfarin may be started postoperatively and should be continued for at least 6 months. A postoperative echocardiogram should be performed to assess for a proximal source. If the patient is not in atrial fibrillation and there is no clear etiology on transthoracic echocardiogram, a transesophageal echocardiogram may be beneficial.

Routine follow-up with history and physical examination is needed, but no specific imaging protocol is required for the affected and contralateral limb. Standard risk factor modification therapies should be pursued. The most common cause of death in patients with ALI is due to medical comorbidities, reflecting their generalized ill condition.

TAKE HOME POINTS

- Initiate anticoagulation with full-dose heparin as soon as the clinical diagnosis of ALI is made.
- Proceed with operative intervention early especially in patients with evidence of severe limb ischemia.
- CTA and echocardiogram may serve as useful adjuncts in patients with an unclear etiology of ischemia.

SUGGESTED READINGS

Andersen LV, Mortensen LS, Lindholt JS, et al. Upper-limb thrombo-embolectomy: national cohort study in Denmark. *Eur J Vasc Endovasc Surg.* 2010;40(5):628-634.

Andersen LV, Mortensen LS, Lip GY, et al. Atrial fibrillation and upper limb thromboembolectomy: a national cohort study. *J Thromb Haemost.* 2011;9(9):1738-1743.

Gossage JA, Ali T, Chambers J, et al. Peripheral arterial embolism: prevalence, outcome, and the role of echocardiography in management. *Vasc Endovascular Surg.* 2006;40(4):280-286.

Licht PB, Balezantis T, Wolff B, et al. Long-term outcome following thromboembolectomy in the upper extremity. *Eur J Vasc Endovasc Surg.* 2004;28(5):508-512.

Rittoo D, Stahnke M, Lindesay C, et al. Prognostic significance of raised cardiac troponin T in patients presenting with acute limb ischaemia. *Eur J Vasc Endovasc Surg.* 2006;32(5):500-503.

Schmid S, Heiss P. Embolic occlusion of forearm arteries: percutaneous embolus aspiration via antegrade brachial access. *Cardiovasc Intervent Radiol.* 2011;34(suppl 2):S312-S314.

Zaraca F, Ponzoni A, Sbraga P, et al. Does routine completion angiogram during embolectomy for acute upper-limb ischemia improve outcomes? *Ann Vasc Surg.* 2012;26(8):1064-1070.

CLINICAL SCENARIO CASE QUESTIONS

1. What is the appropriate step in the management of a patient with severe upper extremity limb ischemia?

   a. Operative embolectomy
   b. Anticoagulation alone
   c. Echocardiogram
   d. Computed tomography angiography
   e. Magnetic resonance angiography

2. You are called by an outside emergency department that is 1 hour away with a patient who has evidence of a brachial embolus secondary to atrial fibrillation. What is the next best step in management?

   a. Warfarin 5 mg PO
   b. Heparin bolus followed by a drip
   c. Enoxaparin 40 mg SQ
   d. Computed tomography angiography
   e. Dabigatran 150 mg PO

24 Buerger's Disease

PARTHY SHAH and SANJAY RAJAGOPALAN

Presentation

A 43-year-old man who is an assembly line worker presents with pain and discoloration in all four extremities. He previously noted a discolored area in the tip of his right fourth and fifth fingers approximately a month ago. He also previously noted pain in his feet bilaterally with exertion that seems to have worsened over the last several weeks with cessation with rest. He has not been able to work the last 2 weeks owing to these symptoms. On further questioning, he notes increasing cold intolerance in his upper and lower extremities over the last 2 years, which he attributes to his age. Past medical history is unremarkable for prior medical illness or rheumatologic disease. He smoked two to three packs of cigarettes a day for the past 25 years and cannot quit. His medications currently include Tylenol with codeine. There is no history of migraine medication or ergot-type derivative use. Although he has worked as an assembly line worker, his job does not include exposure to vibratory tools. There is no family history of premature atherosclerotic vascular disease or death. On physical examination, the patient is afebrile with normal blood pressures in the upper extremities. Examination of the right upper extremities reveals a healed ulcer measuring 2 mm on the tip of the right fourth digit. Radial pulses are normal. Allen's test reveals severe blanching of the right hand on occlusion of the ulnar artery, suggesting occlusion of the radial artery at the wrist. No Osler nodes or Janeway lesions are noted. Examination of the lower extremities reveals normal femoral, popliteal, and dorsalis pedis pulses but an absent posterior tibial artery pulse on the left lower extremity. Cardiac examination is normal, with no murmurs or rubs on auscultation. No bruits are appreciated.

Differential Diagnosis

The presentation is one of an individual with advanced signs of ischemia in his lower and upper extremities and Raynaud's symptoms. These symptoms are concerning for small vessel disease involvement in both upper and lower extremities and are therefore suggestive of a systemic process. The presence of a healing ulcer in the upper extremity (evidence of tissue loss) rules out primary Raynaud's syndrome. The differential diagnosis includes diseases that involve small and medium vessels of both the upper and lower extremities. Consideration should also be given to infectious etiologies (e.g., infective endocarditis) or intracardiac sources of embolism. Table 1 lists potential considerations.

Workup

A complete evaluation is ordered, including laboratory studies as outlined in Table 2 and Figure 1.

Evaluation Report

Complete blood counts, total cholesterol, lipid profile, and homocysteine levels are normal. A workup for collagen vascular disease and hypercoagulability (including antiphospholipid antibodies, antithrombin III, protein C,

and protein S activities) are normal. Erythrocyte sedimentation rate (ESR) is 15 mm/h, and the level of C-reactive protein (CRP) is low.

A transthoracic echocardiogram followed by a transesophageal echocardiogram does not reveal a cardiac or aortic (ascending arch and portion of descending) source.

Segmental pressures in the upper extremity reveal symmetric diminution in pressures at the level of the fingers with a decrease in pressures in most fingers of both upper extremities (40 mm in the right fourth and fifth digits), with damped waveforms in these digits. normal finger pressures should be greater than 80 mm Hg.

Upper extremity duplex testing reveals patent brachial and axillary arteries without evidence of aneurysm or occlusion.

An ankle-brachial index (ABI) and segmental pressures of the lower extremity revealed an index of 0.9 in the right and 0.9 in the left. Toe brachial indices were 0.3 bilaterally with monophasic waveforms in all digits of the feet.

Recommendations

A three-dimensional contrast-enhanced magnetic resonance arteriography (MRA) is ordered of the abdomen and lower extremities to rule out concomitant large

TABLE 1. Etiologic Considerations

Large Vessel Obstructive Disease	Small Vessel Obstructive Disease	Vasospasm
Atherosclerotic • Aneurysmal • TOS • Traumatic • Kawasaki's • FMD Vasculitis • Giant cell (Takayasu's) • Radiation	Blood dyscrasias • Cryoglobulins • Myeloproliferative disease • Multiple myeloma (especially Waldenström's macroglobulinemia) Buerger's disease Embolic • Atheromatous plaque • Heart, innominate, subclavian • Aneurysms Innominate, subclavian, axillary, brachial, ulnar Henoch-Schönlein purpura Hypercoagulable states • Antiphospholipid syndrome • AT-III, protein C, S deficiency • Lupus anticoagulant • Heparin induced thrombocytopenia Vasculitis • Scleroderma • CREST • Rheumatoid arthritis • Systemic lupus erythematosus • Polymyositis/dermatomyositis • MCTD Miscellaneous • Frostbite	Large vessel vasospasm • Cocaine • Ergotamine • Methamphetamine • Cannabis Small vessel vasospasm • Primary Raynaud's • Secondary Raynaud's

AT-III, anti-thrombin III; CREST, calcinosis, Raynaud's phenomenon, esophageal involvement, sclerodactyly, telangiectasia (syndrome); FMD, fibromuscular dysplasia; MCTD, mixed connective tissue disease; TOS, thoracic outlet syndrome.

vessel disease in the pelvis and thighs. MRA of the lower extremities did not reveal large vessel occlusive disease (iliac and femoral arteries were patent bilaterally). However, it did reveal occlusion of the left posterior tibial artery bilaterally at its origin with reconstitution at both ankles by collaterals. Disease of the tibioperoneal system was noted bilaterally with incomplete visualization of the pedal vessels bilaterally. The pedal vessels were poorly visualized bilaterally.

Diagnosis

This man has systemic disease that selectively affects small and medium vessels of the upper and lower extremities. The patient also has symptoms suggestive of Raynaud's syndrome. The major etiologies to consider in this case are related to infectious, embolic, and vasculitic causes, and Buerger's disease. Specific aspects of this case that are of interest and enable one to arrive at the diagnosis are as follows. *Unilateral versus bilateral symptoms*: Bilaterality of symptoms and signs (asymptomatic involvement of digits) suggests a systemic process. *Tissue necrosis in the upper extremity* excludes primary Raynaud's, which is intermittent and shows complete resolution in between attacks. Moreover, the lower extremity symptoms in this case are suggestive of a systemic diagnosis. Digital ulcerations are most commonly caused by vasculitis (50% to 75% of all cases); half of the vasculitis cases are caused by primary Sjögren's syndrome (PSS); the syndrome of calcinosis, Raynaud's phenomenon, esophageal involvement,

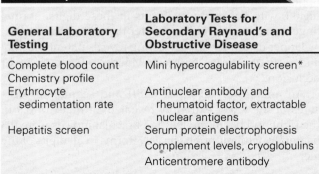

TABLE 2. Laboratory Testing in Patients with Suspected Small Vessel Disease

General Laboratory Testing	Laboratory Tests for Secondary Raynaud's and Obstructive Disease
Complete blood count Chemistry profile	Mini hypercoagulability screen*
Erythrocyte sedimentation rate	Antinuclear antibody and rheumatoid factor, extractable nuclear antigens
Hepatitis screen	Serum protein electrophoresis
	Complement levels, cryoglobulins
	Anticentromere antibody

*Mini hypercoagulability screen includes antiphospholipid antibodies, lupus anticoagulant, antithrombin III, protein C (activity) and protein S levels, factor V Leiden, and prothrombin gene mutation.

For large artery obstruction, one may consider performing this workup in addition, when appropriate.

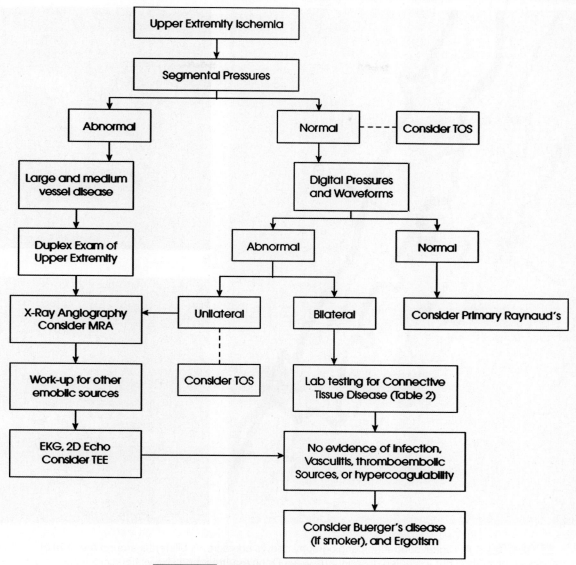

FIGURE 1 • Upper extremity ischemia algorithm.

sclerodactyly, and telangiectasia (CREST); Buerger's; and complications of atherosclerosis (e.g., embolism). The presence of foot claudication suggests small vessel involvement often seen in Buerger's disease. However, foot claudication is by no means specific for Buerger's disease (it may also be seen with thromboembolization). Smoking history is almost invariably present, and the absence of smoking should render the diagnosis of Buerger's disease suspect.

Discussion

Buerger's disease (thromboangiitis obliterans) is a non-atherosclerotic segmental peripheral arterial disease primarily affecting small- and medium-sized vessels of the arms and legs. It is strongly associated with current or recent tobacco use and appears to be more common in countries with heavier tobacco use. The disease has a male predominance with an onset before age 45 to 50 years. Affected patients often first notice dysesthesias, Raynaud's

phenomenon, and pedal claudication. Ischemic rest pain, ulceration, superficial migratory thrombophlebitis, and digital gangrene are characteristics of disease progression. Multiple limbs are nearly always involved, even in cases where clinical signs and symptoms exist in a single limb. Hence, an Allen test may be positive even in the setting of only lower extremity pain and ulceration.

Diagnosis is by exclusion, as detailed above. Commonly measured markers for inflammatory disease (ESR, CRP) and autoantibodies (antinuclear antibody, rheumatoid factor) are usually normal or negative. Proximal sources of emboli should be considered as part of the differential diagnosis and may be evaluated by transthoracic or transesophageal echocardiogram, depending on clinical suspicion. Arteriography typically shows segmental occlusive lesions of distal vessels surrounded by "corkscrew" or "tree-root" collateral vessels in the absence of atherosclerosis (Fig. 2). These findings are suggestive

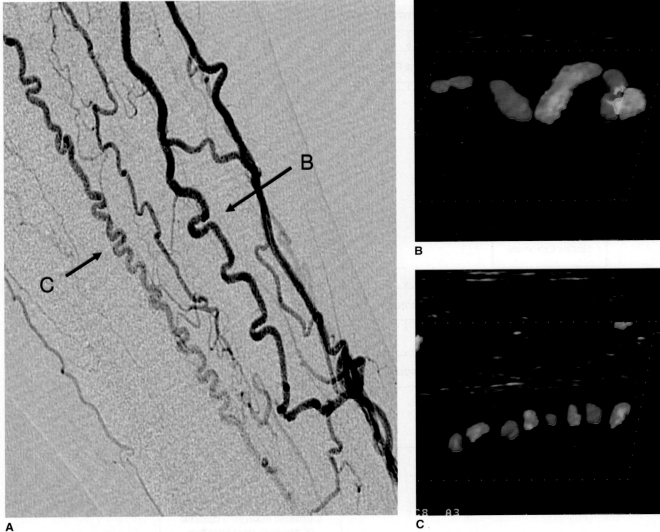

FIGURE 2 • **A:** Digital subtraction angiography shows corkscrew collaterals around the area of occlusions in the right lower leg. Continuous-wave Doppler ultrasound shows corkscrew collaterals as color Doppler flows of a snake sign (**A** [*arrow* B] and **B**) and a dot sign (**A** [*arrow* C] and **C**). (From Fujii Y, Nishioka K, Yoshizumi M, et al. Corkscrew collaterals in thromboangiitis obliterans (Buerger disease). *Circulation.* 2007;116:e539-e540, with permission.)

but not pathognomonic. An excisional biopsy is rarely needed but can be obtained from amputations or acute superficial phlebitis for confirmation of the diagnosis. Histopathologic analysis of an acute phase lesion may demonstrate the classic findings of inflammatory cellular thrombi, with relative sparing of the vessel wall and preservation of the internal elastic lamina. Chronic lesions are characterized by organized thrombus and fibrosis.

The following clinical criteria are used most commonly for the diagnosis: (1) age younger than 45 years and current (or recent past) history of tobacco use; (2) presence of distal extremity ischemia (claudication, rest pain, ischemic ulcers, or gangrene) documented with noninvasive vascular testing; (3) laboratory tests to exclude autoimmune diseases, hypercoagulable states, and diabetes mellitus; (4) exclusion of a proximal source of emboli by means of echocardiography and arteriography; and (5) consistent arteriographic findings in the involved and clinically noninvolved limbs.

Recommendations

Treatment approaches in Buerger's disease are outlined in Table 3. The initial approach in this patient should be the complete cessation of tobacco use, including smoking, chewing, or using nicotine replacement products. A large majority of patients who quit smoking will avoid disease progression and amputations. If he continues to have active disease, despite reports of tobacco cessation, testing for urinary nicotine or cotinine should be considered prior to evaluation for other less definitive medical or surgical therapies.

TABLE 3. Treatment Approaches in Buerger's Disease

General Recommendations
Smoking cessation
Exercise
Avoid trauma
Treat infection with antibiotics

Local Wound Care
Lubricate skin with lanolin-based cream
Lamb's wool between toes in case of ulcers or gangrene

Medical Treatment
Control pain (narcotics may be needed)
Calcium channel blockers (amlodipine or nifedipine) if severe Raynaud's
Aspirin and/or clopidogrel
Iloprost
Spinal cord stimulator
Endoscopic sympathectomy

Surgical
Infrainguinal bypass with vein
Surgical sympathectomy

Pain Control

In patients with intractable pain due to lower or upper extremity involvement, sympathectomy (thoracic or lumbar) using endoscopic means may be considered. Spinal cord stimulator treatment may also be of benefit in patients with recalcitrant pain.

Concomitant Medical Therapy

Although no prospective evidence exists regarding the benefit of therapies such as antiplatelet agents, statins, or anticoagulation in patients with Buerger's disease, antiplatelet therapy with aspirin and/or clopidogrel is probably reasonable. In this patient, who has a severe vasospastic component, a calcium channel antagonist was initiated (amlodipine 5 to 10 mg/d). If ongoing tissue loss occurs, treatment with prostaglandin analogues, such as iloprost, may be beneficial. Oral iloprost has not been demonstrated to be as effective, thus obligating patients to intravenous therapy. There are also limited data on the use of angiogenic growth factors, such as vascular endothelial growth factor (VEGF), in these patients.

Revascularization

Surgical revascularization is rarely performed because of poor target vessels and the diffuse distal predilection of the disease, as seen in this patient, and because of the usually good response following tobacco cessation. Vascular reconstruction may be considered in patients with bypassable disease and severe non-healing ulcers or ischemic rest pain who have quit smoking. Infrainguinal bypass using autogenous vein grafts from a series in Japan revealed 5-year patency rates of less than 50% in patients with Buerger's disease, with patency rates directly related to smoking continuation.

Sympathectomy

As there are often no reconstructive options in patients with Buerger's disease, lumbar sympathectomy remains a feasible option for patients with refractory pain and lower extremity ischemia despite maximal medical therapy. Sympathectomy removes the vasoconstriction effect in the area of interest and causes increase in the blood flow to cutaneous vascular beds but not significant increase in the blood flow to the muscles. Thus, this is reserved only for patients who have superficial ulceration or vasospastic manifestations and not in patients with claudication. Once performed, the effects may only last for a few months to 1 to 2 years. This, however, may be sufficient time to allow for wound healing.

Amputation

According to the Cleveland Clinic experience, amputations were rarely required for those patients who stopped smoking. Those who did not adhere to smoking cessation frequently required amputation. Most amputations are distal, infrapopliteal. However, if Buerger's disease is diagnosed early and the patient completely avoids tobacco products, amputations can be avoided.

TAKE HOME POINTS

- Buerger's disease (thromboangiitis obliterans) is a nonatherosclerotic segmental peripheral arterial disease primarily affecting small- and medium-sized vessels of the arms and legs.
- Smoking or chewing tobacco is the most common and strongest risk factor for Buerger's disease.
- Diagnosis is based on clinical manifestation. Ischemic rest pain, ulceration, superficial migratory thrombophlebitis, and digital gangrene are characteristics of disease progression.
- Arteriography typically shows segmental occlusive lesions of distal vessels surrounded by "corkscrew" or "tree-root" collateral vessels in the absence of atherosclerosis.
- The cornerstone to treatment of Buerger's disease is complete cessation of tobacco use, including smoking, chewing, or using nicotine replacement products.

SUGGESTED READINGS

Dilege S, Aksoy M, Kayabali M, et al. Vascular reconstruction in Buerger's disease: is it feasible? *Surg Today.* 2002;32:1032-1047.

Joyce JW. Buerger's disease (thromboangiitis obliterans). *Rheum Dis Clin North Am.* 1990;16:463-470.

Mills JL, Porter JM. Buerger's disease (thromboangiitis obliterans). *Ann Vasc Surg.* 1991;5:570-572.

Olin JW. Thromboangiitis obliterans (Buerger's disease). *N Engl J Med.* 2000;343:864-869.

Olin JW, Young JR, Graor RA, et al. The changing clinical spectrum of thromboangiitis obliterans (Buerger's disease). *Circulation.* 1990;82(suppl IV):3-8.

Piazza G, Creager MA. Thromboangiitis obliterans. *Circulation.* 2010;121(16):1858-1861. Review.

Rajagopalan S, et al. *Manual of Vascular Diseases.* Philadelphia, PA: Lippincott Williams & Wilkins; 2011.

Sasajima T, Kudo Y, Dhaba M, et al. Role of Infra-inguinal bypass in Buerger's disease: an eighteen year experience. *Eur J Vasc Endovasc Surg.* 1997;13(2):186-192.

CLINICAL SCENARIO CASE QUESTIONS

1. Biopsy of the vessel wall in Buerger's disease is likely to demonstrate all of the following except:
   a. In situ thrombus
   b. T-cell infiltration of the vessel wall
   c. Sparing of the internal elastic lamina
   d. Collaterals

2. The following clinical criteria are used most commonly for the diagnosis except:
   a. Age older than 45 years
   b. Current (or recent past) history of tobacco use
   c. Presence of distal extremity ischemia (claudication, rest pain, ischemic ulcers, or gangrene) documented with noninvasive vascular testing
   d. Laboratory tests to exclude autoimmune diseases, hypercoagulable states, and diabetes mellitus
   e. Consistent arteriographic findings in the involved and clinically noninvolved limbs

25 Hypothenar Hammer Syndrome

HARI R. KUMAR and HERON E. RODRIGUEZ

Presentation

A 60-year-old man presents to the emergency department with 10 days of pain and bluish discoloration of the third to fifth digits of his right hand. He is right hand dominant and works as a mechanic. He frequently gets small cuts on his hand and has noticed difficulty healing these wounds on the distal aspects of his fourth and fifth digits. He denies any previous episodes of symptoms or recent major trauma to the extremity. There are no paresthesias in the affected area. The bluish discoloration was not preceded by any other color changes. The patient is a nonsmoker. A hand x-ray is negative for acute fracture.

Differential Diagnosis

Ischemia of the hand has a broad differential diagnosis. The most common etiology is embolization from a proximal source including the heart or upper extremity arterial system. Cardiac sources include emboli from atrial fibrillation or ventricular aneurysm, as well as mycotic emboli from endocarditis. Proximal arterial sources can include plaque from the aortic arch or emboli from a subclavian aneurysm due to thoracic outlet syndrome. Thrombosis from a hypercoagulable state should be considered as well.

Small vessel pathologies can affect the hand and include primary and secondary Raynaud's phenomenon and thromboangiitis obliterans (Buerger's disease). Vasculitis causing upper extremity ischemia can be associated with autoimmune or connective tissue disorders, such as scleroderma, systemic lupus erythematosus, rheumatoid arthritis, or Sjögren's syndrome.

Other causes of hand ischemia include steal syndrome from a proximal arteriovenous fistula/graft, iatrogenic arterial injury, radiation arteritis, injury due to intravenous drug abuse, and occupational repetitive injury. In this latter category, hand-arm vibration syndrome, thenar hammer syndrome, and hypothenar hammer syndrome (HHS) should be considered in manual laborers.

Workup

While the differential for hand ischemia is quite broad, a thorough history and physical can help to narrow the list. The inciting factors for ischemia, such as cold temperature, should be documented. Any changes in the color of the hand, such as the typical pallor, cyanosis, and rubor known as Raynaud's phenomenon, should be documented. Specific questions should also be asked about the type of work done with hands, including repetitive striking of the palm or use of vibratory tools. The use of tobacco products or intravenous drugs should be documented.

The vascular exam of the hand should include bilateral palpation and auscultation of the brachial, radial, ulnar, and digital arteries and the superficial palmar arch. An Allen's test should be performed to look for ulnar artery occlusion. Vascular laboratory studies to document digital waveforms and pressures should be obtained.

The chest should be auscultated for abnormal heart sounds or rhythms. Cardiac studies should include an EKG to evaluate for arrhythmia and an echocardiogram to evaluate for sources of embolus.

Laboratory tests for thrombophilia and autoimmune disease should be ordered if hypercoagulability or vasculitis is suspected.

Imaging of the arteries from the aortic arch to the digital arteries should be obtained. Although conventional digital subtraction angiography remains the gold standard, magnetic resonance and computed tomography angiography provides an excellent level of anatomical detail and is the study of choice in many centers. Adequate visualization of the arteries of the hand is essential in operative planning.

Diagnosis

This patient presents with symptoms of hand ischemia and an occupational history of repetitive striking of his hands. He states that in his work as a mechanic, he repeatedly strikes objects with his hand. He is a nonsmoker. He has no history of Raynaud's or any autoimmune disorder. Physical examination and noninvasive flow showed normal flow to the wrist with evidence of ischemia in the digital arteries of the third to fifth fingers. The Allen's test is positive. His workup did not demonstrate a proximal embolic source. An angiogram demonstrated embolic occlusion of multiple digital arteries and an ulnar artery aneurysm (Fig. 1). All of these findings are consistent with *hypothenar hammer syndrome*.

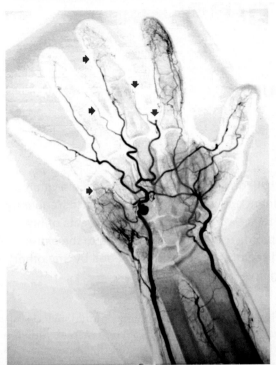

FIGURE 1 • Selective arteriogram of the hand showing a saccular aneurysm of the distal portion of the ulnar artery. There is embolic occlusion of multiple digital arteries (*arrows*).

Discussion

The ulnar artery is vulnerable to injury at the hypothenar eminence. Distal to the wrist, the ulnar artery passes through Guyon's canal bound by the pisiform and hamate bones. Here, the ulnar artery is in a superficial location and cushioned only by skin, subcutaneous tissue, and the thin palmaris brevis muscle. Repetitive use of the palm of the hand as a "hammer" compresses the unprotected ulnar artery against the nearby hook of the hamate bone, which serves as an "anvil."

Previous reports of the disease exist, but it was Conn and Bergan who, in 1970, first recognized the anatomic mechanism and coined the term "hypothenar hammer syndrome." The incidence of the disease is low, with HHS seen in only 1.1% to 1.6% of referrals to tertiary centers for hand ischemia; however, the condition is likely underreported, as Little and Ferguson's study of 79 mechanics showed 14% had ulnar artery occlusion, but none experienced symptoms severe enough to seek out medical attention.

Both aneurysm formation and occlusive disease can be seen with the disease and depend upon the type of injury to the arterial wall. Damage to the intimal layer can cause vasospasm and platelet aggregation leading to thrombus formation. Damage to the medial layer can cause aneurysm formation, which can also be a nidus

for distal emboli. Histologic examination of the resected ulnar artery specimens shows disruption of the internal elastic lamina and hyperplastic proliferation of the intima or media. There is currently debate whether the pathophysiology represents changes from repetitive trauma or if there is a coexistent focal arterial pathology, such as fibromuscular dysplasia to which the repetitive trauma is superimposed.

Patients may present with Raynaud's phenomenon. However, several features can distinguish HHS from other syndromes. The patient demographic is mostly male manual laborers with a history of repetitive striking of the hand. The dominant hand is the most affected one, and there is a lack of symptoms in the lower extremity. The three fingers on the ulnar side are the most affected. The thumb is usually spared. Cyanosis and pallor can occur, but the hyperemic rubor seen with Raynaud's phenomenon tends to be absent. A positive Allen's test, indicating ulnar artery occlusion, can be present. A pulsatile mass overlying the hypothenar eminence can indicate an aneurysm.

Treatment

Patients with mild symptoms and without an aneurysm can be treated nonoperatively. Padded hand protection and avoidance of further repetitive trauma is associated with significant clinical improvement. Tobacco cessation should be recommended if applicable. Medical therapies can include calcium channel blockers, antiplatelet agents, and/or anticoagulation. Thrombolysis can be used in the acute setting in cases of distal embolization. Surgical intervention is indicated in patients with an aneurysm or severe hand ischemia. Surgical intervention can include simple ligation of the aneurysm if there is adequate collateral circulation; typically, resection of the affected segment with reconstruction is required. Previous treatment modalities have included thoracic sympathectomy, in an attempt to increase skin perfusion. The results from this approach have been disappointing.

In the case of this patient who presented with an aneurysm and severe hand ischemia, surgical treatment was recommended. A positive Allen's test and arterial noninvasive studies consistent with ischemia would preclude simple ligation of the aneurysm. The patient was offered resection with reconstruction.

Surgical Approach

The procedure is performed in the operating room and can be done under general anesthesia or axillary block. The patient is placed in the supine position with arm abducted. The surgical field is prepped and draped in a sterile fashion (Fig. 2).

A slightly oblique, longitudinal incision is made over the hypothenar eminence of the hand just distal to the

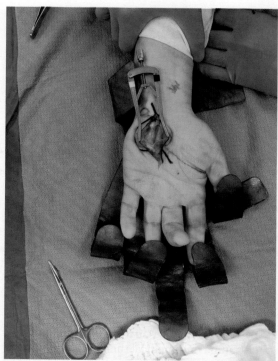

FIGURE 2 • Operative exposure is obtained with the arm abducted and the fingers extended. An incision is made over the hypothenar eminence of the hand just distal to the wrist crease and is carried into the mid palm.

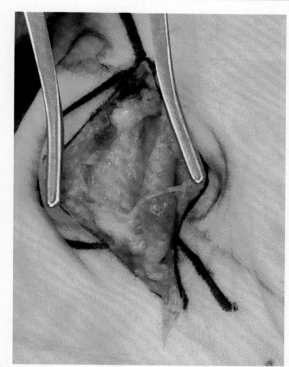

FIGURE 3 • The distal portion of the ulnar artery is exposed by retracting the palmaris brevis muscle. The origin of the fifth digital branch is exposed at the most distal portion of the field.

wrist crease and carried to the mid palm. The subcutaneous tissue and palmaris brevis muscle are divided and retracted (Fig. 3).

The artery will be identified at the proximal edge of the palmaris brevis muscle and can be traced distally. The dissection must proceed carefully in order to preserve the numerous small branches that originate from the artery and to avoid injuring the ulnar nerve that lies on the ulnar side of the artery. The artery can be followed distally where the fifth digital branch arises, and the artery then becomes the superficial palmar arch.

The diseased portion of the artery is removed and sent to pathology for further analysis (Fig. 4). If the resection is less than 2 cm, a primary anastomosis may be attempted. A longer resection will likely require reconstruction. Numerous conduits have been used that are appropriate size matches. Venous conduits have included the greater or lesser saphenous vein below the knee or superficial forearm veins. Arterial conduits have included the descending branch of the lateral femoral circumflex artery and branches of the thoracodorsal artery. Studies have shown that bypass patency is reduced when length of the bypass is increased, so dedicated effort is required to minimize the length of the bypass.

In the case of our patient, a descending branch of the lateral femoral circumflex artery was harvested by dissecting in between the rectus femoris and the vastus

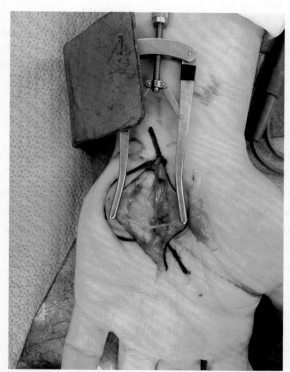

FIGURE 4 • The aneurysmal segment of the ulnar artery has been excised. The cut ends of the proximal and distal ulnar artery are prepared for revascularization.

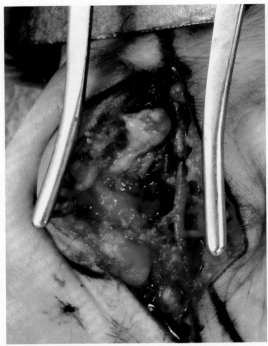

FIGURE 5 • The descending branch of the lateral femoral circumflex artery has been interposed via end-to-end anastomosis to the ulnar artery. Note that a branch was used to perform a separate anastomosis to the fifth digital artery.

lateralis. The conduit was anastomosed in an end-to-end fashion for both anastomoses using interrupted 8-0 Prolene sutures (Fig. 5).

Once the bypass is completed, flow is then reestablished and hemostasis confirmed. The bypass is auscultated with a Doppler to confirm excellent flow. The palm incision is closed in layers with interrupted nylon sutures used for the skin (Table 1).

Case Conclusion

The patient is maintained on lifelong antiplatelet therapy (aspirin 81 to 325 mg/day). Vascular lab flow studies including digital waveforms and pressures are obtained prior to discharge. Surveillance duplex and flow studies are performed every 6 to 12 months to evaluate patency and monitor for evidence of stenosis or aneurysm of the graft.

TAKE HOME POINTS

- HHS is a rare cause of hand ischemia.
- Distinguishing features include tendency toward male gender, a history of manual labor involving repetitive striking of the hand, predominantly affecting the dominant upper extremity, and lack of involvement of the thumb.

TABLE 1. Hypothenar Hammer Syndrome

Key Technical Steps

1. Longitudinal incision over the hypothenar eminence.
2. Divide the subcutaneous tissue and palmaris brevis muscle.
3. Resect the affected segment of the artery.
4. If resection is <2 cm, primary anastomosis may be performed.
5. If resection is >2 cm, reconstruct with either arterial or venous conduit of appropriate size.
6. Venous conduits are typically reversed, and the anastomosis is performed in an interrupted fashion.

Potential Pitfalls

- Avoid injury to ulnar nerve or numerous small arterial branches.
- Minimize the length of resected artery in order to improve patency of bypass.

- Mild symptoms may be treated with avoidance of further trauma and medical therapy.
- Indications for surgical intervention include aneurysm or severe ischemia.

SUGGESTED READINGS

Conn J, Bergan JJ, Bell JL. Hypothenar hammer syndrome: post-traumatic digital ischemia. *Surgery.* 1970;68:1122.

Dethmers RS, Houpt P. Surgical management of hypothenar and thenar hammer syndromes: a retrospective study of 31 instances in 28 patients. *J Hand Surg [Br].* 2005;30(4): 419-423.

Eskandari MK, Kumar HR. Occupational vascular problems. In: Cronenwett JL, Johnston KW, eds. *Rutherford's Vascular Surgery.* 8th ed. Philadelphia, PA: Elseveir and Saunders; 2014:Chapter 123.

Ferris BL, Taylor LM Jr, Oyama K, et al. Hypothenar hammer syndrome: proposed etiology. *J Vasc Surg.* 2000;31:104.

Kleinert HE, Burget GC, Morgan JA, et al. Aneurysms of the hand. *Arch Surg.* 1973;106:554.

Larsen BT, Edwards WD, Jensen MH, et al. Surgical pathology of hypothenar hammer syndrome with new pathogenetic insights: a 25-year institutional experience with clinical and pathologic review of 67 cases. *Am J Surg Pathol* 2013; 37(11):1700-1708.

Lifchez SD, Higgins JP: Long-term results of surgical treatment for hypothenar hammer syndrome. *Plast Reconstr Surg.* 2009;124:210-216.

Little JM, Ferguson DA. The incidence of the hypothenar hammer syndrome. *Arch Surg.* 1972;105:684.

Marie I, Hervé F, Primard E, et al. Long-term follow up of hypothenar hammer syndrome: a series of 47 patients. *Medicine (Baltimore).* 2007;86:334.

Pineda CJ, Weisman MH, Bookstein JJ, et al. Hypothenar hammer syndrome: form of reversible Raynaud's phenomenon. *Am J Med.* 1985;79:561.

CLINICAL SCENARIO CASE QUESTIONS

1. Which of the following symptoms is *not* consistent with the diagnosis of hypothenar hammer syndrome?

   a. The thumb is asymptomatic
   b. The Allen's test is positive
   c. A history of manual labor with repetitive striking of the palm of the hand
   d. Bilateral hand involvement
   e. The presence of an ulnar artery aneurysm

2. In a patient who presents with an ulnar artery aneurysm and evidence of acute hand ischemia, which of the following treatments should *not* be performed?

   a. Counseling on avoidance of further hand trauma
   b. Counseling on smoking cessation
   c. Ligation of the aneurysm
   d. Resection with reconstruction
   e. Thrombolysis

26 Innominate Artery Disease: Open Surgery

AMANI D. POLITANO and KENNETH J. CHERRY

Presentation

A 76-year-old male presents with a 2-year history of recurrent transient ischemic attacks (TIAs) and cerebral vascular accidents (CVAs) despite combination therapy with aspirin, clopidogrel, and warfarin. He has residual right-sided weakness and right eye blindness from a CVA 2 years ago. His medical history is significant for prostate cancer with urinary retention, hypertension, dyslipidemia, and rectal prolapse for which he underwent a Hartmann's procedure. Current medications include aspirin, clopidogrel, warfarin, lovastatin, losartan, and terazosin. His mother has a history of a stroke, and his father died of a myocardial infarction. He is a former 40-pack-year smoker and does not drink. On physical examination, his vital signs are notable for a sinus heart rate of 77 beats per minute, blood pressure of 148/82 mm Hg, and no murmurs on auscultation. Peripheral pulses are intact and equal bilaterally. His carotid arteries are notable for an absence of bruits. He has decreased strength in his right arm and leg, but is otherwise neurologically intact.

Differential Diagnosis

Multiple and recurrent TIAs or CVAs are concerning for an embolic phenomenon rather than a hemorrhagic one. Common etiologies include atheroembolism from calcific plaques, embolic events from atrial thrombus in the setting of atrial fibrillation or from systemic venous thrombus via a septal defect, or inflammatory arteritis. The persistent deficits help to localize the potential source, as distal emboli or inflammatory conditions are more likely to be bilateral. The absence of other symptoms associated with arteritis also makes the latter less likely.

Case Continued

Further questioning reveals no prior fevers, fatigue, weight loss, or arthralgia. He has no history of prior radiation exposure or vasculitis, nor any family history of vasculitis. Aside from the residual weakness and right eye blindness, he demonstrates no neurologic deficits.

Workup

Evaluation of a cardiac or distal embolic source can be accomplished with an electrocardiogram (EKG) to assess for atrial fibrillation or other arrhythmia and an echocardiogram to detect mural thrombus or septal defects. Imaging studies including duplex ultrasound or cross-sectional imaging (computed tomography angiography [CTA] or magnetic resonance angiography [MRA]) with intravenous contrast enhancement are also of benefit in identifying an offending stenotic plaque or ulceration.

Duplex ultrasound of the bilateral carotid arteries and their bifurcations will detect narrowing of these vessels, most commonly at the internal carotid artery. However, added value is obtained from imaging the origins of these vessels and the aortic arch, as arteriosclerotic disease at this location can contribute to the above symptoms and are best identified prior to planning any operative intervention. Angiography for evaluation of carotid or aortic arch disease can be done if other imaging modalities are inconclusive. However, it should not be the first-line assessment tool as it carries the risk of showering emboli distally with wire and catheter manipulation. With cross-sectional or angiographic techniques, the images should be extended cephalad to capture the circle of Willis, as its patency may affect operative planning, especially if the carotid or vertebral circulation is affected by arteriosclerosis.

Case Continued

The patient underwent an EKG and echocardiogram that demonstrated normal sinus rhythm, an ejection fraction of 60%, and no evidence of septal defects or valve disease. In addition, a dobutamine cardiac stress test showed a mild reversible defect in the anterior left ventricle. A CTA of the head and neck revealed 50% stenosis of the left internal carotid artery with an irregular lumen concerning for ulcerated plaque (Fig. 1A). The dominant left vertebral artery demonstrated distal stenosis, as did the basilar artery. Several old and small embolic infarcts were

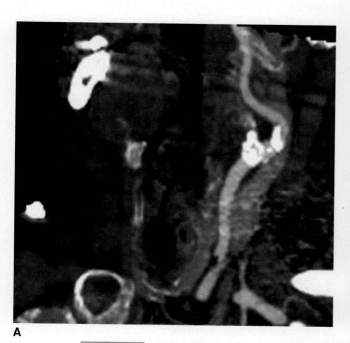
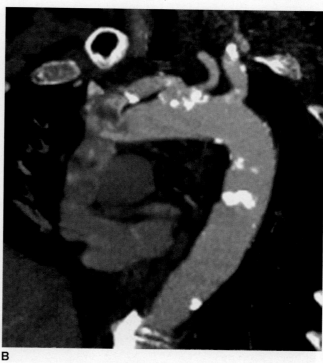

FIGURE 1 • CTA of the great vessels demonstrating significant calcific deposits in the LCC artery (**A**) and at the bovine-variant origin of the innominate and LCC arteries (**B**).

seen. Evaluation of the aortic arch demonstrated bovine-type anatomy with a shared origin of the brachiocephalic and left common carotid (LCC) arteries rife with calcific changes and a high-grade stenosis (Figs. 1B and 2). The right carotid system demonstrated minimal atherosclerotic changes without narrowing.

Diagnosis and Treatment

Arteriosclerosis of the great vessels is the most common pathology requiring intervention, followed by Takayasu's arteritis and radiation-induced arteritis. Still, the vessels of the root of the arch are involved in only 7.5% of cases, far less commonly than the carotid arteries at their bifurcation or the vertebral arteries. The prevalence of arteriosclerosis is greater in men and in younger persons with a median age of 50 to 61 years. Operative planning should include examination and planned repair of multiple supra-aortic lesions, as these can be seen in 60% to 80% of patients with innominate disease.

Symptomatic lesions manifest as either cerebral or upper extremity ischemic episodes and warrant repair. Asymptomatic lesions of the common carotid arteries may be repaired using the same criteria as for bifurcation disease. If upper extremity arterial insufficiency due to stenosis hinders formation or function of dialysis access or extra-anatomic bypass grafts, repair may also be considered. Finally, correction of otherwise asymptomatic lesions should be considered if a sternotomy is required for treatment of alternate pathology to avoid reentering the field at a later time. However, as the perioperative morbidity for this operation is not small, the risks must be weighed carefully, and surgical intervention for asymptomatic lesions in the absence of the above caveats is not recommended.

Options for repair of the great vessels include direct reconstruction and extra-anatomic bypass. Extra-anatomic procedures, including subclavian-carotid, carotid-subclavian, carotid-carotid, and axillary-axillary bypasses, were developed as alternates to the perioperative morbidity and mortality of a median sternotomy. However, the improved outcomes of sternotomy and direct repair and concerns about long-term patency of extra-anatomic repairs other than the carotid-subclavian or subclavian-carotid bypasses have shifted interest back toward direct arch repair.

Case Continued

The presenting symptoms in this case may be related to either the left carotid bifurcation disease or the ulcerated plaque at the bovine origin of the innominate and LCC. Both can be addressed with a single operative approach. As a part of the preoperative workup, coronary artery disease was evaluated. Should the patient have significant coronary lesions, coordination of repair in conjunction with coronary bypass or angioplasty may be necessary. For this patient, this is not necessary, and proceeding to operative repair is appropriate.

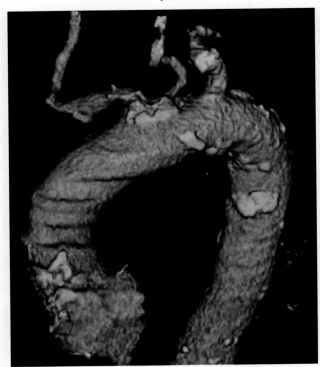

FIGURE 2 • Three-dimensional computed tomography color vessel reconstruction of the aortic arch demonstrating heavy calcification of the bovine-variant common origin of the proximal innominate and LCC arteries.

Surgical Approach

Patient positioning optimizes exposure. After appropriate monitoring devices and access are obtained, the patient is placed in supine position with the arms tucked to allow surgeon access to the operative field. A roll placed vertically between the shoulder blades aids with exposure and allows extension of the head. Rotation of the head is dictated by the planned procedure; access to the innominate, right common carotid, and right subclavian arteries can be accomplished with the head rotated to the left slightly, whereas access to the left-sided vessels requires the head be prepped in order to be rotated intraoperatively. The sterile field should extend to the upper abdomen.

The decision to shunt during the procedure can be made based on preoperative imaging of the circle of Willis. Alternatively, intraoperative adjuncts, such as electroencephalography, cerebral oximetry, or carotid artery stump pressures, may guide decision making. Criteria similar to that used during carotid endarterectomy should be employed. The use of neuroprotective anesthetics may also be desired. If bilateral carotid artery repair is indicated, the more diseased vessel should be repaired first to preserve intracranial blood flow.

A midline incision with partial or complete sternotomy is performed and is extended in a hockey stick fashion along the anterior boarder of the right sternocleidomastoid muscle to expose the bifurcation of the innominate artery. A sternal retractor is placed. If the procedure requires access to the right carotid bifurcation, the incision can be extended superiorly. The LCC artery may be accessed through the primary incision, while access to the bifurcation is obtained via a separate incision. Exposure of the innominate artery and its branches can be accomplished with either division or mobilization of the left brachiocephalic vein.

Initial anastomosis to the ascending aorta begins with placement of a side-biting clamp as far laterally as is possible. A vertical aortotomy is made, and an 8- or 10-mm Dacron graft is spatulated and anastomosed with a running suture. If a branched configuration is necessary, side-arms can be added to the graft intraoperatively with a similar or smaller graft. This serves to reduce mediastinal bulk that can result from prefabricated branched grafts with larger proximal components and allows optimal positioning of the side-arm. Relaxation of the sternal retractor allows visualization of the mediastinum as it will lie upon closure. Once the proximal anastomosis is complete, the graft is occluded and the aortic clamp is carefully released. Hemostasis can be aided by placement of simple interrupted sutures. Once this is satisfactory, the patient is systemically heparinized.

Construction of the distal anastomosis begins with clamp placement on the innominate branches prior to placing the proximal clamp to prevent distal embolization. Preoperative imaging and intraoperative palpation of the arteries help to identify suitable sites for clamp placement. The graft may be tunneled posterior to the left brachiocephalic vein if left intact. In addition, branching grafts to the left carotid bifurcation may be tunneled anterior to the common carotid artery. If both carotid arteries require reconstruction, preference is given to the more stenotic lesion.

Once the anastomoses are complete, clamps are released beginning with the subclavian, then the aortic, and finally the carotid. This minimizes risk of emboli to the cerebral circulation. Heparin may be reversed. Closure proceeds with hemostasis and placement of chest or mediastinal tubes as indicated, followed by sternal reapproximation with wire and layered closure of the soft tissues and skin.

During dissection, care must be taken to identify and preserve the vagus, recurrent laryngeal, and phrenic nerves. While direct injury is less common, stretch injury of the brachial plexus can occur with improper patient positioning. Pneumothorax of hemothorax may occur if the thoracic cavity is violated during the procedure. Lymphatic structures, particularly the thoracic duct, deserve careful attention, as lymphatic leak and chylothorax may result. Additional consideration for clamp placement is needed in patients who have undergone coronary artery bypass grafting with the use of the internal mammary artery. Careful dissection and clamp placement can reduce the risk of distal emboli from plaques.

Similarly, thoughtful release of clamps can reduce the risk of showering debris to the cerebral circulation.

Case Continued

The patient was taken to the operating room, and a sternotomy with a hockey stick extension along the right sternocleidomastoid muscle was made. A second incision along the anterior left sternocleidomastoid muscle was also created. A 10-mm Dacron graft was anastomosed in an end-to-side fashion from the ascending aorta, and an 8-mm Dacron side-arm was added.

In consideration of the significant calcific disease of the left carotid system, this was addressed first. The internal and external branches of the carotid artery were clamped prior to dissecting the tunnel and bringing the graft into the lateral incision to prevent distal embolization of the friable plaque. The proximal carotid was then clamped, the internal carotid artery was dissected off of the plaque, which really encompassed most of the common and external branches, and a graft to artery anastomosis was performed in an end-to-end manner.

Next, the innominate artery and its branches were controlled, and the graft was sewn to the spatulated distal innominate artery, again in an end-to-end configuration (Fig. 3). The proximal innominate artery was clamped, transected, and oversewn in two layers with a horizontal mattress followed by a running over-and-over

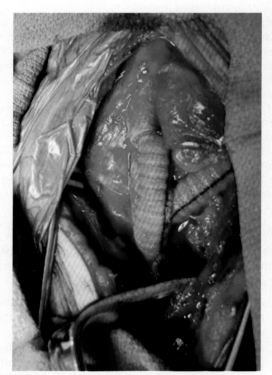

FIGURE 3 • Branching graft from the ascending aortic arch (AA) to the innominate artery (IA) and the left common carotid (LCC) artery.

TABLE 1. Innominate Artery Disease: Open Surgery

Key Technical Steps

1. Review preoperative imaging studies to determine the extent of disease and the optimal locations for clamp placement and anastomoses.
2. Position the patient supine with arms by the side, a shoulder roll in place, and the neck extended and slightly rotated. Prepare the sterile field from the neck to the upper abdomen.
3. Perform a median sternotomy with extension along the anterior right sternocleidomastoid. Extension of the incision can expose the right carotid bifurcation, while the left carotid bifurcation may require a counter incision. The left brachiocephalic vein may be divided or mobilized.
4. Expose the right common carotid artery and the right subclavian artery, preserving the vagus, recurrent laryngeal, and phrenic nerves.
5. Select and prepare the graft. Bifurcated grafts with side-arms of a similar or smaller diameter graft can be constructed intraoperatively.
6. Place a side-biting clamp in the lateral ascending aorta and fashion a vertical aortotomy. Perform the proximal anastomosis between the aorta and the spatulated limb of the graft with a 3-0 or 4-0 Polypropylene suture. Clamp distally on the graft and gently release the aortic clamp. Ensure hemostasis, utilizing simple repair sutures as necessary.
7. Systemically anticoagulate the patient.
8. Place distal clamps on the subclavian and common carotid arteries prior to the proximal innominate artery to prevent distal embolization.
9. Fashion distal anastomosis to spatulated distal innominate artery in end-to-end manner. If the left brachiocephalic vein is intact, tunnel the graft posterior prior to anastomosis. Ensure hemostasis. Remove clamps from the subclavian artery, the proximal graft, and finally the carotid artery.
10. Resect the bypassed portion of the innominate artery and oversew the proximal stump.
11. Ensure hemostasis of the operative field, place chest tubes or mediastinal tubes as needed, reapproximate the sternum with wire, and close the subcutaneous tissues and skin in layers.

Potential Pitfalls

- Injury to the vagus, recurrent laryngeal, or phrenic nerves or the brachial plexus
- Lymphatic leaks from injury to the thoracic duct or other lymphatic vessels
- Distal embolization of plaque during dissection or clamp placement
- Compression of the graft upon closure of the sternotomy

suture. The wound was closed over mediastinal drains. The patient underwent neurologic evaluation following extubation and remained intact (Table 1).

Special Intraoperative Management

Mediastinal crowding with graft compression upon closure of the sternotomy is a concern. Steps to minimize this include lateral placement of the origin of the graft on the ascending aorta, avoiding the more bulky prefabricated branch grafts and relaxing the sternal retractor during placement of side-arms to optimize positioning when the chest is closed. Resection of the bypassed segment of the innominate artery also permits more optimal lie of the graft. If there is still impingement of the graft on closure of the chest, the posterior sternoclavicular joint can be excised with rongeurs.

In treating lesions of the great vessels, it is important to be familiar with the standard branching configuration, as well as common variants, for appropriate surgical planning. Aberrant origin of the right subclavian artery, for example, can alter the course of the right recurrent laryngeal nerve. The vagus nerve within the carotid sheath and the phrenic nerve along the anterior scalene should be identified and preserved if the field of dissection extends into their territory. Finally, the brachial plexus posterior to the subclavian artery may be at risk from either direct injury or stretch injury related to patient positioning. Lymphatic structures, particularly the thoracic duct, also warrant careful attention and ligation (Table 1).

Postoperative Management

Following surgery, patients should be awakened from anesthesia and undergo a full neurologic evaluation and pulse examination. As is done following carotid procedures, strict blood pressure control with the aid of vasoactive medications may be necessary to reduce the risk of reperfusion syndrome. Patients with chest or mediastinal tubes in place should undergo a postoperative chest radiograph and should have the tubes removed when drainage is reduced. Patients should also receive physical therapy and instruction for poststernotomy precautions. Clinical follow-up occurs at 6 weeks, 6 months, and then annually. While CT angiography may help evaluate the repair, a more cost-effective alternative is the combination of duplex ultrasound and bilateral upper extremity blood pressure measurements.

Case Conclusion

The patient was recovered overnight in a monitored unit, with available vasoactive medications administered as needed. A neurologic exam revealed only the preoperative deficits. The mediastinal tubes were removed on postoperative day 2, and follow-up chest roentgenography revealed no accumulation of fluid or pneumothorax. Physical therapy instructed him on appropriate poststernotomy activities. He was discharged without incident, and at his 6-week follow-up, he was event free with patent vessels and graft on follow-up CTA.

TAKE HOME POINTS

- Evaluation of embolic neurologic events should include evaluation of the aortic arch in addition to the carotid bifurcations.
- Indications for intervention include symptomatic presentation, asymptomatic lesions that limit flow to dialysis access or extra-anatomic bypasses, inability to reliably measure blood pressure, or if sternotomy is otherwise being performed in patients with great vessel disease.
- Asymptomatic common carotid disease can be treated using the same criteria as for bifurcation disease.
- Multiple supra-aortic lesions can be addressed at the same procedure. If bilateral carotid arteries require intervention, the more diseased side is addressed first.
- Lateral placement of the graft on the aorta and the construction of side-arms intraoperatively allow optimal positioning of the graft within the mediastinum.
- Clamp placement and removal should proceed in a neuroprotective order to prevent distal embolization.

SUGGESTED READINGS

Berguer R, Morasch MD, Kline RA. Transthoracic repair of innominate and common carotid artery disease: immediate and long-term outcome for 100 consecutive surgical reconstructions. *J Vasc Surg.* 1998;27(1):34-41.

Cherry KJ Jr, McCllough JL, Hallett JW Jr, et al. Technical principles of direct innominate artery revascularization: a comparison of endarterectomy and bypass grafts. *J Vasc Surg.* 1989;9(5):718-723.

Crawford ES, Stowe CL, Powers RW Jr. Occlusion of the innominate, common carotid, and subclavian arteries: long-term results of surgical treatment. *Surgery.* 1983;94(5):781-791.

Kieffer E, Sabatier J, Koskas F, et al. Atherosclerotic innominate artery occlusive disease: early and long-term results of surgical reconstruction. *J Vasc Surg.* 1995;21(2):326-336.

Reul GJ, Jacobs MJ, Gregoric ID, et al. Innominate artery occlusive disease: surgical approach and long-term results. *J Vasc Surg.* 1991;14(3):405-412.

Tracci MC, Cherry KJ. Surgical treatment of great vessel occlusive disease. *Surg Clin North Am.* 2009;89(4):821-836, viii.

Wylie EJ, Effeney DJ. Surgery of the aortic arch branches and vertebral arteries. *Surg Clin North Am.* 1979;59(4):669-680.

CLINICAL SCENARIO CASE QUESTIONS

1. Which of the following patients with radiographic evidence of great vessel arteriosclerosis does not warrant operative intervention?

    a. A 76-year-old woman with end-stage renal disease and a poorly functioning right upper extremity arteriovenous fistula

    b. A 47-year-old male with three-vessel coronary disease being scheduled for a coronary-artery bypass graft with a heavily calcified origin of the innominate artery

    c. A 68-year-old male with a recent cerebrovascular accident

d. A 59-year-old female with a calcified innominate artery and no neurologic symptoms

e. A 72-year-old male with a 90% stenosis of the proximal left common carotid artery

2. Which intraoperative maneuver will reduce bulk within the mediastinum and allow appropriate graft positioning?

a. Use of a prefabricated bifurcated graft

b. Resecting the bypassed segment of artery and oversewing the proximal stump

c. Placing the graft on the anterior surface of the ascending aorta

d. Widening the sternal retractor during the procedure to allow more room for the repair

27 Endovascular Management of Innominate Artery Disease

MARTYN KNOWLES and CARLOS H. TIMARAN

Presentation

A 69-year-old male presents with right arm weakness and difficulty performing routine tasks. He also endorses a transient episode of left arm and leg numbness and weakness several weeks ago, and episodes of near-syncope and vertigo. His past medical history includes hypertension, peripheral vascular disease, chronic obstructive pulmonary disease (COPD), diabetes mellitus, and coronary artery disease requiring coronary artery bypass grafting (CABG) 9 years before presentation. He has been a heavy smoker for most of his life. On physical examination, he is neurologically intact and has a right carotid bruit. His blood pressure is 80/54 mm Hg in the right arm and 167/76 mm Hg in the left arm. He has a palpable pulse in the left arm but not in the right. A carotid duplex ultrasound is ordered.

Differential Diagnosis

The differential diagnosis includes stroke or transient ischemic attack (TIA), degenerative joint disease, musculoskeletal disease, thoracic outlet syndrome, occlusive brachiocephalic vessel disease, and vertebrobasilar insufficiency (VBI).

Workup

A complete duplex ultrasound is obtained; no prior study is available for comparison. The ultrasound shows a peak systolic velocity (PSV) of 284 cm/s in the right internal carotid artery (ICA), a PSV of 100 cm/s in the right common carotid artery (CCA), and an end-diastolic velocity (EDV) of 186 cm/s in the ICA, yielding an ICA/CCA ratio of 2.8. The vertebral artery on the right is occluded. On the left, there is a PSV of 103 cm/s in the ICA, a PSV of 54 cm/s in the CCA, and an EDV of 53 cm/s, yielding an ICA/CCA ratio of 0.8. Interpretation: right carotid artery severe stenosis, 80% to 99%; his right vertebral is occluded, left carotid artery mild stenosis, 1% to 49%; the left vertebral is blunted.

A magnetic resonance (MR) angiogram is obtained and reveals severe innominate artery stenosis greater than 90%, left proximal subclavian artery occlusion, left proximal CCA stenosis greater than 90%, and severe right internal carotid stenosis (greater than 70%) just distal to the bulb.

Discussion

The brachiocephalic branches of the aorta include the innominate artery, the left CCA, and the left subclavian artery. Congenital variations are not infrequent and include a bovine arch with a common orifice for the innominate artery and left CCA and an aberrant takeoff of the right subclavian artery. The brachiocephalic arteries, also known as the great vessels, supply the upper extremities and the brain. The great vessels are frequently affected by atherosclerotic disease, which accounts for 70% of cases, which can cause flow-limiting stenoses or embolism. Atherosclerotic disease can cause single or multivessel disease in 60% and 40% of patients, respectively.

Symptoms of severe atherosclerotic disease of the great vessels include stroke, TIA, upper extremity ischemia, and VBI. Single-vessel carotid disease is more likely to cause symptoms of a stroke or TIA. Innominate artery disease can cause stroke, TIA, upper extremity ischemia, or a combination of these symptoms. Occlusion of the proximal subclavian artery can cause a steal syndrome involving the vertebral arteries. VBI is more likely in, but not exclusive of, multivessel disease. Symptoms of VBI include vertigo, diplopia, dizziness, drop attacks, and ataxia. Lesions involving the subclavian or innominate arteries can cause upper extremity claudication, embolism, or distal ischemia. There are other diseases that can cause brachiocephalic disease including giant cell arteritis, Takayasu's disease, aneurysm, dissection, infections (syphilis and tuberculosis), radiation-induced injury, and trauma.

The diagnostic evaluation of patients with presumed brachiocephalic disease should start with a complete physical examination. Assessment of the upper extremity pulses and blood pressures should be performed and documented. The carotid arteries should be evaluated for bruits. Complete duplex ultrasonography is usually recommended as the initial imaging modality. Careful

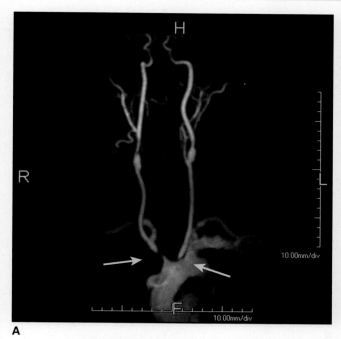 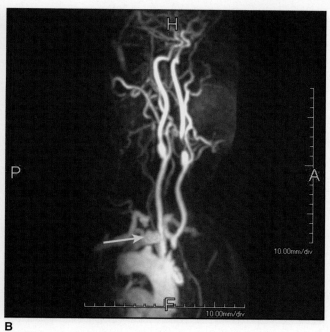

A   **B**

FIGURE 1 • MR angiogram showing severe innominate artery stenosis, left subclavian occlusion, and proximal left CCA stenosis. (arrows, lesions in sequential order from left to right).

examination of the carotid, vertebral, and subclavian arteries should be sought. Demonstration of poststenotic flow or reversal of flow should raise suspicion for occlusive disease. Computerized tomography (CT) and MR angiography can provide excellent imaging of the aorta and brachiocephalic vessels and have mostly replaced the need for angiography. Detailed images with 1-mm or finer cuts can accurately be used for careful case planning. Angiography should, however, be used if there is any question of severity or location of disease and for the assessment of flow dynamics or collateral flow (Figs. 1 and 2).

Indications for repair include symptomatic lesions (VBI, stroke, TIA, and upper extremity symptoms). Asymptomatic subclavian-vertebral or subclavian-carotid steal from innominate artery stenosis is not an indication for repair. Severe stenosis of the proximal left subclavian artery, even if asymptomatic, should be pursued if the patient has current or future plans for use of the left internal mammary artery for bypass in CABG (Fig. 3).

Diagnosis and Treatment

Diagnosis of severe symptomatic brachiocephalic occlusive disease with severe stenosis of the innominate artery, proximal left CCA, and right ICA requires prompt surgical intervention. Options for brachiocephalic atherosclerotic arterial occlusive disease include both open and endovascular revascularization. In the current case, an endovascular option is sought due to the high morbidity and mortality associated with open surgical

revascularization. The patient has severe COPD, history of CABG, and multivessel disease that would require a redo sternotomy (Fig. 4).

Options for Surgical Repair

Options for open repair of brachiocephalic atherosclerotic arterial occlusive disease include transthoracic

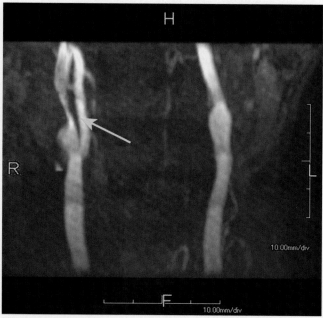

FIGURE 2 • MR angiogram showing severe right ICA stenosis just distal to the bifurcation (*arrow*).

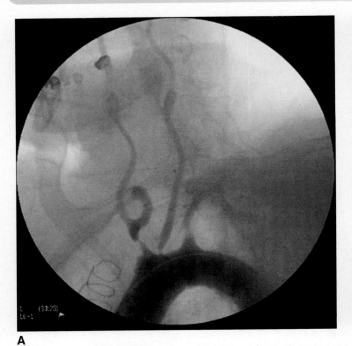

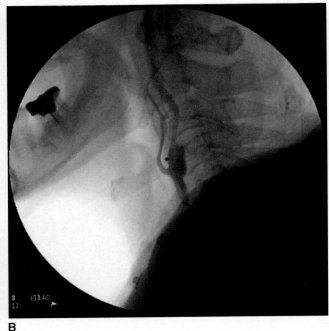

FIGURE 3 • Intraoperative angiography showing: **(A)** Severe stenosis of the proximal left CCA and innominate artery, and left subclavian artery occlusion. **(B)** Severe stenosis of the right ICA distal to the bifurcation.

repair and extra-anatomic repair. Transthoracic repair involves a bypass from the ascending aorta or proximal arch to the involved vessels distal to the disease or endarterectomy. Results after transthoracic repair include an operative mortality of 3% to 13%, stroke risk of 2.9% to 8%, with excellent 88% to 96% patency at 10 years.

Extra-anatomic repair is typically used for single vessel disease, such as subclavian artery disease, especially in high-risk patients. Carotid-subclavian artery transposition or bypass is performed with minimal morbidity, with patency rates of carotid-subclavian artery bypass of 82% to 96% at 5 years.

Endovascular management of brachiocephalic disease should be considered in patients who are high risk for open repair or those who have lesions amenable to endovascular techniques and has become more popular over recent years. Careful planning is required for interventions, especially evaluation of the aortic arch for significant disease and plaque that could be dislodged during manipulation. Meticulous examination of preoperative imaging relating to anatomy, lesion location, and case planning is imperative.

Endovascular Approach

Arch anatomy is critical for procedural planning and assessing the difficulty in cannulating vessels, particularly because of the likelihood of a proximal vessel stenosis and elongation of the arch with deeper origin of the great vessels. In most cases, the brachiocephalic vessels come off the aorta at the most superior part of the arch; difficulty arises if the great vessels arise on the ascending portion of the arch with a steep angle.

Crossing the lesion in the presence of proximal stenosis of the great vessels adds additional difficulty to the case, with the chance of embolism with successive attempts. Most endovascular failures for the treatment of brachiocephalic lesions are related to inability to cross the lesion. Once across, consideration should be given to placing a filter for embolic protection during manipulation of the lesion with ballooning and stenting. Most practitioners will perform percutaneous transluminal angioplasty (PTA) with stenting; however, results of PTA alone are reasonable. Balloon-expandable covered stents, such as the iCAST (Atrium, Hudson, NH), may also be used. Description of techniques for cannulation of the specific brachiocephalic vessels may be complex and discussed in depth elsewhere. In addressing the subclavian vessels, particularly the left subclavian after previous CABG, careful consideration must be given to the avoidance of covering the vertebral and internal thoracic or mammary artery. In difficult arch anatomy or a tight proximal lesion in the subclavian or innominate artery, brachial artery access is a useful adjunct. When intervening on the common carotid arteries, cerebral protection should be considered. When antegrade great vessel cannulation is difficult,

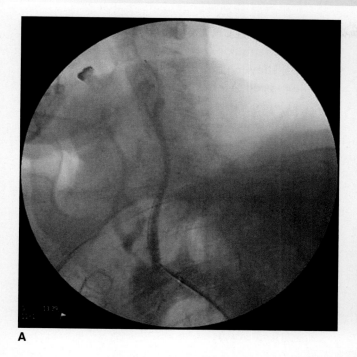

A

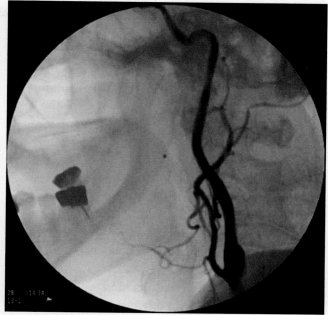

B

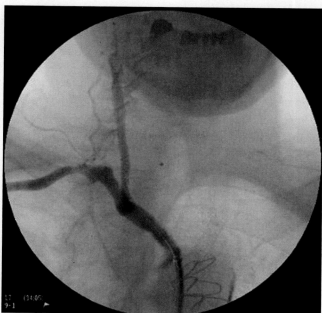

C

FIGURE 4 • Completion angiography following stenting of **(A)** the left common carotid, **(B)** right internal carotid and **(C)** innominate arteries with excellent result and minimal residual stenosis.

retrograde access via an open exposure should be entertained.

Patency after endovascular brachiocephalic intervention appears to be approximately 75% to 90% at 5 years, fairly durable when it comes to endovascular repair but appears to be inferior to open bypass. However, given the much improved morbidity and mortality compared to open repair, especially in high-risk patients, endovascular management remains a good option.

Case Conclusion

The patient is brought to the operating room, and arterial monitoring via a radial arterial line is obtained. He is currently on dual antiplatelet therapy with aspirin and clopidogrel. During endovascular brachiocephalic intervention, the patient receives minimal sedation so as to converse with the surgery team for continued neurologic exams. The groins are prepped and draped. Ultrasound-guided access, after local anesthetic infiltration, is accomplished and a 5-French sheath is placed. A femoral arteriogram is performed ensuring anterior access over the femoral head above the bifurcation. If incorrectly placed, the sheath is pulled and pressure held prior to heparin administration. Once systemic heparinization is accomplished, activated clotting time are monitored and maintained greater than 300 seconds. A Glidewire (Terumo Medical Corporation, Somerset, NJ) is placed and advanced into the aorta, and a flush catheter is then placed over the wire.

A left anterior oblique orientation with the c-arm is accomplished to open up the arch; preoperative imaging with 3D reconstruction allows determination of the correct angle without the use of fluoroscopy. An arch angiogram is performed for vessel location and to confirm the presence of a critical proximal stenosis of the left CCA. A 7-French sheath is advanced to the distal arch, and cannulation of the left CCA is performed. An 8-mm balloon expandable stent is placed over a support working wire. Completion angiogram shows minimal residual stenosis with good apposition. The wire is pulled out into the arch, exchanged for a Glidewire, and the innominate artery is then cannulated. Selected catheterization of the right CCA is performed. The Glidewire is exchanged for a stiff wire, and balloon angioplasty of the lesion is performed with a 7-mm balloon followed by placement of a 9-mm balloon expandable stent, with excellent result.

The 7-French sheath is then advanced into the right CCA, and an Accunet (Abbott, Abbott Park, IL) filter is carefully tracked into the right ICA, past the tight stenosis, after cervical angiograms are performed for roadmapping. The filter is placed in the distal ICA and deployed, followed by balloon angioplasty with a 5-mm balloon. Careful monitoring of the heart rate is performed during ballooning, ensuring no bradycardia. Subsequently, a 7-mm tapered Acculink (Abbott, Abbott Park, IL) stent is placed from the internal

carotid into the CCA. Completion angiograms in multiple orientations show no evidence of residual stenosis, showing no need for reballooning, and the filter is collapsed and removed. Completion cervical and cerebral angiograms are performed showing excellent collateral intracerebral flow and no evidence of embolism. The filter is flushed and shows no evidence of embolic debris. The patient remained neurologically intact throughout the procedure. The heparin is not reversed, and a vascular closure device is used for arterial puncture closure. After pressure was held and there was no hematoma, sterile dressings were applied, and the patient was moved to the intensive care unit whilst remaining flat. Careful monitoring of the blood pressure and neurologic status was continued overnight (Table 1).

TABLE 1. Innominate Artery Disease—Endovascular Approach

Key Technical Steps

1. The patient is placed on dual antiplatelet therapy with aspirin and clopidogrel.
2. During endovascular brachiocephalic intervention, the patient receives minimal sedation so as to converse with the surgery team for continued neurologic exams.
3. Ultrasound-guided access, after local anesthetic infiltration, is accomplished and a sheath is placed.
4. Once systemic heparinization is accomplished, activated clotting time are monitored and maintained >300 seconds.
5. A left anterior oblique orientation with the c-arm is accomplished to open up the arch; preoperative imaging with 3D reconstruction allows determination of the correct angle without the use of fluoroscopy.
6. An arch angiogram is performed for vessel location and to confirm the presence of a critical proximal stenosis of the innominate artery.
7. A 7-French sheath is advanced to the distal arch, and cannulation of the innominate artery with a Glidewire is performed. Selected catheterization of the right CCA is performed. The Glidewire is exchanged for a stiff wire, and balloon angioplasty of the lesion is performed with a 7-mm balloon followed by placement of a 9-mm balloon expandable stent, with excellent result.
8. Completion angiograms in multiple orientations show no evidence of residual stenosis, showing no need for reballooning, and the filter is collapsed and removed.

Potential Pitfalls

- Careful monitoring of the heart rate is performed during ballooning, ensuring no bradycardia.
- Careful monitoring of the blood pressure and neurologic status is continued overnight to prevent hyperperfusion syndrome in this patient with multivessel cerebrovascular occlusive disease.

Postoperative Management

The patient is discharged on aspirin for life and clopidogrel for 1 month. Duplex ultrasonography should be obtained after 1 month and followed every 6 months for 2 years, then yearly thereafter. Ensuring smoking cessation is imperative as well as maintaining lifelong statin therapy.

TAKE HOME POINTS

- Patients with unequal upper extremity blood pressure should raise concern for brachiocephalic occlusive disease.
- Symptoms of brachiocephalic disease depend on whether one or more vessels are involved and can include stroke, TIA, upper extremity ischemia, and vertebrobasilar insufficiency.
- Atherosclerosis is the most common pathology; however, Takayasu's disease, giant cell arteritis, trauma, dissection, infection, dissection, and aneurysms can all cause brachiocephalic disease.
- Asymptomatic disease, with the exception of proximal left subclavian disease in patients with presence or need for CABG with left internal mammary artery bypass graft, is treated conservatively.
- Options for repair include open repair via a sternotomy and bypass or endovascular stenting.

SUGGESTED READINGS

AbuRahma AF, Bates MC, Stone PA, et al. Angioplasty and stenting versus carotid-subclavian bypass for the treatment of isolated subclavian artery disease. *J Endovasc Ther.* 2007;14(5):698-704.

Berguer R, Morasch MD, Kline RA. Transthoracic repair of innominate and common carotid artery disease: immediate and long-term outcome for 100 consecutive surgical reconstructions. *J Vasc Surg.* 1998;27(1):34-41; discussion 42.

Berguer R, Morasch MD, Kline RA, et al. Cervical reconstruction of the supra-aortic trunks: a 16-year experience. *J Vasc Surg.* 1999;29(2):239-246; discussion 46-48.

Schneider PA. Brachiocephalic interventions. In: *Endovascular Skills: Guidewire and Catheter Skills for Endovascular Surgery.* 3rd ed. New York: Informa Healthcare; 2009: 381-402.

Woo EY, Fairman RM, Velazquez OC, et al. Endovascular therapy of symptomatic innominate-subclavian arterial occlusive lesions. *Vasc Endovascular Surg.* 2006;40(1): 27-33.

CLINICAL SCENARIO CASE QUESTIONS

1. Symptoms of brachiocephalic disease can present with which symptoms?
   a. Stroke
   b. TIA
   c. Upper extremity ischemia
   d. Vertebrobasilar insufficiency
   e. All of the above

2. The most common pathology causing brachiocephalic disease is:
   a. Atherosclerosis
   b. Takayasu's disease
   c. Giant cell arteritis
   d. Trauma
   e. Dissection

28 Neurogenic Thoracic Outlet Syndrome

ROBERT W. THOMPSON and CHANDU VEMURI

Presentation

A 28-year-old female postal clerk presents to your office with a 3-year history of left hand, arm, and neck pain. She also experiences left upper extremity numbness and tingling that are aggravated by use, especially with the arm elevated, as well as occipital headaches. All of these complaints began several months after an automobile collision in which the patient suffered a hyperextension strain to the neck but had no definitive cervical spine injury. Her symptoms did not improve with several courses of physical therapy, and she was advised to continue working despite the discomfort. Over the past year, she eventually found it too painful to work; her symptoms progressed to the extent that she often has difficulty sleeping at night. The patient has seen seven different physician specialists over the past 2 years without insight into the cause of her symptoms, and she has not experienced any symptomatic improvement with a variety of different treatment modalities. Previous evaluations have included cervical spine and shoulder radiographs, computed tomography (CT) and magnetic resonance imaging (MRI) of the head and neck, and nerve conduction and electromyography studies. The results from all of these tests have been described as normal.

Differential Diagnosis

A large number of conditions have to be considered in the initial differential diagnosis of this patient's symptoms. This list includes cervical spine arthritis, degenerative disc disease or spinal stenosis, posttraumatic cervical spine strain, and fibromyalgia of the trapezius muscles. Shoulder tendinitis or other degenerative joint conditions should also be considered, along with acromioclavicular impingement syndrome, epicondylitis, ulnar nerve (cubital tunnel) entrapment syndrome, and median nerve (carpal tunnel) compression syndrome. The diffuse and nonspecific nature of her complaints might also make it necessary to consider a peripheral neuropathy or multiple sclerosis. Given the frequent lack of objective findings on previous evaluations, it is also important to include even psychogenic causes of her symptoms and the possibility of secondary gain.

Diagnostic Testing

Most of the entities in this differential diagnosis can be evaluated either by specific elements of the physical examination or by diagnostic tests that yield positive findings in the presence of the condition. For example, the presence of degenerative cervical spine disease or disc herniation on CT scan or MRI could provide definitive evidence of these conditions. Alternatively, negative test results can also definitively exclude some of the diagnoses in question; thus, the absence of focal slowing of nerve conduction over the wrist excludes carpal tunnel syndrome. In this case, the results of previous evaluations have effectively eliminated a problem restricted to the cervical spine, the shoulder joint, or a single peripheral nerve distribution. In this situation, a diagnosis of neurogenic thoracic outlet syndrome (TOS) begins to emerge as a distinct possibility.

Neurogenic TOS is an uncommon condition often not considered until other entities have been excluded, and there is ongoing symptomatic deterioration. Unfortunately, there are no single aspects of the physical examination or specific diagnostic tests that can confirm or exclude a diagnosis of neurogenic TOS. Establishing a diagnosis of neurogenic TOS thereby depends on a constellation of subjective symptoms and corroborative findings on physical examination that fit into a typical clinical pattern, combined with the exclusion of other, more common conditions.

Case Continued

Physical examination reveals a cool left hand without signs of ischemia, thromboembolism, or venous congestion. The left arm has a full range of motion with pain, numbness, and tingling induced by abduction to 180 degrees. There is tenderness upon palpation of the left supraclavicular space with reproduction of left hand symptoms. Muscle spasm is detectable along the border of the left trapezius and sternocleidomastoid muscles. There are pain and tenderness along the medial border of the scapula.

In performing the Adson's test, the left radial artery pulse is not easily palpable with the arm at rest but is present. The pulse seems to dampen with the arm positioned at 90 degrees abduction or higher. The right radial pulse is also diminished at rest but is palpable in all arm positions. The patient is unable to complete a 3-minute elevated arm stress test (EAST), due to the development of severe left arm and hand pain within 10 seconds of arm elevation. Examination of the right upper extremity is completely normal.

On moderate palpation of the left infraclavicular subcoracoid space, the patient reports a reproduction of symptoms similar to those aggravated by repetitive use of the arm. Furthermore, with the patient's hand pressed against yours and flexion of the pectoralis major muscle, the symptoms induced by subcoracoid palpation are relieved.

Diagnosis

The most probable diagnosis is left neurogenic TOS with brachial plexus compression at the level of the scalene triangle and the subcoracoid (pectoralis minor) space. The factors supporting the diagnosis are the history of previous neck trauma and progressive symptoms affecting the entire arm and hand. The absence of a previous diagnosis despite multiple tests and evaluations is also supportive of neurogenic TOS. Although numbness and tingling in the hand are often considered worrisome symptoms, pain is the most disabling and predominant symptom for which treatment is directed. The findings on examination that support neurogenic TOS include localized muscle spasm and tenderness over the left scalene triangle and pectoralis minor tendon, with reproduction of hand symptoms on palpation. Although positional ablation of the radial pulse suggests compression of the subclavian artery within the scalene triangle, this is a common finding even in asymptomatic individuals; the positional pulse examination therefore offers little insight into the nature or cause of the symptoms. The most important finding is difficulty completing the EAST: a positive test is highly suggestive of neurogenic TOS, whereas a negative result calls the diagnosis into question.

Neurogenic TOS is thought to arise as a result of variations in individual anatomy that predispose to neurovascular compression, combined with some form of trauma to the scalene and/or pectoralis minor muscles. One of the anatomical factors associated with TOS is the presence of a congenital cervical rib. Radiographs should be inspected to evaluate whether such an anomaly is present, because it may help to solidify the diagnosis and influence management decisions.

Radiographs
Radiology Report
Normal radiographs of the upper chest and cervical spine, with no evidence of cervical rib.

Discussion

In some cases where TOS is suspected, one must consider the possibility of subclavian artery compression resulting in formation of a poststenotic subclavian aneurysm. These lesions are usually clinically silent until they produce thromboembolism with occlusion of distal vessels within the upper extremity. Because the clinical presentation of this complication may be subtle, the examiner must be sure that any changes in perfusion of the hand do not represent ischemia. When physical examination is equivocal or in cases where a cervical rib is present, it is useful to consider magnetic resonance (MR) angiography as a noninvasive test by which to rule out the presence of a subclavian aneurysm.

Magnetic Resonance Angiography
MRA Report
A contrast-enhanced MR angiogram was performed to evaluate the left subclavian artery (*arrow*) at the level of the thoracic outlet. With the arms at rest, the subclavian arteries exhibit a normal contour and luminal caliber, without signs of occlusive disease or aneurysm dilatation (Fig. 1A). With the arms elevated above the head, the subclavian arteries remain patent without signs of positional occlusion (Fig. 1B). The results of this study are normal.

Recommendation

A trial of physical therapy specifically targeted toward relief of neurogenic TOS is recommended. Although the patient has not improved with previous courses of therapy, it is unlikely that these efforts were undertaken with the specific diagnosis of TOS. Because therapy for TOS differs from that given for other related conditions, this treatment should be conducted by a therapist with expertise, interest, and experience in management of TOS. Adjunctive measures should be recommended, including use of anti-inflammatory medications and muscle relaxants. Use of narcotic pain medications is not recommended.

Case Continued

After 8 weeks of physical therapy, the patient has had no change in symptoms. The therapist reports that the patient has made minimal improvement in pain-free range of motion and that her progress is limited by ongoing pain with activity. At this point, she returns to clinic to consider evaluation for surgical intervention. Following the visit, she undergoes an anterior scalene and pectoralis minor muscle block with local anesthetic under imaging guidance, which results in complete relief of symptoms for several hours.

Diagnosis and Recommendation

This patient may be considered to have neurogenic TOS refractory to conservative treatment, and surgical decompression is recommended. The patient is

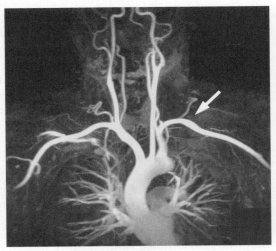

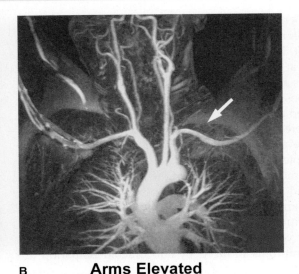

A   **Arms at Rest**   B   **Arms Elevated**

FIGURE 1 • **A:** A contrast-enhanced MR angiogram was performed to evaluate the left subclavian artery (*arrow*) at the level of the thoracic outlet. With the arms at rest, the subclavian arteries exhibit a normal contour and luminal caliber, without signs of occlusive disease or aneurysm dilatation. **B:** With the arms elevated above the head, the subclavian arteries remain patent without signs of positional occlusion.

informed that a substantial improvement in symptoms can be expected in approximately 85% to 90% of patients following appropriate surgical treatment but that complete long-term relief of all symptoms (i.e., "cure") is unlikely. It is emphasized that ongoing physical therapy and rehabilitation will remain an essential part of her overall treatment. Potential complications of surgery are discussed, including nerve or vascular injuries and temporary dysfunction of the phrenic and/or long thoracic nerves, with an incidence in experienced hands of less than 2%. The positive response to the localized muscle block is a very strong predictor of symptom relief following surgery.

Surgical Approach

The patient has compression in both the supraclavicular space and the infraclavicular subcoracoid space requiring surgical decompression in both areas. The recommended approach to this problem is supraclavicular exploration with complete resection of the anterior and middle scalene muscles, first rib resection, and brachial plexus neurolysis, along with pectoralis minor tenotomy. During dissection and resection of the anterior scalene muscle, care is taken to identify and preserve the phrenic nerve, brachial plexus nerve roots C5-T1, and the subclavian artery. Similarly, during dissection and resection of the middle scalene muscle, one must identify and preserve the long thoracic nerve as well as the brachial plexus (Fig. 2). Any associated fibrous bands and muscle anomalies within the scalene triangle are also resected. Complete brachial plexus neurolysis is included to remove any associated fibroinflammatory tissue that may be contributing to nerve irritation. It is recommended

that first rib resection be included in most decompression procedures, although some specialists avoid resection of the first rib if they believe that adequate decompression has been accomplished by scalenectomy alone. The first rib is resected posteriorly to its junction with the C7 transverse process, with clear visualization and protec-

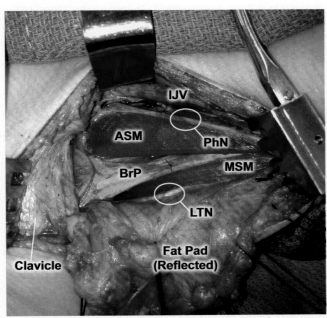

FIGURE 2 • Sample operative image of the critical view of the essential structures in a standard supraclavicular thoracic outlet decompression. IJV, internal jugular vein; ASM, anterior scalene muscle; PhN, phrenic nerve; BrP, Brachial plexus; MSM, middle scalene muscle; LTN, long thoracic nerve.

tion of the C8 and T1 nerve roots, and anteriorly to a level just medial to the scalene tubercle, underneath the clavicle. Following supraclavicular decompression, the brachial plexus nerve roots are wrapped with an absorbable polymeric film in an effort to reduce postoperative adhesions. A closed-suction drain is placed into the pleural space and is removed several days later. Two small multihole perfusion catheters are placed within the resection bed and connected to an osmotic pump, which will provide continuous infusion of local anesthetic for the first three postoperative days.

Pectoralis minor tenotomy has emerged as an important surgical adjunct in the treatment of neurogenic TOS in patients with evidence of nerve compression in the subcoracoid space and can be readily performed at the same time as supraclavicular decompression. A vertical incision is made adjacent to the deltopectoral groove in the lateral infraclavicular space. Dissection is carried down to the pectoralis major muscle, which can then be retracted medially to expose the underlying pectoralis minor muscle. The pectoralis minor tendon is dissected circumferentially and then divided with the cautery at its insertion onto the coracoid process (Fig. 3).

Discussion

The central goal of thoracic outlet decompression is to remove the structural elements that contribute to brachial plexus nerve root compression and irritation. This has traditionally been focused on resection of the first rib at the base of the scalene space. However, greater appreciation for the role of the anterior and middle scalene muscles has led to renewed emphasis over the past

decade on the need for scalenectomy, with or without rib resection. It has also become appreciated that scar tissue surrounding the brachial plexus nerve roots may play an important role in nerve irritation.

Several different operative approaches for thoracic outlet decompression have been described including (1) transaxillary first rib resection, (2) supraclavicular scalenectomy with or without first rib resection, and (3) posterior thoracotomy with first rib resection. Although the transaxillary approach allows removal of the first rib, it is usually not feasible to perform complete scalenectomy, brachial plexus neurolysis, or vascular reconstructions, if necessary, without repositioning the patient and using an alternate incision. In contrast, all of these procedures can be performed through the supraclavicular approach. Although there is not yet clear evidence that outcomes are different with any of these approaches, the risks of injury, incomplete decompression, and recurrence appear to be lowest with supraclavicular exploration. Supraclavicular exploration also has the advantage that any associated procedures involving the subclavian artery or vein can be readily performed through the same exposure.

The importance of evaluation and surgical treatment of compression of the brachial plexus in the subcoracoid space has long been recognized. Recent evidence has shown that some patients only have nerve compression in this anatomic area, in which case pectoralis minor tenotomy alone may provide relief of symptoms. Therefore, it is imperative to assess and treat this anatomic area of potential compression as well as that related to the scalene triangle (Table 1).

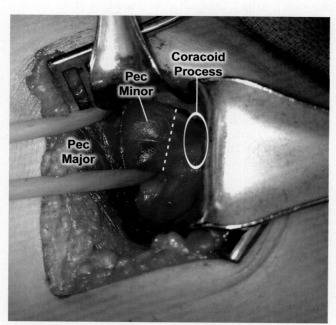

FIGURE 3 • Sample operative image of the pectoralis minor tendon before transection.

TABLE 1. Neurogenic Thoracic Outlet Syndrome

Key Technical Steps

1. Supraclavicular incision with mobilization of the scalene fat pad
2. Resection of the entire anterior scalene muscle
3. Resection of the middle scalene muscle
4. Resection of the first rib from its junction with the C7 transverse process to beyond the scalene tubercle
5. Complete neurolysis of the brachial plexus
6. Placement of absorbable anti-adhesion film, closed-suction pleural drain, and anesthetic perfusion catheters
7. Pectoralis minor tenotomy in select cases

Potential Pitfalls

- Injury to the subclavian artery during division of the anterior scalene muscle
- Injury to the phrenic nerve during division of the anterior scalene muscle or long thoracic nerve during resection of the middle scale muscle
- Injury to C8-T1 nerve roots during division of the posterior aspect of the first rib
- Injury to the thoracic duct
- Injury to the brachial plexus
- Incomplete decompression resulting in persistent symptoms

Postoperative Management

Use of the affected extremity is not restricted following operation, and physical therapy begins on postoperative day 1 with increasing activity over the first few postoperative weeks. The continuous bupivacaine perfusion catheters are removed on postoperative day 3. The closed suction pleural drain is removed in clinic the day following discharge, and a postprocedure chest x-ray is completed.

These patients have usually had a long history of procedures, treatments, and medications before their treatment of TOS. Thus, pain control can be challenging, and it is critical to evaluate their pain and provide appropriate analgesia given their level of tolerance. A side effect of the narcotic regimen is constipation, and thus a strict bowel regimen must be set in place.

Patients will often complain of mild paresthesias in the distribution of C8-T1. Traction injury to the phrenic nerve frequently results in an elevated hemidiaphragm on the surgical side. The partial paralysis can result in dyspnea on exertion. Injury to the long thoracic nerve can result in winging of the scapula. The resolution of neurologic symptoms is related to the degree of injury at initial operation. Simple traction injuries resolve over time, while more severe nerve injuries or transections may require intervention for symptom relief.

While major vascular injuries are uncommon in high-volume centers, thoracic duct injuries can occur. This is most common with operations on the left side. The management is similar to that of thoracic duct injury from other operations.

Patients with nTOS require long-term follow-up. While their immediate postsurgical issues resolve by 4 to 6 months, they require additional evaluation for continued physical therapy, medication alteration, and evaluation for persistent or recurrent symptoms.

Case Conclusion

The patient underwent successful left supraclavicular thoracic outlet decompression with scalenectomy, brachial plexus neurolysis, and first rib resection, along with concomitant pectoralis minor tenotomy. The hospital stay was 4 days with no complications, and the supraclavicular drain was removed in the office on postoperative day 6. She began a focused program of postoperative physical therapy 4 weeks after operation and returned to work, with restrictions, at 6 weeks. Over the next 2 months, she continued to increase activity with the left arm and work restrictions were gradually lifted. By 16 weeks, she had minimal and easily managed symptoms, had discontinued all medications, and was considered to have had an excellent outcome from surgical treatment. Periodic office visits for follow-up continued over the following year, during which she remained well.

TAKE HOME POINTS

- Neurogenic TOS is a diagnosis of exclusion, and all other more common etiologies of extremity symptoms must be ruled out.
- Physical examination can aid in diagnosis, and reproduction of symptoms with palpation of the scalene triangle or infraclavicular subcoracoid space supports the diagnosis.
- Response to scalene and/or pectoralis minor nerve blocks indicates a higher likelihood of symptom relief with surgery.
- Complete surgical decompression of the supraclavicular and subcoracoid spaces can provide lasting relief in the majority of patients.
- Patients require a planned regimen of pre- and postoperative physical therapy with long-term follow-up.

SUGGESTED READINGS

Cheng SW, Reilly LM, Nelken NA, et al. Neurogenic thoracic outlet decompression: rationale for sparing the first rib. *Cardiovasc Surg.* 1995;3:617-624.

Hempel GK, Shutze WP, Anderson JF, et al. 770 consecutive supraclavicular first rib resections for thoracic outlet syndrome. *Ann Vasc Surg.* 1996;10:456-463.

Juvonen T, Satta J, Laitala P, et al. Anomalies at the thoracic outlet are frequent in the general population. *Am J Surg.* 1995;170:33-37.

Lindgren KA, Oksala I. Long-term outcome of surgery for thoracic outlet syndrome. *Am J Surg.* 1995;169:358-360.

Novak CB. Conservative management of thoracic outlet syndrome. *Semin Thorac Cardiovasc Surg.* 1996;8:201-207.

Reilly LM, Stoney RJ. Supraclavicular approach for thoracic outlet decompression. *J Vasc Surg.* 1988;8:329-334.

Sanders RJ. *Thoracic Outlet Syndrome: A Common Sequelae of Neck Injuries.* Philadelphia, PA: JB Lippincott; 1991.

Sanders RJ, Jackson CG, Banchero N, et al. Scalene muscle abnormalities in traumatic thoracic outlet syndrome. *Am J Surg.* 1990;159:231-236.

Sanders RJ, Raymer S. The supraclavicular approach to scalenectomy and first rib resection: description of technique. *J Vasc Surg.* 1985;2:751-756.

Thompson RW, Petrinec D. Surgical treatment of thoracic outlet compression syndromes. I. Diagnostic considerations and transaxillary first rib resection. *Ann Vasc Surg.* 1997;11:315-323.

Thompson RW, Petrinec D, Toursarkissian B. Surgical treatment of thoracic outlet compression syndromes. II. Supraclavicular exploration and vascular reconstruction. *Ann Vasc Surg.* 1997;11:442-451.

Urschel HC Jr. The transaxillary approach for treatment of thoracic outlet syndromes. *Semin Thorac Cardiovasc Surg.* 1996;8:214-220.

Vemuri C, Wittenberg AM, Caputo FJ, et al. Early effectiveness of isolated pectoralis minor tenotomy in selected patients with neurogenic thoracic outlet syndrome. *J Vasc Surg.* 2013;57: 1345-1352.

CLINICAL SCENARIO CASE QUESTIONS

1. In postoperative clinic, you have the patient stand and push against you with both hands. You notice that her scapula protrudes from her back during this test. Her exam is otherwise unremarkable. Which nerve was likely injured?

   a. Phrenic
   b. Long thoracic
   c. Vagus
   d. Hypoglossal
   e. Lateral pectoral

2. During division of the posterior aspect of the first rib, which nerve roots are at risk of injury and therefore must be clearly visualized?

   a. C2-C3
   b. C4-C6
   c. C5-C7
   d. C8-T1
   e. T1-T3

Venous Thoracic Outlet Syndrome

LOUIS L. NGUYEN

Presentation

An 18-year-old right-hand dominant high school basketball player presents with acute swelling of his right arm. He has no other medical history. His vital signs are normal. On physical examination, he has a circumferentially enlarged right arm with prominent chest varicosities. He has palpable brachial and radial pulses bilaterally. No motor or sensory deficits are noted. He has no family history of clotting disorder.

Differential Diagnosis

Acute swelling in the arm most likely represents a deep venous thrombosis (DVT). When upper extremity DVT occurs in young, active persons, the cause is presumed to be effort thrombosis (Paget-von Schrötter syndrome), where structures of the thoracic outlet contribute to the stenosis and compression of the subclavian vein. Other causes of upper extremity DVT include the presence of intravenous catheters, external venous compression from trauma, and congenital or acquired hypercoagulable states, including malignancy. Most often, venous TOS (VTOS) occurs in the dominant arm, though nondominant VTOS can occur in persons who participate in bilateral arm sports (kayaking, swimming, weightlifting) or occupations (package handlers, retail shelf stockers).

Workup and Initial Treatment

Confirmation of the DVT and assessment of the extent of thrombosis can be made on venous duplex. Patients with acute DVT should be started on systemic anticoagulation unless otherwise contraindicated. A plain chest x-ray can evaluate for bony abnormalities, such as a cervical rib, a hypoplastic rib, and prior rib or clavicular fractures with a large bone callus. If the patient has symptoms of dyspnea or hypoxia, a computed tomography angiogram (CTA) of the chest can evaluate for pulmonary embolism.

In addition to prompt systemic anticoagulation, patients with VTOS should be considered for catheter-based thrombolysis of the DVT. This is performed via access of the basilic or cephalic vein in the upper arm under ultrasound guidance, followed by an attempt to cross the subclavian thrombosis and presumed stenosis with wires and catheters (Fig. 1). Successful mechanical and pharmacologic thrombolysis will reveal a stenosis at the proximal portion of the subclavian vein where the clavicle and first rib cross. Balloon angioplasty of the stenosis with a high-tensile strength balloon will help improve venous flow in the vein. Completion venograms in the arms-down and arms-up positions will demonstrate the dynamic compression of the vein at the thoracic outlet (Fig. 2). After successful thrombolysis, patients can be discharged on anticoagulation for subsequent VTOS decompression surgery after 2 weeks to allow for resolution of edema and inflammation.

Surgical Approach

In order to access the supra- and infraclavicular spaces as well as the affected arm, the patient is placed in the semi-Fowler's position (supine with back of bed up at 30 degrees) with the head turned slightly away from the affected side. The ipsilateral neck, anterior chest, and arm are prepped. A sterile arm sleeve is placed around the hand and forearm to allow for complete mobility of the arm.

A supraclavicular incision is made lateral to the sternal head of the sternocleidomastoid muscle (SCM) and carried through the platysma. The clavicular head of the SCM is divided to reveal the underlying internal jugular vein (IJV). The supraclavicular fat pad is mobilized laterally to expose the underlying anterior scalene muscle (ASM) and phrenic nerve. The phrenic nerve is carefully mobilized laterally to allow for circumferential dissection of the ASM insertion on the first rib. The ASM is sharply divided off the rib, and a 1- to 2-cm segment of the ASM is resected to reduce the chance of distal reattachment.

Next, the subclavian artery and roots of the brachial plexus are mobilized medially to expose the middle scalene muscle (MSM) as it attaches to the first rib. A periosteal elevator is used to lift the MSM off the rib, taking care to avoid the long thoracic nerve lying posterior and lateral to the MSM. The first rib is then cut at the MSM insertion site.

A medial infraclavicular incision is then made over the first rib and lateral to the sternal border. The dissection is carried down to the pectoralis fascia and then to the rib. A periosteal elevator is used to circumferentially

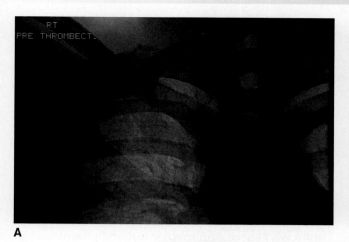

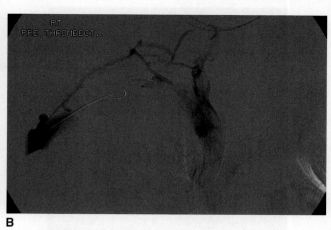

A

B

FIGURE 1 • **A, B:** Initial subclavian venogram showing thrombosis.

free the rib from the surrounding intercostal muscles. The first rib is then divided just lateral to the sternal border and removed for inspection. The rib specimen should contain the subclavian artery and vein grooves as well as the costoclavicular ligament (Fig. 3). The proximal subclavian vein is mobilized, and any external fibrous bands are removed to allow the vein to fully fill. Care is taken to fully visualize the junction of the subclavian vein and IJV to assure that there is no longer any compression from a retained rib segment or fibrous scar.

After an intraoperative venogram (Table 1), the operative field is inspected for sources of hemorrhage and lymphatic leak. Typically, the pleura is entered during the rib resection, and a small chest tube is placed for postoperative drainage.

Special Intraoperative Considerations

While some surgeons perform subclavian venogram days or weeks after rib resection, there are several advantages in performing intraoperative venogram. First, the patient is already under anesthesia and prepped and draped, saving time and resources. Secondly, a venogram

showing persistent subclavian vein compression can be corrected with additional resection of a residual rib segment or releasing more fibrotic bands around the vein. Finally, if the subclavian vein is ruptured during intraoperative balloon angioplasty, it can be more readily repaired.

Open subclavian vein endarterectomy with patch angioplasty has been described by some surgeons as an adjunct to improve vessel patency. This procedure is technically difficult because of the limited accessibility of the superior vena cava without a sternotomy. However, this author finds that external venolysis and intraoperative balloon angioplasty with high-pressure balloons yield excellent results without the need for open patch angioplasty.

Postoperative Management

Because of the significant symptoms from the cut rib, pain management is one of the key objects of postoperative care. The chest tube is quickly advanced to water seal and maintained until the patient has eaten a fatty meal and no lymph leak is seen. Patients are encouraged

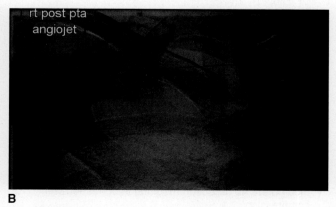

A

B

FIGURE 2 • Subclavian venogram showing **(A)** patency in the arm-down position and **(B)** cessation of flow due to TOS compression in the arm-up position.

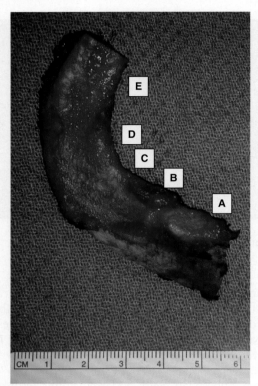

FIGURE 3 • Right rib specimen with key landmarks (medial to lateral) (*A*) costoclavicular ligament, (*B*) subclavian vein groove, (*C*) anterior scalene muscle insertion site, (*D*) subclavian artery groove, and (*E*) middle scalene muscle insertion.

TABLE 1. Venous Thoracic Outlet Syndrome

Key Technical Steps

1. Setup the patient to allow supra and infraclavicular access, as well as mobile access of the affected arm
2. Through a supraclavicular incision, identify the insertion of the ASM and the overlying phrenic nerve
3. Divide the ASM at the first rib insertion and resect a segment of the muscle
4. Mobilize the subclavian artery and brachial plexus medially to expose the insertion of the MSM
5. Divide the MSM off of the first rib, with care to avoid the long thoracic nerve laterally
6. Divide the first rib at the MSM insertion site
7. Through a medial infraclavicular incision, circumferentially clear the first rib at the sternal junction
8. Clear the pericostal muscle above and below the first rib
9. Cut the first rib through the infraclavicular incision and remove the rib
10. Perform an external venolysis of the proximal subclavian vein
11. Access the left arm for an intraoperative subclavian venogram and balloon angioplasty
12. Check for residual compression with a venogram in the arms-down and arms-up positions

Potential Pitfalls

• Injury to the phrenic and long thoracic nerve
• Incomplete rib resection resulting in continued vein compression
• Postoperative hematoma from pericostal muscle bleeding

to use their arm during the recovery period but to avoid heavy lifting or prolong elevation of the arm above the shoulder. If the intraoperative venogram shows minimal residual subclavian vein stenosis or thrombosis, patients are only given aspirin and not anticoagulation, which significantly reduced their chance of postoperative bleeding. Patients are liberalized to full unrestricted activity at 4 weeks and followed with venous ultrasound annually.

Case Conclusion

The patient underwent right upper extremity venogram with successful mechanical and pharmacologic thrombolysis. A subclavian stenosis was seen and balloon dilated. Venogram with the arm up showed cessation of venous flow at the proximal subclavian vein, confirming the diagnosis of VTOS. The patient was discharged home on fractionated heparin. He returned 2 weeks later for successful VTOS decompression with intraoperative venogram and balloon angioplasty (Fig. 4). He was discharged on postoperative day 4 and resumed competitive basketball at 30 days.

TAKE HOME POINTS

• Effort thrombosis (Paget-von Schrötter syndrome) is a relatively rare condition that requires prompt recognition and referral to experienced clinicians.

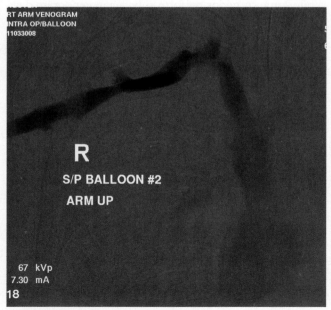

FIGURE 4 • Intraoperative venogram showing patency in the arm-up position after rib resection.

- Early thrombolysis, followed by TOS decompression and intraoperative venogram with angioplasty, can result in restoration of venous patency, arm functionality, and patient quality of life.

SUGGESTED READINGS

Schneider DB, Dimuzio PJ, Martin ND, et al. Combination treatment of venous thoracic outlet syndrome: open surgical decompression and intraoperative angioplasty. *J Vasc Surg.* 2004;40(4):599-603.

Taylor JM, Telford RJ, Kinsella DC, et al. Long-term clinical and functional outcome following treatment for Paget-Schrotter syndrome. *Br J Surg.* 2013;100(11):1459-1464.

Thompson RW, Petrinec D, Toursarkissian B. Surgical treatment of thoracic outlet compression syndromes II. Supraclavicular exploration and vascular reconstruction. *Ann Vasc Surg.* 1997;11(4):442-451.

CLINICAL SCENARIO CASE QUESTIONS

1. Rib resection for VTOS occurs immediately deep to the:
   a. Anterior scalene muscle
   b. Middle scalene muscle
   c. Phrenic nerve
   d. Long thoracic nerve
   e. Pectoralis major muscle

2. In what position is the patient placed into in order to access the supra- and infraclavicular spaces?
   a. Greenfield's position
   b. Cherry's position
   c. Semi-Fowler's position
   d. Wylie's position
   e. Mannick's position

30 Arterial Thoracic Outlet Syndrome

MARGARET CLARKE TRACCI

Presentation

A 47-year-old woman with a history of smoking presents to the emergency department with a cool, painful right hand and bluish discoloration of several fingertips. She has had several episodes of coolness and tingling of her fingertips with associated discoloration over the past several months, although these have previously resolved on their own. Physical examination reveals a cool hand with dusky color changes to several fingertips. Radial and ulnar pulses are not palpable. A proximal brachial pulse is palpable, as is the subclavian just above the clavicle.

Differential Diagnosis

The differential diagnosis for upper extremity ischemia includes atherosclerotic disease, embolic phenomena, and vasculitis. Atherosclerotic disease most commonly presents as chronically progressive fatigue with activity, typically related to a proximal lesion of the subclavian or innominate artery. Atherosclerotic lesions, which tend to be proximal in location, may also serve as a nidus for distal emboli.

Other proximal sources of emboli include the heart and aneurysms of the subclavian or innominate arteries. Aneurysms in this position may be associated with atherosclerosis, connective tissue disorders, anatomic anomalies such as an aberrant right subclavian artery, or represent poststenotic dilatation distal to extrinsic compression within the thoracic outlet. Larger emboli lodging in brachial, radial, and ulnar arteries may present more dramatically, with the sudden onset of ischemic symptoms, though the rich collateralization of the upper extremity often protects patients from critical ischemia even with complete occlusions of these vessels. Microemboli may present much more subtly, with recurrent episodes ranging from painful, markedly ischemic fingertips to an asymmetric Raynaud's phenomenon.

Less frequently, ischemia of the upper extremity may be related to large (Takayasu's), medium (thromboangiitis obliterans or Buerger's disease), or small vessel (ANCA-associated) arteritides. Functional disorders resulting in very distal ischemia include Raynaud's phenomenon or rarer vasomotor phenomena, such as erythromelalgia.

Workup

The patient undergoes CT angiography (CTA) for further evaluation of her upper extremity ischemia, which reveals a thrombus-lined aneurysm of the midsubclavian artery, occlusion of the brachial artery, and evidence of embolization to the digital arteries of the hand. A right cervical rib is noted with a prominent synostosis with the first rib (Figs. 1,2 to 3).

CTA offers several advantages in the diagnosis of arterial thoracic outlet syndrome (aTOS). While catheter-based angiography remains the gold standard for fine resolution imaging of the distal arteries of the hand and digits, it may not fully demonstrate a thrombus-lined aneurysm. CT offers excellent 3D renderings of both the vascular system and of the surrounding musculoskeletal structures that create compressive syndromes of the thoracic outlet. MR angiography (MRA) does not yet offer sensitivity equal to CTA for arterial thoracic outlet syndrome. Plain chest radiographs may demonstrate bony abnormalities such as cervical rib, anomalous transverse process, or a callused fracture of the clavicle that are classically associated with aTOS.

Noninvasive vascular laboratory studies are of somewhat limited diagnostic utility. Traditionally, maneuvers intended to elicit compression of the subclavian artery have been performed, with examination for changes in flow velocity or diameter by duplex ultrasound or waveform with pulse volume recordings. However, there is a significant rate of false-positive results, with nearly 20% of asymptomatic patients demonstrating some degree of arterial compression with abduction maneuvers. Duplex may be useful in identifying aneurysm disease, intraluminal thrombus or injury, and patency of distal vessels. Pulse volume recordings with segmental pressure measurements are useful in the identification and quantification of digital embolization.

Laboratory evaluation is typically useful only to the extent that it may identify or rule out conditions, such as vasculitis or thrombophilia in the differential diagnosis of upper extremity ischemia.

Diagnosis and Treatment

The presentation, clinical examination, and imaging studies are consistent with arterial thoracic outlet syndrome with aneurysm degeneration of the artery distal to the site of extrinsic compression and presenting with

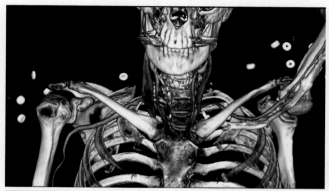

FIGURE 1 • 3D CT reconstruction demonstrating right cervical rib.

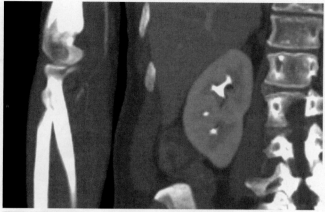

FIGURE 3 • CT image demonstrating brachial artery occlusion.

distal embolization of aneurysm thrombus. These patients typically present with microembolization to the digits but may suffer from larger emboli resulting in brachial artery occlusion or present with exertional pain that is either subtle and positionally related or more severe and related to aneurysm thrombosis, compressive symptoms related to aneurysm growth, or asymmetric Raynaud's phenomenon.

While arterial, venous, and neurogenic thoracic outlet syndrome all involve compression of structures passing through the confines of the thoracic outlet, presentation, the location of extrinsic compression, and management differ significantly. Arterial thoracic outlet syndrome is the least common of the three, representing 1% to 6% of patients in large series of thoracic outlet decompression. The source of compression in this syndrome is most frequently a cervical rib, which is present in this case, but may also be an anomalous first rib, fibrocartilaginous bands, prior clavicular fracture with associated bony callus, or an elongated C7 transverse process. Where a cervical rib is present, the artery is

typically high riding and easily palpable well above the clavicle (Figs. 4 and 5).

The mainstay of treatment of symptomatic aTOS is treatment of distal emboli, if present, coupled with generous resection of bony, fibrocartilaginous, and muscular structures contributing to compression within the thoracic outlet and reconstruction of an injured or aneurysmal

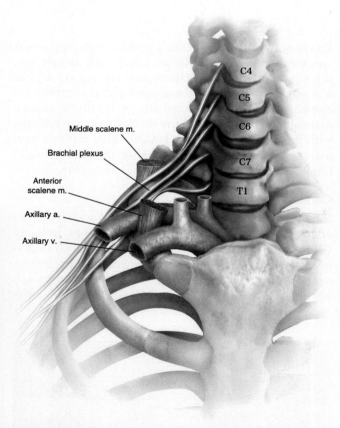

FIGURE 4 • Anatomic relationships at the thoracic outlet. (From Tracci MC. Thoracic outlet syndrome: transaxillary approach. *Op Tech Thorac Cardiovasc Surg.* 2011;16(4):267-277, with permission.)

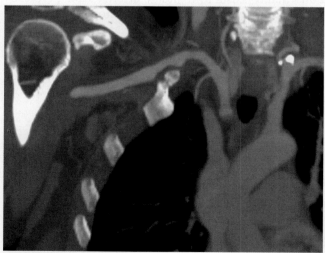

FIGURE 2 • CT image demonstrating thrombus-lined subclavian artery aneurysm.

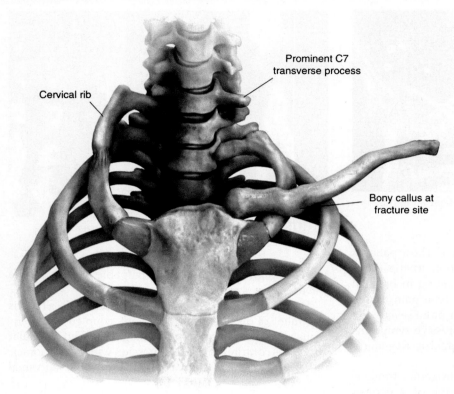

FIGURE 5 • Bony anomalies associated with thoracic outlet compression. (From Tracci MC. Thoracic outlet syndrome: transaxillary approach. *Op Tech Thorac Cardiovasc Surg.* 2011;16(4): 267-277, with permission.)

subclavian artery. In general, a patient with only minor abnormalities of the subclavian artery, such as mild stenosis or poststenotic dilatation, may not require arterial reconstruction but may be managed with decompression alone. Any significant irregularity or aneurysm change mandates reconstruction of the subclavian artery, typically with an interposition graft. Finally, distal embolization may necessitate thrombolysis and/or thromboembolectomy in addition to decompression and reconstruction.

Case Continued

It was determined that the hand was not acutely threatened. Catheter-directed thrombolysis was initiated with resolution of brachial occlusion and much of distal occlusion. If the hand were immediately threatened, surgical thromboembolectomy via a brachial approach would be appropriate. Thrombolysis, where possible,

may offer an advantage with regard to resolution of distal, small vessel occlusions of the hand and digits (Figs. 6 and 7).

Surgical Approach

Surgical therapy of aTOS requires decompression of the thoracic outlet, with resection of cervical ribs or other culprit bony or ligamentous anomalies, where present, as well as resection of the anterior scalene and first rib. The key decision point is whether sufficient arterial abnormality exists to mandate arterial repair, typically by replacement with synthetic or autogenous interposition graft. The Scher system of classification of aTOS may be helpful in guiding therapy and determining the extent of operation. In this case, arterial reconstruction is mandatory due to the presence of a thrombus-lined aneurysm of the subclavian artery (Tables 1 and 2).

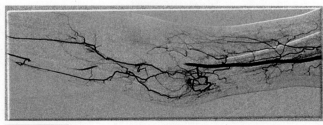

FIGURE 6 • Prethrombolysis image of brachial artery occlusion.

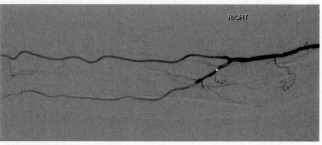

FIGURE 7 • Postthrombolysis image of patent brachial artery.

TABLE 1. Supraclavicular Approach (Preferred Surgical Approach Where Arterial Reconstruction Is Indicated)

Key Technical Steps

1. Supine positioning, roll between the shoulders.
2. Prep neck, shoulder, and arm, with stockinette over the hand to facilitate mobilizing arm.
3. Supraclavicular incision.
4. Scalene fat pad mobilized.
5. Phrenic nerve identified/mobilized on anterior surface of anterior scalene.
6. Anterior scalene generously resected.
7. Middle scalene attachments to first rib divided, with identification and protection of long thoracic nerve.
8. First rib resected from lateral to anterior scalene insertion to medial to the vein.
9. Subclavian artery mobilized proximal and distal to injured/aneurysmal segment.
10. Infraclavicular counterincision may be required for distal control.
11. Administer systemic heparin.
12. Control subclavian proximally and distally, as well as major branches, such as the thyrocervical trunk.
13. Resect affected portion and replace with choice of conduit (ringed PTFE, polyester, or saphenous or femoral vein). Anastomoses are performed in an end-to-end fashion using a running monofilament polypropylene suture.
14. If length of lesion requires passing the graft from the supraclavicular to infraclavicular incision for distal anastomosis with the axillary artery, ensure that there is no external compression within the tunnel. This may require limited bony resection of the posterior clavicle if it is prominent and impinges on the graft.
15. Assess graft and arterial patency, including evaluation of brachial, radial, and ulnar pulses.

Potential Pitfalls

- Inadequate bony resection
- Failure to resect ligamentous attachments
- Inadequate scalene resection
- External compression of completed graft
- Lymphatic injury and leak
- Pleural entry
- Distal embolization
- Nerve injury (phrenic, brachial plexus, long thoracic)

TABLE 2. Transaxillary Approach (Cervical and First Rib Resection Only)

Key Technical Steps

1. Supine positioning with roll beneath operative shoulder to raise 20–30 degrees
2. Shoulder, arm, and axilla prepped with arm stockinette to facilitate abduction
3. Avoid hyperabduction or extension that would place undue traction on brachial plexus, maintain elbow bend, return to neutral position every 20 minutes
4. Transverse incision just below the axillary hairline
5. Carry dissection to chest wall
6. Identify and protect thoracodorsal and long thoracic nerves
7. Expose first rib
8. Identify and mobilize phrenic nerve
9. Resect anterior scalene muscle
10. Middle scalene attachments to the first rib divided, with identification and protection of long thoracic nerve
11. First rib resected from lateral to middle scalene insertion to near the costochondral junction
12. Assess arterial patency, including evaluation of brachial, radial, and ulnar pulses

Potential Pitfalls

- Inadequate bony resection
- Failure to resect ligamentous attachments
- Inadequate scalene resection
- Lymphatic injury and leak
- Pleural entry
- Nerve injury (phrenic, brachial plexus, long thoracic, thoracodorsal)

Special Intraoperative Considerations

Be attentive to lymphatics, particularly during the mobilization of the scalene fat pad. These should be carefully ligated with ties or hemoclips, rather than suture ligation. Nerve injury may be avoided by careful identification and mobilization of nerve structures with scrupulous attention to avoiding excessive traction or transmitted energy from electrocautery. The transaxillary approach mandates careful management of positioning, with avoidance of excessive tension on the brachial plexus and periodic relaxation of the arm. When dividing the first rib, the pleura may be gently mobilized from the posterior rib using blunt dissection. If the pleura is entered, it should be carefully closed and catheter drainage of both wound and pleura considered. If there is a question of pleural entry or air leak, this may be assessed at the conclusion of the case by instilling sterile saline solution in conjunction with 30 mm Hg of sustained positive pressure ventilation. Pleural injury becomes apparent either through drainage into the pleural space or bubbles rising from the space. Sustained bubbles suggest a possible air leak. When completing the arterial graft, careful assessment for external compression may be necessary. On occasion, a rongeur may be used to perform limited bony resection of the posterior clavicle if it is prominent and impinges on the graft.

Case Conclusion

The patient undergoes successful catheter-directed TPA thrombolysis of her right brachial artery.

She then undergoes resection of the cervical rib and bony prominence of the first rib, anterior scalenectomy, and reconstruction of the aneurysmal portion of the subclavian artery using an 8-mm ringed PTFE graft via supraclavicular and infraclavicular incisions. There is no evidence of pleural entry with the Valsalva maneuver prior to closing. A 15-Fr Jackson Pratt drain is left in place and removed on postoperative day 1 with less than 30 mL of total serosanguineous drainage. The patient is instructed by physical therapy on gradual advancement of range-of-motion exercises for the shoulder and is discharged home on postoperative day 2.

Postoperative Management

1. Consider placement of drains
2. Consider postoperative heparin in patients with emboli
3. Serial physical examination, including vascular and neurologic examinations
4. Adequate analgesia: may include oral or intravenous narcotics, nonsteroidal anti-inflammatory drugs, and muscle relaxants
5. Range-of-motion exercises
6. Physical therapy
7. Graft surveillance

TAKE HOME POINTS

- Arterial thoracic outlet compression is a relatively uncommon cause of upper extremity ischemia being less common than neurogenic or venous TOS.
- Arterial TOS may present with effort-related ischemic symptoms or with emboli, typically in the setting of a partially thrombosis aneurysm.
- Bony abnormalities, such as a cervical rib, prominent C7 transverse process, or prominent bony callus following clavicular injury, are typically associated with this compressive syndrome.
- Arterial TOS may be caused by fibrous bands or other nonbony structures.
- Embolization may require urgent treatment with thrombolysis or surgical embolectomy.
- Significant arterial abnormalities necessitate subclavian artery reconstruction, while milder arterial injury may be treated with thoracic outlet decompression alone.
- The supraclavicular approach is generally preferred where arterial reconstruction is indicated, for better access to the subclavian artery. Either supraclavicular or transaxillary approach is appropriate for decompression alone without arterial repair.

- Endovascular therapy, typically covered stent repair of subclavian aneurysm paired with surgical thoracic outlet decompression, has been reported, but long-term results are not yet available. Stent thrombosis prior to decompression has been reported.

SUGGESTED READINGS

Bower TC, Pairolero PC, Hallett JW Jr, et al. Brachiocephalic aneurysm: the case for early recognition and repair. *Ann Vasc Surg.* 1991;5(2):125-132.

Brooke BS, Freischlag JA. Contemporary management of thoracic outlet syndrome. *Curr Opin Cardiol.* 2010;25(6):535-540.

Roos DB. Congenital anomalies associated with thoracic outlet syndrome. Anatomy, symptoms, diagnosis, and treatment. *Am J Surg.* 1976;132:771-778.

Scher LA, Veith FJ, Haimovici H, et al. Staging of arterial complications of cervical rib: guidelines for surgical management. *Surgery.* 1984;95:664-669.

Smith ST, Valentine RJ. Thoracic outlet syndrome. In: Cronenwett JL, Johnston KW, eds. *Rutherford's Vascular Surgery.* 7th ed. Philadelphia, PA: Saunders Elsevier; 2010:Chapter 124.

Thompson RW, Petrinec D. Surgical treatment of thoracic outlet compression syndromes: diagnostic considerations and transaxillary first rib resection. *Ann Vasc Surg.* 1997;11:317-323.

CLINICAL SCENARIO CASE QUESTIONS

1. Which of the following is the favored diagnostic modality for identification of arterial thoracic outlet syndrome?
   a. Duplex ultrasound with provocative maneuvers
   b. Catheter angiography
   c. Magnetic resonance angiography
   d. CT angiography
   e. Electromyelography

2. Arterial thoracic outlet syndrome presenting with embolization from a subclavian artery aneurysm is most appropriately treated by:
   a. Anticoagulation
   b. Transaxillary resection of the scalene muscle, first rib, and cervical rib, if present
   c. Supraclavicular resection of the scalene muscle, first rib, and cervical rib, if present
   d. Supraclavicular resection of the scalene muscle, first rib, and cervical rib, if present, with graft replacement of aneurysmal segment of the subclavian artery
   e. Covered stent graft treatment of the subclavian artery aneurysm

31 Vascular Access Evaluation

ANNA SATTAH and WORTHINGTON SCHENK III

Presentation

A 71-year-old right-handed male is referred for evaluation for arteriovenous (AV) fistula creation for dialysis access. He had a right-sided Cimino radiocephalic wrist fistula created at an outside hospital 3 months ago, which has failed to mature. He is not currently on dialysis; however, his estimated GFR is 16 mL/min/1.7 m², down from 20 prior to his last operation. His past medical history is significant for hypertension, insulin-dependent diabetes, peripheral vascular disease, and recurrent foot infections resulting in a left below-knee amputation (BKA). He denies any history of central lines in the neck but does report having had a right-sided peripheral inserted central catheter (PICC) line for intravenous (IV) antibiotics. On physical examination, the incision over his Cimino fistula is well healed, but there is no thrill. He has a scar on his right upper arm, which he confirms is from his prior PICC line. He has no other visible scars on his arms or neck. His BKA site is well healed. His pulse exam reveals normal radial and brachial pulses bilaterally. Allen's test is normal bilaterally.

Imaging

A duplex ultrasound including vein mapping of both arms is obtained. On the *right*, a thrombosed radiocephalic fistula is seen in the forearm. Flow remains intact in the radial artery distal to the fistula. At the antecubital fossa, the brachial artery internal diameter measures 3.2 mm without evidence of calcifications, and the median antecubital vein measures 3.6 mm. In the upper arm, the cephalic vein measures 2.8 mm. The basilic vein measures 3.4 to 3.9 mm with a focal stenotic lesion narrowing to 2.2 mm corresponding to the site of his prior PICC line. On the *left*, see Figure 1: in the forearm, the radial artery measures 1.8 mm, and the cephalic vein measures 1.6 mm. At the antecubital fossa, the brachial artery measures 4.2 mm without calcifications, and the median cubital vein measures 4.0 mm. In the upper arm, the cephalic vein measures 2.8 mm. The basilic vein measures 4.6 to 5.5 mm without focal stenoses and remains separate from the deep brachial system into the axilla.

It is useful to perform an ultrasound evaluation at the initial office visit, which allows for the opportunity to depict the size, course, and location of branches of the veins as well as the size, course, and character of the flow signal of the arteries (Fig. 1). Venous branches near the proposed anastomosis are important to identify for two reasons. First, they can be used to form a Carrel patch when creating an anastomosis. Second, large intact branches may form alternate venous drainage sites and lead to nonmaturation of the fistula.

Recommendations

While there are no well-established evidence-based ultrasound criteria for successful fistula construction, adequate flow through the fistula must be established in order to dilate the venous channel. Suggested sonographic exclusion criteria for creation of autologous fistulas are listed in Table 1. When patients do not fit criteria for a fistula, a PTFE graft should be considered in order to avoid permanent percutaneous catheters.

Based on his preoperative ultrasound, there are no appropriate autologous options in the right upper extremity. In the forearm, the Cimino fistula has failed. In the upper arm, the cephalic vein is only 2.8 mm, and the basilic vein is small and has a stenotic lesion from a prior PICC line.

On the left, in the forearm, the radial artery is only 1.8 mm, and in the upper arm, the cephalic vein is only 2.8 mm. The basilic vein, however, looks good (greater than 4.5 mm). These ultrasound evaluations can be done by the surgeon or by a trusted vascular lab and are recommended for preoperative planning. This patient is not yet on dialysis but has progressive stage IV chronic kidney disease (CKD). Based on the National Kidney Foundations 2006 Kidney Disease Outcomes Quality Initiative (KDOQI) guidelines (Table 2), he is appropriate for surgical evaluation and angioaccess construction. He has a reasonable conduit for creation of a basilic vein transposition, and he is scheduled for surgery.

Discussion

The National Kidney Foundation published the KDOQI guidelines in 2006 for the creation of AV fistulas in patients with CKD (Table 2). Their goal is for patients to have a working permanent vascular access in place prior to initiation of dialysis and to avoid the need for percutaneous catheters. They set a goal to have 66% of patients dialyzed through AV fistulas and to reduce the number of patients using permanent cuffed catheters to less than 10%. In order to achieve these goals, patients should be

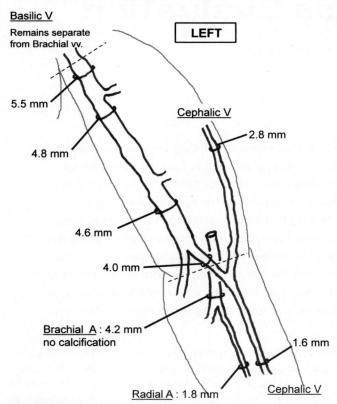

Basilic V
Remains separate
from Brachial vv.

LEFT

5.5 mm

Cephalic V

4.8 mm

2.8 mm

4.6 mm

4.0 mm

Brachial A: 4.2 mm
no calcification

1.6 mm

Radial A: 1.8 mm

Cephalic V

FIGURE 1 • Preoperative sonographic evaluation. A Cimino fistula in the left forearm appears a poor choice due to small size of both artery and vein. An upper arm brachiocephalic fistula is possible but runs a substantial risk of nonmaturation due to the small size of the cephalic vein. The anatomy looks favorable for a one-stage basilic vein transposition: the vein diameter is favorable, the antecubital branch (4.0 mm) can be included to gain additional length, and the basilic vein remains separate from the brachial veins.

TABLE 1. Sonographic Exclusion Criteria for Fistula Construction[a]	
Forearm/Wrist Fistula	
Cephalic Vein in Forearm:	Absent
	Smaller than 2.5 mm ID
	Deeper than 7 mm
	Sclerotic, discontinuous, or skip areas
	No outflow at antecubital level
Radial Artery in Forearm:	Smaller than 2.5 mm
	Significantly calcified
	Abnormal flow signal
Antecubital/Above Elbow Fistula	
Cephalic Vein in Upper Arm:	Absent
	Smaller than 3.5 mm
	Sclerotic, discontinuous, or skip areas
	Deeper than 7 mm (secondary transposition may be considered)
Brachial Artery:	Smaller than 3.0 mm
	Abnormal flow signal
Basilic Vein Transposition	
Basilic Vein in Upper Arm:	Absent
	Smaller than 4.5 mm in proposed usable area. A short zone of minimum 3.5 mm at distal end is acceptable
	Inadequate length at proximal end: junction of basilic and brachial veins must be near anterior axillary line or higher
	Inadequate length at the distal end: a branch of the basilic vein at least 3.5 mm must extend to antecubital crease or below
Brachial Artery:	Smaller than 3.0 mm
	Abnormal flow signal

[a]This table represents an example of sonographic exclusion criteria, intended as an illustration only, not as a recommendation. The criteria are guidelines only and not based on evidence-based data.

referred to a surgeon in advance of dialysis initiation and with sufficient lead time to allow for maturation of the fistula and correction of any problems in advance of dialysis. This patient clearly meets those criteria. He should be fully evaluated with a complete history and physical examination with attention to any history of prior central lines or pacemakers as well as the expected timing before progression to end-stage renal disease and initiation of dialysis.

Preoperative Imaging

Patients should undergo a thorough duplex evaluation of upper extremity arterial and venous anatomy. Important factors include any sign of arterial inflow obstruction, stenotic lesions, or calcified areas, particularly in diabetic patients. Venous mapping should be performed with attention to diameter, compressibility, and venous outflow. Veins can be traced by ultrasound back to the axillary, sometimes distal subclavian veins. If a patient has a history of ipsilateral central lines/pacemakers, an evaluation of his or her central veins should be considered with a CO_2 venogram or an MR venogram to look specifically for central venous stenosis. Iodinated contrast is generally avoided in patients

with stage IV or V renal failure to avoid hastening the onset of dialysis. The intended venous conduit needs to lie superficial enough to allow for cannulation and in reasonable proximity to the artery to create an anastomosis. If not, there needs to be adequate length to allow for dissection and mobilization of one or both vessels. The basilic vein, which typically lies too deep to cannulate, will generally require transposition to a more superficial location.

Preoperative Planning

Distal fistulas are considered preferable because they preserve more proximal autologous options for future access sites. That said, it is not worth creating a distal fistula that is unlikely to mature, particularly if the patient is already on dialysis. This is only likely to subject the patient to additional surgery and prolong the length of time he or she dialyzes through a percutaneous catheter.

TABLE 2. National Kidney Foundation 2006 KDOQI Guidelines for the Creation of AV Fistulas in Patients with Chronic Kidney Disease

CKD stage 4 GFR <30	• Nephrology referral • Discussion of renal replacement options (HD, PD)
CKD stages 4 and 5	• Surgical referral and evaluation of dialysis access options • Protect forearms from venipuncture • Avoid subclavian lines PICCs • AVF candidates—surgery 6 mo in advance of anticipated need for HD to allow time for maturation • AV graft candidates—surgery 3–6 wk in advance of anticipated need for HD; no need to wait for maturation • PD candidates—PD catheter placement 2 wk in advance of anticipated need for dialysis • Goal to have functional permanent access in place prior to initiation of dialysis

Access options (in order of preference)	• Fistulas (distal is better)
	   ○ Radiocephalic
	   ○ Brachiocephalic
	   ○ Transposted brachiobasilic
	• Grafts
	• Percutaneous central lines—should be avoided

Preoperative evaluation	• History and physical • Duplex ultrasound of upper extremity arteries and veins • Central venous evaluation in patients with h/o prior central lines or pacemakers

Autologous fistulas are preferred to grafts due to their decreased risk of infection; however, if a patient does not have any reasonable autologous conduits, a PTFE graft is still a superior option to a tunneled catheter.

The fact that this patient has already had one failed access is not an uncommon scenario. Primary failure is defined as fistulas which never develop sufficiently to be used for dialysis access. This can be due to thrombosis or to nonmaturation of the fistula. This is frequently secondary to an inadequate conduit, that is, small veins or focal stenoses secondary to frequent phlebotomy, or to central stenosis from prior central lines.

Other considerations include the time it takes for an access to mature. AV fistulas may take 6 to 12 weeks or longer and may require additional interventions/revisions if they fail to mature. PTFE grafts are typically ready for use in 4 to 6 weeks. AV fistula primary failure rates vary widely and range between 20% and 50%. Not surprisingly, radiocephalic fistulas have higher rates of nonmaturation than more proximal brachiocephalic fistulas. It is also preferable to use the nondominant extremity if feasible.

However, if the only autologous option is on the dominant side, that is generally the favored approach. Finally, upper extremity access is better than lower extremity options. Thigh grafts are harder to access and more likely to become infected or develop hematomas or venous stenosis that can be very hard to treat.

Special Considerations for Basilic Vein Transpositions

These fistulas can be created in either one or two stages. If the venous conduit appears marginal, consider a two-stage approach. Here, an anastomosis is created at the first stage, and the vein is allowed to arterialize. The vein is then transposed to a more superficial location at a second stage. For patients with a better conduit, both steps can be performed in a single operation.

The second decision to consider is whether to use one long incision or several shorter ones. The latter allows for preservation of skin bridges between the incisions and fewer wound complications while maintaining adequate access to dissect the vein (Fig. 2). The vein is then tunneled in an arc superficially and away from the incisions.

Adequate length of the conduit must be assured. In an obese patient, that may mean transposing the vein more than 2 cm superficially. Adequate length permits

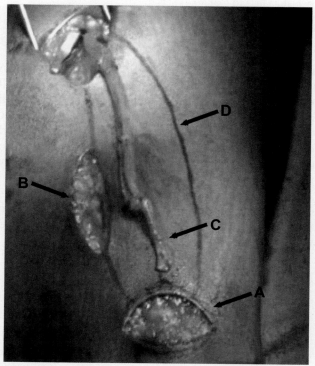

FIGURE 2 • Intraoperative preparation of the basilic vein for transposition. (*A*) Transverse incision in the antecubital fossa for dissection of the antecubital branch of the basilic vein and exposure of the brachial artery. (*B*) Vein harvest incision, leaving skin bridges. (*C*) The antecubital branch of the vein, although slightly smaller in diameter, adds enough length to the harvested conduit to reach the artery in the antecubital fossa. (*D*) The planned course of the transposition.

TABLE 3. Vascular Access Evaluation

Key Technical Steps

1. An autologous fistula should be possible in most patients; the accepted benchmark is 66%.
2. The critical step to success is pre-op planning, with primary reliance on ultrasound.
3. Choice of anatomic site is more critical to success than technical expertise.
4. The pre-op screening should be done well in advance of requiring dialysis—this then allows better timing and protection of the intended venous conduit.
5. When evaluating by ultrasound, while the diameter of artery and vein at the proposed site of fistula construction is important, it is the condition/size of the conduit in the proposed puncture zone that is critical, that is, the conduit that will be used for needle access.
6. If the ultrasound screening is not done by the surgeon, it should be done by a technician who understands the anatomic options and other relevant surgical relationships.
7. Even with the best pre-op planning and intra-op technique, some primary failures will still be seen. A primary failure rate of 10%–15% may indicate an aggressive approach toward fistula construction, rather than technical imperfection.
8. Regarding the basilic vein transposition option, adequate length of the basilic vein is critical to allow both transposition to a more superficial location, as well as displacement to a more accessible location.

Potential Pitfalls

- Fistula fails to mature.
- Development of steal syndrome.
- Central vein stenosis.

tunneling the vein from its origin deep in the axilla to a superficial location accessible to cannulation and still reach the brachial artery, preferably in the antecubital fossa. In patients with an antecubital branch of the basilic vein at least 3.5 mm in diameter, this branch can be used for additional conduit length. The added length also allows for greater flexibility to tunnel the vessel laterally over the biceps to a more easily accessed position.

Fortunately, basilic vein transpositions have the shortest maturation time of all the AV access options. The vein begins as a larger conduit and avoids the delay associated with encapsulation required for a PTFE graft (Table 3).

Case Conclusion

The patient underwent a basilic vein transposition without complication. He progressed to end-stage renal failure and was initiated on dialysis 2 months later. He was successfully able to dialyze through his fistula and did not require the placement of a percutaneous catheter.

TAKE HOME POINTS

- Work with nephrologists to get renal failure patients educated and evaluated prior to requiring dialysis.
- The critical step to success is thorough preoperative evaluation, relying heavily on duplex ultrasound, to identify the best anatomic option.
- Allow for maturation time; neither autologous nor prosthetic access can be used immediately.
- General anesthesia is rarely required; typically local anesthesia with sedation for fistulas, regional block for grafts, and transpositions.

SUGGESTED READINGS

Huber TS, Ozaki CK, Flynn TC, et al. Prospective validation of an algorithm to maximize native arteriovenous fistulae for chronic hemodialysis access. *J Vasc Surg.* 2002;36(3):452-459.

National Kidney Foundation. NKF KDOQI Guidelines. In http://www.kidney.org/professionals/kdoqi/guideline_upHD_PD_VA/index.htm. 2006.

Schenk WG III. Improving dialysis access: regional anesthesia improves arteriovenous fistula prevalence. *Am Surg.* 2010;76(9):938-942.

Schild FA, Collier PS, Fuller JC. Vascular access surgery: an emerging specialty. In: Cameron JL, Cameron AM, eds. *Current Surgical Therapy.* 10th ed. Philadelphia, PA: Elsevier Saunders; 2011:861-867.

CLINICAL SCENARIO CASE QUESTIONS

1. An autologous AV fistula is preferable to a prosthetic AV graft for dialysis because:
   a. It requires fewer interventions to maintain.
   b. It has lower (better) primary failure rate.
   c. It has better early reliability.
   d. It has more available anatomic sites for construction.
   e. All of the above.

2. Duplex ultrasound evaluation for dialysis access:
   a. Should only be done by certified ultrasound technologists
   b. Involves evaluation of veins, not arteries
   c. Should be done prior to initiation of dialysis
   d. Should only evaluate the nondominant upper extremity
   e. Has well-established exclusion criteria for each fistula anatomic site

AV—Access Forearm Graft

RANDALL SUNG and SETH WAITS

Presentation

A 67-year-old male with a history of end-stage renal disease (ESRD) from non–insulin-dependent diabetes mellitus presents to clinic for ongoing management of his dialysis access. He now undergoes dialysis three times per week through a temporary dialysis catheter. Two weeks ago, he underwent placement of forearm loop graft with polytetrafluoroethylene (PTFE). He is now experiencing hand stiffness, pain, and ulceration of his distal thumb on the ipsilateral hand.

Differential Diagnosis

Several etiologies should be considered for the new complaints in this patient. Although ischemic neuropathy and venous hypertension could cause pain and tissue loss in severe cases, the most likely diagnosis in this patient is arterial steal.

Several risk factors have been associated with the development of arterial steal. Diabetes is present in nearly 80% of patients with this diagnosis, and older women are at particularly high risk. Several preoperative hemodynamic parameters have been suggested to be anticipatory as well, with digital-brachial indices (DBI) of less than 0.6 and digital cuff pressures of less than 50 mm Hg being the most common. It is likely that an inability to increase arterial inflow is the precipitating cause for many patients.

Case Continued

The patient states that the symptoms started 2 days after placement of his graft. He experiences pain continuously, and his wife states that his hand is almost always cold. He had none of these symptoms prior to graft placement.

Workup

A thorough history and physical examination are the mainstay for diagnosis of arterial steal. Upon questioning, symptoms related to arterial steal may have begun early following placement of a fistula or graft. Because grafts tend to have greater flow early after placement than fistulas due to physiologic fistula maturation, symptoms of steal often occur earlier in grafts, while they may take several weeks to develop for fistulas. The patient will frequently complain of hand stiffness or pain, coolness, and tissue loss may occur in the affected extremity. On physical examination, compression of the fistula or graft will relieve ischemic-related symptoms in most patients. Additionally, some patients will demonstrate augmentation of the radial pulse distal to the takeoff of the fistula or graft.

Digital-brachial index can be a reliable adjunct to history and physical examination. Measurements should normalize with occlusion of the arteriovenous (AV) fistula or graft, and a DBI of less than 0.45 is suggestive of arterial steal. Additionally, photoplethysmography (PPG) will demonstrate augmentation of monophasic or flat waveform contours that occur with arterial steal (Fig. 1).

Diagnosis and Treatment

For the majority of patients without rest pain or tissue loss, watchful waiting is the mainstay of therapy. Debate exists as to the most appropriate treatment for severe cases. Ligation of the fistula or graft will provide the greatest likelihood of success. However, this approach must be balanced with the need to maintain dialysis access in these fragile patients. Losing dialysis access means that the patient must find a new site for dialysis, often a limited prospect.

Increasing resistance within the fistula or graft has been a widely used method for treatment of ischemic steal syndrome. This can be accomplished through a combination of banding, partial clipping, or lengthening of the graft. Intraoperative Doppler flow measurements can assist in titrating the flow to achieve maximal results. Loss of thrill over the fistula or graft can indicate over-restriction of blood flow and the need for intraoperative revision. Data supporting the use of restrictive procedures is mixed, with many authors believing that this procedure leads to an unacceptably high rate of thrombosis. It is the authors' belief that when done correctly, this procedure can lead to satisfactory results.

Several other surgical options have been described in the literature. Distal revascularization with interval ligation (DRIL) bypasses the AV fistula or graft takeoff location and prevents the retrograde flow that is often associated with arterial steal. The DRIL procedure is best suited for proximal fistulas or grafts and relieves symptoms in over 80% of patients, while maintaining patency in greater than 95% of patients at 1 year. Ligation of the radial artery distal to the fistula or graft takeoff has also been reported in the literature. After assurance of ulnar collateral flow, this procedure reverses retrograde flow and provides symptomatic relief while maintaining the integrity of the AV fistula or graft.

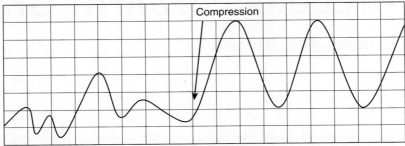

FIGURE 1 • Dampened digital photoplethysmography (PPG) waveforms of a patient with radiobasilic arteriovenous fistula and arterial steal. With manual compression, the waveform returns to normal contours.

Case Continued

Following history and physical examination, the patient is diagnosed with arterial steal related to his recent AV graft placement. He scheduled for elective banding of his fistula.

Surgical Approach

Anesthesia can be provided by regional nerve block or general anesthesia. The AV graft is accessed through an incision over the prior access point. After proximal and distal control has been obtained, options for ligation include simple suture ligation or division of the fistula or graft. The latter is generally regarded as having better outcomes in diabetic patients.

When performing flow-limiting procedures, such as banding, partial ligation, or hemoclip placement, intraoperative Doppler measurements or blood flow probes may be used. After exposure and control of the artery and fistula or graft, a self-made restrictive band is fashioned out of a piece of 6-mm PTFE. In general, a section that can sufficiently cover 2 cm (length) of AV graft circumferentially is preferable. Alternatively, the access can be narrowed with sequential ligatures spaced several millimeters apart. While intermittently monitoring the graft and distal takeoff artery with Doppler or blood flow probe, the band is placed just distal to the anastomosis and sequentially tightened to achieve maximal flow in both vessels.

In the case of proximal arm grafts or fistulas, the DRIL procedure is frequently cited as the best option for reversal of arterial steal. In the first phase of this procedure, a reversed saphenous vein graft is used to fashion an arterial bypass from the brachial artery (above the antecubital fossa) to the distal brachial artery. The second phase of the procedure involves ligation of the brachial artery proximal to the distal anastomosis. Technical precision is critical as thrombosis of the bypass graft can be limb threatening.

Endovascular approaches are gaining popularity in the treatment of arterial steal. If proximal arterial stenosis is found to be the cause of arterial steal symptoms, balloon angioplasty may correct the arterial steal. Additionally, selective stent placement can be used to cover the graft outflow if ligation is desired or stent the residual arterial stenosis (Table 1).

Special Intraoperative Considerations

1. Several attempts may need to be made to achieve the proper balance between access flow and flow to the extremity.
2. Priority should be given to ensuring enough flow in the extremity to alleviate the steal, and assessment of arterial in-flow (subclavian-brachial) is essential.
3. If restriction does not augment arterial flow, a distal stenosis should be suspected and the distal anastomosis and artery should be evaluated.

Postoperative Management

Despite revision of the AV graft, complete resolution of symptoms is not ensured. Several series report improvement in steal symptoms in 70% to 80% of patients with reversal of tissue loss and improvements in hemodynamic parameters. Close follow-up of ischemic-related complications is recommended, and monitoring for signs of thrombosis is advised. A classification scheme for arterial steal is summarized in Table 2.

TABLE 1. AV-Access Forearm Graft

Key Technical Steps

1. Anesthetic technique can be provided via local nerve block or general anesthesia.
2. Proximal exposure of the graft is obtained through the previous incision.
3. A suitable segment of PTFE graft is cut to provide a circumferential wrap around the artery. In general, a segment of PTFE that covers 2 cm in length is preferable.
4. Prolene suture is used to narrow the band in successive increments while the takeoff artery and graft are being monitored for hemodynamic changes.

Potential Pitfalls

- If performing a flow-limiting procedure, overrestriction can lead to thrombosis.
- Insufficient restriction can result in continued symptoms.
- Care should be taken to ensure that a distal stenosis, either anastomotic or otherwise, does not exist. If present, it may be the etiology of the steal and may not resolve following banding.

TABLE 2. Classification Scheme for Severity of Arterial Steal

Grade	Symptoms	Treatment
0	No steal	None
1, Mild	Minimal symptoms, cool extremity	Watchful waiting
2, Moderate	Swelling, intermittent discomfort	Intervention sometimes needed
3, Severe	Ischemic pain at rest, tissue loss	Intervention always needed

Case Conclusion

The patient tolerates the banding procedure and has near-complete reversal of ischemic symptoms. He is able to use his graft immediately following the procedure, and his wounds have fully healed in 4 weeks following the procedure.

TAKE HOME POINTS

- Arterial steal can occur immediately following AV fistula or graft creation and manifests as hand stiffness, cold sensation, or rest pain with tissue ulceration.
- History and physical examination provide the best tools for diagnosis of arterial steal. PPG and DBI are useful adjuncts to diagnosis.
- The mainstay of therapy in mild cases is watchful waiting. Cases involving more severe symptoms may require operative intervention.

- Options for surgical treatment include ligation of the AV fistula, banding or partial suturing, and reconstruction with distal bypass and ligation.
- Endovascular methods are becoming more common for correctable causes of arterial steal including proximal stenosis amenable to balloon angioplasty.

SUGGESTED READINGS

Schanzer H, Eisenberg D. Management of steal syndrome resulting from dialysis access. *Semin Vasc Surg.* 2004;17(1):45-49.

Wilson SE. *Vascular Access Principles and Practice.* 10th ed. Philadelphia, PA: Wolters Kluwer, Lippincott Williams & Wilkins; 2010.

Wixon CL, Hughes JD, Mills JL. Understanding strategies for the treatment of ischemic steal syndrome after hemodialysis access. *J Am Coll Surg.* 2000;191(3):301-310.

CLINICAL SCENARIO CASE QUESTIONS

1. Following placement of a forearm loop graft, what DBI and digital pressure measurement is suggestive of arterial steal?

    a. 0.8 and 80 mm Hg
    b. 0.5 and 40 mm Hg
    c. 1.0 and 60 mm Hg
    d. 1.0 and 120 mm Hg

2. A patient presents with swelling and intermittent discomfort in his ipsilateral hand following forearm loop graft placement. What grade of severity would his ischemic steal symptoms comprise?

    a. 0
    b. 1
    c. 2
    d. 3

33 AV Access (Salvage— Endovascular)

LUKE R. WILKINS and WAEL E. SAAD

Presentation

A 72-year-old woman with end-stage renal disease (ESRD) on hemodialysis (HD) via a left upper extremity brachial-basilic arteriovenous graft presents with a pulsatile graft and a marked decrease in flow rates during most recent dialysis session.

Differential Diagnosis

The differential diagnosis of pulsatile graft with decrease flow rates on HD includes venous outflow stenosis occurring at the venous anastomosis or within the central venous system. Alternatively, an arterial inflow lesion can also cause decreasing flow rates and diminished thrill within the graft.

Workup

A complete medical and surgical history was obtained. The left upper extremity graft was placed approximately 2 years prior to presentation. In addition, the patient previously had a left-sided, tunneled hemodialysis (HD) catheter with access in the left internal jugular vein. After placement of the graft in the left upper extremity, the patient has had multiple prior interventions for recurrent central stenosis of the left brachiocephalic vein. At the most recent intervention, 2 months prior to presentation, the central stenosis required placement of a 20 mm × 40 mm Wallstent that was postdilated with a 16 mm × 4 cm Maxi LD balloon. The patient tolerated dialysis well until presentation when, at scheduled dialysis, a marked decrease in flow rates was identified (less than 400 mL/min). The patient reported no abnormal symptoms during most recent dialysis session. Pertinent negatives include no evidence of steal symptoms and no complaints of upper extremity swelling.

On physical examination, there is a pulsatile graft in the left upper extremity. No definite thrill could be identified. Brachial, ulnar, and radial pulses are palpable. A bedside ultrasound was performed that showed a patent arterial anastomosis with no evidence of stenosis or narrowing (Fig. 1). The venous outflow was also evaluated and showed no evidence of narrowing or stenosis.

On the basis of the ultrasound, the cause for decrease in flow rates is likely secondary to either venous outflow obstruction or central venous disease (CVD). A digital subtraction central venogram was performed via antegrade access in the venous outflow. Images demonstrate previously placed Wallstent in the left brachiocephalic vein with marked degree of narrowing/stenosis at its central-most aspect with extensive collateral vessel formation (Fig. 2).

Diagnosis and Treatment

The diagnosis of CVD may be made on the basis of several clinical and imaging findings. The provided clinical history of prior HD catheter and prior intervention should raise suspicion. Frequently, patients will present with ipsilateral face, neck, breast, or arm edema. In addition, the presence of massive arm edema in the access arm is virtually diagnostic of CVD. However, as can be seen in the provided case, the absence of significant swelling does not preclude the diagnosis. The presence of enlarged collateral veins in the neck, chest, and ipsilateral extremity may also be identified. The diagnosis of CVD may be suggested through findings on duplex ultrasound as absence of normal respiratory variation in the diameter of the central veins and polyphasic atrial waveforms. As demonstrated in the provided case, digital subtraction central contrast venography is the gold standard for the diagnosis of CVD.

Endovascular intervention is the primary treatment consideration for CVD. Current options include percutaneous transluminal angioplasty (PTA), bare-metal stent (BMS) placement, or covered stent (CS) placement. Currently, the Kidney Disease Outcome Quality Initiative (KDOQI) guidelines recommend PTA with or without stent placement as the preferred treatment option for CVD.

PTA is the traditional first-line therapy for CVD. However, most research involving PTA of CVD has lacked clearly defined reporting standards leading to highly variable methodologies and inconsistent conclusions. Generally, PTA has a high technical success with highly variable primary patency rates of 23% to 55% at 6 months and 12% to 50% at 12 months. Multiple repeated interventions with close follow-up are necessary when attempting to maintain patency in CVD patients with PTA.

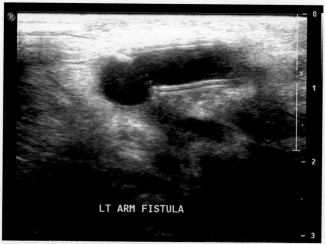

FIGURE 1 • Ultrasound image at level of arterial anastomosis showing no evidence of stenosis or narrowing.

Given efficacy of PTA, a more long-term, durable solution was sought. For this role, BMS have been used for maintenance of patency in CVD. Initial attempts focused on elastic or highly resistant fibrotic lesions. This approach is associated with a high rate of technical success (close to 100%). Primarily, self-expanding stents are utilized in this anatomical region. Balloon-expandable stents are not routinely used as they may deform or migrate. This is particularly evident in the subclavian and left brachiocephalic veins where adjacent osseous structures combined with respiratory motion may cause significant external compression. The first generation of self-expanding stents consisted of the Wallstent (Boston Scientific, Natick, MA). The advantages of this stent are its variability of diameter and lengths combined with its marked radiopacity. Second-generation stents are the nitinol stents. Nitinol is an alloy of nickel and titanium.

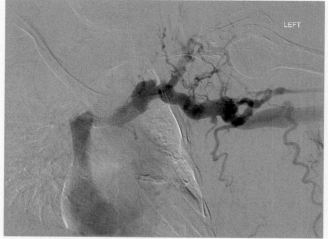

FIGURE 2 • Central venogram via left upper extremity fistula showing Wallstent in left brachiocephalic vein with recurrent stenosis and marked collateral vessel formation.

This material will have a reversible shape transformation at high temperatures (martensitic transformation) that is preset by its nickel and titanium ratio.

While initial technical success is high for BMS in CVD, long-term results remain variable. Primary patency rates range from 63% to 100% at 3 months, 42% to 89% at 6 months, and 14% to 73% at 12 months. Cumulative patency results have ranged 72% to 100% at 3 months, 55% to 100% at 6 months, and 31% to 97% at 12 months. While the current literature demonstrates variable long-term patency results, there is clearly a significant population of CVD patients whose lesions are inadequately treated with PTA and will require BMS for both technical success and better long-term patency.

CS have recently been utilized with varying degrees of success in the treatment of CVD. In theory, CS provide a relatively inert and stable intravascular matrix for endothelialization while providing the mechanical advantages of a BMS. This could decrease the intimal hyperplastic response and reduce the restenosis rate seen after PTA or BMS. However, as with studies evaluating PTA and BMS, the results are varied with nonuniform methodology. Within these limitations, there may be a trend toward improved 3-, 6-, and 12-month patency after CS stent placement. In addition, the cost-benefit analysis of CS placement will need to be studied with long-term follow-up and comparative assessments to delineate the future role of this treatment option.

Lastly, while endovascular treatment is the first-line therapy for CVD, some patients may be refractory to endovascular options. In this patient population, surgical treatments may be the only option. While 12-month patency rates of open surgical management of CVD range from 79% to 86%, the procedure is frequently associated with significant morbidity. A full and complete discussion regarding surgical management of CVD is beyond the scope of this chapter, and the reader is referred to a dedicated text for a more detailed analysis.

Technical Approach

A 0.035 guidewire and angled tip catheter were used to cross the central venous stenosis. Given previously placed stent, great care was taken to ensure that the wire stayed in an intraluminal location without crossing the interstices of the stent (Figs. 3 and 4). Sequential balloon inflations were then performed at the area of stenosis with 6-, 8-, 10-, and 12-mm angioplasty balloons. Despite multiple, prolonged inflations, a marked degree of residual stenosis remained. At this point, the decision was made to extend the left brachiocephalic stent. While in this anatomic location a self-expanding stent is the preferred stent, given the location of the residual stenosis, precise deployment in the left brachiocephalic vein at the junction of the SVC was felt to be of utmost importance. Placement of a self-expanding stent in this location and with this type of lesion may result in stent migration.

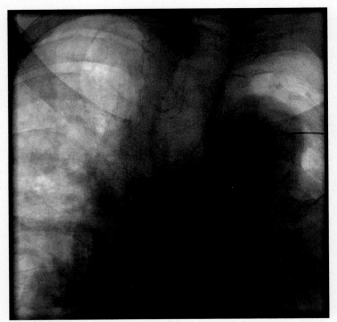

FIGURE 3 • Image demonstrating wire access through existing Wallstent in the left brachiocephalic vein.

Further, the stenotic lesion was in the central-most aspect of the left brachiocephalic vein and posterior to the sternum, thus decreasing the risk for significant compressive forces related to respiratory motion. With these considerations in mind, the decision was made to place a balloon-expandable stent. A 12-French, 40-cm sheath was then advanced through the stent. A 10 × 39-mm Palmaz stent (Cordis, Miami Lakes, FL) was loaded on a 14 × 40 angioplasty balloon. The stent was then deployed within the distal left brachiocephalic vein stent extending just to the junction with the SVC. Repeat fistulogram was performed demonstrating markedly improved flow through

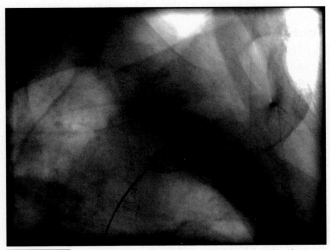

FIGURE 4 • Image obtained in a steep oblique projection verifying intraluminal position of wire access shown in Figure 3.

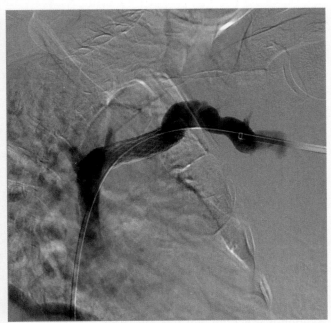

FIGURE 5 • Central venogram following placement of Palmaz stent with no evidence of residual stenosis or collateral vasculature.

the brachiocephalic vein without any filling of the previously noted collaterals along the left chest wall and left upper extremity (Fig. 5). The sheath was removed and a 2-0 purse string suture was then placed at the puncture site to achieve hemostasis Table 1.

Special Intraoperative Considerations

Great care should be taken in the case of restenosis following prior stent placement. As seen in the provided case, the lesion was inadequately treated with a self-expanding stent. While the original treatment was appropriate for the given presentation, now that the vein showed restenosis that was not responding to sequential, prolonged balloon

TABLE 1. AV Access (Salvage— Endovascular)

Key Technical Steps

1. Ultrasound evaluation to determine probable etiology
2. Decide access point on the basis of the US evaluation
3. Obtain central venogram
4. Define lesion and decide optimal treatment (e.g., PTA vs. stent)
5. If stent, determine appropriate type and size on the basis of venogram and anatomic location (see text)
6. Obtain central venogram following treatment to assure resolution of stenotic lesion

Potential Pitfalls

- Inappropriate type or size of stent
- Overly aggressive PTA that can cause acute extravasation
- Inadequate treatment of underlying lesion

inflations, a new approach was warranted. Placement of a balloon-expandable stent in the central venous system should only be performed after careful consideration of the underlying anatomy.

Postoperative Management

The patient should be monitored for a minimum of 2 hours following stent placement for CVD. Close monitoring of vital signs and symptoms of chest pain should be performed. The patient may be discharged without scheduled, routine follow-up. However, close surveillance of access function should be performed in the patient's dialysis center. Any change in access function should warrant repeat evaluation with ultrasound and/or fistulogram.

Case Conclusion

CVD is a frequently seen cause of poorly functioning fistulas or grafts. While PTA with or without self-expanding stent placement is the preferred therapy, alternative treatment methods may be considered in the salvage setting. This should only be done after a thorough evaluation of the lesion, underlying anatomy, and previous treatment methods.

TAKE HOME POINTS

- Evaluation of poorly functioning fistulas or grafts should first include a focused physical examination and ultrasound evaluation.
- A fistulogram should be performed for concern of venous outflow or central venous stenoses.
- For treatment of CVD, PTA with or without stent placement is the preferred therapy.
- Self-expanding stents should be placed in most cases of CVD.

- If a balloon-expandable stent is to be placed, a thorough consideration of underlying anatomy, lesion, and previous treatments is warranted.
- CS show promise in the treatment of CVD, though more research may be needed to justify routine use.

SUGGESTED READINGS

Anaya-Ayala JE, Bellows P, Ismail N. Surgical management of hemodialysis-related central venous occlusive disease: a treatment algorithm. *Ann Vasc Surg.* 2011;25:108-119.

Kundu S, Modabber M, You JM, et al. Use of PTFE stent grafts for hemodialysis-related central venous occlusions: intermediate-term results. *Cardiovasc Intervent Radiol.* 2011;34:949-957.

Modabber M, Kundu S. Central venous disease in hemodialysis patients: an update. *Cardiovasc Intervent Radiol.* 2013;36: 898-903.

Rayner HC, Besarab A, Brown WW, et al. Vascular access results from the Dialysis Outcomes and Practice Patterns Study (DOPPS): performance against Kidney Disease Outcomes Quality Initiative (K/DOQI) Clinical Practice Guidelines. *Am J Kidney Dis.* 2004;44:22-26.

Vesely TM, Hovsepian DM, Pilgram TK, et al. Upper extremity central venous obstruction in hemodialysis patients: treatment with Wallstents. *Radiology.* 1997;204:343-348.

CLINICAL SCENARIO CASE QUESTIONS

1. Current KDOQI recommendations for first-line treatment of CVD involves:
   a. Open surgical management
   b. Initial stent placement
   c. PTA with or without stent placement
   d. PTA with covered stent placement

2. When treating CVD with stent placement, self-expanding stents are often preferred because of what property?
   a. Increased hoop strength
   b. Radial force and noncompressibility
   c. Ease of deployment
   d. Metal fatigue coefficient

34 Arteriovenous Hemodialysis Access—Beyond Traditional

THOMAS S. HUBER

Presentation

A 57-year-old obese female with a history of end-stage renal disease presents to your clinic for permanent hemodialysis access. She has been on dialysis for the past 7 years and is currently dialyzing through a tunneled, cuffed catheter in her right femoral vein. Her end-stage renal disease is secondary to both diabetes and hypertension. She is right handed. She has a complex access history and has had permanent access procedures in both upper extremities including a left brachioaxillary prosthetic arteriovenous access that had to be removed secondary to infection. Most recently, she was dialyzing through a right upper extremity brachial-basilic autogenous access. She has a known axillary/subclavian vein stenosis on the right that was remediated several times with a combination of percutaneous procedures including balloon angioplasty and stenting. The right-sided central vein occlusion, likely the etiology of the most reason access failure, could not be crossed with a wire during the last remedial attempt.

Differential Diagnosis

The patient requires permanent hemodialysis access and has been labeled as "complex" given her prior access history, obesity, and known central vein occlusion. Although most access surgeons have a clinical impression of what constitutes "complex" or "tertiary" problems, the term is poorly defined, and there are no clear recommendations or guidelines from the Kidney Disease Outcome Quality Initiatives (KDOQI), the standard of care for maintaining hemodialysis access. The anatomic and patient comorbidities that complicate the construction of a permanent hemodialysis, potentially leading to the definition of a complex access, are shown in Table 1. Central vein occlusions and/or stenoses are likely the most common complex problem given the widespread use of central vein catheters for both dialysis- and non–dialysis-related indications. Unfortunately, the cohort of patients with complex access problems is likely expanding given the improvements in care for patients with end-stage renal disease, their improved life expectancies, and the reliance on central venous catheters as noted above.

Workup

The initial approach to patients with "complex" access problems is identical to that for those presenting for their first access (Fig. 1). This systematic approach can help identify potential problems or contraindications to an access (e.g., arterial inflow stenosis secondary to subclavian stenosis) and, thereby, suggest solutions or remedial treatments (e.g., subclavian angioplasty). It is based upon the KDOQI guidelines with a strong emphasis on creating autogenous accesses due to their improved patency and decreased infectious complication rates. Constructing a permanent hemodialysis access is similar to a lower extremity bypass procedures and based upon the principles of vascular surgery including adequate inflow, adequate outflow, and a suitable conduit. True complex access problems are not all that common, and it is possible to construct a traditional access in most patients, usually an autogenous access.

The initial approach includes a focused history and physical examination in combination with noninvasive imaging. Special attention should be directed at documenting the access history including procedures, revisions, and associated complications. Physical examination should include a detailed pulse examination with an Allen's test to determine the forearm vessel responsible for the dominant arterial supply to the hand. The noninvasive testing in the diagnostic vascular laboratory includes examination of both the arterial and venous circulation. The arterial studies include blood pressure measurements of the brachial, radial, ulnar, and digital arteries along with the corresponding Doppler waveforms of all but the digital vessels (Fig. 2). Additionally, the Allen's test is repeated, and the diameters of both the radial and brachial arteries are measured at the wrist and antecubital fossa, respectively. Venous imaging includes the interrogation of the cephalic and basilic veins from the wrist to the axilla complete with diameter measurements, similar to the preoperative vein survey obtained prior to infrainguinal arterial revascularization (Fig. 3).

TABLE 1. Anatomic and Patient Comorbidities Complicating Permanent Hemodialysis Access Procedures

Central vein occlusions or stenoses
Obesity
Advanced age
Prior access-related hand ischemia (steal)
Multiple failed prosthetic access procedures
Human immunodeficiency virus
Inadequate arterial inflow
Inadequate peripheral vein (for autogenous access)

An operative plan is then generated based upon the results of the history, physical examination, and noninvasive imaging with a strong emphasis on autogenous access. The objective is to select the combination of the artery and vein that most likely result in a successful arteriovenous fistula (AVF). The usual conventions of using the nondominant > dominant extremity and the forearm > arm are not always pertinent, although I have followed these standard approaches when the choices are equivocal. The criteria for an adequate artery and vein include an adequate diameter, no hemodynamically significant arterial inflow stenoses, no venous outflow stenoses, and a peripheral vein segment of suitable length and diameter (Table 2). My preferences in descending order include the radial-cephalic, radial-basilic, brachial-cephalic, and brachial-basilic autogenous accesses prior to use of prosthetic material (Table 3). Notably, these preferences are consistent with the current KDOQI guidelines.

Contrast arteriography and venography can be used to confirm the preliminary access choice and are particularly helpful for those with complex problems. Similar to most other applications in vascular surgery, the contrast imaging has evolved from catheter-based procedures to computed tomography (CT)-based procedures. CT venography has the potential ability to image the central venous runoff from all four extremities with a single study, although I have experienced some difficult with the timing of the contrast deliver, particularly in patients with limited peripheral venous access.

Case Continued

The patient undergoes noninvasive imaging as outlined above. She is found to have an axillary vein occlusion on right although the axillary vein on the left appears to be patent. She has evidence of a thrombosed brachial-basilic autogenous access on the right and no suitable peripheral veins (i.e., cephalic or basilic) on either side for an autogenous access based upon the criteria outlined above. Her brachial and radial arterial pressures are normal and symmetric bilaterally with the diameter of the brachial arteries both being greater than 4 mm.

Workup (Continued)

The noninvasive imaging suggest that further access attempts are precluded on the right upper extremity based upon the axillary vein occlusion (and the known history of a central vein occlusion based upon previous fistulagram attempts). The left axillary vein appears to be patent and, thus, suitable for a potential access although

FIGURE 1 • An algorithm for patients presenting for permanent hemodialysis access is shown. Note that *Invasive Arterial/venous Imaging* now includes both catheter- and CT-based arteriography and venography. Patients with *No Potential Autogenous Access* due to peripheral veins that are insufficient diameter (less than 3 mm) are either reimaged in the operating room with ultrasound after induction of anesthesia or the veins are dissected and explored directly. *Adjuncts for Autogenous Access* include endovascular treatment of arterial inflow/venous outflow lesions and composite access configurations. (Reproduced from Huber TS, et al. Prospective validation of an algorithm to maximize arteriovenous fistulae for chronic hemodialysis access. *J Vasc Surg.* 2002;36:452-459, with permission.)

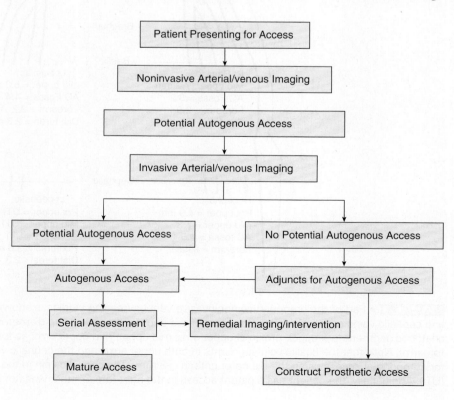

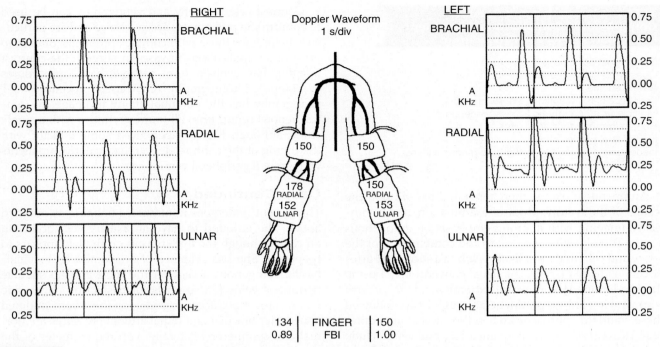

FIGURE 2 • Part of the preoperative noninvasive arterial imaging studies is shown. The brachial, radial, and ulnar arterial pressures (mm Hg) are shown on the diagram of the upper extremities while the finger pressures are shown in the center of the figure at the bottom. The corresponding Doppler waveforms (s/div) are shown for the brachial, radial, and ulnar arteries. The FBI denotes the finger/brachial index and is the ratio of the finger pressure to the ipsilateral brachial artery pressure. Note the symmetric brachial artery pressures and the corresponding normal appearing triphasic Doppler waveforms.

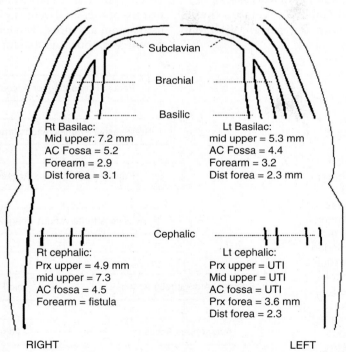

FIGURE 3 • Part of the preoperative noninvasive venous imaging studies is shown. The diameters (mm) of both the basilic and cephalic veins are shown on the diagram of the upper extremities. The diameters are reported for the corresponding anatomic segment (prx upper, proximal upper arm; mid upper, mid upper arm; ac fossa, antecubital fossa; dista forea, distal forearm). Note that the basilic vein segments in both upper arms and the cephalic vein in the right upper arm are suitable for autogenous access using the diameter criteria (≥3 mm). The cephalic vein in the left upper arm was unable to be imaged (UTI). Additionally, the patient has a patent access in the right forearm that was not imaged.

TABLE 2. Critical Steps to Determine Suitability of Artery and Vein for Autogenous Access

Vein
Diameter ≥3 mm without evidence of significant stenosis
Suitable segment from the wrist to antecubital fossa (forearm access) or antecubital fossa to axilla (upper arm access)
Absence of significant central vein stenosis in the ipsilateral extremity

Artery
Diameter ≥2 mm
Absence of hemodynamically significant inflow stenosis[a]
Nondominant radial artery for wrist access

[a]≥15 mm Hg pressure gradient between the brachial arteries for proposed arm accesses or between the ipsilateral brachial and radial arteries for proposed forearm accesses.

ultrasound interrogation of the central veins proximal to the axillary vein is limited due to the bony thoracic cavity. The patient has no suitable peripheral veins for an autogenous access; thus, the only potential traditional access option would be a brachial-axillary prosthetic access with the venous anastomosis site more proximally on the axillary vein than the previous one that became infected, necessitating excision. Further imaging with either a CT venogram or catheter-based venogram is necessary to confirm the patency of the central veins on the left.

Case Continued

The patient undergoes a CT venogram that demonstrates that the internal jugular, subclavian, and brachiocephalic veins are occluded on both sides. The superior vena cava appears to be patent but is filled predominantly from collaterals. There is a crushed, thrombosed stent in the right subclavian vein that extends into the brachiocephalic vein. The axillary vein on the left appears to be patent, as suggested by the noninvasive studies. There is a dialysis catheter in the right common femoral vein that extends into the inferior vena cava. The common femoral, external iliac, and common iliac veins are patent on both sides.

Workup (Continued)

The CT venogram findings suggest that further attempts at an upper extremity access are relatively contraindicated. However, the study suggests that the lower extremity

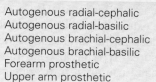

TABLE 3. Hierarchy for Permanent Hemodialysis Accesses Configurations

Autogenous radial-cephalic
Autogenous radial-basilic
Autogenous brachial-cephalic
Autogenous brachial-basilic
Forearm prosthetic
Upper arm prosthetic

central veins are patent and that a lower extremity access may be an option. Similar to my generic access algorithm outlined above, noninvasive imaging of the lower extremities is obtained with ankle/brachial indices and duplex ultrasound of the saphenous and femoral system prior to formulating an initial operative plan.

Case Continued

The ankle/brachial indices are not able to be obtained because the tibial vessels are noncompressible. However, the pedal waveforms are triphasic, and the toe/brachial indices are 0.65 bilaterally. The duplex ultrasound of the lower extremities demonstrates that the saphenous and femoral veins are widely patent bilaterally. The femoropopliteal veins are greater than 7 mm, and the saphenous veins are greater than 3 mm. No evidence of venous reflux is seen in either extremity.

Diagnosis and Treatment

Central vein stenoses or occlusions are likely the most common etiology of patients with complex access issues as noted above. The obvious solution is to simply select an alternative extremity with a patent central vein run-off without evidence of stenosis. However, this is not always an option given the widespread use of tunneled dialysis catheters and the prevalence of central vein lesions. I have strongly favored upper extremity accesses over lower extremity ones given the higher incidence of infectious complications associated with the latter, even when this mandates addressing the central vein lesion. The options for placing an access ipsilateral to a known central vein stenosis or occlusion include bypassing or correcting the lesion at the time of access creation or delaying until when/if the venous hypertension and arm edema become problematic. Notably, it is worth emphasizing that a central vein stenosis or occlusion is only a relatively contraindication to an ipsilateral access. Indeed, there are several patients in my current practice that have known central vein occlusions and a functional access with minimal arm edema, presumably secondary to their significant collateral network. Unfortunately, it is difficult to predict preoperatively which patients will develop sufficient collaterals to overcome any significant stenosis, and, thus, I have favored addressing the lesions preemptively. Importantly, superior vena cava syndrome is an absolute contraindication to an upper extremity access.

There are both open and endovascular options for treating the central vein stenosis or occlusions. Similar to most applications, the endovascular options are less invasive but tend to be less durable. The technical success rates for the endovascular approaches are quite good, provided that the lesion can be crossed with a wire. However, the primary patency rates are only about 50% and 25% at 6 and 12 months, respectively. It is unclear whether stents improve the patency rates associated with angioplasty alone, but they are susceptible to being crushed when placed in the thoracic outlet. The patency rates may be improved with covered stents (compared to bare-metal stents), but they have the potential to compromise the venous return through collaterals or the main channels (e.g., internal jugular vein, contralateral brachiocephalic vein) if maldeployed. Multiple open surgical options have been described including axilloaxillary bypass, axillojugular bypass, jugular vein turndown, axilloatrial bypass, and axillofemoral bypass with the potential options largely dictated by the patent vessels. However, the long-term patency rates of these reconstructions are poorly described given their relative infrequency. I have had a modest amount of success with the axillojugular bypass (i.e., ipsilateral) although it is rarely an option since the jugular vein is the preferred site for tunneled dialysis catheters and usually occluded by the time patients are referred to my clinic for their complex access issues.

The HeRO (Hemosphere, Inc., Minneapolis, MN) is a hybrid graft/catheter composed of a 6-mm PTFE graft and a 5-mm (i.d.) nitinol-reinforced silicone catheter that may be useful in the setting of central vein stenoses or occlusions. The system is essentially a prosthetic graft that is connected to central venous catheter that functions similar to a prosthetic access from a patient standpoint. The catheter component is mated to the graft component with a coupling mechanism and serves to provide the outflow from the graft into the atrium or superior vena cava, overcoming the central vein stenosis or occlusions. Insertion of the device requires passing the catheter component (19 French, 6.3 mm o.d.) through the stenotic or occluded central veins. The initial report documenting the outcome of the device reported primary and secondary patency rates of 39% and 72%, respectively, at a mean follow-up of 8.6 months with a bacteremia rate of 0.70/1000 days. It has been my anecdotal impression that the infectious complication rates are significantly higher and the patency rates are lower, but I would readily concede that I have only used the device in a very complex group of patients with extremely limited options, and, thus, my poor results may reflect patient selection rather than limitations of the device.

The permanent hemodialysis access options in the lower extremity are somewhat limited and associated with a higher incidence of ischemic and infectious complications. The most common configuration is a prosthetic thigh loop based off the femoral vessels. I prefer to use the common femoral artery and vein, but others have reported various combinations of the vessels, including the superficial femoral artery and saphenous vein. A recent large series reported primary and secondary patency rates at 12 months of 54% and 75%, respectively, with an infectious complication rate of 27%. Notably, the ischemic complication rate in this series was only 2%, but the low rate likely reflects the authors' selection criteria. Notably, other authors have reported that infectious complication rates for the lower extremity prosthetic accesses are so high that a tunneled dialysis catheter is a better, safer long-term option. The

autogenous options include using either the saphenous vein or the femoropopliteal vein. Although there are several early reports, the saphenous vein is rarely an option. The wall of the saphenous vein is relatively thick (compared to the cephalic and basilic vein), and, thus, it does not dilate much in response to the hemodynamic forces associated with the arteriovenous fistula. Furthermore, it is rarely large enough in terms of diameter (i.e., 5 or 6 mm) to sustain effective dialysis. The femoropopliteal vein can be mobilized and used for an autogenous access, but the wound and ischemic complications are prohibitive and likely exceed those for the prosthetic alternatives.

A number of exotic access configurations have been reported (e.g., axillary artery–renal vein prosthetic access), and, theoretically, it is possible to construct a prosthetic arteriovenous access given a suitable arterial inflow and venous outflow. The long-term durability of these exotic options remains undefined but is likely somewhat limited.

Case Continued

The patient undergoes a left common femoral artery–common femoral vein prosthetic access with 6-mm PTFE.

Surgical Approach

The surgical approach for the femoral-based prosthetic access is fairly straightforward and familiar to most vascular surgeons. I prefer a vertical incision over the femoral artery and try to keep it caudal to the inguinal crease. Some surgeons prefer a transverse or oblique incision, believing that it is associated with a lower incidence of wound complications, although it is my impression that the exposure with the transverse is inferior, particularly for reoperations. The common femoral artery and vein are dissected free sufficiently to apply a side-biting or partially occluding clamp (e.g., Satinsky clamp). In the presence of significant calcification in the common femoral artery, it may not be possible to use a side-biting clamp, necessitating dissecting and occluding the common, profunda, and superficial femoral arteries individually. As noted above, I prefer to site the venous anastomosis on the common femoral vein based upon the logic that it facilitates the largest venous outflow for the anastomosis and, thus, is less likely to develop significant intimal hyperplasia that threatens the graft. The proposed course of the loop graft is marked on the skin, and a separate stab wound is made at the 6 o'clock position to facilitate passing the graft. Alternatively, two separate incisions (i.e., 4 and 8 o'clock) may be made to facilitate tunneling the graft with the choice based upon the patient's body habitus. The graft is tunneled using a curvilinear tunneling device. The tunnel should be created immediately deep to the dermis throughout the extent that will be used for cannulation but sufficiently deep to the soft tissue in the groin to facilitate wound closure. I typically use a 6-mm PTFE graft but will occasionally use an 8-mm graft in patients with larger femoral vessels and no evidence of arterial occlusive disease, based upon the impression that the patency rates are better. The arterial and venous anastomoses are performed in a standard end-side fashion.

Case Continued

The patient returns to clinic on her 7th postoperative day with some mild redness and swelling at the site of her surgical incision. Ultrasound of her groin demonstrates a small amount of fluid surrounding the graft.

Postoperative Management—Initial

Patients are routinely seen in clinic 2 weeks after their procedure or earlier as dictated by any active access-related issues. Patients with prosthetic access are subsequently seen approximately 30 days after their procedure, and their access is cleared for cannulation provided that there are no new issues. I have generally waited 4 to 6 weeks before cannulating prosthetic accesses although it is likely safe to cannulate them a bit earlier, and this situation occasionally arises in patients who are having difficulties with their tunneled catheters. There are a variety of "early cannulation" grafts commercially available that afford the theoretical appeal of eliminating or reducing the need for tunneled catheters. However, most patients cannot tolerate the discomfort of having their graft cannulated early secondary to the pain and trauma related to the incision and tunneling process. As noted above, infectious complications are common after lower extremity access procedures, albeit usually related to cannulation, and I have taken an aggressive approach in terms of initiating antibiotic treatment. It is common to develop seromas or fluid collections around PTFE grafts. These seromas can lead to graft infections, but they are usually self-limited.

Case Conclusion

The patient's mild cellulitis resolves in response to the antibiotics. Her access is cleared for cannulation at 4 weeks, and a diagram, with instructions, is sent to her dialysis center.

Postoperative Management—Long Term

The role of postoperative access surveillance and remediation remains unresolved. The dialysis access should be assessed by physical examination with each dialysis session and most dialysis units employ some type of monthly assessment (e.g., blood flow monitoring, static venous dialysis pressures, duplex ultrasound). Several randomized trials have failed to demonstrate a benefit for surveillance and preemptive intervention (e.g., angioplasty) in patients with prosthetic grafts despite the widespread application of this approach. Admittedly, these trials were performed in patients with more straightforward access procedures, and the findings may not be applicable to patients with complex access issues. I have not committed my patients to any type of surveillance protocol but have taken an aggressive approach in terms of access interrogation and remediation when/if any access dysfunction is identified during dialysis, particularly in patients with complex access problems.

The long-term success rates for many of the procedures outlined for patients with complex access procedures are likely somewhat limited. However, the patient's life expectancies are also likely compromised, and it is the underlying hope that some type of access can be maintained to assure effective dialysis. Accordingly, preventative strategies to preserve all potential access options should be initiated including engaging patients about the importance of preserving all peripheral veins for potential autogenous access, limiting the use of percutaneously inserted central catheters (PICC lines), avoiding central vein catheters (particularly subclavian lines), optimizing the use of autogenous access procedures, and sustaining each permanent access as long as possible. Furthermore, options for transplantation and peritoneal dialysis should be explored as alternative renal replacement therapies in these patients with limited hemodialysis access options.

Discussion

Although central vein occlusions and stenoses were the focus of the case presentation, other conditions that complicate the construction of a permanent hemodialysis access merit further discussion.

The epidemic of obesity in our country has impacted all access of health care including the incidence of end-stage renal disease and the construction of permanent hemodialysis accesses. The fundamental problem with obese patients from an access standpoint is that the "superficial veins" (i.e., cephalic, forearm basilic) tend to run "deep" due to the overlying fat and subcutaneous tissue. Somewhat surprisingly, obese patients have a comparable number of autogenous access options on preoperative noninvasive imaging. Due to the depth of the overlying tissue, the "superficial" veins usually need to be elevated, similar to the scenario of patients undergoing a two-stage brachiobasilic autogenous access. My preferred approach is to make a longitudinal incision over the vein and then "elevate" it by simply closing the underlying soft tissue with a series of interrupted sutures. Other authors have proposed "elevating" the vein by excising the subcutaneous tissue using a series of transverse "skip" incisions. A forearm prosthetic (e.g., brachial-median antecubital) and chest wall axillary-axillary loop are both viable options in obese patients. Notably, their forearms tend to be relatively spared by the subcutaneous fat relative to the upper arm. Lastly, I have favored the two-stage brachial-basilic approach over the single stage for obese patients since the extensive dissection (and potential wound complications) is not performed unless the vein has dilated and, thus, is likely to be suitable for cannulation after elevation.

Advanced patient age is relevant to the choice of access configuration for several reasons including the presence of other comorbidities, limited life expectancy, and "thin" skin. Although there is no clear cutoff in terms of when a patient is not a candidate for a permanent access procedure (or renal replacement therapy), I have modified my emphasis on autogenous access in elderly patients with the primary goal to establish a functional access with limited complications. It is not clear that the purported advantages of autogenous accesses are relevant for elderly patients, particularly given the potential for a prolonged maturation period, and, thus, a prosthetic access may be a better choice for many patients. Prosthetic accesses should be tunneled deeper in the subcutaneous plane in patients with "thin" skin, if at all possible, in an attempt to provide an additional biologic tissue layer between the skin and the graft.

Patients with a history of access-related hand ischemia or "steal" syndrome are at increased risk for further events with each subsequent access procedure, and this should be factored into the preoperative evaluation. Arterial noninvasive imaging with pressure measurements and Doppler waveforms should be obtained along with a CT- or catheter-based arteriogram. All inflow lesions should be corrected. A lower extremity vein survey should be obtained to identify a suitable segment of saphenous vein for a potential distal revascularization and interval ligation (DRIL) procedure. Strategies to reduce the incidence of hand ischemia should be implemented at the time of the procedure including siting the anastomosis as proximal on the arterial tree as possible (i.e., proximal brachial artery vs. brachial artery at the antecubital fossa), and a remedial plan should be generated preoperatively to address any postoperative ischemia.

There appears to be a subset of patients who have limited patency with prosthetic accesses. The obvious solution in this situation is to create an autogenous access, and the outlined algorithm can help identify possible configurations. In patients who do not have a suitable upper extremity vein for an access, the femoropopliteal vein can be translocated and used in a brachial-axillary configuration. Indeed, I have had very good results with this procedure, albeit a major undertaking with a significant incidence of perioperative complications.

Give the advances in retroviral therapy, HIV has evolved into a chronic illness with a reasonable life expectancy. However, patients with HIV are at a higher risk of infections complications and, accordingly, are better suited for autogenous accesses given the higher risk of infectious complications associated with prosthetic accesses.

The principles of access surgery are the same as those for the broader discipline of vascular surgery and contingent upon adequate inflow, adequate outflow, and a suitable conduit as outlined above. Patients with an arterial inflow lesion that precludes using the extremity for the access, commonly a subclavian artery stenosis or occlusion, can be treated with a remedial endovascular or surgical bypass to correct the lesion. Patients with an adequate caliber vein (i.e., greater than 3 mm diameter) that is not sufficiently long to be used for an autogenous access can have composite configuration using another segment of arm or leg vein. Those with inadequate vein that require an autogenous conduit can have translocated femoropopliteal vein access as detailed above. Admittedly, patients with an inadequate vein can have prosthetic access in most situations, but the autogenous options are worth considering given the major emphasis on autogenous configurations in the national guidelines.

TAKE HOME POINTS

- The approach to patients with "complex" access problems is identical to those presenting for their initial procedure.
- The approach to patients with "complex" access problems is based upon the principles of vascular surgery—adequate arterial inflow, adequate venous outflow, suitable conduit.
- Noninvasive and invasive imaging will help identify the potential access options.
- It is possible to correct the underlying problem leading to the designation of "complex" access in many cases.
- Preventative strategies should be implemented to preserve and maintain all potential access options.
- Maintaining hemodialysis access is a complex problem that requires a lifelong plan with committed providers.

SUGGESTED READINGS

Agarwal AK. Central vein stenosis. *Am J Kidney Dis.* 2013; 61:1001-1015.

Bronder CM, Cull DL, Kuper SG, et al. Fistula elevation procedure: experience with 295 consecutive cases during a 7-year period. *J Am Coll Surg.* 2008;206:1076-1081.

Feezor RJ. Approach to permanent hemodialysis access in obese patients. *Semin Vasc Surg.* 2011;24:96-101.

Geenen IL, Nyilas L, Stephen MS, et al. Prosthetic lower extremity hemodialysis access grafts have satisfactory patency despite a high incidence of infection. *J Vasc Surg.* 2010;52:1546-1550.

Huber TS, Ozaki CK, Flynn TC, et al. Prospective validation of an algorithm to maximize native arteriovenous fistulae for chronic hemodialysis access. *J Vasc Surg.* 2002;36:452-459.

Huber TS, Seeger JM. Approach to patients with complex permanent hemodialysis access problems. In: Zelenock GB, Huber TS, Lumsden AB, et al., eds. *Mastery of Vascular and Endovascular Surgery.* 1st ed. Philadelphia, PA: Lippincott; 2006:689-698.

Katzman HE, McLafferty RB, Ross JR, et al. Initial experience and outcome of a new hemodialysis access device for catheter-dependent patients. *J Vasc Surg.* 2009;50:600-607.

National Kidney Foundations. KDOQI 2006 Vascular Access Guidelines. *Am J Kidney Dis.* 2006;48:S177-S322.

Scali ST, Huber TS. Treatment strategies for access-related hand ischemia. *Semin Vasc Surg.* 2011;24:128-136.

CLINICAL SCENARIO CASE QUESTIONS

1. The approach to patients with "complex" hemodialysis access problems outlined in the chapter includes all but the following:

   a. The outlined algorithm for patients with "complex" access problems is identical to those presenting for their initial procedure.

   b. Patients with a history of multiple prosthetic access failures are at prohibitive risk for any future permanent access procedure and are best treated with tunneled dialysis catheters.

   c. The approach to patients with "complex" access problems is based upon the principles of vascular surgery—adequate arterial inflow, adequate venous outflow, suitable conduit.

   d. Noninvasive and invasive imaging will help identify the potential access options.

2. The management of patients with central vein stenoses or occlusions presenting for permanent hemodialysis access includes all but the following:

   a. The superior vena cava syndrome is an absolute contraindication to an upper extremity permanent hemodialysis access.

   b. CT- or catheter-based venography can help identify the patent central veins and is an important component of the diagnostic algorithm for patients with known central vein stenoses or occlusions.

   c. The HeRO catheter may play a role for patients with upper extremity central vein occlusion or stenoses provided the central vein lesion can be crossed with a wire and the catheter component.

   d. Central vein stenosis and occlusions are rarely encountered in clinical practice and do not present much of a problem in terms of establishing permanent hemodialysis access.

35 Open Abdominal Aortic Aneurysm Repair

WILLIAM FORREST JOHNSTON and GILBERT R. UPCHURCH Jr

Presentation

A 65-year-old woman is referred to the office for evaluation of a pulsatile abdominal mass. She states that she first felt the mass 2 years ago, and after telling her primary care physician about it, she was recommended to consult with a vascular surgeon. The mass does not cause her any pain and feels slightly larger to her now than when she initially recognized it. Her past medical history includes hypertension that is well controlled on hydrochlorothiazide and lisinopril and hyperlipidemia controlled with simvastatin. She is a former 40-pack-year smoker that quit 5 years ago. Her past surgical history consists of laparoscopic appendectomy 10 years ago and tonsillectomy when she was a child. On physical examination, she is well appearing with regular heart sounds and bilaterally clear chest sounds. Her abdomen is thin with a nontender pulsatile mass just above the umbilicus. She has 2+ femoral pulses and 1+ dorsalis pedis and posterior tibial pulses with no lower extremity edema.

Differential Diagnosis

Given the pulsatile nature of the abdominal mass, one must consider abdominal arterial pathology. An abdominal aortic aneurysm (AAA) is the most likely cause, although a normal aorta may be palpated in thin patients. Consideration should also be given to malignancy, pancreatic pseudocyst, and liver enlargement from right-sided heart failure. All of the above possibilities can be evaluated with appropriate imaging.

Workup

During the workup of an abdominal mass, an abdominal x-ray is often performed. If the aorta has a calcified wall, an AAA may be apparent on x-ray (Fig. 1A). However, further workup with cross-sectional imaging is needed to confirm an AAA and rule out other causes of pulsatile abdominal masses. Computed tomography (CT) angiography (Fig. 1B) is frequently the preferred imaging modality because it provides high-resolution arterial imaging with contrast delivered through a large-bore peripheral intravenous line. Unlike traditional angiography, no

arterial access is required. The most significant limitation of CT angiography is the risk of contrast-induced nephropathy, especially in patients with preexisting renal insufficiency. Contrast-induced nephropathy is the third leading cause of hospital-acquired renal failure. Hydration prior to contrast exposure with bicarbonate solution and administration of N-acetylcysteine may help to prevent renal damage with minimal risk for adverse effects. If the patient has a contrast allergy, she may be pretreated with steroids and diphenhydramine or evaluated with magnetic resonance angiography (MRA). MRA frequently employs gadolinium-based contrast, which is associated with nephrogenic systemic fibrosis (less than 1%) in patients with renal insufficiency. Given the risks of both CT angiography and MRA with gadolinium in patients with renal insufficiency, consideration should be given to imaging patients with baseline renal insufficiency using time-of-flight MRA, diagnostic CO_2 angiography, or duplex ultrasound.

The maximal aortic diameter should be measured orthogonal to the aortic long axis. This is most easily performed on cross-sectional imaging with fine cuts to allow

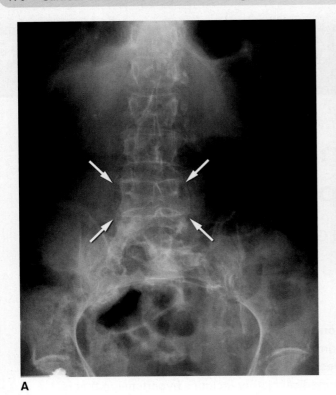

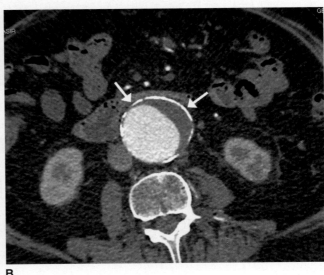

B

FIGURE 1 • **A:** Abdominal plain film demonstrating a calcified aortic shadow consistent with an AAA (*arrows*). **B:** CT angiography demonstrates an AAA with a calcified aortic wall (*white arrows*) and adjacent mural thrombus.

A

centerline measurements of aortic diameter, aneurysm length, angularity, extent of calcification, aortic thrombus, and iliac vessel tortuosity. Aortic diameter should be measured perpendicular to the aortic centerline long axis to prevent overestimation of aortic diameter (Fig. 2). In addition to cross-sectional imaging to determine arterial and venous anatomy, the workup of a patient with a suspected AAA should include evaluation of renal and hepatic function, as well as coagulation studies. All patients should receive an EKG to evaluate cardiac function and provide a baseline comparison for postoperative studies. Eagle's criteria can be applied to determine if further cardiac assessment is indicated. If the patient is not over 70 years old and does not have a history of Q waves on EKG, angina, ventricular ectopy requiring treatment, or diabetes mellitus, he or she is considered low risk for a perioperative cardiac event and no further cardiac evaluation is necessary.

Case Continued

Since the patient has no baseline renal insufficiency, CT angiography is performed and demonstrates an AAA with a maximal aortic diameter of 7.2 cm and a large amount of mural thrombus (Fig. 3). The aneurysm extends proximally and is within 5 mm of the origin of the renal arteries (Fig. 4). No other abdominal pathology is identified on CT. She has normal renal function, electrolytes, liver function tests, hematocrit, and coagulation studies. Since

she does not meet any Eagle's criteria, an EKG is sufficient cardiac evaluation, and she is started on β-blockers to decrease her perioperative cardiac risk.

Diagnosis and Treatment

An AAA is defined as enlargement of the aorta to 1.5 times the normal diameter, which is approximately 2 cm (range = 1.9 to 2.3 cm in men, 1.7 to 1.9 cm in women). Therefore, an AAA has been conventionally defined as an aortic diameter greater than 3 cm. AAA repair is intended to prevent aortic rupture, which carries a 75% to 90% risk of mortality. The risk of rupture increases dramatically with increasing aortic size with an aortic diameter of 3 to 4 cm having nearly no risk of rupture, 4 to 5 cm associated with 0.5% to 5% annual rupture risk, 5 to 6 cm associated with 3% to 15% rupture risk, and greater than 8 cm associated with 30% to 50% rupture risk. Since the risk of mortality during open AAA repair is approximately 1% to 5%, elective repair is reserved for an aortic diameter of greater than 5.5 cm in men. Women have smaller aortic diameters at baseline, and a diameter of 5.0 cm may be a more suitable indication for elective repair for women. Most AAAs will progress over time, averaging 0.3 cm/year of expansion. A more rapid expansion rate would prompt earlier consideration for repair, as rapid expansion is associated with an increased risk of rupture. Additional risk factors for aortic rupture include female gender, hypertension, current smoking,

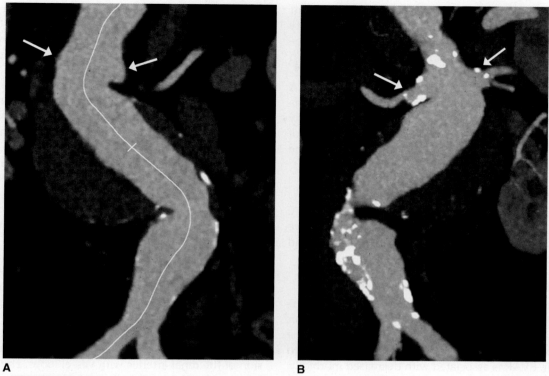

A   B

FIGURE 2 • Coronal view of the abdominal aorta from CT angiography showing a juxtarenal AAA using (**A**) centerline measurement compared to (**B**) multiplanar resolution. Renal artery origin is shown with *arrows*.

chronic obstructive pulmonary disease (COPD), and a family history of AAAs.

If the AAA measures less than 5.5 cm in a man or less than 5.0 cm in a woman, the patient may be conservatively followed with close observation, annual imaging, smoking cessation, and medical treatment of

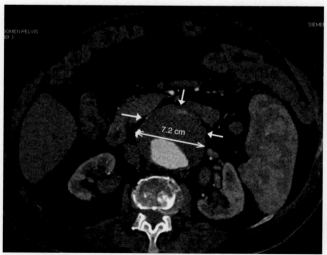

FIGURE 3 • Axial image of CT angiography demonstrates a 7.2-cm AAA with extensive mural thrombus (*arrows*).

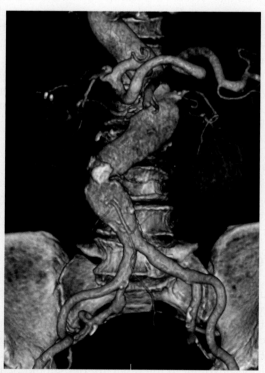

FIGURE 4 • Three-dimensional reconstruction of a CT angiogram showing a juxtarenal AAA.

hypertension and hyperlipidemia. While our patient presented with a pulsatile abdominal mass, the majority of AAAs are diagnosed incidentally on diagnostic imaging performed for other reasons. Physical examination alone has a positive predictive value of 15% for diagnosing an AAA greater than 3.5 cm. Regarding AAA screening, population screening with duplex ultrasound decreases AAA-related mortality and is currently an included Medicare benefit for all men over the age of 65 years old who have ever smoked as well as anyone with a family history of AAAs.

Case Continued

The patient is diagnosed with a 7.2-cm juxtarenal AAA. Since her risk of rupture exceeds her risk of operative mortality, she is offered AAA repair. Endovascular and open options are discussed.

Open or Endovascular Approach

Once a patient meets size criteria, he/she should be evaluated for repair with either endovascular aneurysm repair (EVAR) or open repair. EVAR has rapidly become the standard of care for infrarenal aneurysms. Compared to open repair, EVAR is associated with decreased morbidity, operative times, ICU length of stay, and perioperative mortality. Despite the success of EVAR, open repair remains a valuable adjunct to the treatment of patients with AAAs and is indicated in patients with small diameter or severely angulated iliac vessels that cannot accommodate sheath placement, a severely angulated proximal aortic neck, an aortic neck length less than 7 to 15 mm (until fenestrated or multibranch EVARs are approved in the United States), aortoiliac occlusive disease in the distal aorta, a large inferior mesenteric artery (IMA) appearing as the dominant blood supply to the colon, or according to patient preference. Some surgeons also prefer open repair in younger patients under the age of 65 years old since the long-term durability of EVAR remains unknown.

Case Continued

After extensive discussion regarding EVAR compared to open repair, the patient decides to pursue open repair due to the angulation of her aortic neck and the proximity of the renal arteries to the aneurysm.

Surgical Approach

Prior to making an incision, careful review of the preoperative imaging should be performed to determine where aortic clamps will be placed. The proximal clamp may be infrarenal, suprarenal, supramesenteric, or supraceliac depending on the proximal extent of the aneurysm and the amount of calcifications. The duration of aortic occlusion proximal to the renal arteries should be minimized to decrease renal ischemic injury. The infrarenal abdominal aorta may be approached either transabdominal through a midline incision or retroperitoneal from the patient's left side.

Using a transabdominal approach, a midline laparotomy is performed with reflection of the transverse colon superiorly and retraction of the small bowel to the patient's right side after division of the ligament of Treitz. Exposure is facilitated with the assistance of a self-retaining retractor system. The posterior peritoneum is incised longitudinally from the iliac arteries to the inferior aspect of the pancreas. Routine preservation of sexual function includes careful retraction of the autonomic nerves coursing on top of the left iliac artery. Additionally, the left ureter may be identified crossing the iliac bifurcation and avoided. The left renal vein is dissected free and may be retracted superiorly to fully identify the aneurysm neck. If needed, the left renal vein may be divided at its junction with the IVC to maintain collateral flow through the left lumbar, gonadal, and adrenal veins.

Once the aorta is dissected, disease-free proximal aorta and iliac arteries should be identified for cross-clamping, avoiding the risk of distal embolization with clamping atherosclerotic plaque. Heparin is given for anticoagulation at a dose of 50 to 100 U/kg. First, vascular clamps are placed across the common iliac arteries. Next, a proximal vascular clamp is placed in the suprarenal position after occlusion of the renal arteries with vessel loops. The aneurysm is incised longitudinally with care taken to avoid the origin of the IMA. Any thrombus or debris is removed from the aortic lumen, and the proximal aorta is fashioned with a horizontal incision just below the renal artery origins for proximal anastomosis. Back bleeding lumbar arteries are encountered posteriorly and ligated with figure-of-eight sutures. The IMA has moderate back bleeding and is oversewn. The proximal anastomosis is performed in end-to-end fashion using polypropylene sutures with large aortic bites and smaller bites on the prosthetic graft. A felt pledget ring may be incorporated into the anastomosis for reinforcement. Once the proximal anastomosis is complete, the proximal clamp is released to check for hemostasis at the suture line. If adequate, the vascular clamp is moved down to the proximal portion of the graft and flow is reestablished to the renal arteries. The proximal anastomosis should be done in the timely fashion, preferable less than 20 to 30 minutes. If distal anastomosis is planned for the terminal aorta, a similar technique is used to attach a graft to the aorta above the bifurcation. Frequently, aneurysm disease will extend to the iliac arteries, requiring placement of a bifurcated graft sutured to disease-free iliac vessels.

After adequate perfusion of the intestines and lower extremities is confirmed, heparin anticoagulation is reversed with protamine sulfate. The anterior arteriotomy is closed over the graft, followed by closure of the retroperitoneum to provide a barrier to the intestines. The small bowel and colon are placed back in their normal position, and the anterior abdominal wall is closed in standard fashion.

If preferred, retroperitoneal exposure may be performed through a midline incision or via a left retroperitoneal incision along the 10th to 12th ribs with the patient rotated onto his right side. The retroperitoneal approach

TABLE 1. Open AAA Repair

Key Technical Steps

1. Exposure from above the aneurysm neck to the iliac bifurcation
2. Clamp placement across noncalcified aorta
3. Longitudinal arteriotomy preserving the IMA
4. Evacuation of thrombus
5. Oversewing lumbar vessels
6. Evaluate IMA for reimplantation
7. Anastomose proximal followed by distal graft
8. Close aneurysm sac and retroperitoneum for graft coverage

Potential Pitfalls

- Embolization of atheromatous plaque to the renal vessels or lower extremities
- Postoperative renal insufficiency from prolonged suprarenal aortic clamping
- Injury to the pelvic autonomic nerves leading to retrograde ejaculation in males
- Injury to the ureter as it crosses the iliac artery bifurcation
- Incorrect management of colon and pelvic perfusion

may be associated with decreased postoperative ileus. Dissection is performed in the retroperitoneal plane and may be continued either anterior or posterior to the left kidney. If carried posterior to the kidney, the lumbar vein must be identified and ligated. The ureter is retracted medially with the kidney. Exposure of the right renal artery and right iliac artery can be performed once the aneurysm is entered. Repair is otherwise similar to the transabdominal approach in Table 1.

Case Conclusion

The patient does well postoperatively until she becomes mildly tachycardic on the afternoon of postoperative day 1. On evaluation, her heart rate is in the 130s and regular with a blood pressure of 90/60 mm Hg. Her abdomen is distended and diffusely tender. Peripheral pulses are intact. With a concern for bleeding, labs are immediately drawn and reveal a stable hematocrit, elevated white blood cell count, and elevated lactic acid. With hemorrhage ruled out, exam findings are concerning for colonic ischemia since the patient's IMA was ligated. A flexible sigmoidoscopy is performed at the patient's bedside and confirms colonic ischemia with frank necrosis of the sigmoid and descending colon. The patient is taken immediately to the operating room, and a left colectomy with end transverse colostomy is performed. The distal rectal stump is stapled and ligated (Hartmann's procedure). Afterward, the patient slowly recovers without further complication.

Special Intraoperative Considerations

During AAA repair, pelvic blood flow must be evaluated to prevent possible colon or spinal ischemia from chronic thrombus or embolic disease. The quality of the internal iliac arteries and mesenteric arteries, including the IMA, should be evaluated on preoperative imaging. Perfusion through one patent internal iliac artery is often adequate to prevent pelvic ischemia. However, if the common iliac arteries are diseased and distal iliac graft limbs are implanted onto the femoral or external iliac arteries, consideration should be given to performing an additional bypass to an internal iliac artery to maintain pelvic perfusion.

The decision to ligate or implant the IMA is made once the aortic graft is in place and flow to the pelvis is reestablished. If the IMA is small caliber with adequate back bleeding and a healthy colon, the IMA may be suture ligated. Indications to implant the IMA include poor back bleeding of the IMA, a large caliber IMA with diseased celiac, superior mesenteric, or internal iliac arteries, or a poorly perfused colon based on examination. Implantation accomplished by forming a Carrel patch with the wall of the aorta surrounding the origin of the IMA and anastomosing patch to graft in an end-to-side fashion.

Postoperative Management

Postoperative management of patients is aimed at early detection of complications. The most common complications following open AAA repair are pulmonary dysfunction (15%), renal failure (10%), myocardial infarction (2% to 8%), deep venous thrombosis (5%), wound infection (1% to 5%), distal embolization (1% to 4%), colonic ischemia (1%), ureteral injury (less than 1%), and spinal ischemia (less than 1%). If the patient develops metabolic acidosis or guaiac-positive stools, flexible sigmoidoscopy is performed to evaluate the colonic mucosa. If necrotic, a left colectomy with end colostomy should be performed to prevent graft infection. If dusky but viable, emergent reimplantation of the IMA can be attempted.

Following discharge, patients are seen in 2 to 4 weeks for evaluation of their repair and incision (Fig. 5). Afterward, aortic imaging can be performed every 5 years to look for metachronous aneurysms. Minimal follow-up and infrequent imaging is one of the benefits of open repair compared to rigorous follow-up required after EVAR. Open repair is considered more durable than EVAR because open repair has decreased need for aortic reinterventions and decreased long-term rupture rate. However, laparotomy-related interventions are more common following open repair, including repair of abdominal wall hernias and bowel resection secondary to adhesive obstructions.

TAKE HOME POINTS

- Open AAA repair still has a valuable role in modern vascular surgery in younger patients, as well as older patients who will physiologically tolerate open surgery and cannot receive EVAR due to arterial anatomy or patient preference.

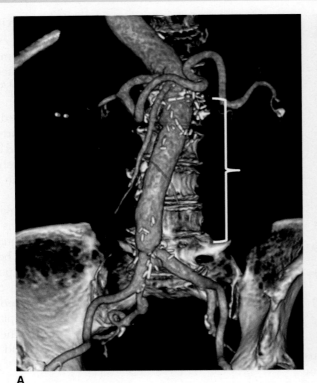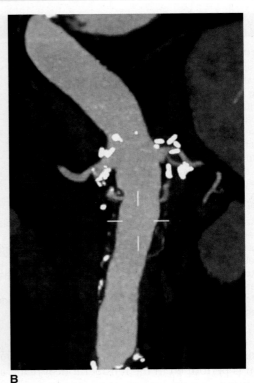

A   B

FIGURE 5 • **A:** Three-dimensional reconstruction demonstrating placement of an aortic tube graft from the level of the renal arteries to the aortic bifurcation (*bracket*). **B:** Both renal arteries remain patent.

- Open AAA repair is still preferred in most patients with connective tissue disorders.
- Preoperative planning of clamp sites and minimizing suprarenal clamping are essential.
- Postoperative management should be aimed at early detection of complications.

SUGGESTED READING

Ailawadi G, Eliason JL, Upchurch GR Jr. Current concepts in the pathogenesis of abdominal aortic aneurysm. *J Vasc Surg.* 2003;38:584-588.

Chaikof EL, Brewster DC, Dalman RL, et al. The care of patients with an abdominal aortic aneurysm: the Society for Vascular Surgery practice guidelines. *J Vasc Surg.* 2009;50:S2-S49.

Dimick JB, Upchurch GR Jr. Measuring and improving the quality of care for abdominal aortic aneurysm surgery. *Circulation.* 2008;117:2534-2541.

Eagle KA, Coley CM, Newell JB, et al. Combining clinical and thallium data optimizes preoperative assessment of cardiac risk before major vascular surgery. *Ann Intern Med.* 1989;110:859-866.

Eliason JL, Upchurch GR Jr. Endovascular abdominal aortic aneurysm repair. *Circulation.* 2008;117:1738-1744.

Schermerhorn ML, O'Malley AJ, Jhaveri A, et al. Endovascular vs open repair of abdominal aortic aneurysms in the Medicare population. *N Engl J Med.* 2008;358:464-474.

Thompson SG, Ashton HA, Gao L, et al. Final follow-up of the multicentre aneurysm screening study (MASS) randomized trial of abdominal aortic aneurysm screening. *Br J Surg.* 2012;99:1649-1656.

CLINICAL SCENARIO CASE QUESTIONS

1. Open repair is indicated in which of the following patients?

   a. Nine-millimeter iliac arteries bilaterally
   b. Aortic angulation of 50 degrees
   c. A 40-year-old man with a mycotic aneurysm
   d. Aortic neck length of 25 mm

2. All of the following are signs of colonic ischemia *except*:

   a. Tachycardia
   b. Abdominal pain
   c. Primary metabolic acidosis
   d. Guaiac positive stool
   e. Anemia

36 Open AAA Repair for Rupture

ANDREW LEAKE and RABIH A. CHAER

Presentation

A 68-year-old male presents to the emergency department (ED) for evaluation of back pain. He describes a syncopal event 4 hours prior, with the onset of severe pain (8/10). The pain is in the midback area, is constant, and is not positional. He denies a history of trauma and any gastrointestinal complaints. His past medical history is significant for coronary artery disease, hyperlipidemia, and hypertension. His father had an aneurysm, but does not recall the details. He denies a history of prior back pain and has not previously been evaluated for an abdominal aortic aneurysm (AAA). His current medications are metoprolol, simvastatin, and aspirin. He currently smokes 1 pack per day of cigarettes, with a 60-pack-year history. In the ED, his vital signs are as follows: temperature, 37.9°C; blood pressure, 110/62 mm Hg; heart rate, 110 beats per minute; respiratory rate, 19 per minute; and saturations, 98% on 2 L nasal cannulas. He appears uncomfortable but is mentating appropriately. Abdominal examination reveals midabdominal tenderness with guarding, but no peritoneal signs. Deep palpation in the periumbilical area identifies a pulsatile mass. No abdominal or inguinal hernias are appreciated. Femoral, popliteal, and pedal pulses are normal in both extremities.

Differential Diagnosis

The initial presentation of a patient with a ruptured AAA is variable, and the differential diagnosis is broad (Table 1). The most common chief complaints are abdominal, back, or groin pain. Identified factors that predispose a patient to the development of an AAA include male gender, increasing age, family history, hypertension, hyperlipidemia, and smoking. Smoking is the strongest risk factor for AAA development. This patient presents with multiple risk factors, and a high clinical suspicion is necessary for early recognition.

Workup

The clinical triad of sudden onset of abdominal (or back) pain, hypotension, and pulsatile abdominal mass is characteristic of a ruptured AAA. It is present in less than 50% of the patients with ruptured AAAs. With this constellation of symptoms, ruptured AAA must be considered among the most likely diagnoses and must be ruled out.

Management options at this point are dictated by the hemodynamic stability of the patient. The unstable patient with a high clinical suspicion for a ruptured AAA should be transported emergently to the operating room for surgical intervention. At medical facilities unable to offer urgent surgical repair, rapid stabilization and transport to an appropriate institution should be expedited. Resuscitation until definitive repair should allow permissive hypotension. Aggressive resuscitation with crystalloid should be avoided, as it has been shown to increase bleeding and worsen coagulopathy. Resuscitation goals are aimed at maintaining cerebral and myocardial perfusion by monitoring consciousness and ST changes on cardiac monitoring (systolic blood pressure 70 to 80 mm Hg).

In a patient with stable vital signs, computed tomography (CT) imaging is critical for accurate diagnosis. Prior to any transportation, large-bore peripheral IVs should be placed and a blood sample sent for cross-matching. The abdominal/pelvic CT scan should be obtained using a 3-mm (thin)-cut protocol with intravenous contrast, to assess for possible endovascular repair (EVAR). Oral contrast is not indicated, as it may degrade the image quality of vascular structures due to artifact and carries the risk of delaying intervention. Continuous monitoring and supervision by the surgical team is essential prior to definitive repair.

Case Continued

The patient is alert and remains hemodynamically stable, and a CTA is immediately obtained.

Diagnosis and Treatment

The CT scan shows a ruptured AAA, requiring immediate repair (Fig. 1). Current repair options for ruptured AAA include either an open standard repair (OSR) or an EVAR. Widely accepted exclusion criteria for EVAR include proximal neck length less than 10 mm, proximal neck diameter greater than 32 mm, neck angulation greater than 60 degrees, and external iliac diameter of less

TABLE 1. Differential Diagnosis for Back, Abdominal, and Groin Pain in Patients Presenting to an Emergency Room

	Presenting Symptom		
	Back Pain	Abdominal Pain	Groin Pain
Cardiac		Inferior MI	
Gastrointestinal	Pancreatitis	Perforated viscus	Inguinal hernia
	Perforating duodenal ulcer	Mesenteric ischemia	
	Strangulated hernia		
	Acute cholecystitis		
	Ruptured appendicitis		
	Diverticulitis		
Genitourinary	Ureteral calculus		Testicular torsion
	Pyelonephritis		Epididymitis
Vascular	Ruptured AAA	Ruptured AAA	Ruptured iliac artery aneurysm
	Symptomatic AAA	Symptomatic AAA	
	Aortic dissection		
Musculoskeletal	Paravertebral muscle spasms		
	Vertebral fracture		
Neurologic	Lumbar radiculopathy		

AAA, abdominal aortic aneurysm.

than 6 mm. This patient is excluded from EVAR because of short proximal neck length and will require an OSR.

Surgical Approach

Prior to the initial arrival of the patient with a suspected ruptured AAA, the operating room staff is contacted to begin preparations including cross-matching of blood products and assembly of a cell-scavenging system. Before induction of general anesthesia, prophylactic antibiotics are administered and the patient

is prepped and draped from his nipples to his knees. Immediately upon induction, the operation is initiated through either a transperitoneal or retroperitoneal incision. Our preference is a transperitoneal incision through a vertical midline abdominal incision, extending from the xiphoid process to just below the umbilicus. Proximal aortic control is the first critical step. In the unstable patient, supraceliac control and clamping can be done quickly (Fig. 2). A nasogastric tube can be placed to avoid esophageal injury while resecting the left crus of

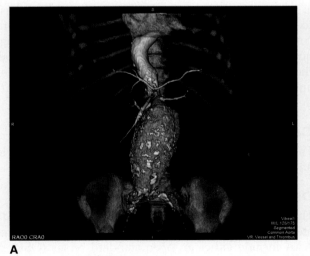

A

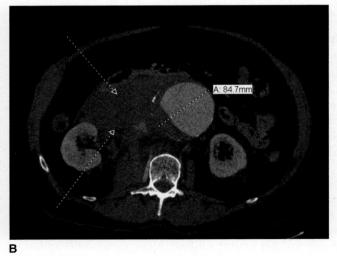

B

FIGURE 1 • CT scan. CT scan shows an AAA from the renal arteries to the aortic bifurcation **(A)**, with a maximum diameter of 8.4 cm **(B)**. There is a large right-sided retroperitoneal hematoma (*arrows*). Detailed examination of the infrarenal aorta demonstrates a proximal neck diameter of 32 mm, a proximal neck length of 5 mm, with 30-degree angulation. Common iliac arteries are 15 mm bilaterally (from personal patient file).

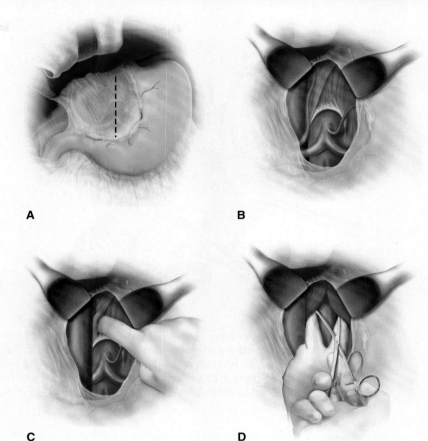

A   B

C   D

FIGURE 2 • Supraceliac control, exposure of the supraceliac aorta. **A:** Lesser sac is entered by incising the gastrohepatic ligaments (*dotted line*). **B:** The diaphragmatic crura is now visualized. **C:** The crus is either sharply or bluntly opened to gain access to the supraceliac aorta. **D:** After blunt dissection on both sides of aorta to the spine is accomplished, the clamp is placed. (From Mulholland MW, ed. *Operative Techniques in Surgery*. Philadelphia, PA: Wolters Kluwer Health; 2015.)

the diaphragm. If the patient remains stable, the aortic clamp is not applied; however, it may be left in position in case the patient decompensates during dissection of the aneurysm. Supraceliac aortic clamping is associated with increased ischemic injury to liver, bowel, and kidneys and should be moved to an infrarenal location when appropriate. Alternative proximal control measures include an aortic compressor, which is used to compress the aorta against the spine, or an intra-arterial occlusion balloon. Once proximal control is achieved, the anesthesia team may maximize their resuscitation efforts in anticipation of subsequent blood loss.

Distal control of either the aorta or common iliac arteries is the next critical step. This can be difficult, as it requires opening of the retroperitoneum. Vascular clamps may be placed if the distal aorta or iliac arteries are well visualized. Dissection should be limited, and circumferential control is not needed. In addition, blind placement of vascular clamps may lead to iliac vein injury and should be avoided.

The abdominal aorta exposure is facilitated by the use of retractors, such as the Omni track retractor (Fig. 3). The retroperitoneal hematoma is entered, and the infrarenal aorta is visualized. Oftentimes, the hematoma dissects the tissue planes and allows visualization of the renal vessels. If possible, the supraceliac aortic clamp is

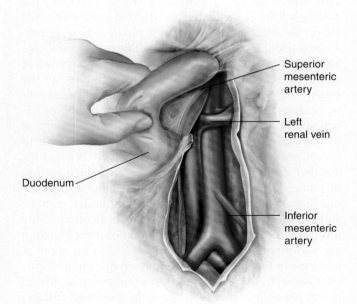

Superior mesenteric artery

Left renal vein

Duodenum

Inferior mesenteric artery

FIGURE 3 • Abdominal aorta exposure. The infrarenal aorta is exposed by reflection of the transverse colon cephalad and the small bowel to the right upper quadrant (not shown). Mobilization of the duodenum to the patient's right allows visualization of the retroperitoneum. (From Mulholland MW, ed. *Operative Techniques in Surgery*. Philadelphia, PA: Wolters Kluwer Health; 2015.)

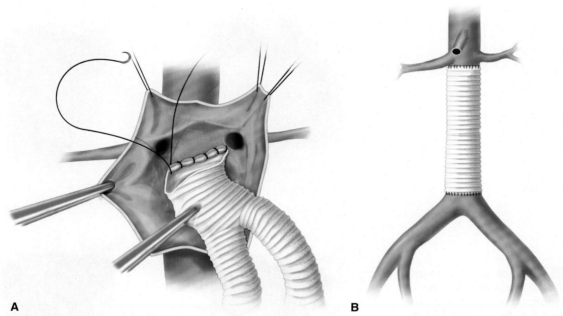

A   **B**

FIGURE 4 • Operative steps. The aneurysm sac is entered sharply and mural thrombus removed. Bleeding lumbar vessels are oversewn from within the aneurysm sac (not shown). Both anastomoses are performed in an end-to-end configuration, with a running permanent monofilament suture **(A)**. Once adequate hemostasis is ensured **(B)**, the aortic sac and retroperitoneum is approximated over the graft. (From Mulholland MW, ed. *Operative Techniques in Surgery*. Philadelphia, PA: Wolters Kluwer Health; 2015.)

moved to the infra- or suprarenal aorta. If the left renal vein cannot be safely mobilized to gain access to the aortic neck, it can be ligated and divided to expeditiously clamp the infrarenal aorta. Aortic repair is quickly performed using a Dacron tube graft. Bifurcated grafts take longer to implant and have been shown to have worse outcomes (Fig. 4). If the aneurysm extends close to the origin of the renal arteries with minimal infrarenal aortic neck, a suprarenal clamp is required and the proximal suture line can be taken across the inferior edge of the orifice of the renal arteries, with extra care not to compromise their patency. Systemic heparin is generally avoided during ruptured aneurysms to reduce further bleeding; however, local heparinized saline and vigorous flushing should be performed to minimize embolization. After completion, a systematic evaluation of the retroperitoneum and vascular anastomoses for bleeding are performed. Inspection of the abdomen for signs of ischemia or bowel edema is completed prior to abdominal closure. In some patients, primary abdominal closure is not possible and may be done in a delayed fashion (Table 2).

Special Intraoperative Considerations

Rarely, profuse venous bleeding can be from a ruptured AAA into the iliac veins or the inferior vena cava, causing an aortocaval fistula. Manual control/compression of the cava with sponge sticks is recommended rather than

dissection and clamping of venous structures. The fistula is best repaired primarily from within the aneurysm sac. Venous abnormalities, such as a retroaortic or circumaortic renal vein, can be encountered in up to 3% of patients. Care must be taken during the dissection of the pararenal aorta and in placing the proximal aortic clamp to avoid

TABLE 2. Open AAA Repair for Rupture

Key Technical Steps

1. Midline laparotomy
2. Obtain proximal aortic control, supraceliac control if unstable
3. Obtain distal control with iliac clamping or occlusion balloons once aneurysm open
4. Enter aneurysm sac; oversew bleeding lumbar arteries
5. If possible, move aortic clamp to infra- or suprarenal aorta
6. Perform proximal anastomosis with permanent monofilament suture
7. Move clamp onto aortic graft
8. Perform distal anastomosis
9. Vigorously flush proximal and distal anastomosis with heparinized saline
10. Close aortic sac and retroperitoneum over aortic graft

Potential Pitfalls

- Difficult proximal control
- Injury to iliac veins during distal control

venous injury. Circumferential dissection of the aortic neck is best avoided as a matter of routine and is not required for aortic control.

Case Conclusion

The patient underwent a tube graft repair of his ruptured infrarenal AAA. His abdomen was primarily closed, and he had palpable distal pulses at completion. He was transported to the intensive care unit intubated and hemodynamically stable.

Over the next 48 hours, he had intermittent episodes of hypotension that respond to bolus administration of intravenous crystalloids. On postoperative day 2, the patient started developing worsening lactic acidosis and passing moderate amounts of maroon-colored stool. A sigmoidoscopy demonstrated patchy areas of mucosal ischemia within the sigmoid colon. He was placed on broad-spectrum antibiotics with the presumptive diagnosis of ischemic colitis with plans for operative intervention should his condition deteriorate. Over the next several days, his acidosis and melena resolved.

The patient was transferred out of the ICU on postoperative day 8 to a monitored surgical floor. His diet was slowly advanced, and physical therapy was initiated. He was discharged to a rehabilitation unit on postoperative day 15 in stable condition.

Postoperative Management

Mortality rates for *elective* AAA repair range from 2% to 5%, but mortality rates following OSR of a *ruptured* AAA range from 45% to 70%. The morbidity of ruptured AAA is equally significant. The most frequent postoperative complications include respiratory failure (48%), renal failure (42%), and myocardial infarctions (24%). One of the most lethal complications is ischemic colitis, with an incidence of 38%. Occurring early in the postoperative period, clinical findings include bloody diarrhea, metabolic acidosis, and sepsis. Diagnosis is usually confirmed by flexible sigmoidoscopy, and evaluation for transmural ischemia is critical in the decision-making process. Although ischemic injury isolated to the mucosa can initially be treated nonoperatively, close observation and systemic antibiotics are warranted. The development of transmural ischemia, worsening sepsis, or peritoneal signs requires a prompt surgical intervention with resection of involved colon.

TAKE HOME POINTS

- Ruptured AAA has a 50% mortality rate following open surgical repair.
- CT scan is the diagnostic test of choice in stable patients.
- Decision of open versus EVAR is evolving, but absolute exclusion criteria for EVAR include infrarenal neck length less than 10 mm, aortic neck diameter greater than 32 mm, neck angulation greater than 60 degrees, and external iliac diameters less than 6 mm.
- Proximal control is the most critical portion of the operation.

SUGGESTED READINGS

Cho JS, Kim JY, Rhee RY, et al. Contemporary results of open repair of ruptured abdominal aortoiliac aneurysms: effect of surgeon volume on mortality. *J Vasc Surg.* 2008;48(1):10-17.

Johansen K, Kohler TR, Nicholls SC, et al. Ruptured abdominal aortic aneurysm: the Harborview experience. *J Vasc Surg.* 1991;13:240-245.

Mehta M, Byrne J, Darling RC, et al. Endovascular repair of ruptured infrarenal abdominal aortic aneurysm is associated with lower 30-day mortality and better 5-year survival rates than open surgical repair. *J Vasc Surg.* 2013;57(2):368-375.

Meissner MH, Johansen KH. Colon infarction after ruptured abdominal aortic aneurysm. *Arch Surg.* 1992;127:979-985.

Saqib N, Park SC, Park T, et al. Endovascular repair of abdominal aortic aneurysm does not confer survival benefits over open repair. *J Vasc Surg.* 2012:56(3):614-619.

CLINICAL SCENARIO CASE QUESTIONS

1. A 75-year-old male with known AAA presents after a syncopal episode to the emergency department. His blood pressure is 70/40 mm Hg and heart rate is 120 beats per minute. He is arousable but lethargic. His abdomen is distended and tender, with a pulsatile aneurysm. What is the best next step in management?

   a. Aggressive IV fluids
   b. Immediate surgical repair of suspected ruptured AAA
   c. High-resolution CT scan with IV contrast
   d. Emergent intubation in the ER

2. A 82-year-old female is postoperative day 7 from an open AAA repair for rupture. Her course has been complicated by hypotension and persistent acidosis. She now has peritonitis on her abdominal exam with a WBC of 30,000. What is the best next step in management?

   a. Initiate antibiotics and observe for 24 to 48 hours
   b. Sigmoidoscopy
   c. Emergent abdominal reexploration, for suspected ischemic colitis
   d. Check bladder pressure to rule out abdominal compartment syndrome

37 Elective Endovascular Repair of Abdominal Aortic Aneurysm

REID A. RAVIN and PETER L. FARIES

Presentation

The patient is a 77-year-old man who was discovered to have an abdominal aortic aneurysm (AAA) by ultrasound performed for evaluation of intermittent right upper quadrant discomfort. The ultrasound demonstrated no cholelithiasis, thickening of the gallbladder wall, or dilatation of the common bile duct and was not remarkable for findings other than an AAA. A subsequent computed tomography (CT) scan is ordered. The CTA confirms the presence of a 7.9 cm AAA (Figure 1).

Differential Diagnosis

The diagnosis of an asymptomatic AAA has been established using radiographic studies. There is no evidence of rupture or acute expansion. Further decisions regarding treatment must now incorporate evaluation of the patient's overall condition, ability to tolerate surgery, life expectancy, and likelihood of aneurysm rupture. Given the large size of the aneurysm, rupture within 12 months is likely. Intervention is therefore indicated for the prevention of rupture, if the patient does not have a terminal illness and if he is able to tolerate surgical repair.

Workup

The patient's ability to tolerate conventional open aneurysm repair should be evaluated. History and physical examination should focus on assessing functional status, and identifying factors that may complicate a surgical approach, as well as any comorbid conditions that may affect a patient's long-term prognosis or perioperative morbidity and mortality. Particular attention should be directed at evaluating a patient's cardiac and pulmonary status as these diseases are commonly comorbid with AAA. Renal function should also be assessed. According to AHA guidelines, patients with multiple risk factors and poor functional capacity who require vascular surgery should undergo noninvasive stress testing prior to surgery. For patients with a known pulmonary condition or in whom there is suspicion of undiagnosed pulmonary disease, pulmonary function testing is justified.

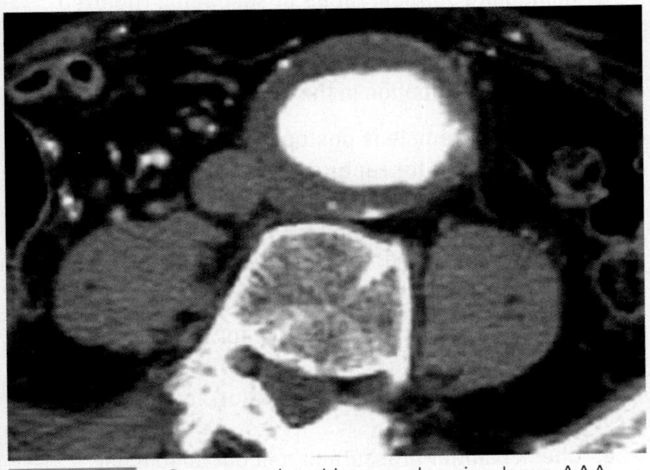

Case Continued

Upon obtaining additional history, it is determined that the patient requires elevation of his head on two pillows to sleep at night, he cannot ascend a flight of stairs due to the onset of significant dyspnea, and he awakens two to three times a night to urinate. He has a 45 pack-year history of smoking but discontinued smoking 10 years ago. Physical examination demonstrates an 8-cm pulsatile abdominal mass that is nontender. He has normal femoral pulses bilaterally. His colostomy site from his prior abdominoperineal resection is intact and functioning well, and his prior abdominal surgery did not significantly limit his ambulation. He has 2+ pedal edema without ulceration or evidence of venous insufficiency. Further cardiac and pulmonary evaluation is ordered.

Report of Diagnostic Tests

An echocardiogram and adenosine thallium stress test are performed. The patient is demonstrated to have global ventricular hypokinesis with a markedly reduced ejection fraction of 35%. There are fixed myocardial perfusion defects in the left anterior and lateral wall regions, but no reversible perfusion defects.

FIGURE 1 • Cross sectional image showing large AAA.

Pulmonary function tests indicate significantly reduced pulmonary capacity and functional reserve with forced expiratory volume in 1 second (FEV$_1$) of 0.9 L.

Diagnosis and Treatment

Several factors suggest that this patient will be at significantly increased risk for morbidity and mortality if conventional AAA repair is performed. His cardiac and pulmonary capacity is considerably reduced. In addition, the presence of a stoma and the loss of abdominal domain make his a "hostile" abdomen and increase the difficulty of conventional repair and increased potential for prosthetic graft infection. Therefore, this patient should be considered for endovascular aneurysm repair (EVAR) using a stent graft.

Anatomic evaluation is performed to determine if a stent graft will be successful in excluding the aneurysm from the arterial circulation, thereby preventing aneurysm rupture. To achieve aneurysm exclusion, undilated arterial areas must be present proximal and distal to the aneurysm. These fixation zones in the immediate infrarenal aorta proximally and common iliac arteries distally allow for sealing of the aneurysm and prevent arterial flow into the aneurysm sac. An undilated aortic segment at least 10 mm in length should be present distal to the renal arteries for successful repair. Excessive angulation of the pararenal aorta may also prevent adequate stent graft fixation and sealing. A distal region of nonaneurysmal artery must also be present to achieve fixation and sealing. Typically, this occurs in the common iliac arteries; however, stent grafts may be extended into the external iliac if the common iliac is dilated. Extension into the external iliac arteries requires occlusion of the internal iliac arteries, which may be associated with ischemic complications of the pelvis and gluteal region. Preoperative embolization of the internal iliac arteries prior to EVAR is being done with increasing frequency and is associated with a significant incidence of postoperative buttock claudication, as well as rare, but serious ischemic complications to the lower gastrointestinal tract. Bypass to the internal iliac arteries at the time of EVAR can be performed if it is essential to preserve arterial perfusion. Alternatively, newer branched iliac devices are currently being evaluated for use in aneurysms involving the iliac bifurcation. Finally, the vessels used to access the aorta must also be of an adequate caliber to allow passage of the endovascular stent graft. Typically, this is carried out from the femoral arteries through the external iliac arteries.

The current patient undergoes a contrast-enhanced spiral CT scan with images obtained at 2.5-mm intervals to allow measurement of the proximal aortic and common iliac artery diameters. Three-dimensional reconstruction and center line calculations obtained from the CT scan can be used to determine the length of the arterial segment that is to be excluded by the stent graft. That is the distance from the distal-most renal artery to the bifurcation of the common iliac arteries bilaterally. These measurements are used to determine the length of the stent graft.

CT Scan and Angiogram

CT Scan

The proximal aortic fixation zone is determined to be 25 mm in diameter and 18 mm long. The common iliac arteries are 14 mm in diameter, and the distance from the renal ostia to the iliac bifurcations is 147 mm on the right and 152 mm on the left.

Case Continued

The most appropriate course of management for this patient is endovascular AAA repair. His anatomy will allow successful exclusion of the aneurysm by placement of a stent graft. He exhibits multiple factors that would place him at increased risk for conventional repair. He has a large AAA and no terminal conditions, so he is likely to die from aneurysm rupture if repair is not performed.

Surgical Approach

Repair is performed in the operating room on a radiolucent table. The patient may receive local, epidural, or general anesthesia. Because he exhibits significant pulmonary disease, regional anesthesia without the requirement for intubation is preferable. The abdomen and legs are prepared in a sterile manner in the event that conversion to open repair becomes necessary. The stoma site is excluded from the sterile field. Exposure of the common femoral arteries is performed bilaterally, and an angiographic guidewire is introduced into the abdominal aorta. Alternatively, percutaneous access can be obtained to the femoral arteries using the preclose technique, wherein two perclose devices (Proglide, Abbot Vascular, Redwood City, CA) are deployed in the femoral arteries prior to advancing large sheaths and/or delivery catheters. The perclose devices, which contain sutures and preformed slip knots, are typically deployed medially and laterally at 45-degree angles. The sutures are then tagged and placed aside for the duration of the intervention, and the artery is closed at the end of case by pushing down the preformed knots on to the artery after the delivery devices/catheters are removed.

After access is obtained using percutaneous access or femoral cut down, a flush catheter is placed in the aorta over the wire to allow the performance of angiography. A stiff guidewire is placed through a selective angiographic catheter from the ipsilateral femoral artery. After administration of systemic anticoagulation, the main body of the stent graft is brought into position in the aorta over the stiff guidewire and deployed in the infrarenal aorta. The short contralateral gate of the main body of the stent graft is then cannulated from the contralateral femoral access site using a guidewire. A pigtail catheter is tracked over the guidewire and spun within

TABLE 1. Elective Endovascular Repair of AAA

Key Technical Steps

1. Obtain access to both femoral arteries via percutaneous technique or open exposure.
2. Aortogram is performed with a sizing flush catheter, and stiff guidewires are introduced into both femoral arteries.
3. The main body of the graft is brought into position and deployed in the infrarenal aorta.
4. The short contralateral gate of the graft is cannulated from the contralateral femoral access site, and a pigtail catheter is used to confirm intraluminal position.
5. The contralateral limb is advanced over a stiff glide wire via the contralateral femoral artery and deployed.
6. Completion angiography is performed.
7. Closure of the arteriotomies via direct repair or percutaneous closure device is performed.

Potential Pitfalls

- Injury to the iliac vessels during delivery of the endovascular graft.
- Coverage of the renal or visceral branches.
- Inadequate graft seal with persistent endoleak.

the stent graft to confirm intraluminal position. A second stiff guidewire is then brought through the short contralateral gate, and the contralateral iliac delivery system is tracked into position through the contralateral femoral arteriotomy site. After deployment of the contralateral iliac limb, completion angiography is performed to ensure complete exclusion of the aneurysm Table 1.

Special Intraoperative Considerations

Due to the availability of high-quality preoperative CT and conventional angiography, major deviations in operative plan should be rare during endovascular repair, particularly if 3D reconstruction and sizing of endovascular devices occur preoperatively. However, the presence of highly tortuous iliac vessels and narrow aortic bifurcations can complicate passage of the endograft delivery system and the cannulation of the short contralateral gate of the stent graft. Different combinations of angled catheters and wires should be employed first, but when this fails, a catheter can be placed from the ipsilateral graft limb or the upper extremity and used in combination with a snare to obtain wire access into the contralateral gate.

Case Conclusion

The patient tolerates the procedure well. Completion angiography demonstrates no evidence of aneurysm perfusion or endoleak, and the patient is discharged to home on the first postoperative day. He is enrolled in a standard follow-up imaging

protocol as described below. His follow-up CTAs at 30 days and 6 months were unremarkable. The 1-year follow-up scan is depicted in Figure 2.

CT Scan

CT Scan Report

At 1-year follow-up, contrast is seen perfusing the aneurysm sac.

Postoperative Management

Standard follow-up protocol following EVAR consists of contrast CT scans to be obtained within 30 days, at 6 months, at 1 year, and annually thereafter. If surveillance imaging demonstrates arterial flow into the aneurysm sac, additional measures must be taken to determine the source of the continued perfusion. The CT scan may suggest the location of the source of the endoleak, with small endoleaks located posteriorly being suggestive of a lumbar arterial source. Endoleaks that originate from patent collateral branches of the aneurysm, including the lumbar and inferior mesenteric arteries, generate retrograde perfusion and have been classified as type II endoleaks.

Contrast that can be traced to the proximal or distal fixation sites of the stent graft may be more suggestive of an attachment site endoleak. Perfusion that originates from incomplete fixation or incomplete sealing at the attachment site results in antegrade flow into the aneurysm. These endoleaks have been classified as type I endoleaks. Antegrade endoleaks may also originate from the junction site between stent graft components. These are classified as type III endoleaks.

Antegrade endoleaks (types I and III) result in the transmission of systemic pressure to the aneurysm sac and lead to continued aneurysm expansion and rupture. Therefore, they mandate treatment at the time of diagnosis. The pressure and force generated by retrograde-collateral endoleaks (type II) is not known, and their

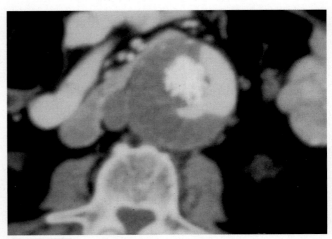

FIGURE 2 • Endoleak following EVAR.

natural history is not well established. However, most investigators recommend correction if they are persistent and are associated with continued aneurysm growth.

With the appearance of a new endoleak, steps should be taken to determine its source. These may include duplex ultrasound, time-resolved magnetic resonance imaging (MRI), and contrast angiography. Duplex ultrasound may be useful to confirm the presence of flow in the aneurysm and often may suggest the likely source of the flow. Time-resolved MRI is a relatively novel technique that allows the gadolinium contrast bolus to be followed, to determine the source and direction of arterial flow. Definitive establishment of the source of an endoleak may frequently require performance of a contrast arteriogram.

Angiography can also be used as a therapeutic modality, particularly in cases of retrograde endoleaks. In these cases, coil embolization or other occlusive measures may be used to thrombose the source vessel of the endoleak. Type II endoleaks require both an inflow and an outflow collateral branch vessel, so efforts should be made to identify and treat these multiple aneurysm side branches. Coil embolization of type I endoleaks has also been reported; however, it is unclear that this is effective in eliminating arterial pressure or the risk of aneurysm rupture.

Angiogram

Angiogram Report

Anterior-posterior (Fig. 3A), lateral (Fig. 3B), and selective (Fig. 3C) angiograms demonstrate continued arterial perfusion originating from the proximal attachment site, a proximal type I endoleak.

Diagnosis and Treatment (continued)

Antegrade endoleaks (types I and III) may be successfully treated by placement of an extension stent graft. In this case, there is sufficient undilated aorta distal to the renal ostia to allow successful placement of a proximal extension stent graft. This is the best treatment for this elderly patient with multiple comorbid illnesses. If a sufficient proximal aortic fixation region is not present, then conversion to standard aneurysm repair must be considered as the definitive treatment. Use of embolic material to seal proximal endoleaks has not been demonstrated to be effective in preventing aneurysm rupture and cannot be recommended.

TAKE HOME POINTS

- Patients with aneurysms greater than 5.5 cm should undergo repair.
- Patients should be considered for open or endovascular repair. Factors favoring endovascular repair instead include preoperative comorbidities and the presence of factors complicating traditional repair (e.g., hostile abdomen, presence of stoma).
- This case demonstrates the importance of postoperative surveillance for the detection of endoleaks.
- Type I endoleaks typically need repair, and extension of graft limbs is a common treatment.

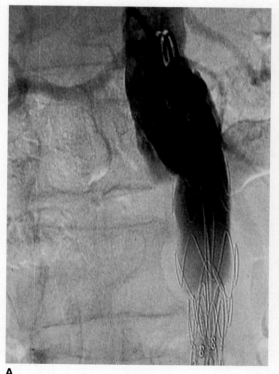

A

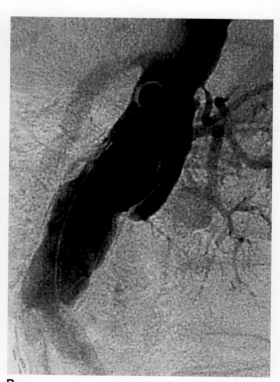

B

FIGURE 3 • Type 1 endoleak following EVAR **(A, B)**. Direct injection of type 1A endoleak **(C)**.

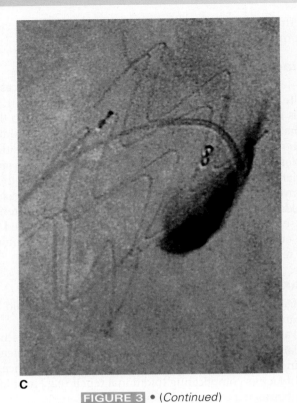

C

FIGURE 3 • (Continued)

SUGGESTED READINGS

Bernhard VM, Mitchell RS, Matsumura JS. Ruptured abdominal aortic aneurysm after endovascular repair. *J Vasc Surg.* 2002;35:1155-1162.

Fransen GA, Vallabhaneni SR, van Marrewijk CJ. Rupture of infra-renal aortic aneurysm after endovascular repair: a series from EUROSTAR registry. *Eur J Vasc Endovasc Surg.* 2003;26:487-493.

Gioacchino C, Gennai S, Saitta G, et al. Treatment of ruptured abdominal aortic aneurysm after endovascular aneurysm repair: a comparison of patients without prior treatment. *J Vasc Surg.* 2009;49:582-588.

Kelso RL, Lyden SP, Butler B, et al. Late conversion of aortic stent grafts. *J Vasc Surg.* 2009;49:598-95.

Lyden SP, McNamara JM, Sternbach Y. Technical considerations for late removal of aortic endografts. *J Vasc Surg.* 2002;36:674-678.

Mehta M, Paty PS, Roddy SP, et al. Treatment options for delayed AAA rupture following endovascular repair. *J Vasc Surg.* 2011;53:14-20.

CLINICAL SCENARIO CASE QUESTIONS

1. Which of the following anatomical features is a contraindication to endovascular aneurysm repair?

   a. Fifteen degrees of cranial-caudal angulation at the infrarenal aorta
   b. A 4-mm infrarenal neck
   c. A 9-mm common femoral artery
   d. A 7.2-cm aneurysm with intraluminal thrombus

2. Which of the following is true regarding endoleaks after endovascular aneurysm repair?

   a. Type II endoleaks have never been associated with aneurysm expansion or rupture.
   b. Type III endoleaks virtually always require open repair.
   c. Type I and III endoleaks result in pressurization of the aneurysm sac.
   d. Embolic glue is the standard of care in repairing type III endoleaks.

38 Rupture EVAR

MEHDI J. TEYMOURI, PHILIP K. PATY, PHILIP S. K. PATY, and MANISH MEHTA

Presentation

A 69-year-old man presents to the emergency room with sudden onset of abdominal pain and near syncope. His past medical history is significant for hypertension, coronary artery disease, hyperlipidemia, and smoking. On presentation to the emergency room, the patient has complaints of abdominal pain, is diaphoretic, and is hypotensive (BP: 82/50 mm Hg). He denies any prior similar episodes and denies any chest or back pain. Physical examination does not indicate any murmurs, pulses are faint and normal, abdomen is distended with a pulsatile mass, femoral pulses are intact, and his feet appear well perfused.

Differential Diagnosis

Patients with a ruptured abdominal aortic aneurysm (r-AAA) typically present with abdominal and/or back pain, hypotension with or without syncope, and a pulsatile abdominal mass. The presence of all three findings is considered diagnostic for r-AAA. Rupture of AAA remains a lethal condition and had an expected overall mortality of nearly 50% nearly a decade ago. Over the past decade, with the evolution of endovascular aneurysm repair (EVAR) from elective to emergent r-AAA has had a significant impact in improving patient survival with most studies reporting an expected rupture EVAR mortality in proximity of 20%. The implications of improvements in our technical ability to offer rupture EVAR are significant: To date, no other therapy has offered such a survival advantage to these high-risk patients presenting with r-AAA.

Workup

An emergency room FAST exam (Focused Assessment with Sonography in Trauma) can be extremely helpful in making the diagnosis of r-AAA. The hemodynamic status of the ruptured AAA patient generally dictates the need for a preoperative CT scan, and although while planning for this emergent open surgical repair, a preoperative CT is not considered a necessity, while planning an emergent EVAR, its critically important to obtain a preoperative CT scan for evaluating the feasibility of EVAR as well as for stent graft sizing. Adequate resuscitation of patients with r-AAA is vital to a successful outcome. As long as the patients maintain a measurable blood pressure, the techniques of "permissive hypotension" by limiting the resuscitation to maintain a detectable blood pressure can help minimize ongoing hemorrhage.

When considering these endovascular techniques for treating r-AAA, one has to prepare for the challenges of streamlining patient care from the emergency room (ER) to the operating room (OR) and the subsequent endovascular

procedure that often requires a multidisciplinary approach and a change in paradigm and local cultures. Furthermore, there is a need for adequate fluoroscopic equipment, trained personnel, and a variety of available stent graft, and ancillary equipment.

Collectively, worldwide experience demonstrates that an increasing number of r-AAAs are being treated by EVAR. The endovascular approach is less invasive, eliminates laparotomy, eliminates aortic cross clamping, decreases surgical bleeding and possibly general anesthesia, and has been shown to decrease the mortality of r-AAA repair with fewer complications, shorter hospital length of stay, and more patients being able to return home rather than going to institutional care after these emergent procedures. An understanding of the context in which the r-AAA patients were treated, the underlying patient selection, and the local, regional, and national influences in offering endovascular treatments to r-AAA patients is of critical importance when evaluating the evidence in favor of or against of r-EVAR.

Endovascular Approach

There remain several fundamental concerns regarding EVAR for ruptured AAA that include anatomical suitability for EVAR, the availability of dedicated staff and equipment to perform emergent EVAR at all hours, feasibility of treating hemodynamically stable and unstable patients by EVAR, and the surgeon/interventionist's ability to manage unexpected scenarios under emergent circumstances. Many of the high-volume institutions have adopted a standardized protocol-based approach that includes a heightened awareness among the ER staff to suspect the diagnosis of ruptured AAA and notify the on-call vascular surgeon and the OR staff.

Since not all patients with ruptured AAA can undergo endovascular repair, all OR/hybrid endovascular OR suites should be setup to facilitate EVAR, as well as open surgical repair. Depending on the size of the room and the fluoroscopic equipment that can be fixed or portable with viewing screens and power injectors, one has to customize the layout of the OR suite that is conducive for endovascular and open surgical repair; we have found it best to set up the room for endovascular repair with standard needles, wires, catheters, and sheaths open on a sterile table, have the surgical instruments in the room if needed, situate the patient on the OR table, and as the anesthesiology team prepares the patient, set up the fluoroscopic equipment and supplies (Table 1).

The patient is prepped and draped in supine position. Via a percutaneous or femoral artery cut-down, ipsilateral access is obtained using a needle, floppy guidewire, and a guiding catheter. The floppy guidewire is exchanged for a super-stiff wire that can be used to place a large sheath (12 –14 French × 45 cm length) in the ipsilateral femoral artery and the sheath advanced up to the juxtarenal abdominal aorta, so it is ready to be used to deliver and support the aortic occlusion balloon (AOB) if needed. A compliant occlusion balloon should always be available in these procedures, and in hemodynamically unstable patients, the occlusion balloon is advanced through the ipsilateral sheath over the super-stiff wire into the supraceliac abdominal aorta under fluoroscopic guidance, and the balloon is inflated as needed. Contralateral femoral access is subsequently obtained via percutaneous or cut-down approach in a similar fashion and a "marker flush-catheter" advanced to the juxtarenal aorta for an arteriogram.

The placement of the stent graft main body is planned based on the aortoiliac morphology that is best suited for EVAR. Unless prohibitive, *in hemodynamically stable patients*, following the initial arteriogram, the AOB is removed from the initial ipsilateral side and the stent graft main body advanced under fluoroscopic guidance; this limits the number of catheter exchanges. *In hemodynamically unstable patients* who require inflation of the AOB, the "marker flush-catheter" is exchanged for the stent graft main body that is delivered up to the aortic neck. An arteriogram is done via the sheath that is used to support the AOB, the tip of the stent graft main body is aligned with the lowermost renal artery, the occlusion balloon is

subsequently deflated and withdrawn back with the delivery sheath into the AAA, and the stent graft main body deployed. The remainder of the EVAR procedure is performed similar to as in elective circumstances: (1) the tip of the stent graft main body aligned with the lowermost renal artery, (2) the contralateral gate aligned to facilitate expeditious "gate cannulation," and (3) the ipsilateral and contralateral iliac extensions planned and deployed as needed.

Special Intraoperative Considerations

The proportion of r-AAA patients that are suitable for EVAR is variable and on the basis of two meta-analysis ranges from 47% to 67%. r-EVAR patients with hostile aortic necks had a significantly higher incidence of female gender, mean maximum AAA diameter, abdominal compartment syndrome (ACS), Type I endoleaks, and the need for all secondary interventions.

Depending on one's comfort level and the logistics, EVAR for rupture can be performed under local anesthesia via percutaneous approach to general anesthesia and femoral artery cut-down. The potential benefits of local anesthesia/conscious sedation and percutaneous approach is that it might avoid the loss of "sympathetic tone" in the compromised ruptured AAA patients. One has to be comfortable with obtaining percutaneous access and using closure devices in patients who might be hemodynamically unstable with difficult to palpate femoral pulses. Although the advantage may be significant, it must be balanced by the potential difficulties encountered during these emergent procedures, as the patient might not be coherent and cooperative enough to lie still.

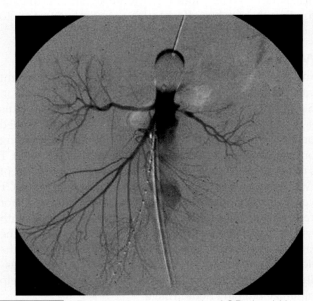

FIGURE 1 • The sheath supporting the AOB should be advanced and supported fully into the aortic neck to prevent downward displacement and prolapse of the occlusion balloon into the abdominal aortic aneurysm. (From Mehta M. Endovascular aneurysm repair for ruptured abdominal aortic aneurysm: the Albany Vascular Group approach. *J Vasc Surg.* 2010;52(6):1706-1712.)

TABLE 1. Rupture EVAR

Key Technical Steps

1. Percutaneous vs. femoral artery cut-down
2. Use of AOB
3. Stent graft contralateral gate cannulation
4. Managing type I endoleaks
5. Potential stent graft coverage of one renal artery
6. Diagnosing abdominal compartment syndrome

Potential Pitfalls

- Hemodynamically unstable patient
- Inability to cannulate the stent graft contralateral gate
- Type I endoleak
- Conversion to open surgical repair

The appropriate use of AOBs in hemodynamically unstable patients is vital to the success of EVAR. Access for AOBs can be obtained via the brachial or the femoral artery. There are several advantages of the femoral approach: (1) it allows the anesthesia team to have access to both upper extremities for arterial and venous access, (2) the patients who require the AOB are often hypotensive, and, in these patients, percutaneous brachial access can be more cumbersome and time consuming than femoral cut-down, and (3) the currently available AOBs require at least a 12–14 French sheath, which requires a brachial artery cut-down and repair, and stiff wires and catheters across the aortic arch without prior imaging under emergent circumstances might lead to other arterial injuries and/or embolization causing stroke.

Several important points should be considered during placement of the AOB. The sheath supporting the balloon should be advanced and supported fully into the aortic neck prior to inflation of the occlusion balloon as this will prevent downward displacement and prolapse of the occlusion balloon into the AAA (Fig. 1). Inability to fully engage the sheath into the aortic neck due to the presence of significant aortoiliac stenosis, calcifications, or tortuosity might result in downward displacement of the inflated occlusion balloon; this often required forward traction on the inflated balloon catheter to maintain adequate position at the suprarenal/supraceliac aorta (Fig. 2A–C). If inflation of the aortic balloon is required to maintain a viable blood pressure, just prior to deployment of the stent graft main

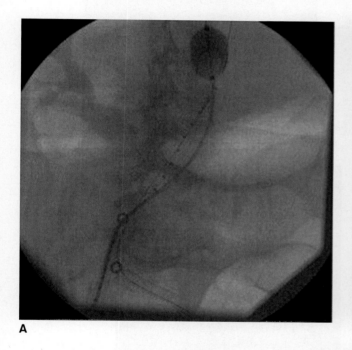
A

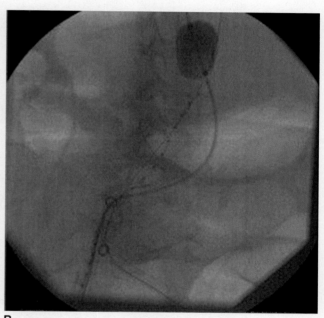
B

C

FIGURE 2 • A–C: Inability to fully engage the sheath into the aortic neck due to the presence of significant aortoiliac stenosis, calcifications, or tortuosity might result in downward displacement of the inflated occlusion balloon. This often requires forward traction on the inflated balloon catheter to maintain adequate position at the suprarenal/supraceliac aorta. (From Mehta M. Endovascular aneurysm repair for ruptured abdominal aortic aneurysm: the Albany Vascular Group approach. *J Vasc Surg.* 2010;52(6):1706-1712.)

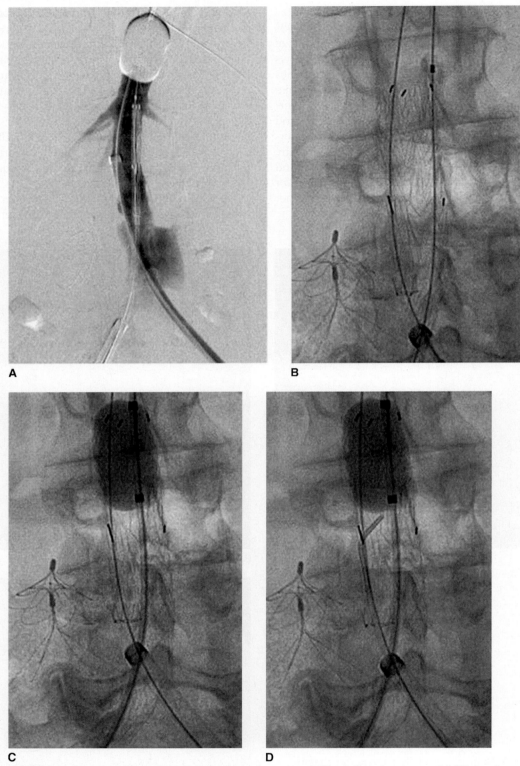

FIGURE 3 • **A–E:** Managing the AOB during stent graft deployment. **A:** The inflated suprarenal AOB is advanced through the left femoral approach, the stent graft main body is advanced through the right femoral approach, and the arteriogram is done through the left femoral sheath supporting the occlusion balloon. **B:** The AOB is deflated and retracted back from the aortic neck, and the stent graft main body is subsequently deployed. This avoids trapping of the compliant AOB between the aortic neck and the stent graft. **C:** In hemodynamically unstable patients, the occlusion balloon can be redirected into the aortic neck from the side ipsilateral to the stent graft main body and reinflated at the infrarenal aortic neck within the stent graft main body before contralateral gate cannulation. **D:** After the occlusion balloon is reinflated in the stent graft main body in hemodynamically unstable patients, the contralateral stent graft gate can be cannulated, and contralateral stent graft extensions are placed as needed.

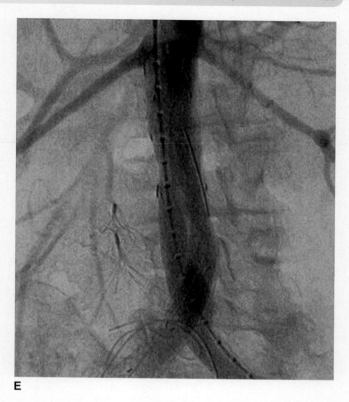

E

FIGURE 3 • (*Continued*) **E:** After contralateral iliac extension and ruptured abdominal aortic aneurysm exclusion, the occlusion balloon can be removed, as shown in the completion arteriogram. (From Mehta M. Endovascular aneurysm repair for ruptured abdominal aortic aneurysm: the Albany Vascular Group approach. *J Vasc Surg.* 2010;52(6):1706-1712.)

body, the AOB should be deflated from the suprarenal level and withdrawn. The stent graft main body is subsequently deployed; this will avoid trapping the compliant AOB between the aortic neck and the stent graft. This temporary deflation of the AOB rarely results in hemodynamic collapse and usually is of little consequence. In hemodynamically unstable patients, the occlusion balloon can be redirected into the aortic neck from the side ipsilateral to the stent graft main body and reinflated at the infrarenal aortic neck within the stent graft main body; this allows for aortic occlusion and does not interfere with the remainder of the endovascular procedure (Fig. 3A–E).

The pathophysiology of ACS after EVAR for ruptured AAA is multifactorial: (1) the retroperitoneal hematoma is a space-occupying lesion and a significant factor contributing to intra-abdominal hypertension, (2) ongoing bleeding from lumbar and inferior mesenteric arteries into the disrupted aneurysm sac in the setting of severe coagulopathy might be a contributing factor, and (3) the shock state associated with r-AAA is associated with alterations in microvascular permeability that can lead to visceral and soft tissue edema. Patients with ACS following ruptured EVAR have increased mortality of greater than 50%, and factors such as the need for AOB, need for massive blood transfusions, coagulopathy, and hemodynamic instability have been implicated with increased risk for ACS following ruptured EVAR. ACS requires prompt recognition and treatment, which includes decompression laparotomy.

When on-table surgical conversion is needed, the use of AOB can be extremely valuable in maintaining hemodynamic stability; the techniques of AOB have been discussed above. In addition, during the time of laparotomy and open surgical conversion, it is crucial to maintain the position of the AOB and its delivery sheath; failure to do so might result in AOB prolapse into the AAA and loss of aortic occlusion. If open surgical conversion is needed subsequent to stent graft deployment, the exact approach should be tailored to the type of stent graft, the type of proximal and distal fixation including suprarenal versus infrarenal stents and barbs.

Postoperative Management

Patients typically are admitted to the ICU for at least 1 day following ruptured EVAR, depending on their clinical status. Patients require close monitoring of their hemodynamic status and assessment of multisystem organ dysfunction. Patients should be assessed for the development of ACS, and for the first 24 hours frequent abdominal exams, and bladder pressure measurements. The incidence of ischemic colitis is nearly 10% with ruptured EVAR, and sigmoidoscopy/colonoscopy should be used judiciously when indicated, particularly in patients with bloody bowel movement, abdominal pain out of proportion, and unexplained leukocytosis. Patients with persistent or recurrent hypotension should be evaluated for ongoing retroperitoneal bleeding from endoleaks. A CTA can be diagnostic for Type I endoleak (from proximal or distal stent graft attachment sites) or Type III endoleak (from stent graft component separation), both require immediate reintervention. Type II endoleaks (retrograde flow into the aneurysm sac or retroperitoneum from inferior mesenteric or lumbar arteries) can be treated by crystalloid/colloid resuscitation, and PRBC transfusion depending on the clinical scenario.

Following discharge from the hospital, the postoperative surveillance of rupture EVAR patients is similar to elective EVAR patients, and generally includes yearly clinical exam and CTA.

Case Conclusion

The 74-year-old patient with a presumed diagnosis of ruptured AAA underwent a CTA that indicated a ruptured 7.4-cm AAA and a retroperitoneal hematoma. He was emergently taken to the hybrid endovascular suite and underwent percutaneous ruptured EVAR with local anesthesia. His blood pressures were labile, and AOB was needed prior to stent graft deployment. The remainder of the EVAR procedure was uneventful, and the patient was discharged home on postoperative day 2. Follow-up CT scans out to 18 months have indicated complete aneurysm exclusion and no endoleaks, and AAA sac size has decreased to 4.5 cm.

TAKE HOME POINTS

- In appropriately selected patients, EVAR for rupture offers a survival advantage when compared to the traditional open surgical repair.
- Percutaneous rupture EVAR with local anesthesia is feasible and might have the greatest benefit for hemodynamically unstable patients.
- The use of AOB is needed in approximately 20% of rupture EVAR patients, and in the vast majority of these patients, AOB retrieval prior to stent graft deployment is well tolerated. In patients with sustained hemodynamic collapse, after stent graft main body deployment, the AOB can be repositioned and inflated from the ipsilateral side within the stent graft main body until the contralateral gate is cannulated and AAA excluded.
- Risk factors for development of ACS after ruptured EVAR include the use of AOB, massive blood transfusion requirement, and coagulopathy. Early diagnosis and decompression laparotomy are critical for patient survival.
- Following rupture EVAR, all patients should be thoroughly evaluated for the presence of Type I and III endoleaks, which require treatment. Type II endoleaks can be managed conservatively.

SUGGESTED READINGS

Fillinger MF, Racusin J, Baker RK, et al. Anatomic characteristics of ruptured abdominal aortic aneurysm on conventional CT scans: implications for rupture risk. *J Vasc Surg.* 2004;39(6):1243-1252.

IMPROVE trial investigators, Powell JT, Hinchliffe RJ, Thompson MM, et al. Observations from the IMPROVE trial concerning the clinical care of patients with ruptured abdominal aortic aneurysm. *Br J Surg.* 2014;101(3):216-224; discussion 224. doi: 10.1002/bjs.9410.

McPhee J, Eslami MH, Arous EJ, et al. Endovascular treatment of ruptured abdominal aortic aneurysms in the United States (2001–2006): a significant survival benefit over open repair is independently associated with increased institutional volume. *J Vasc Surg.* 2009;49(4):817-826.

Mehta M, Byrne J, Darling RC III, et al. Endovascular repair of ruptured infrarenal abdominal aortic aneurysm is associated with lower 30-day mortality and better 5-year survival rates than open surgical repair. *J Vasc Surg.* 2013;57(2):368-375.

Mehta M, Darling RC III, Roddy SP, et al. Factors associated with abdominal compartment syndrome complicating endovascular repair of ruptured abdominal aortic aneurysms. *J Vasc Surg.* 2005;42:1047-1051.

Mehta M, Paty PSK, Byrne J, et al. Hemodynamic status impacts outcomes of endovascular aneurysm repair for rupture. *J Vasc Surg.* 2013;57:1255-1260.

Mehta M, Paty PSK, Roddy SPR, et al. Treatment options for delayed AAA rupture following endovascular repair. *J Vasc Surg.* 2011;53:14-20.

Mehta M, Taggert J, Darling RC III, et al. Establishing a protocol for endovascular treatment of ruptured abdominal aortic aneurysms: outcomes of a prospective analysis. *J Vasc Surg.* 2006;44:1-8.

Van Beek SC, Conijn AP, Koelemay MJ, et al. Endovascular aneurysm repair versus open repair for patients with a ruptured abdominal aortic aneurysm: a systematic review and meta-analysis of short-term survival. *Eur J Vasc Endovasc Surg.* 2014;47(6):593-602. doi:10.1016/j.ejvs.2014.03.003.

CLINICAL SCENARIO CASE QUESTIONS

1. A 68-year-old man presents with a ruptured AAA, is hemodynamically unstable, and undergoes ruptured EVAR. He requires an aortic occlusion balloon during the procedure, 8 units of PRBC transfusion, and 4 L of crystalloids. During the postoperative period, the patient is hypotensive (BP 78/55 mm Hg) and oliguric, his abdomen is distended, and the ventilator peak and plateau pressures are elevated. The most likely diagnosis is:

   a. Type I endoleak
   b. Ongoing retroperitoneal bleeding from Type II endoleak
   c. Abdominal compartment syndrome
   d. Contrast-induced acute tubular necrosis

2. Ruptured AAA patients

   a. Present with syncope, abdominal pain, and pulsatile abdominal mass the vast majority of times
   b. Should all undergo EVAR
   c. Require aggressive fluid resuscitation with a target systolic BP of >100 mm Hg
   d. Have a significantly higher incidence of ischemic colitis when compared to elective AAA patients.

39 Rupture after EVAR from Endoleak

DANIEL FREMED and PETER L. FARIES

Based on chapter in previous edition by Peter L. Faries, Rajeev Dayal, Scott Hollenbeck, Albeir Mousa, and K. Craig Kent

Presentation

The patient is a 72-year-old man who complains of increasing left-sided abdominal pain of 48 hours' duration. He had undergone elective endovascular aneurysm repair (EVAR) 2 years prior but has since been lost to follow-up. On physical examination, the patient is in visible discomfort. His blood pressure is 115/35 mm Hg with a heart rate of 110 beats per minute. His abdomen is distended with a palpable, tender, left-sided pulsatile mass. There is no flank ecchymosis. There are well-healed transverse groin incisions bilaterally. Peripheral pulses are palpable. The patient denies chest pain, shortness of breath, or syncopal episodes.

Differential Diagnosis

The patient presents with tachycardia, acute abdominal findings, and a pulsatile mass; however, he reports having undergone prior endovascular abdominal aortic aneurysm (AAA) repair. The differential should therefore include ruptured abdominal aortic aneurysm but should also include diverticulitis, renal lithiasis, intestinal perforation, pancreatitis, and spontaneous retroperitoneal hematoma. The differential diagnosis may also include rare aneurysms, including splenic and other visceral artery aneurysms, as well as para-anastomotic aneurysms with or without infection. In this instance, physical examination is consistent with a ruptured AAA despite prior EVAR.

Workup

The most accurate method of diagnosing ruptured AAA is computerized tomography (CT) with intravenous contrast. CT findings consistent with rupture include extravasation of contrast outside of the aorta, retroperitoneal hematoma, and retroperitoneal stranding. In patients with a history of EVAR, CT may provide the etiology of likely endoleak. Imaging may reveal endograft position in relation to native aorta, presence of significant lumbar arteries or patent inferior mesenteric artery (IMA), and degree of component overlap in multibody devices. In addition to making the diagnosis of rupture, CT scan can be used to evaluate multiple organ systems to exclude other diagnoses in the differential (Fig. 1).

Diagnosis and Treatment

Based on history, physical exam, and CT findings of retroperitoneal bleeding in the setting of aortic disruption, the most likely diagnosis is ruptured AAA despite prior EVAR.

The goal of treatment is identification and exclusion of the source of rupture. Continued arterial perfusion of the aneurysm sac after endovascular repair has been termed an *endoleak*. Endoleaks result in continued pressurization of the aneurysm sac. The significance of the continued perfusion is determined by the source of the endoleak. Endoleaks that result in direct arterial flow into the aneurysm sac cause systemic pressurization of the aneurysm. These leaks may occur at the sites of attachment of the stent graft to the native arterial wall, the seal, or implantation zones (type I endoleak). Direct antegrade endoleaks may also occur at junction sites between different endovascular stent graft components (type III endoleak). Types I and III endoleaks are the most common causes of rupture after EVAR (Fig. 2).

Surgical Approach

When an untreated or unrecognized endoleak results in aneurysm rupture, immediate surgical intervention is necessary to prevent exsanguination and death. Several approaches may be used, including placement of an occlusion balloon in the aorta proximal to the aneurysm, immediate standard surgical repair, and endovascular aneurysm repair. The choice is based on anatomic suitability of the aorta on CTA, as well as surgeon comfort with each type of intervention.

Open Approach

Patients presenting with rupture are taken to the operating room emergently. The patient is prepped and draped in the supine position prior to induction general

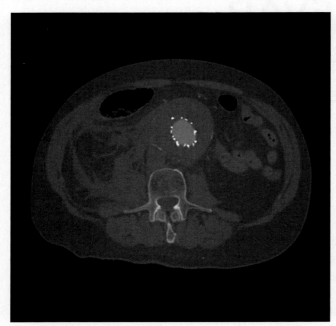

FIGURE 1 • CT image of infrarenal aortic endograft with evidence of rupture.

anesthesia. The aorta is exposed via a traditional transperitoneal or retroperitoneal approach.

The site of proximal cross-clamping is dependent on the type of previously placed endograft. Infrarenal clamping of the aorta is preferred in endografts without suprarenal fixation. The aorta may be clamped above the renal arteries in the presence of suprarenal endograft fixation. Distal control is obtained bilaterally by cross-clamping the iliac arteries.

Once systemic anticoagulation is achieved, proximal and distal control is obtained. The sac is opened via a longitudinal incision exposing the endograft. The endograft is then carefully removed. If the barbs of the device are well incorporated in the aortic wall, the lateral wall can be longitudinally incised with or without endarterectomy. Once the graft is explanted, a traditional unibody

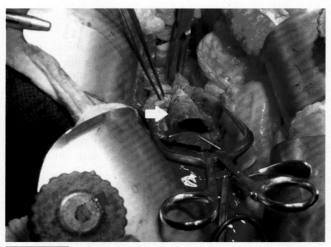

FIGURE 2 • Exposure of aneurysm sac revealing embedded endovascular stent graft (*arrow*).

TABLE 1. Rupture after EVAR from Endoleak

Key Technical Steps

1. Exposure of abdominal aorta via transperitoneal or retroperitoneal approach
2. Clamp proximal aorta relative to graft; may need supraceliac control if suprarenal fixation is present
3. Open sac via longitudinal incision to expose endograft
4. Explant endograft, including barbs
5. Sew in traditional graft to healthy vessel
6. Reestablish blood flow through graft, obtain hemostasis
7. Close sac over new graft
8. Close abdomen, check distal pulses

Potential Pitfalls

- Scarring and incorporation of endograft into aortic wall
- Retained nitinol shrapnel
- Damage to healthy vessel lumen upon explantation
- Prolonged suprarenal cross-clamping

or bifurcated graft is sewn into nondiseased portions of proximal and distal vessel. In cases where complete graft removal is not feasible, the standard graft may be sewn to residual well-incorporated endograft. To do so, the stent graft may be divided sharply and the suprarenal component incorporated with the proximal suture line. Similarly, the distal iliac limbs may not be readily amenable to removal without causing injury to the iliac arteries. In such instances, the bifurcated aortic graft may be sewn to the iliac limbs of the stent graft.

Proximal and distal clamps are removed, and suture lines are inspected for hemostasis. The fascial layers of the abdomen are closed in usual fashion provided there is little tension. The abdomen may be left open if closure proves difficult or results in abdominal compartment syndrome (Table 1).

Endovascular Approach

The patient is prepped and draped in supine position. A femoral artery cutdown is performed, and ipsilateral access is obtained with a needle, floppy guidewire, and guiding catheter. Alternatively, percutaneous access to the femoral arteries can be obtained under ultrasound guidance. The guidewire is exchanged for a stiff wire that can accommodate and exchange for a large sheath (12 to 14 French). The sheath is advanced up to the juxtrarenal aorta should an aortic occlusion balloon be needed. Contralateral access is then obtained either via cutdown on percutaneous approach. A marker flush catheter is advanced to the juxtarenal aorta for an arteriogram.

The mode of endovascular therapy is based on the etiology of rupture. CTA and intraoperative angiography can determine if stent graft extensions are necessary proximally, distally, or within the endograft. A Palmaz stent may be needed to facilitate treatment at the proximal neck of a type IA endoleak.

The stent graft main body is delivered through the initial ipsilateral side. In hemodynamically unstable patients where an aortic occlusion balloon is required, the marker

TABLE 2. Endovascular Repair of Ruptured AAA after EVAR ("Redo EVAR")

Key Technical Steps

1. Ipsilateral femoral artery cutdown
2. Arterial access via needle, guidewire, and guide catheter
3. Exchange guidewire for super stiff wire
4. Advance large French sheath over stiff wire to the juxtarenal aorta
5. Obtain contralateral access via cutdown or percutaneous approach
6. Send marker flush catheter to the juxtarenal aorta via the contralateral femoral artery
7. Perform angiogram to identify leak
8. Stent graft extensions or small covered stents based on etiology of endoleak
9. Completion angiogram after deployment of new stent graft
10. Repair groins, check pulses

Potential Pitfalls

- Hemodynamic collapse upon induction of general anesthesia
- Scarred groins from previous EVAR
- Hemodynamic instability after deflation of the aortic occlusion balloon
- Development of abdominal compartment syndrome requiring laparotomy
- Renal compromise from ischemia, contrast nephropathy, hemodynamic fluctuations/hypoperfusion

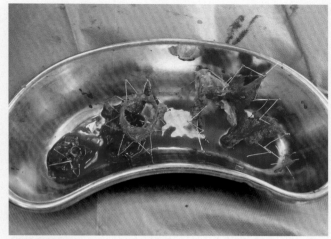

FIGURE 4 • Explanted endovascular stent graft.

flush catheter on the contralateral side may be exchanged for the main body.

After stent graft deployment, angiography is performed to ensure exclusion of the endoleak. Groin cutdowns are repaired primarily, and peripheral pulses are checked (Table 2).

Special Intraoperative Considerations

Periaortic scarring or well-incorporated grafts may complicate explantation. Wire cutters may be necessary to free the graft from well-embedded barbs or stents. In cases where complete explantation of the stent graft is not feasible, a "hybrid" approach may be utilized by sewing the new graft to segments of well-embedded stent graft at the proximal or distal anastomosis (Figs. 3 and 4).

Postoperative Management

All patients undergoing repair of ruptured AAA should be transferred to the intensive care unit postoperatively. The most common postoperative complications after rupture from EVAR include MI, acute kidney injury, and abdominal compartment syndrome. Demand ischemia, suprarenal cross-clamping, and massive retroperitoneal hemorrhage are major risk factors for developing these complications. The patient should remain on telemetry monitoring with diligent monitoring of renal function. Although a less invasive procedure, redo EVAR for rupture still carries these risks postoperatively.

Patients undergoing redo EVAR should follow-up with CT angiography at 1, 6, and 12 months postoperatively with annual scans afterward to ensure no new endoleaks or migration of new stent graft extensions.

Case Conclusion

The patient undergoes successful open repair. The old endograft is successfully explanted and replaced with a Dacron bifurcated graft. Upon closing, the patient's abdominal wall demonstrates significant tension and is left open. He remains stable and is brought back to the operating room for abdominal wall closure with mesh on postoperative day 4. He is discharged 10 days later and remains symptom free at outpatient follow-up.

TAKE HOME POINTS

- The most common causes of rupture after EVAR are types I and III endoleaks.
- Most incidences of rupture after EVAR occur in patients lost to follow-up surveillance.

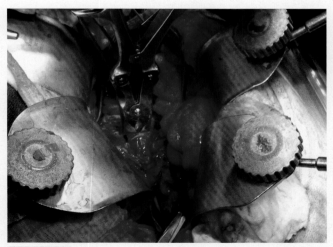

FIGURE 3 • Wire cutters may be required to successfully explant old stent graft.

- Rupture after EVAR can successfully be managed by open surgical conversion or redo EVAR.
- The level of proximal aortic cross-clamping depends on the type of original endograft.
- Replacement with new graft may involve sewing to stubborn well-embedded stent graft.
- Patients must be monitored postoperatively for cardiac and renal complications.

SUGGESTED READINGS

Bernhard VM, Mitchell RS, Matsumura JS. Ruptured abdominal aortic aneurysm after endovascular repair. *J Vasc Surg.* 2002;35:1155-1162.

Fransen GA, Vallabhaneni SR, van Marrewijk CJ. Rupture of infra-renal aortic aneurysm after endovascular repair: a series from EUROSTAR registry. *Eur J Vasc Endovasc Surg.* 2003;26:487-493.

Gioacchino C, Gennai S, Saitta G, et al. Treatment of ruptured abdominal aortic aneurysm after endovascular aneurysm repair: a comparison of patients without prior treatment. *J Vasc Surg.* 2009;49:582-588.

Kelso RL, Lyden SP, Butler B, et al. Late conversion of aortic stent grafts. *J Vasc Surg.* 2009;49:598-95.

Lyden SP, McNamara JM, Sternbach Y. Technical considerations for late removal of aortic endografts. *J Vasc Surg.* 2002;36:674-678.

Mehta M, Paty PS, Roddy SP, et al. Treatment options for delayed AAA rupture following endovascular repair. *J Vasc Surg.* 2011;53:14-20.

CLINICAL SCENARIO CASE QUESTIONS

1. What is the most frequent cause of AAA rupture after EVAR?

   a. Type I endoleak
   b. Type II endoleak
   c. Type III endoleak
   d. Type IV endoleak
   e. a and c

2. What is the most effective method of preventing AAA rupture after EVAR?

   a. Routine CT surveillance after initial EVAR to ensure the integrity of the repair
   b. No follow-up, have the patient return as needed
   c. Strict antiplatelet regimen

40 Inflammatory Abdominal Aortic Aneurysm

RODNEY P. BENSLEY Jr and MARC L. SCHERMERHORN

Presentation

A 67-year-old man presents to the emergency department with complaints of abdominal pain. He reports intermittent sharp pain over the past several months that has become increasingly more intense in character over the past several days. The pain is centrally located with radiation to his midback. He denies alleviating or exacerbating characteristics. He also reports occasional low-grade fevers and a 10-pound weight loss over the past few months. He smokes heavily and has marginally controlled hypertension. He does have a family history of abdominal aortic aneurysms in his mother. On physical examination, he is afebrile, hemodynamically stable, and in moderate discomfort. His blood pressure is equal bilaterally, and pulses are fully palpable in all extremities. His abdomen is moderately tender in the periumbilical region without peritoneal signs. He has mild costovertebral angle tenderness.

Differential Diagnosis

The differential diagnosis for this clinical presentation is broad. The initial focus should be on potentially life-threatening conditions. In addition to the obvious vascular conditions, such as a ruptured abdominal aortic aneurysm (AAA) or acute aortic dissection, other intra-abdominal conditions, such as mesenteric ischemia, intestinal volvulus, or a perforated viscus, need to be considered. Other conditions that are not immediately life threatening include neoplastic causes, pyelonephritis, nephrolithiasis, and ureterolithiasis. An inflammatory AAA is realistically very low on the differential. Inflammatory AAAs constitute 3% to 10% of all AAAs.

Discussion

This patient's presentation requires a high index of suspicion and an aggressive diagnostic workup to rule out a potentially life-threatening diagnosis. In addition to timely laboratory studies, the current speed and detail of spiral computed tomography (CT) scanners make an intravenous contrast scan the imaging modality of choice. An intravenous CT scan can rule out an immediately life-threatening aortic condition. In addition to evaluating the vasculature, the CT scan can reveal any other intra-abdominal pathology that may be causing this patient's symptoms. Magnetic resonance arteriography (MRA) is superior in diagnosing periaortic inflammation; however, its availability and the time required to obtain the images favor obtaining a CT scan at most institutions.

Workup
Laboratory Tests

Laboratory testing should be broad and include a complete blood count (CBC), basic metabolic panel, and liver function tests. Other tests that may be helpful include a coagulation profile, an erythrocyte sedimentation rate (ESR), C-reactive protein, and a urinalysis. This patient's CBC is normal. His blood urea nitrogen is 34 mg/dL and creatinine is 1.2 mg/dL. His ESR is elevated at 101 seconds.

CT Scan

This patient's CT scan demonstrates a 4.8 × 4.2-cm infrarenal AAA with significant fat stranding and wall thickening of the anterior and lateral aortic wall at the inferior portion of the AAA. The posterior wall of the aorta is relatively spared. There is mural thrombus but no evidence of aortic sac hemorrhage or extravasation. The ureters were of normal caliber and uninvolved. There were no other intra-abdominal abnormalities (Fig. 1). Note the inflammatory rind involving the anterior and lateral wall of the AAA. The posterior wall is spared.

Diagnosis and Treatment
Diagnosis

Inflammatory Abdominal Aortic Aneurysm

The leading diagnosis in this patient is an inflammatory AAA. Patients with inflammatory AAAs frequently present with abdominal and back pain, an elevated ESR denoting a generalized inflammatory state, and imaging

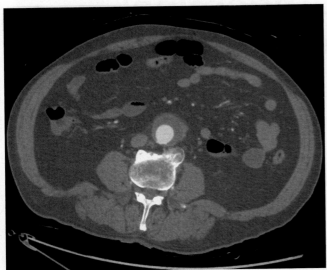

FIGURE 1 • CT scan demonstrating an infrarenal abdominal aortic aneurysm with an inflammatory rind involving the anterior and lateral walls of the aneurysm. Note that the posterior wall is spared.

revealing a thickened aortic wall with inflammation of surrounding structures, such as the retroperitoneum, kidney and ureter, inferior vena cava, and duodenum. The ureters are involved in approximately 25% of cases. Weight loss is often present as well. Aneurysm development is multifactorial in nature with both a genetic predisposition and environmental factors contributing to aneurysmal degeneration of the aorta.

Inflammatory AAAs were first described in 1972. At the time, they were thought to be an entirely separate entity from noninflammatory AAAs; however, current understanding favors an inflammatory process similar to typical aneurysms, but with an advanced degree of inflammation.

Treatment

The decision to treat inflammatory AAAs should be based on the same criteria used to treat patients with degenerative-type aneurysms. The estimated rupture risk, operative risk, and life expectancy will all influence the decision to intervene. Concerning aortic characteristics, such as periaortic edema, pain, and involvement of surrounding structures, may prompt a more aggressive management strategy. Many inflammatory aneurysms are repaired urgently or emergently due to the inability to rule out acute expansion and imminent rupture.

This patient's CT scan and laboratory values indicate the presence of an inflammatory aneurysm without involvement of the ureters and secondary hydronephrosis. Although the aneurysm does not appear to be leaking at this time, the progressive nature of his abdominal pain is of concern. If all other potential sources of his pain can be ruled out, it is reasonable to recommend an urgent repair

of his inflammatory aneurysm. The operative approach to patients with inflammatory AAAs should have two primary objectives: (1) to effectively replace the aneurysm with a prosthetic conduit and (2) to manage the secondary fibrotic complications if present. In this patient, there are no fibrotic complications present.

Surgical Approach

Prior to the introduction of endovascular AAA repair, open AAA repair was the only feasible approach to aneurysm replacement. Open repair of inflammatory AAAs is technically demanding. Repair of inflammatory AAAs has been shown to have significantly increased operating room time and requirement of blood product transfusion as compared to open repair of noninflammatory AAAs. A retroperitoneal approach is recommended due to the extensive inflammation that often affects the anterior and lateral surfaces of the aorta. This approach attempts to minimize dissection through the surrounding dense fibrotic tissue. The limitations of this approach include the limited accessibility of the right ureter, right iliac artery, and duodenum. The dense fibrotic tissue may provide a good substance to the aortic wall to hold sutures; however, dehiscence of the anastomosis is a concern, and reinforcement of the anastomosis with Teflon pledgets or polytetrafluoroethylene strips can be performed. Early reports of open repair of inflammatory AAAs showed increased perioperative mortality and complications, but more contemporary series have demonstrated that the perioperative mortality and complications are comparable to open repair of noninflammatory AAAs. In situations where acute expansion or impending rupture is suspected, an anterior approach may also be employed, but the retroperitoneal approach is quite feasible for urgent AAA repair as well.

The endovascular approach to inflammatory AAAs is appealing as it obviates the need for difficult dissection through fibrotic tissue and the pitfalls of performing a hand-sewn anastomosis to tissues of questionable quality. There have been numerous reports in the literature describing successful endovascular approaches to these aneurysms. As mentioned, it obviates the need for difficult dissection through fibrotic tissue and its accompanying risk of injury to surrounding structures. There have been reports that the endovascular approach is not associated with the degree of resolution of the inflammation that is seen with open repair. In a study by Stone et al., there was a decrease in the inflammatory rind by 51% after endovascular repair of inflammatory AAAs.

Ureteral obstruction is seen in approximately 25% of these patients and is due to the periaortic and retroperitoneal fibrosis. If there is significant hydronephrosis and deterioration of renal function, ureteral stents can be placed perioperatively to relieve the acute obstruction and to act as a guide to identifying the ureters intraoperatively.

TABLE 1. Open Repair of Inflammatory AAA

Key Technical Steps

1. Left retroperitoneal incision
2. Can place ureteral stents preoperatively if needed
3. Careful dissection of periaortic tissue
4. Obtain proximal and distal control of the aorta (and iliac arteries if necessary)
5. Isolate healthy aortic tissue to perform the anastomoses
6. Reinforce anastomoses with pledgets

Potential Pitfalls

- Injury to surrounding structures (ureters, renal vein, duodenum)
- Failure to recognize injury to surrounding structures at the time of injury
- Anastomotic dehiscence

After repair of the inflammatory AAA, the fibrosis usually resolves along with the ureteral obstruction. If symptoms of obstruction persist, additional intervention may be necessary, such as ureterolysis, ureteral stent placement, or lysis of intra-abdominal adhesions. Appropriate follow-up is necessary to prevent long-term complications of end-organ damage, such as renal atrophy from chronic ureteral obstruction.

This patient was not a candidate for an endovascular approach secondary to anatomic considerations nor did he have any ureteral involvement based on CT scan or deterioration of renal function based on laboratory values, so ureteral stents were not placed. Therefore, a left retroperitoneal approach was utilized to expose the aneurysm. Minimal dissection was needed around the ureters and duodenum. Proximal and distal control were obtained, and an infrarenal cross-clamp was applied. Healthy aortic tissue was isolated to perform the anastomosis. Teflon pledgets were used to reinforce the anastomosis. The remainder of the procedure followed standard aortic surgery techniques.

Pitfalls of open repair of inflammatory AAAs included injury to surrounding structures such as the ureter, kidney, and duodenum. The dense fibrotic tissue that is often present makes dissection difficult and challenging. The aortic tissue used in the anastomosis can be of questionable quality so reinforcement with pledgets can be performed to decrease the risk of dehiscence. Persistent ureteral obstruction and periureteral inflammation can increase the likelihood of injury to the ureter during dissection. Placement of ureteral stents can serve as a guide in identifying the ureter during dissection (Table 1).

Special Intraoperative Considerations

Certain intraoperative clinical findings can change the intraoperative management of inflammatory AAAs. One situation that may be encountered is the finding of an aortoenteric fistula. In this situation, the goal of surgery would be to obtain vascular control of the aorta, restore vascular continuity in the form of an extra-anatomic bypass, resect the aortoenteric fistula, and to debride and close the bowel. Another potential finding would be the identification of a periaortic abscess likely from a case of perforated appendicitis or diverticulitis.

Postoperative Management

Postoperative complications after repair of inflammatory AAAs are similar to complications that can develop after repair of noninflammatory AAAs. Myocardial infarction, respiratory failure requiring reintubation, pneumonia, colonic ischemia, renal failure, and thrombosis are all common complications after repair of inflammatory AAAs. Renal failure is of particular interest because its cause can be multifactorial. Intraoperative hypotension and a prolonged suprarenal clamp time are common causes of acute renal failure after open repair of AAAs. With inflammatory AAAs, the retroperitoneal fibrosis and inflammation often involves the ureters causing an acute ureteral obstruction. This can be treated with the placement of ureteral stents (or if stenting is not feasible, nephrostomy may be performed) either pre- or postoperatively depending on the clinical situation. It may even require more invasive management with ureterolysis or lysis of intra-abdominal adhesions.

Endovascular repair of inflammatory AAAs is associated with the same complications that can be seen after endovascular repair of noninflammatory AAAs. Renal failure is of particular concern here as well as there is the added component of retroperitoneal fibrosis and inflammation.

Case Conclusion

Due to this patient's worsening abdominal pain and CT findings concerning for an inflammatory AAA, with no other identifiable cause for his pain, he was taken to the operating room for an endovascular aortic aneurysm repair. Postoperatively he did well and experienced no complications. He was discharged home from the hospital on postoperative day 2. His 1-month postoperative CT scan showed a near-complete resolution of the inflammatory rind around the AAA.

TAKE HOME POINTS

- You need to have a high index of suspicion when making the diagnosis of an inflammatory AAA.
- Inflammatory AAAs constitute 3% to 10% of all AAAs.

- Ureteral involvement and impairment of renal function is seen in up to 25% of patients with inflammatory AAAs.
- Open surgical repair used to be the mainstay of treatment, but with the advent of endovascular techniques, endovascular repair is preferred.
- A left retroperitoneal approach is recommended to avoid dissection through dense fibrotic tissue unless there is concern for acute expansion or impending rupture, at which point a transabdominal approach may be more appropriate for those unfamiliar with an emergent retroperitoneal approach.
- Reinforcement of the anastomosis with pledgets is often performed to decrease the risk of dehiscence, as the quality of the aortic tissue can be questionable.
- The fibrosis and inflammation usually resolve after repair but to a lesser degree with an endovascular repair.
- Postoperative follow-up is necessary to ensure that no long-term end-organ complications develop such as renal atrophy from chronic ureteral obstruction.

SUGGESTED READINGS

Deleersnijder R, Daenens K, Fourneau I, et al. Endovascular repair of inflammatory abdominal aortic aneurysms with special reference to concomitant ureteric obstruction. *Eur J Vasc Endovasc Surg.* 2002;24:146-149.

Lange C, Hobo R, Leurs LJ, et al.; on behalf of the EUROSTAR Collaborators. Results of endovascular repair of inflammatory abdominal aortic aneurysms. A report from the EUROSTAR database. *Eur J Vasc Endovasc Surg.* 2005;29:363-370.

Pennell RC, Hollier LH, Lie TJ, et al. Inflammatory abdominal aortic aneurysms: a thirty-year review. *J Vasc Surg.* 1985;2:859-869.

Sterpetti AV, Hunter WJ, Feldhaus RJ, et al. Inflammatory aneurysms of the abdominal aorta: incidence, pathologic, and etiologic considerations. *J Vasc Surg.* 1989;9:643-650.

Stone WM, Fankhauser GT, Bower TC, et al. Comparison of open and endovascular repair of inflammatory aortic aneurysms. *J Vasc Surg.* 2012;56:951-956.

Tang T, Boyle JR, Dixon AK, et al. Review: inflammatory abdominal aortic aneurysms. *Eur J Vasc Endovasc Surg.* 2005;29:353-362.

CLINICAL SCENARIO CASE QUESTIONS

1. A 77-year-old man presents with increasing abdominal pain that radiates to his back. Imaging is consistent with a 5.8-cm inflammatory aortic aneurysm associated with severe bilateral hydroureteronephrosis. His creatinine is 2.3 mg/dL. Anatomic characteristics are not favorable for an endovascular approach. He will undergo an open repair. What is the next appropriate step in management of his ureteral obstructions and renal function impairment?

   a. Do nothing
   b. Repair the inflammatory AAA
   c. Place bilateral ureteral stents
   d. Place bilateral percutaneous nephrostomy tubes
   e. Place a Foley catheter for decompression

2. Which of the following is true regarding inflammatory abdominal aortic aneurysms?

   a. They are not amenable to endovascular repair.
   b. The associated retroperitoneal fibrosis does not resolve after repair.
   c. They have similar operative time and transfusion requirements as open repair of noninflammatory AAAs.
   d. Twenty-five percent of patients have concomitant ureteral obstruction with evidence of renal function impairment.

41 Acute Type B Dissection without Malperfusion

AMANI D. POLITANO and GILBERT R. UPCHURCH Jr

Presentation

A 51-year-old female presented to the emergency department with several days of chest pain that she describes as sharp and stabbing. Her past medical history is remarkable for hypertension for which she is on hydrochlorothiazide. She is a current 1-pack-per-day smoker with a 30-pack-year history. On examination, her vital signs are significant for a blood pressure of 170/74 mm Hg, a heart rate of 91 beats per minute, and moderate anxiety. Her physical examination demonstrates a nontender abdomen and equal bilateral radial, femoral, and distal pulses. She has well-healed scars from a prior cholecystectomy. She is retired, volunteers locally, and walks 3 days a week.

Differential Diagnosis

The acute onset of back pain can have several etiologies, including musculoskeletal, cardiac, vascular, or gastrointestinal. Characteristics of the presentation should help to guide further evaluation and workup. Acute life-threatening conditions include myocardial infarction and aortic dissection or aneurysm rupture, and therefore, these entities should be evaluated promptly. Further history of genetic disorders (Marfan, Ehlers-Danlos, and Loeys-Dietz syndromes) or inflammatory syndromes may also aid with diagnosis and help to predict which patients are predisposed to an increased risk of dissection.

Case Scenario

Further inquiry reveals no history of reflux or peptic ulcer disease. The patient denies any prior similar pains or history of angina. As she has already had a cholecystectomy and does not drink, the likelihood of pancreatitis, which can also cause back pain, is low. However, it is worth evaluating these scenarios, as well as aortic pathology, since they can present without prodrome.

Workup

An electrocardiogram and laboratory assessment including complete blood count, chemistry panel, amylase, lipase, and troponin should be obtained. An intravenous contrasted cross-sectional imaging study in arterial phase, such as computed tomography (CT) or magnetic resonance imaging, is obtained. Additionally, evaluation of delayed contrast phases can elicit evidence of venous pathology or delayed renal or gut perfusion. Even in the absence of clinical signs of malperfusion, careful evaluation of the appearance of splanchnic vessels on imaging can indicate involvement that may be more concerning for impending malperfusion and warrant more aggressive therapy.

Case Scenario

The patient demonstrated normal values for all of the above and an electrocardiogram (EKG) documented sinus tachycardia. A CT scan demonstrates a type B aortic dissection just distal to the ligamentum arteriosum (Fig. 1). The dissection continues through the thoracic and abdominal aorta and terminates within the right common iliac artery. The celiac trunk, superior mesenteric artery, and bilateral renal arteries arise from the true lumen (Fig. 2). There is no mesenteric thickening to suggest ischemia. An accessory right renal artery arises from the false lumen. The inferior mesenteric artery is also patent. Multiple fenestrations are present in the thoracic aorta. Delayed imaging demonstrates appropriate contrast filling of the renal collecting system and bladder. The maximal aortic diameter is 4.0 cm.

Diagnosis and Treatment

Aortic dissections remain the most common vascular injury with potentially catastrophic consequences. The incidence is difficult to capture due to immediately fatal cases, but ranges from 2.5 to 30 cases per million persons per year. The presentation can be defined as hyperacute (less than 24 hours), acute (24 hours to 2 weeks), subacute (2 to 6 weeks), or chronic (greater than 6 weeks). The pathophysiology involves a disruption of the intima and subsequent separation of the intima and media by tracking blood into a dissection plane. Further anatomic definition is traditionally reported as either the DeBakey (type I-IIIa/b) or Stanford (type A/B) classification systems. In either case, dissections that involve the

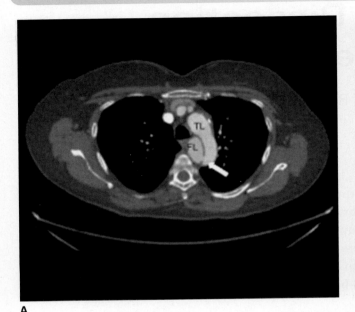

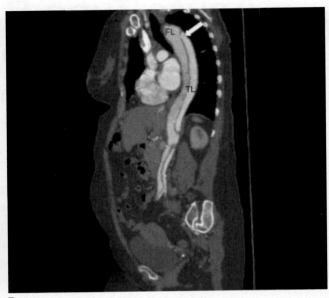

FIGURE 1 • Aortic dissection originating distal to left subclavian artery, demonstrating true lumen (TL), false lumen (FL), and fenestration (*arrow*, **A**). Longitudinal view demonstrates proximal fenestration (*arrow*) and extent of dissection into right common iliac artery **(B)**.

ascending aorta are considered surgical emergencies and warrant rapid intervention.

Acute type B aortic dissection presents most commonly with the sudden onset of back, chest, or abdominal pain, or a combination thereof. Abdominal pain or peripheral numbness in the absence of chest or back pain is indicative of end-organ pathology. Absence of distal pulses is also quite concerning and can be confused with other etiologies, such as embolic or thrombotic events.

Acute type B dissections can be designated uncomplicated or complicated based on evidence of malperfusion, size greater than 5.5 cm maximal diameter, annual increase in size by 4 mm, or aortic rupture. Patients with otherwise uncomplicated features of their dissection who cannot obtain blood pressure control on three or more agents should be considered refractory to medical management and treated as a complicated dissection. Conversely, presentation associated with hypotension (systolic blood pressures less than 90 mm Hg)

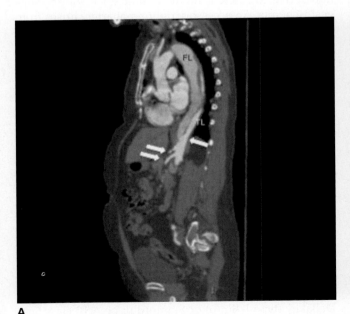

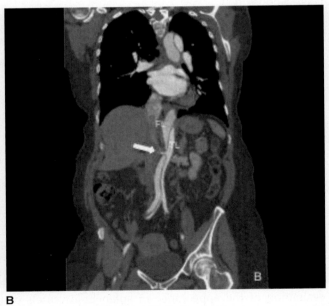

FIGURE 2 • Sagittal images demonstrating distal fenestration (*single arrow*, **A**). Celiac and superior mesenteric arteries (*double arrow*, **A**) and right renal artery **(B)** originate from the true lumen.

is concerning for rupture, malperfusion, cardiac involvement, or intra-abdominal catastrophe and should also be treated aggressively.

Initial therapy should begin with admission to the hospital, strict blood pressure control via intravenous medications, and careful monitoring, including an arterial line. Heart rate control with the use of beta-blockade or calcium channel blockers should precede any vasodilitory agents to avoid reflex tachycardia, which can increase stress on the aortic wall. If this is insufficient to reduce systolic blood pressure below a target of at least 120 mm Hg, addition of angiotensin-converting enzyme inhibitors and vasodilatory medications should be employed. Serial laboratory examinations to evaluate renal function and bowel perfusion should be followed. If there are any signs of malperfusion in the early presentation, conversion to endovascular or operative intervention should be pursued.

Case Continued

The patient is admitted, and with the aid of intravenous esmolol and nicardipine infusions, her heart rate decreases to near 60 beats per minute and her blood pressure remains under 120 mm Hg systolic. Her CT scan is repeated at 24 hours with no change in the aortic diameter and no extension of the dissection. Serial laboratory values demonstrate stable creatinine, amylase and lipase, and lactic acid. Her physical examination, particularly the abdominal and distal pulse exams, remains stable and uncompromised. She is then transitioned to oral medications to maintain the goal parameters.

Discussion

Studies have shown that beta-blockade is associated with improved survival for all patients with aortic dissections, and calcium channel blockers are associated with improved survival in patients with type B dissections treated with best medical management (Table 1).

Postoperative Management

Several studies have shown no survival advantage to endovascular intervention over medical management for uncomplicated type B dissections. Early mortality from medical management of uncomplicated type B dissections has been estimated at 6.4%, with early stroke and spinal cord ischemia rates of 4.2% and 5.3%, respectively. Five-year survival ranges between 70% and 89%. In comparison, patients treated with thoracic endovascular repair (TEVAR) have an early mortality rate of 10.2%, early stroke and spinal cord ischemia rates of 4.9% and 4.2%, respectively, and survival rates ranging from 56.3% to 87% at 5 years.

In a recent study comparing medical management versus TEVAR for uncomplicated subacute or chronic type B dissections, 1-year survival was comparable with medical management versus endovascular repair (97.0% ± 2.1%

TABLE 1. Acute Type B Dissection without Malperfusion

Key Technical Steps
1. Identify complicated vs. uncomplicated dissection at presentation.
    a. Complicated type B dissections should receive optimal intervention (endovascular vs. surgical repair as indicated by patient characteristics).
    b. Uncomplicated type B dissections should undergo optimal medical therapy and close observation.
2. Obtain heart rate control (goal 60 beats per minute) and blood pressure control (systolic blood pressure <120 mm Hg).
3. Repeat imaging studies at 24 hours, 7 days, prior to discharge, and 6 weeks.
4. Appropriate therapy involves conversion to interventional approach for any dissection that becomes complicated during the course of medical management or in which the blood pressure or pain is refractory.
 	
Potential Pitfalls
• Failure to recognize signs of complicated type B dissection early can result in end-organ damage, neurologic compromise, or death.
• Patient education regarding the importance of medical compliance, routine surveillance, and vigilance regarding signs or symptoms of progression is paramount.

vs. 94.2% ± 2.8%, respectively). The risk of conversion to endovascular therapy in this setting was not associated with increased procedural complications and therefore should be considered if a patient converts to a complicated dissection. TEVAR does demonstrate improved survival over open intervention and should be employed when feasible.

Case Conclusion

The patient was placed on an oral beta-blocker and a calcium channel blocker with appropriate response. Repeat imaging revealed a stable dissection at 7 days, and she was discharged home. She was scheduled for repeat evaluation in clinic and by contrast-enhanced imaging at 6 weeks, and then annually.

TAKE HOME POINTS

• Uncomplicated type B aortic dissections present without signs of end-organ malperfusion or impending rupture and are small (less than 5.5 cm) on imaging.
• Complicated dissections present with evidence of malperfusion syndromes, impending rupture, size greater than 5.5 cm, or growth of more than 4 mm per year or are refractory to blood pressure control with three or more agents.

- Preferred treatment for uncomplicated type B dissections involves best medical therapy with heart rate and blood pressure control.
- Routine early surveillance consists of repeated aortic imaging at 24 hours, 7 days, at the time of discharge, and again at 6 weeks.
- Initial medical management for type B dissections with beta-blockade and calcium channel blockers has demonstrated survival advantage.
- Careful evaluation for the conversion from uncomplicated to complicated dissections should prompt change in management to intervention as appropriate.

SUGGESTED READINGS

Fattori R, Cao P, De Rango P, et al. Interdisciplinary expert consensus document on management of type B aortic dissection. *J Am Coll Cardiol.* 2013;61(16):1661-1678.

Hiratzka LF, Bakris GL, Beckman JA, et al. American College of Cardiology Foundation/American Heart Association Task Force on Practice Guidelines; American Association for Thoracic Surgery; American College of Radiology; American Stroke Association; Society of Cardiovascular Anesthesiologists; Society for Cardiovascular Angiography and Interventions; Society of Interventional Radiology; Society of Thoracic Surgeons; Society for Vascular Medicine. ACCF/AHA/AATS/ACR/ASA/SCA/SCAI/SIR/STS/SVM guidelines for the diagnosis and management of patients with thoracic aortic disease. *Circulation.* 2010;121(13): e266-e369.

Nienaber CA, Kische S, Akin I, et al. Strategies for subacute/chronic type B aortic dissection: the Investigation of Stent Grafts in Patients with type B Aortic Dissection (INSTEAD) trial 1-year outcome. *J Thorac Cardiovasc Surg.* 2010;140 (6 suppl):S101-108; discussion S142-S146. doi: 10.1016/j.jtcvs.2010.07.026.

Suzuki T, Isselbacher EM, Nienaber CA, et al. IRAD Investigators. Type-selective benefits of medications in treatment of acute aortic dissection (from the International Registry of Acute Aortic Dissection [IRAD]). *Am J Cardiol.* 2012;109(1):122-127.

CLINICAL SCENARIO CASE QUESTIONS

1. Patients who may be candidates for medical management of an acute type B aortic dissection include:

   a. A patient presenting with abdominal pain and tenderness on examination with evidence of aortic rupture

   b. A patient with radiographic evidence of periaortic hematoma and splanchnic vessel compromise

   c. A patient with an aortic diameter of 5.8 cm, equal pulses on examination, and continued back pain despite initiation of blood pressure control

   d. A patient who achieves a systolic blood pressure of 130 mm Hg and a heart rate of 65 beats per minute after initiation of intravenous beta-blockade and calcium channel blockade with relief of pain

2. Which of the following is *not* appropriate for the treatment of uncomplicated acute type B dissections?

   a. Initiation of heart rate and blood pressure control with beta-blockade, calcium channel blockade, or renin-angiotensin inhibitors

   b. Serial examination and laboratory assessment to aid in early detection of complications

   c. Cross-sectional contrast-enhanced imaging at presentation, 24 hours, and 6 weeks

   d. A patient who demonstrates an 8-mm enlargement of the aorta upon repeat imaging within 6 months

42 Pararenal Abdominal Aortic Aneurysm—Open Repair

BO WANG, ARASH BORNAK, ATIF BAQAI, JORGE REY, and OMAIDA C. VELAZQUEZ

Presentation

A 62-year-old woman is seen in the emergency room (ER) for acute onset of lower abdominal pain radiating to the left flank. A quick chart review reveals that the patient has an abdominal aortic aneurysm (AAA) discovered incidentally 3 years prior to this visit and diagnosed during a sigmoid diverticulitis workup. At that time, the aneurysm measured 4.6 cm (AP) in maximum diameter, limited to the infrarenal aorta with a 1.8-cm neck. The patient was discharged after a course of antibiotics and never followed up with vascular surgery. In the ER, an aortic ultrasound reveals an AAA approximately 6.9 cm in diameter. Vascular surgery is consulted for a symptomatic AAA. The patient's past medical history also includes a myocardial infarction that occurred 4 years ago. She had drug-eluting stents placed on that occasion. Her past surgical history includes perforated diverticulitis, followed by a Hartmann's procedure and a colostomy reversal. She has a 50-pack-year history of smoking and is currently a smoker. Her current medications include aspirin, simvastatin, and Lopressor. On physical examination, the patient is hypertensive (178/96 mm Hg) with a tender pulsating epigastric mass. The patient's femoral and pedal pulses are palpable. The rest of her physical examination is unremarkable. Her medical records also note the result of a recent Persantine stress thallium test indicating a myocardial scar involving the inferolateral region of the left ventricle, but no evidence of reversible myocardial ischemia.

Differential Diagnosis

AAAs are often diagnosed incidentally on computed tomography (CT) scan performed for other abdominal pathologies. Occasionally, an abdominal x-ray may reveal the calcified rim of the aneurysmal aorta prompting further workup. Most AAAs remain asymptomatic until they present with acute symptoms indicating impending, contained, or free rupture. Free rupture is commonly associated with sudden severe abdominal or back pain, syncope, and death.

Aortic aneurysms may become symptomatic with abdominal, back, groin, or flank pain. Such nonspecific signs and symptoms may be related to other abdominal pathologies ranging from a simple urinary tract infection to pancreatitis, diverticulitis, or other inflammatory processes involving the abdominal viscera. Therefore, the workup should not only include an accurate anatomical evaluation of the abdominal organs by radiologic means but also a complete laboratory exam including a full metabolic panel, pancreatic enzymes, and urinary sample. Two other problematic key differential diagnoses should be considered during workup: aortic dissection and acute myocardial infarction.

Diagnosis and Treatment

A computed tomography angiography (CTA) is the most frequent and accurate radiologic imaging that can be obtained for suspected symptomatic aneurysm. Two characteristic findings are worth mentioning in the case of symptomatic aneurysms, which make the diagnosis highly probable. First, on physical exam, the aortic aneurysm is exquisitely tender on palpation. The sensitivity depends, however, on the size of the aneurysm and patient's body habitus. Second, in hypertensive patients, lowering the systemic blood pressure may alleviate the pain. If a symptomatic aneurysm is suspected, an arterial line should be placed, permissive hypotension should be allowed, and/or the patient's blood pressure should be pharmacologically decreased and controlled during workup completion.

Workup
CT Angiogram of the Abdomen

The laboratory results are all normal including blood urea nitrogen (BUN) of 14 mg/dL and creatinine level of 0.56 mg/day and no anemia.

The above case presents a stable patient with evidence of an expanding symptomatic AAA on ultra-

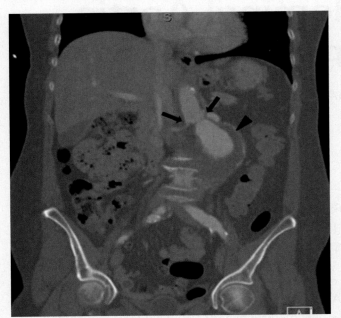

FIGURE 1 • CTA coronal view of the aneurysm and aortic branches. *Black arrows*: origin of the renal arteries. *Arrowhead*: mural thrombus. Mural thrombus is visible between the contrast in the lumen and aortic wall calcification.

sound that will most likely require surgical repair. A high-resolution (1.5- to 3-mm thin sections) CTA including the thorax, abdomen, and pelvis should be performed to provide an accurate anatomic detail of the

aneurysm. It will reveal any involvement of the visceral aorta and iliac arteries, guiding the treatment options for either an endovascular or open repair. To further guide the surgical treatment, the surgeon can also appreciate severe angulations and identify the location and distances between renal and visceral vessels, as well as the presence of coexistent occlusive disease in the iliac, renal, and splanchnic vessels (Figs. 1 and 2). The 3D-reconstructed images (Fig. 2) are very helpful in treatment planning, allowing a spatial understanding of the aneurysm and aorta.

The sudden onset of abdominal pain may also represent a contained rupture, aortic dissection, aneurysm/aortic inflammation, or even infection. All these entities would be evaluated on CTA.

As an alternative to CTA imaging, magnetic resonance angiography (MRA) can be performed in order to avoid exposure to iodinated products. This modality is lengthy, can overestimate stenotic lesions, and does not reliably depict calcifications. Moreover, for patients with baseline chronic renal insufficiency, the predisposition for gadolinium-associated nephrogenic systemic fibrosis has made this modality less attractive than in the past.

CTA Report

There is a fusiform pararenal AAA measuring up to 6.4 cm in maximum diameter, with extensive mural thrombus (Fig. 1) and with no rupture, dissection, or

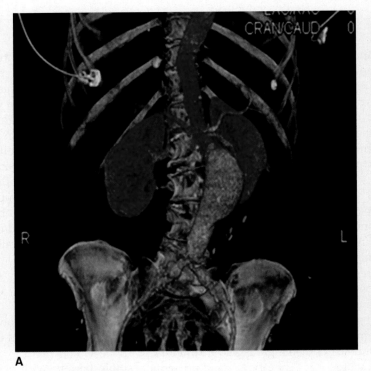

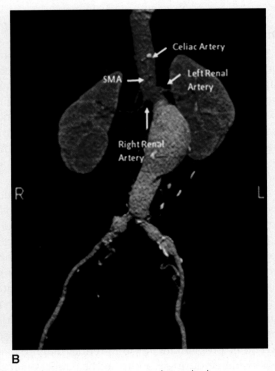

FIGURE 2 • **A and B:** 3D reconstruction images help delineate the aneurysm sac, renal arteries' location, and visceral arteries.

inflammation. The right renal artery is noted to be lower than the left renal artery. The aorta is tortuous deviating to the left of midline. The aneurysm extends from the lower end to the left renal artery to the iliac bifurcation. Extensive mural atherosclerosis extends into the bilateral iliac arteries and branches. The origins of the celiac trunk and superior mesenteric artery (SMA) are patent, while the inferior mesenteric artery (IMA) is thrombosed. Focal stenosis of the proximal common iliac arteries is noted with some poststenotic dilatation. This is a pararenal AAA, specifically a juxtarenal (not suprarenal) AAA.

Case Continued

The patient's blood pressure is decreased and controlled with a labetalol intravenous drip, and her pain is thus resolved. You inform the patient of the findings and her surgical options. The patient inquires whether she is a candidate for "stent graft" repair of her AAA. The patient's workup has shown a 6.4-cm juxtarenal AAA. The renal arteries and visceral branches are not involved.

Because the aneurysm extends to the level of the left renal artery, the patient is not a good candidate for an endovascular AAA repair using currently available endografts approved by the U.S. Food and Drug Administration (FDA). An open repair should be planned. Customized fenestrated and branched devices are currently under investigation in the United States and used electively in surgically high-risk patients in a few centers. Outside companies' Instructions for Use (IFU) and other endovascular options are available. In urgent and emergent situations, surgeon-modified fenestrated endografts have been used in extremely high-risk patients. Other endovascular alternatives including "chimney" or "snorkel" endografting have been used in order to preserve visceral perfusion.

The patient presents with signs of impending rupture, which represents a surgical urgency. The patient should be admitted and medical management optimized. Given her past cardiac history, a baseline echocardiogram should be obtained to guide intra-anesthetic management that carefully balances hydration versus pressors. This is not an elective case; thus, an extensive preoperative workup is not required in this setting.

Test Report

Echocardiogram

Hypokinetic area visualized in the left ventricle with an ejection fraction of 40%. This is essentially unchanged since her last cardiac workup.

Surgical Approach

This is a high-risk surgery in a surgically high-risk patient given her cardiac comorbidities. A left retroperitoneal (RP) approach is chosen. RP exposure is in particular indicated in patients with multiple previous intraperitoneal procedures or infections because of the adhesions generated by these processes, as well as in patients with abdominal wall stomas, ectopic kidneys, or inflammatory aneurysms. The left RP approach, with or without mobilization of the left kidney anteriorly, facilitates exposure of the suprarenal aorta and visceral arteries; it is also associated with lower perioperative pulmonary complications.

Because of the extent of the aneurysm, a clamp above the renal arteries will be necessary. This will allow the surgeon to perform a proximal graft anastomosis to the short aortic stump below the renal arteries. Occasionally, intraoperative palpation of the aorta may reveal extensive calcification of the aorta just above the renal arteries and a supraceliac clamp may be necessary.

Operative Details

The patient is placed in a right lateral decubitus position with the left side of the torso rotated approximately 45 degrees. The patient is positioned on a beanbag to maintain this posture, and the table is flexed optimally with the kidney rest elevated (Fig. 3). A left RP incision starts at the lateral border of the left rectus muscle midway between the pubis and umbilicus. It extends superiorly (5 cm medial to the anterior-superior iliac spine), curving upward and laterally at the costal margin to follow the course of the 10th interspace. Incisions centered lower, onto the 11th or 12th rib, offer less exposure to the suprarenal aorta. The left ureter should be identified immediately and protected. Ligation of the junction of the gonadal vein with the left renal vein provides the exposure needed to appropriately isolate the infrarenal neck (Fig. 4). Superior mobilization of the left renal vein facilitates exposure of the aortic neck up to the level of the left renal artery. An alternative approach is to mobilize the left kidney anteriorly and medially, a maneuver that is required for adequate exposure of suprarenal aortic pathology. A large lumbar vein that drains into the posterior wall of the left renal vein should be ligated early to avoid avulsion. Visible lumbar arteries are clipped behind the aneurysm. The left crus of the diaphragm is divided for exposure up to 4 to 6 cm above the celiac axis. The next step is to expose the distal anastomotic site at the level of the bifurcation of the aorta. Common iliac arteries are exposed. Before cross-clamping, systemic heparinization is initiated. The iliac arteries are clamped, first distally and then the aorta is clamped proximally in order to prevent embolization. The aneurysm is opened, the thrombus is evacuated, and any bleeding lumbar arteries are suture ligated from within the aneurysmal sac. An end-to-end anastomosis between the prosthetic graft and the aorta is performed proximally first, then the clamp

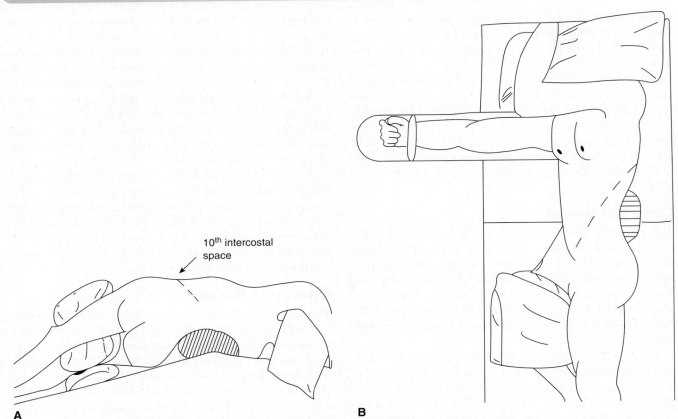

10th intercostal space

A

B

FIGURE 3 • **A and B:** The patient positioned for a left retroperitoneal (RP) approach.

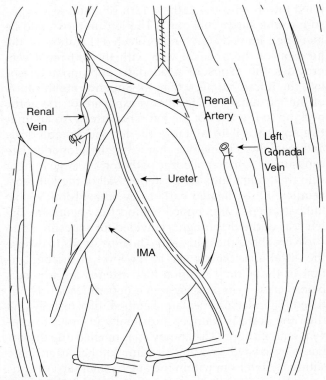

Renal Vein

Renal Artery

Left Gonadal Vein

Ureter

IMA

FIGURE 4 • Left ureter and gonadal vein are identified. Gonadal and lumbar veins are ligated to facilitate the mobilization of the left kidney and get access to the aortic neck.

is released, and the graft is clamped below the renal arteries. Hemostasis is obtained, and distal anastomosis is then performed. The distal anastomosis may be to the aortic bifurcation (tube graft) or to the iliac arteries (bifurcated graft). Before releasing the clamps, back bleeding and forward bleeding are allowed, the graft is flushed profusely with heparin saline solution and anastomosis completed. Communication with the anesthesiologist before releasing the clamps is important to adjust blood pressure and avoid sudden hypotension. In patients with stenotic/occlusive disease of the celiac axis, SMA, and/or internal iliac arteries, reimplantation of the IMA should be considered in order to avoid bowel and pelvic ischemia (Table 1).

Special Intraoperative Considerations

One easily overlooked site of bleeding is inadvertent splenic injury caused by retractor placement. From an RP approach, splenic hemorrhage is difficult to recognize. Keep in mind this is a differential diagnosis: the patient appears to be suffering from hypovolemia, which cannot be explained by the degree of blood loss in the surgical field. It may be necessary to open the peritoneum to inspect the abdominal cavity for bleeding.

TABLE 1. Pararenal Abdominal Aortic Aneurysm—Open Repair

Key Technical Steps

1. Left RP incision starts at the lateral border of the left rectus muscle and extends superiorly, curving laterally at the 10th costal interspace.
2. Identify the left ureter and protect it.
3. Identify the left gonadal vein. Ligation at the junction of the gonadal vein with the left renal vein.
4. Mobilization of the left renal vein to facilitate anterior rotation of the left kidney to adequate expose suprarenal aortic pathology.
5. Distal exposure of the bifurcation of the aorta and common iliac arteries.
6. Heparinization before cross-clamping.
7. Achieve distal and then proximal control (Fig. 4).
8. Enter into aneurysm sac, evacuation of thrombus.
9. Ligation of lumbar arteries within the aneurysmal sac.
10. End-to-end anastomosis proximally and then distally with running polypropylene suture.
11. Communication with anesthesiologist before releasing the clamp to avoid large shifts in blood pressure.

Potential Pitfalls

- The periureteral vascular plexus should be carefully preserved during dissection to avoid devascularization of the ureter and resultant fibrosis.
- During common iliac artery exposure, close attention to the location of the pudendal nerves is important to avoid postoperative sexual dysfunction.
- Careful selection of the cross-clamping location is needed to avoid embolic events.
- Inadequate collateral circulation may result in ischemic colon. Patients at risk include those with celiac/SMA occlusive lesions, previous bowel resection, significant pelvic occlusive disease, and hypotension in the perioperative period.
- Lumbar arteries may not be actively bleeding when the aneurysm sac is initially inspected while the proximal clamp is in place. Careful inspection of the posterior aspect of the aneurysm sac at the conclusion of the procedure is essential to avoid lumbar arteries bleeding.
- If the anastomosis is performed to the common iliac artery, every attempt to preserve at least one internal iliac artery should be made.

Case Conclusion

Lower extremity pulses need to be evaluated before and after operation. A reduced pulse needs to be monitored carefully in the following hours to ensure return of adequate perfusion in order to rule out embolization or iliac artery clamp site dissection. Decreased lower extremity perfusion during period of cross-clamping can be a risk factor for arterial thrombosis formation.

The patient needs to be on a continuous cardiac monitor. Beta-blockade should be continued in the postoperative period if the blood pressure allows.

Colon ischemia and infarction may occur and are associated with up to 50% mortality. The degree of ischemia may vary from mucosal injury that can be managed with aggressive fluid resuscitation and antibiotics to full-thickness necrosis in which case emergent laparotomy and colon resection should be performed emergently. For elective aneurysm surgery, the rate of colon ischemia is between 0.6% and 3%.

Spinal cord ischemia is a rare complication secondary to embolization or direct blood supply interruption. Symptoms may range from mild transient paraparesis to permanent flaccid paralysis.

TAKE HOME POINTS

- CT angiogram of the aorta is required to evaluate the extent of the AAA and involvement of branches of the aorta for surgical planning and suitability for an endovascular approach.
- 3D reconstruction image can help delineate aortic angulation as well as spatial relation between aneurysm and aortic branches.
- Symptomatic aneurysms are urgent, and extensive preoperative workup is not required and should not delay intervention.
- A left RP approach is the preferred surgical approach for pararenal and suprarenal AAA. It allows easy and adequate exposure to suprarenal aorta and mobilization of left kidney without sacrifice of the renal vein.
- Special care need to be taken when choosing the location of aortic and iliac level cross-clamp to avoid unnecessary complications.
- Coordination with anesthesiologist needs to be carried out during clamping and declamping in order to avoid large shift of blood pressure and cardiac preload.

SUGGESTED READINGS

Patel VI, Cambria RP. Abdominal aortic aneurysm: open repair. In: *Current Surgical Therapy*. 10th ed. Philadelphia, PA: Elsevier; 2012.

Rubin BG, Sicard GA. Abdominal aortic aneurysms: open surgical treatment. In: *Rutherford's Vascular Surgery*. 7th ed. Philadelphia, PA: Elsevier; 2010.

Darling C, Shah DM, Chang BB, et al. Current status of the use of retroperitoneal approach for reconstructions of the aorta and its branches. *Ann Surg*. 1996;224(4):501-508.

Messina LM. Pararenal aortic aneurysms: the future of open repair. *Cardiovasc Surg*. 2002;10(4):424-433.

Resch J. Pararenal aneurysms: currently available fenestrated endografts. *J Cardiovasc Surg*. 2013;54:27-33.

Schneider JR, Gottner RJ, Golan JF. Supraceliac versus infrarenal aortic cross-clamp for repair of non-ruptured infrarenal and juxtarenal abdominal aortic aneurysm. *Cardiovasc Surg.* 1997;5(3):279-285.

West CA, Noel AA, Bower TC, et al. Factors affecting outcomes of open surgical repair of pararenal aortic aneurysms: a 10-year experience. *J Vasc Surg.* 2006;43(5):921-927; discussion 927-928.

CLINICAL SCENARIO CASE QUESTIONS

1. When applying super celiac cross-clamp, what strategies can be used to reduce the patient's cardiac stress?

    a. Volume loading with crystalloid before clamp; vasodilator after clamp

    b. Mannitol diuresis before clamp; vasopressor after clamp

    c. Volume loading with mannitol diuresis before clamp; vasodilator after clamp

    d. Vasodilator before clamp; diuresis after clamp

2. Which of the following is not an advantage of the use of retroperitoneal approach?

    a. Reduced pulmonary comorbidities

    b. Preferred exposure during ruptured AAA

    c. Reduced fluid requirement during surgery

    d. Ease of supraceliac exposure

43 Infected Abdominal Aortic Aneurysm

MARTYN KNOWLES and J. GREGORY MODRALL

Presentation

A 76-year-old male cattle farmer with a history of hypertension, diabetes, and coronary artery disease presented to the emergency room with a 12-day history of abdominal pain, malaise, recurrent fevers to 102°F, and chills. Vital signs included a temperature of 101.3°F, heart rate of 107 bpm, and blood pressure of 138/78 mm Hg. He is tender to palpation in the epigastrium, and has palpable pedal pulses bilaterally. Laboratory studies revealed a white blood cell count of 17×10^9/L and a serum creatinine of 1.57 mg/dL. A noncontrast computed tomogram of the abdomen was obtained (Fig. 1).

Differential Diagnosis

The differential diagnosis for an abdominal aortic aneurysm (AAA) with constitutional symptoms includes an infected AAA, aortic pseudoaneurysm (noninfected), penetrating atherosclerotic ulcer, aortic dissection, and noninfected degenerative AAA. Particular attention should be paid to an AAA that develops or changes quickly, exhibits saccular morphology, produces constitutional symptoms, or exhibits stranding around the aneurysm on computed tomography (CT) scan. Any aneurysm associated with these findings on history or CT scan should be assumed to be infected.

Workup

Appropriate imaging should include a CT angiogram with appropriate thin cuts (<3 mm), but a noncontrast CT scan of the abdomen and pelvis was obtained in this case due to the elevated serum creatinine. The CT scan revealed a 5-cm saccular infrarenal AAA near the inferior mesenteric artery with periaortic stranding (Fig. 1). Even without contrast, one can make out the calcification of the aortic wall with the presence of loss of distinct margins of the aorta, periaortic thickening, and stranding. Laboratory evaluation with blood cultures demonstrated Salmonella growth in the blood.

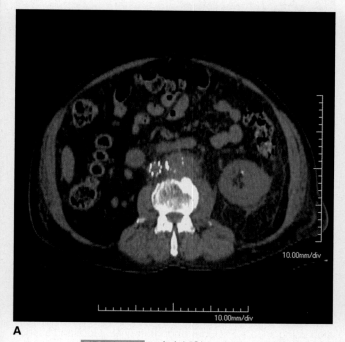
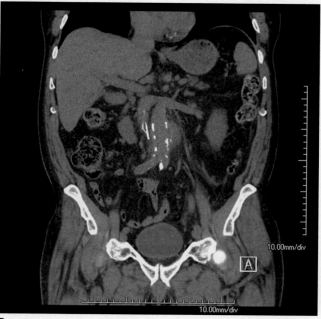

FIGURE 1 • Axial (**A**) and coronal (**B**) cut of a CT scan showing a saccular infrarenal AAA with periaortic stranding.

Discussion

Infected AAA refers to several pathologic conditions that lead to the presence of infection in an AAA. Examples of infected AAAs include mycotic aneurysms due to endocarditis, microbial arteritis (from bacteremia) with aneurysm formation, infection of a preexisting AAA, and posttraumatic infected false aneurysms of the aorta. In most infected AAAs, the infection causes degeneration of the aorta to produce an aneurysm. Fewer than 5% of infected AAAs result from infection of a preexisting AAA. The most common site for an infected AAA is the infrarenal aorta (70%), but infected AAAs occasionally occur in the suprarenal or thoracic aorta.

Diagnosis of an infected AAA usually involves a high index of suspicion and imaging studies suggestive of the diagnosis. Clinical scenarios that should arouse suspicion for an infected AAA include the presence of positive blood cultures in a patient with a known AAA, identification of a new AAA after a septic episode, and concurrent AAA and lumbar vertebral erosions. An antecedent history of a septic episode may be identified in approximately 61% of cases but is not a requirement for the diagnosis. The most common presenting symptoms of an infected AAA are abdominal pain (92%), fever (77%), leukocytosis (69%), positive blood cultures (69%), palpable abdominal mass (46%), and rupture (31%).

Radiographic imaging should include both a contrast-enhanced CT scan and an arteriogram. CT findings suggestive of an infected AAA include the presence of a saccular aneurysm, evidence of partial aortic disruption or frank rupture, contiguous inflammatory changes, fluid collections, or air adjacent to an AAA. The vast majority of infected AAAs are saccular aneurysms, although infection of an existing aneurysm typically occurs in a fusiform aneurysm because most AAAs have a fusiform morphology. Arteriography often aids in the diagnosis by demonstrating saccular aneurysm morphology and facilitates operative planning. A high-quality CT arteriogram (CTA) with three-dimensional reconstruction may obviate the need for arteriography.

Treatment

The presence of an infected AAA obligates urgent repair. The risk of rupture is greater with the findings of symptoms, CT evidence of surrounding stranding, saccular nature of the AAA, or rapid growth. In addition to systemic antibiotics, the mainstay of treatment is aneurysm resection and debridement of the retroperitoneum. The options for aortic reconstruction include aortic ligation with extra-anatomic bypass, in situ placement of rifampin-soaked Dacron graft, cryopreserved arterial allograft, or femoropopliteal vein (FPV). In the case above, the patient developed chest pain at admission and was found to have an ST elevation inferior

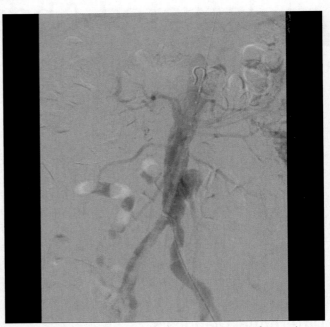

FIGURE 2 • Aortogram showing a saccular infrarenal aneurysm.

wall myocardial infarction and was taken urgently for percutaneous coronary intervention. The patient was taken subsequently for an aortogram (Fig. 2) and temporary repair with endovascular aortic aneurysm repair (EVAR) (Fig. 3) under local anesthesia to mitigate the risk of AAA rupture. The patient was then placed on culture-directed antibiotic coverage.

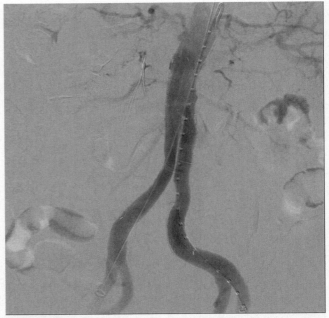

FIGURE 3 • Infected AAA treated with temporary exclusion using a Gore Excluder endograft (W.L. Gore and associates, Flagstaff, AZ).

Options for Surgical Repair

The mainstay of treatment of infected AAAs is excision of all grossly infected aortic and retroperitoneal tissue. It is not necessary to debride to microscopically uninfected tissue, but generous debridement is thought to decrease the risk of recurrent infection of the aorta or aortic reconstruction. Reconstruction of the aorta may be accomplished with either extra-anatomic bypass or in situ interposition grafting. The clinical outcomes for each of these options are summarized in the Table 1 below. Extra-anatomic bypass with an axillobifemoral bypass, followed by removal of the infected aneurysm and aortic stump ligation, is the most commonly performed reconstruction. However, this option carries a significant risk of stump blowout (approximately 20%), reinfection of the graft in 3% to 15%, and a mortality rate between 10% and 25%. This option is most appropriate for patients who are deemed high risk for in situ reconstruction. Unfortunately, the patency of these extra-anatomic repairs is relatively poor (as low as 45% at 3 years).

In situ reconstruction is an alternative approach to revascularization of the lower extremities after resection of an infected AAA. In unstable patients or those infected with a relatively low virulence organism, such as *Staphylococcus epidermidis*, use of an in situ prosthetic graft has yielded acceptable clinical results in several series. Some authors view this approach as the treatment of choice for infected AAAs due to its relative simplicity and the absence of a ligated aortic stump at risk for blowout. Use of a rifampin-bonded Dacron graft and the liberal use of omental coverage of the graft are reasonable adjunct procedures to attempt to minimize the risk of graft infection. Rifampin bonding of a Dacron graft is accomplished by bathing the graft with rifampin (1200 mg in 20 mL normal saline) for 15 minutes prior to implantation. This approach is the mainstay of treatment for infected paravisceral or thoracic aortic aneurysms for which extra-anatomic reconstruction is not a reasonable option. The principal risk of this approach relates to the

risk of graft infection when placing a prosthetic graft into an infected operative field, upward of 10%. Alternative approaches may be advisable in more aggressive infections, especially those infections attributed to gram-negative or fungal species.

Cryopreserved arterial allograft is another option for an in situ repair. The advantage of this repair is the avoidance of prosthetic in an infected field and elimination of time required to harvest an autogenous conduit. The disadvantage of cryopreserved arterial conduit is the cost, approximately $10,000 to 18,000 per segment, and the risk of aneurysmal degeneration and graft disruption with hemorrhage (3% to 9%).

In situ aortic reconstruction with FPV offers several potential advantages over prosthetic reconstruction. As an autogenous conduit, FPV is resistant to recurrent infection and provides excellent long-term patency. In addition, FPV provides a reasonable size match to the typical infrarenal aorta. Chronic venous morbidity is minimal, as one third of patients have minor leg swelling, and no venous ulceration or venous claudication has been described after FPV harvest. However, approximately one in five limbs will require fasciotomy after FPV harvest. The principle disadvantage of using FPV for in situ aortic reconstruction relates to the time required for harvesting this vein (>120 minutes or more). A detailed description of the technique for FPV harvest is provided elsewhere. Preoperative duplex ultrasonography of the FPV should be employed to confirm patency, absence of thrombus, and document adequate size (at least 6.0 mm) of this vein.

Endovascular management of mycotic and infected aneurysms has been described recently in case reports and small, single-center series. Endografting may be a reasonable option in some cases with a low risk of rupture in the short term, but little is known about the long-term durability of this treatment. Currently, we view endografting as a temporizing measure until a more definitive repair can be accomplished. Endovascular repair is also a reasonable option if a patient is medically unfit for either extra-anatomic or in situ repair. In these patients, CT-guided drainage of the abscess and long-term antibiotic coverage are important adjuncts to help manage the risk of reinfection of the endograft.

Surgical Approach

The operative approach is dictated primarily by the clinical presentation. The classic approach in the stable patient with a nonruptured infected AAA is to perform a preemptive extra-anatomic bypass, usually via an axillobifemoral bypass, followed by excision of the infected AAA, wide debridement of the retroperitoneum, and "triple ligation" of the infrarenal aortic stump. "Triple ligation" of the aortic stump consists of a two-layer

TABLE 1. Infected Abdominal Aortic Aneurysm

Key Technical Steps
1. Perform a preemptive extra-anatomic bypass, usually via an axillobifemoral bypass
2. Excision of the infected AAA
3. Wide debridement of the retroperitoneum
4. "Triple ligation" of the infrarenal aortic stump

Potential Pitfalls
- The most dramatic potential complication of aortic ligation is aortic stump blowout, which is almost universally lethal.
- The relatively poor long-term patency of axillofemoral bypass grafts and the potential for prosthetic graft infection are additional pitfalls of this approach.

closure of the aorta (horizontal mattress and simple running suture lines) with monofilament polypropylene suture, followed by stump coverage with a vascularized omental pedicle flap. When the diagnosis of an infected AAA is certain, the potential for bacterial seeding of the bypass graft may be minimized by completing all "clean" portions of the operation, including application of occlusive dressings, prior to initiating exposure of the infected AAA. Frank aortic rupture or uncertainty regarding the presence of infection will alter the operative sequence, as the aortic component of the operation is addressed first in such cases. Rupture may also be managed with endografting, followed by definitive repair with extra-anatomic or in situ reconstruction. The most dramatic potential complication of aortic ligation is aortic stump blowout, which is almost universally lethal. The relatively poor long-term patency of axillofemoral bypass grafts and the potential for prosthetic graft infection are additional pitfalls of this approach. As discussed previously, in situ repair with rifampin-impregnated Dacron, cryoarterial allograft, or FPV is the approach of choice in most centers unless a particularly virulent organism is suspected (Table 1).

Postoperative Management

Culture-directed antibiotic coverage is paramount in any repair that is undertaken for an infected AAA. Although there are no data to support a particular duration of antibiotics, most clinicians with experience with this condition favor a full 6 weeks of antibiotics with a longer course advisable if in situ prosthetic graft is used for reconstruction or a virulent organism (gram negative or fungal species) is identified.

Case Conclusion

In the case above, in situ reconstruction was contraindicated due to the patient's high cardiac risk following a severe myocardial infarction. Thus, infrarenal aortic ligation and extra-anatomic bypass was the only viable option for this patient. Due to the recent myocardial infarction, definitive repair was delayed for 6 weeks after endografting.

Because the diagnosis of an infected AAA was not in question, an axillofemoral bypass was performed as the initial step in the operation. After skin closure, occlusive dressings were applied prior to proceeding with a laparotomy. At laparotomy, proximal control of the aorta was obtained initially at the supraceliac aorta, because infected AAAs are prone to disruption with excessive operative manipulation. In this case, the infrarenal endograft precluded infrarenal aortic clamping.

Distal control was achieved at the common iliac arteries. After systemic anticoagulation, clamps were applied, and the infrarenal aorta was opened. The endograft was explanted, and the aorta was debrided and sent for culture. The supraceliac clamp was then moved to an infrarenal position. The aorta was debrided to healthy tissue before closing the infrarenal aortic stump in three layers, as described above. The origins of the common iliac arteries are ligated from within the aorta. Postoperative antibiotic coverage was tailored to cultures obtained at surgery to minimize the risk of aortic stump or prosthetic graft infection.

TAKE HOME POINTS

- Evidence of an AAA with evidence of systemic infection or a previous septic episode should raise concern for an infected AAA.
- The findings of a saccular aneurysm, periaortic stranding, or rapid growth confer a higher risk of rupture.
- An endovascular repair, CT-guided drainage, and antibiotic coverage may be used as a temporizing measure in high-risk patients.
- Definitive treatment involves extra-anatomic bypass and aortic stump ligation versus in situ reconstruction with rifampin-soaked Dacron, cryopreserved arterial allograft, or FPV.
- Culture-directed antibiotic coverage helps lessen reinfection.

SUGGESTED READINGS

Ali AT, Modrall JG, Hocking J, et al. Long-term results of the treatment of aortic graft infection by in situ replacement with femoral popliteal vein grafts. *J Vasc Surg.* 2009;50(1): 30-39.

Brown KE, Heyer K, Rodriguez H, et al. Arterial reconstruction with cryopreserved human allografts in the setting of infection: a single-center experience with midterm follow-up. *J Vasc Surg.* 2009;49(3):660-666.

Chung J, Clagett GP. Neoaortoiliac system (Nais) procedure for the treatment of the infected aortic graft. *Semin Vasc Surg.* 2011;24(4):220-226.

Kan CD, Yen HT, Kan CB, et al. The feasibility of endovascular aortic repair strategy in treating infected aortic aneurysms. *J Vasc Surg.* 2012;55(1):55-60.

Oderich GS, Bower TC, Hofer J, et al. In situ rifampin-soaked grafts with omental coverage and antibiotic suppression are durable with low reinfection rates in patients with aortic graft enteric erosion or fistula. *J Vasc Surg.* 2011;53(1):99-106, 07e1-7; discussion 106-107.

Reddy DJ, Shepard AD, Evans JR, et al. Management of infected aortoiliac aneurysms. *Arch Surg.* 1991;126(7):873-878; discussion 78-79.

Seeger JM, Pretus HA, Welborn MB, et al. Long-term outcome after treatment of aortic graft infection with staged extra-anatomic bypass grafting and aortic graft removal. *J Vasc Surg.* 2000;32(3):451-459; discussion 60-61.

CLINICAL SCENARIO CASE QUESTIONS

1. The options for aortic reconstruction include all of the following except:

   a. Aortic ligation with extra-anatomic bypass
   b. In situ placement of rifampin-soaked Dacron graft
   c. Cryopreserved arterial allograft
   d. Femoropopliteal vein (FPV)
   e. Femoropopliteal artery (FPA)

2. Evidence of an infected AAA include all of the following except:

   a. A saccular aneurysm
   b. A fusiform aneurysm
   c. Periaortic stranding
   d. Rapid aortic growth

AAA with IVC Fistula

KOTA YAMAMOTO, TETSURO MIYATA, and ALAN DARDIK

Presentation

An 82-year-old man presents with dyspnea that started suddenly several months prior to the visit. He has a history of coronary intervention after myocardial infarction 6 years ago. On abdominal examination, a pulsatile mass is noted with continuous murmur. He has no history of abdominal or back pain. Edema and varicose veins of the left lower extremity are seen, but distal pulses are palpable. Plain chest x-ray shows pulmonary vascular congestion, cardiomegaly, and a small right pleural effusion. His EKG reveals P pulmonale and left ventricular hypertrophy.

Differential Diagnosis

There are three conditions to consider. Each of them is fairly simple to diagnose, but the problem with this patient is to evaluate if they are independent or related conditions. If related, then what is the pathophysiology?

1. Congestive heart failure

   The dyspnea with x-ray and EKG findings show that this patient has congestive heart failure. Further workup is needed to evaluate its severity, as well as its etiology. Previously undiagnosed congenital abnormalities, such as patent foramen ovale, or central malignancies may contribute to the circulatory overload and heart failure.

2. Abdominal aortic aneurysm (AAA)

   Pulsatile abdominal mass is a straightforward clue to the presence of an AAA. Workup is needed to differentiate AAA from an abdominal mass, such as a tumor. In addition, aneurysm size and shape need to be evaluated to plan treatment strategies.

3. Lower limb venous congestion

   Lower limb edema accompanied with varicose veins is suggestive of venous congestion. The finding that the edema is unilateral, without any manifestations on the contralateral limb, suggests that the edema may be secondary to mechanical obstruction, such as deep venous thrombosis. Although edema may not be life threatening, further workup is needed to determine its etiology.

Workup

This patient undergoes contrast-enhanced CT scan of the abdomen (Fig. 1). This study shows an aneurysm involving the left common and internal iliac artery. In addition, contrast is seen in the inferior vena cava (IVC) (venous enhancement in the arterial phase), demonstrating the presence of a fistula between the artery and the vein (arteriovenous fistula [AVF]). The exact location of the AVF may be difficult to locate with the CT scan, but the continuous murmur located at the abdominal mass suggests that the AVF is probably located at the aneurysm.

Although not always necessary, angiograms can also be performed to evaluate the fistula (Figs. 2 and 3) The angiogram shows that this patient has a duplicated IVC, and the flow through the fistula goes directly into the left IVC. Angiogram of the left lower limb shows that the flow from the AVF refluxes retrogradely into the left lower limb veins.

As preparation for surgery, systemic workup is necessary. Cardiac evaluation is especially necessary not only to understand the degree of heart failure but also to

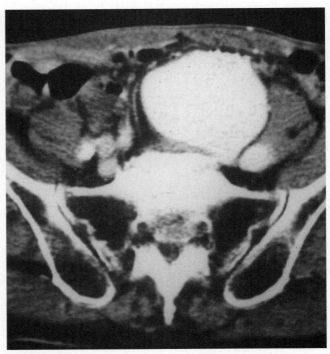

FIGURE 1 • Contrast-enhanced CT. The vein (left-sided IVC) is enhanced at the same time as the iliac aneurysm.

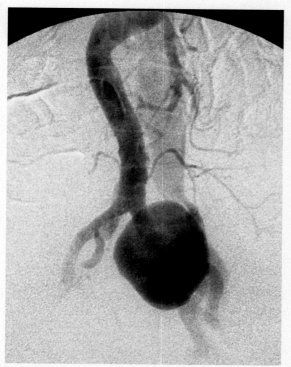

FIGURE 2 • Angiogram showing the iliac aneurysm. A left-sided IVC is also detected as soon as the iliac aneurysm is seen.

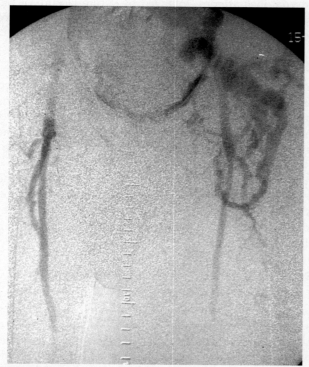

FIGURE 3 • Angiogram of the lower limb. Left iliac and femoral veins can be seen as the distal retrograde flow below the fistula.

anticipate and prepare for potential physiologic changes that may occur after closure of the AVF.

Diagnosis and Treatment

Based on the information obtained from the CT scan and the angiogram, the primary diagnosis is the left common iliac artery aneurysm extending into the internal iliac artery. The aneurysm is likely to have ruptured into the left iliac vein forming an AVF between the iliac arteries and veins. This enormous flow through the AVF led to the precardiac overload upstream of the AVF and congestion of the left lower limb veins downstream of the AVF.

Aneurysmectomy accompanied with AVF closure is the best treatment that is a durable solution for all the pathophysiology. Recent advances in vascular surgery allow us to choose between two treatments for abdominal aortic aneurysmal repair.

One treatment option is endovascular aneurysmal repair (EVAR) using stent grafts. For EVAR in this patient, all the branches of the internal iliac artery would need to be embolized using coils and then the stent graft placed to cover the inflow into the internal iliac artery. After placement of the stent graft, the presence of an endoleak would suggest persistence of the fistula that should be considered for additional treatment; placement of a covered stent inside the caval side of the fistula may be a potential solution. However, prophylactic placement of a venous covered stent prior to aneurysm repair could potentially induce aneurysm rupture.

The other treatment option is open iliac artery aneurysm repair. In the open procedure, direct AVF closure can be performed in addition to aneurysmectomy with a graft replacement. The superiority between EVAR and open has been debated; surgeons are advised to take into account the benefits and risks of each procedure for individual patients.

Surgical Approach

Open repair of the iliac aneurysm with AVF closure is chosen for this patient. EVAR is not chosen to prevent the possibility that if the branches of the internal iliac artery were imperfectly occluded, residual type 2 endoleak could drain through the AVF, continuing potential for precardiac fluid overload and residual congestive heart failure. Open repair affords the ability for direct AVF closure but has the risk of performing open surgery on an octogenarian.

Under general anesthesia, a midline laparotomy is followed by full exploration of the abdomen. The bowels are set aside to the right side revealing the aorta and the iliac arteries. Inspection of the aneurysm leads us to decide that the terminal aorta and the right common iliac artery will be the proximal clamping sites. As for the distal clamping sites, the left external artery is soft, but the aneurysm precludes assessment of the internal iliac artery and will need to be occluded with a balloon catheter after opening the aneurysm. We also decide not to reconstruct the internal iliac artery. Arteries are mobilized and controlled; prior to clamping, a pneumatic tourniquet is applied to the left lower limb to decrease the venous inflow.

Opening the aneurysm reveals an AVF (25 × 10 mm) with tremendous back bleeding of venous blood. Immediately, large Foley balloon catheters are inserted through the AVF to control the bleeding from the common, external and internal iliac veins (Fig. 4). This internal iliac vein catheter is also used to occlude the main trunk of the internal iliac artery. Another option to control back bleeding is the use of two sponge-sticks, controlling the venous flow above and below and allowing oversewing of the fistula.

Back bleeding from the branches within the aneurysm are controlled with sutures. Direct closure of the AVF is performed, and the Foley catheters are removed just before completion of the closure. Although the time to oversew a fistula is typically short, the massive back bleeding that may occur prior to fistula control may contribute to low cardiac output after repair. To avoid massive bleeding, some surgeons prefer to isolate and control the IVC or iliac veins prior to aneurysm opening; we do not perform this due to the risk of injuring the vein, which is usually intimately adherent to the aneurysm secondarily to the chronic inflammation of the aneurysm and the fistula.

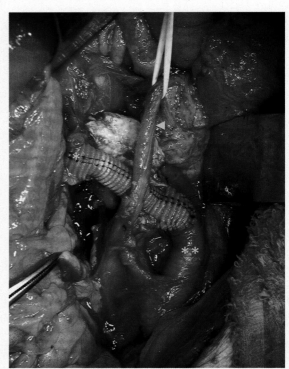

FIGURE 5 • After reconstruction. (*, Left common iliac artery; **, left external iliac artery, *arrowhead*: left ureter.)

A prosthetic graft is placed between the common and external iliac arteries, followed by suture closure of the internal iliac artery (Fig. 5). After final confirmation of hemostasis, the abdomen is closed.

Discussion

For this procedure, several issues need to be considered carefully. First, if it is difficult to clamp arteries and veins prior to opening of the aneurysm, balloon catheters must be ready to occlude the vessels from inside the aneurysm. Second, after closure of the AVF, intraoperative decrease of the cardiac preload leading to a decrease in blood pressure may occur. It is very important that the anesthesiologist is aware of every step that the surgeon is performing. Finally, one must be aware of the ureter adjacent to the aneurysm and take care not to injure it (Table 1).

Special Intraoperative Considerations

If the aneurysm has floating intramural thrombus or a diseased clamping site due to atherosclerosis, precaution is needed to avoid intraoperative pulmonary embolism. Although intraoperative arterial embolism to the lower extremities may be treated after the aortic surgery, pulmonary embolism may be life threatening. Take care when controlling or clamping the arteries. If there is a high risk of embolism, placement of a temporary IVC filter may lower the chances of lethal pulmonary embolism.

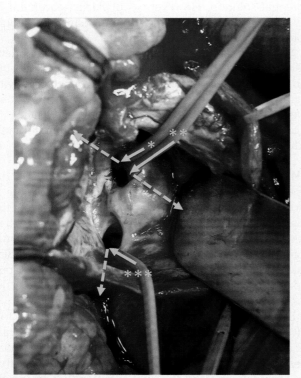

FIGURE 4 • The AVF is confirmed after opening of the aneurysm. Through this fistula, three balloon catheters are inserted to occlude the iliac veins. The dashed arrow shows the direction of the veins that each catheter is placed. (*, Left common iliac vein; **, left external iliac vein; ***, left internal iliac vein.)

TABLE 1. AAA with IVC Fistulae

Key Technical Steps

1. Midline laparotomy and full exploration
2. After exposure of the arteries, proximal and distal clamping sites are controlled
3. Application of pneumatic tourniquet to control venous inflow
4. Opening of the aneurysm
5. Immediate control of bleeding using catheters
6. Closure of the AVF
7. Prosthetic graft replacement of the aneurysm

Potential Pitfalls

- Prepare balloon catheters for occlusion of vessels
- Be aware of circulatory changes after AVF closure
- If there is an iliac aneurysm, be careful of injuries to the ureter

Postoperative Management

The most important postoperative management specific to aneurysm repair associated with AVF is the close monitoring of the hemodynamic status. Low cardiac output heart failure from acute myocardial infarction or acute renal failure can also occur following any aneurysm repair. The patient is kept in the intensive care unit for a few days, using a Swan-Ganz catheter to monitor his cardiac output.

Case Conclusion

Due to the close monitoring and intensive care, the patient recovered uneventfully and was discharged from the hospital several days after surgery.

TAKE HOME POINTS

- AAA with associated IVC fistula is an unusual complication of AAA, occurring in approximately 1% of asymptomatic and 3% to 4% of symptomatic aneurysms.
- Symptoms and findings include abdominal or back pain (73% to 100%), continuous murmur (61% to 83%), pulsatile abdominal mass (40% to 58%), congestive heart failure (CHF) (37% to 58%), lower limb edema and/or varicose veins (22% to 34%), and hematuria (22% to 30%).
- The initial diagnostic test is usually an imaging study, either ultrasound, CT scan, or magnetic resonance imaging (MRI), to confirm the presence of the aneurysm.
- Simultaneous opacification of the contrast in the aorta and the IVC is usually indicative of the fistula. In patients with normal anatomy, a typical CT appearance may look like Figure 6.
- Echocardiography can determine cardiac function and hemodynamics, as well as demonstrating the fistula.
- Aneurysm repair and closure of the fistula are needed to prevent additional complications of the high-output shunt.

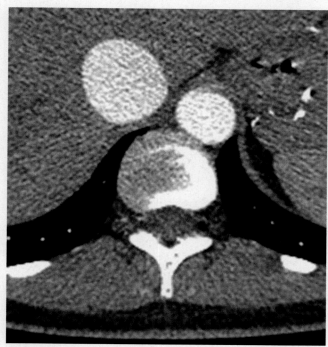

FIGURE 6 • Typical CT appearance of an AAA-IVC fistula with contrast present in the IVC during the arterial phase.

- Repair in the setting of CHF and renal failure has been associated with higher mortality than standard elective repair without an aortocaval fistula, at least as high as 50%; ideally aortocaval fistulae are repaired prior to permanent cardiac or renal damage.
- The hemodynamic consequences of AAA-IVC fistula repair should be anticipated intraoperatively.
- Although the time to oversew a fistula is typically short, the massive back bleeding that may occur prior to fistula control may contribute to low cardiac output after repair.

SUGGESTED READINGS

Bednarkiewicz M, Pretre R, Kalangos A, et al. Aortocaval fistula associated with abdominal aortic aneurysm: a diagnostic challenge. *Ann Vasc Surg.* 1997;11:464-466.

Dardik H, Dardik I, Strom MG, et al. Intravenous rupture of arteriosclerotic aneurysms of the abdominal aorta. *Surgery.* 1976;80:647-651.

Lau LL, O'Reilly MJ, Johnston LC, et al. Endovascular stent-graft repair of primary aortocaval fistula with an abdominal aortoiliac aneurysm. *J Vasc Surg.* 2001;33:425-428.

McKeown BJ, Rankin SC. Aortocaval fistulae presenting with renal failure: CT diagnosis. *Clin Radiol.* 1994;49:570-572.

Naito K, Sakai M, Natsuaki M, et al. A new approach for aortocaval fistula from ruptured abdominal aortic aneurysm. Balloon occlusion technique under echogram guidance. *Thorac Cardiovasc Surg.* 1994;42:55-57.

Schmidt R, Bruns C, Walter M, et al. Aortocaval fistula: an uncommon complication of infrarenal aortic aneurysms. *Thorac Cardiovasc Surg.* 1994;42:208-211.

CLINICAL SCENARIO CASE QUESTIONS

1. What is the likely cause of contrast in veins during arterial phase?

    a. Misunderstanding which vessels are the arteries and veins

    b. Arteriovenous fistula

    c. Retrograde flow

    d. Calcification of veins

2. What is the most critical change that occurs after closure of a large arteriovenous fistula?

    a. Lower limb swelling

    b. Hypertension

    c. Low cardiac output

    d. High cardiac output

45 Primary Aortoenteric Fistulae

CARLA C. MOREIRA and JAMES T. MCPHEE

Presentation

A 74-year-old male active smoker with a history of chronic obstructive pulmonary disease (COPD), hypertension, and hyperlipidemia complains of 1 week of malaise, low-grade fevers, and chills. He has a family history of a father with an "aneurysm" and a brother who died suddenly at age 70. He presents to the emergency department after an episode of vomiting bright red blood twice at home. He denies abdominal pain, back pain, flank pain, or dysuria. Physical examination is notable for temperature of 99.9°C, heart rate of 115 bpm, blood pressure of 110/80 mm Hg and 90/70 mm Hg on right and left arms, respectively. He is somewhat pallid in appearance and has mild mid-abdominal tenderness without guarding or rebound, and a pulsatile abdominal mass is found. He has 2+ femoral pulses bilaterally. Electrocardiogram (EKG) and chest x-ray (CXR) are unremarkable. Gastroenterology consultants perform an esophagogastroduodenoscopy (EGD) through the second portion of the duodenum and find no evidence of gastritis, peptic ulcer disease (PUD), or hemobilia. A nasogastric tube (NGT) is left in place. Next, a computed tomography (CT) angiogram is performed.

Differential Diagnosis

The differential diagnosis for upper gastrointestinal (GI) bleed includes PUD, gastritis, esophageal varices, esophagitis, gastritis, neoplasms, hemobilia, and aortoenteric fistula (AEF).

Case Continued

CT angiogram demonstrates a 5.2-cm infrarenal abdominal aortic aneurysm (AAA) (Fig. 1). Concern is raised for primary AEF due to air bubbles within the aortic wall and within the mural thrombus. Additionally, stranding of the retroperitoneum and loss of the fat plane between the fourth portion of the duodenum and the aortic wall are noted. Intravenous (IV) access is obtained, and a rapid blood sample is sent to the blood bank. The patient has ongoing bleeding from the NGT and receives two units of packed red blood cells (PRBC).

Diagnosis

Despite technologic advances, the cornerstone of diagnosing AEF continues to be high index of clinical suspicion. The classic triad of GI bleeding, sepsis, and abdominal pain is rarely found in a single patient. The initial bleeding is usually minor and self-limiting. Additionally, the interval between this "herald bleed" and massive subsequent rebleeding is unpredictable, occurring hours to months later, and is a major cause of delay in making the definitive diagnosis.

CT scanning has been advocated as the preferred initial diagnostic test for patients with AEF, with a reported sensitivity of up to 93% in some series. The presence of a pulsatile abdominal mass, fever, hematemesis, and air within the wall of an aneurysmal aorta are indicative of primary AEF. The diagnosis can be confirmed by EGD performed by an experienced endoscopist who is able to examine the entire duodenum and localize the small defect in the wall with a 25% to 83% success rate. Angiography should be reserved for patients in whom the diagnosis of AEF is unclear to help determine a source of bleeding and aid in planning arterial reconstruction.

Recommendation

The patient is prepared for emergent surgery. Adequate IV access is obtained, resuscitation efforts are undertaken and communication with the blood bank regarding the potential for massive transfusion is initiated. Broad-spectrum antibiotics are initiated as well, and the patient is monitored in appropriate setting, commonly the intensive care unit (ICU). A frank discussion with the patient and family regarding the grave nature of the condition will appropriately set the stage for a likely complicated postoperative course with high rates of major morbidity and mortality.

On occasion, appropriately informed patients and caregivers may not be desirous of major complex surgery and/or may be of prohibitive risk (advanced age, advanced cancer, or severe comorbidity) and may opt for comfort measures only. Preoperative cardiology assessment is unnecessary in this setting, and the surgeon and anesthesiologist may proceed if they deem the

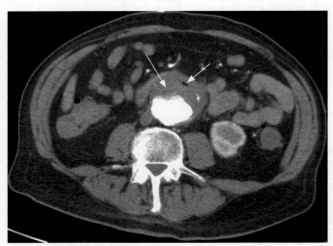

FIGURE 1 • CT angiogram with air within the aortic thrombus, highly suggestive of aorto-enteric fistulae.

patient to be of acceptable risk. Preoperative bilateral arm blood pressures should be performed, as well as a thorough lower extremity pulse exam. The surgical approach will be dictated by the patient's hemodynamic stability, aortic aneurysm anatomy (infrarenal, juxtarenal, or pararenal), conduit availability, and surgeon preference. The tenets of repair are proximal aortic control, debridement of nonviable or infected tissue, intestinal repair, and establishment of distal perfusion by either in-line reconstruction or extra-anatomic means.

Surgical Approach

The surgical strategy used in the treatment of AEF depends primarily on two things, whether the patient is hemodynamically stable at the time of surgery and whether infection is present in the aortic bed. In an actively bleeding, unstable patient, expeditious aortic control is imperative. The abdomen is usually explored through midline incision, allowing for full exposure and examination of the intestine and aorta. Supraceliac aortic control should be established by either isolating the aorta through the crus of the diaphragm or by medial visceral rotation. Left retroperitoneal approach has been advocated in cases where the proximal aorta may be difficult to access because of a short infrarenal neck. However, the major disadvantage of this approach is that it offers less favorable exposure of the duodenum and limited exposure of the right iliac artery.

After establishing proximal control, the abdomen should be carefully explored and distal control established by clamping of the iliac vessels or by means of occlusion balloon catheters. Careful dissection of the adherent bowel to the diseased aorta allows proper identification of the fistula. Gross spillage from the bowel can be quickly temporized and bowel repair deferred until after the aortic pathology is addressed using the strategies discussed in detail below. The enteric fistula can be treated with a simple primary repair by transverse closure, resection and anastomosis, or Roux-en-Y reconstruction depending on anatomic limitations. Gastrostomy and feeding jejunostomy tubes are generally placed to aid in postoperative feeding, as these patients usually have a prolonged postoperative course.

Extra-Anatomic Bypass

The most expeditious means of accomplishing revascularization is extra-anatomic bypass through uninfected tissue. Axillobifemoral bypass is the option of choice if the infected AAA is truly infrarenal, as oversewing of the aortic stump should not impinge upon the renal arteries. This can be performed in a staged manner, depending on the hemodynamic stability of the patient.

In a two-stage procedure, the diagnosis of AEF has been made in a stable patient who is not actively bleeding. During the first operation, which can be the same day or a day before, a standard axillobifemoral bypass is performed using externally supported (ringed) polytetrafluoroethylene (PTFE). If the infection has extended to the femoral arteries, which would be quite rare for primary AEF, bilateral axillounifemoral grafts tunneled laterally to the available superficial femoral, profunda femoris, or popliteal arteries may be required. At the second operation, laparotomy, aneurysmectomy with debridement of aorta and infected tissue, intraoperative cultures are sent, and two-layer aortic closure and omental buttress of aortic stump are performed.

Alternatively, in an unstable or bleeding patient, this is performed as a one-stage procedure. The first step entails laparotomy, debridement, aortic and bowel repair, and abdominal closure. The patient is then reprepped and redraped, and new set of instruments are used for the axillobifemoral bypass. Tunneling of the left extra-anatomic bypass may be problematic if a left retroperitoneal approach was used. A proposed solution is the use of composite graft; the synthetic extra-anatomic graft is tunneled in noncontaminated tissue plane, and an autogenous graft is tunneled in potentially contaminated field. Care must be taken to avoid contamination of the synthetic component. More commonly, a right axillobifemoral bypass will be used, specifically in this case where the right arm pressure was 20 mm Hg higher than the left.

The operating surgeon should be familiar with techniques, such as rotation of a sartorius muscle flap, to provide adequate soft tissue coverage of the femoral vessels. The biggest risk associated with this technique is stump blow-out, especially if tissue margins are positive for bacteria. Appropriate antibiotic coverage is important to minimize the risk of seeding the extra-anatomic bypass graft, which can occur in approximately 15% to 25% of patients. The advantage of preemptive extra-anatomic bypass is the elimination of lower extremity ischemia and decreasing risk of subsequent amputations in these patients.

In-line Reconstruction

Primary AEF is a distinct and separate clinical entity than secondary AEF. In the absence of gross evidence of infection, some authors have advocated repair of the duodenum and in situ aortic reconstruction with a standard synthetic prosthesis in selected patients. The involved aorta and surrounding tissues are debrided. Care must be taken to avoid contamination by intestinal content at the time of surgery to minimize risk of infecting the aortic prosthesis. Well-vascularized, healthy tissue should be positioned between the repaired bowel and the prosthetic graft. This approach obviously requires sound clinical judgment. The same authors advocating this treatment strategy have also advocated close follow-up and long-term antibiotics because up to 30% of aneurysms associated with primary AEF formation may prove to be infected.

Some recent studies have shown promising results with variety of conduit options, such as antibiotic-bonded/soaked synthetic grafts (i.e., rifampin-soaked and silver-coated Dacron grafts), as a reasonable option for treatment of abdominal aortic infections. Cryopreserved arterial homograft (CAH) is also considered a suitable conduit in the setting of arterial infection and has shown favorable outcomes even against highly virulent microorganisms. The availability of these grafts and the relatively low rates of secondary procedures have been listed as their important advantages. Again, careful patient selection and clinical judgment are paramount if these treatment options are undertaken. These conduits may be associated with early and late complications, such as aneurysm degeneration, occlusion, and reinfection.

Neo-Aortoiliac System

Clagett et al. described an innovative approach to revascularization of the lower extremities by using the femoral veins to reconstruct an autogenous neo-aortoiliac system (NAIS) in the setting of an infected aortic prosthesis. A similar approach may be considered in the setting of primary aortic infection. This approach allows in situ vascular reconstruction with completely autologous tissue, and it has been shown to be effective and durable. The primary disadvantage of this procedure is that its time consuming, which can be problematic in the setting of hemorrhage, hemodynamic instability, and prolonged lower extremity ischemia. An additional consideration is the risk of postoperative leg swelling. In selected patients, this situation may be ameliorated if multiple surgical teams are available to permit simultaneous vein harvest. Experience with the NAIS procedure in the setting of primary AEF is limited.

Endovascular Stent Graft "Bridging"

The use of endovascular stent grafts in secondary AEF, where a new stent graft is deployed into a previously placed stent graft, has been described as a quick method to control bleeding and facilitate aortic control by several authors. However, this method is not typically a viable

---

TABLE 1. Primary AEF

Key Technical Steps

1. High index of suspicion needed for early and proper diagnosis of AEF.
2. The classic triad of abdominal pain, palpable mass, and GIB occurs in a small minority of patients.
3. The time interval between a "herald bleed" and massive GIB can be hours, days, weeks, or even months.
4. In an actively bleeding or unstable patient with known history of AAA, diagnostic images should not delay a trip to the OR for abdominal exploration.
5. The outcome depends on the timeliness of diagnosis, the patient's general state, the degree of contamination, and the anatomic site of the aorta involved.
6. The surgical approach is dictated by the patient's hemodynamic stability, aortic anatomy, conduit availability, and surgeon preference.
7. The tenets of repair are proximal aortic control, debridement of nonviable or infected tissue, intestinal repair, and establishment of distal perfusion by either in-line reconstruction or extra-anatomic bypass.

Potential Pitfalls

- In the setting of duodenal stump blowout, if a graft has been used in the same bed, graft contamination may occur.
- Long period of time prior to re-establishing blood flow to legs can cause significant ischemia reperfusion injury.
- In the long term, extra-anatomic bypass may thrombose and lead to limb loss.

AEF, aortoenteric fistula; GIB, gastrointestinal bleed; AAA, abdominal aortic aneurysm; OR, operating room.

---

long-term option for two main reasons: (1) the enteric fistula is not repaired leading to persistent infection and possibly bleeding from the injured bowel mucosa and (2) aortic and retroperitoneal debridement is not possible, again leading to chronic infection and eventual contamination of the newly placed stent graft. Another limitation is that standard anatomic endograft restrictions apply, thus an adequate infrarenal seal zone of healthy aorta as well as adequately sized access vessels are necessary to consider this temporizing technique. Currently, this technique should be reserved for life-and-death scenarios to quickly to address ongoing hemorrhage. Still, some authors advocate the use of this procedure as a "bridge to surgery"; either carried out simultaneously with preparation for laparotomy or in a delayed fashion with semielective graft explant and extra-anatomic bypass in a timely fashion (Table 1).

Discussion

Primary AEF is a rare disease entity that occurs spontaneously in association with either aortic or GI disease. The pathogenesis of primary AEF is thought to be related to mechanical compression of the bowel by the enlarging aorta, coupled with local inflammatory changes, and primary aortic infections leading to spontaneous communication between the aorta and the bowel lumen.

The vast majority of cases are due to an aortic aneurysm, which erodes into the intestinal wall after degeneration of the aortic wall. Other causes include aortitis or mycotic aneurysms attributed to *Staphylococcus*, *Salmonella*, and *Klebsiella* infections, erosion of GI neoplasm, tuberculous mesenteric lymphadenitis, and PUD. Radiation injuries, and intra-abdominal infections due to appendicitis, diverticulitis, etc., are other rare causes.

The prevalence of primary AEF is low, estimated to be between 0.04% and 0.07% based on autopsy studies. The clinical presentation can be subtle and nonspecific, and a high clinical index of suspicion is required to make prompt diagnosis and initiate treatment. Mortality from untreated primary AEF is almost 100% while survival after surgery ranges from 18% to 93%. Treatment options depend on patient stability, presence of infection, patient comorbidities, and availability of suitable conduits. Management goals are to control hemorrhage, control infection, and to maintain adequate distal perfusion. This can be achieved through variety of surgical techniques as previously detailed. In cases of gross contamination, infected AAA, positive intraoperative cultures, and placement of synthetic graft material, 4 to 6 weeks of organism-specific antibiotics is advocated.

Case Conclusion

An EGD with the pediatric colonoscope showed fresh blood in the distal duodenum without clear source of bleeding. No further testing was undertaken because the patient's condition quickly deteriorated, and he was taken immediately to the operating room for surgical intervention. Midline laparotomy was performed, and an EAF was found between the fourth portion of the duodenum and the proximal infrarenal aortic aneurysm. Proximal infrarenal aortic control was obtained above the site of the fistula and distal control at the level of the iliac bifurcation. There was no evidence of infection or gross contamination. The AAA was repaired with a Dacron tube graft, the duodenum was closed in two layers, and the omentum was mobilized placed between the aorta-graft anastomosis and duodenum.

The patient did well after surgery and was discharged from the hospital to home on postoperative day 12 on oral Bactrim as prophylaxis. Intraoperative cultures were all negative, but given the placement of prosthetic graft, it was felt safer to maintain the patient on long-term antibiotics to minimize the risk of graft infection. At 1-year follow-up, the patient was alive and well.

TAKE HOME POINTS

- Primary AEF is a very rare disease entity.
- A high index of suspicion is needed in making prompt diagnosis and treatment plan.
- Do not go to the operating room to pursue diagnostic testing in a unstable patient.
- CT angiogram is the best imaging modality for diagnosis of EAF.
- Many options for repair and distal revascularization are now available.

SUGGESTED READINGS

Alzobydi AH, Guraya SS. Primary aortoduodenal fistula: a case report. *World J Gastroenterol.* 2013;19(3):415-417.

Batt M, Jean-Baptiste E, O'Connor S, et al. Early and late results of contemporary management of 37 secondary aortoenteric fistulae. *Eur J Vasc Endovasc Surg.* 2011;41:748-757.

Biancari F, Romsi P, et al. Staged endovascular stent-grafting and surgical treatment of a secondary aortoduodenal fistula. *Eur J Vasc Endovasc Surg.* 2006;31:42-43.

Bisdas T, Wilhelmi M, et al. Cryopreserved arterial homografts vs silver-coated Dacron grafts for abdominal aortic infections with intraoperative evidence of microorganisms. *J Vasc Surg.* 2011;53(5):1274-1281.

Burks JA, Faries PL, et al. Endovascular repair of bleeding aortoenteric fistulas: a 5-year experience. *J Vasc Surg.* 2001;34:1055-1059.

Cho YP, Kanq GH, Han MS, et al. Staged surgery for chronic primary aortoduodenal fistula in a septic patient. *J Korean Med Sci.* 2004;19:302-304.

Clagett GP, Valentine RJ, Hagino RT. Autogenous aortoiliac/femoral reconstruction from superficial femoral-popliteal veins: feasibility and durability. *J Vasc Surg.* 1997;35:255-270.

Delgado J, Jotkowitz AB, Delgado B, et al. Primary aortoduodenal fistula: pitfalls and success in the endoscopic diagnosis. *Eur J Intern Med.* 2005;16:363-365.

Honjo O, Yamada Y, Arata T, et al. A primary aorto-duodenal fistula associated with an inflammatory abdominal aortic aneurysm: a case report. *Acta Med Okayama.* 2005;59:161-164.

Kakkos SK, Antoniadis PN, Klonaris CN, et al. Open or endovascular repair of aortoenteric fistulas? A multicenter comparative study. *Eur J Vasc Endovasc Surg.* 2011;41:625-634.

Kashyap V, O'Hara PJ. Chapter 42—Local complications: Aortoenteric fistulae. In: *Rutherford's Vascular Surgery.* 7th ed. Philadelphia, PA. Saunders Elsevier; 2013.

Kelliher C, Kavanagh DO, Belton F, et al. Primary aortoduodenal fistula following staphylococcal septicaemia. *Eur J Vasc Endovasc Surg.* 2004;27:679-681.

Lawlor DK, DeRose G, Harris KA, et al. Primary aorto/iliac-enteric fistula: report of 6 new cases. *Vasc Endovascular Surg.* 2004;38:281-286.

Lemos DW, Raffetto JD, Moore TC, et al. Primary aortoduodenal fistula: a case report and review of the literature. *J Vasc Surg.* 2003;37:686-689.

Pirard L, Creemers E, Van Damme H, et al. In situ aortic allograft insertion to repair a primary aortoesophageal fistula due to thoracic aortic aneurysm. *J Vasc Surg.* 2005;42:1213-1217.

Reckless JPD, McColl I, Taylor GW. Aorto-enteric fistulae: an uncommon complication of abdominal aortic aneurysms. *Br J Surg.* 1972;59:458-460.

Saers SJ, Scheltinga MR. Primary aortoenteric fistula. *Br J Surg.* 2005;92:143-152.

Sweeney MS, Gadacz TR. Primary aortoduodenal fistula: manifestations, diagnosis and treatment. *Surgery.* 1984;96:492-497.

Tambyraja AL, Murie JA, Chalmers RT. Ruptured inflammatory abdominal aortic aneurysm: insights in clinical management and outcome. *J Vasc Surg.* 2004;39:400-403.

Vogt PR, Pfammatter T, et al. In situ repair of aortobronchial, aortoesophageal, and aortoenteric fistulae with cryopreserved aortic homografts. *J Vasc Surg.* 1997;26:11-17.

Voorhoeve R, Moll FL, de Letter JA, et al. Primary aortoenteric fistula: report of eight new cases and review of the literature. *Ann Vasc Surg.* 1996;10:40-48.

CLINICAL SCENARIO CASE QUESTIONS

1. What is the single best diagnostic test to rule out the presence of an aortoenteric fistula?
   a. Upper endoscopy
   b. Computerized tomography (CT)
   c. Aortic angiography
   d. Magnetic resonance imaging (MRI)
   e. None of the above

2. Which part of the bowel is involved in an aortoenteric fistula?
   a. Duodenum.
   b. Jejunum.
   c. Ileum.
   d. Appendix.
   e. Any of the above could be involved.

Acute Limb Ischemia after Open AAA Repair

T. KONRAD RAJAB and MATTHEW T. MENARD

Presentation

A 75-year-old obese male presents to the emergency department with the acute onset of abdominal pain. He is a smoker with a known abdominal aortic aneurysm (AAA). The patient collapses on the way from the triage area to his assigned stretcher and requires cardiopulmonary resuscitation for approximately 20 minutes. Following return of spontaneous circulation, a computed tomographic angiogram (CTA) is performed and demonstrates a ruptured AAA. The aneurysm extends into both common iliac arteries and is felt not to be suitable for endovascular stent grafting given the absence of a suitable proximal landing zone. The patient is taken emergently to the operating room, where laparotomy reveals a small amount of free peritoneal blood. The decision is made not to administer heparin prior to supraceliac cross-clamping. The aneurysm is repaired using an aortobifemoral graft with 10-minute supraceliac and 30-minute infrarenal clamp times. Following construction of the distal anastomoses, the patient is hemodynamically stable with systolic blood pressure of 104 mm Hg on a 5 mcg/min Levophed infusion. On inspection of the lower extremities, however, the left foot is noted to be pale and cooler than the left. Femoral pulses are palpable bilaterally. The patient had faintly dopplerable pedal signals bilaterally prior to induction, and currently, there are strongly biphasic right pedal Doppler signals. The left popliteal and pedal pulses and Doppler signals are absent.

Differential Diagnosis

The incidence of acute limb ischemia after open AAA repair is approximately 5%. The differential diagnosis depends on whether one or both legs are affected. Acute ischemia affecting both legs can be caused by a technical issue with the proximal anastomosis, thrombus formation within the aortic tube graft or within the main body of a bifurcated graft, distal thromboembolism to both graft limbs or lower extremities, atheroembolism, or systemic hypotension.

Acute limb ischemia affecting just one leg only usually results from a technical problem with the distal anastomosis, thromboembolism, atheroembolism, or in situ thrombosis of the ipsilateral graft limb. One generally has a suspicion as to which among these diagnostic possibilities is most likely given the intraoperative conduct of the procedure.

Workup

While thromboembolism is the most frequent cause for acute limb ischemia after AAA, this patient also has risk factors for technical complications at the anastomoses, in situ thrombosis, and hypotension. Technical complications are more likely during urgent and emergent cases when expedient operative conduct is necessary, and a less-than-perfect technical result may be accepted in interest of shortening operative time. Additionally, standard heparinization dosing is often modified in the setting of a ruptured aneurysm or actively bleeding patient, raising the risk of in situ thrombosis. High blood loss also puts the patient at risk for systemic hypotension and further increases the risk of graft or outflow thrombosis.

Evaluation should begin by evaluating the patient's hemodynamic status. Hypotensive patients are aggressively resuscitated. Next follows a full vascular examination of the lower extremities, focused on assessment of the peripheral pulses and Doppler signals. Hematomas at the operative site should raise concern for a technical complication at the anastomosis and possible graft compression. In the event of acute limb ischemia, platelet counts should be checked to rule out heparin-induced thrombocytopenia, and creatinine kinase should be monitored given the risk of ischemia-induced rhabdomyolysis.

Diagnosis and Treatment

The diagnosis of acute limb ischemia after AAA repair is usually made relatively easily by routine postoperative physical examination. This is best done while the surgical team remains scrubbed, to allow for immediate treatment of any identified problem (Table 1).

As mentioned, the most common etiology of acute limb ischemia following AAA repair is either embolism of

TABLE 1. Acute Limb Ischemia after Open AAA Repair

Key Technical Steps

1. The surgical team remains on standby until routine assessment of pedal perfusion is performed. If lower extremity ischemia is detected, then the patient is immediately reheparinized.
2. The graft is inspected for kinks or compression, and distal anastomotic sites are assessed.
3. After reclamping, the distal anastomosis is opened and inspected for intimal flaps and other technical errors.
4. The site of a directed arteriotomy or graftotomy is guided by the presence or absence of iliac or femoral pulses in the affected limb.
5. Fogarty thrombectomy catheters are passed proximally and distally to clear thromboembolic material.
6. A completion angiography is performed unless palpable pedal pulses or baseline distal perfusion are restored.
7. If necessary, the popliteal artery is explored.

Potential Pitfalls

- Failure to identify heparin-induced thrombocytopenia
- Failure to perform timely fasciotomies
- Unrecognized narrowing at site of longitudinal arteriotomy closed primarily

disrupted plaque or chronic thrombus or new thrombus formation. In a study of 100 consecutive patients undergoing open AAA repair, 6 out of 7 patients who developed acute limb ischemia had sustained distal embolization of thrombus and debris. Atheroembolization is frequently caused during clamping, and as such, this risk can be reduced by careful assessment of all potential clamp sites prior to clamp placement. This should entail both a thorough review of all possible clamp sites on any available preoperative CT imaging and intraoperative palpation. Thrombus formation can also occur during the period of diminished limb perfusion when the arterial clamps are in place, with subsequent embolization following clamp release. This can potentially be avoided by adequate anticoagulation during clamping, frequent flushing during construction of the anastomoses, adequate forward and back bleeding during final flushing maneuvers, and efforts to minimize clamp times. Appropriate monitoring of the activated clotting time can be of particular help in gauging the degree to which ongoing prophylactic heparinization is successful. Attention to detail in constructing the anastomosis, with particular focus on removing or tacking any areas of disrupted intima, is a further important safeguard. The factors that raise suspicion for a thromboembolic etiology in the patient discussed above are the unilateral leg involvement and the reduced level of heparin utilized prior to cross-clamping.

Formal angiography can be used to confirm suspected acute limb ischemia and also to help in determining the etiology. Ideally, this is performed expeditiously in the operative suite using the fixed imaging of a hybrid operating room or a portable C-arm.

Once acute limb ischemia is diagnosed, the patient is immediately reheparinized to prevent further propagation of occlusive thrombus, and preparations are made for emergent surgical reintervention.

Surgical Approach

Maintaining a sterile field, sterile instruments, and a scrubbed surgical team until adequate distal perfusion is confirmed is standard practice after open aortic surgery and will serve to minimize any delay until necessary reintervention can be performed. Physical examination findings dictate the strategic approach to the reintervention.

Following exploration of the wound, any obvious technical problems, such as kinking of the graft or compression of a graft limb by the inguinal ligament, are addressed. If there is an absent pulse in either the proximal native common iliac artery (in the event of initial reconstruction with a tube graft) or the proximal limb of a bifurcated graft, one may elect to reapply clamps and perform a unilateral limb graftotomy or iliac arteriotomy. This may result in identification of a focal raised intimal flap or thromboembolic plug, lending itself to a relatively easy surgical fix.

Alternatively, one can initially utilize a common femoral artery approach, particularly if the common femoral artery was already dissected during an aortobifemoral reconstruction or in the setting of a palpable femoral pulse in the ischemic limb. Depending on the degree of suspicion of the underlying cause, either a transverse or longitudinal graftotomy or arteriotomy can be carried out, or the entire distal anastomosis can be taken down. Any technical errors are corrected, and the intima is carefully inspected. Simply tacking down an intimal plaque may be sufficient, or performing a more extensive endarterectomy may be required. Once technical problems with the anastomosis are excluded, the antegrade flow is evaluated by releasing the proximal clamp. Fogarty catheters are passed retrograde to remove any proximal thrombus; typically, a 4- or 5-French Fogarty balloon will be used for a graft limb or the native iliac artery. A 3-French Fogarty balloon is also passed distally to clear any thrombus or embolic debris from the profunda femoral and superficial femoral arteries as well. At this point, the femoral access is closed and distal perfusion assessed. If insufficient, further angiography may be undertaken to identify the location of any remaining distal thrombotic material, or a below-knee popliteal exploration can be carried out. Extending the dissection to expose the origins of each of the tibial vessels and performing a longitudinal arteriotomy rather than a transverse arteriotomy allow directed passage of a 2-French Fogarty balloon into each of the tibial runoff vessels. A longitudinal incision typically mandates patch angioplasty to avoid stenosis. After adequate backflow is obtained, the arteriotomies are closed. Attention is paid to the order of removal of the clamps during closure of the arteriotomy. Attention should be given to adequate flushing of both the inflow and the outflow vessels prior to completing the arteriotomy closure by transiently releasing the proximal and distal clamps; detection of any fresh thrombus during this step would typically indicate an insufficient level of heparinization. Finally, the distal perfusion should be reassessed to confirm adequate restoration of flow to the ischemic limb. A completion angiogram is recommended at this point to ensure that the thrombectomy was technically successful. While it is appropriate in certain circumstances to defer on further treatment of a small amount of residual thrombus that does not appear to be causing hemodynamic compromise, it is important to be aware that remnant thrombus may serve as a nidus for subsequent recurrent thrombotic complications.

In instances when extraction of in situ thrombus or emboli proves prohibitive, a definitive salvage bypass procedure around the obstruction may prove necessary. This will typically be in the setting of chronic multilevel atherosclerotic occlusive disease, in patients in whom important collaterals have been affected by the acute process or in whom the profunda femoral artery proves insufficient to sustain ongoing patency of the inflow graft. While any such infrainguinal graft is ideally performed with saphenous vein, the importance of timely restoration of distal perfusion may render a prosthetic conduit the better choice. Similarly, if efforts at the iliac or femoral level fail to reestablish adequate aortoiliac inflow, an expeditious femorofemoral bypass is usually the most appropriate bailout maneuver. Alternatively, intraoperative endovascular balloon angioplasty or stent placement is an acceptable and potentially time-saving salvage option. If the ischemic time is relatively short, then lower extremity fasciotomies are not necessary. However, close postoperative observation with serial neurovascular examinations and compartment checks are mandatory in the event they are deferred.

Special Intraoperative Considerations

While a rare event in the current era, falling platelet counts and the presence of white-colored thrombus formation in the operative field should raise suspicion for heparin-induced thrombocytopenia. If identified, intravenous heparin should be discontinued and substituted with bivalirudin or an equivalent alternative. Any heparin-coated central lines should also be replaced.

Postoperative Management

The risk of compartment syndrome following acute limb ischemia after AAA repair obligates serial neurovascular examination for evidence of developing ischemia and close monitoring for rhabdomyolysis. Additional postoperative management efforts include appropriate wound care and the maintenance of ongoing anticoagulation. Open fasciotomy wounds can be managed by vacuum sponge dressings until subsequent secondary operative closure, eventual outpatient resolution or split thickness skin grafting. If no technical complication explaining the thrombosis is found, the patient should be considered for evaluation of a hypercoagulable disorder.

TAKE HOME POINTS

- Lower extremity ischemia is an early complication of open AAA repair.
- Maintaining an adequate level of systemic anticoagulation, performing antegrade and retrograde flushing maneuvers and noting appropriate forward and back bleeding prior to completing the distal anastomoses, and vigilant attention to tacking areas of disrupted intima to avoid intimal flaps are all critical steps in preventing acute limb ischemia during AAA repair.
- Diagnosis is most frequently made by physical examination. Peripheral pulses are checked after completion of the distal anastomosis while the surgical team remains on standby.
- Treatment of lower extremity ischemia after open AAA repair involves immediate reheparinization and surgical exploration.
- Postoperatively, patients require serial pulse exams and compartment checks.

SUGGESTED READINGS

Ameli FM, Provan JL, Williamson C, et al. Etiology and management of aortofemoral bypass graft failure. *J Cardiovasc Surg.* 1987;28:695-700

Cronenwett JL, Johnston KW, Rutherford RB. *Rutherford's Vascular Surgery*. Philadelphia, PA: Saunders/Elsevier; 2010:1966.

Hirsch AT, et al. ACC/AHA 2005 Practice Guidelines for the management of patients with peripheral arterial disease (lower extremity, renal, mesenteric, and abdominal aortic): a collaborative report from the American Association for Vascular Surgery/Society for Vascular Surgery, Society for Cardiovascular Angiography and Interventions, Society for Vascular Medicine and Biology, Society of Interventional Radiology, and the ACC/AHA Task Force on Practice Guidelines. *Circulation.* 2006;113(11):e463-e654.

Imparato AM. Abdominal aortic surgery: prevention of lower limb ischemia. *Surgery.* 1983;93:112-116.

Imparato AM, Berman IR, Bracco A, et al. Avoidance of shock and peripheral embolism during surgery of the abdominal aorta. *Surgery.* 1973;73:68-73.

Jang IK, Hursting MJ. When heparins promote thrombosis: review of heparin-induced thrombocytopenia. *Circulation.* 2005;111(20):2671-2683.

Starr DS, Lawrie GM, Morris GC Jr. Prevention of distal embolism during arterial reconstruction. *Am J Surg.* 1979;138:764-769.

Tchirkow G, Beven EG. Leg ischemia following surgery for abdominal aortic aneurysm. *Ann Surg.* 1978;188:166-170.

Towne JB, Bernhard VM, Hussey C, et al. Antithrombin deficiency: a cause of unexplained thrombosis in vascular surgery. *Surgery.* 1981;89:735-742.

CLINICAL SCENARIO CASE QUESTIONS

1. Acute limb ischemia after open AAA repair is most frequently diagnosed by:
   a. Physical examination
   b. Duplex ultrasound
   c. Computed tomography
   d. Angiography

2. The initial step in the treatment of acute limb ischemia after open AAA repair are:
   a. Readministration of heparin
   b. Immediate reexploration
   c. Intra-arterial thrombolysis
   d. Observation in the ICU with serial exams and creatine kinase measurements

47 Intestinal Ischemia after AAA Repair

ENJAE JUNG and PATRICK J. GERAGHTY

Presentation

A 78-year-old man with history of diabetes, hypertension, and significant tobacco use is transferred from an outside hospital with a computed tomography (CT) confirming a diagnosis of a ruptured abdominal aortic aneurysm (AAA). On initial presentation to the outside hospital, he was hypotensive with systolic blood pressure of 55 mm Hg. He is transfused two units of packed red blood cells and transferred to your institution. On arrival to the emergency department, his vital signs are as follows: temperature 37.1°C, heart rate 110 bpm, and blood pressure 73/39 mm Hg. He is awake and alert and complains of back pain. Review of his CT again confirms a contained ruptured infrarenal AAA with a moderate-sized left retroperitoneal hematoma. His aneurysm anatomy is suitable for an endovascular aneurysm repair (EVAR), and he is taken emergently to the operating room. He undergoes an uncomplicated EVAR under local anesthetics with a modular, bifurcated graft from his infrarenal aorta to the iliac artery bifurcation. Both of his internal iliac arteries are diseased but patent and preserved. Postoperatively, he is taken to the surgical intensive care unit, where he remains hemodynamically stable. However, several hours later, you receive a call from his nurse that his urine output has decreased. He is also complaining of acute abdominal pain and a distended abdomen.

Differential Diagnosis

The differential diagnosis for decreased urine output in a postoperative patient is broad and includes bleeding, hypovolemia, cardiogenic shock, and sepsis. However, in the immediate postoperative period following an AAA repair, intestinal ischemia should be high on the differential. In addition, since this patient presented with a ruptured aneurysm, abdominal compartment syndrome from the hematoma and resuscitation should also be considered.

Workup

You go to examine the patient. He remains afebrile, and his vital signs are stable. He has a mildly distended abdomen that is tender to palpation especially in the left lower quadrant with voluntary guarding, but his abdomen is soft, and his bladder pressure is 8 mm Hg. Rectal exam is negative for gross blood, but a stool sample is guaiac positive. Laboratory testing is significant for a serum lactate level of 3.1 mmol/L and a leukocytosis of 16,000 cells/mL.

Discussion

No laboratory tests are pathognomonic of intestinal ischemia, and a high index of suspicion is essential. Findings potentially suggestive of ischemic colitis include persistent acidosis, leukocytosis, elevated lactate levels, and fluid sequestration. Patients may also have diarrhea or bloody bowel movement, but the classic finding of bloody diarrhea in the early postoperative period occurs in only about 30% of cases. Early identification is essential because progression to full-thickness necrosis is associated with a high mortality rate.

Fiberoptic colonoscopy is the diagnostic modality of choice to confirm the diagnosis and is important in guiding subsequent treatment since the severity of the ischemic insult widely varies. The mildest form of ischemic colitis results in ischemia limited to the colonic mucosa and submucosa. Patients may have symptoms of abdominal pain, ileus, distention, or bloody diarrhea and on endoscopy display patchy mucosal erythema, pallor, or ecchymosis. This is the most common form, and the disease resolves with adequate resuscitation and bowel rest alone. Extensive changes of mucosa with large confluent areas of involvement may indicate a more moderate form of ischemia. This involves ischemia of the muscularis and may eventually result in ischemic stricture formation. The most severe form of colonic ischemia involves transmural ischemia and colonic infarction. Fortunately, this is the least common form of colonic ischemia. Endoscopic changes include a flaccid or rigid colonic segment with mucosal friability, ulceration, and fissures (Fig. 1). Severe ischemic colitis requires resection of the infarcted bowel.

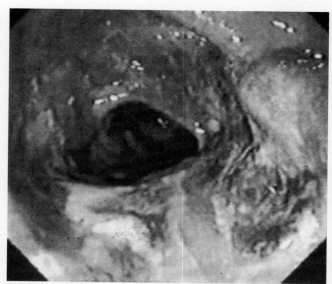

FIGURE 1 • Endoscopic changes of severe ischemic colitis with evidence of mucosal friability and ulceration as well as patchy areas of necrosis.

Diagnosis and Treatment

The patient undergoes a bedside flexible sigmoidoscopy that shows boggy, erythematous mucosa with dusky patches circumferentially throughout the sigmoid colon, and rectum suggestive of mild to moderate ischemic colitis.

In elective open aortic reconstructions, clinically evident ischemic colitis develops in 1% to 3% of patients. Clinically insignificant colonic ischemia occurs more frequently. Routine endoscopic surveillance studies have reported an incidence of 4.5% to 11.4% in patients after elective AAA repair, whereas biopsy of the mucosa has identified ischemic changes in 30% of patients after aortic surgery, with half the patients having no macroscopically apparent ischemic changes. Fortunately, severe colon ischemia is rare after AAA repair, occurring less than 1% of the time, but it carries a high degree of morbidity and a significant mortality rate. Aneurysm rupture significantly increases the incidence of this complication, with as many as 60% of survivors demonstrating endoscopic evidence of colonic ischemia. Other risk factors for development of colonic ischemia after open aneurysm repair include hypotension, hypoxemia, prolonged aortic cross-clamp time, and operative trauma to the colon. Unlike open repair in which the onset is thought to occur from a global physiologic insult, the pathogenesis of colonic ischemia after endovascular repair is thought to be due to atheromatous embolization to the mesenteric microvasculature. Bilateral internal iliac artery occlusion and other factors, such as intraoperative hypotension, may have a possible secondary role.

In all forms of colonic ischemia, broad-spectrum antibiotic therapy is routinely initiated. Mild ischemic injury isolated to the mucosa can initially be treated nonoperatively with bowel rest, broad-spectrum antibiotics, and

TABLE 1. Colon Ischemia after AAA Repair

Key Technical Steps

1. No laboratory tests are pathognomonic of intestinal ischemia, and a high index of suspicion is essential.
2. Findings potentially suggestive of ischemic colitis include persistent acidosis, leukocytosis, elevated lactate levels, and fluid sequestration. Patients may also have diarrhea or bloody bowel movement, but the classic finding of bloody diarrhea in the early postoperative period occurs in only about 30% of cases.
3. Early identification is essential because progression to full-thickness necrosis is associated with a high mortality rate.
4. Fiberoptic colonoscopy is the diagnostic modality of choice to confirm the diagnosis and is important in guiding subsequent treatment since the severity of the ischemic insult widely varies.
5. The most severe form of colonic ischemia involves transmural ischemia and colonic infarction. Severe ischemic colitis requires resection of the infarcted bowel.

Potential Pitfalls

- Aneurysm rupture significantly increases the incidence of this complication, with as many as 60% of survivors demonstrating endoscopic evidence of colonic ischemia.
- Other risk factors for development of colonic ischemia after open aneurysm repair include hypotension, hypoxemia, prolonged aortic cross-clamp time, and operative trauma to the colon.
- Bilateral internal iliac artery occlusion and other factors, such as intraoperative hypotension, may have a possible secondary role.
- Development of transmural ischemia, worsening sepsis, or peritoneal signs all require prompt surgical intervention.

fluid resuscitation, but close observation is warranted. Development of transmural ischemia, worsening sepsis, or peritoneal signs all require prompt surgical intervention (Table 1).

Surgical Approach

When suspected, intestinal ischemia is confirmed by endoscopy. Severe ischemia warrants an early return to the operating room for bowel resection with fecal diversion, creation of an ostomy, and washout of the abdomen. Colonic ischemia after aortic surgery sufficient to require reoperation predicts 50% mortality, and this mortality rate increases if perforation with contamination has occurred. At the time of reexploration, diverting ostomies at the appropriate level and mucous fistula or Hartmann's pouch are preferred to primary anastomosis. Colostomy reversal should await full recovery from the initial surgical procedure(s).

Other Considerations

Several studies advocate for attempting to maintain adequate colonic and pelvic blood supply after aortic reconstructive procedures. Zelenock et al. demonstrated that an aggressive algorithm for pelvic revascularization (i.e., inferior mesenteric artery reimplantation, direct bypass to internal iliac artery) at the time of open aortic reconstruction can limit the occurrence of colonic ischemia. Similarly, in endovascular repair, all attempts should be made to preserve pelvic perfusion by maintaining antegrade flow to at least one patent internal iliac artery.

Case Conclusion

After endoscopy, the patient was placed on bowel rest with broad-spectrum antibiotics and underwent serial abdominal exams. Over the next several hours, his serum lactate level normalized, and his abdominal exam improved over the next 24 to 48 hours. He was eventually started on an oral diet that he tolerated well and was discharged from the hospital on the 8th postoperative day.

TAKE HOME POINTS

- Colon ischemia after aortic surgery is uncommon, but it carries a high mortality and morbidity rate mandating a high index of suspicion and low threshold for action.
- Endoscopy is typically the diagnostic test of choice.
- Global physiologic insult is thought to be the pathogenesis of colonic ischemia after open AAA repair, while atheromatous embolization to the mesenteric microvasculature is thought to be the cause of colonic ischemia after EVAR.
- Aggressive attempts should be made to maintain colonic and pelvic perfusion either by reimplantation or by revascularization in open surgical repair or by maintaining antegrade flow to at least one patent internal iliac artery during EVAR.
- Patients should be placed on bowel rest, given fluid resuscitation, and broad-spectrum antibiotics as soon as possible.
- Patients with evidence of severe colonic ischemia should be taken promptly to the operating room for bowel resection with diverting ostomy.

SUGGESTED READINGS

Fanti L, Masci E, et al. Is endoscopy useful for early diagnosis of ischaemic colitis after aortic surgery? Results of a prospective trial. *Ital J Gastroenterol Hepatol.* 1997;29:357-360.

Geraghty PG, Sanchez LA, et al. Overt ischemia after endovascular repair of aortoiliac aneurysms. *J Vasc Surg.* 2004; 40(3):413-418.

Meissner MH, Johansen KH. Colon infarction after ruptured abdominal aortic aneurysm. *Arch Surg.* 1992;127:979-985.

Tollefson DF, Ernst CB. Colon ischemia following aortic reconstruction. *Ann Vasc Surg.* 1991;5:485-489.

Welborn MB, Seeger JM. Prevention and management of sigmoid and pelvic ischemia associated with aortic surgery. *Semin Vasc Surg.* 2001;14(4):255-265.

Zelenock GB, Stodel WE, et al. A prospective study of clinically and endoscopically documented colonic ischemia in 100 patients undergoing aortic reconstructive surgery with aggressive colonic and direct pelvic revascularization, compared with historic controls. *Surgery.* 1989;106:771-779.

CLINICAL SCENARIO CASE QUESTIONS

1. A patient develops abdominal pain, leukocytosis, and bloody diarrhea after an uneventful, elective open abdominal aortic aneurysm repair. You suspect ischemic colitis. What is the best diagnostic test?

    a. Serum lactate level
    b. Barium enema
    c. Sigmoidoscopy or colonoscopy
    d. Computed tomography of the abdomen and pelvis

2. A patient with suspected ischemic colitis undergoes flexible sigmoidoscopy, which reveals mucosal erythema as well as patchy areas of ecchymosis. He is otherwise hemodynamically stable except for mild tachycardia. What is the next course of action?

    a. Bowel rest, intravenous hydration, and antibiotics in preparation for the operating room for bowel resection
    b. Bowel rest, intravenous hydration, and antibiotics with plans for operating room only if the patient's exam worsens
    c. Immediate colon resection
    d. Start a bowel prep followed by colon resection

48 Small Abdominal Aortic Aneurysm

G. MATTHEW LONGO and B. TIMOTHY BAXTER

Presentation

A 73-year-old male is referred to the vascular surgery clinic for evaluation of a small abdominal aortic aneurysm (AAA). He received a CT scan of the chest/abdomen/pelvis for follow-up of his asbestosis. On the CT scan, it was appreciated that there was a 4.4-cm infrarenal AAA. His past medical history is significant for hypertension, hypercholesterolemia, atrial fibrillation, a transient ischemic attack, and asbestosis. He previously smoked 0.5 to 1.0 packs of cigarettes/day for 60 years. He denies any history of abdominal or back pain and continues working as an administrator. His physical examination reveals palpable femoral, popliteal, and tibial pulses bilaterally. There is no palpable abdominal mass or tenderness.

Differential Diagnosis

Small AAAs are often recognized incidentally by ultrasound or CT scan. These studies are performed for other abdominal/back complaints or as part of a screening program, when the discovery of an aneurysm is made. An AAA is defined as an abnormal dilatation of the aorta, with an increase in diameter of 50% or greater compared to its baseline size. Due to the fact, the baseline size is difficult to ascertain, a maximal measurement of ≥30 mm is frequently utilized to define an AAA.

AAA prevalence increases with age, and studies have revealed that they are present in up to 9% of men over the age of 55. Besides male gender, other risk factors include a history of smoking and a family history of AAA in a first-degree relative. Physical examination is notoriously unreliable for detection of AAA. However, both abdominal ultrasound and CT angiography exhibit a high degree of accuracy in detection. Ultrasound is generally regarded as the screening study of choice, due to cost, a relatively high specificity and sensitivity for detection, and its noninvasive nature.

Workup

On initial presentation, the most important elements of the workup include a complete history and physical examination and a discussion with the patient regarding the diagnosis of an AAA and what this entails. The vast majority of individuals presenting with a small AAA have no symptoms that can be attributed to the aneurysm. At this point, patients are understandably concerned about this new diagnosis. Thus, a definition of an aneurysm, coupled with a discussion of the natural history of the disease process, and time points for intervention are generally provided. Conveying the gradual progression of the disease and the ability to safely monitor growth are helpful in allaying anxiety. The patient also needs to know the signs and symptoms of an expanding or rupturing aneurysm.

After obtaining a detailed history and physical, a review of the available imaging is done. If there has not been a CT angiogram performed, this is usually advisable since it removes the size variability of ultrasound measurements and enables the surgeon to evaluate the branch vessels of the aorta and the extent of the aneurysm. CT also will better define the relationship to the renal arteries and demonstrate internal iliac aneurysms that may not be found on ultrasound. A compete blood count and basic metabolic profile allow for assessment of renal function and hemoglobin, platelet, and electrolyte abnormalities.

Other important elements of the workup involve a discussion with the patient regarding long-term follow-up. It is known that AAAs enlarge over time, with pooled estimates of AAA growth of about 2.5 mm/year. However, among individual patients, there is marked variation. Baseline diameter (smaller aneurysms grow at slower rates) is the most important determinant of growth rate. Continued smoking increases growth rate by approximately 10%/year, while diabetes is associated with slower growth. Since the aneurysm will remain asymptomatic even as it expands, both the patient and the physician need to remain committed to a long-term follow-up plan.

In the present case of a 74-year-old male with a 4.4-cm AAA, his CT scan demonstrates a fusiform, 4.4-cm infrarenal AAA (Fig. 1). The size of the aneurysm indicates that it has a low risk of rupture, and the recommendation is for surveillance. The rates of progression of AAA were discussed, as were the various treatment

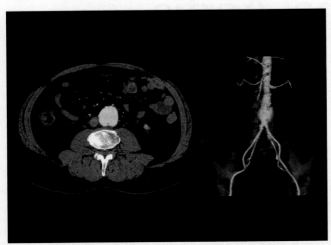

FIGURE 1 • Axial cut of a CT scan documenting an infrarenal AAA and 3D reconstruction.

options if his aneurysm grew to a size warranting repair. A long-term surveillance program was also explained to him. He was also informed of the signs and symptoms of aortic rupture.

Treatment

Although AAA can, on rare occasion, cause pain from nerve compression or erosion into the spine, or present with leg pain from embolization of thrombus, rupture is the major risk. Mortality from rupture is reported as high as 90% prior to reaching a hospital and as high as 70% with emergency aneurysmorrhaphy depending to some extent on the patient's comorbidities. The risk of rupture is correlated with aneurysm size, female gender, smoking, uncontrolled hypertension, and chronic obstructive pulmonary disease (COPD). Thus, working with a patient to quit smoking and control blood pressure has theoretical benefit.

Current recommendations are to repair aneurysms once reaching a size of 5.5 cm in maximal diameter or in situations where the aneurysm has grown greater than 1 cm in year. Women appear to have a higher rupture rate when compared to men with equivalent sized aortas. A recommendation has been made by the joint council of the American Association for Vascular Surgery and the Society of Vascular Surgery to use a lesser diameter as a threshold for repair in women; however, this is not backed by randomized trial evidence.

There are investigations ongoing for the medical treatment of small aneurysms. These are not widespread, and none has yet shown positive results. However, the potential of decreasing the growth rate of an aneurysm offers the promise of both reducing the mortality from rupture and decreasing the number of patients requiring operative repair.

Case Continued

In the clinical scenario, our patient was offered the opportunity to participate in a pharmacologic trial for the treatment of his small aneurysm. He accepted and was then followed according to the treatment protocol of the trial. If he had declined trial participation, he would have entered a long-term surveillance program of clinic visits coupled with ultrasound or CT scan every 6 months. Contrast is not necessary for follow-up CT scans assessing changes in aneurysm size.

Recommendation

There have been four randomized trials looking at both open and endovascular repair of small aortic aneurysms versus surveillance: the UK Small Aneurysm Trial (UKSAT), the Aneurysm Detection and Management Trial (ADAM), the Comparison of Surveillance Versus Aortic Endografting for Small Aneurysm Repair (CAESAR), and the Positive Impact of Endovascular Options for treating Aneurysms Early trial (PIVOTAL). These studies compared survival benefit in patients with early surgery (surgery for aneurysms less than 5.5 cm) versus those placed in surveillance programs. The results of all four trials suggest no overall benefit from early surgery, and that early surgery could potentially expose patients to unnecessary risks; the approach of early repair clearly results in higher health care costs since many patients with small aneurysms die of other causes before reaching the size threshold for repair.

Research is still needed to validate repair at smaller diameters for women, especially considering the high operative risks for women. Similarly, patients with severe COPD may have a higher rupture risk but also have higher morbidity and mortality for AAA repair. Whether there are better plasma or morphologic (aneurysm shape, volume, thrombus content) markers that predict growth rate or rupture risk are areas of ongoing research. Since smaller aneurysms grow slower and will take longer to reach standard repair thresholds, it has been suggested that surveillance intervals be increased. Extending this interval beyond a year is typically unsettling to patients and risks loss to follow-up since some EMR systems are not setup for follow-up appointments beyond 12 months.

Case Conclusion

The patient has continued in both the surveillance program and the pharmacologic trial for small aortic aneurysms. After 18 months of follow-up, there has been no change in his aneurysm size or shape.

TAKE HOME POINTS

- Upon initially evaluating a patient with a small aneurysm, a complete history and physical and high-quality radiologic imaging of the aneurysm are necessary.
- For aneurysms less than 5.5 cm, surveillance has demonstrated equivalent survival rates compared to early repair.
- Patients require regular surveillance imaging for an aneurysm less than 5.5 cm.

SUGGESTED READINGS

Filardo G, Lederle FA, Ballard DA, et al. Immediate open repair vs. surveillance in patients with small abdominal aortic aneurysms: survival differences by aneurysm size. *Mayo Clin Proc.* 2013;88(9):910-919.

Filardo G, Powell JT, Martinez MAM, et al. Surgery for small asymptomatic abdominal aortic aneurysms. *Cochrane Database Syst Rev.* 2012;(3):CD001835. doi: 10.1002/14651858. CD001835.pub3.

Lederle FA. The rise and fall of abdominal aortic aneurysm. *Circulation.* 2011;124(10):1097-1099.

Lederle FA, Freischlag JA, Kyriades TC, et al. Open Versus Endovascular Repair (OVER) Veterans Affairs Study Group; Outcomes following endovascular vs open repair of abdominal aortic aneurysm: a randomized trial. *JAMA.* 2009;302(14):1535-1542.

RESCAN Collaborators. Surveillance intervals for small abdominal aortic aneurysms. *JAMA.* 2013;309(8):806-813.

Rughani G, Robertson L, Clarke M. Medical treatment for small abdominal aortic aneurysms. *Cochrane Database Syst Rev.* 2012;(9):CD009536. doi: 10.1002/14651858.CD009536. pub2.

CLINICAL SCENARIO CASE QUESTIONS

1. Optimal treatment of a 4.5-cm infrarenal AAA in a healthy 65-year-old female consists of:

   a. Open aneurysmorrhaphy, due to her age and known higher rupture rates in women with small aneurysms

   b. Aortic endografting, because of the lower morbidity and mortality of endografting compared to open repair of the aneurysm

   c. Routine surveillance with clinic visits and aortic imaging

   d. Assurance that the rupture risk in this aneurysm is small, thus no treatment or long-term follow-up is necessary

2. Most small aneurysms are discovered at what time?

   a. Upon rupturing and presentation to the emergency department

   b. Incidentally, during evaluation for another complaint requiring abdominal or spinal imaging

   c. During the initial Medicare history and physical, as part of its screening program

   d. At autopsy

49 Isolated Iliac Artery Aneurysm

CALOGERO DIMAGGIO, EVAN J. RYER, and JAMES R. ELMORE

Presentation

A 76-year-old male presents to his primary care physician for his routine annual physical examination. He has been in his usual state of health but reports mild right lower abdominal and groin discomfort for the last 3 weeks, which he attributes to overexertion. He denies any recent weight loss, change in bowel habits, dysuria, urgency, or frequency. His medical history is significant for ongoing tobacco use, coronary artery disease, hypertension, chronic kidney disease, and dyslipidemia. His medications include aspirin, simvastatin, hydrochlorothiazide, and carvedilol. On physical examination, blood pressure is 163/95 mm Hg and heart rate is 82 bpm. His abdominal examination reveals no palpable masses or surgical scars. His femoral pulses are 2+, and he has 1+ dorsalis pedis and posterior tibialis pulses bilaterally.

Differential Diagnosis

The differential diagnosis for right lower quadrant and groin discomfort is quite broad. A palpable pulsatile abdominal mass on exam is classic for an abdominal aortic aneurysm (AAA). In an obese patient, an abdominal aneurysm may not be felt, and in a very thin patient, one is expected to palpate a normal-sized aorta. Physical examination is unreliable when it comes to detecting isolated common iliac aneurysms due to their location deep in the pelvis. Computed tomography (CT) scans are the imaging modality of choice for intra-abdominal processes, including aneurysmal disease. Duplex ultrasound screening of the lower extremities should be performed to rule out any peripheral artery aneurysm, particularly femoral and popliteal artery aneurysms, especially in the setting of prominent peripheral pulses.

Workup

As part of his outpatient workup, a CT scan of the abdomen and pelvis was obtained that revealed an isolated 5.2-cm right common iliac artery (CIA) aneurysm (Fig. 1). No evidence of AAA or other gross intra-abdominal pathology was noted (not shown). Serum laboratory studies revealed a hemoglobin level of 13 g/dL, a normal platelet count, a normal prothrombin time, and a serum creatinine of 1.5 mg/dL (glomerular filtration rate [GFR] 47 mL/min).

Diagnosis and Treatment

An iliac artery aneurysm (IAA) is any permanent, localized dilation of the iliac artery measuring larger than 1.5 cm in maximal diameter. Many others consider an aneurysm to be a localized expansion of an artery, iliac included, greater than 50% of the normal caliber of the artery. Multiple reports have demonstrated that IAAs most commonly occur in the presence of AAAs. Alternatively, isolated iliac artery aneurysms (iIAAs) are rare and account for less than 3% of all intra-abdominal aneurysms. In approximately 70% of iIAAs, the CIA is involved, followed by the internal iliac artery in 25% of cases. Rarely, isolated external IAAs are encountered. Like AAA, iIAAs are more common in men (5 to 16× more common depending on the series) with most patients presenting after age 65. The natural history of iIAAs, similar to AAA, is one of continued expansion with the potential for life-threatening rupture. In fact, approximately 30% of patients with iIAAs present with rupture accounting for mortality rates as high as 60%, whereas the mortality for elective repair is less than 5%.

Although the clinical presentation of iIAAs is variable, most patients are asymptomatic and are diagnosed after an incidental discovery on imaging studies for unrelated indications. In symptomatic iIAAs, the size and location often dictate the clinical presentation. Very large aneurysms (greater than 5 cm) detected late are more likely to be associated with local compressive symptoms or rupture resulting in hemodynamic collapse. Compression of surrounding structures may include the ureters resulting in hydronephrosis, nerve compression leading to neurogenic pain, bowel compression resulting in intestinal obstruction, or iliac vein compression leading to edema or a venous thromboembolic event. As previously mentioned, the natural history of iIAAs is one of expansion over time with the rate of expansion directly related to iliac artery diameter on initial diagnosis. iIAAs less than 3 cm have demonstrated expansion rates of approximately 1 mm/year, whereas aneurysms greater than 3 cm are estimated to expand by approximately 2.5 mm/year. The average size of ruptured isolated IAAs is between 5 and 7 cm. With the high mortality associated with rupture, current recommendations favor intervening when

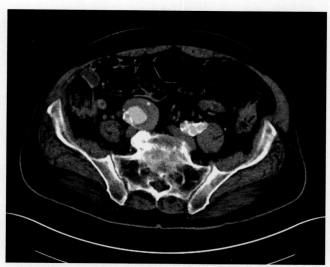

FIGURE 1 • CT scan of the abdomen and pelvis with intravenous contrast: 5.2-cm right common IAA. No evidence of AAA or left iliac aneurysm (not shown).

iIAAs reach 3.5 cm. For iIAAs less than 3 cm, annual duplex ultrasonography is recommended. For those aneurysms greater than 3 cm, but less than the 3.5 cm threshold, serial imaging at 6 months or elective repair for carefully selected cases such as those with continued aneurysm expansion is recommended.

Surgical Approach for Endovascular Iliac Aneurysm Repair

A thorough understanding of the aneurysm's anatomic characteristics is paramount when planning repair and is achieved only by meticulous review of fine-cut (1-mm) CT scans with sagittal and coronal reconstructions. As in endovascular AAA repair, adequate proximal and distal landing seal zones are critical. Although no formal criteria for adequate neck length exist, a minimum of 1.0 cm length has been recommended for iliac arteries. In addition to adequate neck length, the aneurysm's anatomic location also factors into the surgeon's decision making. Unilateral repair is appropriate in individuals with a normal caliber (nonaneurysmal) proximal CIA, but implantation of a bifurcated aortic stent graft is necessary when the proximal CIA is aneurysmal. Aneurysms that extend to the common iliac bifurcation often require internal iliac artery coil embolization with coils or an excluding plug (i.e., Amplatzer plug [AGA Medical Corp, Plymouth, MN]) to prevent retrograde perfusion and a potential type 2 endoleak.

Preparation of the patient for endovascular repair of IAAs is done in a similar fashion to endovascular AAA repair. The procedure can be performed under general, regional, or local anesthesia with sedation if necessary. With the patient supine in the hybrid operating room suite, percutaneous access is obtained using a micropuncture needle. Using the standard Seldinger technique, a guidewire is passed under fluoroscopic guidance.

After the appropriate-sized sheath is placed, a marker catheter is passed over the wire and an abdominal/pelvic aortogram obtained. Systemic anticoagulation is next administered. Coil embolization of the internal iliac artery is performed with standard coils or plugs delivered to the origin of the internal iliac artery (Fig. 2). The proximal and distal extent of the CIA aneurysm is identified, and measurements are obtained. Next, the appropriate stent is selected, opened, and prepared for use. Under fluoroscopy, the stent graft device is delivered over the wire to planned graft deployment site. Of note, with regard to stent sizing, a 10% to 20% CIA and 10% external iliac artery oversizing is recommended. Placement is confirmed with retrograde sheath angiogram. Postdeployment stent graft dilation performed to ensure optimal apposition of vessel wall and graft. Finally, perform completion angiogram to assess for endoleak(s).

Recent advances have led to the development of branched iliac artery stent grafts. This technology allows the surgeon to extend a conventional endovascular stent graft repair (i.e., endovascular aneurysm repair [EVAR]) into the external iliac artery while preserving flow into the ipsilateral internal iliac artery. Current literature provides little information about the safety and efficacy of these devices. Additionally, these devices are currently limited to use within clinical trials within the United States. As experience grows, these devices may alter current treatment algorithms. Chimney grafts were intentionally omitted from this chapter as the authors believe

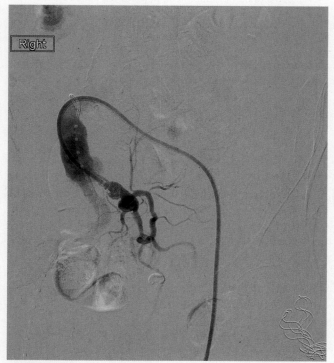

FIGURE 2 • An occluding plug placed in the internal iliac artery prior to stent graft occlusion of the iliac bifurcation.

TABLE 1. Endovascular Iliac Artery Aneurysm Repair

Key Technical Steps

1. Study preoperative CT imaging to ensure suitable anatomy for endovascular intervention.
2. Determine need for internal artery embolization to achieve complete aneurysm exclusion.
3. Based on preoperative imaging, select appropriately sized stent graft with approximately 10%–20% oversizing.
4. Obtain percutaneous common femoral artery access or perform open surgical exposure, as indicated.
5. Administer systemic heparin to achieve a therapeutic activating clotting time (ACT).
6. Insert appropriate-sized sheaths, guidewires, and catheters for pelvic angiography and endovascular stent graft insertion.
7. Perform internal iliac artery embolization, if indicated.
8. Advance stent graft over stiff guidewire into position.
9. Confirm positioning with retrograde sheath angiogram.
10. Deploy stent under fluoroscopic guidance.
11. Angioplasty proximal and distal seal zones.
12. Perform completion angiogram to rule out endoleak(s).
13. Withdraw guidewires/catheters/sheaths and achieve open or percutaneous closure of arteriotomies, as appropriate.
14. Administer protamine.
15. Check distal pulses prior to leaving the operating room.

Potential Pitfalls

- Iliac artery injury or dissection while traversing aneurysm
- Lower extremity ischemia due to emboli
- Progressive enlargement of aneurysm from incomplete exclusion
- Buttock claudication, impotence or bowel ischemia following internal iliac artery embolization
- Graft thrombosis
- Access site complication (i.e., hematoma, pseudo aneurysm, or dissection)

this technique is only suitable for very select cases who are not candidates for traditional open or endovascular repair. In the future, it is anticipated that the branched iliac stent grafts will replace the chimney grafts for this iliac aneurysmal disease (Table 1).

Surveillance Following Endovascular Iliac Artery Aneurysm Repair

Initial imaging should include a CT scan to document exclusion of the aneurysm and serve as a baseline study for future reference. Future imaging can then be performed with aortic duplex depending on image quality. CT scan can subsequently be used selectively for evaluation and detection of suspected migration, new endoleaks, or an enlarging aneurysm sac. Future imaging is also important to detect other aneurysms.

Surgical Approach to Open Iliac Artery Aneurysm Repair

Before endovascular repair was available, IAAs were repaired using open surgical techniques. Similar to endovascular repair, the traditional open surgical approach is dictated by the location and extent of the aneurysm. Open repair is typically performed under general anesthesia. The use of a self-retaining retractor is recommended to facilitate open surgical exposure. Most commonly a midline (i.e., transperitoneal) or retroperitoneal approach is used; however, the incision and extent of vascular exposure are dictated by the extent of the aneurysmal degeneration. If the abdominal aorta is normal and CIA involvement is unilateral, simple interposition graft placement via a transperitoneal or retroperitoneal approach is warranted. If the abdominal aorta is abnormal or iliac involvement is bilateral, a transperitoneal approach is preferred. If both common iliac arteries are involved and require replacement, it is essential to preserve perfusion to at least one internal iliac artery. This is especially important in cases in which the inferior mesenteric artery is chronically occluded as colonic perfusion may be dependent on collateral pathways. In the presence of early aneurysmal degeneration of the aorta (i.e., ectasia), it is recommended that both the aorta and iliac artery be replaced, as continued aortic expansion is likely.

To perform retroperitoneal exposure of a unilateral iliac artery, an oblique incision is made in the lower quadrant of the abdomen. The incision is started near the pubic tubercle with extension obliquely and lateral, staying medial to the anterior superior iliac spine. The external oblique aponeurosis, the internal oblique, and the transversus abdominis muscles are divided in the direction of the incision, and the preperitoneal space is entered. The peritoneum, along with the ureter, are pushed medially to expose the external iliac artery. Exposure of the CIA requires extension of the incision proximally and laterally. The surgeon must be careful to not injure the ilioinguinal or genitofemoral nerves during exposure or retraction. Their location on the anterior surface of the psoas muscle puts them at significant risk for injury.

To perform transperitoneal exposure of the infrarenal aorta and proximal common iliac arteries, a midline abdominal incision from the xiphoid to symphysis pubis is used. The peritoneal bands holding the duodenum to the aorta are divided. The duodenum is retracted laterally. The retroperitoneum overlying the infrarenal aorta is divided. When dissecting distally along the abdominal aorta, one should proceed slightly on the vena cava side to avoid interrupting the inferior mesenteric artery and its branches. Next, the surgeon must identify the aortic bifurcation and expose the common iliac arteries from the midline. The midline approach decreases the chance of a ureter injury. The surgeon must also take care to avoid injuring the sympathetic nerve fibers that course over the left CIA in males, as this can result in erectile dysfunction and retrograde ejaculation. As the dissection moves distally, the external iliac arteries are exposed by incising along the white line of Toldt and mobilizing the sigmoid colon toward the midline. Graft limbs coursing out to this level should be passed under both the colonic mesentery and ureter.

After gaining proper exposure, proximal and distal control of the IAA (or accompanying aortic aneurysm) is obtained using vessel loops and atraumatic vascular clamps once the patient is given heparin. Again, several repair options exist depending on the clinical presentation, extent and location of aneurysm, and overall hemodynamic status. For large common IAAs with compressive symptoms, the aneurysm should be opened, decompressed, and repaired directly (endoaneurysmorrhaphy) with an interposition graft. It is imperative to avoid any unnecessary dissection in an effort to minimize iatrogenic injury to adjacent structures. This is particularly true with regard to the ureter that can be adherent to the aneurysm. For similar reasons, resection of aneurysm sac is usually not necessary. If the aneurysm involves the internal iliac artery, it must be ligated. Ligation of the internal iliac artery is usually performed from within the common iliac aneurysm sac. If the internal iliac artery is aneurysmal itself, the incision should be extended into this aneurysm as well until the distal neck of the internal iliac artery is exposed. Once the neck is exposed, it can be oversewn without much difficulty. An appropriately sized prosthetic graft (Dacron or polytetrafluorethylene [PTFE]) is typically used for the iliac artery interposition graft. After achieving exposure of normal proximal and distal arteries, the proximal and distal anastomoses are performed with monofilament suture (i.e., polypropylene) in a standard fashion. Prior to completion of the final anastomosis, the graft is flushed with heparinized saline, backbled, and flow restored. Once hemostasis is secured and distal limb perfusion adequate, the heparin is reversed. The aneurysm sac is closed over the prosthetic graft. The distal pulses are checked prior to the patient leaving the operating room.

Special Intraoperative Consideration to Open Repair

During the course of open repair of IAA, significant atherosclerotic disease of the iliac vessels may be encountered. As such, clamping vessels with extensive atherosclerotic plaque is fraught with significant risk of embolization with resultant lower extremity ischemia. In these circumstances, obtaining proximal and distal control using intraluminal balloon catheters may be necessary. In cases of ruptured internal IAAs, in which the patient may be hemodynamically unstable or in extremis, simple ligation may be the most expeditious and prudent approach. Simple ligation has the advantage of limited pelvic dissection. However, if this approach is undertaken, each of the internal iliac artery branches must be individually ligated to avoid the back bleeding.

Postoperative Management

The incidence of complications during open or endovascular repair, excluding cardiopulmonary morbidity, ranges from 5% to 25%. The most common complications associated with endovascular intervention are endoleaks

TABLE 2. Open Iliac Artery Aneurysm Repair

Key Technical Steps

1. Lower midline/retroperitoneal incision.
2. Use of self-retaining retractor to facilitate exposure.
3. Isolate aneurysm proximally and distally.
4. Heparinize to achieve an ACT >250 seconds.
5. Control vessels with atraumatic clamps.
6. Open aneurysm sac longitudinally.
7. Select appropriate-sized prosthetic graft.
8. Perform proximal and distal anastomoses in standard fashion.
9. Flush graft with heparinized saline; forward/back bleed graft prior to completion of the final anastomosis.
10. Ensure hemostasis and adequate distal limb perfusion; give protamine.
11. Close aneurysm sac over prosthetic graft.
12. Close abdominal incision.
13. Check distal pulses prior to leaving the operating room.

Potential Pitfalls

- Iatrogenic injuries to adjacent structures during dissection of aneurysm sac
- Lower extremity ischemia from emboli during clamping
- Difficulty in obtaining distal control of aneurysm—may require intraluminal balloon occlusion or femoral exposure

(occurring in approximately 5% to 7%) and access site complications (infection, hematoma, pseudoaneurysm, arteriovenous fistulas). Additionally, complications associated with either open or endovascular repair include lower extremity ischemia from stent graft thrombosis, distal embolization, and pelvic ischemia thus mandating careful neurovascular monitoring in the immediate postoperative period and at regular intervals upon discharge. Finally, in cases of ruptured IAAs, patients are typically transferred to the ICU postoperatively for close monitoring and ongoing resuscitation. Aggressive measures to reverse hypothermia, coagulopathy, and acidosis are critical. Serial labs, including coagulation profile and renal function, should be closely monitored for the initial 24- to 48-hour period (Table 2).

Case Conclusion

This patient was noted to have a right CIA isolated aneurysm with a maximum diameter of 5.2 cm that extended to the origin of the internal iliac artery mandating the need for embolization plug occlusion of the right internal iliac artery (Fig. 2). This was followed by right CIA aneurysm exclusion using a bifurcated aortic stent graft (Fig. 3). Completion angiogram demonstrated successful exclusion of aneurysm without endoleak, and the patient was discharged home on POD #1. Postoperative surveillance imaging has revealed an intact repair with no evidence of enlargement or endoleaks (Fig. 4).

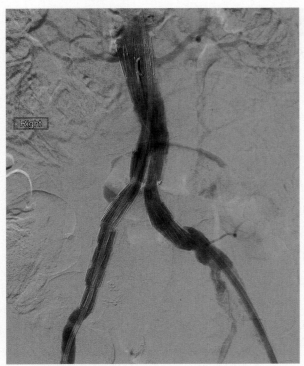

FIGURE 3 • Completion angiogram following right internal iliac artery embolization and endovascular exclusion of an isolated right common IAA.

TAKE HOME POINTS

- iIAAs are exceedingly rare and often discovered incidentally.
- Although data on overall natural history are largely unknown due to their rarity, most experts would agree that asymptomatic aneurysms greater than 3.5 cm require repair.
- Other indications for repair include ruptured or symptomatic aneurysm regardless of size or aneurysm greater than 3 cm with documented continued growth.

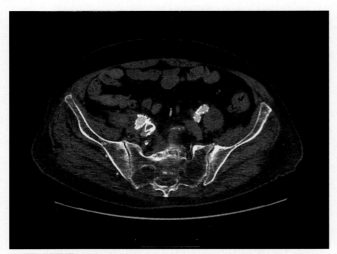

FIGURE 4 • Postoperative CT scan (1-year follow-up), axial image—demonstrating successful exclusion of right CIA aneurysm and significant aneurysm sac shrinkage.

- Rupture is associated with high mortality rates, while elective repair is associated with a mortality rate of less than 5%.
- Preoperative imaging is essential to planning an effective repair.
- Endovascular repair of iIAAs has become the preferred treatment in individuals with favorable anatomy.
- Traditionally, the open surgical repair involves endoaneurysmorrhaphy with interposition grafting.
- Both open and endovascular repair have comparable durability rates with respect to patency.
- Postoperative image surveillance at regular intervals is mandatory.

SUGGESTED READINGS

Buckley CJ, Buckley SD. Technical tips for endovascular repair of common iliac artery aneurysms. *Semin Vasc Surg.* 2008;21:31-34.

Chaer RA, et al. Isolated iliac artery aneurysms: a contemporary comparison of endovascular and open repair. *J Vasc Surg.* 2008;47:708-713.

Huang Y, et al. Common iliac artery aneurysm: expansion rate and results of open surgical and endovascular repair. *J Vasc Surg.* 2008;47:1203-1211.

Krupski W, et al. Contemporary management of isolated iliac aneurysms. *J Vasc Surg.* 1998;28:1-13.

Pitoulias GA, et al. Isolated iliac artery aneurysms: endovascular versus open elective repair. *J Vasc Surg.* 2007;46:648-654.

Sandu RS, Pipinos II. Isolated iliac artery aneurysms. *Semin Vasc Surg.* 2005;18:209-215.

Santilli SM, et al. Expansion rates and outcomes for iliac artery aneurysms. *J Vasc Surg.* 2000;31(1 Pt 1):114-121.

CLINICAL SCENARIO CASE QUESTIONS

1. When compared to open repair, all of the following are true with regard to endovascular repair of isolated iliac artery aneurysm except:

   a. Endovascular repair is associated with decreased operative time, shorter length of stay, and decreased need for blood transfusion.

   b. Endovascular repair is associated with higher rate of secondary interventions to maintain stent graft patency.

   c. Endovascular repair is associated with lower long-term patency rates.

   d. Lifelong surveillance is necessary for patients treated with endovascular and open surgical techniques.

2. A 72-year-old man is undergoing stent graft repair of a right common iliac artery aneurysm. CT scan shows evidence of 3.6-cm AAA and 3.6-cm right iliac aneurysm with a 1.5-cm distal common iliac landing zone. What type of stent graft should be planned?

   a. Right iliac stent graft; the AAA is too small to repair.

   b. AAA and iliac stent graft; might as well do both.

   c. Iliac branched device to preserve flow to the internal iliac.

   d. Cannot do a stent graft in this patient.

50 Diagnosing and Managing Internal Iliac Artery Aneurysms

RAFAEL D. MALGOR and GUSTAVO S. ODERICH

Presentation

A 72-year-old male patient with hypertension, hyperlipidemia, colonic diverticulosis, constipation, and benign prostatic hyperplasia (BPH) is referred for evaluation of left lower extremity edema, cyanosis, and left lower abdominal discomfort that have gradually worsened over the past 2 weeks. The patient denied history of traumatic injuries or prior venous thrombosis. When questioned about similar symptoms in the past, he recalled an episode of urinary retention that resolved after urinary catheterization. A month prior to presentation, the patient underwent a transurethral resection of prostate (TURP) and cystoscopy, which was negative for any masses. His last month digital rectal exam was unremarkable for any gross abnormalities except prostate enlargement compatible with BPH; his prostate-specific antigen was within normal limits. The patient also denied any previous episodes of diverticulitis. He had no fever, chills, weight loss, and changes in bowel habitus, blood per rectum, hematuria, or dysuria. His surgical history was notable for open appendectomy, laparoscopic cholecystectomy, left great saphenous vein stripping, open abdominal aortic aneurysm repair, and right total knee replacement. The patient states that he only drinks alcohol on special occasions and that he had a 65-pack-year smoking history but has recently quit. He denied intravenous drug abuse. His father and mother had passed away of causes that were unknown to him.

At presentation, the patient is not in any acute distress. Positive findings of physical examination are a left lower quadrant machinery-type bruit radiating to the left groin but no abdominal tenderness to palpation. The abdomen was not distended, and no ecchymosis or mottling was noted. No abdominal pulsatile mass was felt, and lower extremity pulses were easily palpable throughout the lower extremities. Engorged veins were easily seen in the groin and proximal thigh area. There was a palpable thrill in the left groin. Significant edema in the entire left lower extremity along with modest cyanosis was clearly noted compared to his right lower extremity (Fig. 1). Laboratory test results, such as complete blood count, coagulation, and chemistry panel, were within normal limits.

Differential Diagnosis

The differential diagnosis of left lower extremity edema is broad, but machinery-type bruit and left lower quadrant discomfort are strongly suggestive of an arteriovenous fistula (AVF). The most common causes of acquired AVFs are traumatic injuries, such as penetrating or blunt trauma, prior endovascular procedures, and abdominal, pelvic, or spine surgery. On rare occasions, patients with aortic or iliac artery aneurysms can present with contained rupture of the aneurysm into a large vein causing a spontaneous AVFs. The most common location is an aortic aneurysm associated with aortocaval fistula. Our patient denied any traumatic injuries or spine surgery. His only pelvic procedure was TURP for BPH.

A rare complication of TURP is the occurrence of an AVF associated with the procedure, but this is extremely rare. Lower extremity edema can be found in this particular scenario, but it is often seen in patients with sizeable, high-flow AVFs. Another symptom often associated with AVF secondary to TURP is hematuria. Deep vein thrombosis (DVT) should be in the differential diagnosis of any patient with asymmetric lower extremity edema. Often, DVT is associated with lower extremity pain, which is not present in this scenario. Other classic predisposing

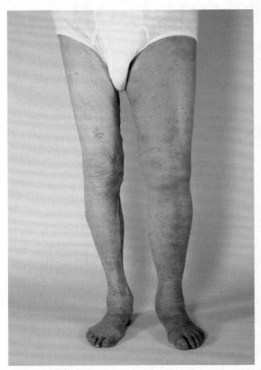

FIGURE 1 • 72 year-old male with left lower extremity edema and audible left lower quadrant machinery-type bruit.

factors for DVT, such as major surgery, multiple trauma, hip or knee surgery, prolonged immobility, or known malignancy, are not present. Most importantly, the presence of a left lower quadrant bruit favors the diagnosis of an AVF over DVT.

Workup

A duplex ultrasound of lower extremity veins was obtained that revealed no evidence of DVT but arterial waveforms consistent with AVF. A computed tomography angiography (CTA) of the abdomen and pelvis was performed. It is not infrequent that a CT with oral contrast is performed to rule out intra-abdominal inflammatory or infectious disease, such as diverticulitis or infectious colitis, in a patient who presents with abdominal discomfort of unknown cause. In this patient with a bruit suggestive of AVF, a CTA with lower extremity runoff is the most appropriate imaging study, providing detailed imaging for diagnosis and therapeutic planning. In addition, helical CTA provides small cuts (≤3 mm) and delineate the vascular anatomy in preparation for potential endovascular treatment. If a patient with suspected large-volume AVF involving the aorta or iliac arteries, or in those with symptomatic aneurysm disease, a CTA should be obtained.

Lower extremity venous duplex ultrasound in patients with lower extremity edema is an excellent screening study. Advantages include low cost, portability, safety to use, ease of repetition, and noninvasive features. In this

patient, a DU was obtained, confirming the diagnosis of AVF and no evidence of DVT. However, the study is limited in its ability to provide enough anatomical information for definitive diagnosis and therapeutic planning. It can be limited in some patients because of bowel gas and body habitus. In this particular scenario, there was no contraindication for CTA that is a more complete and detailed study especially to rule out an AVF in the pelvis. Further, CT is not operator dependent, and it can be obtained in a very expeditious manner.

Workup (CTA of the Abdomen and Pelvis)

A CT of the abdomen showed an AVF between a 4-cm left internal iliac artery (IIA) aneurysm and the left internal iliac vein (Fig. 2). The right CIA and IIA were patent and nonaneurysmal. Colonic diverticulosis, but no inflamed diverticula, was also noted.

Diagnosis and Treatment

The diagnosis is a symptomatic AVF between a left internal iliac artery aneurysm (IIAA) and left internal iliac vein. Nonetheless, the majority of IIAAs are first diagnosed incidentally by abdominal imaging (CT or ultrasound) performed for other reasons. Up to one third of patients with AAAs have an iliac artery aneurysm. On the other hand, 70% to 80% of patients with iliac artery aneurysms have AAAs. The estimated incidence of isolated iliac artery aneurysms, which most commonly involves the common iliac artery, is only about 2% of all intra-abdominal aneurysms. Of those isolated iliac artery aneurysms, approximately 20% are confined to the IIA. Overall, isolated IIAAs occur in approximately 0.3% to 0.5% of patients with intra-abdominal aneurysms. The majority of patients with IIAA are male with a mean age of 72 years, which is compatible with our case.

The natural history of IIAAs still remains unknown. The vast majority of patients remain asymptomatic. In contemporary reports, most patients with IIAAs are asymptomatic and treated in conjunction with concomitant aortic or common iliac artery aneurysms. Nonetheless, IIAAs can cause complications by rupture or local compression of adjacent organs. Patients with IIAAs can present with urinary symptoms, renal failure, lumbosacral, groin, hip or buttock pain, rectal bleeding, constipation, or DVT. Similar to our case, urinary symptoms are often obstructive in nature due to compression of the bladder by the aneurysm or caused by ureteric compression with subsequent hydronephrosis, pyelonephritis, and renal failure. Intermittent hematuria secondary to a ruptured IIAA into the bladder has been reported associated or not with scrotal ecchymosis. Left lower quadrant discomfort is usually secondary to compression or deviation of the sigmoid colon and rectum by the aneurysm causing worsening of constipation, tenesmus, and rectal pain. Due to its pelvic location, neurologic symptoms related to nerve

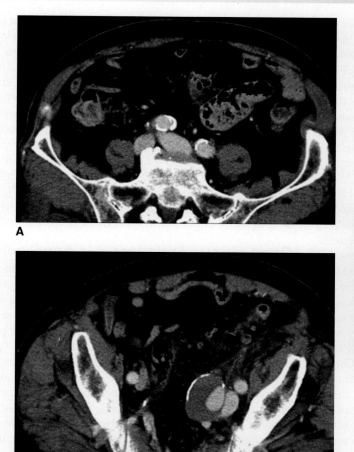

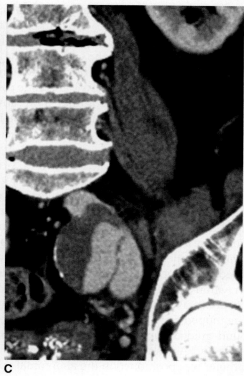

FIGURE 2 • **A:** This CTA of the abdomen shows simultaneous contrast enhancement of both common iliac artery and vein. **B** and **C:** An arteriovenous fistula is suspected between a 4cm-IIAA and the iliac vein. The communication between the IIAA and the vein can be clearly identified.

compression, such as ipsilateral leg pain, paresis, sciatic neuralgia, and lumbosacral pain secondary to compression of the pelvic and lumbosacral nerve roots, have also been reported.

There are several potential treatment options for patients with IIAAs. The relationship between IIAA size and rupture has not been well established. Current recommendations for repair include presence of rupture, symptoms, or a size diameter of 3 to 4 cm in asymptomatic patients. In the patient herein described, treatment is recommended independent of the size of the aneurysm. Nonetheless, most patients with symptoms have large aneurysm, as exemplified by this case. Treatment selection should take into consideration the size, extent of disease in the contralateral IIA, involvement of other aortic segments, and patency of IIA branches. A critical question is the presence of bilateral IIA involvement or adequacy of the contralateral IIA. Preservation of pelvic flow is important to prevent ischemic complications. In patients with unilateral IIAAs, surgical ligation or more frequently IIAA catheter embolization can be performed with low rate of severe ischemic complications because of rich cross-pelvic collateral network. In

these patients, embolization of distal branches is more frequently associated with ischemic symptoms as compared to exclusion of the main trunk of the IIA. One exception is patients with aortic disease affecting the thoracic or thoracoabdominal segments. In these patients, preservation of any IIA flow is critical to help prevent spinal cord injury; embolization of IIA should therefore be avoided whenever possible.

Bilateral involvement of the IIA can be challenging, particularly if the aneurysm involves the distal branches. Exclusion of both IIA can be performed but carries a higher risk of serious ischemic complications, such as ischemic colitis, buttock muscle, or pelvic ischemia. More frequently, patients may notice erectile dysfunction and/or buttock claudication. In these patients, preservation of at least one of the IIAs is recommended.

Endovascular interruption of the IIA can be performed using several techniques. Most often this is done with coil embolization, placement of endovascular plugs, stent graft coverage, or a combination of these. In this patient with AVF, it is critical to eliminate inflow into the fistulous communication. Because the right IIA was patent, exclusion of the left IIA was the least invasive and most straightforward alternative. This was done by placement of coils and Amplatzer plugs into the distal branches of the IIA along with coverage of the proximal IIA inflow by placement of a stent graft from the left CIA to the EIA.

Open repair remains an option but carries higher risk of complications in a patient with AVF and large collateral veins adjacent to the aneurysm. Other more advanced endovascular and hybrid techniques are available if preservation of IIA flow is indicated or warranted (see below).

Case Continued

All potential risks including, but not limited to major bleeding, buttock claudication, erectile dysfunction, colonic ischemia requiring colectomy and colostomy creation, myocardial infarction, stroke, and death and the benefits of excluding the left common and IIAAs were discussed at length with the patient. Three units of pack red blood cells were typed, and prophylactic antibiotics were ordered to be given within an hour prior to starting the procedure.

The patient was then taken to a hybrid operating room that is equipped with wall-mounted fluoroscopy unit. Ultrasound-guided puncture of the right common femoral arteries (CFAs) was performed. A 5-French Omni-flush catheter was positioned in the abdominal aorta. An aortogram with iliac angiography was obtained to delineate the anatomy and obtain measurements of proximal and distal landing zones in the common and external iliac artery anatomy. Using contralateral right femoral

access, a 45-cm long, 6-French sheath was advanced up an over the aortic bifurcation into the left IIA. Selective catheterization of the IIA divisional branches was performed using a 100-cm, 5-French angled catheter. After selective angiography of each branch, coil embolization was performed using 0.035-inch coils to exclude the IIAAs outflow (Fig. 3A). Access from the left CFA was obtained and a 12-French sheath was advanced over an Amplatz wire into the left common iliac artery. After exclusion of the IIAA, a Gore Excluder stent graft limb was deployed from the left common to the external iliac artery covering the origin of the left IIA (Fig. 3B). Both femoral punctures were closed using a preclose technique with Perclose devices with no complications (Table 1).

Open versus Endovascular Approach

Open iliac artery aneurysm repair can be challenging in a patient with IIAA involving distal branches. In this particular patient with an AVF originating from the left IIA, the risk of bleeding from the internal iliac vein or collaterals is significant, particularly if dissection is carried deep in the pelvis. Significant inflammatory reaction and the limited operative field in a narrow pelvis make an open procedure even less desirable. Several studies have compared the results of endovascular and open surgical repair for iliac aneurysms. In most studies, the most common open surgical strategy is aneurysm exclusion by ligation. Mortality rate is similar between elective open and endovascular repair,

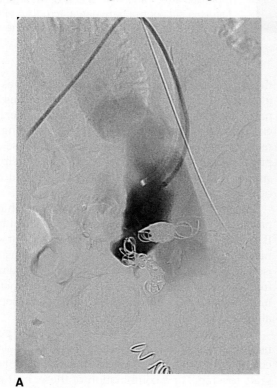
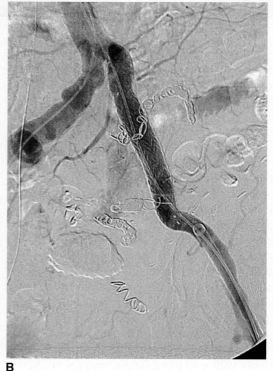

A   **B**

FIGURE 3 • Endovascular repair of left IIAA. **A:** Selective coil embolization of left IIAA via contralateral (up-and-over) approach. **B:** Iliac artery stenting with a 16x18x124 mm endograft limb across the IIA takeoff. Completion angiogram showing complete resolution of AVF.

TABLE 1. Diagnosing and Managing of IIA Aneurysm Workup and Endovascular Treatment

Key Technical Steps

1. A CTA of the abdomen should be obtained to further delineate the anatomy of iliac arteries and to measure the IIAA.
2. Preoperative planning includes evaluation of contralateral internal iliac flow to ensure that exclusion of the affected IIA can be done without compromising the pelvic flow.
3. Obtain ultrasound-guided contralateral femoral artery access.
4. Using up-and-over technique, park a guiding sheath at the orifice of the affected IIA to provide support during IIAA treatment.
5. Decision whether a Amplatzer plug or coils should be used to embolize an IIAA relies on operator's preference as patient-important outcomes are fairly similar.
6. Once exclusion of the IIAA is performed, an endograft may be placed across the orifice of IIA to limit flow to the affected IIA
7. Obtain a completion angiogram to evaluate for any endoleak

but endovascular therapy is associated with significantly less blood loss, shorter operative time, shorter hospital stay, and lower short-term morbidity rates than open repair. Pelvic flow preservation is often challenging or not possible with open repair, it makes logical sense to use a less invasive alternative to exclude flow into the IIA.

Treatment of iliac aneurysms is evolving rapidly. Hybrid repair can be performed using exposure of the IIA via a flank incision to perform bypass into the IIA, followed by placement of stent grafts. Endovascular strategies have also been widely adopted in most centers. Iliac branch devices are available to treat common iliac aneurysms using a side branch to preserve flow into one or both IIAs. In these cases, the anterior divisional branch is typically excluded by coil embolization, and the iliac branch is placed into the posterior divisional branch preserving flow into the gluteal artery. Currently, there have been more than 6000 patients treated by iliac branch devices using one of the three designs by Cook Medical Inc. (straight, helical, or bifurcated-bifurcated design). The Cook Iliac branch device and Gore iliac branch device are under clinical investigation in the United States.

Other endovascular strategies include the use of parallel stent grafts, also known as "sandwich" stent grafts. Limitations of this technique include compression of one of the side limbs with occlusion or endoleak via gutters. External to IIA stenting with femoral crossover grafts can also be performed.

Special Preoperative and Intraoperative Considerations

Preoperative planning based on patient's anatomy is critical to optimize technical result and outcomes. Some important hints include the presence of excessive iliac

tortuosity, calcification or stenosis, and involvement of the distal portion of the IIA by aneurysm. This results in inadequate distal landing zone for IIA preservation and requires extension of the repair into one of the IIA branches. If the IIA needs to be preserved because of contralateral occlusion or aneurysm, preservation of one of the internal iliac branches is a reasonable option to avoid pelvic ischemic complications. The anatomic criteria for use of internal iliac branch devices continue to evolve. These devices are typically indicated in patients with common iliac artery aneurysms with diameter greater than 20 mm who are not ideal candidates for endovascular repair with preservation of IIA flow using conventional techniques. Requirements include a 20-mm-long distal landing zone in the EIA, EIA diameter between 8 and 12 mm, CIA length of 50 mm, and the IIA with nonaneurysmal segment (fixation site) of greater than 10 mm length and inner wall diameter of 6 to 10 mm. The presence of IIA stenosis is not a contra-indication but increases technical difficulty.

Postoperative Management

The machinery-type bruit resolved immediately after IIAA repair, and the patient was able to ambulate on the same day. The puncture sites were clean and intact, renal function remained unchanged, and he was dismissed home on the first postoperative day. His left lower extremity edema significantly improved within a few days following the procedure. Repeat CTA revealed no evidence of endoleak and resolution of the AVF.

Imagining surveillance is warranted after exclusion of an IIAA. The most common complication is persistence of a type II endoleak via retrograde filling of an IIA branch. This is not infrequent due to significant collateralization that occurs after IIAA exclusion. Persistent type II endoleak should be treated by additional coil embolization if there is further aneurysm enlargement. Because inflow to the aneurysm has been often excluded, access into the aneurysm sac is difficult. This can be done via direct aneurysm puncture or using transarterial catheterization via profunda branches or contralateral IIA. Rarely, migration of coils can occur.

Open conversion after endovascular repair is rarely needed. This may be indicated in the patient with recalcitrant compression type symptoms despite endovascular treatment or for treatment of endoleaks that are not suitable to percutaneous intervention. Open surgical ligation of IIA branches is perhaps the only feasible option.

Imaging surveillance protocol includes CTA at 1 to 4 months, every 6 months in the 1st year and yearly thereafter. Nonetheless, if the aneurysm is successfully excluded in the first follow-up CTA and there is no evidence of endoleak, follow-up with yearly duplex ultrasound is adequate. CTA is recommended only if there is questionable growth or endoleak.

Case Conclusion

IIAAs are rare, but they can be associated with high mortality rates if rupture occurs. In this clinical scenario, we highlighted an usual and challenging case of IIAA. However, it is important to remember that IIAAs are often incidentally found rather than being associated with symptoms. The endovascular treatment of IIAAs follows the tenets of saccular arterial aneurysm embolization and its exclusion from systemic circulation. As depicted in this case, the best treatment option for IIAAs is now endovascular therapy.

TAKE HOME POINTS

- Isolated IIAAs are rare; half of the patients with IIAA also have a CIA aneurysm.
- CTA remains the most valuable preoperative imaging modality prior to open or endovascular treatment.
- IIAAs are often found in imaging studies obtained for other reasons (incidental finding).
- Other symptoms related to IIAAs are abdominal pain; urinary symptoms; lumbosacral, groin, hip or buttock pain; constipation; and rectal bleeding.
- All symptomatic IIAA must be treated expeditiously. The indications for IIAA treatment in asymptomatic patients remain debatable. Several specialists would recommend repair for an IIAA with diameter greater than 3.5 cm; however, the relationship between size and risk of rupture has not yet been established for this aneurysms.
- Potential complications of IIAA exclusion without pelvic revascularization are from the most to the least common complication, buttock claudication, erectile dysfunction, and colonic ischemia.
- Pelvic revascularization by endovascular means in patients with single, patent IIAA can be accomplished using iliac artery bifurcation devices or iliac sandwich or parallel stent grafts. External to IIA stenting with femoral crossover bypass has also been described.
- Endovascular therapy is associated with less blood loss, shorter operative time, shorter hospital stay, lower short-term morbidity rates but similar mortality rates when compared to open repair in patients with asymptomatic iliac artery aneurysms.

SUGGESTED READINGS

Fatima J, Correa MP, Mendes BC, et al. Pelvic revascularization during endovascular aortic aneurysm repair. *Perspect Vasc Surg Endovasc Ther.* 2012;24(2):55-62.

Huang Y, Gloviczki P, Duncan AA, et al. Common iliac artery aneurysm: expansion rate and results of open surgical and endovascular repair. *J Vasc Surg.* 2008;47(6):1203-1210.

Pitoulias GA, Donas KP, Schute S, et al. Isolated iliac artery aneurysms: endovascular versus open elective repair. *J Vasc Surg.* 2007;46:648-654.

Rana MA, Kalra M, Oderich GS, et al. Outcomes of open and endovascular repair for ruptured and nonruptured internal iliac artery aneurysms. *J Vasc Surg.* 2014;59(3):634-644.

Rayt HS, Bown MJ, Lambert KV, et al. Buttock claudication and erectile dysfunction after internal iliac artery embolization in patients prior to endovascular aortic aneurysm repair. *Cardiovasc Intervent Radiol.* 2008;31(4):728-734.

CLINICAL SCENARIO CASE QUESTIONS

1. While treating a patient with bilateral IIAA, the operator must be aware of which potential complications?
   a. Buttock claudication that is the least common complication.
   b. Erectile dysfunction that is usually transitory and occurs in less than 1% of patients with bilateral IIA embolization.
   c. Colonic ischemia that is the most common complication afflicting 10% of the patients who undergo isolated left IIA embolization.
   d. Open and endovascular iliac artery aneurysm treatment have similar operative time, length of hospital stay, and short-term morbidity rates.
   e. Regardless of the treatment modality, mortality rate is similar in patients who undergo open or endovascular treatment of an asymptomatic iliac artery aneurysms.

2. A 72-year-old morbidly obese man presents to the emergent department with lower abdominal pain. He is alert and talks coherently, his pulse is 136 bpm, and his BP is 100/65 mm Hg after 1 L of saline bolus given in the ED. Comorbidities are significant for coronary artery disease with previous coronary bypass done 7 years ago, diabetes, hyperlipidemia, and COPD on home oxygen. A CT scan shows a contained ruptured right IIAA with no concomitant CIA aneurysm. At this point, the best treatment for this patient is:
   a. Open repair with IIA branch ligation
   b. Iliac branch device to ensure pelvic flow
   c. Iliac sandwich or parallel stent grafts to avoid colonic ischemia
   d. Right internal iliac artery coil embolization
   e. External to internal iliac artery stenting with femoral crossover graft due to his advanced age

51 Thoracoabdominal Aortic Aneurysm

DONALD G. HARRIS and ROBERT S. CRAWFORD

Presentation

A 65-year-old woman with hypertension and a 30-pack-year smoking history presented to the emergency department with acute chest pain, dyspnea, nausea, and diaphoresis. The pain was sharp and radiated to her back and was associated with EKG changes and a mildly elevated troponin. An emergent left heart catheterization was negative for coronary artery disease. A chest x-ray showed a widened aortic silhouette.

Differential Diagnosis

Acute chest pain mandates evaluation for cardiac ischemia, and given this patient's history and high-risk findings, a cardiac evaluation was warranted. However, for any patient with new chest pain, acute aortic syndrome remains in the differential, especially if back pain or abdominal symptoms are present. Acute aortic events include dissection, intramural hematoma, penetrating ulcer, and aneurysm instability or rupture, all of which can be readily diagnosed by CT. Other conditions that should be considered and ruled out include pulmonary embolism, pneumothorax, and esophageal perforation.

Most thoracoabdominal aneurysms (TAAAs) are asymptomatic and are diagnosed incidentally. Alternatively, TAAA expansion with compression of neighboring structures may result in nonspecific complaints including back pain, hoarseness, or respiratory symptoms without causing acute aortic syndrome. These symptoms may mimic a variety of cardiopulmonary or abdominal conditions, such as musculoskeletal disease, pancreatitis, or nephrolithiasis. Because these conditions are relatively more common, even if TAAA is confirmed radiographically, they should be excluded by routine testing.

Workup

TAAAs can be readily diagnosed and classified by CT. To completely define the extent of the aneurysm and the anatomy of the carotid, visceral, and iliofemoral vasculature, a CT of the neck, chest, abdomen, and pelvis with contrast arteriography should be obtained. Because patients often have comorbid chronic kidney dysfunction, IV hydration should be given with contrast studies to prevent nephropathy. Alternatively, magnetic resonance aortography is an option if contrast and radiation exposures are of concern. Once defined, the proximal and distal extent of the lesion dictates how the aneurysm is resected and reconstructed, and the aneurysm can be classified according to the Crawford scheme (Fig. 1).

Most TAAAs are due to degenerative aortic disease, which is often associated with hypertension, atherosclerosis, and smoking. As such, patients considered for elective surgery should undergo cardiac risk stratification and pulmonary function testing, with appropriate management as indicated.

Discussion

This patient had a negative cardiac catheterization, but a chest x-ray was suggestive of aortic disease. As such, a contrast CT was obtained and demonstrated diffuse, multilevel aortic degeneration consistent with a Crawford type II aneurysm (Fig. 2). As part of her preoperative cardiac evaluation, a transthoracic echocardiogram was performed, which demonstrated normal left ventricular function and an ejection fraction of 65%.

Diagnosis and Treatment

This patient has a symptomatic Crawford type II TAAA complicated by acute aortic syndrome. Her cardiac workup demonstrates acceptable risk for surgery, but the urgent nature of her presentation precludes pulmonary preconditioning and smoking cessation. For asymptomatic patients, repair should be performed if the aneurysm diameter is ≥6 cm (or ≥5 cm with Marfan's disease) or increases by ≥1.0 cm/year. The patient's large, symptomatic TAAA and acceptable cardiac risk warrant operative repair to prevent progression to frank rupture.

Surgical Approach

Repair techniques have evolved over time. Although a major advance at the time, the "clamp-and-sew" technique is associated with significant mortality and paraplegia rates, despite improvements in technique and perioperative care. Clamp and sew remains appropriate for type IV lesions where proximal aortic clamping poses decreased risk for spinal ischemia.

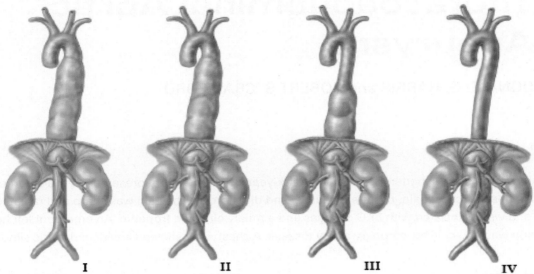

FIGURE 1 • Crawford classification of thoracoabdominal aneurysms. (From Cambria RP, Crawford RS. Thoracoabdominal aortic aneurysm repair. In: Jones DB, Pomposelli FB, Upchurch GR, eds. *Fischer's Mastery of Surgery*. 6th ed. Philadelphia, PA: Lippincott Williams & Wilkins; 2011:2203, Chapter 217.)

More recently, segmental clamping with distal perfusion has become the standard of care for type I to III lesions. Using this method, the aneurysm is clamped, resected, and sequentially reconstructed proximally to distally. Distal arterial perfusion is maintained via full cardiopulmonary bypass, left atriofemoral bypass, or a temporary axillofemoral bypass, which maintains visceral and pelvic perfusion, improves spinal blood flow, and reduces complication rates. The addition of cerebrospinal fluid (CSF) drainage further minimizes the risk of spinal cord ischemia. Finally, intraoperative motor evoked potentials enable monitoring for neurologic deficits and guide reimplantation of intercostal and lumbar arteries if needed.

The details of aortic resection and reconstruction vary depending on the TAAA extent. Generally, a CSF drainage catheter is placed in the lumbar spine subarachnoid space prior to surgery, and right-sided radial and femoral arterial catheters enable monitoring of systemic and distal perfusion, respectively. The patient is placed in a right lateral decubitus position. To facilitate maximal thoracic and visceral exposure, left shoulder is flexed with the arm placed across the table, and the right anterior superior iliac spine is positioned at the break of the table. Appropriate padding is required to prevent skin breakdown at pressure points during these long procedures.

The level of the initial left thoracoabdominal incision is dictated by the proximal aneurysm extent. For type I and II aneurysms, incision through the fourth to sixth intercostal space facilitates proximal and distal exposure, while for type III lesions, a lower incision may suffice. The standard incision for a type IV repair is a thoracoabdominal incision through the ninth inter-

space. The incision is carried distally along the lateral rectus border to limit functional impairment from rectus transection. Medial visceral rotation is performed to expose the abdominal aorta, which is then dissected inferiorly and superiorly from the left renal artery origin. The left diaphragm is divided circumferentially to spare the phrenic nerve and avoid postoperative paralysis of the hemidiaphragm.

After exposure of the aneurysm, a Dacron graft is sized to the patient's anatomy and customized for the specific reconstruction. For distal perfusion using left atriofemoral bypass, a circuit is established by cannulating the left atrium via the left inferior pulmonary vein and bypassing blood to the left common femoral artery. Alternatively, a temporary right axillo-femoral bypass can provide distal perfusion. Next, the thoracic aorta is clamped proximal to aneurysm. Retrograde distal aortic perfusion is then established and distal pressure confirmed through a right femoral arterial catheter. The aneurysm is opened, and bleeding intercostal arteries are ligated or occluded with Fogarty balloon catheters for possible later reimplantation.

The proximal anastomosis is performed. Depending on the quality of the proximal aorta, pledgets can be fashioned to provide a secure proximal suture line. The clamps are moved distally and the aorta opened through the visceral segment. The renal arteries are perfused with cold perfusate to limit warm ischemia. The anastomosis of the visceral patch that includes the celiac, superior mesenteric, and right renal arteries is performed in a circumferential fashion. Special attention is paid to the posterior suture line as bleeding from this segment can be difficult to control. The left renal artery is reconstructed separately using an end-to-end PTFE graft.

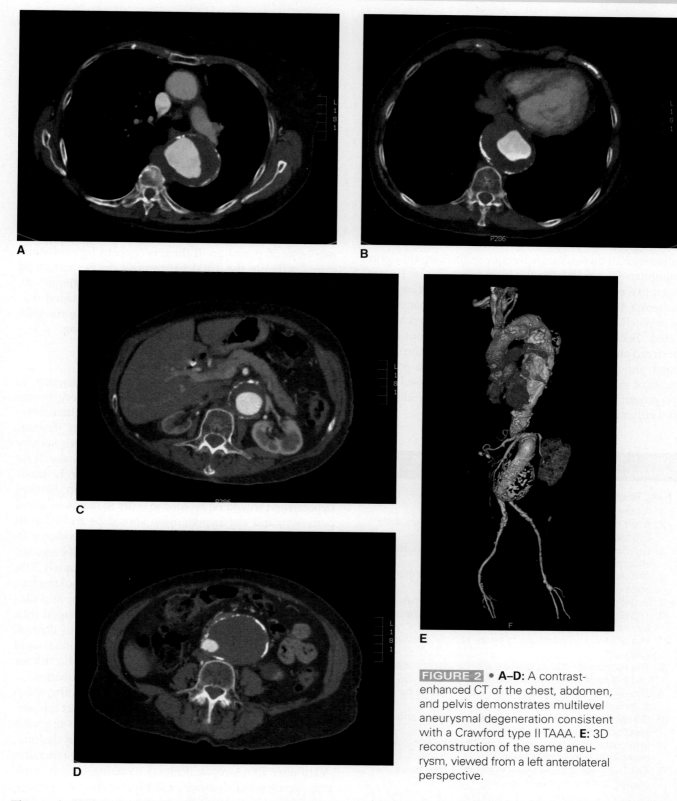

FIGURE 2 • **A–D:** A contrast-enhanced CT of the chest, abdomen, and pelvis demonstrates multilevel aneurysmal degeneration consistent with a Crawford type II TAAA. **E:** 3D reconstruction of the same aneurysm, viewed from a left anterolateral perspective.

This is fashioned with a gentle curve from the aortic prosthesis to avoid kinking. Alternatively, the renal artery can be reimplanted directly onto the Dacron graft with a Carrel patch. If motor evoked potentials dictate, spinal arteries can be reimplanted.

Finally, the distal aortic anastomosis is performed in an end-to-end fashion. For type I repairs, the anastomosis can be beveled to include the visceral vessels. Perfusion of the legs and visceral arteries is confirmed by palpation and Doppler ultrasound. The aneurysm sac is closed over the graft, the diaphragm is reconstructed, and a left chest tube is placed. Complete hemostasis is ensured, the incision is closed, and the patient is transferred to the intensive care unit.

Potential Pitfalls

Due to frequently comorbid tobacco use and lung disease, these patients are at significant risk for postoperative pulmonary complications. Hemidiaphragm paralysis can be avoided by circumferential, as opposed to radial, division during exposure. This reduces postoperative lung collapse and its associated complications. If there is an inflammatory component to the aneurysm, dissection of the thoracic aorta may be complicated by adhesions to the lung or other mediastinal structures. In this situation, adherence to meticulous technique with sharp dissection minimizes bleeding from the lung parenchyma. If intraoperative evoked motor potential signals indicate spinal ischemia, the critical T9-L1 arteries can be reconstructed as a patch, or individual segments reimplanted as indicated. Because residual aortic tissue can continue to undergo aneurysmal degeneration, the size of the visceral patch should be kept to a minimum. Finally, a potential cause of major postoperative bleeding is a missed patent intercostal or lumbar artery, which should be identified and either ligated or reimplanted (Table 1).

TABLE 1. Open Thoracoabdominal Aortic Aneurysm Repair

Key Technical Steps

1. A lumbar CSF drainage catheter is placed.
2. A left thoracoabdominal incision is made to adequately expose the TAAA.
3. Left medial visceral rotation is performed to expose the abdominal aorta.
4. The diaphragm is circumferentially divided and thoracic aorta exposed.
5. Distal perfusion is provided via atriofemoral bypass.
6. The proximal aorta is clamped and opened; spinal arteries are ligated or occluded.
7. The proximal anastomosis is sewn, and distal control is obtained.
8. The remaining TAAA is opened and the visceral island and left renal anastomoses performed.
9. The distal anastomosis is made, which may be beveled to include visceral vessels.
10. Complete hemostasis is achieved and visceral and leg perfusion ensured.
11. Intercostal arteries are reimplanted if dictated by changes in evoked potentials.
12. The TAAA sac is closed over the graft, a chest tube is placed, and the incision is closed.

Potential Pitfalls

- Radial division and subsequent paralysis of the diaphragm
- Missed back bleeding from patent spinal arteries
- Renal artery impingement by the visceral patch anastomosis
- Excess aneurysmal tissue in implanted patches

Special Intraoperative Considerations

Impingement of the right renal artery from the visceral patch anastomosis or kinking of the reconstructed left renal artery can cause postoperative renal dysfunction or failure, so the anastomoses should be constructed to ensure patency and blood flow verified prior to closure. If there is significant right renal artery atherosclerosis, intraoperative angioplasty and stenting can be performed. Antegrade visceral perfusion off the bypass circuit can be used to maintain visceral perfusion during reconstruction. If the visceral patch or island is not possible, or if the quality of the patch is in question, the visceral vessels can be individually bypassed. In this situation, exposure of the proximal celiac and superior mesenteric arteries can facilitate rapid aortomesenteric bypass if required to salvage visceral perfusion. If there is concern for prolonged spinal ischemia, the distal anastomosis can be performed before the left renal anastomosis. Finally, in patients with concomitant iliac aneurysmal disease, a bifurcated iliofemoral graft can be sewn to the distal main aortic graft and used to anastomose distal to the obstruction.

Postoperative Management

Postoperative care requires ongoing management to prevent spinal cord ischemia. Early after surgery, hourly neurologic monitoring is required and can facilitate interventions to improve spinal ischemia if deficits develop. Spinal drainage is continued for 48 hours after surgery with protocolized measurement of hourly drainage. If no deficits develop, the drain can be clamped for 12 hours and removed if no neurologic deficits develop. Further, hypotension should be avoided in order to maintain spinal perfusion, and any hypertension should be treated with short-acting agents. Finally, there is limited evidence to support intravenous naloxone as a neuroprotective adjunct.

Pulmonary complications occur in approximately 50% of patients and are due to a combination of smoking history and/or chronic lung disease, thoracotomy, and diaphragm dissection. These can typically be managed with judicious ventilator weaning, appropriate pain control, and aggressive pulmonary toilet. Special attention should be paid following chest tube removal due to the risk for atelectasis, pneumonia, and the need for reintubation.

Because of potential postoperative coagulopathy, reversal of anticoagulants, platelet, and blood product replacement is often necessary to limit bleeding. Postoperative acute kidney injury is common, and severe renal dysfunction is one of the strongest predictors of postoperative death after TAAA repair. Patients requiring dialysis while undergoing spinal drainage or in the presence of a postoperative neurologic deficit should undergo continuous venovenous hemodialysis to minimize potential spinal ischemia. Ultimately, although perioperative mortality after TAAA repair has historically been around 5% to 10%, rates as low as 2% have been reported by incorporating distal pelvic and visceral perfusion and optimal perioperative care.

Case Conclusion

The patient was transferred to the intensive care unit, where she was extubated on postoperative day 2. She tolerated clamping and subsequent removal of her CSF drain without complication and was discharged for brief inpatient rehabilitation. By 6 months, she was near her functional baseline, and follow-up imaging demonstrated a satisfactory reconstruction.

TAKE HOME POINTS

- TAAAs may be diagnosed incidentally or may result in mild symptoms or acute aortic syndrome.
- Symptomatic TAAAs generally cause nonspecific symptoms, but can be readily diagnosed by CT.
- Patients with symptomatic or large TAAAs should undergo repair.
- Repair with CSF drainage and distal perfusion improves surgical outcomes.
- Perioperative care requires diligent management of cardiopulmonary and renal dysfunction.

SUGGESTED READINGS

Cambria RP, Crawford RS. Thoracoabdominal aortic aneurysm repair. In: Jones DB, Pomposelli FB, Upchurch GR, eds. *Fischer's Mastery of Surgery*. Philadelphia, PA: Lippincott Williams & Wilkins; 2011.

Conrad MF, Crawford RS, Davison JK, et al. Thoracoabdominal aneurysm repair: a 20-year perspective. *Ann Thorac Surg.* 2007;83:S856-S861.

Conrad MF, Ergul EA, Patel VI, et al. Evolution of operative strategies in open thoracoabdominal aneurysm repair. *J Vasc Surg.* 2011;53:1195-1201.

Coselli JS, LeMaire SA, Koksoy C, et al. Cerebrospinal fluid drainage reduces paraplegia after thoracoabdominal aortic aneurysm repair: results of a randomized clinical trial. *J Vasc Surg.* 2002;35:631-639.

Odero A, Arici V, Bozzani A. Clinical presentation and evidence-based indications to treat. In: Chiesa R, Melissano G, Zangrillo A, eds. *Thoraco-Abdominal Aorta: Surgical and Anesthetic Management*. Milan, Italy: Springer; 2011.

CLINICAL SCENARIO CASE QUESTIONS

1. Which of the following is not a component of limiting spinal ischemia during extensive TAAA repair?

   a. Spinal CSF drainage
   b. Distal pelvic perfusion
   c. Systemic anticoagulation
   d. Avoiding intra- and postoperative hypotension

2. Which of the following is not an acceptable way to reconstruct the visceral arteries?

   a. As a celiac, superior mesenteric and right renal arterial patch or island
   b. A circumferential cuff incorporating the spinal, renal, and visceral arteries
   c. A beveled patch incorporated into the distal anastomosis
   d. Individual grafts from the aortic prosthesis to the visceral arteries

52 Hybrid Thoracoabdominal Aortic Aneurysm Repair

JEFF MATHEW, PRAVEEN C. BALRAJ, and LOAY S. KABBANI

Presentation

A 65-year-old female, who is a 50-pack-year smoker, is referred by her primary care physician who felt a pulsatile abdominal mass. The patient is not experiencing pain and has no complaints other than some back discomfort. A review of the patient's past medical history reveals poorly controlled hypertension and chronic obstructive pulmonary disease (COPD). The patient is partially dependent on 2 L/min of oxygen at home. She can walk up one flight of stairs, but gets dyspneic. She did not have any previous abdominal surgeries. Physical examination reveals a nontender abdomen, with a pulsatile epigastric mass left of midline.

Differential Diagnosis

The most common etiology of a pulsatile epigastric mass is aortic aneurysm. Much less common is superior mesenteric aneurysm. Other entities that transmit the aortic pulse to the abdominal wall and can mimic abdominal aortic aneurysms are tumors, pancreatic pseudocysts, hepatomegaly secondary to right heart failure, and an enlarged spleen. Keep in mind, though, that in a thin patient, a normal aorta can be palpated and mistaken for an abnormal pulsating mass. Conversely, the aneurysm cannot be palpated in 24% patients with a greater than 5 cm abdominal aneurysm.

Workup

The patient's serum creatinine is 0.9 mg/dL. A cardiac stress test was performed 6 months prior to admission for atypical chest pain and revealed no significant ischemia. Pulmonary function tests report an FEV1 of 1.2 L/min (30% predicted), an FVC of 1.7 L (35% predicted), an FEV1/FVC of less than 0.7, and a 20% improvement after using bronchodilators.

CT Scan

A thin-slice (1.5 mm) CT angiogram (CTA) is ordered. A 7.0-cm nonruptured thoracoabdominal aneurysm (TAAA) is seen, extending from the midthoracic aorta to the level of the renal arteries (type V) (Fig. 1). There is a moderate amount of intraluminal thrombus in the aneurysm sac. The ostium of the superior mesenteric artery (SMA) has moderate amount of atherosclerotic disease, but no stenosis. The celiac artery has a high-grade stenosis at its origin, and the inferior mesenteric artery (IMA) is occluded. Both renal arteries are patent. The femoral and iliac arteries are of good caliber.

Discussion

Unfortunately, very few patients with aortic aneurysms present with symptoms prior to an acute aortic event, with most events occurring in the absence of heralding symptoms. Symptoms may include a dull abdominal or thoracic pain or pressure, or, in the event of rupture, patients may experience an acute tearing or stabbing chest or back pain. As with other forms of aortic aneurysms, TAAAs are usually detected during an examination for other conditions. When working up the patient, it is important to perform a comprehensive history and physical examination and investigative studies. Of particular importance is assessment of cardiac, respiratory, and renal function (Fig. 2).

CTA is an expedient and extremely accurate way to diagnose aortic aneurysms. When performing imaging for a suspected aortic disease, it is important to delineate the whole thoracic and abdominal aorta and to rule out other areas of aneurysmal dilation (found in up to 12% of patients). Renal function must be evaluated prior to imaging with intravenous contrast. CTA provides most of the diagnostic information needed; it can reveal the presence of hostile angles, atherosclerosis of branch vessels, and the presence of thrombus in the aorta. It can also provide measurements for endovascular repair planning, in terms of landing zones, location of branch vessels, size of endografts needed, and whether access vessels are of sufficient size to permit endograft deployment. CTA can also provide valuable information for open repair, such as optimal location for aortic clamping, and location/patency of branch vessels. Such knowledge gained preoperatively can transform a "hostile terrain" into a more manageable one.

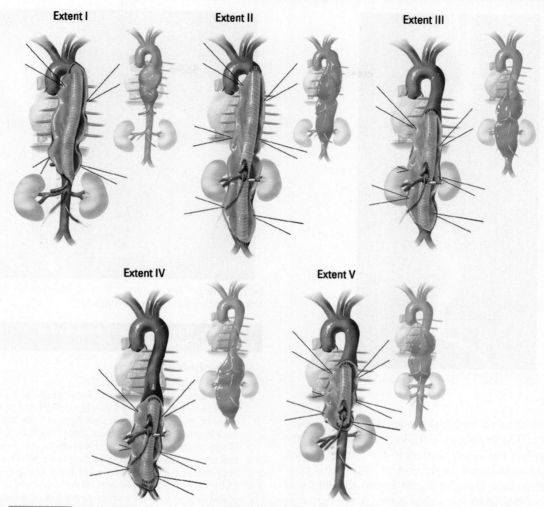

FIGURE 1 • TAAAs, classified by the proximal and distal extent of the aortic aneurysm. (Adapted from Frederick JR, Woo YJ. Thoracoabdominal aortic aneurysm. *Ann Cardiothorac Surg.* 2012;1(3): 277–285.) Type I involves most of the descending thoracic aorta from the origin of the left subclavian to the suprarenal abdominal aorta. Type II is the most extensive, extending from the subclavian to the aortoiliac bifurcation. Type III involves the distal thoracic aorta to the aortoiliac bifurcation. Type IV is limited to the abdominal aorta below the diaphragm. Type V extends from the distal thoracic aorta including the celiac and superior mesenteric origins, but not the renal arteries.

Size of the aneurysm and rate of growth are important predictors of rupture. Size criteria for repair of TAAA are not as clearly defined as for infrarenal AAA. Adjustment for body surface area needs to be incorporated into the decision making when it comes to the optimal time for repair. Most surgeons would consider repairing a TAAA in an average-sized patient when it reaches 6 to 6.5 cm in diameter, with a lower threshold for aneurysms in patients with connective tissue disorders. According to Elefteriades, a descending thoracic aorta that has reached 6 cm maximal diameter faces the following yearly rates of devastating adverse events: rupture (3.6%), dissection (3.7%), and death (10.8%). A 7-cm aneurysm has a lifetime rupture risk of 43%. Overt symptoms and yearly aneurysm growth (greater than 10 mm/year) are other indications for repair. Aortic

rupture is a catastrophic event with extremely high morbidity and mortality.

The treatment of TAAA is contingent upon the balance between the risk of rupture and the risk associated with operative repair. Treating TAAA is more complicated than is managing infrarenal aortic aneurysms, because the mesenteric and renal vessels are contained within the repair zone. There are three operative approaches to consider: open, endovascular, and hybrid repair.

Open surgical repair is the traditional modality and the gold standard for managing this aneurysm. However, the thoracoabdominal incision carries significant morbidity and is associated with a high mortality rate in a patient who has significant pulmonary insufficiency.

Use of fenestrated endografts provides an alternative option. It avoids a large, traumatic incision and may

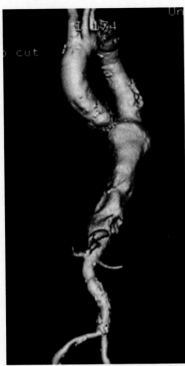

FIGURE 2 • CTA showing TAAA.

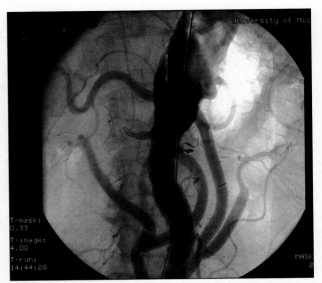

FIGURE 3 • Angiogram following four-vessel debranching documenting patency of bypasses.

be better tolerated in high-risk patients. This approach, however, is still in its infancy. Fenestrated endografts are offered in only a few select centers in the United States, though more centers are beginning to utilize this procedure. Our patient has significant mural thrombus in the vicinity of her SMA, her celiac artery is severely diseased, and her IMA is not patent. There is a serious risk of embolizing thrombus into the SMA while attempting to cannulate the SMA and placing the covered stent, making an endograft a less attractive alternative (Fig. 3).

The third option for this patient is a hybrid approach (hybrid open endovascular repair [HOER]). This divides the operation into two stages. The first stage creates landing zones for an endoprosthesis, which is accomplished by bypassing visceral vessels (debranching) in a retrograde or antegrade fashion. The second stage is placement of an endograft, to exclude the diseased aneurysmal aorta from the systemic circulation. By eliminating aortic cross-clamping, avoiding a thoracoabdominal incision that would require division of the diaphragm, and decreasing intraoperative ischemia, a hybrid repair is thought to improve operative survival and reduce morbidity, compared with conventional open surgery.

The two stages of the hybrid repair may be performed during the same operation, though separating the procedures may improve outcomes.

Treatment

The patient is offered a hybrid repair with visceral debranching through a midline laparotomy, followed by endograft repair of her TAAA.

TABLE 1. Key Technical Steps and Potential Pitfalls

Key Technical Steps

1. Perform midline laparotomy.
2. Celiac artery exposure; first, dissect out the suprarenal aorta by taking down the triangular ligament of the liver, entering the lesser sac and taking down the crus of the diaphragm. The celiac trunk is identified after dissection of the neural tissue around the aorta.
3. The SMA is exposed by retracting the transverse colon cephalad and small bowel to the right. The proximal SMA (up to middle colic and ileocolic branch) is palpated at the root of the mesentery to the left of the superior mesenteric vein. The origin of the SMA may be exposed through a left medial visceral rotation in mesentery to the right of the fourth portion of the duodenum.
4. The right renal artery is exposed by a right medial visceral rotation or just off the aorta below the left renal vein.
5. The left renal artery is exposed by a left medial visceral rotation or just off the aorta below the left renal vein.
6. On the back table, make a Y graft using a 7- or 8-mm ring thin-walled PTFE graft and a 5- or 6-mm ring thin-walled PTFE graft for the renal bypasses.
7. The bypass to visceral vessels is taken off the distal aorta or iliac artery. The grafts are tunneled through the retroperitoneal space.
8. Visceral bypasses should be constructed in a "lazy C" configuration to avoid kinking.
9. Placement of an endograft is performed during the primary procedure or during a follow-up secondary procedure.

Potential Pitfalls

- Kinking of grafts postoperatively can cause mesenteric ischemia or renal artery occlusion.
- Spinal cord ischemia can result from the thoracic endograft covering the intercostal arteries/artery of Adamkiewicz (the risk of spinal cord ischemia can be decreased by increasing spinal perfusion pressure; this is achieved by draining CSF, preventing hypotension, and, if necessary, medically inducing hypertension).
- Ligate the proximal end of the native arteries to prevent endoleaks.

Operative Details

The patient is brought to the operating room, where the anesthesiologist placed a spinal drain. A midline incision is performed. The celiac axis, SMA, and bilateral renal arteries are dissected out (Table 1). A retrograde anastomosis is created using a branched PTFE graft from the right external iliac artery to the right renal artery and SMA. Another branched PTFE graft is taken off the left external iliac artery and anastomosed to left renal and celiac arteries. A lazy C configuration is created to prevent kinking of the grafts. The aortic stent graft is placed via a standard femoral artery approach.

Postoperative Management

It is important to be vigilant in detecting spinal cord ischemia. If there is evidence of motor function loss postoperatively, a spinal drain (if not previously placed) should be inserted and the mean arterial pressure elevated to increase spinal perfusion pressure. Also, these patients may develop renal failure and mesenteric ischemia.

Case Conclusion

The patient was seen 6 weeks postoperatively and is recovering well. Her CTA (Fig. 4) revealed no endoleaks, and all of her bypasses were patent.

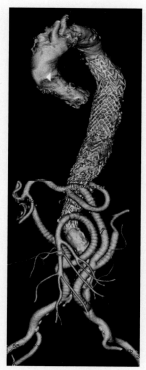

FIGURE 4 • CTA at follow-up following four-vessel debranching and endovascular stent graft placement.

TAKE HOME POINTS

- The goal of surgical repair of TAAAs is to prolong the patient's life and avoid the morbidity and mortality due to dissection or rupture.
- CTA is the imaging modality of choice.
- There are three operative approaches: open, endovascular (fenestrated or branched endografts), and a hybrid approach.
- Hybrid approaches still carry significant mortality and morbidity, but theoretically offer a less traumatic approach. Given the right indications, they are a good treatment option.

SUGGESTED READINGS

Biasi L, Ali T, Loosemore T, et al. Hybrid repair of complex thoracoabdominal aortic aneurysms using applied endovascular strategies combined with visceral and renal revascularization. *J Thorac Cardiovasc Surg.* 2009;138:1331-1338.

Drinkwater SL, Bockler D, Eckstein H, et al. The visceral hybrid repair of thoracoabdominal aortic aneurysms—a collaborative approach. *Eur J Vasc Endovasc Surg.* 2009;38(5):578-585.

Elefteriades JA, Botta DM Jr. Indications for the treatment of thoracic aortic aneurysms. *Surg Clin North Am.* 2009;89(4):845-867.

Kabbani LS, Criado E, Upchurch GR Jr, et al. Hybrid repair of aortic aneurysms involving the visceral and renal vessels. *Ann Vasc Surg.* 2010;24(2):219-222.

Moulakakis KG, Mylonas SN, Avgerinos ED, et al. Hybrid open endovascular technique for aortic thoracoabdominal pathologies. *Circulation.* 2011;124(24):2670-2680.

Quinones-Baldrich W, Jimenez JC, DeRubertis B, et al. Combined endovascular and surgical approach (CESA) to thoracoabdominal aortic pathology: a 10-year experience. *J Vasc Surg.* 2009;49(5):1125-1134.

CLINICAL SCENARIO CASE QUESTIONS

1. Concerning the optimal size to repair a thoracoabdominal aneurysm (TAAA):
   a. 5.0 to 5.5 cm has been shown to be the most suitable size to repair TAAA.
   b. Due to the high complication rate and risk of spinal cord ischemia, TAAA repair is best performed when the patient becomes symptomatic.
   c. Optimal size recommended to repair a TAAA depends on the patient's body size.
   d. Connective tissue disorders do not play a role in the decision with regard to the optimal size recommended to repair a TAAA.
   e. Saccular and fusiform aneurysms are treated similarly in terms of the size recommended to repair them.

2. Type I TAAA:
   a. Is an aortic aneurysm extending from the innominate artery to just below the visceral vessels

b. Involves the descending thoracic aorta from the origin of the left subclavian to the suprarenal abdominal aorta

c. Extends from the subclavian artery to the aortoiliac bifurcation

d. Involves the distal thoracic aorta and extends to the aortoiliac bifurcation

e. Extends from the distal thoracic aorta to the celiac and superior mesenteric artery origins, but not the renal arteries

53 Endovascular Thoracoabdominal Aortic Aneurysm Repair

GUILLERMO A. ESCOBAR

Presentation

A 65-year-old male presents to the emergency room with a 3-month history of progressive back pain that was unrelieved by oral pain medications and multiple visits to a chiropractor. He also states he has had progressive, painless dysphasia that was evaluated at an outside hospital with an upper endoscopy and was found to be negative for malignancy or hernia. He has lost approximately 10 kg of weight over the last 2 months and complains of significant overall deconditioning and weakness. His past medical history is notable for smoking 40 pack-years, hypertension, and coronary artery disease treated with the stenting 2 years ago. He has a previous open repair of an infrarenal abdominal aortic aneurysm 5 years ago. While currently unable to do so now, he walked on a treadmill 1 mile a day prior to this event.

Differential Diagnosis

Dysphasia can be characterized by either obstructive or functional diseases of the esophagus. With the combination of back pain and dysphasia in a 65-year-old male, malignancy should be considered first. However, a negative endoscopy increases the odds of an extrinsic esophageal compression or a functional disorder of the esophagus. Hiatal and diaphragmatic hernias may also present with dysphasia and intermittent back pain mostly associated with eating. Malignancies originating from the pulmonary or intrathoracic lymphatic systems can also encase the esophagus.

Vascular causes for dysphasia would include extrinsic compression from dysphagia lusoria or intrathoracic aneurysm disease. Dysphagia lusoria occurs when the right subclavian artery has an anomalous origin on the left side of the aortic arch, wraps behind the esophagus, and compresses it against the trachea. Aneurysms of the aortic arch, great vessels, or descending thoracic aorta may all compress the esophagus. These aneurysms may be primary, mycotic, or associated with a chronic dissection, and they can even erode into the esophagus leading to aortoesophageal fistulae.

Progressive back pain can be a primary disease of the musculoskeletal system or referred pain from a large variety of intrathoracic etiologies. Because extrinsic compression of the esophagus will generally lead to chronic dilatation, progressive back pain would not be expected unless there was an esophageal leak and mediastinitis. While acute aortic dissection could manifest with back pain, unless there was also an aneurysm, dysphasia would not be present as in this case.

A CTA would be the best step to distinguish the possible etiology of this patient. If negative, one would evaluate for esophageal dysmotility using a barium swallow. Because the barium would negate the visibility of the CT scan from scatter artifact, this should be done after the CTA if necessary (Fig. 1).

CTA Report

A 13-cm fusiform thoracoabdominal aortic aneurysm involving the distal third of the thoracic aorta, that includes both mesenteric and renal arteries. The aneurysm ends just before an aortobiiliac bypass graft. There is no evidence of malignancy in the chest or abdomen. There is no evidence of inflammation in the mediastinum. The celiac artery appears occluded at its origin with a well-developed gastroduodenal artery. All three branches of the celiac are patent.

Discussion

Of all aneurysms of the thoracic aorta, the most common are ascending aortic aneurysms (40%), while thoracoabdominal aneurysms (TAAAs) only account for 10%. Almost 25% of patients with thoracic aortic aneurysms also have an abdominal aortic aneurysm. The shape of the aneurysm can help the clinician anticipate additional challenges. Most TAAAs are fusiform, and while penetrating ulcers and saccular aneurysms may be atherosclerotic, approximately 93% of mycotic aneurysms are saccular.

According to the Crawford classification of TAAAs, Crawford extent (type) IV aneurysms are limited to the aorta below the diaphragm and above the iliac bifurcation

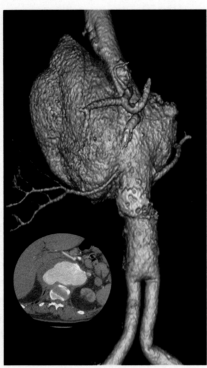

FIGURE 1 • 3D reconstruction of a large type IV TAAA. **Inset** is an axial cut demonstrating the largest portion of the TAAA. Note the aortobiiliac graft in the distal aorta.

and are the most common (52%). Extent II TAAAs are the next most common (23%) and begin at the left subclavian artery down to the iliacs. Those beginning in the mid-thoracic aorta and extending through the mesenteric and renal vessels are "extent III" and account for 15%. Type I (9%) TAAAs are limited to the intrathoracic aorta from the left subclavian artery to the diaphragm.

Case Continued

His vital signs on presentation are blood pressure 180/90, heart rate 92, temperature 37.5, respiratory rate 18, and an oxygen saturation of 90% on room air. He is thin, and visibly uncomfortable due to his back pain. His chest is barrel shaped and clear to auscultation bilaterally. Abdominal exam reveals a scaphoid abdomen with a well-healed midline scar. There is a palpable pulsatile mass in the epigastrium. He has palpable pulses in all four extremities. His laboratory workup is notable for a creatinine of 1.3 mg/dL, blood urea nitrogen of 40 mg/dL, and a hemoglobin of 14 g/dL.

Discussion

For every increase of 1 cm above a 5-cm descending thoracic aorta, there is almost a doubling of the rupture risk. Within 2 years of diagnosis, a TAAA greater than 5.6 cm has a risk of death from rupture of approximately 25%. Generally, because patients with these aneurysms tend to have other significant comorbidities, a predicted survival greater than 25% at 2 to 4 years from other causes

needs to be established prior to considering open repair. Crawford and DeNatale followed 94 patients who were not candidates for surgery, and 80% of those that ruptured had COPD.

This patient is relatively young but has become significantly deconditioned, malnourished, and dehydrated (elevated BUN and creatinine) from incapacitating back pain and dysphasia. His relatively low oxygen saturation suggests COPD in association to his smoking history. The very large size of his aneurysm and his progressive back pain are highly suggestive of imminent rupture, and a mycotic etiology must be considered. The combination of clinical findings is concerning for a poor outcome for traditional open surgery; however, conservative management is also very high risk for rupture and death.

Alternative options for managing this aneurysm would include endovascular approaches or hybrid (aortic debranching) techniques. The latter would still require an open abdominal exposure and bypasses to all four visceral vessels, in the setting of a previous abdominal aortic aneurysm repair. Avoiding any open procedure so as to limit further deconditioning makes endovascular a more attractive option. Four-vessel, totally endovascular management of a thoracoabdominal aneurysm is not available in the United States outside of investigational studies. Therefore, this only leaves physician-modified fenestration/branching of endografts or the use of parallel grafts (snorkels, chimneys, periscopes, and "sandwich" techniques) to maintain perfusion into the renal and mesenteric vessels, while excluding the thoracoabdominal aortic aneurysm.

Case Conclusion

A long discussion was had with the patient regarding his options, and appropriate institutional review board approval was obtained to perform an endovascular treatment for his thoracoabdominal aortic aneurysm. Access was obtained via cutdown of bilateral common femoral arteries, and a "preclose technique" was used to access his left axillary artery. The right lower extremity access was used to cannulate the left renal artery. This was aided by slowly injecting contrast while gently pulling back a cobra catheter on the aneurysm wall until the vessel was identified. The right renal artery was accessed via the left lower extremity, and the superior mesenteric artery was cannulated via the left axillary artery access. Rosen wires were placed inside of the visceral vessels, and subsequently, long sheaths were inserted into each. In a separate site on the right common femoral artery, a large sheath was placed inside of the abdominal aorta in order to deploy the thoracic stent graft. The aortic stent graft was advanced and put into position such that the distal portion would end approximately 5 mm before the bifurcation of his previously placed bifurcated Dacron graft. Fifteen-cm-long covered stent grafts (Gore Viabahn) were first deployed into the visceral vessels, and this was followed by placement of long angioplasty balloons into all three of the visceral vessels. These were insufflated while simultaneously deploying the thoracic aortic endograft (Gore cTAG). Using an aortic balloon, we expanded the aortic endograft while simultaneously insufflating the balloons in our visceral vessels. We determined that the overlap in the thoracic aorta was insufficient for an adequate seal between it and the superior mesenteric artery stent graft. Therefore, an additional aortic stent graft and covered stent graft was deployed into both the thoracic aorta and SMA, respectively, to extend the proximal seal zone. Simultaneous ballooning of the SMA and aortic grafts was again performed. Completion angiogram demonstrated no endoleak (Table 1).

The patient's dysphasia and back pain resolved immediately after the procedure. A CTA was obtained within 48 hours demonstrating a seal and no endoleak. At 1 month, a site where the renal stent grafts crossed over each other seemed to compress one another against the aortic wall and the aortic endograft. Despite the patient not demonstrating hypertension or changes in creatinine, we reinforced this stent graft with a balloon-expandable stent at the site of compression. Six months later, the aneurysm sac decreased to approximately 4 cm in maximum diameter (Fig. 2) without endoleak. The patient's creatinine was unchanged, and he continues to live independently.

Discussion

We elected to access the right and left renal arteries from the contralateral femoral access due to the very large aortic lumen. In order to access the renal arteries from the ipsilateral femoral artery, we would have needed to have a nearly 180-degree turn on our wire while inside a massive aortic lumen. When the sheaths and long stent grafts would have been advanced, they may have pulled out our wire despite stiffness or length. The downside was that there was an "X" formed by the renal stent grafts and they

TABLE 1. Endovascular TAAA Repair

Key Technical Steps

1. Ensure that there at least 5 cm of nonaneurysmal aorta where the aortic and visceral grafts can overlap to minimize the risk of endoleaks.
2. Obtain enough stock of covered stents to extend or replace a stent graft.
3. Gain vascular access via both femoral arteries and at least one upper extremity when positioning/prepping.
4. Confirm access vessels are of adequate size for introducing the sheaths necessary. Generally, open arterial exposures are best, especially when using large or parallel sheaths. "Preclosing" failures can ruin an otherwise successful procedure and prolong an already long procedure.
5. Inflate long balloons in the visceral stents to maintain stability and stent expansion during any manipulation of the aortic stent graft (insertion, deployment, or balloon expansion).
6. Ensure enough long balloons sized appropriately for each stent graft are available.

Potential Pitfalls

- Cannulating renal arteries that lie further lateral than the origin of the iliac arteries can be very difficult and/or lead to unstable positioning of sheaths and stents when done from the ipsilateral femoral artery. Using the contralateral can aid access and maintain a more stable sheath position.
- Identifying the origin of visceral vessels in large aneurysms can be aided by dragging a catheter along the aortic wall and slowly injecting contrast.
- If there is difficulty advancing a sheath into a visceral branch due to angulation or stiffness of the introducer, using a long balloon instead of the introducer can help. Access can be obtained by inflating the balloon by hand with a regular syringe and pushing the sheath over the balloon while gently deflating it.
- Don't be afraid to expand the seal zones proximally or distally in order to avoid type I endoleaks (have more stent grafts available than you should need). 5 cm of overlap is a minimum, sometimes you may need much more to get a good seal.
- Make sure the branch endografts stick out beyond the aortic graft to allow access to them later, and to ensure they are fully expanded.

ultimately got compressed between the aortic stent graft and the aortic wall/Dacron. We anticipated this consequence and identified it on a CTA and treated it preemptively with a balloon-mounted stent.

Some publications recommend deploying the aortic graft prior to the visceral stent grafts. The reasoning is that advancement of the stent graft into the aorta may pull out the visceral stents and that the visceral stent grafts will adapt better to the aorta-aortic stent graft interface than the aortic graft having to adapt to a fully deployed visceral stent—and thus obtain a better seal. After doing this both ways, I find that having long balloons inside of the deployed visceral stent grafts maintains good stability when manipulating the aortic graft;

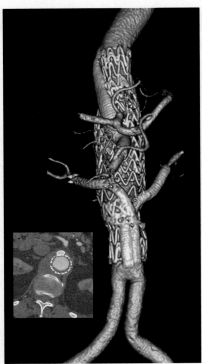

FIGURE 2 • 3D reconstruction of the TAAA 6 months after treatment, without endoleak and all grafts patent. **Inset** is an axial cut demonstrating the largest portion of the TAAA. Note the dramatically reduced diameter of the aneurysm sac (4 cm).

however, when the aortic stent graft is deployed first, the visibility for positioning and accurately deploying multiple visceral stent grafts becomes severely impaired due to the abundant overlapping radiopaque materials (aortic stent graft, sheaths, wires, visceral stent grafts). In addition, advancing and deploying the aortic graft can also pull out the visceral sheaths because they have minimal friction holding them in place. Modern, conformable aortic stent grafts adapt rather nicely around the visceral stent grafts and may even minimize the need for "eye of the Tiger" techniques to avoid endoleaks.

In order to minimize the risk of "gutter" type I endoleaks, at least 5 cm of nonaneurysmal aorta should be used. Ideally, no more than two visceral stent grafts should run parallel to and aortic graft, and combining upward-facing and downward-facing visceral grafts is preferable to an uncontrolled type I endoleak.

TAKE HOME POINTS

- Endovascular management for thoracoabdominal aneurysms is not standard therapy and requires "off-label" use of stents and endografts. This also demands a high level of endovascular experience and usually requires at least two primary operators.
- You will generally use it in patients who have inordinate risks to open repair. Care must be taken to ensure adequate credentialing and meticulous documentation of consent prior to attempting.

- The use of snorkel, chimney, periscope, and parallel stent grafts ("CHIMPS") has good medium-term outcomes when compared to other off-label techniques; however, endoleaks and stent patency can be long-term problems. Its primary benefit is that it can usually be done with materials available in-house in an emergent setting.
- Ensure at least 5 cm of nonaneurysmal aorta is available to minimize the risk of leakage between the aortic and visceral stent grafts. In addition, ensure that the visceral stent graft is neither shorter than the aortic graft nor too redundant to avoid occlusion.
- Surgeon-modified endografts is another technique, which also requires specific knowledge and experience. Despite its own pitfalls (time-consuming preparation for fenestrations and branching, failure to line up fenestrations with the visceral orifice, difficulty deploying), this technique can allow for similar outcomes to commercially made branched/fenestrated grafts.
- Meticulous follow-up imaging is critical to ensure visceral stent grafts remain patent, as their occlusion can lead to morbid or lethal consequences.

SUGGESTED READINGS

Escobar GA, Upchurch GR Jr. Management of thoracoabdominal aortic aneurysms. *Curr Probl Surg.* 2011;48(2):70-133.

Lachat M, Veith FJ, Pfammatter T, et al. Chimney and periscope grafts observed over 2 years after their use to revascularize 169 renovisceral branches in 77 patients with complex aortic aneurysms. *J Endovasc Ther.* 2013;20(5):597-605.

Lobato AC, Camacho-Lobato L. Endovascular treatment of complex aortic aneurysms using the sandwich technique. *J Endovasc Ther.* 2012;19(6):691-706.

Oderich GS, Ricotta JJ II. Modified fenestrated stent grafts: device design, modifications, implantation, and current applications. *Perspect Vasc Surg Endovasc Ther.* 2009;21(3):157-167.

Pecoraro F, Pfammatter T, Mayer D, et al. Multiple periscope and chimney grafts to treat ruptured thoracoabdominal and pararenal aortic aneurysms. *J Endovasc Ther.* 2011;18(5):642-649.

CLINICAL SCENARIO CASE QUESTIONS

1. What is the most common type of thoracoabdominal aortic aneurysm (Crawford type)?

   a. I
   b. II
   c. III
   d. IV
   e. V

2. What medical comorbidity is most associated with rupture of untreated thoracoabdominal aneurysms?

   a. COPD
   b. Gender
   c. Atherosclerosis
   d. High cholesterol
   e. Low HDL

54 Isolated Thoracic Aortic Aneurysm (Open)

GUIDO H. W. VAN BOGERIJEN and HIMANSHU J. PATEL

Presentation

A 67-year-old female with a history of tobacco use (current smoker, 50 pack-years), hypertension, depression, chronic sinusitis, history of colon cancer status post colectomy, and breast cancer with lumpectomy and radiation therapy is referred to your office by her primary care physician. The patient experienced an allergic reaction to Allegra and underwent evaluation of the chest. An x-ray demonstrated abnormal findings suggestive for a left thoracic mass. On initial questioning, the patient denies any pain or other symptoms. Her medications include loperamide, atenolol, lisinopril, aspirin, and sertraline. Physical examination reveals no abnormalities.

Differential Diagnosis

Considering patient age, history of tobacco use, and the abnormal chest x-ray, a lung mass is an important concern. To rule out a lung mass, further evaluation of the chest is indicated through CT imaging. Taking into account the abnormal chest x-ray, also a mediastinal mass should be considered. To further evaluate a possible mediastinal mass, which is most commonly of thymic or lymph node origin, further evaluation with CT imaging is warranted. An asymptomatic descending thoracic aortic aneurysm (TAA) is frequently an incidental finding detected during evaluation of the chest performed for another medical purpose. Descending thoracic aneurysms occur most commonly in the sixth and seventh decades of life, and hypertension is an important risk factor that is seen in greater than 60% of the TAA patients. To detect a TAA, total aorta CT imaging is indicated.

Workup

CT imaging should be performed to further evaluate the left thoracic mass detected on the chest x-ray. A total aorta CT scan, with thin 1-mm cuts, including the chest, abdomen, and pelvis, is performed and reveals an atherosclerotic thoracoabdominal aorta with a distal arch and descending TAA with a maximum diameter at the mid–descending aorta of 6.5 × 7.4 cm (Fig. 1). Also, the ascending aorta and abdominal aorta are dilated as demonstrated in Figure 2.

This patient has an aneurysm (defined as having an aortic diameter of greater than 50% larger than normal), with the normal thoracic descending aortic diameter being 2.5 to 3.0 cm. The aortic diameter is frequently assessed to determine the risk for rupture or dissection and also important when describing indications for intervention.

Although the patient is female in this particular case, TAA is two to four times more prevalent in males. Patients with a large TAA have approximately a 25% probability of coexisting abdominal aortic aneurysm and a higher probability of other aortic/arterial pathologies, suggesting that these patients should undergo a CT of the total aorta.

The patient was encouraged to quit smoking immediately as this increases her chance for rupture. Further questioning reveals a negative family history for TAA, Marfan's syndrome or other connective tissue diseases, and aortic dissection. Serum laboratory studies include hemoglobin of 15 g/dL, normal platelet count, and creatinine of 0.7 mg/dL.

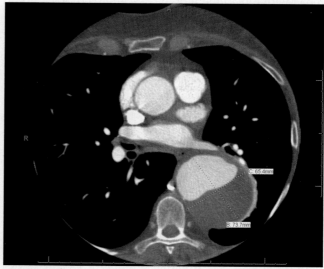

FIGURE 1 • TAA with maximum diameter at the mid–descending thoracic aorta (6.5 to 7.4 cm).

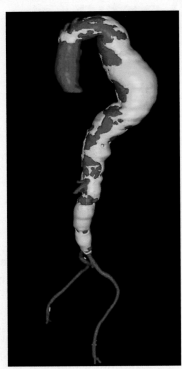

FIGURE 2 • 3D reconstruction of the total aorta CT. TAA of the distal arch and total descending aorta is demonstrated; also dilation of the ascending and the atherosclerotic abdominal aorta is present.

Diagnosis and Treatment

TAA repair is indicated in this patient. In general, recent guidelines suggest that a TAA greater than 5.5 to 6.0 cm or a TAA greater than 5.0 to 5.5 cm with a positive family history for TAA, Marfan's syndrome, or aortic dissection should be repaired. This 67-year-old female with a large aneurysm of the distal arch and total descending thoracic aorta has met the requirements for thoracic aortic repair with replacement of the descending thoracic aorta, with a maximum diameter of 6.5 to 7.4 cm. Therefore, the options for open TAA repair as well as thoracic endovascular aortic repair (TEVAR) were discussed with the patient and family.

A number of tests were performed to be certain that she is an appropriate candidate for one or both of these options. These tests include a right and left heart catheterization, transesophageal echocardiography (TEE), carotid duplex scanning, pulmonary function testing 6 weeks following her smoking cessation, and ankle-brachial indices. All test outcomes are unremarkable with the exception of identification of mild COPD (FEV1 60%, DLCO 65%) and are adequate enough to proceed with either open or endovascular TAA repair.

In this particular case, an open approach was performed because it became quite apparent that in order to perform TEVAR, she would also require exposure of her infrarenal aorta to deliver the stent graft, as well as the coverage of the left subclavian artery. In our institution

for these latter circumstances, we routinely revascularize the left subclavian artery by extra-anatomic bypass from the left carotid artery in order to provide potential persistent collateral blood flow to the spinal cord and the posterior circle of Willis. Given this extensive associated need for other procedures, it was felt that at her relative young age of 67, an open operation may be a more suitable choice. After discussion and consideration of the treatment options with the patient and her family, the patient prefers to be treated with open TAA repair.

Surgical Approach

In case more than the proximal third is resected, adjunctive cerebrospinal fluid drainage via placement of a lumbar drain is accomplished just after induction of anesthesia. In this particular case, hypothermic circulatory arrest was also identified as an important adjunct given the extent of the TAA into the distal arch as well as the need to resect the total descending aorta (i.e., additional neuroprotective strategy).

The standard operative approach for isolated TAA is as follows. The patient is placed in the right lateral decubitus position with the left chest up and is widely prepped and draped. A standard left posterolateral thoracotomy is performed. The left femoral vessels are cannulated via a transverse infrainguinal incision, and the thoracic descending aorta is mobilized for planned resection.

After withdrawal of 2 to 3 units of autologous blood for later reinfusion, the patient is then systemically heparinized and under TEE guidance, a venous cannula is inserted via the left common femoral vein into the right atrium. The left femoral artery is isolated via a transverse arteriotomy, and an 8-mm Dacron graft is sewn in an end-to-side fashion for arterial return. The patient is placed on cardiopulmonary bypass, and the patient is then actively cooled to circulatory arrest to eventually reach a temperature of 18°C. During cooling, the intercostal vessels, which will not be preserved, are externally ligated and divided down. When the patient reaches 18°C, systemic potassium is administered to arrest the heart. Cardiopulmonary bypass is then discontinued, and the patient is drained of volume. A cross clamp is applied at the level of T4 with the flow reduced to half from the femoral artery to keep the lower body perfused. The proximal incision in the descending thoracic aorta is performed, and the proximal anastomosis is created using external felt reinforcement with a running 4-0 polypropylene suture, which is constructed to a Dacron graft with a single prefabricated side branch. Following completion of this anastomosis, the prefabricated side branch is cannulated for cardiopulmonary bypass and flow is then reinstituted to the upper body. The aorta is de-aired out through the open distal end of the graft, and the proximal clamps are placed distal to the prefabricated side branch to restore flow to the upper body and heart.

Attention is then focused on the distal thoracic aorta, where the aorta is mobilized and circumferentially encircled. The distal clamp is placed beyond the location of the intended anastomosis. Flow is maintained to the lower body via the left femoral artery. Active rewarming to normothermia is initiated, and the descending TAA specimen is removed. The Dacron graft is sized to an appropriate length, and the distal anastomosis to the distal descending thoracic aorta is constructed, again using external felt reinforcement. The clamps are released with adequate de-airing maneuvers, and the patient is then separated from cardiopulmonary bypass when normothermic. The patient is decannulated during rewarming from the left groin, and the left femoral artery is then primarily repaired. Protamine sulfate and autologous blood are administered to reverse the coagulopathy. At this point, hemostasis is assured in the aneurysm bed as well as at the anastomoses. Chest tubes are placed. The main thoracotomy and left groin wounds are closed routinely. The wound is dressed at this point, and the patient can be transported back to the intensive care unit (Table 1).

Special Intraoperative Considerations

If intraoperative examination reveals a calcified arch or proximal descending aorta, and the original intent was to use left heart bypass, the strategy may need to change to use of hypothermic circulatory arrest. When mobilizing a big aneurysm containing debris, retrograde embolization of atheroma to the head can occur, thus suggesting that a "no touch" technique until the time of circulatory arrest is appropriate. Furthermore, minimal manipulation of the left lung is mandatory during the procedure to avoid intraparenchymal hemorrhage, particularly when fully heparinized for cardiopulmonary bypass.

Postoperative Management

Adequate postoperative management to prevent major complications is essential. The most common complication after open TAA repair is postoperative respiratory failure. Predictive factors to develop respiratory insufficiency are active cigarette smoking, baseline COPD (especially in those with significant reduction of FEV_1), and cardiac, renal, or bleeding complications. Risk factor modification with smoking termination and bronchodilator therapy for COPD patients is essential for acceptable outcomes. In this particular case, the patient is encouraged to quit smoking postoperatively for a minimum of 6 to 8 weeks to decrease her probability of having respiratory insufficiency.

In recent years, improvements in operative care, in particular increased care of intercostal artery preservation and the implementation of protective agents, have led to decreased risks for spinal cord ischemia (SCI). Cerebrospinal fluid drainage is recommended in those patients at high risk of SCI, and the lumbar drain is left in place for 48 to 72 hours postoperatively. During open TAA repair, different adjunctive techniques to increase the tolerance of the spinal cord to impaired perfusion, such as hypothermic circulatory arrest, distal perfusion, epidural irrigation with hypothermic solutions, and high-dose systemic glucocorticoids, can be performed in patients at high risk for SCI. In addition, neurophysiologic monitoring can be used to detect SCI and can guide the preservation of intercostal arteries and the hemodynamic optimization to prevent and treat SCI, though we have not found these helpful. Maintaining moderate systemic hypothermia during open repair and spinal cord

---

TABLE 1. Open Descending Thoracic Aortic Aneurysm Repair

Key Technical Steps

1. Perform left posterolateral thoracotomy.
2. Expose left femoral vessels for cannulation via transverse infrainguinal incision.
3. Mobilize the affected aortic segment.
4. Insert venous cannula through the femoral vein into the right atrium.
5. Perform a transverse arteriotomy with sewing an 8-mm polyester graft in an end-to-side fashion for arterial return and start cardiopulmonary bypass.
6. Cool the patient to circulatory arrest; after cooling to 18°C, administer systemic potassium to arrest the heart (cardioplegia).
7. Place the proximal clamp at T4 (with the flow reduced to half from the femoral artery to keep the lower body perfused), and incise the proximal aortic segment and perform proximal anastomosis to a Dacron graft.
8. Reinstitute flow to the upper body through the prefabricated side branch.
9. Incise the distal aortic segment and remove the specimen.
10. Size the Dacron graft to the right length and perform distal anastomosis.
11. Rewarm to normothermia and separate patient from cardiopulmonary bypass.
12. Decannulate the left groin and repair the left femoral artery primarily.
13. Administer autologous blood and protamine.
14. Place chest tubes.
15. Close thoracotomy and infrainguinal incisions.

Potential Pitfalls

- Vagus and left recurrent laryngeal nerve damage. Entrapment of the vagus nerve/left recurrent laryngeal nerve in the aortic aneurysm with involvement and adherence to the adventitia can make its dissection and preservation difficult.
- If aortic insufficiency is moderate or severe, for an elective descending thoracic aortic repair with adjunctive hypothermic circulatory arrest, the patient may need prophylactic aortic valve repair or replacement. If emptying of the heart is difficult and the patient has aortic insufficiency, a left ventricular vent may need to be placed via the left inferior pulmonary vein.
- In case of entering the right pleural space during mobilization of the aorta, a right chest tube is inserted postoperatively.
- To prevent chyle leak, the thoracic duct may need to be ligated in multiple locations in the distal thorax.

perfusion pressure optimization in the early postoperative phase is vital to prevent SCI.

To preserve the renal function, preoperative hydration and intraoperative mannitol administration are helpful approaches.

Case Conclusion

The patient undergoes successful distal hemiarch and total descending aortic replacement with a #28 Dacron graft using deep hypothermic circulatory arrest and repair of the left common femoral artery. She is discharged from the hospital on the 12th postoperative day. The postoperative course is unremarkable for major complications. She developed postoperatively dehiscence of the groin incision, which was successfully treated with continued Clorpactin dressing changes and doxycycline. Surveillance CT imaging after 3 months and 1 year shows stable condition of the aortic size and no postsurgical complications (i.e., leak and infection).

TAKE HOME POINTS

- TAAs are frequently incidentally discovered on CT imaging performed for workup of another problem.
- A TAA may be suspected on base of a routine chest radiograph, and subsequently CTA or MRA is the gold standard to detect TAA.
- Surgery for TAA repair is indicated when the diameter is larger than 6.0 cm, the aneurysm is rapidly expanding, or there is a positive family history for Marfan's syndrome, other connective tissue disease, or aortic dissection.
- It is important to give the patient a broad perspective of treatment options available and their concomitant risk, considering patient age, additional procedures, and risk for major complications.
- Open repair can be the preferred treatment option if the patient is younger (less than 55 years of age), if the patient has a connective tissue disorder, if extensive additional procedures need to be performed next to TEVAR, or if the anatomy is not suitable for endovascular repair.
- Pre-, intra-, and postoperative care is vital to prevent major postoperative complications, such as respiratory insufficiency, SCI, and renal failure. Preoperative cardiac evaluation is also mandatory.

SUGGESTED READINGS

Conrad MF, Cambria RP. Contemporary management of descending thoracic and thoracoabdominal aortic aneurysms: endovascular versus open. *Circulation.* 2008;117(6):841-852.

Coselli JS, LeMaire SA. Left heart bypass reduces paraplegia rates after thoracoabdominal aortic aneurysm repair. *Ann Thorac Surg.* 1999;67:1931-1934; discussion 1953-1958.

Coselli JS, Lemaire SA, Köksoy C, et al. Cerebrospinal fluid drainage reduces paraplegia after thoracoabdominal aortic aneurysm repair: results of a randomized clinical trial. *J Vasc Surg.* 2002;35:631-639.

Crawford ES, Crawford JL, Safi HJ, et al. Thoracoabdominal aortic aneurysms: preoperative and intraoperative factors determining immediate and long-term results of operations in 605 patients. *J Vasc Surg.* 1986;3(3):389-404.

Crawford ES, Svensson LG, Hess KR, et al. A prospective randomized study of cerebrospinal fluid drainage to prevent paraplegia after high-risk surgery on the thoracoabdominal aorta. *J Vasc Surg.* 1991;13:36-45.

Estrera AL, Miller CC III, Chen EP, et al. Descending thoracic aortic aneurysm repair: 12-year experience using distal aortic perfusion and cerebrospinal fluid drainage. *Ann Thorac Surg.* 2005;80(4):1290-1296; discussion 1296.

Hiratzka LF, Bakris GL, Beckman JA, et al. 2010 ACCF/AHA/AATS/ACR/ASA/SCA/SCAI/SIR/STS/SVM Guidelines for the diagnosis and management of patients with thoracic aortic disease. A Report of the American College of Cardiology Foundation/American Heart Association Task Force on Practice Guidelines, American Association for Thoracic Surgery, American College of Radiology, American Stroke Association, Society of Cardiovascular Anesthesiologists, Society for Cardiovascular Angiography and Interventions, Society of Interventional Radiology, Society of Thoracic Surgeons, and Society for Vascular Medicine. *J Am Coll Cardiol.* 2010;55(14):e27-e129.

Patel HJ, Shillingford MS, Mihalik S, et al. Resection of the descending thoracic aorta: outcomes after use of hypothermic circulatory arrest. *Ann Thorac Surg.* 2006;82(1):90-95; discussion 95-96.

Svensson LG, Hess KR, D'Agostino RS, et al. Reduction of neurologic injury after high-risk thoracoabdominal aortic operation. *Ann Thorac Surg.* 1998;66:132-138.

CLINICAL SCENARIO CASE QUESTIONS

1. In which of the following patients with descending thoracic aortic aneurysm is intervention indicated?

   a. A 55-year-old female patient is referred to you by her primary care physician for an abnormal x-ray suggestive for a left thoracic mass. She denies any pain or other symptoms and is a former smoker, and medical history includes hypertension. Her family history is negative for TAA, Marfan's, and aortic dissection. CT imaging reveals isolated fusiform descending thoracic aortic aneurysm with a maximum diameter of 5.0 cm.

   b. A 65-year-old male patient is referred to you by his primary care physician for an abnormal x-ray suggestive for a left thoracic mass. He denies any pain or other symptoms and is a current smoker, medical history includes hypertension, and the family history is positive for aortic dissection, but negative for TAA and Marfan's. CT imaging reveals a penetrating aortic ulcer of the descending thoracic aorta with maximum diameter of 3.7 cm (total aortic diameter).

c. A 65-year-old female patient presents to your office with thoracic pain since a week. She is a current smoker, and medical history includes hypertension. Family history is negative for TAA, Marfan's, and aortic dissection. CT imaging reveals an atherosclerotic thoracoabdominal aorta and a distal arch and fusiform descending thoracic aortic aneurysm with a maximum diameter of 5.0 cm at the mid–descending aorta.

d. A 55-year-old male patient presents to your office with thoracic pain since a week. He is a nonsmoker, and medical history includes hypertension. Family history is negative for TAA, Marfan's, and aortic dissection. CT imaging reveals an atherosclerotic thoracoabdominal aorta and a saccular distal arch aneurysm with a maximum diameter of 5.0 cm at the distal arch.

2. For which of the following adjuncts there has been shown level of evidence supporting spinal cord ischemia prevention?

a. Hypothermic circulatory arrest
b. Intercostal artery reattachment
c. Distal perfusion
d. Permissive hypertension
e. Lumbar spinal drain

55 Isolated Thoracic Aortic Aneurysm: TEVAR

JULIA SARAIDARIDIS and MARK CONRAD

Presentation

A 70-year-old male with a past medical history of hypertension and smoking is referred to your office for discussion of a descending thoracic aortic aneurysm (DTA) that was identified as an incidental finding on a chest computed tomography (CT) scan obtained during an emergency department workup of a minor motor vehicle accident. He denies any history of chest or back pain. His past medical and surgical history is remarkable for mild COPD, a left hip replacement, hyperlipidemia (on statin therapy), and hypertension that is well controlled on two agents. He is a former smoker with a 40 pack-year history. On physical examination, he has normal vital signs, clear lungs, a soft abdomen, and a normal pulse exam. His labs show no significant findings, and the CT scan he brings to clinic shows an aneurysmal dilation of the descending thoracic aorta with greatest diameter of 7.0 cm by center-line measurement.

Differential Diagnosis

The majority of DTAs are asymptomatic and are often identified as incidental findings on imaging studies obtained for other indications. On the other hand, a ruptured, expanding, thoracic aortic aneurysm will often present as an acute aortic syndrome whose symptoms include sudden, sharp, tearing chest or back pain. The experience of these symptoms usually prompts the patient to seek emergent medical attention. The differential diagnosis of acute aortic syndrome is a ruptured/expanding aortic aneurysm, acute aortic dissection, aortic intramural hematoma, penetrating aortic ulcer, myocardial infarction, pulmonary embolism, or pneumothorax. For a patient in whom a DTA is discovered incidentally on imaging, the differential diagnosis includes a variety of aortic pathologies including aortic dissection, ascending aortic aneurysm, or thoracoabdominal aortic aneurysm.

Workup

All patients in whom endovascular repair of a thoracic aortic aneurysm (TEVAR) is considered should undergo a CT angiography (CTA) of the chest, abdomen, and pelvis with fine (≤5 mm) cuts. From this scan, a three-dimensional model can be constructed to aid in preprocedural planning (Fig. 1). The chest portion of this study provides information regarding the aortic arch anatomy, the diameter and length of potential seal zones, the relationship of the aneurysm to the left subclavian and celiac arteries, and the presence of intraluminal thrombus. The abdominal and pelvic portions of the CTA are essential for evaluation of calcification and tortuosity of the abdominal aorta. In addition, the scan is necessary to assess adequacy of the iliac arteries as conduit vessels

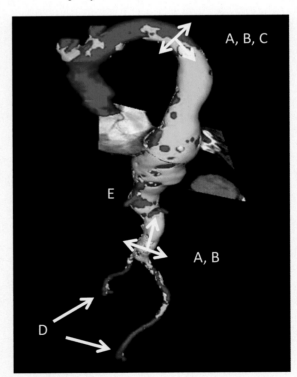

FIGURE 1 • Three-dimensional reconstruction of DTA should be used for preoperative planning. Important measurements to obtain: (*A*) Proximal/distal seal zones length, (*B*) Diameter of seal zones, (*C*) Relationship to left subclavian/celiac artery, (*D*) Access vessels' diameter/calcification, (*E*) Tortuosity.

through which to insert large-diameter sheaths, which are necessary to deliver an endograft into the thoracic aorta (Fig. 1).

Although TEVAR is much less invasive than is open repair of a thoracic aortic aneurysm, the procedure is still associated with significant morbidity and mortality. It is essential for elective patients to undergo a full preoperative assessment. Risk factors, such as coronary artery disease, renal dysfunction, and poor functional status, need to be identified prior to operation. A preoperative chest radiograph (CXR) and electrocardiogram (EKG) should be obtained in all patients. In addition, all patients should undergo a cardiac risk assessment, and, for those who are high risk, a nuclear stress test is indicated.

Diagnosis and Treatment

DTAs are rare with an incidence between 5 and 10 cases per 100,000 patient-years. They are often associated with other aortic degenerative diseases: aortitis (giant cell arteritis), genetic connective tissue disorders (Marfan's, Ehlers-Danlos, and Loeys-Dietz syndromes), and otherwise unidentified familial predispositions to large-vessel aneurysms. When a familial predisposition to aneurysm degeneration is identified, members of that family should be closely followed with a surveillance program aimed at identifying patients prior to the point where their aneurysm has reached accepted size thresholds for elective repair. For all patients, the decision to electively repair a DTA in the hopes of preventing future rupture is dependent upon the location, size, and shape of the aneurysm. Overall, it is agreed that a thoracic aortic aneurysm expands slowly over time with the risk of rupture increasing significantly when the aneurysm reaches a diameter of 6.0 cm. Therefore, 6.0 cm has become the recommended size threshold for elective repair for patients who are of appropriate operative risk. However, patients with a symptomatic aneurysm or rapid growth of the aneurysm (>0.5 cm in 6 months) may be repaired at a smaller size.

Evolution of TEVAR

DTAs have been repaired operatively since the 1950s. In 1994, Dake et al. reported the first successful exclusion of a DTA with an endovascular device. Following this innovation, it quickly became clear that TEVAR was a viable alternative to open repair as this procedure appeared to avoid much of the significant morbidity associated with the requisite thoracotomy and aortic cross-clamping of an open repair. The Food and Drug Administration (FDA) approved the first commercially available TEVAR device in the United States in 2005, and, currently, there are five devices approved by the FDA for use in the United States for the endovascular repair of isolated DTA. Over the last 10 years, industry-sponsored device trials and large case series have provided medium- and long-term outcome data following TEVAR (Table 1). It is clear that the perioperative mortality (3% vs. 10%) and perioperative morbidity including stroke (5% vs. 6%), paraplegia/paraparesis (5% vs. 13%), and cardiac complications (15% vs. 32%) are either equivalent or less for TEVAR than historical data for open surgical repair. As a result, for anatomically appropriate candidates, TEVAR has become the preferred method of DTA repair.

TABLE 1. List of Industry-Sponsored Trials/Sizable Case Series of TEVAR for DTA

Type of Graft	No. of Patients	Years Covered	30-Day Mortality	30-Day Paraplegia/ Paraparesis	30-Day CVA	30-Day Endoleak
Gore TAG	140	1999–2001	1.5%	2.8%	3.5%	3.6%
Cook (TX2)	160	2004–2006	1.9%	5.6%	2.5%	4.8%
Medtronic talent (VALOR I)	195	2003–2005	2.1%	8.7%	3.6%	25.9%
Medtronic valiant (VALOR II)	160	2006–2009	3.1%	2.5%	2.5%	15.8%
Bolton Relay (RESTORE)	304 (all aortic pathology)	2005–2009	7.2%	3.9%	1.6%	4.9%
EUROSTAR	249 (out of 443)	1997–2003	5.3% for elective	4.0%	2.8%	9.2%
Walsh et al.	538	1991–2007 (publications)	5.57%	5.4% (major neurologic)	—	—
Cheng et al.	5888	1990–2009 (publications)	5.8%	3.4%	5.0%	12.1%
Conrad et al.	3529	2004–2007	5.2%	—	—	—

Surgical Approach

Preoperative Planning

The key to successful exclusion of a DTA with TEVAR is in the preoperative planning. A fine-cut CTA should undergo three-dimensional modeling in order to ensure that accurate center-line measurements are obtained: several platforms exist to accomplish this task, and it is important to become facile with one of them. There are several anatomic factors that must be met in order to successfully perform TEVAR for DTA (Table 2). First, it is of utmost importance to choose appropriate proximal and distal seal zones for the graft. The aortic arch has been divided into five proximal landing zones that by virtue of their anatomic characteristics alter the ability and ease of successful deployment in that zone (Fig. 2). In general, a proximal seal in zones 0 to 2 is associated with a higher complication rate compared to zones 3 and 4. Because of the intense physiologic environment of the thoracic aorta, the length of the proximal seal is important, and although a 2-cm seal is adequate in most cases, in the face of a tortuous vessel, a longer seal zone may be necessary. Ideally, the 2-cm proximal seal zone is distal to the takeoff of the left subclavian artery (zones 3 and below). However, in 20% of patients, coverage of the left subclavian artery (zone 2) is required to obtain an adequate length of seal. In emergent situations, the left subclavian artery can be covered with minimal morbidity. However, a left carotid to subclavian bypass should be considered in patients who are at high risk of arm ischemia, spinal cord ischemia (SCI), or cerebral malperfusion (those who have undergone coronary artery bypass graft with use of the left internal mammary artery, those with a dominant left vertebral artery, those with an aberrant right subclavian artery, those with a hypoplastic right vertebral artery, those with an anomalous origin of the left vertebral artery, and those who have increased risk of paraplegia secondary to extensive coverage of the thoracic aorta). Finally, the diameter of the seal zone is currently limited to 42 mm, but grafts this size should be used with caution, as placing a graft in an aneurysmal aorta often leads to further degeneration of the aortic wall with subsequent loss of proximal seal.

For the distal landing zone, coverage of the celiac axis is usually tolerated given the extensive collaterals between the superior mesenteric artery (SMA) and celiac axis.

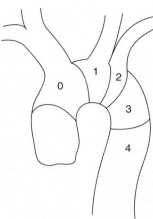

FIGURE 2 • Proximal landing zones: zone 0 involves the takeoff of the innominate artery; zone 1, the origin of the left common carotid artery; zone 2, the origin of the left subclavian artery; zone 3, the proximal descending thoracic aorta down to the T4 vertebral body; and zone 4, the remainder of the descending thoracic aorta.

However, on preoperative imaging, if the SMA appears threatened or if there is a dearth of collaterals, a celiac bypass should be performed prior to TEVAR.

The large diameter of sheaths used to deliver a thoracic endovascular device (up to 25 French) makes access selection an important part of preoperative planning. The external iliac artery must be of adequate caliber (7 mm for a 21-French delivery sheath and 8 mm for a 24-French sheath) to allow passage of the delivery system without injury. Up to 20% of patients have either an inadequate diameter of the iliac arteries or excessive calcified plaque precluding access to the aorta. In this situation, creation of an open iliac conduit (usually a 10-mm graft) through a small retroperitoneal incision or an endoconduit via placement of a 10-mm covered stent within the external or common iliac arteries will allow endograft delivery. The decision to place a conduit and which type to use is best made in the preoperative planning stage rather than in an emergent situation after the iliacs have been injured.

Graft Selection

The specific endograft to be used will be based upon surgeon preference, diameter of the aneurysm, and length of the aneurysm. There are five devices that are currently approved in the United States for treatment of descending thoracic aneurysms including the GORE TAG (Flagstaff, AZ), Cook Zenith TX2 (Bloomington, Indiana), Medtronic Talent (Santa Rosa, California), Medtronic Valiant (Santa Rosa, California), and Bolton Relay (Sunrise, Florida) devices. Endografts should be oversized by 10% to 20% for optimal seal.

Procedure

The primary access vessel is chosen based on preoperative imaging, and this common femoral artery is exposed via standard operative technique. We have transitioned from

---

TABLE 2. Anatomic Requirements for TEVAR

1. Seal zone length: 2 cm
2. Seal zone diameter: 42 mm for a 46-mm graft
3. Minimal angulation/tortuosity of the abdominal aorta and iliac vessels
4. Access needs: >8-mm external iliac artery with minimal atherosclerosis
5. Relative contraindications: aneurysm extending to the left common carotid artery or extending below the celiac artery

a longitudinal incision to a transverse incision because it has decreased wound complications to nearly zero. The contralateral artery is accessed percutaneously, and an angiographic catheter is advanced to the level of the aortic valve. It is important to fully anticoagulate the patient prior to placing wires or hardware across the arch vessels in order to decrease the risk of perioperative stroke. Aortography is performed to further delineate aortic anatomy including proximal and distal landing zones, aortic tortuosity, and the location of mesenteric vessels. For optimal visualization, it is important to angle the image intensifier to open up the aorta to a "candy cane" view. This usually requires at least 30 degrees of left anterior oblique (LAO) view. A stiff wire is advanced to the aortic valve. This wire will be used to deliver the device. Once the landing zones are visualized, the endograft is carefully introduced under fluoroscopic guidance. Extreme care in the arch should be taken not to cause undo manipulation of the wire, which will increase the risk of plaque embolism or dissection.

The details of graft deployment are particular to each commercial stent graft, and the surgeon should be aware of the peculiarities of each device prior to its use. Care should be taken to deploy the graft carefully in the landing zones chosen preoperatively; however, at the same time, deployment must be done quickly and efficiently so as to reduce wind socking (placement of the graft more distally than intended). Because thoracic aortic aneurysms are often longer than available components, numerous components may be required to exclude the aneurysm sac. In this circumstance, the grafts should be placed from smallest diameter to largest regardless of the direction of the taper. Once the grafts are deployed, the distal seal zone and overlapping zones are posted with a compliant balloon. We rarely balloon the proximal seal zone unless there is a type I endoleak on completion angiogram to reduce the risk of embolic stroke. A completion angiogram is performed at the conclusion of the case. If they are present, type I and III endoleaks should be corrected at that time with graft extensions and additional ballooning. The delivery sheath should be removed carefully from the artery after which the groin is closed surgically.

Pitfalls

There are a multitude of potential pitfalls that can face the vascular surgeon performing TEVAR. Many of these pitfalls can be controlled and reduced with careful preoperative planning and fastidious surgical technique; however, some pitfalls are known complications of this complex procedure. Immediate intraoperative and perioperative pitfalls of endovascular repair of a DTA include stroke, endoleak, injury to the iliac arteries, and SCI.

Stroke

The risk of perioperative stroke is approximately 2% to 5% following TEVAR. This is comparable to rates of stroke from open surgical repair of DTA. The strokes encountered following TEVAR are embolic in origin and, as predicted by aortic arch anatomy, can occur in both the anterior distribution and posterior distribution. The risk of perioperative stroke is increased with proximal deployment of the graft (proximal landing zone 0, 1, or 2), end stage renal disease (ESRD), mobile atheromata in the arch, and prior stroke. Most procedural and perioperative strokes are discovered within 24 hours of operation and have an associated in-hospital mortality of 10% to 30%. Therefore, all efforts at reducing undo manipulation of equipment in the arch should be attempted.

Endoleak

The incidence of perioperative endoleak following TEVAR is estimated to range from 3% to 25%. As with EVAR, a type 2 endoleak can be observed if not contributing to progressive sac enlargement. However, if a type I endoleak or type III endoleak is apparent during completion angiogram, all efforts must be made to repair it at that time with either additional graft components or angioplasty. Because of the continued long-term risk of endoleak or stent migration, patients who undergo TEVAR must undergo lifelong radiographic surveillance to assess for the development of endoleak. Most secondary interventions (endovascular or open) performed subsequent to TEVAR are performed to address persistent endoleak.

Injury to the Iliac Artery

Vascular injury complications including injury to the iliac arteries occur approximately 5% to 10% of the time in TEVAR. Up to 20% of patients lack the iliac diameter to accommodate the device delivery sheaths and will require an iliac conduit. If there is any concern regarding inadequacy of the iliacs to handle the delivery system, an iliac conduit (either open or endovascular) should be created prior to device delivery.

Spinal Cord Ischemia

One of the major pitfalls of both open and endovascular repairs of DTAs is the development of SCI. The spinal cord is perfused through small arteries coming off the thoracic aorta and a complex system of collaterals that come from the hypogastric and subclavian arteries. When a stent graft excludes these arteries, SCI is possible. Rates of SCI for open repair were historically as high as 10%. For TEVAR, that rate is lower, approximately 3% to 5%. For that reason, the precautions previously taken during open procedures (ubiquitous CSF drainage through a preoperatively placed spinal drain at L3-L4) are necessary only when the patient is at high risk for SCI. Patients who are at high risk for SCI include those with ESRD, planned long coverage of the thoracic aorta, previous coverage of the infrarenal aorta (previous EVAR), and an intact left internal mammary artery (LIMA) conduit for previous coronary artery bypass graft. These patients should all undergo preemptive spinal drainage and have the spinal drain maintained for 48 hours postoperatively.

In addition, for those high-risk patients, all efforts should be made to preserve collateral flow to the spinal cord through both preservation of the hypogastric arteries and through a left carotid to subclavian bypass if coverage of the left subclavian artery is planned. Hypotension should also be avoided during the operation and in the immediate postoperative recovery period so as to maintain an adequate spinal perfusion pressure.

SCI can be either immediate or delayed. Patients will either wake up from anesthesia with symptoms of paraplegia/paraparesis or develop it in a delayed fashion over the ensuing postoperative days. Regardless of the time of presentation, efforts at improved spinal cord perfusion (spinal drain placement, increase of mean arterial pressure) often result in clinical improvement, such that most patients who experience paraplegia/paraparesis following TEVAR make a partial to complete neurologic recovery.

Special Intraoperative Considerations

With appropriate preoperative assessment of aortic anatomy, there should be no surprises in the operating room. However, if the aneurysm extends into the arch or below the celiac axis, the suitability of an endovascular repair is called into question. If that is the case, a potential option is to perform a hybrid procedure in which the arch or visceral vessels are bypassed with an open procedure to allow subsequent placement of an endograft with appropriate seal. Hybrid procedures have significantly increased mortality and morbidity over standard TEVAR and should be reserved for patients who absolutely cannot tolerate an open thoracotomy or circulatory arrest (Table 3).

TABLE 3. TEVAR for Descending Thoracic Aortic Aneurysm

Key Technical Steps

1. Preoperative planning: seal zone, size, graft selection.
2. Prepare and drape the chest, abdomen, and bilateral groins to the midthigh.
3. Operative exposure of femoral artery on chosen side (if femoral/iliacs inadequate create iliac conduit).
4. Percutaneous access to opposite femoral artery.
5. Systemic heparinization.
6. Aortography.
7. Introduction of device through femoral artery or iliac conduit (over stiff wire).
8. Deployment of device (under fluoroscopy).
9. Post the overlapping and distal seal zones with a compliant balloon.
10. Completion angiography.
11. Removal of delivery system.
12. Pelvic angiography (not always done).
13. Closure of groin.

Potential Pitfalls

- Endoleak
- Stroke
- Injury to iliac artery
- Spinal cord ischemia

Postoperative Management

Most TEVAR patients require 3 to 7 days in the hospital postoperatively (longer if there is a hybrid component to their case or if complications are encountered). The medium- and long-term morbidity and mortality of TEVAR have been shown to be better or equivalent to open procedures. However, endovascular repairs require lifelong imaging surveillance due to the continued risk of endoleak and sac enlargement. Secondary intervention rates for endoleak range from 5% to 10%. Patients will require a CTA at 1 month, 6 months, and then yearly for the rest of their lives to assess for endoleak and stent migration.

Case Conclusion

After review of the patient's CTA, his anatomy was deemed suitable for a TEVAR, which he underwent without complication.

TAKE HOME POINTS

- DTAs should undergo repair once they reach the size threshold of 6 cm.
- Open and endovascular repair of DTA is possible.
- Endovascular repair has decreased perioperative morbidity and mortality compared to open repair.
- Endovascular candidacy is based on whether the patient has appropriate landing zones and conduit.
- If there are inadequate landing zones available, visceral and arch debranching can be performed in a hybrid procedure.

SUGGESTED READINGS

Cheng D, Martin J, Shennib H, et al. Endovascular aortic repair versus open surgical repair for descending thoracic aortic disease. *J Am Coll Cardiol.* 2010;55:986-1001.

Conrad MF, Ergul BS, Emel A, et al. Management of diseases of the descending thoracic aorta in the endovascular era: a Medicare population study. *Ann Surg.* 2010;252(4):603-610.

Fairman RM, Criado F, Farber M, et al. Pivotal results of the medtronic vascular talent thoracic stent graft system: the VALOR trial. *J Vasc Surg.* 2008;48(3):546-554.

Fairman RM, Tuchek JM, Lee WA, et al. Pivotal results for the medtronic valiant thoracic stent graft system in the VALOR II trial. *J Vasc Surg.* 2012;56(5):1222-1231.

Kilic A, Shah AS, Black JH, et al. Trends in repair of intact and ruptured descending thoracic aortic aneurysms in the United States: a population-based analysis. *J Cardiovasc Surg.* 2014;147(6):1-6.

Leurs LJ, Bell R, Degrieck Y, et al. Endovascular treatment of thoracic aortic diseases: combined experience from the EUROSTAR and United Kingdom thoracic endograft registries. *J Vasc Surg.* 2004;40:670-680.

Makaroun MS, Dillavou ED, Kee ST, et al. Endovascular treatment of the thoracic aortic aneurysms: results of the phase II multicenter trial of the GORE TAG thoracic endo-prosthesis. *J Vasc Surg.* 2005;41:1-9.

Matsumara JS, Cambria RP, Dake MD, et al. International controlled clinical trial of thoracic endovascular aneurysm repair with the zenith TX2 endovascular graft: 1 year results. *J Vasc Surg.* 2008;47:247-257.

Riambau V, Zipfei B, Coppi G, et al. Final operative and mid-term results of the European experience in the RELAY endovascular registry for thoracic disease (RESTORE) study. *J Vasc Surg.* 2011;53(3):565-573.

Walsh SR, Tang TY, Sadat U, et al. Endovascular stenting versus open surgery for thoracic aortic disease: systemic review and meta-analysis of peri-operative results. *J Vasc Surg.* 2008;47:1094-1098.

CLINICAL SCENARIO CASE QUESTIONS

1. What is the size threshold for which descending thoracic aortic aneurysms should be repaired?

   a. 4 cm

   b. 5 cm

   c. 6 cm

   d. 7 cm

2. Intraoperatively, you find that the proximal portion of your endograft covers the left subclavian artery. What should be done?

   a. Left common carotid to subclavian bypass prior to graft deployment

   b. Left common carotid to subclavian bypass in the future if the patient develops symptoms

   c. Balloon occlusion of the left subclavian to ensure collateral flow prior to coverage

   d. Immediate conversion to open repair

56 TEVAR for Type B Dissection with Malperfusion

JIP L. TOLENAAR, SANTI TRIMARCHI, and GILBERT R. UPCHURCH Jr

Presentation

A 49-year-old man, without significant past medical history, presented to an outside emergency room with complaints of acute onset of back pain, which he described as sharp and tearing in nature. The patient is in obvious distress and found to have a blood pressure of 190/85 mm Hg in both arms. Intravenous morphine results in some improvement of pain, but on physical examination, the patient has a mildly distended abdomen with diffuse tenderness to palpation. EKG shows no abnormalities. His laboratories are remarkable for a hematocrit of 38% and no troponin leak.

Differential Diagnosis

The differential diagnosis for a patient presenting with the acute onset of sharp or ripping back pain in a patient with hypertension includes: (1) myocardial infarction, (2) pulmonary embolism, (3) esophageal disease or reflux, and (4) aortic dissection.

Case Continued

The patient undergoes evaluation by CT scan imaging of the chest, abdomen, and pelvis, which demonstrates an acute type B aortic dissection from the left subclavian artery to the iliac arteries. The false lumen extends to the celiac access, and there is a mid-SMA filling defect described as thrombosis with retrograde filling (Fig. 1).

Workup

CTA imaging is the preferred modality for diagnosis in type B aortic dissection and should be used liberally. Identification of the proximal and distal intimal tears is vital for the planning and success of the endovascular procedure. In addition, a transesophageal echocardiogram (TEE) was ordered, which confirmed a type B aortic dissection distal to the origin of the left subclavian artery. The echo also showed normal aortic valves and no wall motion abnormalities. The patient is started on a Nipride drip and transported through MedFlight to your institution.

Discussion

Acute aortic dissection is a life-threatening disease with an increasing incidence, due to aging population and improved imaging modalities. Aortic diseases are currently the 14th leading cause of death in the United States. Acute aortic dissection is defined as a laceration of the intimal layer allowing blood to flow along the medial layer, which will separate both layers of the aorta resulting in a true and false lumen. Prognosis of aortic dissection in untreated patients is poor, with a mortality of 20% to 30% before hospital admission and 50% within the first 48 hours. Important risk factors for aortic dissection include systemic hypertension, increasing age, atherosclerosis, bicuspid or unicommissural aortic valve, and connective tissue disorders (i.e., Marfan's, Ehlers-Danlos, and Loeys-Dietz syndromes).

The most commonly used classification scheme is the Stanford classification, which makes a distinction between dissections that involve the ascending aorta (type A) and those that affect the descending aorta, distal to the subclavian artery (type B). In addition, further descriptions of dissections are based on the time from onset of complaint to diagnosis, so-called acute (less than 14 days) or chronic (more than 14 days).

Males are more commonly affected, typically at middle age. The majority of patients present with an abrupt onset of pain, tearing or ripping in nature and located in the chest and/or back. The disease course can be complicated by shock, cardiac tamponade, cardiac failure, myocardial ischemia/infarction, spinal cord ischemia, cerebrovascular accidents, mesenteric malperfusion, renal failure, pulse deficits, and limb ischemia.

Diagnosis and Treatment

The initial management of patients with aortic dissections should be directed at stabilizing the patient and prevent propagation and rupture of the aorta by adequate blood pressure control. Blood pressure should be maintained between 100 and 120 mm Hg systolic and ≤60 to 70 mm Hg diastolic, with a heart rate of less than 60 bpm. This medical therapy should be continued in acute B dissection, unless there is presence of complications, which require intervention. In patients presenting with malperfusion, endovascular interventions, including fenestration and stent and/or stent graft placement, are preferred as

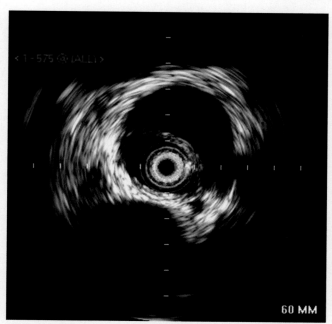

• Intravascular ultrasound (IVUS) to confirm placement of the catheter in the true lumen. Image shows an evident intimal flap between the two lumens with the SMA coming off the false lumen at approximately 3:30.

they convey less invasive and less morbid treatment in order to restore perfusion.

Two principal mechanisms may cause malperfusion, both requiring intervention. A static obstruction, which arises from a dissection flap that directly involves a side branch occluding the lumen, and is usually managed with stent placement into the branch vessel. The other possible cause of malperfusion is a dynamic obstruction, which may originate from obliteration of the side branches by the intimal flap and requires restoration of blood flow in the aortic true lumen and equilibration of blood pressure in both lumens. This usually can be established by covering the proximal entry tear with an aortic stent graft, in order to redirect blood flow to the true lumen, or by creating a hole (fenestration) in the intimal flap, allowing

pressure equilibration and blood flow between the true and false lumen (Fig. 2).

Stent graft placement in aortic dissection is feasible in selected cases, as the landing zone is in the vicinity supra-aortic branches. In 30% to 40% of patients, the subclavian artery must be covered to obtain sufficient proximal aortic neck length. In these cases, carotid-subclavian bypass prior to stent grafting can greatly reduce the risk of mortality and morbidity (i.e., cerebrovascular accidents and paralysis) and should, therefore, be performed routinely in nonemergent cases. Stent graft placement can be considered if the patient has 20 mm of landing zone proximal to the primary entry tear, which is not dissected. In addition, to allow successful device delivery, the iliac/femoral access should be adequate (6 to 8 mm) and without severe tortuosity.

Case Continued

The present patient has a critical indication and meets the criteria for initial endovascular intervention from mesenteric ischemia.

Surgical Approach for Endovascular Repair of Type B Aortic Dissection

A 3D reconstruction of the CT scan is used to select the appropriate-sized endograft, which is usually oversized, in acute B dissection, 0% to 10% compared to the aortic diameter to secure adequate radial force. Spinal cord fluid drainage is placed by the anesthesiologist in order to prevent spinal cord ischemia if greater than 15 cm of aortic dissection needs to be covered. TEVAR is generally performed under general anesthesia, and the patient is prepped from nipples to knees and draped in sterile fashion. Percutaneous ultrasound-guided access was used to access the bilateral common femoral arteries with a 21-gauge needle. An intravascular ultrasound catheter is advanced to confirm placement of the catheter within the true lumen of the aorta throughout its entire course. The location of the guidewire may be confirmed by TEE, which is also important for evidencing the proximal entry tear (Figure 1). An endovascular stent graft is

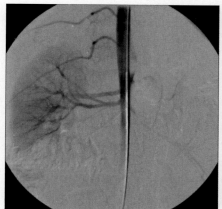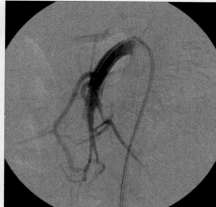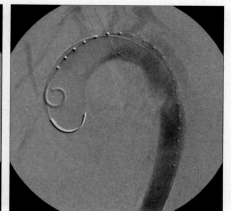

• Angiography during TEVAR procedure. The first image clearly shows obstruction of the SMA and celiac trunk. The second image shows stent placement in the SMA with good distal perfusion. The third image documents stent graft placement in the thoracic aorta excluding the false lumen.

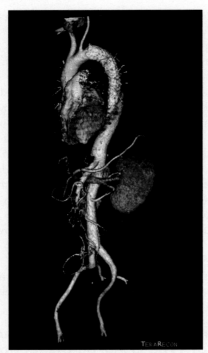

FIGURE 3 • 3D reconstruction of the postoperative CT scan, which shows the thoracic stent graft and stents in the celiac trunk and superior mesenteric artery, with adequate distal perfusion.

then deployed from the origin of the left subclavian to the mid–descending aorta, covering the proximal intimal tear. A post stent graft aortogram is performed to secure satisfactory exclusion of the dissection and no endoleak. To preserve the mesenteric circulation, the superior mesenteric artery is selectively catheterized from the left common femoral access. Angiography is then performed, showing poor flow in the superior mesenteric artery with multiple occluded/dissected branches. After placement of a guidewire, a sheath is advanced, through which a 10 mm × 40 mm SMART stent is deployed across the origin of the superior mesenteric artery. From the left common femoral access, the celiac artery was catheterized and an 8 mm × 17 mm Express stent was deployed in the origin. Post deployment angiography demonstrated appropriate placement of both stents and improved flow in the celiac and superior mesenteric artery. After all catheters and wires are straightened and removed, an Angio-Seal device and Perclose device are used to close the left and right femoral arteries, respectively. Because of concern for small bowel ischemia, an exploratory laparotomy was performed, which showed extensive infarction of the mid small bowel with necrotic segments throughout a length of 210 cm, which was resected (Fig. 3).

Postoperative Management: Surveillance Following TEVAR

Stroke, paraplegia and paraparesis, as well as incidental occlusion of the left subclavian artery are all significant complications of TEVAR. However, retrograde ascending aorta dissection is the most feared complication after TEVAR for type B aortic dissection and might be associated with barbed or uncovered stent grafts, excessive guidewire manipulation, and additional ballooning. During postoperative surveillance, the development of endoleaks and persistent retrograde perfusion of the false lumen may cause dilatation of both the true and false lumens. Current guidelines state that a thoracic and abdominal CT scan with intravenous contrast should be performed at 1, 6, and 12 months following the initial procedure and annually thereafter. In the presence of endoleaks or persistent perfusion of the false lumen, patients should be monitored more closely. An increase in aortic diameter requires intervention, which is most often through an endovascular approach.

Case Conclusion

The patient was admitted to the intensive care unit and started on beta-blockers and Nipride to control his heart rate and blood pressure. Next day, a second look showed viable small intestine, and an anastomosis to the distal limb of the small bowel was performed. The patient remained in the ICU. After 4 weeks in the hospital, the patient was discharged home with adequate hypertensive medications (Table 1).

TABLE 1. TEVAR for Type B Dissection with Malperfusion

Key Technical Steps

1. Choose appropriate endograft based on 3D reconstruction of CT scan.
2. Obtain access to the iliac or femoral artery.
3. Insert sheaths and catheters.
4. Perform aortogram, TEE, and/or IVUS to assure placement of wires and catheters in the true lumen.
5. Insert and deploy stent graft.
6. Perform completion angiogram to determine presence of endoleaks and adequate perfusion of branch vessels.
7. In case of inadequate perfusion of branch vessels, additional endovascular interventions, like fenestration or stent placement, should be performed.
8. Close arteriotomies and groin wounds; check pulses.
9. If there is concern for bowel ischemia, exploratory laparoscopy/laparotomy should be performed.
10. Transport the patient to intensive care.

Potential Pitfalls

- Retrograde ascending aorta dissection, requiring open surgical repair.
- Endoleaks that require additional procedures.
- Assess for iliac artery injury, rupture, and dissection.
- Confirm adequate perfusion to rule out end organ ischemia.

TAKE HOME POINTS

- Type B aortic dissection should be treated medically, unless there is evidence of malperfusion, refractory pain/hypertension, or aortic rupture.
- Endovascular repair, if required, has become the standard of care in all patients that need intervention to cover the primary entry tear in the descending thoracic aorta.
- The type of endovascular intervention depends on the type of obstruction. Dynamic obstruction is caused by the intimal flap itself and can be treated with stent graft placement or fenestration. Static obstruction should be treated by stent placement of the dissected branch vessel.
- Retrograde ascending aortic dissection, endoleaks, and persistent false lumen perfusion are the most common and feared complications after TEVAR.
- Patients require surveillance CTA scans at 1, 6, and 12 months and annually thereafter.

SUGGESTED READINGS

Nienaber CA, Kische S, Ince H, et al. Thoracic endovascular repair for complicated type B aortic dissection. *J Vasc Surg.* 2011;54:1529-1533.

Tolenaar JL, van Bogerijen GHW, Eagle KA, et al. Update in the management of aortic dissection. *Curr Treat Options Cardiovasc Med.* 2013;15:200-213.

Williams DM, Lee DY, Hamilton BH, et al. The dissected aorta: III. Anatomy and radiologic diagnosis of branch-vessel compromise. *Radiology.* 1997;203:37-44.

Williams DM, Lee DY, Hamilton BH, et al. The dissected aorta. Percutaneous treatment of ischemic complications: principles and results. *J Vasc Interv Radiol.* 1997;8:605-625.

CLINICAL SCENARIO CASE QUESTIONS

1. How is the position of the guidewire in the true lumen confirmed?
   a. IVUS
   b. Aortography
   c. TEE
   d. All of the above

2. What is the treatment of static obstruction affecting the visceral vessels?
   a. TEVAR
   b. TEVAR and thoracic fenestration
   c. TEVAR and abdominal fenestration
   d. TEVAR and visceral artery stent

57 Management of Left Subclavian Artery with TEVAR

KRISTOFER M. CHARLTON-OUW and ALI AZIZZADEH

Presentation

An 82-year-old woman complains of left-hand pain after undergoing an urgent TEVAR for a symptomatic descending thoracic aortic aneurysm. A preoperative CT scan showed both saccular and fusiform aneurysms of the descending thoracic aorta without evidence of rupture (Fig. 1A and B). The proximal extent of the aneurysm was near the origin of the left subclavian artery (LSA) and had a maximal diameter of 6.0 cm. Isolation of the aortic aneurysms required two overlapping endografts and coverage of the LSA (Fig. 2A and B). She has palpable right brachial and radial pulses but no palpable left upper extremity pulses. The left hand is slightly cooler than the right. She denies extremity swelling, dizziness, or visual disturbances.

Differential Diagnosis

Coverage of the LSA during TEVAR can cause symptoms of left upper extremity ischemia, such as pain or numbness. In the absence of symptoms, a pulseless left upper extremity does not indicate ischemia by itself. Pulse deficits are common after subclavian artery coverage, but ischemic symptoms are infrequent. Other causes of extremity pain and paresthesia include nerve injury, extremity arterial occlusive disease, and deep vein thrombosis.

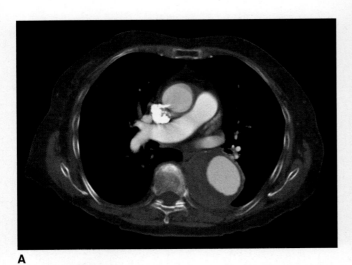
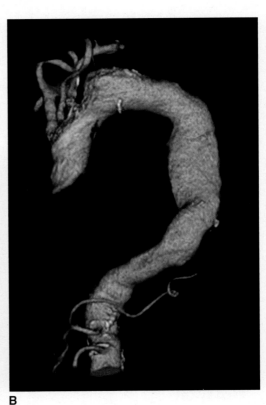

FIGURE 1 • **A:** Preoperative axial CT showing 6.0-cm symptomatic aneurysm of the descending thoracic aorta. **B:** Preoperative 3D reconstruction showing both saccular and fusiform aneurysms with relationship to LSA.

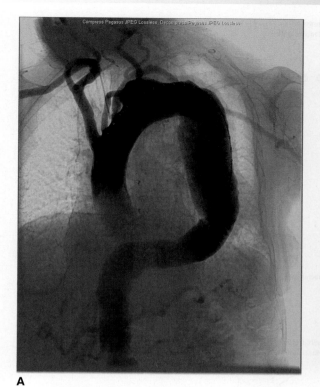
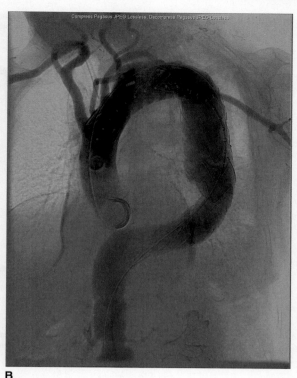

A   **B**

FIGURE 2 • **A:** Initial intraoperative angiogram showing proximity of descending thoracic aortic aneurysm to the LSA. **B:** Completion angiogram after stent graft deployment with uncovered stents over the origin of the left common carotid artery. The graft material covers the origin of the LSA with retrograde filling from the left vertebral artery.

Workup

Carotid duplex ultrasound is recommended in older patients to detect asymptomatic disease of the carotid bulb and internal carotid artery since repair may involve carotid artery clamping. Reversal of flow may be noted in the left vertebral artery. Wrist-brachial indices will be diminished, and segmental arterial waveforms will show attenuation of amplitudes (Fig. 3A and B).

It is prudent to review the patient's pre-TEVAR imaging to insure that there were no missed injuries or additional arterial occlusive disease, such as vertebral, carotid, or subclavian artery dissection or stenoses. If the patient is due for TEVAR surveillance imaging, the chest CTA will typically include enough of the neck and extremity to visualize the proximal to midcarotid and subclavian arteries. If there is doubt about a missed extremity injury or stenoses, dedicated extremity imaging should be obtained. Swelling in the extremity should prompt venous duplex imaging.

Diagnosis and Treatment

The Society for Vascular Surgery consensus guidelines and many authors recommend preoperative subclavian revascularization when coverage is required in elective TEVAR. Preemptive subclavian revascularization may be associated with lower rates of stroke and

spinal cord ischemia. Definitive evidence is difficult to obtain since spinal cord injury occurs in less than 5% of TEVAR procedures. In emergent or urgent cases, such as with traumatic aortic injury, acute complicated aortic dissection, or ruptured aortic aneurysms, preemptive subclavian revascularization is not required. The diagnosis of extremity ischemia after LSA coverage with TEVAR is primarily based on history and clinical exam. Postoperative patients who are asymptomatic, even with flow reversal in the vertebral artery, do not require subclavian revascularization.

The most common method of proximal LSA revascularization is carotid-subclavian artery bypass. Other options include subclavian-carotid artery transposition and laser fenestration of the aortic endograft. With the development of commercial branched thoracic aortic endografts, routine subclavian revascularization will become integrated within the initial endovascular procedure.

Case Continued

Noninvasive imaging, history, and physical exam findings are consistent with left upper extremity ischemia after coverage of the LSA with a thoracic aortic endograft. Revascularization options were discussed with the patient, and the decision was made to proceed with left subclavian-carotid artery transposition.

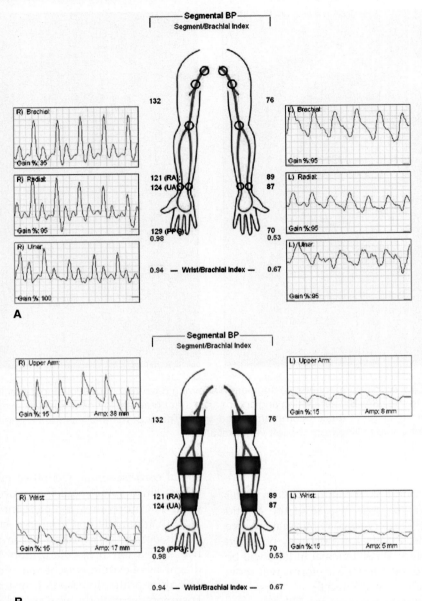

FIGURE 3 • **A:** Wrist-brachial index, segmental waveforms. **B:** Pulse volume recordings after TEVAR with coverage of the LSA.

Surgical Approach

Carotid-subclavian bypass using prosthetic graft is simpler and surgically expedient since it does not require as deep a dissection into the mediastinum. Bypass also preserves flow to the left internal mammary artery since the subclavian artery is clamped distal to the vertebral artery and is a consideration for patients with patent coronary artery bypasses. Transposition requires subclavian clamping proximal to the vertebral and mammary arteries. We prefer bypass when the right vertebral artery is occluded or atretic or if the left vertebral artery is not contiguous with the basilar artery. Patency rates slightly favor transposition over bypass. Five-year patency rates approach 98% for transpositions and 88% for bypass. Complication rates are low in both cases.

The patient is positioned supine with a shoulder roll. The left arm should be tucked at the patient's side. This elevates the subclavian artery superiorly. The neck is slightly extended and rotated to the right.

For a subclavian-carotid transposition, a transverse supraclavicular incision is centered over the sternocleidomastoid muscle. The sternal and clavicular heads are divided at the clavicle and retracted cranially. The omohyoid muscle is divided at the lateral border of the internal jugular vein and retracted laterally. The contents of the carotid sheath are then dissected free; the left internal jugular vein is dissected and retracted laterally; the left common carotid artery is circumferentially dissected; the vagus nerve is identified and protected from excessive retraction. The thoracic duct is ligated with fine silk suture

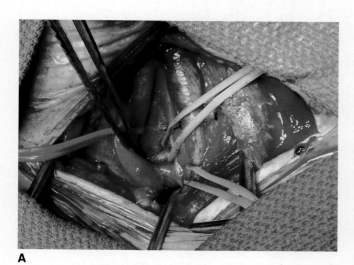

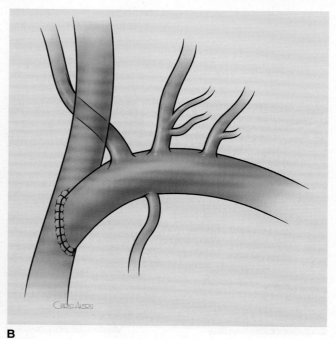

FIGURE 4 • **A:** Intraoperative image of completed subclavian-carotid transposition. The left common carotid artery is retracted medially (red vessel loop), and the vertebral and internal mammary arteries are encircled with blue vessel loops. **B:** Schematic image of transposition with internal jugular vein removed.

at the junction of the internal jugular and subclavian veins. The thoracic duct travels medially from the mediastinum transversely across the neck, anterior to the vertebral artery and superior to the subclavian artery, to enter the confluence of the internal jugular and subclavian veins. The vertebral vein is ligated. The subclavian artery is dissected proximally into the mediastinum and encircled with a vessel loop. Anticoagulation is begun, and the subclavian, vertebral, and internal mammary arteries are clamped. The proximal subclavian artery is ligated with running 4-0 polypropylene suture. The left common carotid artery is clamped, and a longitudinal posterolateral arteriotomy is made for an end-to-side anastomosis. Shunting is cumbersome and usually not needed since the external carotid artery is not clamped. The arteries are allowed to back-bleed before completing the anastomosis and the clamps are released (Fig. 4A and B).

For a carotid-subclavian bypass, a transverse supraclavicular incision is centered over the lateral border of the sternocleidomastoid muscle. The scalene fat pad is elevated superior and laterally. The thoracic duct and lymphatic tributaries are ligated lateral to the left internal jugular vein. The phrenic nerve is dissected off of the anterior scalene muscle and gently retracted medially. The anterior scalene is divided, and the underlying subclavian artery is dissected free. The thyrocervical trunk is divided, if necessary, for full mobilization of the artery. The internal jugular vein is dissected free and retracted laterally to expose the common carotid artery. Anticoagulation is

begun, and an 8- or 10-mm prosthetic graft is selected. Clamps are applied to the subclavian artery, and an end-to-side anastomosis is made. The graft is placed posterior to the internal jugular vein, and the common carotid artery is clamped. A lateral arteriotomy is made for an end-to-side anastomosis (Fig. 5A and B). The scalene fat pad is allowed to fall back over the graft (Table 1).

Special Intraoperative Considerations

Anomalous Origin of Left Vertebral Artery

In 2% of patients, the left vertebral artery originates directly off of the aortic arch just distal to the common carotid artery (Fig. 6). Theoretically, this may predispose patients to left upper extremity ischemia after coverage of the LSA. Consideration should be given to preemptive simultaneous left subclavian and vertebral artery transpositions to the common carotid artery. Cerebral imaging should determine if the left vertebral artery is dominant or terminates in the posterior inferior cerebellar artery. In either case, preemptive revascularization is indicated.

The left vertebral artery can also originate off of the proximal subclavian artery. This is a relative contraindication to subclavian-carotid artery transposition. In such cases, we prefer carotid-subclavian bypass.

Anomalous Origin of the Right Subclavian Artery

In 0.5% of patients, the right subclavian artery originates distal and posterior to the LSA (Fig. 7A and B). A zone 2 proximal thoracic aortic endograft placement would

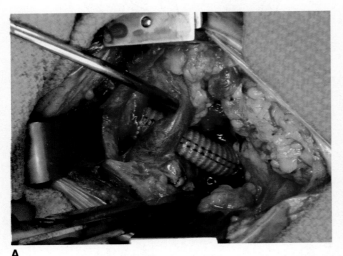

A

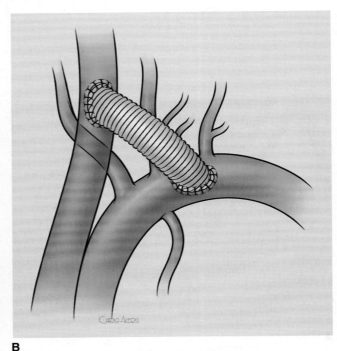

B

FIGURE 5 • **A:** Intraoperative image of completed carotid-subclavian bypass with 8-mm Dacron graft. The right internal jugular vein is retracted laterally to expose the carotid anastomosis. Note the ligated thoracic duct at the inferior internal jugular vein. **B:** Schematic image of bypass with internal jugular vein removed.

then cover both subclavian artery origins. Preemptive subclavian revascularization should attempt to preserve either the dominant or both vertebral arteries.

Concomitant Cervical Spine Injuries

When pre- or postoperative subclavian revascularization is required and the patient has cervical spine injuries, precluding neck extension and rotation, positioning for surgical subclavian revascularization can be difficult. Fenestration of the aortic endograft can be performed via percutaneous brachial or radial access. A 2.0-mm ultraviolet laser catheter (Spectranetics, Colorado Springs, CO)

is advanced over a 0.018-inch wire through a 6-French sheath into the subclavian artery. The tip of the laser is positioned against the aortic endograft, and the laser is

TABLE 1. Carotid-Subclavian Transposition/Bypass

Key Technical Steps

1. Meticulous identification and ligation of lymphatic channels to prevent leak.
2. Identify and preserve key nerves (vagus and sympathetic nerves in transpositions; phrenic nerve in bypasses).
3. The common carotid artery can be rotated medially with clamps to facilitate a lateral arteriotomy.
4. The graft/artery must be the correct length to prevent kinking.

Potential Pitfalls

• For bypasses, prosthetic conduits are preferred, since autogenous grafts are prone to kinking.

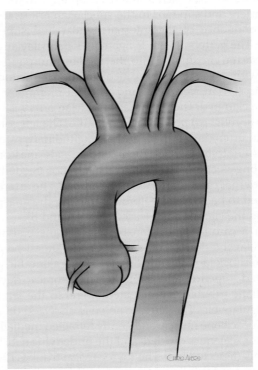

FIGURE 6 • Schematic image of aortic arch origin of the left vertebral artery.

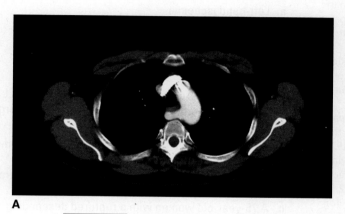

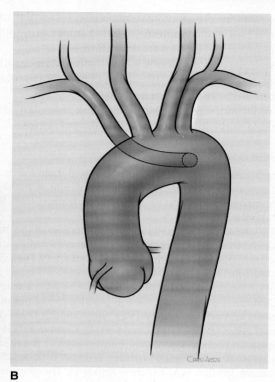

A   **B**

FIGURE 7 • **A:** Axial CT. **B:** Schematic image of aberrant origin of the right subclavian artery.

activated for a few seconds. The wire is advanced through the fenestration and exchanged for a stiff 0.035-inch wire. The fenestration is predilated, and an appropriately sized balloon-expandable covered stent is deployed across the fenestration. The proximal portion of the covered stent inside the aortic endograft can be flared with an oversized balloon.

Case Continued

The patient had an uneventful subclavian-carotid transposition. Her hand pain and paresthesia improved postoperatively, but she complained of chest tightness and shortness of breath. Her oxygen saturation was 90% on room air.

Postoperative Management

The most significant complication is nerve injury (10%). In the case of transpositions, the dissection is medial and the vagus and sympathetic nerves can be injured. With bypasses, the approach is more lateral and injury to the phrenic nerve can occur. Most nerve injuries are due to excessive retraction, and such nerve palsies usually recover after a few months. Elevation of the left hemidiaphragm is common due to phrenic nerve palsy but usually resolves within 6 months. Injury to the thoracic duct or other lymphatic tributaries occurs in 2%. Stroke occurs in less than 2% in most series. Unintentional entry into the pleura can occur during either transposition or bypass. If unrecognized, pleural effusion or pneumothorax may result. The treatment is tube thoracostomy.

Case Conclusion

The patient had a chest radiograph with a moderate hemopneumothorax. A left chest tube was placed, and the patient's symptoms improved. The tube was removed after 2 days and the patient discharged on postoperative day 3.

TAKE HOME POINTS

- Preemptive subclavian revascularization is suggested for most elective cases requiring thoracic aortic endograft coverage of the LSA (zone 2) to prevent stroke and spinal neurologic deficits.
- Preemptive revascularization is required if:
  - There is a patent left internal mammary to coronary artery bypass;
  - The patient has left upper extremity arteriovenous hemodialysis access;
  - The left vertebral artery terminates in the posterior inferior cerebellar artery;
  - The left vertebral artery is dominant or the right vertebral is atretic; or
  - Hypogastric arteries are occluded.
- Selective postoperative revascularization is appropriate in emergent or urgent TEVAR cases, such as with ruptured thoracic aortic aneurysm, traumatic aortic injury, or acute complicated aortic dissection.

- The need for postoperative subclavian revascularization is based on symptoms of either upper extremity ischemia or subclavian steal syndrome.
- Revascularization options include subclavian-carotid transposition, carotid-subclavian bypass, or percutaneous aortic endograft fenestration.
- Complications of surgical subclavian revascularization include nerve injury, lymphatic leak, and stroke.

SUGGESTED READINGS

Chung J, Kasirajan K, Veeraswamy RK, et al. Left subclavian artery coverage during thoracic endovascular aortic repair and risk of perioperative stroke and death. *J Vasc Surg.* 2011;54(4):979-984.

Holt PJ, Johnson C, Hinchliffe RJ, et al. Outcomes of the endovascular management of aortic arch aneurysm: implications for the management of the left subclavian artery. *J Vasc Surg.* 2010;51(6):1329-1338.

Lee WA, Matsumura JS, Mitchell RS, et al. Endovascular repair of traumatic aortic injury: clinical practice guidelines of the Society for Vascular Surgery. *J Vasc Surg.* 2011;53(1):187-192.

Madenci AL, Ozaki CK, Belkin M, et al. Carotid-subclavian bypass and subclavian-carotid transposition in the thoracic endovascular repair era. *J Vasc Surg.* 2013;57(5):1275-1282.

Matsumura JS, Lee WA, Mitchell RS, et al. The Society for Vascular Surgery practice guidelines: management of the left subclavian artery with thoracic endovascular aortic repair. *J Vasc Surg.* 2009;50(5):1155-1158.

Redlinger RE, Ahanchi SS, Panneton JM. In situ laser fenestration during emergent thoracic endovascular aortic repair is an effective method for left subclavian artery revascularization. *J Vasc Surg.* 2013;58(5):1171-1177.

Wilson JE, Galiñanes EL, Hu P, et al. Routine revascularization is unnecessary in the majority of patients requiring zone II coverage during thoracic endovascular aortic repair: A longitudinal outcomes study using United States Medicare population data. *Vascular.* 2014 Aug;22(4):239-45.

CLINICAL SCENARIO CASE QUESTIONS

1. For patients undergoing TEVAR with left subclavian artery (LSA) coverage, preoperative LSA revascularization decreases the risk of all of the following, except:

   a. Left-hand ischemia
   b. Mortality
   c. Paraplegia
   d. Paraparesis
   e. Stroke

2. Preoperative LSA revascularization is required in ALL of the following patients who are scheduled to undergo TEVAR with LSA coverage, except:

   a. A 70-year-old man with previous left internal mammary to coronary artery bypass
   b. A 60-year-old woman with a patent left upper extremity arteriovenous hemodialysis access
   c. A 75-year-old woman with a ruptured descending thoracic aortic aneurysm
   d. A 74-year-old man with left vertebral artery that terminates in the posterior inferior cerebellar artery
   e. A 65-year-old man with a history of an abdominal aortic aneurysm who underwent a previous aortobifemoral bypass

58 Aortic Arch Debranching

JIP L. TOLENAAR, GIANBATTISTA TSHIOMBO, and SANTI TRIMARCHI

Presentation

An 84-year-old female presents to the outpatient ENT clinic with complaints of dysphonia. Direct laryngoscopy shows paralyses of the left vocal cord. A CT scan was obtained to help determine the cause of the vocal cord paralysis (Fig. 1). The patient is referred to you after a diagnosis of a saccular aortic arch aneurysm, 6 cm in diameter, was detected by CTA. On physical examination, a questionable pulsatile abdominal mass is noted. The patient is noted to have normal femoral/popliteal/pedal pulses bilaterally.

Differential Diagnosis

This patient has an extensive and complicated aortic arch aneurysm causing dysphonia. While most of these aneurysms are repaired in good-risk patients using circulatory arrest, a hybrid procedure using aortic arch and stent grafting is preferred in high-risk patients. Typically, this can be performed in either a one- or two-step procedure. Besides degenerative aortic aneurysms, postdissecting aneurysms are a common late complication of a persistent false lumen after type A aortic dissection and some medically treated type B aortic dissections.

Workup

All patients with aortic arch aneurysms should have a CT scan with intravenous agent from the carotid to the femoral arteries. The present patient's CTA (Fig. 1) documents a thoracic aortic arch aneurysm with no abnormalities of the supraaortic brachiocephalic arteries. The use of 3D reconstructions provide a great opportunity to study the morphology of the pathology and to determine whether a direct surgical approach or a hybrid approach with a stent graft and debranching procedure is preferred. Echocardiography showed an ejection fraction of approximately 60%, a cardiac catheterization revealed no significant coronary disease, and her pulmonary function tests are acceptable.

Discussion

Isolated aortic arch disease is relatively uncommon and is usually part of multilevel aortic disease. Treatment of aortic arch disease is challenging and associated with considerable morbidity and mortality, especially in patients older than 75 years of age. A recent large series of open aortic arch repairs reported an early mortality between 4% and 13%, a stroke rate between 1.6% and 9.2%, and spinal cord ischemia ranging from 0% to 13%.

Diagnosis and Treatment

The treatment of aortic arch disease is challenging and associated with considerable morbidity and mortality. The use of selective cerebral perfusion and hypothermic circulatory arrest for brain protection during open surgery for aortic arch disease has considerably improved outcomes, although mortality and morbidity remain substantial. Because of the anatomy of the aortic arch with its side branches, a standard endovascular approach is not yet available in these patients. Therefore, a hybrid approach, which combines debranching of supraaortic arteries with stent graft placement in the thoracic aorta, has become an attractive alternative for high-risk patients. Based on the intended proximal landing zone (LZ) of the stent graft, patients are classified according to the Ishimaru classification. In patients with LZ0, the ascending aorta is used as the proximal LZ and the innominate artery (IA) is covered, requiring revascularization of all supraaortic brachiocephalic branches through a median sternotomy or through extra-anatomic debranching. In case of LZ1, the left common carotid artery (LCCA) and left subclavian artery (LSA) are covered and an extra-anatomic carotid-carotid bypass and revascularization of the left LSA is needed. When only the LSA is covered (LZ2), a left subclavian bypass or transposition is recommended, as this decreases the incidence of spinal cord ischemia and stroke.

Surgical Approach for Thoracic Aortic Arch Debranching

The procedure is performed under general anesthesia, and cerebral monitoring is used throughout the entire procedure. The patient is prepped from head to knees and draped in sterile fashion. A medium sternotomy is performed, and the pericardium is opened. After heparinization, the ascending aorta is tangentially clamped. With the use of a reversed aortobifemoral prosthesis, an end-to-side anastomosis is made between the graft and the ascending aorta. Subsequently, the IA is transected, and after the origin of the IA is clamped and ligated, an end-to-end anastomosis is performed to the graft. Subsequently, the other limb is used to perform an end-to-end anastomosis with the LSA. Depending on the anatomy, the graft is preferably placed deep to

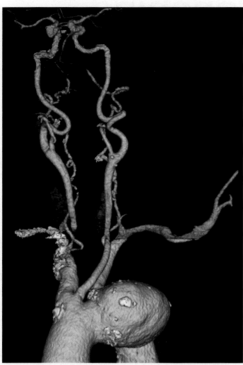

FIGURE 1 • Preoperative CT scan showing saccular aortic arch aneurysm.

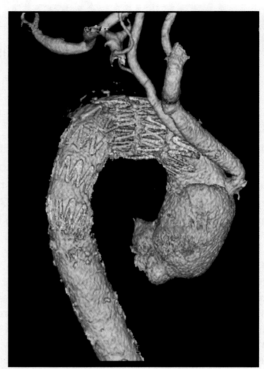

FIGURE 2 • Postoperative CT scan showing total aortic arch debranching and aneurysm exclusion using TEVAR.

the innominate vein, to avoid compression of the vein. Finally, the left common carotid artery is reimplanted in the limb of the prosthesis in an end-to-side fashion. Closure of the chest is performed with sternal wires and the soft tissue closed in multiple layers. The second stage of the procedure, which can be performed in the same setting or during a second procedure, consists of placement of two stent grafts, covering all ligated branches. Postdeployment angiography demonstrated appropriate placement of the stent grafts with aneurysm exclusion and no endoleaks. After all catheters and wires are straightened and removed, an Angio-Seal device is deployed in one groin, and the arteriotomy in the femoral artery is closed. A postoperative CTA showed adequate exclusion of the aneurysm (Fig. 2; Table 1).

Surveillance following TEVAR

Periprocedural stroke and spinal cord ischemia are strongly related to mortality, but are relatively rare as the patency of the supra-aortic grafts is excellent. Extensive experience with TEVAR has shown that neurologic outcome is strongly related to the patency of the LSA, highlighting the necessity for revascularization of the LSA. However, the most disastrous complication is a retrograde type A dissection after stent graft deployment, which should be immediately addressed and treated with open surgical repair. Other complications include chylothorax, chronic lymph fistula, and left laryngeal nerve palsy. Imaging should be performed at 1, 6, and 12 months following the initial procedure and then annually thereafter in order to monitor patency and the presence of endoleak.

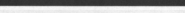

TABLE 1. Aortic Arch Debranching

Key Technical Steps

1. Choose appropriate landing zone based on 3D reconstruction of CT scan.
2. Perform a median sternotomy.
3. Heparinize.
4. Side clamp ascending aorta.
5. Perform an end-to-side anastomosis with a reversed aortobifemoral prosthesis.
6. Dissect the IA, ligate at origin, and perform an end-to-end anastomosis.
7. Dissect LSA, ligate at origin, and perform an end-to-end anastomosis using the other limb prosthesis, preferably deep to the innominate vein.
8. The left common carotid artery is reimplanted into the left limb of the subclavian bypass in an end-to-end fashion.
9. Median sternotomy is closed.
10. TEVAR is performed in normal fashion.

Potential Pitfalls

- Compression/kinking of graft limbs
- Compression of innominate vein
- Retrograde ascending aorta dissection, requiring open surgical repair
- Spinal cord ischemia or stroke

Case Conclusion

The patient was admitted to the intensive care unit, where her hospital course was complicated by atrial fibrillation and pneumonia. After administration of intravenous antibiotics and medical therapy for her arrhythmia, the patient improved slowly and was discharged after a month of hospitalization to a rehabilitation facility.

TAKE HOME POINTS

- Hybrid debranching procedures are reserved for high-risk patients with multisegmental thoracic aortic disease.
- The type of debranching procedure varies from a left subclavian bypass to a total arch debranching, depending on the extent of the disease (Ishimaru classification).
- Patients require surveillance by CTA at 1, 6, and 12 months and annually thereafter.

SUGGESTED READINGS

Cao P, De Rango P, Czerny M, et al. Systematic review of clinical outcomes in hybrid procedures for aortic arch dissections and other arch diseases. *J Thorac Cardiovasc Surg.* 2012;144(6):1286-1300.

Czerny M, Schmidli J, Carrel T, et al. Hybrid aortic arch repair. *Ann Cardiothorac Surg.* 2013;2(3):372-377.

Mitchell R, Ishimaru S, Ehrlich M, et al. First international summit on thoracic aortic endografting: roundtable on thoracic aortic dissection as an indication for endografting. *J Endovasc Ther.* 2002;9(suppl 2):98-105.

CLINICAL SCENARIO CASE QUESTIONS

1. How is a patient with proximal landing zone between the innominate artery and the LCCA classified according the Ishimaru classification?
   a. LZ0
   b. LZ1
   c. LZ2
   d. LZ3

2. What is the most disastrous complication after stent graft placement following an aortic arch debranching?
   a. Type A dissection
   b. Stroke
   c. Spinal cord ischemia
   d. All of the above

59 Type A Aortic Dissection after TEVAR

NICOLAS H. POPE and GORAV AILAWADI

Presentation

A 72-year-old male with a history of hypertension presented to the emergency department complaining of persistent chest pain radiating to the back. CT angiography (CTA) demonstrated a chronic type B aortic dissection with aneurysmal dilatation to 5.8 cm without visceral involvement. He underwent endovascular descending aortic repair (EVAR) with an endograft without complication (Fig. 1). He was seen in clinic and found to be doing well without endoleak or further dilation of his aneurysm. He presented to the emergency department 1 year after his procedure complaining of sudden-onset, persistent chest pain that did not worsened activity. He denied shortness of breath or leg swelling. His heart rate was 110 beats per minute with a blood pressure of 140/80 mm Hg. He was afebrile with an oxygen saturation of 98% on room air and a respiratory rate of 18. His physical examination was unremarkable, and he had 2+ peripheral pulses equally in all four extremities.

Differential Diagnosis

The differential diagnosis includes endoleak causing expansion of the existing false aortic lumen with or without contained aortic rupture, myocardial infarction, pulmonary embolism, and type A aortic dissection. Given the patient's history of type B dissection, further expansion of the false aortic lumen must be high on the differential diagnosis. This may be the result of type I or type II endoleak and may be accompanied by (contained) rupture of the aneurysmal portion of the aorta. A new type A aortic dissection must also be considered. This may be the result of a de novo tear in the ascending aorta or may represent a retrograde dissection related to his previously placed stent graft.

Myocardial infarction (MI) must also be evaluated in this patient. In a patient with a history of aortic dissection, a type A dissection with coronary involvement must also be considered if evidence of myocardial ischemia is present. Pulmonary embolism is unlikely, but should be considered in the differential of acute-onset chest pain.

Workup

History should determine the timing and location of pain and any associated symptoms that may indicate malperfusion. Physical examination should attempt to identify heart murmurs, as new aortic valve insufficiency (AI) as a result of type A dissection or new mitral insufficiency as a result of papillary muscle rupture following MI. Neurologic deficits may indicate arch vessel involvement of a type A dissection.

Workup should include standard laboratory assessment. Cardiac enzymes and an electrocardiogram (EKG) are necessary to rule out myocardial ischemia/infarction. A bedside transthoracic echocardiogram can identify wall motion abnormalities resulting from ischemic areas of myocardium and can often visualize the ascending aorta to evaluate for dissection.

In a hemodynamically stable patient with a thoracic endograft, CTA should be performed early, and is the gold standard to evaluate the position of the graft and look for endoleak and expansion of the false aortic lumen. Chest, abdomen, and pelvis CTA also allows for visualization of the entire aorta and provides important anatomic information to allow for preoperative planning should an aortic repair be required. Ideally, CTA may include the neck to look for extension in the carotid arteries and should be carried as far inferiorly as the femoral vessels to assess their adequacy to support peripheral cannulation (for type A repair) or femoral access for additional stent graft procedures (for endoleak).

Case Continued

Basic laboratory values and cardiac enzymes were normal. EKG showed no ischemic changes, and bedside transthoracic echocardiogram demonstrated no wall motion abnormalities or valvular disease and an ejection fraction of 55% with poor visualization of the ascending aorta. Figure 2 demonstrates significant CTA findings.

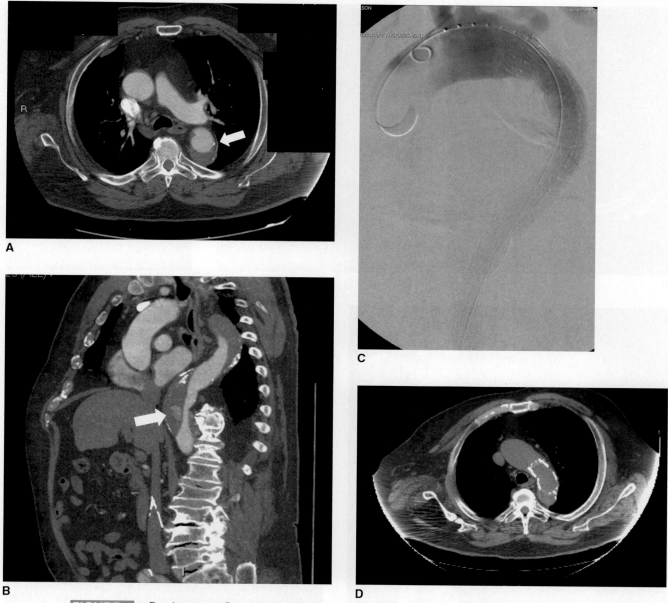

FIGURE 1 • Previous type B aortic dissection seen on CTA (*arrows*) in axial (**A**) and coronal (**B**) views. Completion angiography after placement of a Cook Talent TX2 endograft with no evidence of endoleak (**C**). Noncontrast CT obtained in follow-up demonstrated good position of proximal stent graft without aortic pathology (**D**).

Diagnosis and Treatment

Acute Type A Aortic Dissection

CTA demonstrates a type A aortic dissection extending to the origin of the innominate artery and a moderate pericardial effusion (arrowhead, Fig. 2C). There is no involvement of the arch vessels or evidence of contrast within the false lumen of the previous type B dissection.

The presence of noncovered stent grafts or barbs in the setting of a type B aortic dissection or a thoracic aortic aneurysm may place patients who have undergone TEVAR at increased risk for a retrograde type A dissection. Other risk factors for retrograde dissection following TEVAR include

landing zones in the proximal ascending aorta (zone 0) and an ascending aortic diameter greater than 4.0 cm.

Surgical Approach

Treatment for an acute type A aortic dissection is emergent surgical replacement of the involved aortic segment with exclusion of the entry tear. The specific procedure and the need for deep hypothermic circulatory arrest (DHCA) are dictated by the extent of the dissection flap and the site of the entry tear. Dissection may extend down the aortic root leading to aortic insufficiency occasionally requiring valve replacement. Involvement of arch vessels can typically

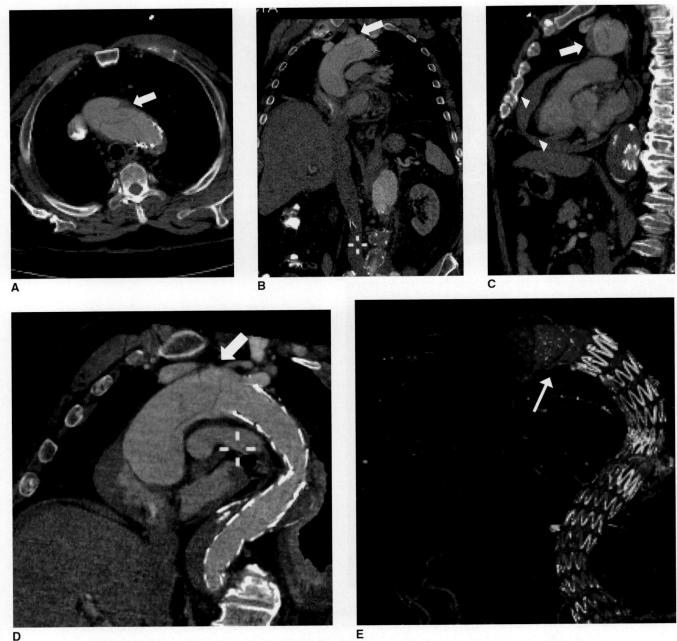

FIGURE 2 • Acute type A dissection following TEVAR. CTA demonstrates acute type A aortic dissection (*arrows*) and pericardial effusion (*arrowhead*) in axial **(A)**, coronal **(B)**, sagittal **(C)**, and multiplane reconstruction, **(D)** three-dimensional reconstruction of the aorta demonstrating intimal tear (*thin arrow*) and aortic endograft **(E)**.

be addressed with a hemiarch replacement; however, an aortic debranching procedure and total arch replacement may rarely be necessary if an arch aneurysm is present, the details of which are beyond the scope of this chapter.

In this patient, the dissection flap appeared to begin at the proximal portion of the existing endograft. Evaluation of the true extent of the dissection flap and whether a complete or partial arch replacement, or an ascending aortic replacement alone must be made intraoperatively, but can be planned based upon the preoperative CTA.

The patient is placed supine with both arms tucked, and a transesophageal echo probe is placed after induction of anesthesia. Exposure of the ascending aorta and arch is achieved through a median sternotomy. The cannulation strategy is aided by the preoperative CTA. Given the involvement of the distal ascending aorta, arterial cannulation is performed through the right axillary artery, the femoral artery, or directly in the ascending aorta proper. In this case, the innominate artery was not dissected, and thus, a right axillary cutdown is performed. Following heparinization, the right axillary artery is clamped and an 8-mm Dacron graft is sewn end to side to the axillary artery to allow for arterial cannulation. A median sternotomy is performed and pericardium opened. In cases of pericardial tamponade, the pericardium is opened gradually to avoid significant hypertension and further injury to the aorta.

Venous cannulation is achieved with a single, multistaged cannula placed in the right atrium. If retrograde cerebral perfusion is planned, a small cannula is placed in the superior vena cava with an umbilical tape placed around the superior vena cava (SVC). Cardioplegia is delivered through a retrograde catheter placed in the coronary sinus. Cardiopulmonary bypass (CPB) is initiated, and the patient is cooled to 18°C to 25°C depending on the planned time for circulatory arrest. The left ventricle is protected from distention with an LV vent placed in the right superior pulmonary vein and across the mitral valve. The appropriate graft size is determined. Once cooling temperature is achieved, the head is packed in ice and the patient's blood volume is emptied out and circulatory arrest initiated. Retrograde cardioplegia is used to arrest the heart. Antegrade (through the innominate artery with partial arterial flow) or retrograde isolated cerebral perfusion (through the superior vena cava) should be considered when the circulatory arrest period is estimated to exceed 30 minutes.

The mid–ascending aorta is then transected and inspected for the entry tear. In this case, the tear lies near the proximal portion of the previously placed endograft. Thus, an ascending aortic replacement with a hemiarch anastomosis is suitable. The distal ascending aortic graft is anastomosed to the aortic arch at the level of the innominate artery in an end-to-end fashion with a Teflon felt strip to reinforce the dissected aorta. The graft is then clamped and CPB is restarted either through the existing arterial cannula or through an arterial cannula is placed through a side arm of the ascending graft, and rewarming is begun. Significant leaks at this anastomosis should be repaired prior to the proximal anastomosis. Proximally, the graft is cut to an appropriate length. The aorta is transected at the sinotubular junction just above the coronary arteries. If the root is dissected (as is typical), a tailored Teflon felt strip is be placed between the layers and secured in place with Bioglue as a sandwich. The aortic valve is resuspended with three pledgeted sutures at the commissures to ensure aortic valve competence.

The proximal graft is then anastomosed to the repaired aortic root. Ventricular pacing wires are placed, and the cross-clamp is removed. The heart function is assessed as the patient is weaned from CPB. The cannulas are removed as protamine is given. The right axillary conduit is oversewn, and the axillary incision is closed. The side arm of the aortic graft is oversewn. The field

TABLE 1. Ascending Aortic Replacement for Type A Dissection

Key Technical Steps

1. Median sternotomy
2. Arterial cannulation through right axillary or femoral artery; venous cannulation via right atrium
3. Cooling to 18°C–25°C and initiation of DHCA
4. Inspection to determine the intimal tear and the extent of the dissection
5. Anastomosis of aortic graft to aorta at level of innominate artery origin; careful consideration for complete arch replacement with anastomosing the graft to the descending stent graft and aorta
6. Placement of arterial cannula in graft side arm and reinstitution of CPB
7. Resection of intimal tear and ascending aorta, +/– aortic root, and/or valve replacement
8. Proper placement of coronary buttons (if root replacement was needed)
9. Repair of aortic root tear with obliteration of the false lumen with felt and Bioglue
10. Aortic valve resuspension with pledgeted sutures above the three commissures
11. Anastomosis of proximal ascending aorta to graft
12. Rewarming and weaning of CPB
13. Cannula removal and oversewing of axillary conduit and aortic graft side arm

Potential Pitfalls

- Inability to locate the site of intimal tear
- Failure to address aortic insufficiency with aortic root or valve replacement
- Coronary buttons placed too far distally, which places them under tension when the heart is filled or with too much redundancy as to allow for kinking in situations where a Bentall or David procedure must be performed
- Significant bleeding at distal or proximal anastomosis requiring more extensive aortic replacement
- Stroke

is inspected for hemostasis, chest tubes are placed, and the chest is closed (Table 1). This patient underwent this procedure as described without any immediate complications.

Potential Pitfalls

As discussed above, consideration of the patient's anatomy when choosing the type of endograft may reduce the likelihood of a new type A dissection. In patients without significant existing coronary disease, time should not be spent obtaining preoperative cardiac catheterization.

Cannulation of the false aortic lumen is best avoided with the use of peripheral arterial cannulation (axillary or femoral) as described above. If the decision is made to cannulate the aorta directly, on-table ultrasound and TEE guidance may help avoid false lumen cannulation. Cannulation of the false lumen can typically be identified by high arterial line pressure, low systemic arterial pressures, and a low flow rate.

Intraoperatively, care must be taken to accurately determine the site of the intimal tear. If the site of the tear cannot be readily identified, the ascending aorta should be replaced as proximally as the sinotubular junction. The conduct of the operation, especially the circulatory arrest portion, must be efficient as prolonged circulatory arrest times are associated with greater incidence of cerebrovascular events.

AI seen on TEE should be addressed. Aortic valve repair/replacement, with or without aortic root replacement, may be considered. Other operations that can be used include a valve-sparing root (David procedure) replacing the entire aorta from just above the valve if the leaflets are normal, to a Bentall procedure where the aortic valve, root, and ascending aorta are replaced. Both of these require reimplantation of the main coronary arteries. When reimplanting coronary ostia, coronary buttons should be reimplanted on the graft such that they are not under excessive tension once the heart is filled, but without laxity, which could result in kinking.

Special Intraoperative Considerations

If anastomosis directly to the previously place endograft is necessary, any proximal wire barbs must first be removed from the endograft with wire cutters. The new Dacron graft may then be anastomosed to both the native aorta and the existing stent graft, again using an onlay technique. We incorporate the descending aorta and a felt strip to minimize risk of bleeding in this case.

Retrograde dissection of one or both coronary ostia requires either local repair or exclusion, and saphenous vein graft may be necessary for revascularization. If the dissection extends around, but does not involve the coronary ostia, reimplantation alone may be sufficient. Several techniques have been described for repair of dissection involving the coronary ostia, including local patch repair or reapproximation of the false to the true lumen.

Postoperative Management

Patients are brought to the cardiac intensive care unit and are typically extubated when hemodynamically stable without signs of ongoing bleeding. Blood pressure is optimized to provide adequate cerebral perfusion without hypertension, which has been shown to increase the need for reoperation for bleeding. Patients should be monitored closely for signs of end organ malperfusion. Malperfusion of the limb or gut must be addressed immediately after reestablishing flow in the true lumen, following type **A** dissection repair.

Case Conclusion

The patient recovered from the procedure without complication. He was discharged on postoperative day 5 and was seen for follow-up 6 weeks after discharge. CTA performed at that time revealed an intact repair with evidence of positive remodeling of the false aortic lumen (Fig. 3).

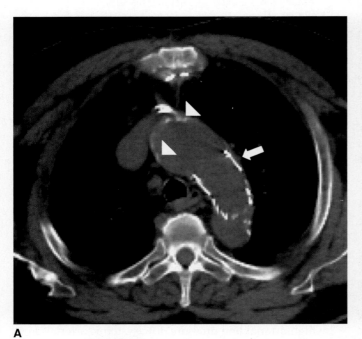
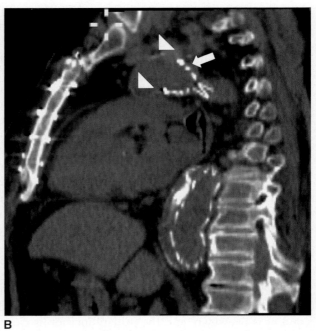

A   B

FIGURE 3 • Aortic arch following repair. Gelweave ascending aortic graft (*arrowheads*) can be seen opposing previous endograft (*arrow*) in axial **(A)** and sagittal **(B)** views.

TAKE HOME POINTS

- Type A aortic dissection represents a surgical emergency and should be treated with emergent aortic repair.
- Placement of a barbed thoracic stent graft in patients with aortic dissection may increase the likelihood of retrograde type A dissection.
- Pre- and postoperative blood pressure and shear force (dp/dt) control reduces the need for reoperation and can be accomplished with short-acting beta-blockers (esmolol) and sodium nitroprusside.
- Acute dissections that involve the arch can typically be treated with hemiarch repair rather than a full arch replacement.
- Dissections that involve the aortic root with normal aortic valve anatomy and coaptation can be treated with valve-sparing root replacement (David procedure), or root reconstruction.
- Patients with a connective tissue disorder and eccentric AI typically require an aortic root without or with valve replacement (Bentall procedure).
- Care must be taken when choosing sites for coronary button reimplantation as to avoid excessive tension or redundancy.
- Systemic hypothermia and antegrade or retrograde cerebral perfusion minimize risk of intraoperative stroke.

SUGGESTED READINGS

Desai ND. Techniques for repair of retrograde aortic dissection following thoracic endovascular aortic repair. *Ann Cardiothorac Surg.* 2013;2:369-371.

Eggebrecht H, Thompson M, Rousseau H, et al. Retrograde ascending aortic dissection during or after thoracic aortic stent graft placement: insight from the European registry on endovascular aortic repair complications. *Circulation.* 2009;120:S276-S281.

Melby SJ, Zierer A, Damiano RJ Jr, et al. Importance of blood pressure control after repair of acute type a aortic dissection: 25-year follow-up in 252 patients. *J Clin Hypertens (Greenwich).* 2013;15:63-68.

Ramanath VS, Eagle KA, Nienaber CA, et al. The role of preoperative coronary angiography in the setting of type a acute aortic dissection: insights from the international registry of acute aortic dissection. *Am Heart J.* 2011;161:790-796; e791.

Williams JB, Andersen ND, Bhattacharya SD, et al. Retrograde ascending aortic dissection as an early complication of thoracic endovascular aortic repair. *J Vasc Surg.* 2012;55:1255-1262.

CLINICAL SCENARIO CASE QUESTIONS

1. Which of the following is NOT true regarding acute aortic dissection?

   a. Acute dissection is defined as onset of less than 14 days prior to presentation.

   b. Type A aortic dissection involving the arch vessels usually requires aortic debranching and full arch replacement.

   c. In patients with suspected acute type A dissection, preoperative cardiac catheterization has not been shown to improve in-hospital or 5-year survival.

   d. Blood pressure and shear force (dp/dt) control postoperatively has been shown to decrease the need for reoperation.

2. Which of the following is true of thoracic aortic endografts?

   a. All retrograde type A dissections have been associated with barbs on the endograft.

   b. All retrograde type A dissections have been associated with a supragraft noncovered stent as part of the endograft.

   c. The Gore TAG endograft utilizes a staged proximal deployment, allowing for more accurate placement in tight landing zones.

   d. Retrograde type A aortic dissection has been reported with all endografts commercially available in the United States.

60 EVAR Removal for Endoleak

NICHOLAS OSBORNE and GILBERT R. UPCHURCH Jr

Presentation

A 77-year-old gentleman, who underwent an endovascular abdominal aortic aneurysm repair with a bifurcated device (Cook Zenith) 3 years ago for a 7.7-cm infrarenal aneurysm on serial CT scan, was found to have an enlarging aneurysm sac. He was thought to have a type II endoleak originating from the left hypogastric branches, and this was embolized. He continued to have aneurysm growth and subsequently underwent embolization of his main left hypogastric artery and extension into the left external iliac artery. Following this, his aneurysm had enlarged to 8.8 cm, and he was referred for a second opinion. When he was seen in the clinic, he was asymptomatic. He had a nonpulsatile abdominal mass in his epigastrium and intact femoral pulses bilaterally. His laboratory studies included a normal white blood cell count of 6.3 and a creatinine of 1.0, and his C-reactive protein (CRP) and erythrocyte sedimentation rate (ESR) were not elevated. An outside hospital CT scan demonstrated a large infrarenal aneurysm with a patent Cook Zenith bifurcated endograft. The left hypogastric artery was occluded with coils in place and the left limb extended into the external iliac artery. He had no evidence of a type I, type II, or type III endoleak on review of previous CT scans. He did not have any stranding around the aorta or in the retroperitoneum.

Differential Diagnosis

An enlarging sac following endovascular abdominal aortic aneurysm repair (EVAR) requires immediate attention to identify the source of the expansion. In general, aneurysm sac expansion can be thought to be due to endoleak (Table 1) or infection. A review of 100 consecutive explants performed at the Cleveland Clinic between 1999 and 2007 reported a temporal relationship to the indication for explant. Early explants (within 1 year of implantation) may be related to endoleak from inadequate seal (38%), less commonly type II (3%) and infection (28%). After the first year, explants are more commonly performed for type I endoleak (35%), type II endoleak (20%), and type III endoleak (24%). After 1 year, infection appears to be a less common indication for explant (7%). After 5 years, type I endoleaks remain the primary indication in over one third of explants (35%). Type III endoleaks are increasingly common (32%) as well as occlusions (9%). In approaching this patient with an endoleak diagnosed after 3 years from this primary EVAR, it is important to rule out not only endoleak but also infection.

Workup

All EVAR patients are followed postoperatively with surveillance imaging to detect sac enlargement and endoleak. Although protocols for surveillance vary from institution to institution, initial CT angiography is the modality of choice to evaluate for an endoleak or sac enlargement in the postoperative period. This patient initially had a stable aneurysm sac following an EVAR with a type II endoleak. Over the course of 2 years, the aneurysm sac appeared to enlarge and he underwent an embolization and extension of endograft limb. When the sac continued to grow, the suspicion for infection was raised. In the absence of an endoleak, an enlarging sac may be due to endotension or infection. The patient underwent CT angiography, which failed to show any stigmata of infection, including any loss of the plane between the aorta and small bowel, stranding in the retroperitoneum or gas in the aneurysm sac (Fig. 1). He was afebrile, and he had a normal WBC count. His inflammatory markers, CRP and ESR, were both normal.

Diagnosis and Treatment

Patients diagnosed with an expanding sac should undergo imaging to identify a cause. In the absence of an identifiable endoleak, the suspicion for infection should increase. Duplex ultrasonography can be employed to follow sac size and to detect evidence of a type I, II, or III endoleak. Although less specific and sensitive, duplex may help to identify gas within the sac or a fluid collection that could be concerning for graft infection. When there is evidence of either sac enlargement of endoleak, a CT angiogram should be performed to further evaluate the repair. CT angiography is the initial diagnostic study of choice due to the high sensitivity and specificity for graft infection and endoleak (Fig. 1). Although the sensitivity for grossly infected grafts may be as high as 95%, CT may

TABLE 1. Types of Endoleaks

Endoleak	Source
Type Ia	Blood flow into the sac due to inadequate seal at the proximal graft seal zone
Type Ib	Blood flow into the sac due to inadequate seal at the distal graft seal zone
Type II	Blood flow into the sac due to collateral vessels (typically lumbar arteries or IMA)
Type III	Blood flow into the sac due to inadequate seal between overlapping stent graft components
Type IV	Blood flow into the sac due to graft porosity
Type V	Expansion of the sac without evidence of ongoing blood flow—described as endotension

be less useful for low-grade indolent infections (sensitivity 50%). In these cases, further imaging with either nuclear medicine tagged white blood cell scan (leukocyte scintigraphy) or FDG-PET scanning may offer higher sensitivities. FDG-PET can be fused with CT imaging and together yields a sensitivity of up to 91% for infections. Leukocyte scintigraphy, long considered the gold standard, offers similar sensitivity, but less exact localization, higher interobserver variability, and more time-intensive preparation (Fig. 2). In addition to imaging, patients with suspicion of a graft infection, either by imaging or an expanding sac without evidence of endoleak, should have routine blood cultures drawn and a CRP and an ESR as well. Although the rate of positive blood cultures is low, the ESR and CRP may be elevated with infection.

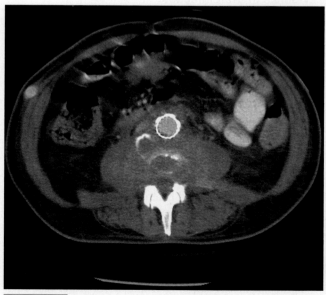

FIGURE 1 • CT angiogram demonstrating a previous aortic endograft and enlarging sac.

When considering treatment strategies for an expanding aneurysm sac, the cause must be evaluated. If there is evidence of a type I, II, or III endoleak, then an endovascular approach may be warranted to seal the sac further. In this patient's case, this was unsuccessful. He had an extension and coiling of his hypogastric artery. In the absence of a potential cause that can be treated with either coiling or extension, most patients will require an explant to treat the expanding sac. Treatment of an expanding sac can be pursued with in-line reconstruction. In the setting of infection, several options for reconstruction exist, including extra-anatomic bypass, in-line reconstruction with an antibiotic-impregnated graft, femoropopliteal vein (neo-aortoiliac system [NAIS]), or cryopreserved aorta.

Surgical Approach

Since there was some concern for graft infection, this patient underwent a WBS scan, which was negative. The patient was considered for explant and reconstruction with a rifampin-soaked Dacron graft. The patient underwent preoperative cardiac clearance and was felt to be an appropriate surgical candidate for explant. The patient was taken to the operating room, and a midline laparotomy was performed. The retroperitoneum was exposed, and the aortic aneurysm was controlled proximally above the renal arteries and the iliac bifurcations controlled distally. Since there was suprarenal fixation in place, care must be taken to expose the suprarenal aorta for the potential to clamp. Since the endograft was potentially infected, all graft material should be removed. A suprarenal clamp was temporarily used to allow for the graft to be completely removed. The suprarenal fixation was cut flush with the graft material, and the grafts were removed. Following this, the clamp was moved down to just below the renal arteries. A rifampin-soaked Dacron graft was then used for in-line reconstruction. The proximal anastomosis was then sewn to the aorta just inferior to the renal arteries, incorporating the suprarenal noncovered stent into the anastomosis. The aneurysm sac and retroperitoneum were irrigated with a pulse irrigator. The omentum was then used to cover the graft. The patient was then closed and maintained on IV antibiotics. The final cultures were negative, and antibiotics were stopped (Table 2).

Special Intraoperative Considerations

Either a transperitoneal or retroperitoneal approach can be used for explant of an endograft. It is important to establish control above the renal arteries in case the aorta is degenerative or tears with endograft removal. Supraceliac and suprarenal control should be obtained ahead of time. Grafts without suprarenal fixation are typically easier to remove with gentle traction. Nitinol stent material will shrink if exposed to ice or cold saline. This may be employed at the time of explant to aid in removal of nitinol-based stent grafts. The suprarenal fixation of some stent grafts (Cook Zenith, Medtronic Endurant, Trivascular Ovation) may be difficult to remove. The bare

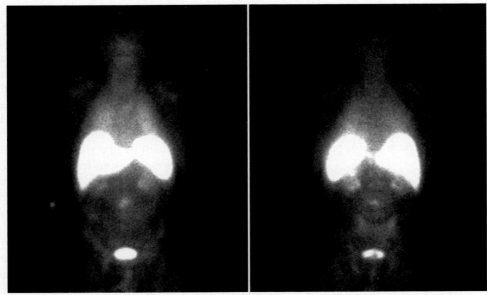

FIGURE 2 • Leukocyte scintigraphy from a different patient demonstrating increased uptake in the region of the aortic graft.

metal can be cut and left behind with little consequence. Removal of the suprarenal fixation in entirety can be accomplished by simply cutting each metal strut with wire cutters and removing each stent segment individually. A cut 60-cc syringe slowly pushed over the stents to collapse the fixation has been described as a method to aid in removal of the suprarenal stent, although the authors have not had much success with this technique. Alternatively, the anterior aorta can be incised vertically to allow for removal of the suprarenal fixation. In most cases, we favor leaving the suprarenal fixation in place unless there is a compelling reason to remove it.

Postoperative Management

Postoperatively, patients should be maintained on antibiotics when there is concern for infection. Since cultures may be negative even in the setting of a positive leukocyte scintigraphy, lifelong antibiotics are required when prosthetic material is employed. Long-term, CRP levels may be useful in surveillance for recurrent graft infection. Cross-sectional imaging can identify perigraft fluid or other associated signs of infection.

Case Conclusion

The patient did well postoperatively. His final culture results remained negative. He was maintained on oral antibiotics for life for a possible graft infection. He is followed in the clinic and was last seen 2 years following his repair with no evidence of graft infection.

TAKE HOME POINTS

- The most common indication for explantation of a previous endograft is persistent sac enlargement.
- Infection should be considered when evaluating patients with a persistent graft infection.
- Suprarenal fixation can be left in place as long as the stent graft material is completely removed. Complete removal of the bare metal stents may be associated with higher morbidity.
- Reconstruction options include in situ reconstruction with a rifampin-soaked Dacron graft or femoropopliteal vein (NAIS), cryopreserved arterial allografts, or extra-anatomic bypass.

SUGGESTED READINGS

Bruggink JL, Slart RH, Pol JA, et al. Current role of imaging in diagnosing aortic graft infections. *Semin Vasc Surg.* 2011;24(4):182-190.

TABLE 2. EVAR Removal for Endoleak

Key Technical Steps

1. Preoperatively, evaluate for evidence of graft infection in the setting of persistent sac growth without evidence of endoleak.
2. Expose and control the suprarenal aorta and potentially supraceliac when explanting an endograft with suprarenal fixation.
3. Suprarenal fixation may be removed completely or cut and incorporated into the suture line. Removing the fixation may result in aortic injury proximal to the graft.

Potential Pitfalls

- In-line reconstructions should be wrapped with omentum when concerned for infection as reinfection is always a risk.
- Stump blowout can occur if the old endograft is entirely removed and an extra-anatomic graft is performed.

Fatima J, Duncan AA, de Grandis E, et al. Treatment strategies and outcomes in patients with infected aortic endografts. *J Vasc Surg.* 2013;58(2):371-379.

Koole D, Moll FL, Buth J, et al. Annual rupture risk of abdominal aortic aneurysm enlargement without detectable endoleak after endovascular abdominal aortic repair. *J Vasc Surg.* 2011;54:1614-1622.

Laser A, Baker N, Rectenwald J, et al. Graft infection after endovascular abdominal aortic aneurysm repair. *J Vasc Surg.* 2011;54:58-63.

Lipsitz EC, Ohki T, Veith FJ, et al. Delayed open conversion following endovascular aortoiliac aneurysm repair: partial (or complete) endograft preservation as a useful adjunct. *J Vasc Surg.* 2003;38:1191.

Mehta M, Paty PS, Roddy SP, et al. Treatment options for delayed AAA rupture following endovascular repair. *J Vasc Surg.* 2011;53:14-20.

CLINICAL SCENARIO CASE QUESTIONS

1. In the early postoperative period, the most common indications for explantation of an aortic endograft are:
   a. Infection
   b. Type I endoleak
   c. Type II endoleak
   d. Type III endoleak

2. The study with the highest sensitivity for graft infection is:
   a. CT angiography
   b. Leukocyte scintigraphy
   c. MRI/MRA
   d. PET scan

3. Leaking from between the components of an endograft is an example of a type _____ endoleak.
   a. Type I
   b. Type II
   c. Type III
   d. Type IV
   e. Type V

61 Pediatric Midabdominal Coarctation

SHIPRA ARYA and DAWN M. COLEMAN

Presentation

A 6-year-old male presents with elevated blood pressure following routine adenoidectomy. On physical examination, his systolic blood pressure measures 180 to 200 mm Hg and diastolic pressures measure 90 to 100 mm Hg in both arms; lower extremity pressures are approximately 95/55 mm Hg. He is admitted for hypertensive urgency and requires four antihypertensive agents for adequate blood pressure control. A vascular surgery consult is obtained. He has an abdominal bruit on auscultation. His bilateral femoral pulses and pedal pulses are nonpalpable, but present on Doppler exam.

Differential Diagnosis

Pediatric abdominal aortic coarctation or middle aortic syndrome (MAS) is an uncommon clinical condition generated by segmental narrowing of the abdominal or distal descending thoracic aorta. Coarctation can involve any portion of the aorta, but most commonly occurs distal to the ductus arteriosus. The abdominal aorta is affected in only 0.5% to 2% of aortic coarctations.

MAS may be acquired (associated with clinical syndromes referenced in Table 1) or congenital, ascribed to a developmental anomaly in the fusion and maturation of the paired embryonic dorsal aortas. Segmental aortic stenosis may be located at the suprarenal (69%), interrenal (23%), and infrarenal (8%) positions, with a high propensity for concomitant stenoses in both the renal (80%) and visceral (60%) arteries.

Hypertension proximal to the aortic stenosis, and relative hypotension distal to it, are characteristic findings in MAS, present in 94% of patients. Changes in pulsatile flow and pressure across renal stenoses or aortic narrowings are responsible for renin-angiotensin system activation and subsequent blood pressure elevations. This form of renovascular hypertension is typically resistant to simple pharmacologic control. Other manifestations including exercise-related lower extremity fatigue or visceral ischemia are less frequent, despite the majority of patients having differential upper and lower extremity blood pressures and associated splanchnic and renal arterial occlusive disease.

Differential diagnoses include essential hypertension, endocrine dysfunction, isolated renal artery stenosis, renal parenchymal disease, Wilms tumor, and neuroblastoma, among others. This patient's medically refractory hypertension despite multiple antihypertensive agents, abdominal bruit, and lack of palpable femoral pulses suggests aortic coarctation.

Workup

Additional clinical history should elicit constitutional symptoms concerning for vasculitis, lower extremity and generalized fatigue with exertion, flank pain, hematuria, and relevant family and birth history. A thorough clinical exam should assess for features suggesting one of the aforementioned clinical syndromes (Table 1), abdominal mass, abdominal bruit, stature, and costal margin. Blood work should be sent to assess renal function (BUN, creatinine), vasculitis (C-reactive protein), and electrolyte levels. Additionally, blood hormone levels may help differentiate the diagnosis in cases of pediatric hypertension. Specifically, high plasma renin activity indicates renovascular hypertension (including MAS), while altered aldosterone and catecholamine levels may indicate endocrine dysfunction (i.e., hyperaldosteronism, pheochromocytoma) or neuroblastoma. Urinalysis will reveal hematuria, concerning for intrinsic renal disease. Fasting lipid panels and oral glucose tolerance tests should be considered to evaluate metabolic syndrome in obese children.

Ultrasonography should be considered the first-line diagnostic imaging modality in patients with renovascular hypertension. Transabdominal aortorenal duplex may reveal abdominal aortic coarctation and renal artery stenosis; additionally, abdominal ultrasonography may reveal tumors and structural anomalies of the kidneys and allow for assessment of renal size, symmetry, and the presence of renal scarring. Echocardiography should be performed to assess for left ventricular hypertrophy (LVH) and ventricular function in addition to surveillance of the thoracic aorta for coarctation. Cross-sectional imaging with computed tomography angiography (CTA) or magnetic resonance angiography (MRA) will provide more specific anatomic information regarding aortic coarctation and any associated renal and visceral

TABLE 1. Associated Clinical Syndromes

Associated Syndromes with MAS

Neurofibromatosis (NF-1)
Williams syndrome
Alagille syndrome
Fibromuscular dysplasia
Retroperitoneal fibrosis
Aortitis
  Takayasu syndrome
  Giant cell arteritis
  Temporal arteritis
Acquired infectious causes
  Rheumatic fever
  Rubella virus
  Syphilis
  Tuberculosis

pathology. MRA is often favored in pediatric patients as it offers diagnostic sensitivity without the associated risks of irradiation. Arteriography with multiplanar and selective views is a helpful adjunct for preoperative planning to define the extent of the coarctation and renal/visceral arterial involvement. Additionally, angiography offers the specificity to identify additional smaller accessory renal arteries or segmental arterial stenoses that might otherwise be missed with traditional cross-sectional imaging. Finally, the adequacy of the iliac arteries for use as conduit can be assessed.

On clinical exam, this patient is of appropriate height and weight for age and has no stigmata concerning for associated syndrome. As referenced above, he has an abdominal bruit, no abdominal masses, and nonpalpable femoral and pedal pulses. Abdominal ultrasound with renal duplex revealed normal renal size, bilateral renal artery stenosis, and aortic narrowing. An echocardiogram revealed mild LVH with preserved function. MRA confirmed midabdominal aortic coarctation extending from the celiac artery to the origin of the inferior mesenteric artery (IMA) with associated superior mesenteric artery (SMA) and bilateral renal artery stenoses (Fig. 1).

Diagnosis and Treatment

Untreated pediatric midabdominal coarctation may result in failure to thrive, hypertensive crisis, stroke, intracranial hemorrhage, renal atrophy, renal insufficiency, progressive LVH with associated heart failure, flash pulmonary edema, and decreased life expectancy (less than 40 years).

Indications for surgical revascularization include medically refractory hypertension (despite three drugs), progressive renal insufficiency, nonischemic cardiomyopathy resulting from concentric LVH, failure to thrive, and lower extremity sequelae (claudication, exertional fatigue, and/or growth disturbance). Often, despite dramatic clinical presentations, even patients with hypertensive emergencies can be managed appropriately medically once the diagnosis of renovascular hypertension secondary to MAS is

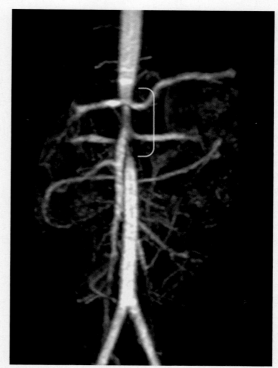

FIGURE 1 • Magnetic resonance angiography revealing midabdominal aortic stenosis and associated superior mesenteric and bilateral renal artery stenoses. (From Stanley JC, Criado E, Eliason JL, et al. Abdominal coarctation: surgical treatment of 53 patients with a thoracoabdominal bypass, patch aortoplasty, or interposition aortoaortic graft. *J Vasc Surg.* 2008;48:1073-1082.)

confirmed. The timing of surgery is especially relevant in pediatric patients given projected axial and vascular growth postrepair and the technical challenges that encompass revascularization in the infant and toddler. As such, at the youthful extreme, it is prudent to allow for growth to at least 3 to 4 years of age is possible, even if this requires a dramatic medication regimen of five to six drugs.

Given this patient's age of 6 years, medically refractory hypertension, and evidence of LVH, revascularization should be considered.

Surgical Approach

Open surgical repair is the primary treatment for abdominal aortic coarctation. Options for revascularization include aortoaortic bypass around the diseased segment, patch aortoplasty, and, less commonly, interposition grafting of the aortic segment. Revascularization of indicated renal artery or mesenteric stenosis should be performed concomitantly as indicated Table 2.

Incision and Exposure (Common to All Open Approaches)

The proximal extent of the coarctation will dictate the surgical approach as either thoracoabdominal or laparotomy. If renal revascularization is intended, a transverse

TABLE 2. Pediatric Aortic Reconstruction for Coarctation

Key Technical Steps

1. Thoracoabdominal incision vs. laparotomy (consider transverse abdominal incision)
2. Medial visceral rotation and aortic exposure from the diaphragm to aortic bifurcation
3. Vascular control (including that of branch vessels) with nontraumatic clamps; consider partial aortic occlusion if appropriate.
4. Appropriate PTFE graft or patch size selection
5. *Patch aortoplasty*
   a. Longitudinal aortotomy
   b. Patch aortoplasty constructed with a circumferential continuous suture line of polypropylene or Teflon suture starting with the most proximal extent
   c. Reposition proximal clamp distal to respective branch vessels as the repair proceeds to limit visceral and renal ischemic time

   Aortoaortic bypass
   a. Creation of retrorenal (left) tunnel if indicated (i.e., thoracoabdominal aortoaortic bypass for long-segment coarctations)
   b. Longitudinal anterolateral aortotomy proximal to coarctation
   c. Bevel graft; creation of end-to-side anastomosis with polypropylene or Teflon suture
   d. Clamp graft and restore aortic flow
   e. Tunnel graft and cut to size
   f. Obtain distal vascular control
   g. Longitudinal aortotomy distal to coarctation
   h. Similar creation of distal anastomosis
6. Restoration of aortic flow and Doppler interrogation
7. Reversal of anticoagulation and closure

Potential Pitfalls

- Injury to the aorta or visceral vessels as vascular tissues are thin and friable in pediatric patients—specifically avoid adventitial hematoma
- Prolonged visceral ischemia
- Injury to the left colon, excessive retraction causing ischemia
- Excessive oversizing or redundancy of graft/patch can cause kinking

laparotomy is favored to facilitate renal exposure for mobilization. Exposure of the suprarenal aorta typically requires medial visceral rotation. Vascular control and anticoagulation should proceed in a standard fashion; additionally, a brisk osmotic diuresis is established with mannitol.

Patch Aortoplasty

Patch aortoplasty is preferred when the coarctation segment maintains adequate diameter to allow completion of the repair without an overlap of suture from the opposing side. A polytetrafluoroethylene (PTFE, Teflon) patch is sized so as to not be constrictive with growth into adulthood, yet not so generous as to risk development of unstable laminar thrombus.

Following anticoagulation and vascular control, a longitudinal aortotomy over the narrowed segment is created sharply and extended accordingly. An appropriately sized patch is then circumferentially sewn in with nonabsorbable Teflon or polypropylene suture placed in a continuous fashion. The proximal extent is typically constructed first permitting replacement of the proximal clamp more distal to relevant visceral/renal branches as the repair proceeds allowing for decreased end organ ischemic time. Following restoration of flow distal aortoiliac, branch vessel and renal parenchymal flow should be confirmed with Doppler interrogation. Anticoagulation is often reversed with protamine, and closure proceeds in the standard fashion.

Aortoaortic Bypass

Aortoaortic bypass is favored for those patients whose coarctation precludes patch aortoplasty secondary to diminutive caliber and in certain complex cases that require concomitant renal and splanchnic reconstruction. The PTFE conduit should be sized at least 60% to 70% the size of the adult aorta to prevent it from becoming an energy-consuming constriction as the aorta matures. This translates into an 8- to 12-mm graft in young children, a 12- to 16-mm graft in early adolescents, and a 14- to 20-mm graft in late adolescents and adults. Graft length should be constructed slightly more redundant in younger children to allow for stretch with axial growth; however, there is minimal axial growth from the diaphragm to the pelvis after 9 to 10 years of age.

Following the guidelines for exposure and vascular control outlined above, the respective aortotomies should be created on the anterolateral aorta sharply and widened with an aortic punch. Thoracoabdominal bypass grafts are typically tunneled posterior to the left kidney. The graft should be beveled accordingly prior to constructing each respective end-to-side anastomosis with Teflon or polypropylene suture. Restoration of flow, hemostasis, and closure should proceed as described above.

Rarely, interposition aortic grafts may be considered to treat short-segment coarctations in the absence of branch vessel involvement. This often permits a more limited exposure. The technical components vary only in that the respective anastomoses are constructed in an end-to-end fashion.

Concomitant Visceral Reconstruction

In the clinical setting of renovascular hypertension, any renal artery stenosis warrants simultaneous revascularization at the time of aortic reconstruction, with the exception being the child at the extremes of youth (i.e., less than 3 years of age). A mandate to visceral reconstruction applies only to the superior mesenteric artery in cases of symptomatic chronic mesenteric ischemia. Nevertheless, a relative indication to prophylactic reconstruction exists when performance of an aortoplasty or renal revascularization would make a subsequent mesenteric revascularization exceedingly difficult. The technical options include direct renal/visceral reimplantation onto the aorta or proper bypass using autogenous conduit. The internal iliac artery is the preferred conduit as saphenous vein is prone to aneurysmal degeneration and prosthetic conduits are more predisposed to restenosis.

Potential Pitfalls

Care must be taken during left colon retraction not to compromise retrograde blood flow through existing mesocolic collaterals arising from the IMA that provide critical blood flow to foregut and midgut structures during the medial visceral rotation. Limit visceral ischemia time during creation of the proximal anastomosis. Meticulous handling of the thin nonsclerotic tissues of pediatric vessels is critical to avoid suture line tears and the need for repair sutures. Avoid excessive oversizing or redundancy as it may lead to kinking of the patched aorta or the bypass graft once the clamps are removed.

Endovascular Therapy

Endovascular therapy may provide a minimally invasive treatment option in abdominal coarctation in young adults when a discrete aortic stenosis fails to involve the mesenteric and renal arteries. However, in light of the frequency with which these branch vessels are involved in MAS, the number of lesions amenable to endovascular repair is limited. Additionally, while available procedural success rates may be encouraging with improvement or cure of hypertension in up to 70% of patients, long-term outcomes remain poorly described. Early and late failures of balloon angioplasty alone suggest that stent placement is necessary to overcome the significant recoil of these often hypoplastic and highly fibrotic aortic narrowings.

Special Intraoperative Considerations

Often, the final surgical procedure is decided upon intraoperatively. As such, the surgeon should be well prepared to transition from intended patch aortoplasty to aortoaortic bypass if the narrowed aorta is not of appropriate caliber. In the case of renal and mesenteric revascularization, direct aortic reimplantation may not be appropriate if it results in undue tension on the anastomosis, despite adequate mobilization of the kidney. This versatility in surgical approach mandates preparation and the availability of conduit—both synthetic and autogenous. Additionally, a midline chevron extension toward the xiphoid may be necessary to facilitate exposure of the supraceliac aorta.

Postoperative Management

Postoperatively, patients are admitted to the intensive care unit for close hemodynamic monitoring. Blood pressure is often elevated postoperatively and intravenous infusions (i.e., nicardipine) may be required. Hypovolemia, hypotension, and vasopressors should be avoided to avoid vasoconstriction of small branch vessel reconstructions. Antiplatelet therapy with aspirin is dosed daily. Electrolytes and renal function should be monitored closely given the tendency toward salt wasting and invariable need for supplementation. Completion imaging to assess a "new baseline" with angiography or CT angiogram is encouraged to facilitate future surveillance. While most patients will transition to an oral antihypertensive regimen prior to discharge, the medication regimen is typically far less than preoperative requirements and typically declines during the first few months postoperatively.

Annual surveillance of lower extremity blood flow with exercise ankle-brachial indices is recommended. Serial MRA/CTA is often performed at 2-year intervals during periods of robust growth and is also indicated to assess for changes in surveillance ankle-brachial indices (ABIs) and acute escalations of blood pressure. Reoperations are infrequent, but may be required for anastomotic narrowings or if a patient outgrows the adequacy of the primary procedure.

Case Conclusion

The patient underwent successful aortoaortic bypass, SMA and right renal artery reimplantations, and left aortorenal bypass using the left internal iliac artery. He was discharged home on postoperative day 7 on two antihypertensive agents. His annual follow-up has since revealed normotension with no antihypertensive requirements, normal growth, and no evidence of anastomotic stenosis by surveillance MRA.

TAKE HOME POINTS

- Pediatric abdominal coarctation is a rare condition with frequent involvement of the splanchnic and renal vessels.
- Hypertension is the most common presentation.
- Decision for surgery depends on degree of hypertension and its complications.
- Open surgery is the preferred approach for revascularization. Surgical options include patch aortoplasty or aortoaortic bypass with concomitant visceral and/or renal reconstruction as necessary.

SUGGESTED READINGS

Delis KT, Gloviczki P. Middle aortic syndrome: from presentation to contemporary open surgical and endovascular treatment. *Perspect Vasc Surg Endovasc Ther.* 2005;17(3):187-203.

Graham LM, Zelenock GB, Erlandson EE, et al. Abdominal aortic coarctation and segmental hypoplasia. *Surgery.* 1979;86:519-529.

Hallett JW Jr, Brewster DC, Darling RC, et al. Coarctation of the abdominal aorta: current options in surgical management. *Ann Surg.* 1980;191:430-437.

Stanley JC, Criado E, Upchurch GR Jr, et al. Michigan Pediatric Renovascular Group. Pediatric renovascular hypertension: 132 primary and 30 secondary operations in 97 children. *J Vasc Surg.* 2006;44(6):1219-1228; discussion 1228-1229.

Upchurch GR, Henke PK, Eagleton MJ, et al. Pediatric splanchnic arterial occlusive disease: clinical relevance and operative treatment. *J Vasc Surg.* 2002;35:860-867.

CLINICAL SCENARIO CASE QUESTIONS

1. What is the most common presentation of pediatric midabdominal aortic coarctation?

   a. Hypertension
   b. Intestinal ischemia
   c. Claudication
   d. Renal failure

2. A 4-year-old presents with hypertensive crisis, absent femoral pulses, and abdominal bruit. The initial diagnostic study of choice is:

   a. Ultrasound
   b. Noncontrast CT of the abdomen
   c. MRA of the chest, abdomen, and pelvis
   d. Diagnostic arteriogram

62 Aortoiliac Occlusive Disease (Open Surgery)

JOHN P. DAVIS and GILBERT R. UPCHURCH Jr

Presentation

A 41-year-old gentleman presents to the clinic with a 24-month history of worsening pain in his buttocks and thighs that is exacerbated by walking or exertion. His pain is worse on the right when compared to the left, and it improves upon resting. The pain is not evident during rest or at night. He has a 26-pack-year smoking history and a past medical history of hyperlipidemia, for which he takes a statin. His surgical and family history are unremarkable. A diminished femoral pulse on the left and an absent femoral pulse on the right are noted on physical examination. Distal pulses are not palpable, but monophasic Doppler signals are evident bilaterally.

Differential Diagnosis

The differential diagnosis of buttock and thigh pain that is exacerbated with exercise is broad. The source of this pain could be neurogenic (spinal stenosis, lumbar disc rupture or bulge, or diabetic neuropathy), musculoskeletal (osteoarthritis of the hip or soft tissue injury), or vascular (arterial insufficiency).

Vascular insufficiency is the most likely origin given the nature of his symptoms and his physical examination findings. More specifically, this patient is likely suffering from aortoiliac disease given his buttock and thigh pain that is easily reproduced and occurs with increasing exertion. Additionally, bilateral diminished femoral pulses are consistent with aortoiliac occlusive disease (AIOD). When there is concern for arterial insufficiency, the examiner must focus on palpation of femoral, popliteal, and distal pulses. Femoral bruits, lower extremity pallor on elevation, hair loss, and thickened toenails are also signs that are indicative of lower extremity arterial insufficiency. Doppler examination is helpful in instances when pulses are abnormal.

Workup

Initial testing includes ankle-brachial indices (ABIs) and pulse volume recordings (PVRs). Additional imaging will be necessary if there are abnormalities in the initial testing.

Ankle-Brachial Indices and Pulse Volume Recordings

ABIs are helpful for determining the degree of arterial insufficiency. An ABI of 0.95 to 1.2 is considered normal, while an ABI of 0.5 to 0.95 is associated with claudication. An ABI of 0.2 to 0.5 is associated with rest pain. An ABI of 0 to 0.3 usually is associated with tissue loss or gangrene. ABIs greater than 1.3 are considered unreliable, as they

are usually a result of calcified noncompressible vessels, which can be seen in patients with diabetes mellitus.

Some patients will give clinical histories and have examinations that support arterial insufficiency, but have normal resting ABIs. These patients benefit from ABI measurements after exercising. A 15% decrease in ABIs after exercising supports the diagnosis of arterial insufficiency.

PVRs indirectly measure the pulsatility of a vessel. These tracings are particularly helpful when evaluating a patient with noncompressible vessels and falsely elevated ABIs. An elevated ABI and attenuated tracings on PVR suggest poor blood flow despite the elevated ABI. Patients with AIOD will have attenuated PVRs throughout the lower extremities (Fig. 1).

Cross-Sectional Imaging

CT Angiography (CTA) is the preferred imaging modality for preoperative evaluation as it allows for visualization of the aorta and the inflow vessels, outflow vessels, and runoff to the lower extremities. This is normally well tolerated in patients with normal renal function. Patients with borderline renal insufficiency are commonly hydrated prior to administration of the intravenous (IV) contrast. Sodium bicarbonate can be administered intravenously for further renal protection, though its efficacy may be in question.

Magnetic resonance angiography with gadolinium administration is an acceptable means of imaging in patients with renal insufficiency. It is usually well tolerated, but patients with renal insufficiency carry an increased risk of gadolinium-induced nephrogenic systemic sclerosis. Cross-sectional imaging gives the surgeon the ability to classify the severity of the disease.

The most commonly utilized classification system is the Trans-Atlantic Inter-Society Consensus (TASCII)

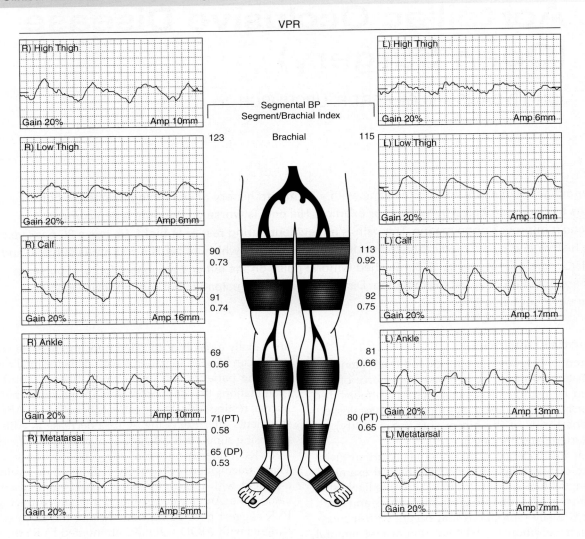

FIGURE 1 • PVR tracings from a patient with AIOD. Note the dampened waveforms in all tracings.

classification (Fig. 2). Classification schemes range from type A to type D lesions, with type A lesions being more isolated and shorter, while type D lesions are more severe and longer. Recently, endovascular therapy is preferred for type A, B, and C lesions, while open surgery is reserved for type D lesions.

Return to Scenario

The patient was referred to the vascular laboratory and underwent ABIs and PVRs. His ABIs were 0.58 on the right and 0.65 on the left. PVRs were obtained, which revealed moderately attenuated waveforms throughout the lower extremities indicative of inflow disease. CTA revealed an approximately 70% stenosis of the aorta secondary to mural thrombus that extended to the renal arteries (Fig. 3A). The renal arteries were patent bilaterally. Additionally, there was segmental occlusion of the right common iliac artery with severe stenosis of the left

common iliac artery secondary to atherosclerotic plaque (Fig. 3B). This patient's imaging was consistent with TASC D classification of disease.

Treatment Options

Medical Therapy

Initiation of risk factor modification and medical therapy is essential in patients with peripheral vascular disease and lower extremity arterial insufficiency. Smoking cessation strategies are essential in this patient population. Antiplatelet therapy with aspirin or clopidogrel is beneficial in patients to reduce the risk of subsequent myocardial infarction and cerebroembolic events. Additionally, statin therapy, angiotensin-converting enzyme inhibitors, and cilostazol have been shown to increase claudication-free walking times at 6 months. Most importantly, a walking regimen for patients with arterial insufficiency promotes collateralization and improves claudication without

Type A lesions

- Unilateral or bilateral stenoses of CIA
- Unilateral or bilateral single short (≤3 cm) stenosis of EIA

Type B lesions:

- Short (≤3 cm) stenosis of Infrarenal aorta
- Unilateral CIA occlusion
- Single or multiple stenosis totaling 3–10 cm involving the EIA not extending into the CFA
- Unilateral EIA occlusion not involving the origins of internal iliac or CFA

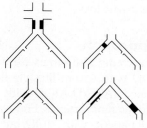

Type C lesions:

- Bilateral CIA occlusions
- Bilateral EIA stenoses 3–10 cm long not extending into the CFA
- Unilateral EIA stenosis extending into the CFA
- Unilateral EIA occlusion that involves the origins of internal iliac and/or CFA
- Heavily calcified unilateral EIA occlusion with or without involvement of origins of internal iliac and/or CFA

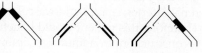

Type D lesions:

- Infra-renal aortoiliac occlusion
- Diffuse disease involving the aorta and both iliac arteries requiring treatment
- Diffuse multiple stenoses involving the unilateral CIA, EIA, and CFA
- Unilateral occlusions of both CIA and EIA
- Bilateral occlusions of EIA
- Iliac stenoses in patients with AAA requiring treatment and not amenable to endograft placement or other lesions requiring open aortic or iliac surgery

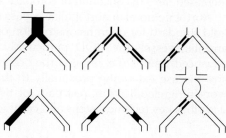

FIGURE 2 • TASC II aortoiliac lesions (Adapted from Bekken JA, Vos JA, Aarts RA, et al. DISCOVER: Dutch Iliac Stent trial: COVERed balloon-expandable versus uncovered balloon-expandable stents in the common iliac artery: study protocol for a randomized controlled trial. *Trials*. 2012;13:215).

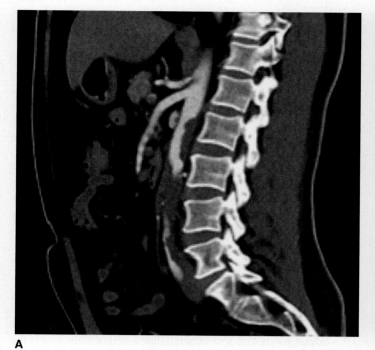

A

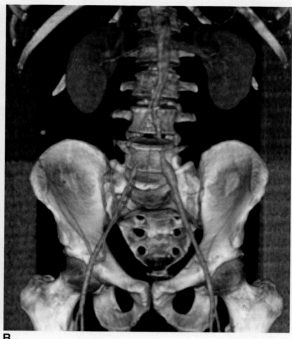

B

FIGURE 3 • **A:** CT imaging revealing a large mural thrombus extending to the level of the renal arteries. **B:** A 3D reconstruction revealing stenosis of the left common iliac artery and complete occlusion of the right common iliac artery.

operative intervention. Medical therapy may be reserved in patients with less severe TASC A or B lesions, while intervention should be considered in patients with advanced lesions resulting in persistent or worsening claudication, rest pain, and/or tissue loss.

Surgical Approach

This patient is a young and otherwise healthy man with significant AIOD with severe lifestyle-limiting claudication. CTA revealed TASC D AIOD with mural thrombus that extended to the renal arteries. Endovascular therapy is considered in all patients with AIOD, but the nature of his disease, particularly the mural thrombus extending to the renal arteries, makes endovascular therapy less attractive. Therefore, this patient would benefit from open aortoiliac reconstruction. In addition to optimization of risk factors and medical therapy, patients with peripheral vascular disease must undergo stringent cardiac risk stratification and screening as patients with peripheral vascular disease have increased rates of concomitant coronary artery disease.

Aortobifemoral or aortobiiliac bypass is considered the gold standard for open reconstruction of the distal aorta and iliac vessels for AIOD, particularly in patients with advanced lesions (i.e., total aortic occlusion with extensive disease extending proximally to the renal arteries), worsening claudication, rest pain, or tissue loss. Table 1 describes key technical steps and common pitfalls.

TABLE 1. Aortiliac Occlusive Disease (Open Surgery)

Key Technical Steps

1. Exposure of bilateral femoral arteries and branches with longitudinal incisions.
2. Midline laparotomy with duodenal reflection and access of retroperitoneum.
3. Transperitoneal incision to expose the aorta to the level of the left renal vein.
4. If ABF is to be undertaken, retroperitoneal tunnels deep to colon and ureters are created.
5. Systemic heparinization and cross-clamping of aorta beneath the renal arteries for proximal and distal control and transection of the aorta.
6. Oversew distal aortic stump, and anastomose graft to proximal aorta.
7. Tunnel femoral limbs of the graft through the retroperitoneum and beneath the inguinal ligament and obtain proximal and distal control of the femoral arteries.
8. Anastomose the femoral limbs to the distal common femoral arteries with evaluation of concomitant femoral endarterectomy/profundaplasty.

Potential Pitfalls

- Improper exposure and control of femoral vessels can lead to troublesome back bleeding.
- Removal of debris from proximal aorta to prevent distal embolization
- Inadequate outflow due to stenotic lesions in the femoral vessels increases risk of graft failure.

First, exposure of the femoral vessels via longitudinal groin incisions is undertaken with care to identify and control the common femoral artery, profunda femoris, and superficial femoral artery. The aorta is exposed to the level of the renal vein by midline laparotomy. Care must be taken with extensive dissection of the distal aorta and left common iliac artery to reduce damage to the nerve plexi that are responsible for sexual function in men. Vessels loops are placed around the bilateral femoral arteries in a Potts fashion. The suprarenal aorta is exposed, and a self-retaining retractor is put in place. If a traditional aortobifemoral bypass (ABF) is to be undertaken, retroperitoneal tunnels are created from the groins to the terminal aorta, being sure to remain deep to the colon and ureters. The patient is systemically heparinized. Depending on the level of atherosclerotic disease, the aorta may be cross-clamped below the renal vessels to obtain proximal control if the pararenal aorta is free of mural thrombus. A decision needs to be made as whether to perform an end-to-end or end-to-side aortic anastomosis. An end-to-end anastomosis is believed to have hemodynamic advantages and to be easier to cover, thus theoretically decreasing the incidence of aortic enteric fistulae. Proponents of an end-to-side proximal anastomosis suggest that this configuration is best used when there is a large inferior mesenteric artery (IMA) or direct in-line flow to the hypogastric arteries is needed. In this patient, an end-to-end configuration was chosen. Following temporary occlusion of the bilateral renal arteries and suprarenal aortic clamping, the infrarenal aorta is transected between the renal arteries and the IMA. An aortic thromboendarterectomy is performed. Control of lumbar arteries is important to minimize back bleeding. A bifurcated Dacron or polytetrafluoroethylene (PTFE) graft is anastomosed to the proximal aorta with a monofilament suture. The surgeon must take care to flush any debris from the proximal aorta to minimize distal embolization once the graft is perfused.

In traditional ABF operations, the distal limbs of the graft are clamped proximally and tunneled beneath the ureter, colon, and inguinal ligament to the groins. The distal limbs of the graft are anastomosed to the distal common femoral artery onto the profunda femoris artery. A femoral endarterectomy or profundaplasty may be warranted prior to performing the distal anastomosis if there is concomitant occlusion of the femoral vessels as inadequate outflow increases the risk of graft thrombosis.

In this particular patient with minimal external iliac artery and femoral artery disease, the decision was made to sew to the common iliac arteries after controlling the bilateral external and internal iliac arteries. This avoids the attendant risk of groin infection that accompanies traditional ABF. This approach also provides for antegrade flow into the internal iliac arteries. Maintaining flow to the internal iliac arteries is especially important in the setting of significant external iliac artery occlusive disease.

Once revascularization is complete, it is necessary to reevaluate the distal pulses or Doppler signals to ensure adequate perfusion. Adequate closure of the retroperitoneum over the graft with consideration of an omentopexy is necessary to prevent fistulization between the graft and bowel.

This modality of repair has an associated 3.3% risk of mortality with primary patency rates ranging from 93% at 2 years to 91% at 5 years. Excellent secondary patency of 100% has also been described at 2 years. Moreover, literature has shown a significant increase in ABIs when using ABF compared with endovascular therapy in patients with advanced AIOD disease. Limb salvage rates approach 90%.

Special Considerations

Other options for AIOD are extraanatomic bypasses, namely, axillofemoral, or thoracofemoral bypass. These procedures are generally reserved for patients who have a higher operative risk, intra-abdominal infection, or an ostomy or who have had multiple previous abdominal operations. Literature regarding axillofemoral bypass has shown a mortality of less than 1%, which is not significantly different when compared to traditional AFB. However, patency rates are lower when compared with AFB at 28 months (primary patency 84.3% vs. 90.5% and secondary patency 81% vs. 92%). Thoracofemoral bypass is another option for distal revascularization with formidable 5-year primary and secondary patency rates (79% and 84%) when compared to axillofemoral bypass. However, patients who undergo this method of distal bypass must be able to tolerate a thoracotomy.

Postoperative Management

Continuation of perioperative beta-blockade and antiplatelet therapy is necessary to decrease the risk of cardiac events, stroke, and overall vascular death. Aggressive pulmonary toilet and early mobilization are necessary to minimize atelectasis and subsequent pneumonia. Furthermore, adequate hydration and avoidance of intraoperative and postoperative hypotension are necessary to preserve adequate renal function. Postoperative diuresis should be considered in order to protect against increased cardiac workload, as fluid shifts occur and to optimize oxygenation after intraoperative fluid administration.

Postoperative follow-up should occur 4 weeks after initial discharge and should include ABIs and a thorough pulse exam. Further follow-up is necessary at 3 months and annually thereafter. Duplex surveillance in addition to ABIs may help to identify graft limbs at risk for thrombosis. The clinician should continue to stress lifestyle modifications, medication compliance, and smoking cessation.

Case Conclusion

The patient underwent an aortobiiliac reconstruction with an uncomplicated hospital stay. During his inpatient admission, he underwent counseling for smoking cessation and was maintained on antiplatelet and statin therapy. At outpatient follow-up at 4 weeks, he was no longer experiencing claudication, and his ABIs were 1.11 on the right (prior 0.58) and 1.06 on the left (prior 0.65) with biphasic Doppler waveforms at the ankles.

TAKE HOME POINTS

- An appropriate clinical history, thorough physical examination, and noninvasive vascular laboratory tests are the initial steps when evaluating arterial insufficiency.
- Smoking cessation; initiation of antiplatelet therapy, statin, or cilostazol; as well as starting a walking regimen are the initial management of lower extremity claudication.
- CTA and MRI/A are accepted imaging modalities to evaluate the aorta, inflow and outflow vessels, and lower extremity runoff vessels during preoperative planning and lesion classification.
- Aortobifemoral or aortobiiliac grafting is the traditional standard of care for extensive TASC D lesions with worsening claudication, rest pain, and tissue loss and offers superior long-term patency when compared to endovascular techniques in patients who can tolerate an open operation.
- Alternatives to aortobifemoral grafting include axillobifemoral and thoracobifemoral grafting, which can be beneficial in select patient populations.
- Full attention should be given to the cardiovascular systems of these patients in the perioperative phase as these patients are at increased risk for myocardial infarction, stroke, and distal embolization.

SUGGESTED READINGS

Bekken JA, Vos JA, Aarts RA, et al. DISCOVER: Dutch Iliac Stent trial: COVERed balloon-expandable versus uncovered balloon-expandable stents in the common iliac artery: study protocol for a randomized controlled trial. *Trials.* 2012; 13:215.

Burke CR, Henke PK, Hernandez R, et al. A contemporary comparison of aortofemoral bypass and aortoiliac stenting in the treatment of aortoiliac occlusive disease. *Ann Vasc Surg.* 2010;24:4-13.

de Vries SO, Hunink MG. Results of aortic bifurcation grafts for aortoiliac occlusive disease: a meta-analysis. *J Vasc Surg.* 1997;26:558-569.

Hans SS, DeSantis D, Siddiqui R, et al. Results of endovascular therapy and aortobifemoral grafting for Transatlantic Inter-Society type C and D aortoiliac occlusive disease. *Surgery.* 2008;144:583-589.

Kashyap VS, Pavkov ML, Bena JF, et al. The management of severe aortoiliac occlusive disease: endovascular therapy rivals open reconstruction. *J Vasc Surg.* 2008;48:1451-1457.

Passman MA, Taylor LM, Moneta GL, et al. Comparison of axil-lofemoral and aortofemoral bypass for aortoiliac occlusive disease. *J Vasc Surg.* 1996;23:263-269.

Rutherford RB. *Rutherford's Vascular Surgery.* 6th ed. Philadelphia, PA : Elsevier; 2005: 1095–1153 (Chapters 78–80).

Sen I, Stephen E, Agarwal S. Clinical profile of aortoiliac occlusive disease and outcomes of aortobifemoral bypass in India. *J Vasc Surg.* 2013;57(2 suppl):20S-25S.

CLINICAL SCENARIO CASE QUESTIONS

1. What is the initial step in the workup for suspected arterial insufficiency with normal resting ABIs?

   a. Two-view lumbar x-ray

   b. Postexercise ABI measurement

   c. CTA of abdomen/pelvis with bilateral lower extremity runoff

   d. Conservative management with medical therapy and smoking cessation

2. Which of the following statements is true regarding aortoiliac occlusive disease?

   a. Aortobifemoral bypass is the stand-alone therapy for aortoiliac occlusive disease.

   b. There is little benefit for endovascular therapy in TASC A or B aortoiliac occlusive disease.

   c. Extra-anatomic bypass offers alternative therapy to distal revascularization of aortoiliac occlusive disease in select patient populations.

   d. There is minimal role for femoral endarterectomy at the time of open aortobifemoral bypass.

   e. The addition of chronic anticoagulation (i.e., Coumadin) is warranted in the medical treatment of aortoiliac occlusive disease.

63 Aortoiliac Occlusive Disease

HUITING CHEN and JONATHAN L. ELIASON

Presentation

A 53-year-old female presents to the clinic for worsening lifestyle-limiting back and thigh pain with ambulation for several years, relieved by rest, and nonhealing ulcers to her lower extremities. Her past medical history includes diabetes mellitus, deep venous thrombosis and pulmonary embolus, hyperlipidemia, hypertension, and pyoderma gangrenosum, with significant wound-healing difficulties. Her medications include daily aspirin 81 mg, a low-dose beta-blocker, Coumadin, and a statin. Her past surgical history includes an angioplasty of her superficial femoral arteries and an inferior vena cava filter. She has a current tobacco use history of two packs per day for 30 years. On physical examination, her blood pressure is 135/58 and her pulse 84. Bilateral femoral and distal pulses are nonpalpable, though distal signals are present by Doppler. Her lower back, buttock, and thighs exhibit multiple shallow coin-sized superficial ulcerations in a bilateral distribution.

Differential Diagnosis

Causes of lower extremity pain with exertion may be arterial, venous, neurogenic, arthritic, or due to diabetic neuropathy. The presentation of symptoms is different for these varied etiologies, and often, the history will allow sufficient narrowing of the differential diagnoses. Arterial claudication is due to demand ischemia with exertion and is classically described as cramping or aching with walking a certain distance, consistently relieved with rest. Venous claudication is due to venous occlusion, with subsequent "bursting" sensation in the legs and associated lower extremity edema. Neurogenic causes of leg pain include sciatic pain from lumbosacral nerve root compression, often presenting with diffuse pain extending from the buttocks to the feet. This pain is classically improved with bending at the waist, which relieves the nerve compression from spinal stenosis. Arthritic pain is experienced at joint spaces and not classically associated with onset of a consistent walking distance. It may be improved with activity and worse just after getting up. Lastly, diabetic neuropathy is often associated with structural foot changes and poorly healing ulcers in the setting of a history of diabetes.

In patients with peripheral arterial disease (PAD) due to inflow insufficiency, the level of disease is found at the aorta or iliac arteries. Patients with aortoiliac occlusive disease (AIOD) will often have diminished or absent femoral pulses and distal pulses possibly only detectable by Doppler.

Diagnostic Tests and Result
Ankle-Brachial Index

The ankle-brachial index (ABI) is easily obtained in a clinical setting by the use of a blood pressure cuff and a Doppler probe. The cuff is affixed to the subject's assessed leg, as close to the ankle as possible. The probe is placed over the location of the dorsalis pedis artery on the dorsum of the foot or over the posterior tibial artery posterior to the medial malleolus while the cuff is inflated above systolic pressure. While the cuff is slowly deflated, the blood pressure for the dorsalis pedis and posterior tibial arteries is measured and recorded when return of arterial Doppler signals is obtained. The higher of these two distal systolic pressures is then divided by the systolic pressure obtained from the brachial artery to obtain the ABI. Normal ABIs range from 0.9 to 1.29, with decreases in value as the severity of PAD increases. Mild to moderate PAD produces ABIs of 0.4 to 0.9. Rest pain, and possibly tissue loss, is typically associated with ABIs less than 0.4. Notably, calcification of the tibial vessels is often seen in diabetic patients, resulting in noncompressible vessels and falsely elevated ABIs. In these patients, often the toe-brachial index (TBI) more reliably reflects the extent of disease, as smaller digital vessels are less affected by the calcification process in diabetes.

Doppler Waveforms

Waveform analysis follows the principle that the waveform produced in a vessel is altered by stenosis in the vessel. Using a Doppler probe, normal waveforms have a triphasic character, with a brisk upstroke in systole, followed by a brief retrograde early diastolic peak, then a smaller antegrade diastolic peak. Mild stenosis produces a biphasic, widened waveform, due to loss of vessel recoil in diastolic flow. Peak systolic velocities also increase with increasing severity of stenosis. Obtaining Doppler waveforms from successive levels in the lower extremity is a useful adjunct in defining the anatomic level of disease.

A monophasic waveform at the groin or femoral level in the right clinical context will strongly suggest the presence of AIOD.

Case Continued

The patient's ABIs were 0.38 on the right and 0.39 on the left. Waveform analysis revealed monophasic morphology in the bilateral femoral arteries and biphasic flow in the tibial and pedal arteries. The combination of findings from physical examination, ABIs, and Doppler waveforms suggests AIOD. In patients whose symptoms are only mild to moderate claudication, conservative management with pharmacology, tobacco cessation, and a supervised exercise program may be attempted first. However, this patient's symptoms are lifestyle limiting, and more extensive diagnostic studies with possible intervention are warranted. A CT angiogram (CTA) is preferred to catheter-based angiography in this nonacute setting, as the CT images the entire aortoiliac system without the risks associated with invasive testing.

CTA Abdomen/Pelvis: CTA from the referring hospital (images not shown) revealed total occlusion of the distal abdominal aorta and common iliac arteries bilaterally extending from just below the inferior mesenteric artery to the common iliac artery bifurcation on both sides. There is reconstitution of both internal and external iliac arteries from collateral vessels.

Diagnosis and Treatment

This patient has clinical symptoms of AIOD confirmed by noninvasive studies including a CTA demonstrating complete occlusion of the aorta and common iliac arteries bilaterally. In addition to a discussion of the risks and benefits of surgery, the critical importance of tobacco cessation is emphasized. The patient agrees to quit smoking and elects to proceed with an intervention.

Approach: Surgical versus Endovascular

The Trans-Atlantic Inter-Society Consensus (TASC) classification of AIOD by lesion morphology recommends endovascular therapy for the treatment of localized disease (TASC A and B), whereas extensive diseases (TASC C and D) are best approached with open reconstruction. Our patient with infrarenal aortoiliac occlusion has a TASC D lesion, which is typically best suited for surgery. The most commonly used and safe surgical approach to this type of TASC D lesion is aortobifemoral bypass. This operation may be performed in an end-to-side or end-to-end fashion for the proximal anastomosis onto the aorta, and distal anastomoses to the femoral arteries are performed in an end-to-side fashion. The distal anastomoses are constructed based upon the pattern of disease and anatomic lie of the graft limbs, with "hooding" the graft limb from the common femoral artery onto the profunda femoris artery being a common and effective reconstructive technique. The durability for this type of bypass procedure is high, with studies commonly reporting greater than 85% primary patency rates at 5 years. It is effective in relieving symptoms due to aortoiliac obstruction. It has long been considered the gold standard for treatment of severe aortoiliac disease.

However, recent advancements in devices and techniques have resulted in admirable outcomes for endovascular approaches to extensive disease. Taurino and colleagues reported that in 50 patients with TASC C or D lesions treated with either a hybrid approach or endovascular only, 100% achieved technical success, with no significant difference in cumulative primary or secondary patency rates between the two approaches. While not stratified by TASC levels, in comparing 118 aortofemoral bypass (AFB) patients with 174 aortoiliac angioplasty and stenting (AS) patients, Burke et al. found no difference in mortality, cerebrovascular accidents, myocardial infarction, or renal failure requiring hemodialysis. More recently in 2013, Sixt et al. evaluated 1184 patients of all four TASC classifications and noted no difference in restenosis, reintervention, or primary and secondary patency rates in the four subgroups at 12 months. While they found that the TASC D group required acute reintervention more often ($p < 0.001$), they concluded that for AIOD, the endovascular approach can be considered for treatment regardless of TASC classification.

In lesions with aortic occlusions, the addition of transbrachial access to standard femoral access has been reported in the literature. Bjorses et al. treated 173 patients of TASC A through D aortoiliac lesions, 11 of whom were recanalized due to aortic occlusions. Similar to our approach, these authors performed bilateral femoral and brachial access for these lesions and reported no statistically significant difference in primary patency between the TASC classes. Lagana and colleagues report endovascular treatment of 19 patients with Leriche syndrome, 5 of which have complete occlusion of the infrarenal aorta and both common iliac arteries. All of these five patients underwent brachial and femoral access; however, crossing of the lesion was not successful in one of these patients, who subsequently underwent an axillobifemoral bypass. Similar access for chronic aortoiliac occlusion by Moise resulted in successful endovascular reconstruction of the occlusion in 29/31 patients. Like Lagana's approach, Moise's patient for which the occluded aorta could not be traversed underwent an axillobifemoral bypass.

While both open and endovascular approaches were offered as treatment options, due to the patient's diagnosis of pyoderma and history of poor wound healing, an endovascular approach was selected.

Endovascular Management

The bilateral common femoral arteries and left brachial arteries were percutaneously accessed under fluoroscopic and ultrasound guidance with a micropuncture needle. Using Seldinger technique, 6-French 25-cm-long Pinnacle sheaths were placed into the common femoral arteries, and a 5-French short Pinnacle sheath was placed in the left brachial artery. The patient was then systemically heparinized.

An aortogram was obtained from antegrade catheter advancement into the abdominal aorta, revealing large paired lumbar arteries providing collateral circulation to the pelvis. The aorta was occluded at the level of the patent origin of the inferior mesenteric artery with a completely occluded terminal aortic segment and bilateral common iliac arteries (Fig. 1). Reconstitution of the iliac arteries occurred at the iliac bifurcation. The length of occlusion was estimated to be between 90 and 100 mm.

Subintimal recanalization of the common iliac arteries was performed in a retrograde fashion to the level of the aortic bifurcation with 5-French glide catheters. The brachial access was then exchanged for a 6-French long sheath and positioned in the abdominal aorta. A 5-French angled 100-cm-long glide catheter over an angled glide wire was used for antegrade recanalization of the terminal aorta to the level of the aortic bifurcation. A snare was advanced through the 5-French catheter, opened within

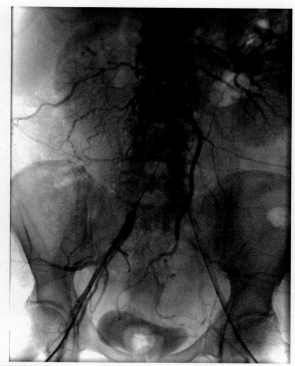

FIGURE 2 • Wire recanalization establishing through-and-through arterial access from the bilateral femoral arteries out the brachial artery facilitates advancement of PTA balloon catheters and/or stents.

the subintimal passage, and used to grasp the guidewire coming up from the left groin. This through-and-through access from the brachial artery to the femoral artery was similarly obtained on the right (Fig. 2).

Both wires were exchanged through catheters for stiff wires, after which the terminal aorta was predilated with percutaneous transluminal balloon angioplasty (PTA), followed by deployment of self-expanding stents. These were deployed from the level of the inferior mesenteric artery to just above the iliac bifurcations bilaterally. After postdilation of the stents with angioplasty balloons (Fig. 3), a completion angiogram was performed from the brachial approach, revealing a patent aortoiliac segment without flow-limiting stenosis. The heparin anticoagulation was reversed with protamine administration, and manual pressure was held at the sheath access sites (Table 1).

Special Intraoperative Considerations

Vessel rupture is a known intraoperative complication of endovascular therapy. The operator must have a high suspicion for rupture and must act quickly. Endovascular therapy or conversions to an open approach are scenario-specific options. Bjorses and colleagues report two ruptures of the external iliac artery of 173 TASC A through D aortoiliac patients treated with kissing stents; both were immediately sealed with covered stents. Their one episode of rupture of the aortic bifurcation resulted in a

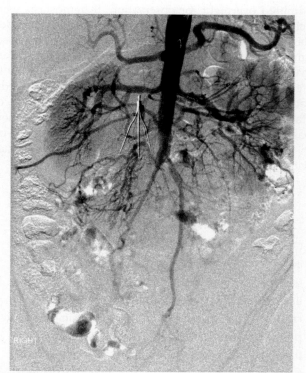

FIGURE 1 • Antegrade transbrachial abdominal aortogram revealing aortic occlusion at the level of the inferior mesenteric artery.

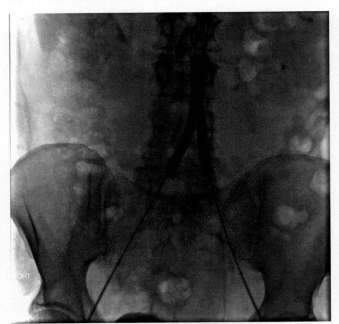

FIGURE 3 • Postdilation of recanalized and stented aortoiliac segment.

slowly growing hematoma, for which the patient underwent an aortobifemoral bypass 41 days postintervention. Moise and associates report vessel rupture in his 1/31 attempted endovascular reconstructions of aortic

TABLE 1. Aortoiliac Occlusive Disease (Endovascular)

Key Technical Steps

1. Obtain brachial and bilateral femoral access with placement of 5- and 6-French sheaths
2. Systemic heparinization
3. Aortogram from the brachial approach
4. Subintimal retrograde recanalization of iliac arteries to the level of the bifurcation
5. Brachial sheath exchange to 6-French long sheath positioned in abdominal aorta
6. Partial recanalization of terminal aorta from an antegrade approach
7. Advance snare through antegrade catheter advanced to the aortic bifurcation
8. Grasp wire from the groin using snare to obtain through-and-through access bilaterally
9. Wire exchange through glide catheters for stiff wires
10. Predilation balloon angioplasty followed by stent and postdilation angioplasty of aortoiliac segment
11. Complication angiogram
12. Hemostasis

Potential Pitfalls

- Vessel perforation with subintimal recanalization or balloon angioplasty
- Reentry into the aorta above the desired level resulting in branch artery occlusion or focal dissection
- Embolization of plaque distally
- Coverage of important branch arteries

occlusion, with no effect in outcome success following treatment with a covered stent. Conversely, treatment of five patients with completely occluded aorta and common iliac arteries by Lagana et al. resulted in no vessel rupture.

Distal embolization of plaque is possible to either the extremities or to the kidneys. In 173 AIOD patients treated with kissing stents, Bjorses et al. report three distal embolizations with one undergoing successful aspiration and one renal embolization without requiring subsequent dialysis. Lagana and colleagues report 11% distal embolisms (2/18). Of Moise's 31 patients with aortic occlusion who successfully underwent endovascular reconstruction, one suffered embolization of a right lower extremity requiring mechanical thrombectomy with successful resolution of his limb ischemia.

Vessel rupture and distal embolization are important intraoperative considerations during manipulation of wires, catheters, and devices through diseased vasculature. Maneuvering past stenoses and occlusions must be performed with finesse and direct visualization. As the literature above suggests, endovascular and open treatment of these complications are both viable options and depend on the clinical scenario.

Postoperative Management

Following stenting of the aortoiliac system, the patient is admitted overnight for observation. If hemostasis were achieved with manual pressure, bedrest is recommended for approximately 6 hours; if a closure device was used, limited or no bedrest is required. The pulses are checked every 4 hours. The patient is treated with Plavix until stent endothelialization occurs. Cardioprotective medications are continued, such as aspirin, beta-blockers, or statins. Prior to discharge, ABIs are repeated for a new baseline, and the patient is scheduled for clinic follow-up in 4 weeks with repeat ABIs. Clinical follow-up is annual, with repeat ABIs at each visit.

Case Conclusion

Our patient has had a relatively stable clinical course following her index intervention. Her ulcers healed within 2 months of the procedure, and her symptoms of claudication completely resolved. She continued to have chronic low back pain. Her primary patency was 4 years, at which time she underwent kissing stent placement to raise the aortic bifurcation. This was performed when symptoms of claudication returned and ABIs were mildly diminished secondary to in-stent

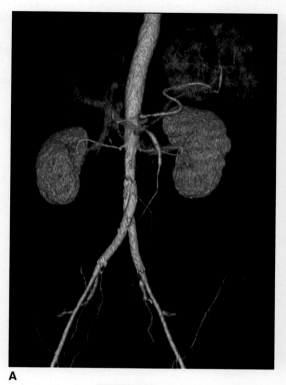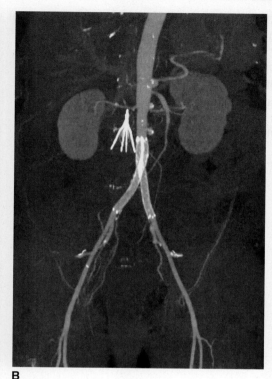

A   B

FIGURE 4 • **A, B:** CTA demonstrating patent recanalized segment.

stenosis bilaterally. Primary assisted patency is now 7 years. She continues to smoke, despite repeated efforts to quit. Recent follow-up CTA reveals a widely patent aortoiliac intervention (Fig. 4A and B).

TAKE HOME POINTS

- History and physical examination are a key initial step in identifying the vasculature affected. Decreased femoral pulses suggest inflow disease.
- CT angiography of the abdomen and pelvis aids in operative planning and in the elective setting is preferred to a diagnostic angiogram.
- The TASC classification is a guideline for operative management of AIOD, but patient-specific factors may influence selection of treatment type.
- When both open and endovascular approaches are options, the intervention must be tailored to the patient.

SUGGESTED READINGS

Bjorses K, Ivancev K, Riva L, et al. Kissing stents in the aortic bifurcation—a valid reconstruction for aorto-iliac occlusive disease. *Eur J Vasc Endovasc Surg.* 2008;36:424-431.

Brewster DC. Clinical and anatomical considerations for surgery in aortoiliac disease and results of surgical treatment. *Circulation.* 1991;83:142-152.

Burke CR, Henke PK, Hernandez R, et al. A contemporary comparison of aortofemoral bypass and aortoiliac stenting in the treatment of aortoiliac occlusive disease. *Ann Vasc Surg.* 2010;24:4-13.

Jongkind V, Akkersdijk GJM, Yeung KK, et al. A systematic review of endovascular treatment of extensive aortoiliac occlusive disease. *J Vasc Surg.* 2010;52:1376-1383.

Lagana D, Carrafiello G, Mangini M, et al. Endovascular treatment of steno-occlusions of the infrarenal abdominal aorta. *Radiol Med.* 2006;111:949-958.

Moise MA, Alvarez-Tostado JA, Clair DG, et al. Endovascular management of chronic infrarenal aortic occlusion. *J Endovasc Ther.* 2009;16:48-92.

Norgren L, Hiatt WR, Dormandy JA, et al. Inter-society consensus for the management of peripheral arterial disease (TASC II). *J Vasc Surg.* 2007;45(Suppl):S5-S67.

Sixt S, Krankenberg H, Mohrle C, et al. Endovascular treatment for extensive aortoiliac artery reconstruction. *J Endovasc Ther.* 2013;20:64-73.

Taurino M, Persiani F, Fantozzi C, et al. Trans-Atlantic Inter-Society Consensus II C and D iliac lesions can be treated by endovascular and hybrid approach: a single-center experience. *Vasc Endovascular Surg.* 2014;48(2):123-128.

CLINICAL SCENARIO CASE QUESTIONS

1. Which of the following is not in the typical differential diagnosis for aortoiliac occlusive disease?

   a. Spinal stenosis

   b. Chronic thigh compartment syndrome

   c. Arthritis

   d. Severe chronic venous insufficiency

2. Trans-Atlantic Inter-Society Consensus (TASC) category D patients with aortoiliac disease are typically considered for open surgical revascularization. If an endovascular approach is considered, key steps include all of the following, except (may not be in order):

    a. Percutaneous or cutdown brachial artery access
    b. Wire recanalization of the occluded aortic and iliac segments
    c. Atherectomy of recanalized channel to facilitate large balloons or stents
    d. Limiting subintimal channel formation to the region of occlusion to preserve branch arteries
    e. Preservation (avoiding coverage) of the internal iliac arteries when possible

64 Acute Aortic Occlusion (Open Surgery)

PANTELIS HADJIZACHERIA, ROBERT S. CRAWFORD, and RAJABRATA SARKAR

Presentation

A 62-year-old man with a history of hypertension, hyperlipidemia, peripheral vascular disease, and a 90-pack-year history of smoking presents to the emergency department with bilateral lower extremity paresthesia, pain, and decreased motor function. He denies back pain or abdominal pain, and has a prior history significant for severe bilateral claudication worsening over the last 2 years and occurring at a distance of less than half a block. His vital signs are normal. Pertinent findings on physical examination are the absence of palpable femoral, popliteal, posterior tibial, and dorsalis pedis arterial pulses bilaterally. He has decreased sensation and strength in both lower extremities.

Differential Diagnosis

The conditions that mimic acute aortic occlusion include arterial dissection, traumatic spinal column/cord injury, lumbar disk herniation, transverse myelitis, acute stroke, and diffuse thromboembolism. In this patient with acute bilateral lower extremity pain and numbness, cardiovascular risk factors, and absent bilateral femoral pulses, the primary diagnosis is acute aortic occlusion until proven otherwise.

Workup

In the evaluation of the patient with acute leg symptoms, the duration and severity of leg symptoms coupled with lower extremity pulselessness points to a vascular cause requiring immediate treatment. The symptoms of aortic occlusion are reflected in the physical findings of lower extremity arterial ischemia and include the "5 Ps": pain, pulselessness, pallor, paresthesia, paralysis, and poikilothermia. Nonvascular causes of similar symptoms listed above in the differential diagnosis will not result in pulselessness, a key differentiator in the evaluation of the patient.

All patients with suspected acute aortic occlusion should be investigated emergently with imaging to define the cause of occlusion and plan revascularization. The following additional studies should be obtained in patients with acute aortic occlusion: electrocardiogram, standard chemistry, complete blood count, prothrombin time, partial thromboplastin time, creatinine phosphokinase, and myoglobin level.

Arteriography is traditionally used for localizing an obstruction and visualizing the distribution of disease before aortoiliac revascularization. However, due to the increased availability, resolution, and speed of computerized tomography (CT), CT angiography (CTA) is the test of choice in the acute setting. Our patient underwent further evaluation with a CT scan that revealed complete occlusion of the infrarenal abdominal aorta and reconstitution of flow at the level of the right and left common femoral arteries (Figs. 1 and 2). However, a major drawback of CTA is the hampered vessel assessment by arterial wall calcifications. Bedside arterial duplex can efficiently detect the femoral or iliac occlusion, which often shows no flow, or monophasic waveforms distally with decreased distal velocities. In the acute setting, the ability of duplex scan to consistently visualize the aorta is poor given bowel gas and other confounding factors. CT scanning is more widely and rapidly available in hospitals and is not operator or patient dependent, making it the ideal test for suspected aortic occlusion.

Discussion

Acute aortic occlusion is a rare occurrence; however, it is a true vascular emergency that requires rapid diagnosis and aggressive surgical intervention to limit poor outcomes. The two main causes for acute aortic occlusion to occur are arterial embolism and thrombosis. Determining associated comorbidities, such as arrhythmias or prior peripheral vascular disease, can help distinguish the two pathologies and guide management. In embolic aortic occlusion, the source of the embolus is almost invariably cardiac in origin and it can be catastrophic because patients tend to lack preexisting collaterals. Patients often recall the exact moment of onset of severe ischemic symptoms. In contrast, the less common acute aortic thrombosis is the result of progressive atherosclerotic narrowing in patients with aortoiliac occlusive disease, with a superimposed acute occlusion when flow decreases below the threshold required to maintain patency. Often, there is

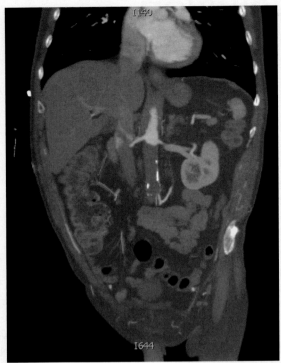

FIGURE 1 • Coronal cut of a CT scan demonstrating complete occlusion of the infrarenal abdominal aorta.

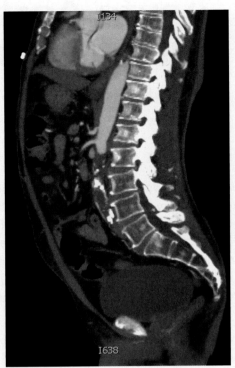

FIGURE 2 • Sagittal cut of a CT scan demonstrating complete occlusion of the infrarenal abdominal aorta.

an antecedent recent history of generalized illness or dehydration that promotes hemoconcentration and hypercoagulability. Because of the prior presence of collateral vessels in long-standing aortoiliac occlusive disease, the clinical manifestations are seldom as dramatic as those of embolization as patients note that symptoms develop gradually over several days.

Diagnosis and Treatment

The most important aspect of diagnosis of acute aortic occlusion is to identify vascular occlusion as the cause of lower extremity neurologic symptoms. The authors have experienced several cases in which the symptoms were attributed to other causes and the aortic occlusion was identified 24 to 72 hours later. These cases uniformly end in bilateral amputation and/or death.

Initial goal of treatment for acute aortic occlusion is to prevent thrombus propagation and worsening ischemia; therefore, intravenous loading dose (100 U/kg) heparin should be administered immediately unless contraindicated. The critical decision in the treatment of acute aortic occlusion was traditionally to determine whether the etiology was an embolus or thrombosis. The rationale for this was that embolus was treated with emergent transfemoral embolectomy and thrombosis required contrast arteriography to define the arterial anatomy. This early distinction has vanished with the widespread use of CTA as described above, which readily distinguishes the two disorders.

The options for open revascularization in patients with aortoiliac occlusion are urgent direct or extra-anatomic arterial revascularization. Selection of the most appropriate method depends largely on the patient's surgical risk, comorbid medical conditions, and degree of extremis. The potential options include direct aortofemoral bypass or extra-anatomic axillobifemoral bypass and femorofemoral bypass. Patients presenting with hypovolemia, acidosis, or oliguria should not be subjected to the greater operative stress of aortofemoral bypass. In selected cases, endovascular revascularization with recanalization, angioplasty, and stenting can be used to rapidly reestablish arterial inflow.

Surgical Approach to Aortofemoral Bypass

In a good-risk patient without evidence of hemodynamic compromise or advanced ischemia, emergent aortofemoral bypass is the procedure of choice for acute aortic occlusion secondary to thrombosis. The patient is widely prepped and draped from nipples to knees. The femoral vessels are preferentially exposed before making the abdominal incision to minimize the length of time that the abdomen is open. The infrarenal abdominal aorta may be exposed using a midline incision; however, a retroperitoneal approach may be employed in obese patients or those with a hostile abdomen.

The groin incisions are extended slightly above the inguinal ligament, and the common femoral, superficial femoral, and profunda femoris arteries are dissected in preparation for clamping, and retrograde retroperitoneal tunnels are begun. A midline abdominal incision is then created extending from the xiphoid to the pubis. After careful exploration of the intra-abdominal organs, the transverse colon and omentum are elevated and retracted cephalad, and the entire small bowel is displaced to the right. A self-retaining retractor is placed. Thereafter, the posterior parietal peritoneum overlying the infrarenal aorta is incised and extended cephalad where the ligament of Treitz is divided. This allows mobilization of the fourth portion of the duodenum off the aorta and facilitates visualization of the left renal vein. The inferior mesenteric vein can be divided if needed, and the aortic dissection is extended distally just beyond the origin of the inferior mesenteric artery. Next, retroperitoneal tunnels are made anterior to the common and external iliac vessels and posterior to the ureter for passage of each graft limb from the aorta to the groins. A Penrose drain or Silastic tubing is drawn through the tunnel.

A prosthetic graft of choice is used for construction of the bypass. For the proximal aortic anastomosis, an end-to-end anastomosis is typically preferred for aortic occlusion and in the setting of concomitant aneurysm disease, juxtarenal aortic occlusion, or the presence of a coral reef aorta. The indications for an end-to-side proximal anastomosis are occluded or severely diseased external iliac arteries, a sizable accessory renal artery arising from the infrarenal aorta, and the presence of a large inferior mesenteric artery. These conditions can be readily discerned on preoperative CTA.

After intravenous administration of heparin (100 U/kg) for an activated clotting time (ACT) greater than 250, appropriate vascular clamps are applied to the aorta just caudal to the renal arteries and immediately caudal or cephalad to the inferior mesenteric artery. For an end-to-end anastomosis, the aorta is transected and a 3- to 4-cm-long segment between the clamps is resected to allow the prosthetic graft to lie without angulation or protrusion in the retroperitoneum. Any patent lumbar artery branches arising from this segment are clamped and ligated. The transected distal aortic end is oversewn in two layers with monofilament suture. Thrombus or debris is removed from the proximal divided end of the aorta, and a proximal anastomosis to the graft is constructed with monofilament suture. Teflon pledgets may be used to bolster the suture. After completion of the aortic anastomosis, the graft is clamped with an atraumatic vascular clamp (Fogarty soft-jawed clamp) and the proximal anastomosis tested by slow release of the proximal aortic clamp. Next, the previously placed Penrose drains in the graft tunnels are elevated, and each graft limb is pulled down through the tunnel ensuring passage of each graft limb posterior to the ureter. The common femoral, superficial femoral, and profunda branches are occluded using appropriate atraumatic vascular clamps. Occasionally, an endarterectomy of the outflow vessels may be required. A standard vascular anastomosis is then performed with monofilament suture to the bilateral femoral vessels. In cases of superficial femoral artery occlusion, the anastomosis should be performed with the hood onto the profunda femoral artery to improve patency.

Blood flow is sequentially restored to the lower extremities to minimize the potential for distal thromboemboli and "declamping hypotension." If necessary, heparin is reversed with protamine sulfate at a dose of 1 mg/100 U heparin. The retroperitoneum is closed over the graft to aid in prevention of aortoenteric fistula. The abdomen and groin incisions are closed in a standard fashion, and the pedal pulses are checked before leaving the operating room. In cases of chronic aortic occlusion, the pedal signals may initially be poor; however, these usually improve over the course of 1 day in the ICU with patient warming. However, the lack of any popliteal Doppler signal following aortic reconstruction is a poor prognostic sign and often portends limb loss without additional infrainguinal revascularization. It is not uncommon for perfusion to continually improve over the course of the first several days, especially in patients with outflow only through the deep femoral artery (Table 1).

Special Intraoperative Considerations for Aortofemoral Bypass

Specific complications related to the aortoiliac bypass include colon/pelvic ischemia, atheroembolization, lower extremity ischemia, male sexual dysfunction, and groin wound complications. Pelvic ischemia is rare; however, it can manifest as colonic ischemia, infarction of the buttock musculature, or cauda equina/lumbar plexopathy with neurologic deficit. Risk factors for this complication include bilateral occlusion of the internal iliac arteries and end-to-end aortic reconstruction with bilateral external iliac artery occlusion. It is generally accepted that maintaining at least one internal iliac artery helps prevent this complication.

Juxtarenal aortic occlusion represents a complete thrombosis of the aorta at the level of the renal artery origin. Several important modifications of the technique are necessary. This problem is best managed by brief suprarenal clamping between the superior mesenteric and renal arteries to allow removal of the juxtarenal thrombus and safe subsequent infrarenal clamping. The approach to the suprarenal aorta remains infracolic, but may require division of the left renal vein near the vena cava to facilitate exposure. Protection of the kidneys by brief renal artery occlusion during removal of thrombus is necessary. The renal arteries can be easily controlled with vessel loops. The infrarenal aorta should never be clamped near the renal arteries until the occluding thrombotic material is removed. After suprarenal clamping, the aorta is divided several centimeters below the renal artery origin and the obstructing thrombus freed

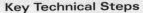

TABLE 1. Acute Aortic Occlusion (Open Surgery)

Key Technical Steps

1. Bilateral groin incisions and exposure of bilateral common femoral, superficial femoral, and profunda femoris arteries
2. Start retrograde retroperitoneal tunnels from each groin incision.
3. Midline subxiphoid to suprapubic incision and abdominal exploration
4. Transverse colon is retracted cephalad, and the small bowel is displaced to the right, and a self-retaining retractor is placed.
5. Posterior parietal peritoneum overlying the infrarenal aorta is incised.
6. Duodenum is dissected off the aorta, and the proximal clamp site is defined at the region where the left renal vein crosses anterior to the aorta just below the renal artery origins.
7. Aortic dissection is extended distally just beyond the origin of the inferior mesenteric artery.
8. Retroperitoneal tunnels are made for passage of each graft limb from the aorta to the groins staying posterior to the ureters.
9. Appropriate graft size is selected, and heparin is administered.
10. Vascular clamps are applied to the aorta just caudal to the renal arteries followed by clamp placement at the level of the inferior mesenteric artery.
11. The aorta is then transected, and a 3- to 4-cm-long segment between the clamps is resected. Patent lumbar arteries are ligated.
12. The transected distal aortic end is oversewn in two layers with monofilament suture.
13. Thrombus is removed from the proximal divided end of the aorta, and the proximal anastomosis to the graft is constructed with monofilament suture.
14. The Penrose drains in the graft tunnels are elevated, and each graft limb is pulled down through the tunnels posterior to the ureters.
15. Distal graft to femoral anastomosis is constructed with monofilament suture.
16. Blood flow is sequentially restored to the lower extremities.
17. Retroperitoneum is closed over the graft.
18. Wounds are closed, and pedal pulses are checked.

Potential Pitfalls

- Proximal graft anastomosis should be placed close to the renal arteries to avoid potential for progression of atherosclerotic occlusive disease
- Passage of the graft anterior to the ureter may lead to compression and obstruction of the ureter with hydronephrosis
- Thromboemboli to the lower extremities
- Ischemia-reperfusion injury

up with an endarterectomy spatula. Following removal of the juxtarenal thrombus, the aorta is clamped infrarenally, renal blood flow is restored, and a standard anastomosis is performed.

Atheromatous debris may embolize at any time during aortofemoral bypass. The most vulnerable time is when the vessels are manipulated such as during dissection or clamp application. The sequelae are dependent upon the size of the debris and the distribution of the involved vessels. Macroscopic particles may occlude the major vessels with the debris frequently lodging at the various bifurcation sites. The majority of these are amenable to removal with a thromboembolectomy catheter. In contrast, the microscopic particles lodge in smaller vessels and are not usually amenable to surgical removal, and antiplatelet and/or anticoagulation therapy is indicated.

Ischemia-reperfusion injury in aortic occlusion transpires in the setting of temporarily diminished or absent blood flow to the lower extremities, followed by the return of oxygenated blood. Reperfusion can result in tissue edema that may progress to compartment syndrome and may be severe enough to require fasciotomy. Reperfusion syndrome may lead to systemic involvement and become life threatening, as profound acidosis, hyperkalemia, myoglobinuria, renal failure, multiple organ dysfunction syndrome, and even death may occur. Therefore, prompt recognition of ischemia-reperfusion injury is essential, and fasciotomy when appropriate can limit the degree of myoglobinuria. Postoperative intubation, sedation, and critical illness often limit the value of physical examination in the determination of subsequent development of postoperative compartment syndrome. It is our practice to perform fasciotomy when severe ischemia is present for 6 hours or more preoperatively. Compartment syndrome occurs more commonly in patients with aortic embolus than aortic thrombosis, presumably due to preformed collaterals as described above in the latter condition. The treatment of rhabdomyolysis should focus on preserving renal function, and the management is supportive with aggressive fluid resuscitation, urine alkalinization, and in the setting of a restored intravascular space, the use of diuretics.

Surgical Approach to Axillobifemoral Bypass

Axillobifemoral bypass has traditionally been regarded as a second-choice alternative to elective aortofemoral reconstruction, but has significant utility in the emergent setting for acute aortic occlusion. It is the procedure of choice in the critically ill patient with aortic occlusion secondary to thrombosis of aortic aortoiliac occlusive disease. Axillobifemoral bypass is also useful in patients with multiple prior abdominal or aortic procedures in which aortofemoral bypass will be a difficult or prolonged operation that will result in delay in reestablishment of lower extremity perfusion.

The patient is placed in the supine position with the donor arm abducted 45 degrees. This minimizes tension on the axillary anastomosis postoperatively and avoids a large deviation in the anatomy of the axillary artery during dissection. General anesthesia with endotracheal intubation is preferred. The supra- and infraclavicular regions, axilla, chest, abdomen, and femoral regions are widely prepped and draped.

The proximal part of the axillary artery is used for the proximal anastomosis because it is relatively fixed in position, is anterior to the brachial plexus, and has a single collateral branch. An incision paralleling the course of the axillary artery is made approximately one to two fingerbreadths below the middle third of the clavicle. The fibers of the pectoralis major muscle are bluntly separated, and the pectoralis minor muscle is mobilized and divided and serves as the lateral border of the dissection. The axillary vein is mobilized and retracted caudally to reveal the axillary artery. Any branches of the vein can be divided to avoid later bleeding during tunneling. The first portion of the axillary artery is dissected and mobilized medial to the thoracoacromial artery for the proximal anastomosis. Next, the femoral arteries are exposed through bilateral groin incisions. The common, superficial, and profunda femoral arteries are exposed and individually controlled in preparation for clamping. Occasionally, an endarterectomy of the outflow vessels may be required.

A subcutaneous tunnel is created at the ipsilateral femoral incision. The tunnel runs medial to the anterior superior iliac spine in the groin, along the midaxillary line laterally, and posterior to the pectoralis minor muscle in the axilla. In some instances, a counterincision is needed to facilitate tunneling; however, it is best to avoid when possible as it is a potential route of graft infection. Thereafter, a subcutaneous, suprapubic, inverted U tunnel is created between the two femoral incisions. This lies anterior to the external oblique and anterior rectus fascia. A prefabricated specialized bifurcated graft (usually 8 mm diameter) is used if available and saves the time of one anastomosis. Alternatively, separate grafts can be used for the axillofemoral and femorofemoral portions of the graft. After completion of the tunnels, intravenous heparin is administered for an ACT greater than 250. The ipsilateral axillofemoral bypass is performed first. A longitudinal arteriotomy is made on the anterosuperior surface of the first part of the axillary artery. The graft is routed parallel to the axillary artery posterior to the axillary vein and pectoralis minor muscle for approximately 5 to 8 cm before forming a gentle curve in the axilla before turning toward its inferior course. This gentle curve protects the proximal anastomosis during extension or raising of the ipsilateral arm. The axillary anastomosis is performed in an end-to-side fashion using monofilament suture. The contralateral side of the femorofemoral graft is clamped with a Fogarty clamp, and the distal end of the axillofemoral graft is anastomosed to the femoral arteriotomy on the ipsilateral side. Blood flow to the ipsilateral lower extremity is restored. The final anastomosis of the femorofemoral bypass is performed as above if required, and blood flow is restored to the contralateral limb. If necessary, heparin is reversed with protamine sulfate at a dose of 1 mg/100 U heparin. All three incisions are closed in the standard fashion, and the pedal pulses are checked before leaving the operating room (Table 2).

TABLE 2. Axillobifemoral Bypass

Key Technical Steps

1. Infraclavicular incision two fingerbreadths below the middle third of the clavicle
2. Fibers of the pectoralis major muscle are bluntly separated
3. Pectoralis minor muscle divided
4. Axillary vein is mobilized and retracted cranially to reveal the axillary artery
5. Circumferentially dissect the first portion of the axillary artery
6. Bilateral groin incisions and exposure of bilateral common femoral, superficial femoral, and profunda femoris arteries
7. Create a subcutaneous tunnel that runs medial to the anterior superior iliac spine in the groin, along the midaxillary line laterally, and posterior to the pectoralis minor muscle in the axilla
8. Create a subcutaneous, suprapubic, inverted U tunnel anterior to the external oblique and anterior rectus fascia between the two femoral incisions
9. Appropriate bifurcated graft size is selected, and heparin is administered
10. The graft is routed parallel to the axillary artery for approximately 5 to 8 cm before forming a gentle curve in the axilla to its inferior course
11. Axillary to graft anastomosis is performed end to side with monofilament suture
12. Bilateral femoral to graft end-to-side anastomoses are created with monofilament suture
13. Wounds are closed, and pedal pulses are checked

Potential Pitfalls

- Proximal axillary anastomotic disruption
- Perigraft seroma
- Thromboemboli to the lower extremities
- Ischemia-reperfusion injury

Special Intraoperative Considerations for Axillobifemoral Bypass

Disruption of the proximal anastomosis of the axillobifemoral grafts occurs in approximately 5% of patients. Perioperative graft disruption is most often associated with forceful arm abduction or shoulder elevation but also occurs in the absence of reported activity. Excessive anastomotic tension can be minimized by division of the pectoralis minor muscle as well as by positioning the anastomosis on the most proximal portion of the axillary artery.

Perigraft seroma is a rare complication following axillobifemoral bypass grafting. It consists of a sterile perigraft fluid collection surrounded by a fibrous pseudocapsule. The cause is unknown, and most cases will resolve with conservative therapy, although the length of time to resolution is variable. In symptomatic patients or persistent seromas, the preferred treatment is complete graft and cyst excision with placement of a new graft of different material in a different tissue plane.

Ischemia-reperfusion injury and thromboemboli to the lower extremities are also potential problems in axillobifemoral bypass and are managed as described in the aortofemoral bypass section.

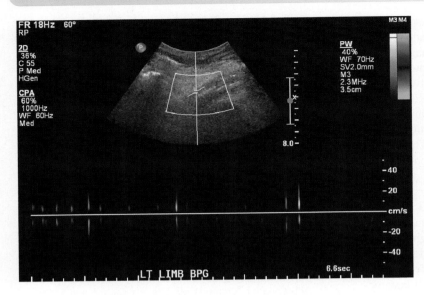

FIGURE 3 • Duplex scan demonstrates occlusion of the left limb of the aortofemoral bypass graft.

Postoperative Management

Patients are usually monitored in the intensive care unit for at least 1 to 2 days, paying particular attention to their volume status, cardiorespiratory and renal function, and their baseline comorbidities. Dysfunction of the pulmonary, cardiac, and renal systems is common in patients with acute aortic occlusion and if severe is the source of the high 30-day mortality (50%) associated with acute aortic occlusion. Frequent physical examination and continuous wave Doppler examination of the dorsalis pedis and posterior tibial arteries assist in determining graft patency. Patients are seen by the physical therapists when they reach the general care floor and are encouraged to start ambulating early. Ankle-brachial indices (ABIs) are obtained in the early postoperative period and at each 6-month follow-up visit.

In aortofemoral bypass, their nasogastric tube is usually removed when bowel function returns. Patients are usually discharged on their sixth or seventh postoperative day. The reported patency rates after aortobifemoral bypass range from 80% to 90% at 5 years. In axillobifemoral bypass, patients are cautioned to avoid placing the donor arm over the head for the first 6 weeks following surgery to avoid excess graft tension and potential axillary anastomotic disruption. The 5-year primary patency of axillofemoral grafts ranges from 69% to 75%. In femorofemoral bypass, the 5-year patency rates range from 60% to 86%.

Case Conclusion

The patient undergoes an emergent aortobifemoral bypass with outflow to the bilateral deep femoral arteries. In the ICU on postoperative day 1, the patient has loss of Doppler signals in the left leg. A bedside duplex scan demonstrates occlusion of the left limb of the aortofemoral bypass graft (Fig. 3). He is taken emergently to the operating room and undergoes an embolectomy of the left limb of the aortobifemoral bypass and a patch angioplasty of the proximal superficial femoral artery (Fig. 4). He is started on a diet on postoperative day 3, and the remainder of his hospital course is uncomplicated. He is discharged home on day 7. Repeat ABIs of the lower extremities in 1 month show no evidence of aortoiliac occlusive disease.

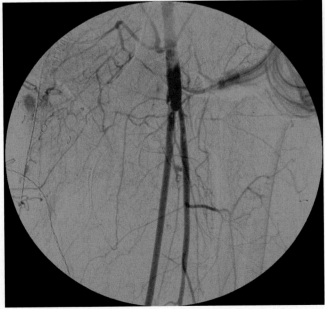

FIGURE 4 • Digital subtraction angiography demonstrating normal flow after embolectomy of the left limb of the aortobifemoral bypass.

TAKE HOME POINTS

- Acute aortic occlusion is a vascular emergency that requires rapid diagnosis and aggressive surgical intervention to limit amputation or death.
- The diagnosis of acute aortic occlusion is easily made with CTA of the abdomen.
- Clinical findings of acute limb ischemia and the finding of absent femoral pulses bilaterally are diagnoses of acute aortoiliac occlusion.
- CT scan can help differentiate aortic embolus from acute thrombosis of aortoiliac occlusive disease.
- Options for open revascularization in patients with aortoiliac occlusion are direct or extra-anatomic reconstruction.
- Aortobifemoral bypass is the procedure of choice in good-risk patients.
- Axillobifemoral bypass is reserved for patients with severe systemic illness with increased operative risk and in patients with a hostile abdomen.

SUGGESTED READINGS

Babu SC, Shah PM, Nitahara J. Acute aortic occlusion: factors that influence outcome. *J Vasc Surg.* 1995;21:567-575.

Dossa CD, Shepard AD, Reddy DJ, et al. Acute aortic occlusion: a 40-year experience. *Arch Surg.* 1994;129:603-608.

Littooy FN, Baker WH. Acute aortic occlusion: a multifaceted catastrophe. *J Vasc Surg.* 1986;4:211-216.

Surowiec SM, Isiklar H, Sreeram S, et al. Acute occlusion of the abdominal aorta. *Am J Surg.* 1998;176:193-197.

CLINICAL SCENARIO CASE QUESTIONS

1. You are called to the emergency department to evaluate a 54-year-old female with a history significant for cardiovascular disease who developed discomfort in her legs while at the grocery store. She states that this rapidly progressed to numbness and weakness in her bilateral lower extremities. On examination, you determine that there are no palpable femoral pulses. The next best step in management is to:

   a. Immediately take the patient to the operating room and perform an aortofemoral bypass
   b. Consult neurology to work up the acute neurologic changes
   c. Order a computer tomography scan
   d. Start anticoagulation with intravenous heparin if there are no contraindications
   e. Perform a preoperative angiography of the lower extremities

2. You are performing an aortofemoral bypass in a 68-year-old male who presented with acute aortic occlusion. At the time of the femoral anastomosis, you find significant profunda and superficial femoral artery atherosclerotic disease. You decide to:

   a. Perform the anastomosis to the common femoral artery
   b. Perform the anastomosis to nondiseased superficial femoral artery
   c. Extend the arteriotomy into the profunda artery and perform an orificial endarterectomy
   d. Extend the arteriotomy into the profunda artery beyond the orificial disease up to normal native profunda artery and perform a profundaplasty
   e. Perform the anastomosis to the common femoral artery and an additional bypass from the common femoral artery to a nondiseased segment of the proximal popliteal artery

65 Acute Aortic Occlusion in a Hostile Abdomen

MARK G. DAVIES

Presentation

A 70-year-old male inpatient complains of sudden onset of paralysis in both his legs for 4 hours. He had been admitted with small bowel obstruction and is 15 days after a laparotomy and lysis of adhesions. This was considered a difficult operation, and the patient has developed a midline enterocutaneous fistula. He has a previous history of an extended left colectomy for Duke's stage C colonic adenocarcinoma 2 years previously and has completed adjuvant chemotherapy. He has a past history of bilateral lower extremity claudication at 100 yards. He has hypertension controlled by two antihypertensive medications, is a non–insulin-dependent diabetic, and has chronic renal insufficiency (eGFR of 58 mL/min/1.73sqm). On examination, the patient is noted to be in mild respiratory distress and unable to move his legs. His upper extremity power and sensation are intact. He is noted to have an irregularly irregular heart rate and to be hypotensive (BP 90/50), tachypneic (30/m), and oliguric (less than 10 mL/hour for the last 4 hours). Examination of the peripheral pulses notes absent pulses in the right and left legs. Femoral pulses were documented as being present, but diminished on his admission physical examination. His legs are cold and pale. He has no motor or sensory function from L1/L2 dermatomes distally. No continuous-wave Doppler signals were identified.

Differential Diagnosis

The differential diagnosis in this case is that of a saddle embolus or acute aortic occlusion. The history of previous claudication would suggest preexisting aortoiliac disease and allow one to suspect acute aortic occlusion rather than saddle embolism. Both require emergent therapy but with different approaches. The presentation is atypical, but is also serious as the patient has paralysis likely due to cauda equina ischemia, and rapid revascularization must be considered.

Workup

This patient is in shock and had very ischemic limbs. An arterial blood gas and a serum chemistry panel are obtained, and an angiogram is arranged. On the blood gas and serum chemistry, the patient has a new-onset metabolic acidosis. This raises the suspicion of mesenteric vessel involvement. Having obtained informed consent, the patient is placed under general anesthesia. In the hybrid operating room, the right arm, right chest, abdomen, and both legs are prepared and draped in a standard fashion to form a sterile field. An angiogram is obtained through a right brachial cut down to ensure no vessel injury and speed closure. The emphasis of the angiogram is to define the visceral vessels, the infrarenal aorta, and bilateral runoff. The angiogram demonstrates intrarenal aortic occlusion with heavy calcifications suggestive of chronic disease. The visceral vessels are intact (Fig. 1). There is reconstitution of the common femoral vessels bilaterally. Prior to right brachial sheath removal, the right subclavian was studied and it was normal.

Case Continued

Prior to and during the angiogram, the patient is resuscitated and prepared for surgery and is heparinized (80 units/kg, IV) to achieve an activated clotting time (ACT) of greater than 250 seconds.

Diagnosis and Recommendation

The patient has a hostile abdomen, an enterocutaneous fistula, and a left colectomy, and as such, a direct transabdominal approach or a retroperitoneal approach would be very difficult. Options in this patient are to attempt endoluminal therapy to reopen one or both iliac vessels. If one iliac is open, a femorofemoral bypass is possible. If this fails, the patient should be considered for axillobifemoral bypass grafting. Acute occlusion of the abdominal aorta due to in situ thrombosis is a relatively rare event with a cumulative incidence of 8% (aortic occlusion due to embolic disease has a relative incidence of 15%). It has a mortality rate of over 50%.

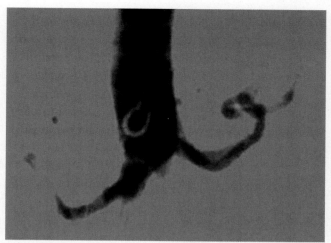

FIGURE 1 • Angiogram of the aorta with AP views demonstrating acute aortic occlusion. A lateral view confirms patent celiac and superior mesenteric vessels.

Case Continued

Under fluoroscopy, percutaneous access is gained into both common femoral arteries, sheaths are placed, and guide wires are passed retrograde into the aorta. The right passed without difficulty, but the left failed to pass. A rheolytic thrombectomy catheter system, initially using bolus instillation of 5-mg tPA in 50 mL to lace the clot with a thrombolytic and then followed by heparinized saline set to standard mode, is performed. The rheolytic thrombectomy catheter is passed over the wire multiple times without adequate restoration of antegrade flow. At this stage, it is decided to stop and pursue open intervention. Primary stenting using covered stents to pave open one iliac system was considered, but risk of thrombus embolization into the visceral vessels was considered to be high (Fig. 2).

Surgical Approach

At this stage, endoluminal intervention cannot be achieved. Bilateral groin cutdowns are performed with care to preserve the femoral artery branches. Following proximal and distal control, Fogarty embolectomies are performed to remove any distal clot and perhaps open up flow proximally to the hypogastric arteries. A right axillobifemoral bypass graft with 8-mm ringed PTFE is performed without difficulty (Table 1). Intraoperative duplex imaging, in order to reduce contrast exposure, confirms adequate distal outflow. The patient receives 25 mg mannitol to induce forced diuresis prior to reperfusion of the lower limbs. Due to the severity of the lower leg ischemia, bilateral four-compartment fasciotomies of the lower extremities are also performed. There are continuous-wave Doppler signals in the anterior and posterior tibial vessels on the foot at the end of the case. Intraoperative labs shows a rising potassium, which peaks at 8.0 and is aggressively treated with fluid diuresis, intravenous glucose, as well as insulin and calcium.

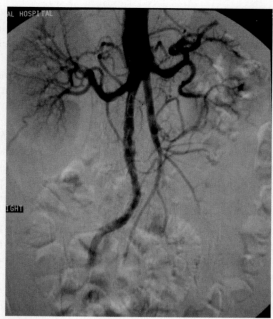

FIGURE 2 • Angiogram of the aorta in an AP view demonstrating a channel in the aorta after rheolytic catheter thrombectomy.

The following potential pitfalls of the operation as it is routinely conducted can be considered (Table 1):

1. *Insufficient laxity in subclavian anastomosis and graft to prevent anastomotic distraction*: When the subclavian anastomosis should be constructed, there will be sufficient laxity to allow for shoulder extension and the graft should be routed laterally before being directed caudally.

TABLE 1. Acute Aortic Occlusion in a Hostile Abdomen

Key Technical Steps

1. Right axillary exposure
2. Bilateral groin exposures through transverse incisions
3. Tunnel with relieving incision on chest to right groin.
4. Perform right subclavian artery graft anastomosis leaving a lazy S of graft to avoid tension on artery.
5. Perform right femoral embolectomy.
6. Perform right femoral artery graft anastomosis, and reestablish flow to the leg and pelvis. Warn anesthesiologist of impending reperfusion.
7. Tunnel femorofemoral graft.
8. Perform left femoral embolectomy.
9. Perform left femoral artery graft anastomosis.
10. Perform graft to graft anastomosis in the right groin.
11. Perform bilateral four-compartment fasciotomies.

Potential Pitfalls

- Insufficient laxity in subclavian anastomosis and graft to prevent distraction
- Not using ringed graft material to prevent compression
- Clamping the left IMA occlusion in a post-CABG patient
- Competitive flow in iliac system resulting in occlusion
- Dissection with Fogarty embolectomy catheter

2. *Not using ringed graft material to prevent compression*: There is a high risk of compression of the graft along the lateral course of the body wall, and as a result, a ringed graft will prevent compression.

3. *Angle of the takeoff of both ends of the femorofemoral graft*: It is important to set up the femorofemoral anastomoses so that there is a downward angle of the anastomoses to prevent preferential flow or steal.

4. *Care to avoid left Internal Mammary Artery (IMA) occlusion in a post-CABG patient*: In left-sided dissections of the subclavian artery, care should be taken to identify and preserve the IMA in patients who are post CABG as occlusion of the vessel can lead to significant myocardial events.

5. *Competitive flow in iliac system resulting in occlusion*: If an axillobifemoral bypass is placed and there is native flow in the iliac system, a competitive flow situation can occur leading to occlusion of the most vulnerable element of the axillobifemoral bypass (the contralateral side).

6. *Dissection with Fogarty embolectomy catheter*: Care should be taken when placing and withdrawing a Fogarty embolectomy catheter as overpressurization of the balloon can lead to intimal dissection or disruption. If there is an inability to access a specific vessel over the wire Fogarty, embolectomy balloons should be considered.

Postoperative Management

The following are considerations in postoperative management:

1. *Postoperative reperfusion injury*: Given the scenario, this patient is assured of experiencing a reperfusion syndrome and will require aggressive therapy to protect his kidneys and control hyperkalemia.

2. *Postoperative cardiopulmonary failure*: In the setting of ischemia and reperfusion, the patient will run the risk of acute myocardial depression and acute lung injury that can worsen preexisting conditions and extend the need for mechanical ventilation.

3. *Subclavian artery anastomosis disruption*: Early aggressive mobilization of the patient can result in an acute disruption of the subclavian artery to graft anastomosis.

4. *Follow-up*: The patient will need close follow-up with office visits at 1, 3, and 6 months. Duplex imaging of the inflow and outflow vessels should be considered. Duplex imaging of the graft itself will not be helpful.

Case Conclusion

The patient remains intubated and is transferred to the surgical ICU. He is continued on anticoagulation with intravenous heparin. Serial serum chemistries demonstrate rising potassium levels to 7.0 and a metabolic acidosis. The patient also develops myoglobinuria. The patient is rehydrated with sodium bicarbonate–supplemented crystalloid solutions. His hyperkalemia is aggressively treated with furosemide and an insulin-glucose infusion. The patient is monitored to ensure forced diuresis. His hyperkalemia and acidosis resolves. He is extubated and discharged from the ICU after 3 days, and on day 7, the patient is returned to the operating room for primary closure of his fasciotomies. He is subsequently returned to the general surgical service for management of his enterocutaneous fistula.

TAKE HOME POINTS

- Endovascular procedures must be able to establish safe inflow without embolization; if this is achieved bilaterally, no further actions are required; if achieved unilaterally, consider femorofemoral bypass.
- Ensure you have an angiogram showing the status of the visceral vessels.
- Right axillary artery is preferred because it less likely to have inflow disease.
- Care should be taken with dissection of subclavian artery and construction of anastomosis.
- Tunnel to ipsilateral groin using ringed graft material
- Ensure you have patent vessels in groin and have runoff.
- Perform axillofemoral first to establish reperfusion.
- Warn anesthesiologist of reperfusion.
- Work on the contralateral side after tunneling.
- Complete graft-to-graft anastomosis last.
- Perform fasciotomies.
- Manage reperfusion syndrome proactively.

SUGGESTED READINGS

Babu SC, Shah PM, Nitahara J. Acute aortic occlusion—factors that influence outcome. *J Vasc Surg*. 1995;21(4):567-572; discussion 573-575.

Davies MG, Lee DE, Green RM. Current spectrum of thrombolysis. In: Moore W, Ahn S, eds. *Endovascular Surgery*. 3rd ed. Philadelphia, PA: WB Saunders; 2001.

Dossa CD, Shepard AD, Reddy DJ, et al. Acute aortic occlusion. A 40-year experience. *Arch Surg*. 1994;129(6):603-607; discussion 607-608.

Haimovic H. Acute arterial thrombosis. In: Haimovic H, Ascher E, Hollier L, Strandness DE, et al., eds. *Vascular Surgery*. 4th ed. Cambridge, MA: Blackwell Scientific; 1996.

Huber TS. Acute aortic occlusion. In: Ernst CB, Stanley JC, eds. *Current Therapy in Vascular Surgery*. 4th ed. St Louis, MO: Mosby; 2001:395.

Naylor AR, Ah-See AK, Engeset J. Axillofemoral bypass as a limb salvage procedure in high risk patients with aortoiliac disease. *Br J Surg.* 1990;77(6):659-661.

Verma H, Baliga K, George RK, et al. Surgical and endovascular treatment of occlusive aortic syndromes. *J Cardiovasc Surg (Torino).* 2013;54(1 Suppl 1):55-69.

CLINICAL SCENARIO CASE QUESTIONS

1. What is the mortality of acute aortic occlusion?

   a. 20%
   b. 40%
   c. 60%
   d. 80%
   e. 100%

2. Which procedure is the least favored option for acute aortic occlusion?

   a. Aortobifemoral bypass graft
   b. Open embolectomies with secondary endovascular interventions
   c. Open embolectomies with secondary axillobifemoral bypass
   d. Primary stenting
   e. Thrombolysis with pharmacomechanical therapy

66 AIOD/PVOD—Critical Limb Ischemia

AMY B. REED

Presentation

A 61-year-old male is referred for evaluation of right lower extremity pain. He has a long-standing history of one-block claudication; however, 2 weeks ago, his right foot developed a bluish discoloration after showering. Since then, he has noted increasing redness upon standing, decreased sensation, and pain in the foot at night. He reports a 60-pack-year smoking history, hypertension, hyperlipidemia, and a history of myocardial infarction treated with percutaneous coronary angioplasty. On physical examination, his blood pressure is 132/80 mm Hg in both arms. The femoral pulses are weakly palpable. The right foot is cool with sluggish capillary refill and a monophasic Doppler signal in the dorsalis pedis (DP). There are no open sores or ulcerations on either lower extremity. Laboratory studies including complete blood cell count, creatinine level, and prothrombin time are normal.

Differential Diagnosis

The differential diagnoses for unilateral lower extremity pain without ulceration include diabetic neuropathy, nerve root compression, reflex sympathetic dystrophy, venous disease, and arterial insufficiency. In this patient with a history of extensive atherosclerosis and lower extremity claudication, which has now progressed to rest pain, critical limb ischemia from atherosclerotic occlusive disease must be considered the primary diagnosis.

Discussion

Critical limb ischemia results from insufficient arterial perfusion to supply the basal metabolic demands of the toes, foot, or ankle. After taking a careful history and performing a thorough physical examination, measurement of the ankle-brachial index (ABI) is a fundamental diagnostic tool for evaluation of lower extremity arterial insufficiency. Many patients, including diabetic patients, will often have heavily calcified arteries, rendering them noncompressible and thus falsely elevating the ABI. Pulse volume recordings (PVRs) and toe pressures are often unaffected by calcification and should be obtained in these patients. Arterial duplex of the aortoiliac vessels and the bilateral lower extremities will be informative in localizing the disease. ABIs less than 0.40, ankle pressures below 50 mm Hg, and toe pressures under 30 mm Hg with monophasic pulse volume recordings are all indicative of critical limb ischemia.

Recommendation

Noninvasive vascular laboratory studies, including ABI and PVRs, and aortography with bilateral lower extremity arteriography are ordered.

Vascular Laboratory Reports

	Right	Left
Brachial	132 mm Hg	132 mm Hg
Thigh	90 mm Hg	104 mm Hg
Calf	62 mm Hg	86 mm Hg
Posterior tibial	38 mm Hg	76 mm Hg
Dorsalis pedis	40 mm Hg	80 mm Hg
Toe	15 mm Hg	45 mm Hg
Ankle-brachial index	0.30	0.61

Pulse volume recordings: Monophasic waveforms are noted at all levels on the right. Waveforms are biphasic at the thigh and calf level on the right and monophasic at all infrageniculate levels on the left.

Arteriography

Aortogram with bilateral lower extremity runoff reveals the following images (Figs. 1 to 4).

Arteriography Report

There is dilation of the infrarenal aorta, suggestive of aneurysmal disease in addition to severe aortoiliac occlusive disease bilaterally. The hypogastric arteries are heavily diseased with the appearance of a prominent middle sacral artery supplying the pelvis. The superficial femoral artery is occluded on the right with single-vessel runoff. The left superficial femoral is diseased, but patent with two-vessel runoff.

Recommendation

Ultrasonography is indicated for follow-up on the arteriographic findings, suggestive of an infrarenal abdominal

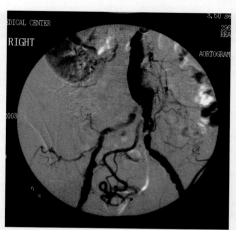

FIGURE 1 • Aortoiliac imaging revealing high grade right common iliac lesion.

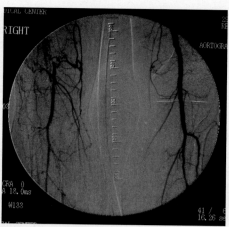

FIGURE 3 • Digital subtraction angiogram demonstrating reconstitution of below knee popliteal segment.

aortic aneurysm (AAA). A computed tomographic (CT) study could also be used; however, this typically requires an additional dye load (150 mL of intravenous contrast on average) on top of the 100 mL utilized for the arteriography and is best avoided.

Ultrasound Report

Ultrasound reveals a heavily calcified 4.0-cm AAA without iliac involvement.

Diagnosis and Recommendation

The patient has a 4-cm AAA with severe bilateral iliac arterial occlusive disease and right superficial femoral artery occlusion with single-vessel runoff to the right foot. This patient is offered an aortobifemoral bypass with possible right femoral to popliteal artery bypass. The presence of aneurysmal disease precludes the use of percutaneous iliac angioplasty and stenting in this patient. It is explained to the patient that the right lower extremity bypass may need to be performed at a later date if the operation is lengthy or significant bleeding is

encountered, but that improving the inflow will be the first step in resolution of his rest pain.

Complications mentioned include bleeding, myocardial infarction, stroke, death, and graft failure requiring further surgery and possible amputation. The patient is instructed to continue all of his preoperative medications up to the day of surgery, particularly beta-blockade and aspirin. Smoking cessation and its importance postoperatively in helping to maintain graft patency is discussed with the patient.

Surgical Approach

Bilateral groin incisions are performed first, taking care to dissect the profunda femoris artery to a soft, nondiseased segment if the superficial femoral artery is occluded. The aorta is dissected free from the surrounding structures at the infrarenal level through a midline incision. After systemic heparinization, the aorta and iliac arteries are clamped. Often, removal of a short segment of infrarenal aorta facilitates the lie of the bypass graft. In this patient, with a 4-cm AAA and severe aortoiliac disease with right

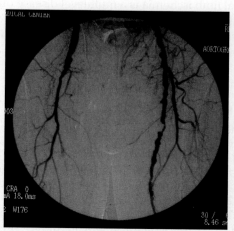

FIGURE 2 • Occluded right superficial femoral artery.

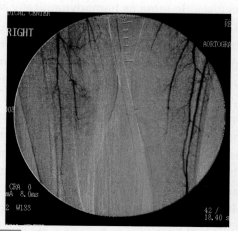

FIGURE 4 • Right tibial level arterial occlusive disease.

lower extremity rest pain, an end-to-end configuration of the proximal anastomosis of the aortobifemoral bypass is necessary to deal with the AAA. A bifurcated prosthetic graft is tunneled anterior to the diseased iliac arteries, making certain the graft lies deep to the ureters. Careful closure of the retroperitoneum is required to avoid development of an aortoenteric fistula in the future.

Case Continued

Upon entering the aorta, there is a significant amount of back bleeding from the prominent middle sacral artery previously noted on arteriography. This vessel, along with several lumbar arteries, is oversewn. Heavy calcification, along with superficial femoral artery occlusion on the right, requires that the distal anastomoses be sewn to the profunda femoris artery. Inspection of the sigmoid colon at this time reveals a pale, grayish color to the serosa with no signals on Doppler insonation.

Approach

Given the extensive occlusive disease of the external and internal iliac arteries, in addition to constructing an end-to-end proximal anastomosis with oversewing of the middle sacral artery, pelvic and distal colonic circulation undoubtedly will be compromised. Reimplantation of the inferior mesenteric artery onto the main body of the prosthetic graft will help improve flow, not only to the colon but also to the pelvic structures. At this time, the patient is cold and has been under anesthesia for nearly 6 hours (Table 1).

Case Conclusion

The patient is transferred to the intensive care unit hemodynamically stable with Doppler signals in the right peroneal and DP arteries, as well as the left posterior tibial and DP arteries. On postoperative day 2, the patient has a guaiac-positive stool with no associated abdominal pain, fever, or leukocytosis. He remains hemodynamically stable with a systolic blood pressure of 130 mm Hg. He has another guaiac-positive stool 2 days later, prompting sigmoidoscopy, which reveals some mild patchy areas of ischemia in the mid–sigmoid colon, but no areas of full-thickness necrosis. By postoperative day 6, he is able to tolerate diet advancement and all preoperative medications are resumed. His feet remain warm with Doppler signals. Repeat noninvasive vascular laboratory studies reveal ABIs of 0.60 on the right and 0.80 on the left, with complete resolution of his right lower extremity rest pain.

TABLE 1. AIOD/PVOD—Combined Rest Pain

Key Technical Steps

1. Bilateral groin incisions are performed first, taking care to dissect the profunda femoris artery to a soft, nondiseased segment if the superficial femoral artery is occluded.
2. The aorta is dissected free from the surrounding structures at the infrarenal level through a midline incision.
3. After systemic heparinization, the aorta and iliac arteries are clamped. Often, removal of a short segment of infrarenal aorta facilitates the lie of the bypass graft.
4. In this patient, with a 4-cm AAA and severe aortoiliac disease with right lower extremity rest pain, an end-to-end configuration of the proximal anastomosis of the aortobifemoral bypass is necessary to deal with the AAA.
5. A bifurcated prosthetic graft is tunneled anterior to the diseased iliac arteries, making certain the graft lies deep to the ureters.
6. Upon entering the aorta, there is a significant amount of back bleeding from the prominent middle sacral artery. This vessel, along with all lumbar arteries, should be oversewn. Heavy calcification, along with superficial femoral artery occlusion, suggests that the distal anastomoses be sewn to the profunda femoris artery.

Potential Pitfalls

- Careful closure of the retroperitoneum is required to avoid development of an aortoenteric fistula in the future.
- Given the extensive occlusive disease of the external and internal iliac arteries, in addition to constructing an end-to-end proximal anastomosis with oversewing of the middle sacral artery, pelvic and distal colonic circulation undoubtedly will be compromised. Reimplantation of the inferior mesenteric artery onto the main body of the prosthetic graft will help improve flow, not only to the colon but also to the pelvic structures.

TAKE HOME POINTS

- Critical limb ischemia is a multilevel disease often including inflow and outflow.
- Revascularization can often be accomplished with a combination of hybrid techniques.
- Cardiac risk factor modification is essential for optimal patient outcome.

SUGGESTED READINGS

Criqui MH, Langer RD, Fronek A, et al. Mortality over a period of 10 years in patients with peripheral arterial disease. *N Engl J Med.* 1992;326:381-386.

de Vries SO, Hunink MGM. Results of aortic bifurcation grafts for aortoiliac occlusive disease: a meta-analysis. *J Vasc Surg.* 1997;26:558-569.

Hirsch AT, Treat-Jacobson D, Lando HA, et al. The role of tobacco cessation, antiplatelet and lipid-lowering therapies in the treatment of peripheral arterial disease. *Vasc Med.* 1997;2:243-251.

Marin ML, Veith FJ, Sanchez LA, et al. Endovascular aortoiliac grafts in combination with standard infrainguinal arterial bypasses in the management of limb-threatening ischemia: preliminary report. *J Vasc Surg.* 1995;22:316-325.

Prendiville EJ, Burke PE, Colgan MP, et al. The profunda femoris: a durable outflow vessel in aortofemoral surgery. *J Vasc Surg.* 1992;16:23-29.

CLINICAL SCENARIO CASE QUESTIONS

1. The differential diagnoses for unilateral lower extremity pain without ulceration include all of the following, except:

   a. Diabetic neuropathy

   b. Nerve root compression

   c. Reflex sympathetic dystrophy

   d. Lymphatic disease

   e. Arterial insufficiency

2. A patient with a combined AAA and aortoiliac occlusive disease (AIOD) can safely undergo:

   a. Endovascular aneurysm repair (EVAR) bifurcated

   b. EVAR aortouniiliac (AUI) and fem-fem bypass graft (BPG)

   c. Open AAA repair with stenting of iliacs

   d. Open AAA with aortobiiliac bypass grafting if externals are not diseased

   e. All of the above

67 Infected Aortic Graft

SUKGU M. HAN, CHARLES M. EICHLER, and CHRISTOPHER D. OWENS

Based on the previous edition chapter written by Christopher Owens and Michael Belkin

Presentation

A 56-year-old man had previously undergone an aortobifemoral Dacron graft placement for claudication due to aortoiliac occlusive disease. In addition, concurrent left femoral to above-knee bypass graft with prosthetic graft was performed for infrainguinal peripheral vascular disease (PVD). He recovered uneventfully and was well until 2 months later when he presented with drainage from left groin incision along with intermittent fevers, fatigue, malaise, and weight loss. He is admitted to the hospital and placed on broad-spectrum intravenous antibiotics. Upon admission, he is noted to have temperature spikes to 102.4°F. His examination is notable for ill-appearing male with purulent drainage from the left groin. He has a well-healed abdominal incision and left groin incision; however, there is a small area of breakdown in the superior pole of his left groin incision with an apparent sinus tract with drainage, and a nontender, nonpulsatile mass is palpable under the draining sinus. Both of his lower extremities are warm and well perfused without ulcers or petechiae. Posterior tibial and dorsalis pedis arteries have multiphasic Doppler signals bilaterally. His white blood cell (WBC) count is 18,100/mm³, and his erythrocyte sedimentation rate is 64 mm/hour. His chemistry panel is normal with the exception that his albumin is 2.2 g/dL. A computed tomography (CT) scan is ordered.

Differential Diagnosis

A pseudoaneurysm must be considered in any patient with a prominent femoral pulse and a known anastomosis in the groin. Ultrasonographic examination is a fast, safe, and reliable method of confirming the diagnosis. The incidence of pseudoaneurysms is reported to be 1% to 5% in the literature, and the femoral anastomosis is most commonly involved in the setting of previous aortobifemoral bypass graft. The common thread among the numerous etiologic factors reported is degenerative changes in the host's arterial wall with dehiscence of the suture line. Because the anastomosis will forever be dependent on the integrity of the suture line, strict adherence to basic vascular surgical principles, such as using nonabsorbable, monofilament suture and taking bites that include all layers of the arterial wall, is essential when sewing prosthetic material to native artery.

Any patient presenting with a pseudoaneurysm should compel the clinician to rule out graft infection. While infectious etiology has been reported in as many as 24% of femoral false aneurysms, pseudoaneurysms occur in approximately 25% of graft infections. Typically, pseudoaneurysms due to graft infections tend to occur earlier than noninfected cases. Furthermore, a pseudoaneurysm in one groin could also herald other graft problems, such as contralateral pseudoaneurysm, and mandates close scrutiny of the entire graft. Finally, a malnourished man presenting with fever of unknown origin and a pulsatile groin mass after aortobifemoral reconstruction has an infected graft until proven otherwise.

CT Scan

CT Scan Report

CT scan demonstrates a peripherally enhancing fluid collection, containing gas, around the left femoral anastomosis (Fig. 1). Superiorly, the fluid collection tracks around the left limb of the aortobifemoral bypass graft above the level of the inguinal ligament. Inferiorly, it is contiguous with the sinus tract out to the skin where purulent drainage was noted on physical examination.

Diagnosis and Recommendation

Findings on this patient's CT scan along with the clinical exam confirm infection involving at least the left limb of the aortobifemoral graft. In general, findings suggestive of graft infection on contrast-enhanced CT include any of the following: loss of normal tissue planes and stranding in the retroperitoneal space, abnormal collections of fluid and gas, focal thickening of the bowel, false aneurysms, vertebral osteomyelitis, and juxta-aortic retroperitoneal

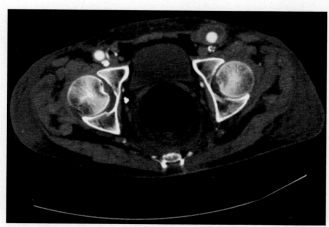

FIGURE 1 • Preoperative CT scan showing a fluid collection over left limb of aortobifemoral bypass graft contiguous with the draining sinus in the groin.

abscess. Postoperative perigraft gas and hematoma are usually absorbed by 3 months. Although computed tomography's diagnostic accuracy has certainly been validated in advanced-stage graft infections, it is inconsistent in low-grade infections with less virulent organisms.

Another modality that can be used in identifying patients with aortic graft infections who do not have obvious findings on the CT scan is imaging techniques using radionuclide scintigraphy. These include indium-labeled WBC, immunoglobin G, or technetium-labeled WBC scans. These methods identify graft infection by radioisotopic imaging of inflammatory sites. They are a useful adjunct in the nonspecific clinical presentation of low-grade graft infections; however, there have been false positives in patients with hematomas or sterile inflammatory processes around the graft. More recently, several fusion imaging techniques have been used to distinguish graft infection from sterile inflammatory response. Particularly, FDG-PET/CT looking at the uptake pattern of radioactive-labeled glucose has been shown to have high positive predictive value for graft infection.

Percutaneous localization of a perigraft cavity by the injection of contrast can be a useful aid in making the diagnosis, although there is a theoretical possibility that it can contaminate an otherwise sterile graft. Culture and Gram stain of the perigraft fluid can often identify the etiologic agent, but failure to do so does not rule out graft infection. A late graft infection, often from a low-virulence microorganism, may only yield WBCs on Gram stain.

Case Continued

The patient is taken to the operating room and undergoes an excision of the infected aortobifemoral and femoropopliteal bypass grafts, with an in situ aortofemoral reconstruction. Initially, the left limb of the aortobifemoral bypass graft is assessed through a small left flank incision. As suspected, the left limb is found to be poorly incorporated and bathed in a purulent fluid collection with Gram stain confirming multiple gram-positive organisms in the perigraft fluid. Bilateral femoral arteries are exposed through longitudinal groin incisions; then, the aorta is exposed through a bilateral subcostal incision. In this patient, with extensive adhesions in the infrarenal aorta, supraceliac exposure is performed with medial visceral rotation. The distal anastomoses are disconnected first, and the surrounding tissue is debrided. The remainder of the graft is removed with a supraceliac clamp. The native aorta is debrided until intact tissue is encountered. An in situ aortofemoral reconstruction is performed with a composite graft using a cryopreserved descending thoracic aorta spliced with a cryopreserved femoral vein. The proximal anastomosis is fashioned end to end, followed by the distal, end-to-side anastomosis to the left common femoral artery. Left to right femoral crossover bypass is constructed using an additional cryopreserved femoral vein (Fig. 2). Left femoral to popliteal bypass graft is completely excised through a medial distal thigh incision. Upon completion of the excision and the in situ reconstruction, the patient is found to have monophasic Doppler signals over the dorsalis pedis and posterior tibial arteries bilaterally. At this point, based on the facts that (1) the patient has undergone an extensive operation with 3.5 L of blood loss, requiring massive transfusion and resuscitation, and (2) left leg is not acutely ischemic after the excision of femoropopliteal vein, the decision is made not to perform a redo femoropopliteal bypass.

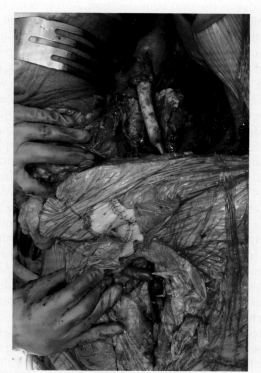

FIGURE 2 • In situ reconstruction using cryopreserved conduit.

The retroperitoneal wound is debrided and cultured. The explanted graft is cultured and yielded *Staphylococcus epidermidis*. Sartorius flaps are performed to provide additional soft tissue coverage over the new grafts in the bilateral redo groin incisions.

Approach

Nowhere in vascular surgery is it more important to have a well thought-out plan than when dealing with a patient with an infected aortobifemoral prosthesis. Consideration of current comorbidities, nutritional state of the patient, and immunocompetence must be weighed before a definitive approach to the patient is carried out. These patients are often immunocompromised and have low albumin. A patient with an indolent infection may benefit from a period of parenteral nutritional supplementation and antibiotics to improve some of these parameters prior to surgery. The patient needs a postoperative care in an intensive care unit (ICU), and the family should be prepared for a long convalescence. Diligent ICU care in the postoperative period is essential to get these critically ill patients through following a large operation.

Surgical Approach

The choices presented to the vascular surgeon contemplating reconstruction of the patient with the infected graft are many and varied. The first is whether an extra-anatomic bypass versus an in situ reconstruction will be performed. If an in situ bypass is chosen, then the choice of conduit is the next consideration. Autogenous femoropopliteal vein, cryopreserved allogenic conduit, and an antibiotic-bonded or antibiotic-soaked prosthetic in the same retroperitoneal bed have all been reported, and all have merit. The conduit of choice at our institution has been cryopreserved allogenic graft, which has yielded acceptable results. At high-volume centers where they are readily available, cryopreserved conduits provide a means to perform the operation without the need for an extensive femoral vein dissection, requiring extended operative time in these critically ill patients. In situ reconstruction is generally avoided in the setting of aorto/graft to enteric fistula or heavy burden of purulence in the retroperitoneum. If an extra-anatomic choice is considered, then what will be the sequence and timing of reconstruction? Removing the infected graft followed by reconstruction may render the legs ischemic for a long time and can subject the patient to complications, such as compartment syndrome, paresis, or amputation. Performing an extra-anatomic reconstruction followed by immediate removal of the infected prosthesis can result in a prolonged operative time with the incumbent fluid requirements, long anesthetic time, and possibly multiple transfusions, all with the attendant physiologic stress on an already debilitated host. It is imperative to isolate infected fields from the extra-anatomic incisions in order to prevent contamination. Staged approach with the initial extra-anatomic reconstruction, followed by removal of the infected prosthesis in a day or two, decreases physiologic stress to the patient, but runs theoretical risk of seeding the new vascular reconstruction.

Case Conclusion

The patient tolerates the procedure well and spends 6 days in the surgical ICU. He is discharged from the hospital on postoperative day 17. Intravenous antibiotics are continued for 2 weeks following the procedure, and the patient is continued on oral antibiotics for the next 3 months. He is followed up every 3 months after discharge and undergoes clinical and noninvasive arterial evaluation (consisting of duplex ultrasonographic surveillance for graft patency). He is discharged on daily aspirin. He is alive and well after the procedure with a patent bypass graft.

Discussion

The reported incidence of aortofemoral graft infection is 0.5% to 3%, making it a rare, but dreaded, complication of reconstructive aortic surgery. Graft infections have been divided at 4 months into early and late. Although less common, early graft infections are caused by more virulent microorganisms, such as *Staphylococcus aureus* or one or more of the gram-negative organisms. These patients are toxic and present in sepsis, which makes the diagnosis straightforward. The imaging modalities (e.g., CT scan) routinely used are more accurate at making the diagnosis in these early infections and often have classic features, such as perigraft abscess or fluid collection.

However, the vast majority of patients with graft infections present late. Late infections can be subtle, often delaying diagnosis and definitive surgical management in a patient who already may be nutritionally and immunologically compromised. For instance, infection several years after implantation or infections caused by less virulent microorganisms may present with nonspecific constitutional symptoms, such as malaise, abdominal pain, or intermittent gastrointestinal bleeding.

A thorough history should be taken, and symptoms such as abdominal pain, recent medical procedures, or illnesses that may result in hematogenous or lymphatic spread should be investigated. Recent nonhealing wounds, foot infections, or urologic manipulations all can contribute to transient bacteremia and possible graft infections. On examination, any pulsatile groin mass should alert the clinician to the presence of pseudoaneurysm due to graft infection. Delayed healing incisions, cellulitis and/or a perigraft mass, or graft cutaneous sinus tract all can be harbingers of an infected graft. The extremities should be carefully examined for septic emboli, which can appear as a cluster of petechiae downstream from the infected anastomosis.

Although several potential etiologic sources of prosthetic infection exist, it is likely from contamination at the time of implantation due to a break in sterile technique. The source can be from the graft itself, the surgical instruments, or the host or a member of the surgical team. The graft itself is an inert material and once contaminated will harbor organisms indefinitely. The porous nature of the woven Dacron fabric may allow sequestration of bacteria in a privileged place, unable to be penetrated by WBCs. The superficial location of the graft in the groin increases its chance of contamination, especially if there is a wound complication or need for re-exploration. Great care must be exercised to avoid contact with the graft and the patient's dermis, especially in the groin areas.

S. aureus, S. epidermidis, and *Escherichia coli* are the causative organisms in 80% of graft infections. Less frequently implicated organisms include *Klebsiella, Proteus, Enterobacter, Pseudomonas,* and nonhemolytic streptococci. While *pseudomonas* is most likely to cause graft anastomotic disruption and hemorrhage, *S. epidermidis* species is especially difficult to detect. Accordingly, the graft infection that is produced includes a sterile exudate, absence of graft incorporation, and a normal WBC count. Methods of tissue culture have been described in graft infections with organisms of low virulence, such as *S. epidermidis,* which improve the chances of identifying the etiologic agent. Different methods of tissue culture, such as tryptic soy broth, and biofilm disruption during processing using sonication or mechanical grinding have been utilized in order to increase the yield.

The surgical goals of managing a patient with infected aortobifemoral prosthesis are twofold: preserve limb viability and function, as well as remove the infected graft. Complete excision of the infected graft and revascularization through a noninfected bed has been the standard treatment of graft infection. However, some advocate newer in situ reconstruction using autogenous, prosthetic, or allograft conduits as a safe and durable alternative. Proponents of this method report that the operation can be performed in selected patients with low-grade infections in whom signs of sepsis are absent with sufficiently low mortality (7.9%) and lower extremity amputation rate (5%). Although these results were encouraging, there was still a sufficiently high complication rate (12.5%) for lower extremity compartment syndrome and recurrent infection rate (10%) to warrant caution. Patient characteristics for which this treatment may be appropriate include presentation of infection months to years after implantation, no clinical signs

TABLE 1. Infected Aortic Graft

Key Technical Steps
1. Unless previously assessed, establish the need for complete excision of the aortic graft by evaluating the limb through a separate incision proximal to the infected groin field.
2. Expose and control common femoral, superficial femoral, and profunda femoris arteries bilaterally. Expose the aortic anastomosis through a transabdominal incision. Supraceliac exposure is often required for proximal control away from the adhesed aortic anastomosis.
3. Excise the infected aortobifemoral bypass graft with debridement of all involved native vessel along with surrounding tissue.
4. Perform an in situ *reconstruction* typically in aortounifemoral with cross-femoral bypass graft configuration.
5. Sartorius flap may be considered for additional soft tissue coverage of the groin incisions.

Potential Pitfalls
- Failing to realize the potential involvement of aortic graft in patients with remote history of aortic graft, who present with indolent infection and drainage from groin wound
- Incomplete debridement of native tissue proximal to the resected graft, leading to pseudoaneurysm development

of sepsis, sterile blood cultures, and inability to culture bacteria from perigraft fluid. These infections are usually found to be due to coagulase-negative staphylococci on graft-biofilm culture.

In contrast, contemporary series of extra-anatomic bypass followed by graft explantation report a mortality rate of 12.5% and a 7% amputation rate. A second operation was required to maintain axillofemoral patency in 14 of 48 survivors (29% incidence), and an aortic stump dehiscence occurred in 1 out of 55 patients. Although these results are sobering, they represent a tremendous improvement over results published just a decade ago and reflect improvements in operative technique, anesthetic care, postoperative ICU care, and infectious disease science.

Few other diseases encountered in vascular surgery can test the creativity and ingenuity of the surgeon like an infected aortobifemoral graft infection. Clearly, no single approach is suitable for all patients, and the contemporary vascular surgeon must be proficient at each of these to tailor the operation to the patient (Table 1).

TAKE HOME POINTS
- Patients with infected aortic graft can present with a wide spectrum of symptoms from local wound drainage to fulminant sepsis.
- CT angiogram is the primary imaging modality of choice to evaluate for abnormal fluid, gas around the graft, retroperitoneal stranding, pseudoaneurysm, or thickened bowel.

- While broad-spectrum antibiotics should be initiated promptly upon diagnosis of aortic graft infection, surgical excision of all involved prosthetic material is the only definitive treatment.
- Reconstructive options are (1) extra-anatomic, using prosthetic graft, most commonly axillobifemoral bypass graft, and (2) in situ, using antibiotic-soaked prosthetic graft, cryopreserved homograft, and autogenous femoral vein conduits.

SUGGESTED READINGS

Bandyk DF, Berni GA, Thiele BL, et al. Aortofemoral graft infection due to *Staphylococcus epidermidis*. *Arch Surg.* 1984;119:102-107.

Bandyk DF, Novotney ML, Back MR, et al. Expanded application of in situ replacement for prosthetic graft infection. *J Vasc Surg.* 2001;34:411-419.

Bruggink JLM, Slart RHJA, Pol JA, et al. Current role of imaging in diagnosing aortic graft infections. *Semin Vasc Surg.* 2011;24:184-190.

Fiorani P, Speziale F, Rizzo L, et al. Detection of aortic graft infection with leukocytes labeled with technetium 99m-hexatazime. *J Vasc Surg.* 1993;17:87-97.

Hodgkiss-Harlow KD, Bandyk DF. Antibiotic therapy of aortic graft infection: treatment and prevention recommendations. *Semin Vasc Surg.* 2011;24:191-298.

Kwaan JHM, Dahl RK, Connolly J. Immunocompetence in patients with prosthetic graft infection. *J Vasc Surg.* 1984;1:45-50.

Lawrence PF. Conservative treatment of aortic graft infection. *Semin Vasc Surg.* 2011;24:199-204.

Reilly LM, Stoney RJ, Goldstone J, et al. Improved management of aortic graft infection: the influence of operation sequence and staging. *J Vasc Surg.* 1987;5:421-432.

Szilagyi DE, Smith RF, Elliott JP, et al. Anastomotic aneurysms after vascular reconstruction: problems of incidence, etiology, and treatment. *Surgery.* 1975;78:800-816.

Yeager RA, Taylor LM, Moneta GL, et al. Improved results with conventional management of infrarenal aortic infection. *J Vasc Surg.* 1999;30:76-82.

CLINICAL SCENARIO CASE QUESTIONS

1. Which of the following organisms is most likely to cause graft anastomotic disruption and hemorrhage?

   a. *Staphylococcus epidermidis*
   b. *Pseudomonas*
   c. *Candida*
   d. *Streptococcus pneumoniae*
   e. All of the above

2. Examples of extra-anatomic bypass include all of the following, except:

   a. Obturator bypass
   b. Axillopopliteal bypass
   c. Axillofemoral bypass
   d. Femorofemoral bypass
   e. Neoaortoiliac system involving femoral vein

68 Aortic Graft Infection with Aortoenteric Fistulae

JOHN B. LUKE and WILLIAM D. JORDAN Jr

Presentation

A 55-year-old male presented to the emergency department with worsening right foot pain for 2 weeks and short distance claudication. The patient had a history of occlusive disease including an aortobifemoral (AoBF) bypass 2 years prior. He also reported lethargy over the past month and intermittent fevers. He experienced one episode of hematemesis 1 week ago, but denied any blood per rectum. On exam, he had blood pressure of 130/85 and HR of 105. There were absent femoral pulses but adequate lower extremity perfusion with no ulcers. Ankle-brachial indices are 0.5 bilaterally. He has tenderness to palpation at epigastrium. Rectal exam identified occult blood.

Differential Diagnosis

In the patient presenting with an aortic graft and gastrointestinal (GI) bleed, a graft enteric fistula is not the most common cause of occult GI bleed; however, it is the most lethal. Thus, graft enteric fistula must be carefully considered for this patient. Although secondary aortoenteric fistula is rare, failure to promptly identify and treat this complication can be a fatal problem. Other common causes of GI bleed include peptic ulcer disease, gastritis, varices, colonic diverticulum, and malignancy. Aside from a GI bleed, other presenting symptoms include fever, lethargy, weight loss, abdominal/back pain, or a pulsatile mass. Lower extremity symptoms secondary to graft thrombosis may also exist.

Case Continued

The patient underwent further evaluation of his AoBF graft with CT angiography (Fig. 1), which reveals an occluded graft that is attached in an end-to-side configuration with periaortic inflammation and air present in the graft limbs. Laboratory values include a leukocyte count of 21×10^3 cc and hemoglobin of 9.2 g/dL.

Workup

In the hemodynamically unstable patient with high index of suspicion of graft enteric fistula, there may be limited time for a complete workup. Diagnosis is confirmed at time of emergency exploration.

In the stable patient, initial laboratory evaluation should include a leukocyte count along with differential. Baseline hematocrit is imperative when graft enteric fistula is suspected. ESR and CRP are nonspecific; however, they may be useful adjuncts to aid in the overall workup process. Further diagnostic tools should be considered based on the clinical condition of the patient.

The duodenum is the most common location of graft enteric fistula; thus, upper GI endoscopy should be performed early in the workup process. This will potentially diagnose a fistula with visualization of adherent clot or even graft in the duodenum. Endoscopy can also aid in ruling out items mentioned above in the differential diagnosis such as varices, gastritis, and peptic ulcer disease. It is important to examine the entire duodenum as a fistula will most commonly develop at the third or fourth portion. A smaller endoscope along with the patient's peristalsis or double-balloon enteroscopy may be necessary for a complete evaluation. Extrinsic compression of the duodenum and pulsatility are clues that the examined portion is overlying the aorta. If an adherent clot is visualized in this area, it should not be disturbed as it may lead to fatal hemorrhage. It is important to note that failure to locate a bleeding source with upper endoscopy does not eliminate aortic graft enteric fistula from the differential as a fistula can occur at any location throughout the GI tract.

Contrast-enhanced CT scan is the mainstay of current radiographic imaging modalities to assist with identification of graft enteric fistula. Common findings include periaortic gas/fluid, anastomotic aneurysm, bowel wall thickening, and other inflammatory changes. Rarely, enteric extravasation of intravenous contrast will be identified.

Catheter-directed arteriography may provide clues, such as anastomotic aneurysm/pseudoaneurysm; however, it provides limited information of graft infection and would only be able to identify a fistula tract if bleeding was evident at a rate of greater than 0.5 mL/minute. It is useful, though, in the preoperative setting to define anatomy in preparation for arterial reconstruction.

Tagged leukocyte (indium-111) scanning is fairly sensitive in detecting aortic graft infection; however, it is ineffective in detecting a graft enteric fistula. Nuclear

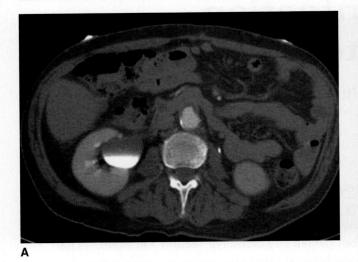

A

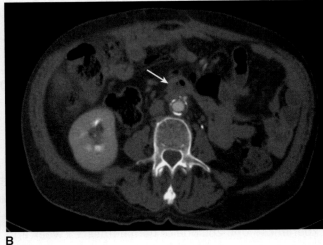

B

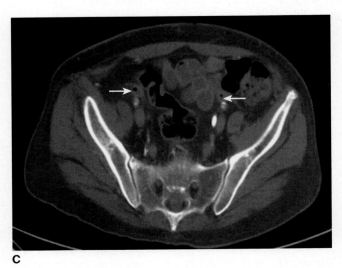

C

FIGURE 1 • CT scan revealing **(A)** patent AoBF graft at proximal anastamosis with end-to-side configuration, **(B)** occluded main body AoBF graft with air in graft (*arrow*), **(C)** occluded graft limbs with air present (*arrows*).

imaging functions best as an adjunct to helical CT imaging. Clinical suspicion along with a positive scan should prompt operative intervention.

Diagnosis and Treatment

Based upon the data available, the leading diagnosis of the above patent is aortic graft enteric fistula.

Nonoperative management is rarely successful in the treatment of aortic graft enteric fistula and is only used in a palliative setting if the patient is unfit for repair. Therapy is centered around repair of fistula and eradication of infection. Broad-spectrum antibiotics are initiated preoperatively. CT imaging is often adequate for operative planning, but assessment of upper extremity perfusion is also important to assess inflow sites if axillofemoral graft is planned. In the hemodynamically unstable patient, control of hemorrhage is the primary goal. Conventionally, this is performed through a midline laparotomy or alternatively through a retroperitoneal approach. Supraceliac clamping may be required for initial control of bleeding

until further dissection is carried out. An alternative to a supraceliac clamp would be balloon occlusion through the existing graft up to the same level. Following vascular control, graft excision along with bowel repair and arterial reconstruction is performed. Due to the nature of an emergency operation, patient morbidity and mortality may be increased due to several factors including preoperative hypotension, necessity of supraceliac clamping for control, and longer-than-usual aortic clamp times. An additional application in the emergency setting of a graft enteric fistula is the use of endovascular stents for fistula coverage. Currently, this option should not be viewed as curative, as the fistulous connection will not be absolved and the endograft will likely become seeded with enteric bacteria. It can, though, be utilized as a temporizing measure prior to a formal repair or a palliative treatment in a terminal patient. This maneuver will allow time for nutritional optimization, antibiotic therapy, and case planning that may include arterial reconstruction prior to graft excision. It should also be considered in those patients

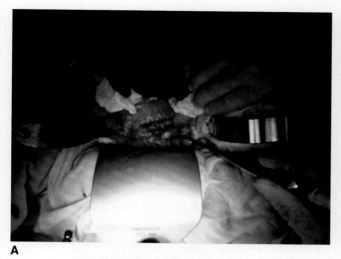
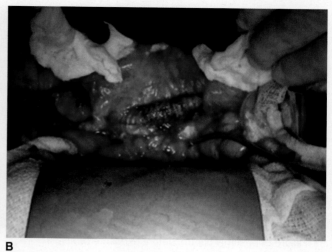

FIGURE 2 • Bile staining of Dacron graft at site of aortic graft enteric fistula. **A:** Shows entire operative filed. **B:** Demonstrates magnified view of bile stained graft.

with overall decline since their initial procedure who may no longer tolerate an open exploration.

In the stable patient, several acceptable alternatives exist for graft enteric fistula repair. Extra-anatomic bypass has been the mainstay of reconstruction in past years. This repair can be either staged with infected graft excision occurring in the following 0 to 3 days or sequential with excision occurring in the same setting. Traditional configuration is an axillary-femoral-femoral bypass with additional outflow options of superficial femoral artery or profunda femoris in the setting of groin involvement. The distal descending thoracic aorta is an alternative inflow source, which would be tunneled in an uninvolved retro-peritoneal plane.

Autogenous tissue in the form of femoral veins has proven in recent years to be a suitable option for reconstruction of a neoaortoiliac system (NAIS). This approach is routinely performed in the same setting of graft excision and can be fairly time-consuming; however, it can be staged with vein exposure left in situ followed by explant and reconstruction in the following day. Construction of NAIS does avoid the decreased long-term patency of certain extra-anatomic configurations and the complications associated with an aortic stump failure. Similarly, cryo-preserved homograft is an available option that allows for in-line aortoiliac reconstruction while eliminating the morbidity associated with a femoral vein harvest. Criticisms of this technique include excessive cost, lack of immediate availability, advanced conduit calcification, and aneurysm degeneration.

An additional option for arterial reconstruction is in the form of rifampin-impregnated Dacron graft. This is an inexpensive option with a fairly high patency rate that is readily available in most institutions. Graft should be soaked in 600-mg rifampin diluted in a saline solution for more than 30 minutes prior to implantation. When used with an omental wrap and long-term anti-biotics in patients without excessive perigraft purulence, rifampin-soaked Dacron is a practical option for reconstruction (Fig. 2).

Surgical Approach

In the hemodynamically unstable patient, the primary goal is control of hemorrhage. Subsequent to this, a complete removal of graft and surrounding infection followed by an expeditious revascularization can be performed if the patient stabilizes and is capable of tolerating further repair. In the stable patient, however, the operative goals of graft removal, bowel repair, removal of all infectious tissue including devitalized aorta, and revascularization can be achieved with various techniques as described above. The decision-making process hinges on physician preference and overall patient status.

In this patient with infected synthetic graft in both groins, we have selected to use autogenous superficial femoral veins for vascular reconstruction. Preoperative superficial femoral vein mapping is performed. Patient is prepped from nipples to toes in supine position. Nasogastric tube should be placed at onset of case. Bilateral superficial femoral veins are harvested with care to not damage the deep femoral veins. Side branches are double ligated. Lower extremity incisions are closed. Groin incisions are opened, and circumferential control of femoral arteries and distal graft is performed. Midline laparotomy reveals a fistula between the third portion of the duodenum and the proximal anastamosis of the aortic graft. Turbid fluid is present surrounding the graft, and intraoperative cultures are taken. Infrarenal aortic control is performed. The entire synthetic graft is removed, and the aorta is debrided back

TABLE 1. Aortic Graft Infection with AEF

Key Technical Steps

1. Harvest length of superficial femoral veins needed, leaving deep femoral veins intact
2. Prepare vein including inversion for valve lysis
3. Laparotomy and tissue cultures
4. Assure proximal aortic control (supraceliac if needed)
5. Identify fistula tract and repair bowel
6. Remove entire graft and surrounding infectious tissue including involved aortic wall
7. Arterial reconstruction (various options for configurations)
8. Omental patch between bowel and arterial reconstruction

Potential Pitfalls

- Failure of proximal control before exposure of fistula
- Injury to ureter
- Failure to remove all infected tissue including involved aortic wall

to normal, healthy-appearing tissue. The defect in duodenum is repaired in two layers. Femoral veins are inverted to facilitate valve lysis. Neoaortic reconstruction is performed from the infrarenal aorta to the bilateral common femoral arteries using the femoral veins in a bifurcated configuration. A pedicle omental patch is placed between the neoaortic reconstruction and the duodenum. Pedal signals are confirmed by Doppler at the conclusion of the procedure (Table 1).

Special Intraoperative Considerations

Several unexpected findings may be encountered at the time of graft enteric fistula repair. First, the most common fistula site is between the duodenum and proximal graft anastamosis. The fistula, though, may be present between any portion of the graft and similarly any portion of the GI tract. If the bowel defect is extensive, resection with anastamosis or Roux-en-Y reconstruction may be required. Also, one may consider placement of distal feeding tube for postoperative nutrition. Second, various degrees of inflammation may be present, making dissection difficult. Some may opt for ureteral stent placement preoperatively. Lastly and most importantly, proximal aortic integrity may be compromised. There must be a plan for supraceliac control if needed and also alternative inflow sites such as the descending thoracic aorta or axillary artery. If extra-anatomic bypass is performed, special care must be taken with aortic stump closure. As previously stated, the aorta is debrided back to normal-appearing tissue. Stump is closed in two layers with polypropylene sutures, and use of pledgets should be avoided as this could be a potential nidus for further infection. Omental patch is placed between stump and bowel.

Case Conclusion

Patients will require an ICU setting in the immediate postoperative course. Early extubation is planned if patient meets criteria. Initial presentation can vary from the stable patient following a herald bleed to the unstable patient with active hemorrhage. Patients may suffer from varying degrees of sepsis, organ system failure, or poor resuscitation. The mainstay of immediate care is supportive with antibiotics and sufficient volume. NG tube should be left in place until bowel function begins to return. It is not unreasonable to obtain UGI study prior to feeding. Lower extremity vascular exam should be followed closely.

In those patients undergoing arterial reconstruction with deep veins, sequential compression devices are used in the immediate postoperative course and prophylactic anticoagulants are implemented soon thereafter when hemostasis is confirmed. These patients can suffer from a significant degree of lower extremity edema and must be monitored for compartment syndrome.

TAKE HOME POINTS

- Patients may present with a "herald bleed," which is self-limited. Aortic graft enteric fistula must be ruled out to avoid a life-threatening hemorrhage.
- Workup may not reveal graft enteric fistula. Clinical judgment and a high index of suspicion play an important role in treatment.
- In the stable patient with graft enteric fistula, operation should be delayed only temporarily to allow for operative planning and patient optimization. Significant delay may result in a hemodynamically unstable patient with an acute bleed.
- In the unstable patient, the primary goal is control of hemorrhage.
- In the stable patient, several options for repair exist consisting of either extra-anatomic bypass or in situ reconstruction with autologous vein, homograft, or antibiotic-impregnated synthetic graft. Extra-anatomic bypass can be performed in a staged procedure 0 to 3 days prior to graft excision or done in the same setting.
- All infected tissue should be removed (including involved aorta). If required, care must be taken for a secure closure of the aortic stump as stump blowout is a fatal complication.
- Patients will need surveillance CT to evaluate for anastomotic aneurysms for those undergoing in situ reconstruction.

SUGGESTED READINGS

Baril DT, Carroccio A, Ellozy SH, et al. Evolving strategies for the treatment of aortoenteric fistulas. *J Vasc Surg.* 2006;44(2):250-257.

Burks JA Jr, Faries PL, Gravereaux EC. Endovascular repair of bleeding aortoenteric fistulas: 5-year experience. *J Vasc Surg.* 2001;34:1055-1059.

Champion MC, Sullivan SN, Coles JC, et al. Aortoenteric fistula: incidence, presentation, recognition, and management. *Ann Surg.* 1982;195:314-317.

Clagett GP, Bowers BL, Lopez-Viego MA. Creation of a neo-aortoiliac system from lower extremity deep and superficial veins. *Ann Surg.* 1993;218:239-249.

Connolly JE, Kwaan JHM, McCart PM, et al. Aortoenteric fistula. *Ann Surg.* 1981;194:402-412.

Gilbert DA, Silverstein FE, Tedesco FJ, et al. The national ASGE survey on upper gastrointestinal hemorrhage. Part III. Endoscopy in upper gastrointestinal bleeding. *Gastrointest Endosc.* 1981;27:94.

Keiffer E, Bahnini A, Koskas E, et al. In situ allograft replacement of infected infrarenal aortic prosthetic grafts: results in forty-three patients. *J Vasc Surg.* 1993;17:349-355.

Kuestner LM, Reilley LM, Jicha DJ, et al. Secondary aortoenteric fistula: contemporary outcome using extra-anatomic bypass and infected graft excision. *J Vasc Surg.* 1995;21:184-196.

Loftus IM, Thompson MM, Fishwick G, et al. Technique for rapid control of bleeding from aortoenteric fistula. *Ann Vasc Surg.* 2000;14:688-696.

Towne JB, Seabrook JR, Bandyk D, et al. In situ replacement of arterial prosthesis infected by bacterial biofilm: long-term follow-up. *J Vasc Surg.* 1994;19:226-233.

CLINICAL SCENARIO CASE QUESTIONS

1. A patient with h/o open AAA repair 3 years prior presents with episode of hematemesis. The patient is hemodynamically stable. EGD reveals adherent clot in the third portion of the duodenum. What is the next step?

   a. BID proton pump inhibitor × 6 weeks
   b. Unroof clot in preparation for epinephrine injection and cautery
   c. CT scan for operative planning followed by exploration
   d. Repeat EGD in 3 months

2. All of the following are common causes of secondary aortoenteric fistulae except:

   a. Duodenal devascularization at original procedure
   b. Pulsatile pressure on the duodenum from an anastomotic aneurysm
   c. Prosthetic infection
   d. Foreign body ingestion

69 Infected Aortofemoral Bypass Limb with Pseudoaneurysm (with Local Flap Coverage)

CYNTHIA K. SHORTELL and KATHARINE L. MCGINIGLE

Presentation

A 60-year-old male smoker underwent aortobifemoral bypass with a bifurcated Dacron graft for claudication due to aortoiliac occlusion. Three weeks later at the postoperative visit, his claudication had resolved, but he reported low-grade fevers for the last 2 to 3 days accompanied by new tenderness at his right groin surgical site. In clinic, he was afebrile with stable vital signs. Cardiopulmonary exam findings were normal, his abdomen was soft with a well-healed laparotomy incision, and his left groin incision was well healed, but his right groin incision had a punctate area of breakdown with turbid drainage (Fig. 1). The remainder of the incision was healed, and there was no cellulitis. He had palpable femoral and pedal pulses. His white blood cell (WBC) count was 9000/mm^3, his chemistry panel was within normal limits with the exception of an albumin of 2.7 g/dL, and blood and urine cultures were negative.

Differential Diagnosis

In this patient with a history of graft placement and new drainage from his right groin incision, superficial surgical site infection (SSI) and prosthetic graft infection should be at the top of the differential diagnosis. The incidence of prosthetic graft infection in aortofemoral bypasses is 0.5% to 3%.

Pseudoaneurysm, infected or sterile, must also be considered in any patient with known vascular anastomosis, especially if there is a prominent femoral pulse or pulsatile mass that is tender to palpation. This diagnosis can be catastrophic if missed. An incidence of pseudoaneurysms in up to 13% of femoral arterial anastomoses (most commonly in aortofemoral grafts) has been reported. Pseudoaneurysm is more likely to occur if there is graft infection. Late presentation is common, and the most likely etiology is degenerative changes in the patient's arterial wall with dehiscence of the suture line. Careful evaluation of both groins is necessary because one third of the patients will have bilateral pseudoaneurysms.

Although this patient presented in the immediate postoperative period, many patients with graft infections present years after their surgery with a fever of unknown origin. Fever of unknown origin is most often the result of infections (tuberculosis, occult abscesses, endocarditis), connective tissue disease (vasculitis, lupus), or malignancy (lymphoma, leukemia). A clue suggesting graft infection may be a history of nonhealing foot wounds, contaminated surgical procedures, or dental or urologic procedures that may lead to a transient bacteremia causing seeding of the graft.

Workup

1. Wound culture and serum markers

   If graft infection or infected pseudoaneurysm is suspected, then Gram stain and culture of the drainage from the wound (or ultrasound-guided sample of perigraft fluid) may be helpful. Often, late graft infections are caused by low-virulence organisms, and Gram stain may only show elevated levels of white cells and no bacteria. Nonspecific serum markers (ESR and CRP) may also be elevated in infection.

2. Ultrasound

   Doppler ultrasound is a fast and reliable method of confirming the diagnosis of pseudoaneurysm and can also characterize the size and presence of thrombus (Fig. 2).

3. CT angiography

   CTA can confirm the diagnosis of pseudoaneurysm (Fig. 3) and also better evaluate the flow lumen, presence of extravasation, presence of perigraft infection, and involvement of the intra-abdominal portion of the graft and contralateral limb. Findings suggestive of infection on CT include loss of normal tissue planes, fat stranding, lymphadenopathy, collections of gas or fluid, pseudoaneurysms (Fig. 3), retroperitoneal abscess, and vertebral osteomyelitis.

4. WBC scan

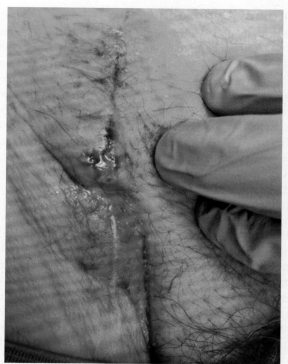

FIGURE 1 • Photograph of right groin following aortobi-femoral bypass with a punctate area of breakdown with turbid drainage. The remainder of the incision was healed, and there was no cellulitis.

If diagnosis is still unclear after ultrasound and CT, then radionucleotide scintigraphy (indium- or technetium-labeled WBC scans) can identify areas of inflammation. These tests may be useful in identifying very low-grade graft infections in patients with nonspecific presentations; however, they have a high false-positive rate since hematomas and sterile inflammatory changes cannot be differentiated with these scans.

Case Continued

Graft infection was suspected in this patient. Gram stain of the right groin drainage showed gram-positive bacteria. ESR was elevated at 30 mm/hour. Ultrasound confirmed the presence of a 5-cm femoral artery pseudoaneurysm in the right groin with active flow within the sack. CTA demonstrated widely patent flow lumen from the aorta into the bilateral extremities, and there was also contrast filling the 5-cm pseudoaneurysm. CT also revealed fluid, fat stranding, and patchy lymphadenopathy around the right limb of the graft in the groin. The abdominal portion and left limb appeared normal and were well incorporated with adjacent tissues, and no surrounding fluid was noted.

Diagnosis and Treatment

Based on the workup, early and localized aortofemoral graft infection with pseudoaneurysm was the confirmed diagnosis and the patient needed to be taken to the operating room. A pseudoaneurysm with active flow requires urgent intervention. While timeliness is important, careful operative planning is needed in the setting of graft infections since there are many variables like the type of organism, extent of infection, presence of systemic disease, and patient's ability to heal that will determine the success of your intervention.

Overall, *Staphylococcus aureus*, *Staphylococcus epidermidis*, and *Escherichia coli* are the causative organisms in 80% of graft infections. Less commonly involved organisms include *Klebsiella*, *Proteus*, *Enterobacter*, *Pseudomonas*, and nonhemolytic streptococci. The most likely etiology of early graft infection is contamination at the time of implantation. The pores of the graft material will harbor organisms indefinitely.

Early graft infections occur within 4 months, and the involved organisms are usually more virulent such as

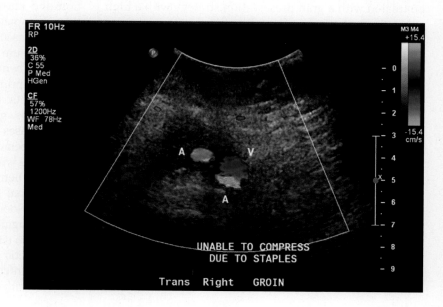

FIGURE 2 • Ultrasound of right groin suggesting the presence of right femoral artery pseudoaneurysm.

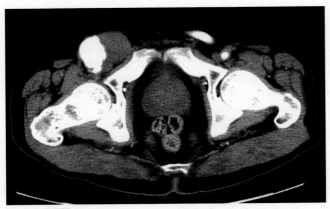

FIGURE 3 • CTA documented right femoral artery pseudoaneurysm following aortobifemoral bypass.

S. aureus or gram-negative organisms. Early infections are less common than are late infections and are usually associated with a postoperative complication such a cellulitis, SSI, or delayed wound healing.

Late graft infections present after 4 months, and the mean time of presentation is 6 years postoperatively. These infections are usually harder to detect as most of them are secondary to organisms with low virulence like *S. epidermidis*. Late infections are more likely to involve the intra-abdominal portion of the graft, and may also present with gastrointestinal bleeding via an enteric fistula. Due to the difficulty of making the diagnosis, these patients often have delay in definitive surgical management, and nutritional compromise and immunologic compromise can be significant factors, also.

Discussion

Gram-positive infections occurring in the early postoperative time period and localized to a single groin can be treated with a graft preservation strategy with a high expectation of success. The patient in this scenario was taken to the operating room for right groin exploration and debridement, primary repair of the pseudoaneurysm, and muscle flap coverage. The right groin incision was reopened with care not to disrupt the tissue around the pseudoaneurysm. There was scant fluid around the graft at the level of the pseudoaneurysm sack. To gain proximal and distal control, vessel loops were passed around the graft, superficial femoral artery, and deep femoral artery. The wound was copiously irrigated with normal saline, and all infected-appearing tissue was debrided. To repair the pseudoaneurysm, the anastomosis was divided and the graft and artery were debrided back to healthy tissue. Only minor debridement was necessary, and tension-free primary reanastomosis was performed without needing an interposition graft. In the setting of graft preservation, we closed the wound with a sartorius muscle flap.

Surgical Approach

The primary goals of the surgical procedure are to address the infected graft and to maintain blood flow to the extremity to preserve limb viability. Within this framework, there are many choices for excision and reconstruction. The first is whether an in situ reconstruction or an extra-anatomic bypass will be performed. Second, especially for in situ reconstruction, one must decide the type of conduit to use. Third, a decision as to whether or not complex wound closure (i.e., muscle flap) is required must be made.

Complete graft excision and revascularization with an extra-anatomic bypass in different tissue planes is the most definitive way to remove the source of infection. Despite the morbidity of abdominal reoperation, if the patient presents with systemic inflammatory response syndrome (SIRS) or sepsis or if there is known gram-negative infection, then complete graft excision and extra-anatomic revascularization is recommended. Complete graft excision is recommended for any graft infected with gram-negative bacteria whether early or late because these infections are more virulent, more likely to involve the whole graft, more likely to result in vascular deterioration (graft blowout), and less likely to respond to conservative treatment.

Most commonly, the extra-anatomic procedure performed is an axillobifemoral graft using ringed 6- or 8-mm polytetrafluoroethylene (PTFE). The sequence and timing of the stages of this operation is important and must be individualized to each patient. Performing an extra-anatomic reconstruction followed by immediate removal of the infected prosthesis increases the risk of seeding the new graft material with the same organism; however, it is generally the preferred approach. Removing the infected graft followed by reconstruction increases the ischemia time to the legs and may increase the risk of complications, such as compartment syndrome, paresis, or amputation.

In patients who are clinically stable with radiographic evidence of retroperitoneal or intra-abdominal infection and known gram-positive or low-virulence infections, complete graft excision is also recommended, but in situ revascularization is possible by creating a neoaortoiliac system (NAIS) using superficial femoropopliteal vein. The benefits of using in situ, autogenous vein are improved primary patency and less reinfection compared to prosthetic material. Performing a NAIS in a patient with sepsis, gram-negative, anaerobic, or fungal infection increases the odds of postoperative 30-day mortality, but has been done successfully by centers with extensive experience with the operation.

The patient in this clinical scenario had a localized infrainguinal infection with a gram-positive organism, negative blood cultures, and no signs of systemic illness, so a less aggressive operation was planned. Local excision and in situ revascularization using autogenous vein or prosthetic conduits has been described with a 10% recurrent infection rate. This option is also appropriate for patients with late infections with only extra-abdominal

TABLE 1. Infected Aortofemoral Bypass Limb with Pseudoaneurysm

Key Technical Steps

1. Reopen groin incision.
2. Obtain vascular control. Retroperitoneal exposure of proximal graft and distal tourniquet may be required.
3. Debride all infected-appearing soft tissue, including artery if pseudoaneurysm is present.
4. Determine if tension-free primary reanastomosis is possible; otherwise, plan for interposition graft.
5. Irrigate, irrigate, irrigate.
6. Divide the sartorius muscle attachments at their insertion on the iliac spine.
7. Mobilize the sartorius laterally, with care not to disrupt its blood supply medially.
8. Rotate the muscle medially as if turning a page in a book.
9. Close in multiple layers over a Jackson-Pratt drain.

Potential Pitfalls

- Bleeding from the pseudoaneurysm prior to securing proximal and distal vascular control
- Arterial dissection

limbs of the bypass affected if there are no clinical signs of systemic infection. Often, these low-virulence late infections only have neutrophils on wound culture, but the excised graft is usually found to have coagulase-negative staphylococci.

In the case of axillofemoral PTFE bypass, it is critical to tunnel the conduit in a new plane away from the contaminated groin sites. Tunneling lateral to the sartorius muscle to approach the mid–deep femoral artery allows for anastomosis creation at a clean site. After graft excision from the groin sites, loosely closing the tissue over a drain and placing a vacuum-assisted wound therapy device are options to promote healing and minimize recurrent SSI. If contaminated sites have to be used, or in case of graft preservation, complex closure with a muscle flap can increase salvage rates. The muscle flap provides healthy, well-vascularized tissue to the area over the vascular graft and fills the soft tissue defect created by the debridement. Rectus femoris, sartorius, and gracilis rotational flaps have all been described as methods of durable coverage in acute graft infections. There is a 5% to 10% rate of persistent/recurrent infection reported after flap closure (Table 1).

Special Intraoperative Considerations

When treating vascular graft infections, a vascular surgeon must be prepared to perform any of the above described operations. With the use of CT scans, the extent of disease is generally known prior to exploration; however, at the time of exploration, if there is fluid around the graft extending into the retroperitoneal space that was unrecognized on CT, then the operative plan may change. The surgeon must be suspicious of infectious involvement of the aortic limb, especially if the patient

had a history of malaise or other constitutional symptoms, and complete excision with extra-anatomic revascularization may be necessary.

Postoperative Management

All patients should be maintained on postoperative intravenous antibiotics. The recommended length of treatment with IV antibiotics for patients with residual graft in place is 6 weeks.

The role of continued antibiotic therapy with oral antibiotics is less clear. Some advocate lifelong suppressive antibiotics as prophylaxis for reinfection. Others limit the length of the course of prophylactic oral antibiotics or chose not to prescribe them at all. The decision to use indefinite suppressive antibiotics can be based on virulence of original organism, resistance pattern of original organism (some resistant infections do not have an oral suppression option), or patient's ability to tolerate the chosen antibiotic. There are no formal recommendations from the Society of Vascular Surgery or the Infectious Diseases Society of America.

Case Conclusion

After right groin exploration and debridement, primary repair of the pseudoaneurysm, and muscle flap coverage, the patient was returned to the floor. He was discharged home 4 days later and was followed closely in clinic until his groin wound fully healed. Two years later, he was still alive and well with a patent aortobifemoral bypass that has allowed for improved exercise tolerance and quality of life.

TAKE HOME POINTS

- *Staphylococcus epidermidis* is the most common pathogen in prosthetic graft infections.
- Pseudoaneurysm occurs in greater than 10% of femoral anastomoses and is more likely with graft infection.
- Graft infections limited to the groin may be treated with local debridement and muscle flap coverage.
- Graft infections involving an intra-abdominal graft are best treated with graft excision and extra-anatomic bypass if the patient can tolerate it.

SUGGESTED READINGS

Ali AT, Modrall JG, Hocking J, et al. Long-term results of the treatment of aortic graft infection by in situ replacement with femoral popliteal vein grafts. *J Vasc Surg.* 2009;50(1):30-39.

Bandyk DF, Berni GA, Thiele BL, et al. Aortofemoral graft infection due to *Staphylococcus epidermidis. Arch Surg.* 1984;119:102-107.

Bandyk DF, Novotney ML, Back MR, et al. Expanded application of in situ replacement for prosthetic graft infection. *J Vasc Surg.* 2001;34:411-419.

Illig KA, Alkon JE, Smith A, et al. Rotational muscle flap closure for acute groin wound infections following vascular surgery. *Ann Vasc Surg.* 2004;18(6):661-668.

Seeger JM, Back MR, Albright JL, et al. Influence of patient characteristics and treatment options on outcome of patients with prosthetic aortic graft infection. *Ann Vasc Surg.* 1999;13(4): 413-420.

Szilagyi DE, Smith RF, Elliott JP, et al. Anastomotic aneurysms after vascular reconstruction: problems of incidence, etiology, and treatment. *Surgery.* 1975;78:800-816.

CLINICAL SCENARIO CASE QUESTIONS

1. A 70-year-old male with history of open infrarenal aortic aneurysm repair presents with a GI bleed and is diagnosed with an aortoenteric fistula at the site of the proximal anastomosis. The most appropriate management is:

   a. Debride and repair fistula primarily, buttress the repair with an omental flap, and put the patient on lifetime suppressive oral antibiotics.

   b. Resect the involved portion of the duodenum, restore GI continuity with gastrojejunostomy, debride and redo the aortic anastomosis, and buttress the repair with an omental flap.

   c. Repair the duodenum primarily, excise the graft, and replace it with in situ Dacron graft.

   d. Repair the duodenum primarily and buttress with omentum, excise the graft, and perform an axillobi-femoral bypass with PTFE.

2. Which of the following statements regarding the diagnosis of graft infection is true?

   a. Perigraft fluid seen on ultrasound or CT 1 month postoperatively is pathognomonic for graft infection.

   b. Gram stain and culture of perigraft fluid are most often negative.

   c. WBC scans are required to confirm graft infection.

   d. White blood cell count is always elevated if infection is present.

70 Renal Artery Fibromuscular Dysplasia

DAWN M. COLEMAN

Presentation

A 29-year-old woman carries a 12-month history of hypertension (HTN). She has been progressively managed medically by her primary care physician and is requiring three drugs presently. She presents with headaches of increasing frequency and intensity. Her review of systems is also notable for new dyspnea on exertion that has been progressive in nature. Exam reveals severe HTN (185/95), a right-sided abdominal bruit, and palpable femoral and dorsalis pedis pulses bilaterally.

Differential Diagnosis

The differential diagnosis for HTN in young adults is broad but should include essential HTN, endocrine dysfunction (i.e., pheochromocytoma, hyperaldosteronism, and hyperthyroidism), renal parenchymal disease, toxins/drugs (i.e., steroid, sympathomimetic drug, and cocaine use), central nervous system pathology and renovascular HTN from aortic coarctation, atheroemboli or renal artery stenosis secondary to atherosclerosis, vasculitis, or fibromuscular dysplasia (FMD). Additionally, given this patient's history of dyspnea on exertion, cardiac dysfunction (and specifically hypertrophic cardiomyopathy) should be considered.

This patient's young age (less than 30 years), three-drug antihypertensive regimen, and bruit should prompt consideration of secondary HTN, and specifically renovascular HTN secondary to renal FMD. Additional indications for diagnostic workup of secondary HTN include sudden acceleration of serum creatinine and HTN, increasing serum creatinine with the administration of angiotensin-converting enzyme (ACE) inhibitors or angiotensin receptor blockers (ARBs), worsening of previously well-controlled HTN, spontaneous hypokalemia, and unexplained (flash) pulmonary edema. Notably, HTN and headache are the most common FMD presenting symptoms, affecting 64% and 52% of patients, respectively,

according to United States Registry for Fibromuscular Dysplasia. Interestingly, headaches are common among patients with isolated renal artery FMD despite well-controlled HTN.

Workup

Additional clinical history should elicit constitutional symptoms concerning for vasculitis and endocrine dysfunction, flank pain, hematuria, and relevant family history. Further symptoms of carotid, mesenteric, and lower extremity FMD might include tinnitus, dizziness, neck pain, flank/abdominal pain, postprandial abdominal pain, claudication, amaurosis fugax, Horner's syndrome, and history of completed myocardial infarction or stroke.

A thorough clinical exam should assess for abdominal bruit, abdominal mass, peripheral pulses and pulse discrepancy across all four extremities, Horner's syndrome (suggesting carotid dissection), neurologic deficit suggesting previous stroke, and a complete cardiopulmonary exam given concerns for hypertrophic cardiomegaly and possible heart failure.

Blood work should be sent to assess renal function (BUN, creatinine), vasculitis (C-reactive protein), and electrolyte levels. Additional blood hormone levels may help differentiate the diagnosis. Specifically, high plasma renin activity indicates renovascular HTN while altered aldosterone, thyroid, and catecholamine levels may indicate endocrine dysfunction. Urinalysis will reveal hematuria or azotemia, concerning for intrinsic renal disease.

Ultrasonography should be considered the first-line diagnostic imaging modality in patients with renovascular HTN. While a high-quality duplex ultrasound examination in an experienced center is extremely accurate for the diagnosis of main renal artery FMD, sensitivity is compromised when surveying branch or parenchymal renal arteries. Ultrasonography allows for determination of renal length and symmetry, the presence of main renal artery stenosis or aneurysm, and the resistive index.

Echocardiography should be performed to assess for left ventricular hypertrophy (LVH) and ventricular function. Computed tomography angiography (CTA) and magnetic resonance angiography (MRA) are both useful adjunctive imaging modalities that will define better focal stenosis, aneurysms, renal infarcts, and dissections. CTA offers excellent spatial resolution, and generated three-dimensional multiplanar images can be very helpful in treatment planning for renal artery aneurysms. CTA, however, is limited in detecting subtle FMD lesions and branch vessel involvement. MRA is often favored in younger patients as it offers diagnostic sensitivity without the associated risks of irradiation.

Catheter-based arteriography remains the gold standard imaging modality for renovascular HTN given its unparalleled spatial resolution and ability to detect reliably branch vessel and parenchymal involvement. Additionally, pressure gradients can be measured across a stenosis (a systolic pressure gradient less than 10 mm Hg is considered normal), intravascular ultrasound may be used to further characterize the renal artery, and any clinically indicated therapeutic interventions can be performed in the same clinical setting.

This patient's electrolytes were normal and creatinine measured 0.7. Renal duplex ultrasound revealed a left renal longitudinal diameter of 11 cm and a right renal longitudinal diameter of 9 cm, a main right renal artery stenosis, and a resistive index of 0.56. Echocardiogram revealed mild LVH with preserved function. An arteriogram revealed alternating stenoses and dilation of the distal two thirds of the main right renal artery producing a "string of beads" appearance (Fig. 1).

Diagnosis and Treatment

This patient has signs and symptoms of renovascular HTN secondary to medial FMD of the right main renal artery. FMD is a nonatherosclerotic, noninflammatory vascular disease that may result in arterial stenosis, occlusion, aneurysm, or dissection. FMD most commonly affects the renal arteries (58% to 75% of FMD cases) followed in frequency by the extracranial carotid and vertebral arteries (32%) and others (including iliac, mesenteric, and intracranial arteries). The prevalence of FMD in the

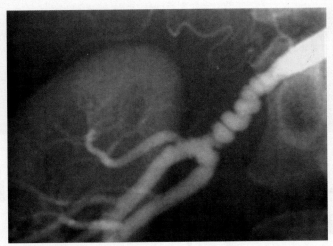

FIGURE 1 • Classic arteriographic appearance of medial fibromuscular dysplasia—alternating stenoses and dilation affecting the distal two thirds of this main renal artery yield a "string of beads" appearance.

general population remains unclear, but it is estimated that 4 in 100 adults are affected by renal FMD. Women are affected more commonly than men by a ratio of 9:1. The etiology remains poorly defined, although evolving data suggests a genetic basis for susceptibility to FMD.

Historically, FMD was classified histopathologically, with medial FMD being the most common histologic variant comprising greater than 90% of cases. Medial FMD includes the following variants: (1) medial fibroplasia (60% to 70%) characterized by deposition of loose collagen in zones of degenerating elastic fibrils in the media resulting in fibromuscular ridges (stenoses) alternating with areas of smooth muscle loss and consequent arterial dilation resulting in a classic "string of beads" angiographic appearance (as described above); (2) perimedial fibroplasia (15% to 25%) characterized by marked fibroplasia of the outer half of the media resulting in irregular luminal narrowing and smaller, less numerous "beads" (or dilated segments) in comparison to medial fibroplasia and obliteration of the elastic lamina; and (3) medial hyperplasia (5% to 15%) characterized by medial smooth muscle hyperplasia without significant collagen deposition such that arterial walls are otherwise well preserved. Intimal fibroplasia and adventitial disease are less common variants of FMD. Most recently, there has been a shift in the classification to radiographic that has been endorsed by the American Heart Association. Specifically, disease is characterized as multifocal (i.e., medial fibroplasia) or focal disease.

Treatment options for renal FMD include medical therapy with surveillance, endovascular therapy, and surgery. First-line antihypertensive agents include ACE inhibitors, ARBs, beta-blockers, calcium channel blockers, and diuretics. ACE inhibitors and ARBs are specifically effective for the treatment of renovascular HTN, and although acute renal insufficiency may occur with administration of renin-angiotensin-aldosterone system–modulating drugs, it is an uncommon complication of therapy and more often to occur in settings of bilateral renal artery stenosis and/or a sodium-depleted state.

This patient has resistant HTN with poorly controlled blood pressure and LVH despite three antihypertensive agents. Indications for renal artery revascularization in the setting of stenosis, dissection, and aneurysm include the following: (1) resistant HTN (failure to reach goal blood pressures in patients on an appropriate three-drug regimen that includes a diuretic); (2) HTN of short duration with the goal of a cure of HTN; and (3) preservation of renal function in a patient with severe stenosis. Percutaneous transluminal renal angioplasty (PTA) has become the treatment of choice for renovascular HTN secondary to FMD, although open surgical reconstructions should be considered for select cases of associated aneurysm, branch vessel disease, and failed PTA.

Surgical Approach—Percutaneous Transluminal Renal Angioplasty

Percutaneous access of the common femoral, brachial, or radial artery should be performed with a micropuncture technique and ultrasound/fluoroscopic guidance. The patient is systemically anticoagulated with Heparin following sheath placement and prior to renal artery selection to decrease the risk of atheroembolism; an activated clotting time greater than 200 should be maintained throughout the procedure. Complete imaging should include aortogram and a full evaluation of the ostia, main renal artery, renal artery branches, and parenchyma of each kidney by way of selective renal arteriography in multiple angles. A trans-lesion pressure gradient evaluation by way of a 4-French catheter or 0.014-inch pressure wire passed into the renal artery will quantify the hemodynamic significance of a radiographic stenosis.

Angioplasty is performed through a guiding catheter or sheath placed at the ostium of the renal artery. Any wire size (0.014 to 0.035 inch) should support balloon delivery and placement across the lesion. Semi-compliant balloon selection is dictated by the diameter of adjacent normal vessel; cutting, scoring, and thermal balloons should be avoided. When the distal artery or its branches are affected, the use of multiple guide wires and a kissing balloon technique may be considered. Completion arteriography and pressure measurements should document procedural success. Primary stenting for renal FMD is not recommended (in contrast to renal atherosclerotic disease) given high rates of in-stent stenosis but may be considered for patients that fail balloon angioplasty or develop a flow-limiting dissection. Endovascular stent grafts may be considered for main renal artery aneurysms, and coil embolization may be considered for branch vessel aneurysms. Anticoagulation should be reversed with protamine prior to sheath removal and manual pressure maintained for hemostasis (Table 1).

TABLE 1. Percutaneous Transluminal Renal Angioplasty

Key Technical Steps
1. Percutaneous access and anticoagulation
2. Renal artery selection
3. Diagnostic angiography, pressure measurements
4. Balloon angioplasty
5. Completion arteriogram

Potential Pitfalls
- Consider premedication with calcium channel blocker and nitroglycerin infusion intraoperatively for vasospasm
- Avoid crossing wires
- Undersize balloons

Potential Pitfalls

As many FMD patients are younger than those with atherosclerotic renal artery stenosis, they demonstrate pronounced vasoreactivity, and vasospasm of the renal vasculature is common. Patients may benefit from premedication with short-acting dihydropyridines (i.e., nifedipine) if not already receiving treatment with calcium channel blockers. Additionally, 0.15 mg of nitroglycerin infused into the renal artery following catheterization may minimize this effect. Additionally, care should be taken to avoid using wires that are designed to cross occlusions as distal advancement into the renal parenchyma may result in perforation. Dissection and arterial rupture are rare with rates approaching 2% to 6%, but care should be taken not to oversize balloons; additionally cutting, scoring, and thermal balloons are not recommended as first-line balloons for angioplasty.

The most common postoperative complications following renal PTA is access site hematoma with an incidence of 3% to 26% necessitating careful placement of the puncture site, utilization of a micropuncture technique, and optimization of compression. Additional major complications are uncommon but can include hemorrhage, dissection, vessel thrombosis, and atheroor thromboemboli (major complication rate up to 6.3%); mortality rate is less than 1%. Patients should receive scheduled daily antiplatelet therapy (i.e., aspirin) postprocedure.

Technical success rates approach 100%. While HTN cure is as low as 6%, HTN is improved in two thirds of patients. Freedom from worsening HTN is 75% at 5 years, and while primary patency is 95% and 71% at 1 and 5 years, respectively, primary-assisted patency approaches 100% out to 9 years. For this reason, judicious surveillance is imperative and recurrent HTN should prompt repeat arteriography and intervention as clinically indicated. Figure 2 demonstrates this patient's completion angiogram following successful right renal PTA.

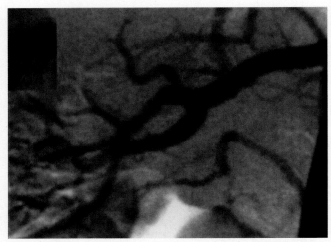

FIGURE 2 • Completion arteriogram following successful percutaneous transluminal renal angioplasty.

Case Conclusion

This patient underwent successful PTA (Fig. 2) with a subsequent decrease in hypertension to only requiring one medication.

TAKE HOME POINTS

- FMD is a nonatherosclerotic, noninflammatory vascular disease that may result in arterial stenosis, dissection, occlusion or aneurysm.
- Medial FMD is the most common histopathologic variant.
- The renal artery is the most common artery affected by FMD.
- HTN is the most common manifestation of renal FMD.
- Catheter-based renal arteriography is the gold standard imaging modality for renal FMD.
- Resistant HTN and preservation of renal function are indications for renal artery revascularization in patients with renal FMD.
- Percutaneous transluminal angioplasty of the renal artery is the procedure of choice for patients with

renal FMD; there are few indications for stenting in this clinical setting.
- Avoid oversizing balloons for angioplasty.
- Antiplatelet therapy and surveillance postoperatively are crucial to maintain primary-assisted patency.

SUGGESTED READINGS

Bonelli FS, McKusick MA, Textor SC, et al. Renal artery angioplasty: technical results and clinical outcome in 320 patients. *Mayo Clin Proc.* 1995;70:1041-1052.

Chobanian AV, Bakris GL, Black HR, et al. The seventh report of the Joint National Committee on prevention, detection, evaluation and treatment of high blood pressure: the JNC 7 report. *JAMA.* 2003;289:2560-2572.

Olin JW, Froehlich J, Gu X, et al. The United States registry for fibromuscular dysplasia: results in the first 447 patients. *Circulation.* 2012;125:3182-3190.

Olin JW, Gornik HL, Bacharach JM, et al. Fibromuscular dysplasia: state of the science and critical unanswered questions: a scientific statement from the American Heart Association. *Circulation.* 2014;129:1048-1078.

Slovut DP, Olin JW. Fibromuscular dysplasia. *N Engl J Med.* 2004;350:1862-1871.

Stanley JC, Fry WJ. Renovascular hypertension secondary to arterial fibrodysplasia in adults: criteria for operation and results of surgery therapy. *Arch Surg.* 1975;110:922-928.

Stanley JC, Gewertz BL, Bove EL, et al. Arterial fibrodysplasia: histopathologic character and current etiologic concepts. *Arch Surg.* 1975;110:561-566.

CLINICAL SCENARIO CASE QUESTIONS

1. What is the most common histopathologic variant of FMD?

   a. Perimedial fibroplasia
   b. Medial fibroplasia
   c. Medial hyperplasia
   d. Intimal fibroplasia
   e. Myointimal hyperplasia

2. Which is the gold standard diagnostic study for renal FMD?

   a. Renal artery duplex ultrasonography
   b. CTA
   c. Catheter-based angiography
   d. MRA
   e. Intravascular ultrasound

71 Renal Artery Stenosis: Surgery

ARSALLA ISLAM and MATTHEW S. EDWARDS

Presentation

A 58-year-old male with a long-standing history of smoking and hypertension is admitted to the hospital with worsening renal function. He is compliant with his four-drug antihypertensive regimen after an episode of flash pulmonary edema that resulted in hospitalization 8 months ago. At that time, his blood pressure was as high as 230/110 mm Hg. His current blood pressure is 150/98 mm Hg. His serum creatinine level is 3.0 mg/dL and was measured at 2.1 mg/dL 6 months ago. His physical examination is unremarkable.

Differential Diagnosis

The differential diagnosis for surgically correctable severe, secondary hypertension includes renovascular hypertension, pheochromocytoma, Conn's syndrome (aldosterone-secreting adenoma), Cushing's syndrome, and coarctation of the aorta.

Discussion

Renovascular disease (RVD, renal artery stenosis [RAS] or occlusion) has a prevalence of approximately 7% in older American adults. The prevalence of RVD is increased in certain patient subgroups. RVD should be suspected as a potential contributory factor in patients with hypertension that is severe, refractory to multidrug therapy, or associated with renal dysfunction. Hypertension that presents at the extremes of age should also be suspected of having a renovascular origin.

Potential findings on history and physical and/or laboratory evaluation include an abdominal bruit, retinopathy, unexplained hypokalemia, or a history of congestive heart failure or pulmonary edema. No single feature or test is diagnostic for RVD-associated hypertension. However, in those patients with the above findings, a noninvasive assessment of the renal vasculature is warranted.

Renal duplex ultrasonography has emerged as the initial diagnostic study of choice for RVD. A renal artery peak systolic velocity (RA-PSV) exceeding 2.0 m/s is associated with stenosis greater than 60% on angiography. The ratio of renal artery to aortic peak systolic velocity is also a useful diagnostic parameter, with a ratio greater than 3.5 strongly associated with stenosis of greater than 60%.

Unfortunately, once RVD is identified in combination with severe hypertension or excretory renal insufficiency, discriminating predictors of blood pressure and renal function response to revascularization therapy are lacking. Renal vein renin analysis and measurement of the renal artery resistive index have been used to try and predict the clinical response to revascularization, but the supporting data for these modalities are inconsistent.

Use of a renal vein systemic renin index has been proposed to predict hypertension response. Lateralizing results from selective renal vein renin assays are useful to guide management in selected cases of unilateral renal artery disease, but this test is poorly tolerated by patients, difficult to standardize and reproduce from a practical standpoint, and extremely expensive. Furthermore, renal vein renin analysis is of no utility in cases of bilateral RVD, which accounts for roughly half of all cases. Given these practical limitations, we rarely use renal vein systemic renin index in our practice.

Renal artery resistive index has also been purported as a predictive tool for functional response following renal revascularization. The renal resistive index (RRI) is calculated as $1 - (RA\text{-}EDV/RA\text{-}PSV)$. Prior published research by our group and others has demonstrated associations between RRI less than 0.8 and favorable blood pressure and renal function responses. Furthermore, RRI greater than 0.8 has been associated with impaired long-term survival and medical/parenchymal disease of the kidney. Unfortunately, the aforementioned data have not been widely reproducible, and the use of RRI as a predictive tool is not an accepted standard of practice.

Renal Duplex Sonography Results

Renal duplex sonography of the patient's left renal artery demonstrates RA-PSV of 2.83 m/s proximal, 0.79 m/s mid, and 0.25 m/s in the distal renal artery with a renal-aortic ratio of 4.6. Right renal artery is occluded. Left kidney measures 12.0 cm in length, and the right kidney measures 5.5 cm in length.

Discussion

In this patient, renal duplex sonography was chosen as the initial diagnostic modality. Depending on available expertise, other modalities can be used in the diagnostic evaluation of RVD, such as renal scintigraphy, magnetic resonance angiography, spiral computed tomographic (CT) angiography, and catheter-based digital subtraction angiography. We strongly feel that catheter-based digital subtraction angiography no longer represents a diagnostic modality, but rather represents part of the therapeutic treatment of RVD, except in cases where a definitive diagnosis of RVD is required and not obtainable using the other described methods.

Renal Arteriography

Renal Arteriography Report

Selective renal artery catheterization with arteriography was then performed for this patient using carbon dioxide as the contrast agent. A single angiogram using dilute iso-osmolar contrast was performed once the optimum image orientation was defined using carbon dioxide. The presented angiographic images demonstrate a left RAS of greater than 80% with a very short main renal artery. An occlusion of the right renal artery was demonstrated without evidence of distal reconstitution or any discernible nephrogram. We did not feel that these findings did not represent appropriate anatomy for endovascular therapy, and the procedure was terminated (Fig. 1).

Discussion

In patients with hypertension and RVD diagnosed by angiography, the decision to proceed with surgical intervention is based on multiple factors: age, anatomic issues, severity of hypertension, medical comorbidities, and presence of ischemic nephropathy. In certain cases, functional studies may be useful in determining the utility of revascularizing kidneys with questionable function. Our group routinely uses nuclear renography to assess small kidneys for the presence of function prior to revascularization. These nuclear studies can be performed using a variety of isotopes. In general, if a small kidney provides less than 10% of the patient's renal function, we do not plan to revascularize. In the patient presented, his right kidney did not demonstrate any significant radioisotope uptake or excretion.

Diagnosis and Recommendations

The options for renal revascularization include percutaneous angioplasty or surgical revascularization in patients with RVD, hypertension refractory to medical management, and/or impaired excretory renal function. In this patient, the decision is made to proceed with surgical revascularization of the left kidney as there was no safe way to perform angioplasty and stenting without risking occlusion of a major branch of the renal artery. Given the proximity of the lesion to the main branch point of the renal artery and the extended warm ischemia time that would have been required if a complex anastomosis or multiple anastomoses were required, a decision was made to proceed with renal artery endarterectomy. This was performed using a left subcostal incision with a medial mobilization of the viscera to broadly expose the aorta, left renal artery, and left kidney. The endarterectomy was performed using a longitudinal arteriotomy extending across the aorta onto the larger of the two main branches of the left renal artery. Following bovine pericardial patch angioplasty of the arteriotomy, an intraoperative duplex exam was performed demonstrating a normal low resistance flow pattern with a RA-PSV of 1.4 m/s and no turbulence (Fig. 2).

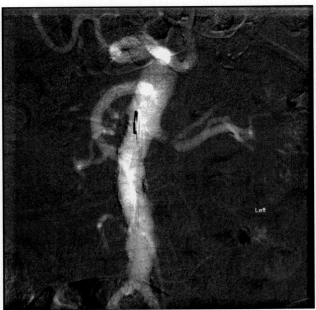

FIGURE 1 • Shows carbon dioxide aortogram with non-visualization of the right renal artery and a left RAS.

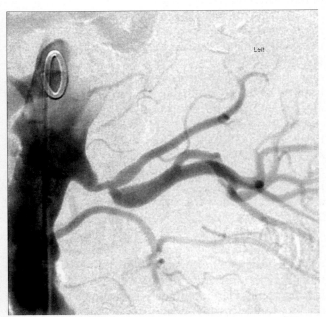

FIGURE 2 • Shows stenosis at the branch point of the early bifurcation of the left renal artery.

Surgical Approach

Multiple surgical options are available to revascularize the kidney, including aortorenal bypass, extra-anatomic bypass, endarterectomy, and reimplantation. A transperitoneal approach utilizing either left or right medial visceral rotation provides adequate exposure of the appropriate renal hilum if a unilateral procedure is planned. For bilateral procedures, a standard anterior approach to the aorta and proximal renal arteries will provide adequate exposure.

Aortorenal Bypass

Aortorenal bypass using autogenous saphenous vein graft or prosthetic material (ePTFE or Dacron) is the most common surgical method of treatment for RVD in adults. In pediatric patients, hypogastric artery conduits are routinely used, as saphenous vein conduits may undergo aneurysmal degeneration over prolonged periods of exposure to the extremely high continuous flow rates of young kidneys.

Extra-anatomic Bypass

The hepatic, splenic, and iliac arteries can be used as alternative sources of inflow for bypasses to revascularize the renal arteries. Saphenous vein and prosthetic conduits can be used for these bypasses, as appropriate. Direct splenic artery to left renal artery bypass can also be performed without the use of additional conduit. Extra-anatomic renal artery bypasses can be used to avoid cross-clamping the aorta in the presence of significant aortic calcification or in patients thought to be poor candidates for the hemodynamic effects of aortic cross-clamping. When using one of its tributaries, the patency of the celiac artery must be confirmed by preoperative imaging.

Thromboendarterectomy

This technique is limited to patients with atherosclerotic RAS. Thromboendarterectomy is frequently performed via a vertical aortotomy, extending from the superior mesenteric artery to the infrarenal aorta, although a transverse arteriotomy extending onto the renal arteries can also be used. This approach is often used because it enables the treatment of multiple renal artery lesions simultaneously.

Nephrectomy

In a minority of patients with RVD, the affected kidney has nonreconstructible vessels and/or contributes only minimally to excretory function. In such patients, nephrectomy is a reasonable option that can provide substantial hypertension benefit. Nephrectomy should only be used in cases of negligible residual renal function in the kidney to be removed. The scenario of planned nephrectomy for hypertension benefit is the only remaining situation in which our group routinely employs renal-vein-systemic renin assays to provide objective data of lateralizing renin overproduction prior to proceeding with surgery.

Key Technical Steps and Potential Pitfalls

The key technical steps to the creation of a renal bypass or renal endarterectomy relate mostly to the exposure. For a unilateral revascularization or a revascularization that may involve the branches, a transverse incision with a medial mobilization of the viscera overlying the target renal vascular structures affords the most versatile exposure. For bilateral revascularization or endarterectomy, a transperitoneal exposure affords the most versatile and easily accomplished exposure in most cases. Mobilization of the venous structures is also essential for visualization. Mobilization of the vena cava in the area of the left renal vein to cava junction at the shoulder is essential to allow retraction of the cava for visualization of the proximal to mid right renal artery for bypass. Similarly, complete mobilization of the left renal vein with division of the adrenal and gonadal branches, as well as any lumbar branches, is essential to being able to manage the proximal portions of both renal arteries and the entire length of the left renal artery. For endarterectomy procedures, it is essential to control the renal arteries well beyond the distal most extension of the plaque to allow for an eversion of the normal renal artery during the endarterectomy to avoid leaving tails of plaque or disrupted intima that can lead to residual stenosis or acute thrombotic failure.

Potential pitfalls include the aforementioned points as well as issues related to management of the aortic side of the anastomosis, selection of revascularization technique, and potential postoperative complications. When creating the aortic anastomosis for the bypass inflow, creation of an aortotomy using an aortic punch maximizes the area of inflow into the bypass conduit. Bypass is an excellent option for normal-sized single renal arteries, but endarterectomy is the best choice for patients with multiple, smaller renal arteries. It is also important to remember that any retraction of tissues cranial and anterior to the left renal vein will involve compression of the pancreas, and it is not uncommon to encounter significant bouts of pancreatitis in the postoperative course if aggressive retraction is required in this area.

Case Conclusion

Patient's course was uncomplicated in the hospital with discharge on postoperative day 4. His renal function improved markedly reaching a stable serum creatinine of 1.7 mg/dL. His blood pressure improved to some degree allowing for elimination of one of his antihypertensive medications. His anatomic and functional results have been durable over 3 years of follow-up.

TAKE HOME POINTS

- No level 1 data currently exist to support open surgical (or endovascular) revascularization versus best medical management in the treatment of renovascular hypertension.
- We recommend reserving renal revascularization for patients with truly refractory, severe hypertension alone or in combination with cardiac disturbance syndrome and/or declining excretory renal function. In such patients, we recommend open revascularization for patients with small renal arteries, multiple renal arteries, patients who are younger, patients who are physiologically fit, patients with concomitant aortic disease requiring address, and for endovascular failures.
- Open surgical bypasses are recommended for single, large renal vessels, and endarterectomy is recommended for patients with multiple, smaller renal arteries. Endarterectomy is also an excellent option for single, large renal arteries as well.
- Extra-anatomic bypasses represent an excellent and durable option in cases where the aorta is hostile or in patients in whom the hemodynamic effects of an aortic cross clamp need to be avoided.
- We strongly recommend the use of completion, intraoperative duplex to ensure that the revascularization is technically sound prior to leaving the operating room. The best time to remediate a poor technical result is at the initial operation.

SUGGESTED READINGS

Islam A, Geary RL. Renovascular disease: general considerations. In: Cronenwett JL, Johnston KW, eds. *Rutherford's Vascular Surgery*. 8th ed. Philadelphia, PA: Saunders Elsevier; 2013:2186-2199.

Hansen KJ, Dean RH. Management of renovascular disease. In: Moore WS, ed. *Vascular Surgery and Endovascular Surgery: A Comprehensive Review*. 7th ed. Philadelphia, PA: WB Saunders; 2006:575-603.

Hansen KJ. Renovascular disease: open surgical treatment. In: Cronenwett JL, Johnston KW, eds. *Rutherford's Vascular Surgery*. 8th ed. Philadelphia, PA: Saunders Elsevier; 2013:2200-2215.

CLINICAL SCENARIO CASE QUESTIONS

1. A 69-year-old white male has moderate, easily controlled hypertension and a serum creatinine of 1.1 mg/dL and an estimated glomerular filtration rate of greater than 60 mL/min. A CT arteriogram demonstrates critical stenosis of the right renal artery and celiac. The preferred mode of management would be:

   a. Common hepatic to right renal artery bypass
   b. Supraceliac aorta to right renal artery bypass
   c. Right renal artery stenting
   d. Transaortic renal endarterectomy
   e. Best medical management and surveillance

2. A 63-year-old white female is currently admitted to the CCU with repeated bouts of pulmonary edema and severe hypertension, which has been poorly controlled with five medications. Her serum creatinine is 1.8 mg/dL. One year ago, her serum creatinine was 1.2 mg/dL. During a cardiac catheterization, she is noted to have an ejection fraction of 60%, no significant obstructive coronary atherosclerosis, and critical stenosis of three of four renal arteries. The best method of revascularization would be:

   a. Bilateral aortorenal bypass
   b. Staged hepatic-to-renal and splenic-to-renal artery bypasses
   c. Transaortic renal endarterectomy
   d. Renal artery stenting
   e. Bilateral iliac artery to renal artery bypasses

72 Renal Artery Stenosis: Endovascular Therapy

VENKATARAMU N. KRISHNAMURTHY and PAULA M. NOVELLI

Presentation

A 62-year-old male presents with a 4-week history of hypertension (210/112 mm Hg). He is a current smoker with a 70-pack-year history of tobacco use. His past medical history is significant for coronary artery disease (CAD), carotid endarterectomy, and peripheral arterial disease (PAD) (aortofemoral bypass surgery for aortoiliac occlusive disease). Initially, he received diuretics and beta-blockers for his hypertension. Because of poor control of hypertension, an angiotensin-converting enzyme (ACE) inhibitor was later added. During this period, his renal function deteriorated (serum creatinine increased from 0.8 to 2.1 mg/dL). The ACE inhibitor was then discontinued with improvement in renal function.

Differential Diagnosis

Essential hypertension is the cause of hypertension in more than 95% of cases. In less than 5% of patients, an underlying cause is identified (Table 1). Renovascular hypertension (RVH) is the most common secondary cause. Nonessential hypertension is usually suspected in patients with recent onset of severe (greater than 200 mm Hg systolic and/or greater than 100 mm Hg diastolic) hypertension. Other indicators of RVH are listed in Table 2. In the current case, RVH is supported by the patient's significant past history of PAD, CAD, and acute deterioration of renal function after administration of an ACE inhibitor.

Discussion

Etiology and Prevalence of RVH

Atherosclerotic renal artery stenosis (ARAS) is the most common etiology (80% to 90% of cases) and is typically ostial (at the ostium and within the proximal 1 cm of the renal artery) (Fig. 1). Major risk factors for ARAS include advanced age, female gender, hypertension, CAD, PAD, chronic kidney disease, diabetes, tobacco use, and hypercholesterolemia. ARAS affects 6.8% of people older than 65 years. Prevalence is higher in patients with congestive heart failure (54.1%), hypertension and diabetes (20%), PAD (25.3%), abdominal aortic aneurysm (33.1%), and end-stage renal disease (40.8%) (Table 1).

Fibromuscular dysplasia (FMD) is the second most common cause (10%) of RVH. FMD is a nonatherosclerotic, noninflammatory disease of medium-sized arteries characterized by fibrodysplastic changes that may cause stenosis, aneurysm, dissection, and/or occlusion. FMD is associated with smoking and is transmitted in an autosomal dominant manner with incomplete penetrance. FMD most frequently occurs in women between the ages of 20 and 60 years. FMD is classified based on the arterial wall layer affected: intima, media, or adventitia. The most common histopathologic type is medial fibroplasia, which angiographically has the classic "string of beads" appearance resulting from alternating areas of stenotic fibrous webs and poststenotic dilatation (Fig. 2).

Other vascular pathologies (vasculitis, neurofibromatosis type 1, aortic wall hematoma, or aortic dissection) account for the remainder 1% to 2% cases of RVH. RAS caused by Takayasu's arteritis is rare in the western world but common in Asia.

Workup of Patients with RVH

Duplex ultrasonography (DU) is the most widely used test in the diagnosis and follow-up of patients with RAS. Major criteria for diagnosis of significant RAS (greater than 60% narrowing) are a peak systolic velocity (PSV) in the main renal artery above 180 cm/s associated with poststenotic turbulence and/or a renal artery to aorta PSV ratio above 3.5. Segmental waveforms within the arcuate vessels such as dampening ("parvus" and "tardus")

TABLE 1. Secondary Causes of Hypertension

- Renovascular hypertension (RVH)
- Endocrine disorders: Conn's syndrome (primary aldosteronism); pheochromocytoma; Cushing's syndrome; thyroid and parathyroid disease (hyper- and hypothyroidism, hyperparathyroidism)
- Chronic kidney disease and obstructive uropathy
- Drug induced (e.g., oral contraceptives, MOA inhibitors, tricyclic antidepressants, steroids, NSAIDs, nasal decongestants, appetite suppressants, heavy alcohol use, and nicotine use)
- Others: coarctation of the aorta; pregnancy; scleroderma; neurofibromatosis

TABLE 2. Clinical Findings Indicative of Renal Artery Stenosis as a Cause of RVH

- Onset of hypertension before age 30 or after age 55; flank or abdominal bruit
- Accelerated, malignant, or resistant hypertension
- New azotemia or worsening of renal function after ACE inhibitor or angiotensin receptor blocker therapy or unexplained renal failure
- Unexplained congestive heart failure/refractory angina or sudden, unexplained "flash" pulmonary edema, especially if patient is azotemic
- Coexisting diffuse atherosclerotic disease (CAD, PAD, or high-grade retinopathy)

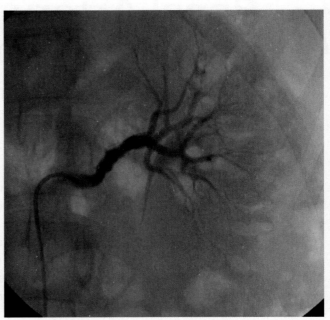

FIGURE 2 • Selective renal arteriogram images of the left renal artery in a young woman with severe uncontrolled hypertension demonstrates classical beaded appearance of the renal arteries consistent with FMD.

and resistive index (relative flow velocities in diastole and systole within small vessels in the kidneys greater than 0.015) provide indirect evidence, but the accuracy is limited. Overall, major limitations of DU are low specificity and accuracy (60% to 90%) as the test is highly operator dependent and difficulties of obtaining adequate studies because of obesity, overlying bowel gas, multiple renal arteries, segmental renal artery/branch stenosis, and renal ptosis.

Computed tomographic angiography (CTA) provides excellent resolution and can outline the vasculature in a manner similar to digital subtraction angiography (DSA). The volume data can be post-processed by multiplanar formatting, maximum intensity projection (MIP), and 3D volume rendering (Fig. 3A and B). CTA has high sensitivity (98%) and specificity (94%) for proximal renal lesions as seen in ARAS. Due to higher resolution capability, CTA is better than is magnetic resonance imaging angiography (MRA) in distinguishing ARAS from FMD. CTA

has the best accuracy among the noninvasive imaging tests in the diagnosis of FMD; reported sensitivity is 64% to 99% and specificity 89% to 98%. Disadvantages are exposure to ionizing radiation, potentially nephrotoxic iodinated contrast medium, and difficulty in assessment of RAS in the presence of heavy calcium burden in the atherosclerotic plaque.

Three-dimensional gadolinium-enhanced MRA, like CTA, is best at evaluating the proximal RAS (83% to 100% sensitivity and 92% to 97% specificity). MRA has an extremely low false-negative rate in determining global renal ischemia (bilateral RAS or RAS in the solitary, functional kidney); therefore, the presence of normal main renal arteries can effectively rule out ischemic nephropathy. Limitations of MRA are its tendency to overestimate the severity of stenosis in the presence of calcified atheromatous plaque, motion artifact due to the patient's inability to hold still due to long scan times or claustrophobia, and presence of metals that disturb the magnetic field such as surgical clips, vascular stents, and prostheses. Another significant disadvantage is the risk of nephrogenic systemic fibrosis (NSF), a debilitating and sometimes fatal skin and muscle condition, associated with the administration of gadolinium-based contrast medium in patients with renal insufficiency. The U.S. Food and Drug Administration has issued a "black box" warning effectively eliminating its use when estimated GFR is below 30 mL/min/1.73 m^2.

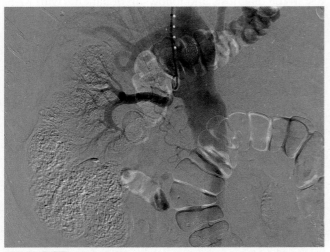

FIGURE 1 • Flush aortogram from brachial approach. Pigtail catheter is seen in the proximal aorta. There is severe ostial stenosis of the right renal artery and nonfilling of the left renal artery. Incidental note made of stent in the celiac artery.

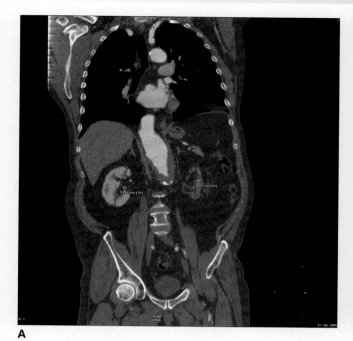

A

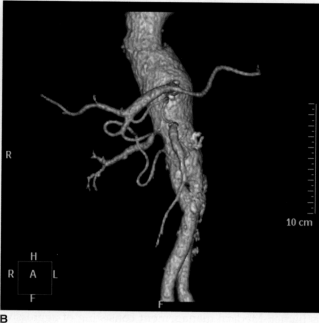

B

FIGURE 3 • **A:** Coronal reformatting of the CT angiogram image from the patient in Figure 1 shows measurements of the kidney lengths. The right kidney demonstrates good enhancement of the cortex, but the left kidney is nonenhancing. **B:** Three-dimensional (3D) volume rendering images from the same patient in anteroposterior and posteroanterior views demonstrate severe renal artery stenosis.

Physiologic and functional studies such as plasma renin activity assay, captopril plasma renin test, renal vein renin assay, and ACE-inhibitor augmented scintigraphy are aimed at detecting the activation of and the resultant effects of the renin-angiotensin system. These studies have the potential to detect hemodynamically and physiologically significant RAS and to predict the clinical response to revascularization. The major limitation is the low accuracy, particularly in the presence of renal insufficiency or bilateral disease and the requirement for the discontinuation of antihypertensive medications affecting the renin-angiotensin system. Therefore, these studies are most appropriate in patients with suspected FMD or uncomplicated ARAS with normal renal function.

Catheter Angiography (DSA) in combination with intra-arterial pressure measurements is an invasive procedure and is considered the gold standard test for evaluation of RAS. DSA has many advantages such as excellent resolution, very high accuracy, and the ability to diagnose and treat RAS during the same session. A ≥70% RAS with a trans-stenotic peak systolic gradient of ≥20 mm Hg is considered hemodynamically significant. Major disadvantages of DSA are its invasive nature, risk of contrast-induced nephropathy (CIN), cholesterol embolization, and high cost.

In patients with renal insufficiency, use of iodinated contrast can potentially be diminished or eliminated by use of carbon dioxide gas as alternative contrast medium (Fig. 4). Intravascular ultrasound (IVUS) may also be used as an adjunct in such situations.

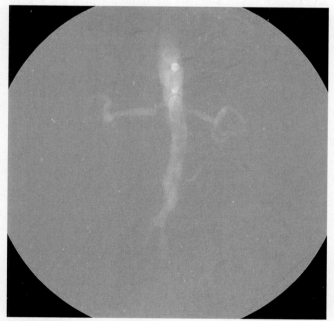

FIGURE 4 • Aortogram using carbon dioxide as contrast agent demonstrates severe focal ostial stenosis of the right renal artery.

Case Continued

A DU evaluation of renal vasculature was unsuccessful due to obesity and bowel gas. CTA was performed demonstrating diffuse atherosclerotic changes in aorta and aortofemoral bypass in the distal aorta (Fig. 3A and B). The right kidney measures 8.9 cm in length, and left kidney is atrophic (6.9 cm).

Recommendation

Catheter angiogram and endovascular revascularization.

Discussion

ARAS: Treatment options for ARAS include medical management and surgical or endovascular revascularization. Most patients can be managed medically without risk of increased mortality or progression to end-stage renal disease. Medical management is also appropriate in older severely atherosclerotic individuals in whom revascularization success is lower and the risk of complications is higher. Medical management consisting of aggressive blood pressure control, lipid-lowering agents, cessation of smoking, and antiplatelet therapy aimed at modifying overall cardiovascular risk factors needs to be applied in all individuals. Renal size and function must be followed very closely while on medical management, particularly in patients with bilateral RAS or RAS stenosis in a solitary kidney. Percutaneous revascularization (percutaneous transluminal angioplasty [PTA] and/or stent placement) is currently the most common method of renal revascularization. Ostial stenosis is primarily stented. Nonostial and branch vessel stenosis are treated with PTA. Open/surgical revascularization is reserved for cases in which endovascular repair has failed or in patients with anatomy-related technical issues or concomitant aortic aneurysms requiring surgical repair.

There is lack of level 1 evidence in support of renal revascularization in ARAS. The majority of randomized trials comparing PTA with best medical management have shown no benefit to invasive therapy over best medical management. Nonetheless, renal revascularization may be justified when there is physiologic evidence of at least partially reversible RVH or ischemic nephropathy on a case-by-case basis. Primary considerations for revascularization are based on the patient's age, anticipated longevity, renal function, ability to withstand a procedural complication, status of the contralateral kidney, and the ease of performance of the procedure. Revascularization is best reserved for patients presenting with a hemodynamically significant ARAS causing (1) unexplained congestive heart failure or sudden unexplained (flash) pulmonary edema; (2) accelerated hypertension, malignant hypertension, or refractory (resistant) despite maximum drug treatment; (3) hypertension due to medication intolerance; (4) ACE inhibitor–induced renal insufficiency with strong clinical reasons to continue

ACE inhibitors; and (5) rapidly deteriorating renal function with adequate renal size.

FMD: Percutaneous endovascular revascularization is considered the first-line treatment option in these patients. PTA is the therapy of choice with stent placement reserved for suboptimal PTA result or post-PTA dissection. Surgical revascularization is reserved for cases of failed of endovascular therapy, and the medical management is reserved for older patients with a prolonged history of hypertension. The technical success of PTA for renal FMD approaches 100% with excellent reported rates of improved or even cured hypertension. PTA of FMD demonstrates 10-year cumulative patency rate of 87%; up to 50% of patients are cured of their hypertension, with the remainder having a reduced drug burden and improved blood pressure control.

Endovascular Technique (Table 3)

1. Preprocedural preparation:
   Adequate hydration (0.45% saline [100 to 150 mL/h] for 12 hours before and 12 hours after intervention) and antiplatelet therapy (loading dose of clopidogrel) should be considered. Review of the relevant anatomy on prior MRA or CTA studies will reduce contrast usage.
2. Procedural steps:
   Femoral arterial approach is the most common route. Brachial or radial artery access can be used if CTA or MRA shows a severe caudal angulation of the renal artery or severely diseased infrarenal aortoiliac segments with marked tortuosity. An aortogram is performed to assess overall anatomy for selection of the appropriate shaped guiding catheter. Intravenous heparin (typically 3000 to 5000 IU) is administered, and if available, activated clotting time (ACT) should be measured to ensure adequate (full) anticoagulation prior to traversing the RAS. The stenosis is traversed with a floppy-tipped guidewire and appropriately shaped (angle tip) catheter. Fluoroscopic road map is

---

TABLE 3. Key Technical Steps and Potential Pitfalls

- Ostial lesions are treated with stents
- Nonostial, FMD are treated with PTA
- Use of guiding catheters
- Low-profile 014/018 platforms are preferable
- Predilate lesions <3 mm to avoid injury to RA
- Stent diameter is matched to the normal renal artery
- Lesions that narrow the vessel cross-sectional area by at least 75% or diameter >50% are considered hemodynamically significant
- Systemic heparin, ACT >250
- Pre- and posthydration is necessary
- Kidney size <8 cm, serum Cr >3.5 mg/dL are poor candidates
- Lifelong ASA
- 1- to 3-month course of clopidogrel

useful for guidance. In the presence of marked aortic atherosclerosis and/or aortic ectasia, the "no-touch" technique may be utilized. In this technique, a guide catheter or guide sheath is advanced with a 0.035-inch J guidewire just beyond its tip. Once just outside the renal artery ostium, blood is aspirated through the guide catheter or guide sheath, which is then flushed. A 0.014-inch floppy tip guidewire and angled catheter are introduced coaxially and passed across the RAS. Upon removal of the J wire, the tip of the guiding catheter or guide sheath engages the renal artery ostium atraumatically. Microcatheters are particularly useful in traversing near-occlusive stenosis.

Traditionally, a "standard platform coaxial" technology (0.035-inch guidewire, 5- to 6-French balloon catheter-stent delivery system and 6- to 7-French guide catheter/sheaths) is used. Current trend is toward using "Small platform" technology (0.014- to 0.018-inch guidewire, coaxial or rapid exchange, 3 to 4-French balloon-stent delivery systems). The latter helps easier crossing of stenosis in caudal angulations and subocclusive, calcified stenosis. It is also expected to decrease local (dissection, embolization) and puncture site complications.

After crossing the stenosis, intraluminal position is confirmed by blood return and contrast injection. In addition, translesional pressure gradient is measured via the catheter and tip of the aortic guide catheter/sheath or using a pressure-sensing wire. If there is a significant translesional gradient (greater than 20 mm Hg), then a vasodilator (approximately 100 to 200 μg of nitroglycerine) is injected directly into the renal arterial bed. The renal arteries, especially in FMD patients, are prone to vasospasm.

The ARAS is treated with primary stent placement. A predilatation using a smaller diameter (3 mm) balloon is recommended to reduce the risk of distal atheroembolism. A balloon-expandable stent is typical stent of choice as they permit greater deployment accuracy and, if needed, can be further expanded by PTA with a larger balloon in order to assure wall apposition and contouring of the stent at the aorto-ostial junction. The stent diameter is matched to that of the normal renal artery segment. The stent length should account for lesion coverage plus 1 to 3 mm on each side. For ostial lesions, the stent should protrude into the aortic lumen by at least 2 mm. When PTA alone is used (e.g., FMD), the balloon should be sized to the diameter of the normal lumen of the uninvolved adjacent renal artery.

Case Continued

The flush aortogram was performed via brachial arterial approach. Severe stenosis of right renal artery noted on CTA was confirmed (Fig. 1). Under fluoroscopic guidance, the stenosis was crossed using a combination of 5F catheter and a 0.035 inch glidewire. The glidewire was exchanged for a 0.035 inch Rosen wire (Fig. 5A). Procedural

imaging shows deployment of balloon expandable stent across the stenosis (Fig. 5B). Completion angiogram demonstrates wide patency of the renal artery (Fig. 5C).

Discussion

Completion renal arteriogram is performed to assess technical success and to exclude complications. Technical success is defined as a residual stenosis of less than 30% and a trans-stenotic peak systolic gradient of less than 10 mm Hg. The success is significantly higher (99%) for primary stenting of ARAS compared to PTA (55% for ostial and 70% for nonostial lesions). The superiority of stents for long-term patency relative to PTA is mostly related to the markedly superior initial success rate and less so to the decreased rate of restenosis.

Upon completion of the revascularization, access site hemostasis may be obtained using manual compression or a vascular closure device. Intravenous hydration is continued for 12 hours, and blood pressure and renal function should be carefully monitored for 24 to 48 hours. Antiplatelet therapy (aspirin, 81 to 325 mg daily) should be given lifelong. If a stent is placed, most advocate the addition of clopidogrel (75 mg daily) for 4 to 6 weeks. Lifelong outpatient follow-up with a renal duplex scan is recommended at 6-month intervals to look for early signs of restenosis.

Discussion

Complications: An overall complication rate of 12% to 36% has been reported, higher in ARAS patients compared with FMD patients. The most common are puncture site trauma and hematoma (approximately 3% to 5%), which are typically managed conservatively (e.g., pressure dressings for hematoma and ultrasound-assisted compression or direct thrombin injection to treat pseudoaneurysm larger than 1 cm in diameter).

Major complications include worsening of renal function (4% to 5%), renal artery occlusion (2% to 3%), segmental infarction (1% to 2%), cholesterol embolization (less than 3%), requirement for surgical intervention for either nephrectomy or salvage (2%), and death (1%). Worsening of renal function may be due to progression of intrinsic disease, CIN, or atheroembolism. CIN presents in the first 24 to 48 hours after the procedure and is usually treated with supportive measures such as IV hydration. Cholesterol embolization is often underdiagnosed with a significant number of patients requiring dialysis within 6 months of diagnosis. It is due to catheter manipulations in the aorta, crossing the stenosis, balloon inflation, stent placement, or more likely a combination of all these maneuvers. Clinical features include insidious onset of symptoms (over 1 to 3 weeks), elevated erythrocyte sedimentation rate (ESR), eosinophilia, and typical livedo reticularis skin rash in lower extremities. It is also treated with supportive measures including systemic anticoagulation. Renal artery injury (perforation or rupture) is a grave complication and is treated by balloon

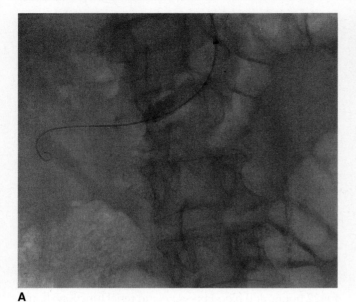

A

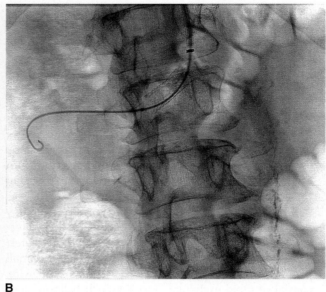

B

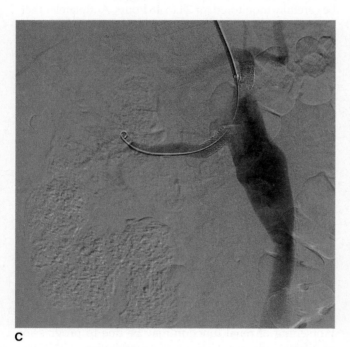

C

FIGURE 5 • **A:** Renal stent placement procedural image demonstrates placement of a Rosen wire in the renal artery and deployment of the balloon expandable stent at the renal ostium. **B:** Renal stent placement procedural image demonstrates fully expanded stent in the renal ostium. **C:** Completion angiogram performed through the injection of sheath demonstrates wide patency of the renal artery.

tamponade and/or stent graft placement. Renal artery dissection and resultant occlusion is treated by stent placement or prolonged balloon inflation. Retroperitoneal (perirenal) hematoma results from capsular perforation by guidewire, and it is managed with supportive care. The perforation is prevented by avoiding stiff-tipped straight guidewires and careful fluoroscopic monitoring of the distal wire tip position. In the event of perforation, transcatheter embolization may be required.

Restenosis is a delayed complication due to development of neointimal hyperplasia. Stents dilated to less than 6 mm diameter, female sex, age greater than 65 years, and smoking are statistically significant independent risk factors for restenosis. Restenosis is usually treated with repeat PTA.

Case Conclusion

The patient was discharged with instructions to maintain a diary of his blood pressure at home twice a day and consult his primary care physician regarding adjustments to his antihypertensive regimen. Antiplatelet therapy was continued with clopidogrel at 75 mg/d for 30 days; the patient was later switched to aspirin 325 mg/d. He was followed up at 1 month and then at 6 monthly intervals for a review of his serial blood pressure records, serum creatinine, and a renal artery duplex scan.

TAKE HOME POINTS

- The suspicion of renal vascular hypertension requires careful analysis of clinical factors.
- Noninvasive imaging modalities are the initial investigative modalities used in patients with high clinical suspicion for RVH.
- Available data from randomized trials to date have not demonstrated a benefit of revascularization over medical therapy. Newer data continue to emerge.
- All patients benefit from aggressive medical therapy aimed at modifying cardiac risk factors.
- Revascularization should be reserved for carefully selected patients with atherosclerotic RVH and as first-line therapy in patients with FMD.

SUGGESTED READINGS

ASTRAL Investigators; Wheatley K, Ives N, et al. Revascularization versus medical therapy for renal-artery stenosis. *N Engl J Med.* 2009;361(20):1953-1962.

Garovic V, Textor SC. Renovascular hypertension: current concepts. *Semin Nephrol.* 2005;25(4):261-271.

Mann SJ, Pickering TG, Sos TA, et al. Captopril renography in the diagnosis of renal artery stenosis: accuracy and limitations. *Am J Med.* 1991;90(1):30-40.

Olin JW, Froehlich J, Gu X, et al. The United States Registry for Fibromuscular Dysplasia: results in the first 447 patients. *Circulation.* 2012;125(25):3182-3190.

Radermacher J, Chavan A, Bleck J, et al. Use of Doppler ultrasonography to predict the outcome of therapy for renal-artery stenosis. *N Engl J Med.* 2001;344(6):410-417.

Slovut DP, Olin JW. Fibromuscular dysplasia. *N Engl J Med.* 2004;350(18):1862-1871.

CLINICAL SCENARIO CASE QUESTIONS

1. The role of renal revascularization in the setting of renal artery stenosis is:
   a. Determined on a case-by-case basis taking into account multiple physiologic and imaging data
   b. Shown to be efficacious in most large trials
   c. Better performed surgically given long-term results
   d. Never indicated in those with diabetes
   e. Only indicated with bilateral renal artery stenosis

2. Renal artery stenosis in a young woman suggests FMD. What is most correct?
   a. This disease is not associated with smoking but is associated with diabetes.
   b. It is best treated with surgical endarterectomy.
   c. It is best treated with angioplasty alone.
   d. It is best treated with angioplasty and stenting.
   e. It is best treated with nephrectomy given long segment disease and arteriolar changes.

73 Concomitant Renal and Aortic Pathology

TIMOTHY K. WILLIAMS and W. DARRIN CLOUSE

Presentation

A 65-year-old male presents to his primary care physician for complaints of recent onset of lower extremity edema, mild shortness of breath, and severe headaches. He has a medical history significant for hypertension, hypercholesterolemia, and a smoking history of 50 pack-years. He quit 5 years ago. There is no history of coronary artery disease, congestive heart failure, or diabetes. Upon further interrogation, the patient reports new-onset dyspnea on exertion and generalized fatigue but denies chest pain.

His current medications include a statin and three antihypertensive medications, including a beta-blocker, diuretic, and angiotensin receptor blocker. Physical exam in the office is notable for a blood pressure of 210/140 mm Hg, whereas previous outpatient encounters have shown good blood pressure control. There are fine crackles at the bilateral lung bases. Auscultation of the abdomen reveals a harsh bruit. The aortic pulsation is easily palpated and seems widened despite mild truncal obesity. There is moderate bilateral lower extremity pitting edema. Peripheral pulses are easily appreciated.

Differential Diagnosis

This patient's presentation is consistent with hypertensive crisis and hyperaldosterone state manifesting with headaches, evidence of pulmonary edema, and volume overload. In this clinical scenario, it is imperative to recognize the acute severity of this condition and need for immediate blood pressure control and expedited evaluation. Hospital admission is appropriate and essential to minimize the risk of end organ dysfunction.

While patients with essential hypertension commonly require several medications for appropriate control, the presence of severe and abruptly worsening hypertension raises concern for secondary etiologies, particularly in the context of continued medication compliance. The differential diagnosis for secondary hypertension includes adrenal cortical tumors, pheochromocytoma, hyperthyroidism, acute cocaine or amphetamine intoxication, and a variety of intrinsic renal pathologies in addition to renovascular disease.

While endocrine diseases and intrinsic renal cortical entities, such as polycystic kidney disease and the spectrum of nephritides and small-vessel vasculitides, are important causes of secondary hypertension, the vascular surgeon's focus in assessing these patients should be the identification of reversible renovascular pathologies requiring intervention. These include atherosclerotic renal artery stenosis, fibromuscular dysplasia, and renal artery dissection, with the former being the more commonly encountered pathology.

In this patient with clear atherosclerotic risk factors, additional physical exam findings suggest complex and/or concomitant vascular pathology. The finding of a harsh abdominal bruit in conjunction with this clinical history strongly suggests the presence of renal artery stenosis. Furthermore, with a strong history of smoking and the presence of an easily palpable aortic pulsation, an abdominal aortic aneurysm should be suspected as well.

Workup

The patient is admitted to the hospital on the medicine service and is placed on intravenous antihypertensive agents, with adequate reduction in his blood pressure. His headache resolves and overall feels better. Echocardiography indicates normal ventricular function with a mildly hypertrophic left ventricular wall. He is managed with volume restriction and gentle diuresis for his pulmonary edema. However, laboratory analysis reveals an elevated serum creatinine at 2.5 mg/dL, increased from his previous baseline of 0.9 3 months ago. Serum and urine markers for various endocrine etiologies of secondary hypertension are obtained, which are unremarkable. Given suspicion for vascular pathology, the vascular surgery service is consulted to evaluate the patient. As the vascular consultant, you are asked to recommend additional diagnostic tests.

There are multiple diagnostic modalities that are useful in the evaluation of patients with suspected renal arterial and aortic pathology. As an initial evaluation, duplex ultrasound has been shown to be both highly sensitive and specific in identifying renal and aortic pathologies, including both aneurysm formation and arterial stenosis. To ensure the highest diagnostic yield, the patient should ideally be fasting overnight prior to evaluation, as bowel gas can easily obscure the images. Direct measurements of the aorta and evaluation of velocities in both the aorta and renal arteries are obtained. Aneurysms are easily identified and diagnosed by size measurements alone.

The presence of renal artery stenosis greater than 60% is based upon an elevation in peak systolic velocity (PSV) on spectral Doppler examination above 180 cm/s, along with a velocity ratio of the renal artery as compared to the aorta of greater than 3.5. In circumstances where the aorta and proximal renal arteries are obscured, the aorta is aneurysmal at the renal origins or has occlusive disease present (PSV ≥100 cm/s), useful data can still be obtained by spectral Doppler waveforms more distally in the renal artery. Blunting of the waveform, increased acceleration times above 100 ms, and spectral broadening/poststenotic turbulence patterns suggest more proximal stenosis. Resistive indices should be obtained, particularly in patients with declining renal function. Generally, a resistive index greater than 0.8 suggests renal parenchymal disease as a potential etiology for impaired renal function.

Computed tomographic angiography (CTA) with intravenous iodinated contrast is commonly utilized in the diagnosis of arterial pathology and serves an important role in case planning, particularly for patients with an abdominal aortic aneurysm (AAA) and/or aortoiliac occlusive disease. Today's available reconstruction software tools make image interrogation much more accurate than in the past. Yet, CTA's major limitation remains dense arterial wall calcification, producing artifact that degrades image quality and accuracy.

Magnetic resonance angiography (MRA) is also commonly utilized in contemporary practice for aortic and renal artery pathologies. While it does have certain advantages over CTA, particularly the lack of ionizing radiation, it does have several notable limitations. As can be seen in other vascular beds, particularly the carotid arteries, MRA tends to overestimate the true degree of stenosis. It also does not demonstrate calcium within lesions, which makes it less useful for operative planning. Even though MRA does not require intravenous contrast through use of specialized protocols such as time-of-flight, the best images are obtained with adjunctive use of gadolinium. This is unfortunately contraindicated in patients with advanced renal dysfunction, as it can cause a severe and life-threatening condition known as nephrogenic systemic fibrosis, making its widespread use limited for patients with suspected renal artery stenosis.

Additional functional and physiologic tests have been described for assessing renal artery stenosis, such as renin selective venous sampling and captopril scintigraphy. These modalities are not commonly utilized in contemporary practice. They are limited by local expertise in the performance and interpretation of these studies, the demanding preparation required, as well as the lack of evidence regarding their impact on renal function and blood pressure outcomes following intervention.

While conventional angiography remains the gold standard diagnostic modality for renal artery stenosis, it is more commonly performed in conjunction with a planned interventional procedure based on results of another noninvasive test. For suspected aortic aneurysms, digital subtraction angiography (DSA) can commonly underestimate the true size of the aorta, given the presence of mural thrombus/atheroma. As such, it is not used as an initial diagnostic modality. Recent interest in catheter-based tools to interrogate hemodynamic significance of renal artery lesions during arteriography has mounted. Technologies such as intravascular ultrasound (IVUS), pressure gradients by wire or catheter, hyperemic gradient induction, and functional flow reserve calculations have all been evaluated. While no absolute consensus exists, it does appear these adjuncts may provide more sensitive and specific renal lesion description than digital subtraction arteriography alone and is the focus of ongoing clinical study.

The patient underwent a screening aortic and renal artery duplex on the ward. Notably, the maximal infrarenal aortic diameter was 7.5 cm. There was a PSV of 400 on the right and 317 on the left (renal artery-to-aorta ratio of 5.3 and 4.2, respectively). Resistive indices were normal bilaterally (Fig. 1). There was notable blunting of bilateral distal renal artery Doppler waveforms with poststenotic turbulence. Following initiation of nephroprotective measures including administration of N-acetylcysteine and infusion of sodium bicarbonate solution, a CTA of the abdomen and pelvis was obtained. This demonstrated favorable anatomy for endovascular aortic repair and again suggested high-grade bilateral renal artery stenosis.

Diagnosis and Treatment

Based on the workup, the patient was found to have high-grade bilateral renal artery stenosis and a large abdominal aortic aneurysm. While the management of patients with abdominal aortic aneurysms is well established, the contemporary management of patients with atherosclerotic renal artery stenosis remains a matter of considerable controversy. Several recent large multicenter trials have suggested minimal clinical benefit in preservation of renal function and control of hypertension following renal artery stenting. However, these trials have been criticized based on poor methodology, leaving the medical community with a lack of resounding support for renal artery interventions. Most vascular specialists would agree that there are a subset of patients who will receive clinical benefit from renal artery intervention, particularly patients with uncontrolled hypertension

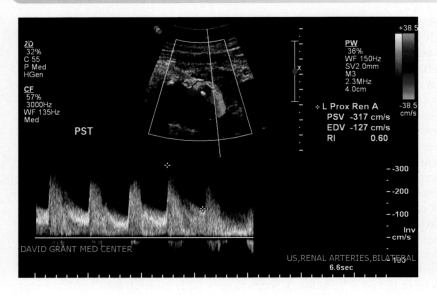

FIGURE 1 • Left renal artery duplex evaluation indicating severe renal artery stenosis with poststenotic turbulence. A normal resistive index does not suggest significant parenchymal disease.

on numerous medications and objective evidence of high-grade renal artery stenosis (particularly bilateral). Additionally, patients with an abrupt decline in renal function with high-grade stenosis are also felt to benefit from intervention either in renal function improvement or slowing of functional deterioration. Additionally, those presenting with acute hypertensive crisis and hyperaldosteronism, as in this clinical scenario, may benefit from renal intervention.

Historically, patients found to have concomitant aortic and renal pathology were managed in an open operative fashion. Given the implications of reoperative surgery, this clinical dilemma drove investigation and the consideration for simultaneous repair. Entering the endovascular era, clinical series of combined open aortic and renal revascularization from centers of excellence did not provide clear consensus. Some indicated similar morbidity and mortality compared with aortic reconstruction alone, yet others showed significantly higher risk of complication and death. These provided a general belief in combined reconstruction in those with absolute renal revascularization indication.

Today, management of patients with abdominal aortic aneurysms and atherosclerotic renal artery stenosis is largely addressed with endovascular techniques. Even patients with anatomy deemed unfavorable for traditional endovascular aneurysm repair (EVAR) are increasingly being treated with endovascular techniques, utilizing FDA-approved or investigational device exemption (IDE)-sponsored fenestrated devices, snorkel, periscope, and sandwich stent graft techniques.

With regard to renal artery stenosis, the overwhelming majority of patients will have anatomy amenable to renal artery stenting (RAS), obviating the need for open revascularization. This shift toward endovascular management creates the practical opportunity for managing concomitant aortic and renal artery pathology in a methodical, staged

fashion. Support for this strategy has been demonstrated by recent data from Protack et al., showing increased periprocedural renal artery complications including functional kidney injury and early vessel occlusion when renal revascularization was performed concomitantly with EVAR as compared to patients undergoing isolated renal artery interventions. Importantly, those patients in the EVAR/RAS and RAS-alone groups faired equally in long-term follow-up in terms of freedom from occlusion and restenosis, renal function, and control of hypertension, when excluding patients with early procedural complications. Even though these data suggest immediate EVAR/RAS renal outcome inferior to singular renal artery intervention, there remains no direct comparison of combined or staged renal artery intervention in those requiring both RAS and either EVAR or aortoiliac intervention. Thus, how this is approached remains dependent upon each disease process indication and clinical judgment.

In light of the favorable anatomy based on CTA, our patient was offered renal artery intervention initially given the acute clinical deterioration and need for renal intervention with plan for staged EVAR within the subsequent few weeks.

Surgical Approach

The details of renal artery interventions, EVAR, and aortoiliac reconstructions are outlined in previous chapters. Percutaneous renal interventions should be considered as first-line therapy in patients undergoing EVAR. When feasible, renal artery interventions should precede EVAR, in an effort to stabilize hemodynamics and optimize renal function. However, the sequence of events does not appear to be particularly important in terms of technical success of either procedure. It has been shown that patients who have previously undergone EVAR can safely undergo renal artery interventions with a high degree of technical success. Therefore, patients in need of EVAR with an equivocal indication for renal artery intervention should have their renal intervention deferred until clinically warranted. The application of open renal artery revascularization in those who are candidates for EVAR or endovascular aortoiliac reconstruction should be reserved for renal artery anatomy not favorable for percutaneous interventions, as well as those failing prior endovascular renal revascularization attempts.

Many patients with juxtarenal aneurysms or aortoiliac occlusive disease managed in an open fashion may still undergo percutaneous renal intervention based on individual anatomy. However, combined open renal and aortic reconstruction should be considered when other indications for open renal revascularization exist, particularly in the context of unfavorable renal artery anatomy and prior failed percutaneous renal intervention. Suprarenal or type IV thoracoabdominal aneurysms repaired via a retroperitoneal approach typically involve a beveled anastomosis with an obligate left aortorenal bypass. Therefore, most ostial left renal artery stenoses will be repaired regardless of their clinical significance. The management of the right renal artery from a retroperitoneal approach can include open stenting or button eversion endarterectomy as clinically warranted. Aortorenal bypass to the right renal artery is possible, but more demanding and requires very proximal disease. When a transabdominal approach is justified, either renal artery can undergo aortorenal bypass, extra-anatomic bypass (splenorenal on left, hepatorenal on right), or transaortic endarterectomy with patch angioplasty based upon lesion characteristics and the clinical circumstance.

Special Intraoperative Considerations

There are very few technical considerations or concerns relevant to combined aortic and renal interventions outside of those related to the individual procedures. It is worth noting, however, that for patients undergoing RAS prior to planned EVAR, care should be taken to avoid significantly extending renal artery stents into the aortic lumen, as these may be vulnerable to damage during EVAR by suprarenal fixation or wire and catheter exchanges. When renal artery intervention occurs after EVAR, arm approaches may provide ease of access and facilitate more robust flaring of the proximal stent, particularly with suprarenal fixation in place. Suprarenal fixation of abdominal aortic endografts and the effects on renal artery anatomy and renal function remain to be more fully defined, let alone how they might affect existing renal artery disease.

Postoperative Management

Management of patients following concomitant or staged aortic and renal intervention largely follows the typical management patterns for the respective procedures. Certainly, careful attention to renal function and close hemodynamic monitoring is more relevant for those patients undergoing concomitant procedures. Furthermore, efforts should be taken to avoid hypotension, maintain adequate hydration and renal perfusion. A minority of patients following renal revascularization, particularly of very high-grade lesions, will undergo a brisk diuresis, which may complicate early postprocedure fluid management. Declining renal function, notable flank pain, or accelerated hypertension early following concomitant procedures or completion of the staged procedures should raise concern for early renal artery occlusion. Postoperative surveillance should proceed as appropriate based on consensus recommendation for the individual procedures. Generally, we obtain an early duplex scan prior to discharge to establish renal artery patency and define initial flow patterns.

Case Conclusion

The patient underwent uneventful percutaneous renal artery intervention, utilizing bilateral 6-mm bare metal stents (Fig. 2). This resulted in normalization of renal function and dramatic reduction in blood pressure, significantly reducing the patient's antihypertensive regimen as well as providing volume overload resolution. Postprocedure duplex revealed normalization of renal artery velocities (Fig. 3). Approximately 1 week later, the patient underwent EVAR with successful exclusion of the aneurysm and no evidence of endoleak. The patient was safely discharged home 2 days later on low doses of only two antihypertensive medications, the beta-blocker and diuretic. In mid-term follow-up, the aneurysm sac remains excluded, and the patient's renal function and blood pressure remain improved and stable (Fig. 4).

TAKE HOME POINTS

- Indications for renal artery intervention in patients needing aortic repair should follow accepted indications for the individual procedures. Avoid renal artery interventions based only on radiographic findings.
- Combined aortic and renal artery pathologies should be managed with endovascular techniques when feasible.
- Repair should proceed in a staged fashion unless both territories clinically require immediate attention.
- EVAR or aortoiliac interventions do not compromise potential for future renal artery interventions; therefore, avoid concomitant renal artery interventions based on equivocal indications.
- Open renal artery reconstruction in those undergoing open aortic surgery is justified in those anatomically unsuitable for endovascular techniques, or failing prior endovascular interventions.

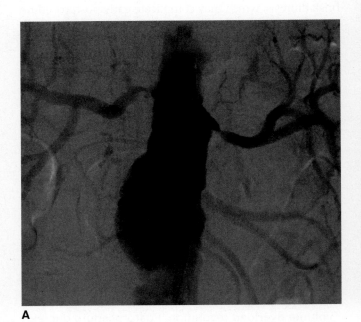

A

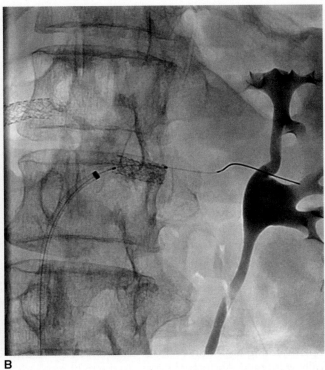

B

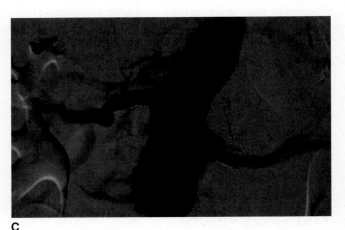

C

FIGURE 2 • **A:** Aortogram confirming severe, bilateral renal artery stenosis. **B:** Placement of bilateral 6 × 16 mm balloon expandable stents including postplacement flaring of the left renal-stent aortic interface. **C:** Postplacement aortogram indicating resolution of severe stenoses.

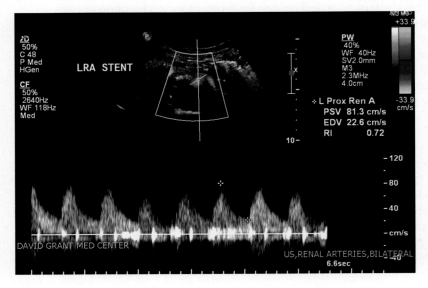

FIGURE 3 • Normalization of renal artery velocities by duplex after renal artery stenting prior to EVAR.

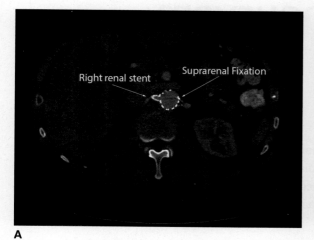
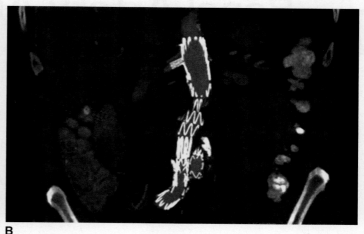

A   B

FIGURE 4 • **A:** Axial and **B:** coronal CTA images revealing the right renal artery stent origin interface with the EVAR suprarenal fixation. This stent was placed in staged fashion prior to the aortic endograft with attention to maintaining proximal renal stent integrity. Stents placed well prior to need for EVAR may occasionally require further endovascular attention at the time of endografting.

SUGGESTED READINGS

Benjamin M, et al. Combined aortic and renal artery surgery. *Ann Surg.* 1996;223(5):555-567.

Bown M, et al. The management of abdominal aortic aneurysms in patients with concurrent renal impairment. *Eur J Vasc Endovasc Surg.* 2005;30(1):1-11.

Cambria RP, et al. Simultaneous aortic and renal artery reconstruction: evolution of an eighteen-year experience. *J Vasc Surg.* 1995;21(6):916-925.

Chaikof EL, et al. Ischemic nephropathy and concomitant aortic disease: a ten-year experience. *J Vasc Surg.* 1994;19(1):135-148.

Jaff MR, et al. Significant reduction in systolic blood pressure following renal artery stenting in patients with uncontrolled hypertension: results from the HERCULES trial. *Catheter Cardiovasc Interv.* 2012;80(3):343-350.

Landry GJ, et al. Adjunctive renal artery revascularization during juxtarenal and suprarenal abdominal aortic aneurysm repairs. *Am J Surg.* 2010;199(5):641-645.

Protack CD, Saad WA, Davies MG. Renal artery interventions during infrarenal endovascular aortic repair: a greater potential of subsequent failure? *J Vasc Interv Radiol.* 2010;21(4):459-464.

Tsoukas AI, et al. Simultaneous aortic replacement and renal artery revascularization: the influence of preoperative renal function on early risk and late outcome. *J Vasc Surg.* 2001;34(6):1041-1049.

CLINICAL SCENARIO CASE QUESTIONS

1. A 65-year-old male presents to your clinic for an incidentally discovered 6-cm infrarenal AAA. The CTA demonstrates high-grade renal artery stenosis bilaterally. His blood pressure is reasonably controlled on three antihypertensive medications, and his serum creatinine is 1.2 mg/dL. What is the best approach to the management of his current clinical presentation?

   a. Perform EVAR, obtain renal artery translesional pressure gradients, with stenting for a systolic blood pressure gradient greater than 40 mm Hg.

   b. Perform bilateral renal artery stenting and EVAR in staged fashion.

   c. Selective venous renin sampling, with renal stenting predicated on these results, and staged EVAR.

   d. EVAR alone.

   e. Fenestrated EVAR with bilateral renal artery stent graft placement.

2. Which of the following statements is true regarding the management of concomitant AAA and renal artery stenosis?

   a. In the presence of high-grade renal artery stenosis, open repair of aortic aneurysms is preferred.

   b. In the presence of high-grade unilateral renal artery stenosis, repair of AAA's 4 cm or greater is justified.

   c. When endovascular therapies are feasible, repair of either pathology should be entertained based on established indications for the respective pathology.

   d. The presence of renal artery stenosis is protective against aneurysm rupture; thus intervention for AAA should be deferred until the aneurysm exceeds 6 cm.

   e. None of the above are correct.

74 Renal Artery Aneurysm

PETER K. HENKE

Presentation

A 45-year-old woman, G6/P5, is evaluated for vague right upper quadrant pain. Past medical history includes hypertension controlled with two medications, including an angiotensin-converting enzyme (ACE) inhibitor and a diuretic. The patient denies any history of tobacco use, diabetes, and hyperlipidemia, and there is no family history of any aneurysmal or other major vascular disease. She is perimenopausal.

CT Scan

CT Scan Report

A computed tomographic (CT) scan shows no evidence of gallbladder or liver pathology, but there is an incidental finding of a right renal artery aneurysm (RAA) approximately 2.5 cm in size, not noted on a prior right upper quadrant ultrasound (Fig. 1), and other mesenteric aneurysms are identified.

Further Diagnostic Workup

No hematuria is detected on urinalysis, and serum creatinine is normal. An arteriogram should be obtained in these patients to delineate the renal anatomy with dedicated catheter injections and multiple projections of both renal arteries. Alternatively, high-resolution CTA can be used with good fidelity for main artery aneurysms, obviating the need for angiogram (Fig. 2).

Arteriogram

Arteriogram Report

A large right RAA at the bifurcation of the main renal artery, and a smaller left RAA in a first-order branch (Fig. 3). No other intra-aortic pathology is identified.

Treatment Considerations

Because this patient is just beyond childbearing age, indications for repair are slightly less compelling than if premenopausal, where repair is definitely indicated. The main risk with RAA is rupture. If this occurs, mortality ranges between 10% and 15%. Rupture risk is higher in premenopausal women, and kidney loss is high in the setting of rupture, ranging between 50% and 100%. Although endovascular repairs have been documented, this does not seem appropriate for most RAA, because they are often fusiform and not amenable to coil embolization. A technical mishap may cause total kidney infarction. Recent reviews suggest that this option is reasonable in high-risk patients, and perhaps better in those with a proximal RAA, that can be treated with a covered stent.

The patient's RAA is a size that is suitable for repair, given that she otherwise has few cardiovascular risk factors. Various methods for repairing these lesions have been described including ex vivo reconstruction with kidney autotransplantation, but it is the author's practice to perform the repair in situ, using aneurysm resection, primary repair, and/or bypass as the individual anatomy dictates.

Surgical Approach

At operation, a lumbar roll is placed to create a lumbar lordosis. A transverse supraumbilical incision allows for excellent exposure of the kidneys. An extensive Kocher maneuver is used to expose the right kidney and renal vasculature. Care must be taken to fully dissect the RAA from surrounding renal venous and hilar structures. A right RAA resection with primary repair is performed.

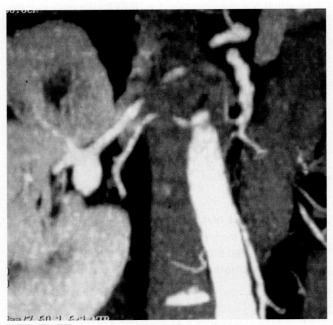

FIGURE 1 • Contrast CTA showing right renal artery aneurysm at bifurcation of main renal artery.

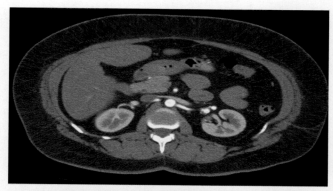
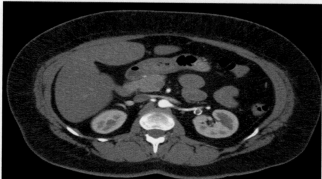

FIGURE 2 • A moderate distal left renal artery aneurysm is found; size is approximately 2.1 cm.

Case Conclusion

The patient's postoperative course is unremarkable, with normal renal function and a technically adequate repair confirmed on arteriogram at postoperative day 7 (Fig. 4). Postoperatively, she requires only one antihypertensive agent. Careful postoperative laboratory follow-up of her creatinine is important as well as blood pressure monitoring. Perioperative intermittent increases in diastolic blood pressure can be a sign for renal arterial stenosis and may signal repair failure.

Long-Term Follow-Up

The patient should undergo close blood pressure evaluation, but screening invasive arteriography is rarely indicated. MRA scanning and/or CT scanning with 3D reconfiguration may be useful as well for following any change in the left RAA size. At this point, the patient has opted to observe the left side, for which the overall rupture risk with RAA less than 2.0 cm is quite low. However, if the left RAA grows in size, an approach similar to the one used on the right side can be performed, though it does necessitate reoperative surgery. Overall, the durability of repair is excellent, with clinical patency at least 95% at 8-year follow-up. Unplanned nephrectomy rates in the settings of

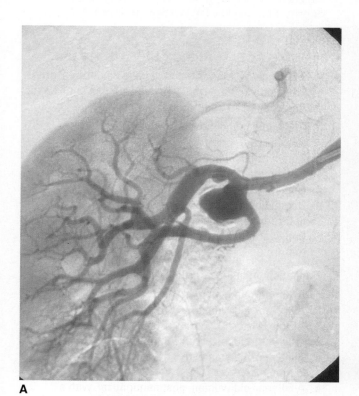
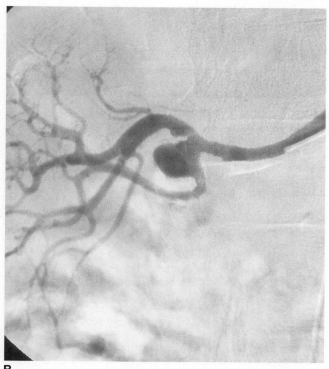

A   B

FIGURE 3 • Contrast arteriogram showing saccular aneurysm at main bifurcation of the right renal artery **(A, B)**.

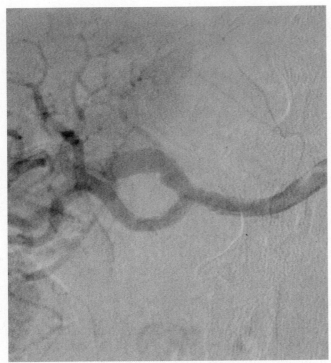

FIGURE 4 • Contrast arteriogram performed on post operative day 7 showing patent arterial system, with no evidence of aneurysm.

repair are very low; however, in one large series, no late dialysis was required in patients who did require an unplanned nephrectomy. Interestingly, hypertension is often improved after RAA repair, though the distinct mechanisms responsible for this observation are not certain (Table 1).

TABLE 1. Key Technical Steps and Potential Pitfalls

Key Technical Steps

1. An upper transverse abdominal incision affords excellent exposure.
2. Take care of the renal vein branches that may be very thin; ligation of most if fine.
3. Reconstruction of the renal artery may be primary, with a vein patch, with resection and interposition grafting—preconsideration is paramount for success.
4. Postrepair evaluation with dedicated angiogram, prior to discharge, is recommend.

Potential Pitfalls

- In patients with numerous small branch aneurysms, take time to fully evaluate and devise plan for reconstruction prior to the OR.
- In distal nonreconstructible RAA, nephrectomy is an option and risk of need for renal replacement therapy is very low.
- In unstable patients with acute rupture, consider endovascular covered stent grafting or direct occlusion to allow patient stabilization.

TAKE HOME POINTS

- Renal artery aneurysms are rare, found often incidentally, and are associated with hypertension.
- Many RAAs can be followed if under 2 cm in men and postmenopausal women.
- Open repair is safe, effective, and with good long-term patency.
- Endovascular repairs should be considered if the patient is too ill for an open repair and the risks of rupture are deemed significant.

SUGGESTED READINGS

Antoniou G, Antoniou S. Endovascular stent graft repair of renal artery aneurysms. *Int Angiol.* 2011;30(5):481-487.

Henke PK, Cardneau JD, Welling TH, et al. Renal artery aneurysms: a 35-year clinical experience with 252 aneurysms in 168 patients. *Ann Surg.* 2001;234:454-463.

Karkos CD, D'Souza SP, Thompson GJ, et al. Renal artery aneurysm: endovascular treatment by coil embolization with preservation of renal blood flow. *Eur J Vasc Endovasc Surg.* 2000;19:214-216.

Pfeiffer T, Reiher L, Grabitz K, et al. Reconstruction for renal artery aneurysm: operative techniques and long-term results. *J Vasc Surg.* 2003;37:293-300.

Schorn B, Valk V, Dalichau H, et al. Kidney salvage in a case of ruptured renal artery aneurysm: case report and literature review. *Cardiovasc Surg.* 1997;5:134.

Stanley JC, Messina LM, Wakefield TW, et al. Renal artery reconstruction. In: Bergan JJ, Yao JST eds. *Techniques in Arterial Surgery.* Philadelphia, PA: WB Saunders; 1990:247.

CLINICAL SCENARIO CASE QUESTIONS

1. A 40-year-old woman is found to have moderate 2 drug hypertension and a 2.1-cm L RAA by a 5-mm cut CT scan for back pain. The appropriate treatment is:

    a. Add additional antihypertensive agent and observe
    b. Obtain renal angiogram and consider covered stent placement
    c. Obtain MRA and consider open repair
    d. Obtain angiogram or high-resolution CTA and consider open repair
    e. Consider primary nephrectomy to prevent rupture

2. The patient at highest risk of RAA rupture would be:

    a. A 75-year-old man with 2-cm RAA
    b. A 35-year-old woman, currently pregnant, with a 1.8-cm RAA
    c. A 60-year-old man with 2.8-cm RAA
    d. A 60-year-old man with 3 drug hypertension and 2.5-cm RAA
    e. A 50-year-old woman, postmenopausal, with a 2.5-cm RAA

75 Acute Mesenteric Ischemia

PRATEEK K. GUPTA and GIRMA TEFERA

Presentation

A 78-year-old woman with known history of atrial fibrillation, on warfarin, presents to the emergency department with a sudden onset of severe abdominal pain and emesis for the past few hours. She has never had similar symptoms. The patient is retired, but fairly active around the house, and able to climb two flights of stairs without shortness of breath. She is a nonsmoker, nonalcoholic, with no prior abdominal operations and has no history of gastric ulcers. On physical examination, she is awake, alert, and oriented. She is tachycardic (heart rate of 111 per minute) with a blood pressure of 89/60 mm Hg. She has abdominal tenderness but no guarding, rigidity, or rebound tenderness. Her peripheral pulses are all palpable.

Differential Diagnosis

The differential diagnosis at this stage includes several etiologies of acute abdominal conditions. These include peptic ulcer disease with and without perforation, acute pancreatitis, acute cholecystitis, acute diverticulitis, acute urologic conditions including infections, acute bowel obstruction, and acute mesenteric ischemia (AMI), besides others.

Workup

In our patient, laboratory findings revealed a normal creatinine, elevated WBC count, and a subtherapeutic INR. CT of the abdomen with IV and PO contrast was obtained to assess for etiology of acute abdomen. This shows (Fig. 1A and B) emboli in the superior mesenteric artery (SMA). The bowel has some wall thickening but no pneumatosis coli, which suggests necrotic bowel. Portal venous gas is also not seen, which would also have been suggestive of bowel necrosis.

Discussion

AMI can be due to an emboli lodging in the SMA (50% of cases), thrombosis of an atherosclerotic lesion at the origin of the mesenteric vessel (20%), mesenteric venous thrombosis (10%), and nonocclusive mesenteric ischemia (20%). Emboli are most commonly from the heart and tend to lodge in the SMA given the angle of its take-off and almost parallel course to the aorta. They tend to progress to 5 to 10 cm beyond the takeoff to the level of the middle colic and jejunal branches where the diameter is narrower (Fig. 1A and B). Thrombus typically forms at the ostia of vessels in the setting of previous chronic mesenteric ischemia resulting in acute-on-chronic mesenteric ischemia (Fig. 2A and B). Rarely, thrombus may form in a setting of dissection into the SMA (Fig. 3).

AMI, if untreated, typically leads to bowel infarction due to compromise in intestinal blood flow. Patients classically present with abdominal pain out of proportion to physical examination. Nausea and emesis are frequent. In patients with SMA emboli, history of atrial fibrillation or heart murmur is frequent, while in thrombotic AMI, patients may have had symptoms of chronic mesenteric ischemia such as postprandial pain, constipation/diarrhea, and weight loss. The abdominal exam is not very impressive in the initial stages; however, peritonitis sets in soon leading to an acute abdomen. Leukocytosis is common. Lactate may be elevated with acidosis and a base deficit in cases of bowel necrosis.

The workup of a patient with acute abdominal conditions includes laboratory investigations, limited abdominal ultrasound (US), and other imaging modalities such as plain abdominal x-rays and computed tomographic scans. The degree of the workup depends on the stability of the patient and presence of acute peritoneal signs. An exploratory laparotomy is warranted in patients with generalized peritonitis, who present with abdominal tenderness and rebound tenderness suggesting generalized peritonitis.

Laboratory investigations such as basic metabolic and hematologic panels are usually very generic and none conclusive; therefore, the results have to be taken within the context of the physical exam. Abdominal US is a readily available, low-cost test that could help screen for acute cholecystitis, appendicitis, renal stones, and hydronephrosis. An abdominal vascular US exam can also be undertaken; however, this can be limited by the presence of bowel gas. A plain abdominal x-ray is a valuable test to identify bowel obstruction or perforated viscus.

In cases of AMI, imaging is needed for confirmation of clinical diagnosis. Abdominal x-ray may show an ileus-like pattern. CT scan with IV contrast is the most

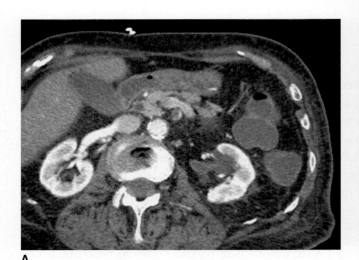
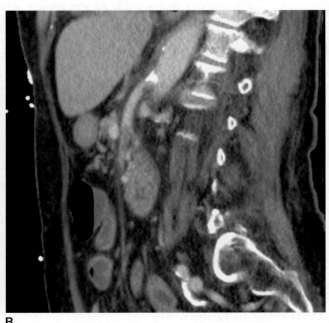

FIGURE 1 • CT scan showing thrombus in proximal SMA by **(A)** coronal and **(B)** sagittal views.

common mode of diagnosis and shows filling defect in the visceral vessels suggestive of thrombosis or embolism. Other imaging modalities may include duplex US and magnetic resonance imaging; however, these are rarely obtained in patients presenting with an acute abdomen. Catheter-based angiography may be needed if CT is not available.

Diagnosis and Treatment

This patient with AMI needs to be resuscitated and started on therapeutic heparin anticoagulation to prevent extension of the clot burden. Nasogastric tube and urinary catheter are placed. Emergent operative intervention is needed to assess the bowel and perform SMA revascularization.

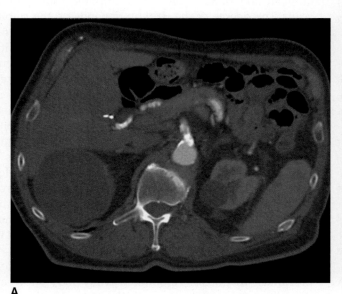
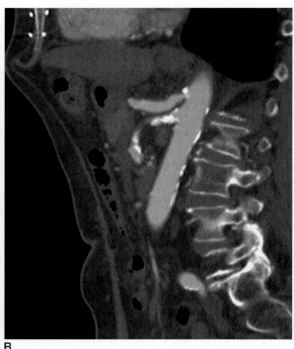

FIGURE 2 • CT scan showing highly calcified proximal SMA with occlusion in **(A)** coronal and **(B)** sagittal views.

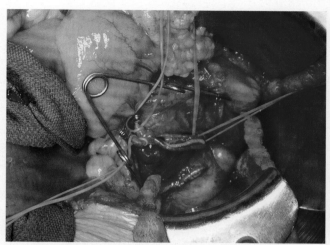

FIGURE 3 • Open surgical exposure of the SMA showing a dissection flap after arteriotomy performed.

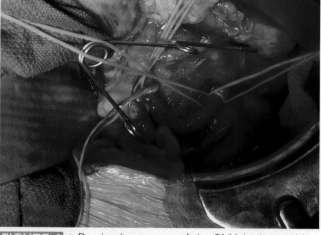

FIGURE 4 • Proximal exposure of the SMA is done with vessel loops, as illustrated here.

In cases of acute-on-chronic mesenteric ischemia that also typically involves the SMA, either retrograde stent through the open abdomen or a bypass, either antegrade from the supraceliac aorta or retrograde from the iliac vessels, is indicated. Rarely, percutaneous lysis is performed in select centers if the disease process is in the early stages without concern for bowel ischemia.

It is important to involve the patient and his or her family in the discussion regarding goals and expectations given the high morbidity and mortality in this disease process. It is imperative to have a clear understanding of patient preferences prior to going to the operating room in case there is large segment of bowel necrosis that would make the patient total parenteral nutrition (TPN) dependent for life.

Surgical Approach

Given the patient has AMI due to an SMA embolus, she is taken to the operating room under general anesthesia and laid supine on the table. If possible, the procedure is performed on a table capable of fluoroscopy in case completion angiogram is needed. The patient is prepped from nipples to knees, taking care to prep a leg in the field, in case saphenous vein needs to be used for a bypass.

The abdomen is opened through a midline vertical incision, and the peritoneum is entered. A self-retaining retractor system is helpful for exposure. The bowel is examined to assess for viability. If a large segment of the bowel is completely necrotic, consideration should be given for stopping the procedure based on the patient's preoperative wishes.

The transverse colon is retracted superiorly and the fourth portion of the duodenum mobilized to the ligament of Treitz. The SMA is identified at the root of the mesentery. If calcified, it may be directly felt; otherwise the middle colic artery can be used to trace down to it; or if the superior mesenteric vein (SMV) is identified, the artery is medial to it. In cases of an embolus, most often the SMA is palpable proximally with a sharp cutoff in pulse present. The vessel

is exposed and controlled at that point using vessel loops (Fig. 4). The branches are also controlled. The patient is therapeutically anticoagulated and activated clotting times checked. In cases of emboli, a transverse arteriotomy is made on the vessel, and balloon catheters are passed both in an antegrade and retrograde fashion until no more clot is retrieved and brisk bleeding is seen. The arteriotomy can then be closed using simple interrupted or mattress stitches. The vessel and bowel mesentery are checked for pulses, and Doppler is used to hear the signals. If there is concern for branch viability due to persisting embolus or dissection due to the embolectomy catheter, an angiogram is helpful in assessing the collaterals and in deciding if the particular branch needs to be revascularized by directly cutting down on it and tacking the dissection flap. The bowel mesentery is then closed with interrupted absorbable stitches. The bowel is reexamined to assess for viability. If necrotic bowel is seen, it needs to be resected and in most cases left in discontinuity. The gallbladder should also be examined to assess for ischemia. Thorough irrigation is performed. Temporary abdominal closure is done with a planned "second-look" operation after 24 hours.

In cases of acute-on-chronic mesenteric ischemia due to an atherosclerotic lesion, the SMA is similarly exposed and controlled with vessel loops. If the preoperative CT shows a focal lesion at the origin of the SMA, consideration may be given to stenting. The SMA is punctured using a needle and a hydrophilic wire passed through the lesion into the aorta. Over this, a long sheath is inserted into the SMA. The long sheath allows wire and catheter manipulation from a distance. A self-expanding bare metal or covered stent may be used with enough projection into the aorta (Fig. 5A and B).

If there is calcific disease in the SMA, local endarterectomy through a longitudinal arteriotomy with patch angioplasty (Fig. 6A and B) and retrograde stenting may be employed. However, another option is to bypass to the nondiseased SMA from the supraceliac aorta or the

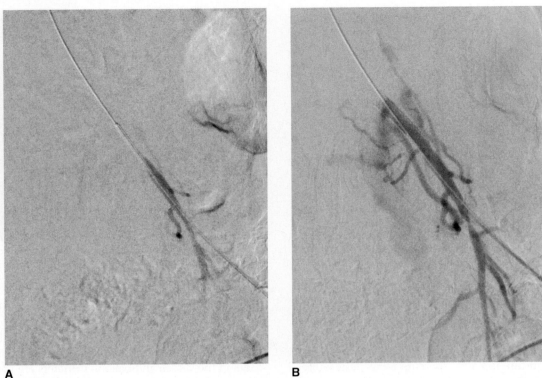

A

B

FIGURE 5 • Contrast arteriography showing high-grade proximal SMA stenosis **(A)** and poststenting with balloon-expandable stent **(B)**.

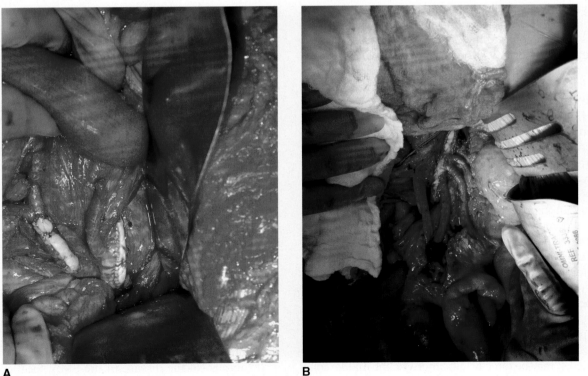

A

B

FIGURE 6 • **A and B:** Open exposure showing postendarterectomized mesenteric arteries with patch angioplasty.

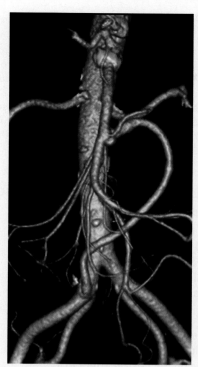

FIGURE 7 • Reformated CTA showing a right iliac to SMA retrograde prosthetic bypass.

iliac vessels. If there is bowel necrosis, saphenous vein may be preferable as a conduit to prosthetic graft. Bypass from the supraceliac aorta involves a supraceliac clamp for which the aorta should be free of significant calcification or thrombus. The conduit is tunneled behind the pancreas. In emergency conditions, we generally prefer a retrograde bypass from the iliac vessels due to lesser morbidity from an infrarenal or iliac artery clamp, provided the iliac vessels are relatively free of occlusive disease. The right common iliac is generally preferred and the conduit fashioned in a gentle C-loop to allow enough laxity for the mesentery (Fig. 7). Another approach in thin patients is to dissect and transect the occluded SMA at its origin from the aorta followed by eversion endarterectomy. The endarterectomized vessel is then reimplanted on to the aorta below the renal arteries (Table 1).

Special Intraoperative Considerations

In case of inadequate preoperative imaging, on opening the abdomen, it is possible to find another source of an acute abdomen with a normal SMA pulse.

Twenty percent of patients have a replaced hepatic artery off the SMA, and this should be kept in mind during the dissection and if placing a retrograde stent. In patients with acute-on-chronic mesenteric ischemia due to atherosclerosis, the patency of the celiac artery and inferior mesenteric artery must be carefully examined on the preoperative CT. Sometimes, it may be possible to revascularize them along with the SMA, which would be protective in case of potential failure of the SMA revascularization.

TABLE 1. Key Technical Steps and Potential Pitfalls

Key Technical Steps

1. Midline laparotomy and insertion of self-retaining retractor.
2. Assess bowel for viability. If extensive necrosis, palliative care may be indicated.
3. Reflect transverse colon superiorly.
4. Identify and expose the SMA.
5. Transverse arteriotomy with embolectomy in case of embolic disease.
6. Longitudinal arteriotomy with patch angioplasty and retrograde stenting in case of thrombotic disease.
7. Antegrade bypass from supraceliac aorta or retrograde bypass from iliac arteries as an alternative in case of thrombotic atherosclerotic occlusive disease.
8. Use of saphenous vein as a conduit may be preferable over prosthetic in case of questionable bowel viability or gross contamination.
9. Reassessment of bowel for viability and resection of nonviable bowel.
10. Resected bowel left in discontinuity with open abdomen and planned "second-look" laparotomy.

Potential Pitfalls

- Prep the leg in the field in case bypass is needed using saphenous vein.
- Dissection of SMA branch vessels while performing embolectomy.
- Make sure that there is adequate forward and back bleeding prior to closure.
- Clamping heavily diseased supraceliac aorta in case of supraceliac aorta to SMA bypass can be a source of major embolization.
- When closing the abdomen with questionably viable bowel, have low threshold for second look.
- Pay attention to not injure superior mesenteric vein.
- Avoid pancreatic injury from retraction.
- Assess for replaced right hepatic artery from the SMA.

Postoperative Management

Postprocedure, the patients typically go to the intensive care unit. Most of the time, due to bowel ischemia and nature of the disease, they are relatively sick, requiring aggressive resuscitation. If bowel resection was performed, a "second-look" operation is common. Due to the nature of the disease, need for multiple operations to assess bowel viability, and the age of these patients, long periods on the ventilator are common. Once on the floor, prolonged ileus is not uncommon, and parenteral nutrition is frequently required. Even later, tube feedings are common as patients may not have enough appetite, especially in cases of acute-on-chronic mesenteric ischemia. Physical therapy is important in getting patients back to their baseline, and most patients get discharged to skilled nursing facilities due to their deconditioning. Imaging in the form of duplex or CT angiogram should generally be performed either prior to discharge or on the first postoperative visit.

Case Conclusion

The patient underwent embolectomy of the SMA with a good result. The bowel was slightly dusky and thus a second look was undertaken the following day at which time all bowel was viable. There was a good pulse present in the bowel mesentery. She was extubated the following day and the diet gradually advanced. She was ultimately discharged to a skilled nursing facility for a week from where she went home.

TAKE HOME POINTS

- Patients classically present with abdominal pain out of proportion to physical examination.
- Early diagnosis with CT angiogram is critical to confirm diagnosis and assess bowel viability and improve survival.
- Open laparotomy with SMA embolectomy/bypass/retrograde stent are the therapeutic options depending upon the etiology.
- Bowel may need to be resected in cases of necrosis.
- Morbidity and mortality are high due to age, comorbidities, and sepsis due to bowel necrosis.

SUGGESTED READINGS

Oderich GS, et al. Comparison of covered stents versus bare metal stents for treatment of chronic atherosclerotic mesenteric arterial disease. *J Vasc Surg.* 2013;58(5):1316-1323.

Oldenburg WA, et al. Acute mesenteric ischemia: a clinical review. *Arch Intern Med.* 2004;164(10):1054-1062.

Wyers MC. Mesenteric vascular disease: acute ischemia. In: Cronenwett JL, Johnston KW, eds. *Rutherford's Vascular Surgery.* 7th ed. New York, NY: Elsevier; 2010:2289-2303, Chapter 149.

CLINICAL SCENARIO CASE QUESTIONS

1. Emboli typically lodge at:
   a. Origin of SMA
   b. 5 to 10 cm beyond takeoff of SMA
   c. Distal SMA branches
   d. The middle colic artery
   e. The gastroduodenal artery

2. SMA can be identified:
   a. By direct palpation if noncalcified
   b. By being lateral to the SMV
   c. By tracing the gastric artery to it
   d. At the base of the inferior mesenteric vein
   e. At the base of the transverse mesocolon

76 Chronic Mesenteric Ischemia: Open Surgical Repair

JESSE MANUNGA and PETER GLOVICZKI

Presentation

A 75-year-old female with cardiovascular risk factors significant for diabetes mellitus, type II; hypertension; hyperlipidemia; peripheral arterial disease; coronary artery disease; and remote history of tobacco abuse presents with complaint of postprandial abdominal pain with weight loss, diarrhea, and inability to eat without pain. Her surgical history is significant for bilateral lower extremity bypasses, cholecystectomy, coronary artery bypass grafting in 1995, and coronary angiography with stenting in 2011. She has diarrhea with five to six loose stools per day and has lost 30 pounds over the last 6 months. She denies bloating and distention, and endorses only minimal intermittent nausea. She is a thin lady in nonacute distress with a loud right carotid and abdominal epigastric bruit. She has 4+ pulses in the upper extremities, 3+ pulses on the right femoral, and 2+ left femoral pulses. She does not have palpable popliteal or distal pulses.

Differential Diagnosis

The diagnosis of chronic mesenteric ischemia requires a high index of suspicion. Because the condition is rare, it is not uncommon for the diagnosis to be delayed by up to a year or more from the onset of symptoms. Common causes of abdominal pain such as cancer, inflammatory bowel disease, malabsorptive disorders, diabetes, chronic pancreatitis, and hyperthyroidism must be ruled out. Patients with chronic mesenteric ischemia usually have disease in other vascular beds, and most would have undergone a battery of tests by the time they are seen by a vascular specialist. Furthermore, it is not uncommon for patients with this condition to undergo a cholecystectomy often without relief of symptoms. Unfortunately, advanced disease at the time of diagnosis adversely affects outcomes.

Workup

Prior to being seen at our institution, the patient had an upper endoscopy that was remarkable only for nonspecific erythema in the antrum. A colonoscopy revealed mild diverticulosis and internal hemorrhoids. A 4-hour gastric emptying scan was normal at 1 hour but delayed at 2 and 4 hours with 79% emptying at that time point. The patient was started on a gastroparesis type of diet without relief. A repeat endoscopy 8 months later was unremarkable for retained food particles in the stomach but revealed an 8-mm clean-based duodenal ulcer that was negative for malignancy. A Botox injection into the antrum made no difference in reliving her symptoms, and a subsequent capsule enteroscopy study was normal.

A fasting duplex ultrasound scan of the abdomen is the initial test to evaluate patients with suspected chronic mesenteric ischemia. Since most patients with this condition may have elements of chronic kidney disease, ultrasound has an added advantage of identifying affected patients without the use of a contrast medium. In patients with no contraindications, a CT angiography of the abdomen and pelvis is done since it helps rule out other causes of abdominal pain and also helps the clinician determine the best way to revascularize the patient.

Compared to superior mesenteric artery (SMA), the celiac access has lower velocity because of fewer branches. Sonographic criteria for diagnosis of greater than 70% stenosis of the celiac artery include the presence of retrograde common hepatic artery flow, peak systolic velocity greater than 200 cm/s, and an end-diastolic velocity greater than 55 cm/s with retrograde common hepatic flow being the most sensitive. Duplex criteria for diagnosis of greater than 70% SMA stenosis correlate best with peak systolic velocity greater than 275 cm/s and an end-diastolic velocity of greater than 45 cm/s.

Our patient underwent a duplex ultrasound at our institution that revealed a velocity of 554 cm/s at the origin of the celiac trunk, 91 cm peak systolic as well as end-diastolic velocities in the SMA, and peak systolic velocity of 425 cm/s in the inferior mesenteric artery (Fig. 1). A CT scan of the abdomen confirmed a high-grade stenosis of the celiac and SMA with extensive calcification of the aorta, iliac, and mesenteric vessels (Fig. 2).

Discussion

Most cases of symptomatic chronic mesenteric ischemia result from ostial atherosclerotic lesions affecting at least two of the three main mesenteric vessels.

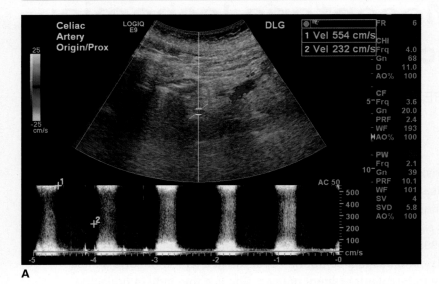

A

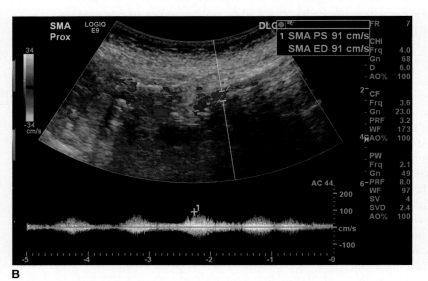

B

FIGURE 1 • Preoperative ultrasound showing a high-grade stenosis of the celiac **(A)** and SMA **(B)**. Note that the peak systolic velocity of the SMA is only 91 cm/s (below the threshold diagnosis of greater than 70% stenosis), but the end-diastolic velocity is higher also 91 cm/s, indicative of greater than 70% stenos.

However, conditions such as fibromuscular disease, aortic dissection, neurofibromatosis, rheumatoid arthritis, Takayasu's arteritis, giant cell arteritis, polyarteritis nodosa, radiation injury, Buerger's disease, systemic lupus, spontaneous mesenteric artery dissection, and drugs (cocaine and ergots) use also account for a handful of cases.

The natural course of asymptomatic mesenteric occlusive disease is unclear. Thomas and associates followed a group of 82 patients found to have, on angiography, 50% stenosis of at least one mesenteric artery. At a mean follow-up of up to 6 years, 10 patients had been lost to follow-up. None of the patients (0/45) with one or two vessel disease developed mesenteric ischemia. Eighty-six percent of the 15 patients with three-vessel disease either developed mesenteric ischemia or had symptoms of abdominal pain. The overall mortality in this cohort was 40%.

Therefore, high-grade stenosis or even occlusion of a single mesenteric vessel rarely results in symptomatic mesenteric ischemia because of the extensive collateral network between the three mesenteric vessels. Even in case of ostial occlusion of the SMA, most of the small bowel can still be perfused via collaterals from the celiac axis via the pancreaticoduodenal artery or inferior mesenteric artery (meandering artery). It is even conceivable for a patient with ostial occlusion of all three mesenteric vessels to be asymptomatic as long as they have a robust network of collaterals.

Oderich et al. in reviewing 229 patients treated for chronic mesenteric ischemia with either an open or endovascular repair at the Mayo Clinic reported that 96% of patients in this cohort presented with complaint of abdominal pain, followed by weight loss in 84% of patients, fear of food in 45%, and diarrhea in 40%, while only 24% of patients with this condition experienced nausea and vomiting.

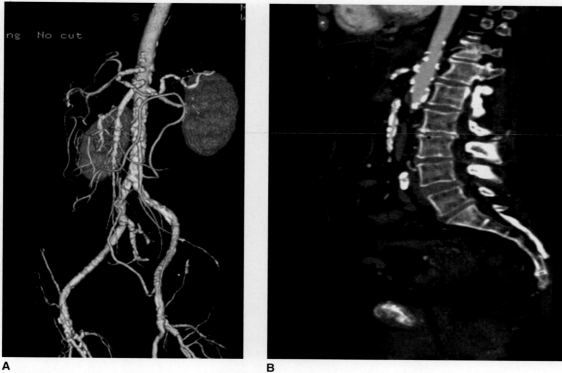

FIGURE 2 • CTA of the abdomen and pelvis showing heavily calcified aorta, celiac, SMA, and iliac vessels. Supraceliac aorta would be the ideal site for inflow, but the patient had severe cardiac disease making supraceliac clamping not ideal. Also, note that the patient is not a good candidate for an endovascular repair because of the long-segment disease in the SMA.

Diagnosis and Treatment

The presence of high-grade stenosis of mesenteric vessels in an otherwise asymptomatic patient does not warrant treatment. However, asymptomatic patients with high-grade three-vessel stenosis should be followed closely. Once symptoms develop, revascularization is necessary because the disease often progresses to acute mesenteric ischemia. Park et al. reported the results of 58 patients treated at the Mayo Clinic from 1990 to 1999. In this series, 65% of patients with acute mesenteric ischemia had history of chronic, recurrent abdominal pain.

Since patients with mesenteric ischemia often have disease in other vascular beds, careful workup is needed prior to subjecting the patient to an open repair. Because of the multiple comorbidities and the advancement in endovascular techniques, mesenteric artery angioplasty and stenting has gained steam as a treatment modality of choice in patients with this condition. However, patients with heavily calcified and long-segment lesions, patients with small-diameter vessels (5 mm or less), those with tandem lesions, and patients with thrombus or debris and those who develop mesenteric ischemia as a result of radiation injury are poor candidates for endovascular repair. In these patients, open revascularization is offered after careful review of CT angiogram

and medical clearance that often include cardiac and pulmonary evaluation.

Our patient's CT angiography showed extensive disease in all three mesenteric vessels with severe calcification of the SMA. She had anatomical limitations making her an unfavorable candidate for an endovascular repair. Unfortunately, she had a markedly positive dobutamine stress test and went on to have coronary angiography with intervention prior to proceeding with open revascularization.

Surgical Approach to Open Repair

For patients who are not candidates for endovascular repair because of anatomical limitations, open repair is considered. Patients must be risk stratified prior to open repair. We find that patients older than 80 years of age, those with severe pulmonary and cardiac dysfunction or renal insufficiency (creatinine > 3.0) have an increased 30-day and 5-year mortality rates following open mesenteric revascularization. We define severe pulmonary dysfunction as $FEV_1 < 800$ mL or $D_{LCO} < 50\%$, resting $PCO_2 > 50$ mm Hg, resting $PO_2 < 60$ mm Hg or on home oxygen. Severe cardiac dysfunction is defined as Left Ventricular Ejection Fraction (LVEF) < 25%, NYHA III or IV angina pectoris, positive cardiac stress test, or myocardial infarction <90 days.

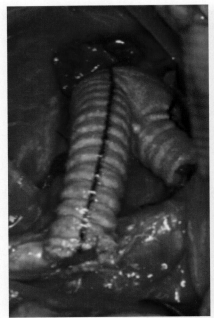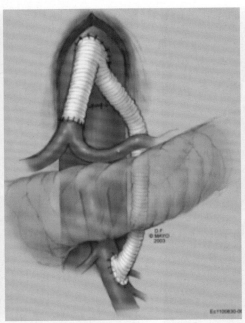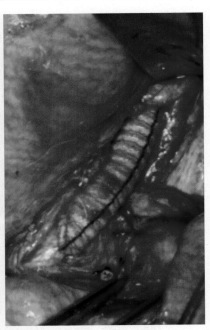

FIGURE 3 • Intraoperative images and sketch of a supraceliac aorta to celiac and SMA bypasses using a bifurcated Dacron graft. Note that the SMA graft is tunneled under the pancreas. Care must be taken not to injure the pancreas during this maneuver.

Our preference in low-risk patients with unfavorable lesions for endovascular intervention is to revascularize two of the three mesenteric vessels. In this case, we usually select the supraceliac aorta as our inflow source and perform a bifurcated graft with one limb to the SMA and the other to the celiac access (Fig. 3). After a careful review of the CT angiography and determination of the aortic clamping site, a midline incision is made from the xiphoid process to the umbilicus. Upon entering the abdominal cavity, the abdominal content is carefully examined, and bowel viability is assessed. Incising the left triangular and the gastrohepatic ligament exposes the supraceliac aorta. Care must be taken not injure any replaced left hepatic artery while dividing the gastrohepatic ligament. The posterior peritoneum is then opened and the median arcuate ligament is divided vertically to expose the aorta. A previously placed nasogastric tube will facilitate the identification of the esophagus, which, along with the lesser curvature of the stomach, is retracted leftward to expose the celiac access and its major branches. Mobilizing the neck of the pancreas and retracting it anteriorly exposes the origin of the SMA. The graft is fashioned, and the SMA limb is tunneled under the pancreas. The patient is systemically heparinized, and anastomoses are completed using running polypropylene sutures (Fig. 3).

In a high-risk surgical patient or those with severe atherosclerotic disease in the aorta preventing clamp placement, our preference is to only treat the SMA and use the right or left iliac artery as inflow source with a C-loop graft configuration as shown in Figure 4. Here, the incision is extended below the umbilicus to expose the iliac arteries and the SMA. The SMA distal to the inferior border of the pancreas is exposed with division of the ligament of Treitz and mobilization of the fourth portion of the duodenum. The SMA is located in the tissue just cephalad to the duodenum, and exposure can be enhanced by gently retracting the inferior border of the pancreas.

Our patient had a strongly positive preoperative cardiac stress test making her an unfavorable candidate for a supraceliac clamp. Additionally, her iliac arteries were heavily calcified (Fig. 2), making them not a good inflow source. Consequently, we decided to use the infrarenal aorta as our inflow source. We proceeded by dissecting out a 6-cm segment of the proximal SMA and performed an anterior SMA endarterectomy after making a longitudinal arteriotomy. We opted to use a 10-mm Hemashield graft that was sutured end-to-side to the SMA using 6-0 Prolene sutures. The aortic anastomosis was performed with 4-0 Prolene sutures (Fig. 5). Every attempt should be made to cover the graft. Our preference is to make a small opening in the mesocolon and bring a tongue of omentum for omentoplasty. The Dacron graft is then wrapped 360 degrees around the greater omentum. For patients with paravisceral atherosclerosis and mesenteric artery ostial lesions, a transaortic thromboendarterectomy with eversion endarterectomy of the mesenteric arteries can be an attractive and effective operative approach (Fig. 6).

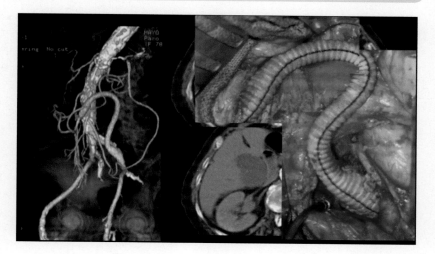

FIGURE 4 • Intraoperative picture and a postprocedure CT angiography showing the C-loop configuration using the right iliac as inflow source. Care is taken to orient the graft in a fashion that will minimize risk of kinking. Meticulous hemostasis is obtained, and the graft is wrapped in omentum, bowel is reexamined, and pulses are checked prior to closing the abdomen.

Special Intraoperative Considerations

Upon entering the abdominal cavity, the small and large bowel viability is assessed prior to proceeding with exposure of vessels. Necrotic bowel needs to be resected. If the bowel is "dusky," one can proceed with revascularization and reevaluate the bowel after adequate blood flow to the intestines is established. If needed, the abdomen can be closed temporarily allowing for a "second-look" laparotomy in 24 to 48 hours. In any of these two instances, autogenous material will need to be used as a conduit. As such, it might prudent to obtain vein mapping prior to taking the patient to the operating suite (Table 1).

Postoperative Management

Because of their high number of comorbidities, we routinely admit these patients to the intensive care unit for least an overnight observation. The nasogastric tube is kept in place, and the patient is kept NPO until there is return of bowel function. The use of incentive spirometer

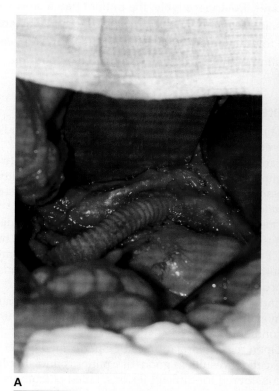

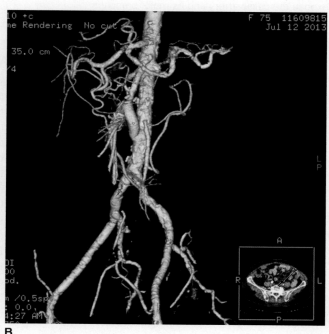

A   B

FIGURE 5 • Intraoperative picture **(A)** and postoperative CT angiography **(B)** of the patient discussed in the chapter. Both images depict the 10-mm Hemashield graft used for the aorto-SMA bypass.

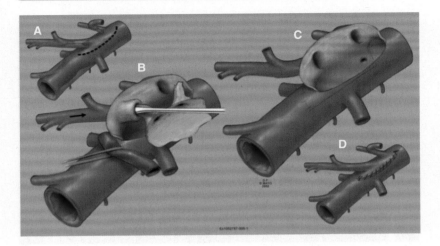

FIGURE 6 • Sketch of the transaortic thromboendarterectomy with eversion endarterectomy of the mesenteric vessels. This technique is ideal for patients with aortic atherosclerotic disease and ostial mesenteric calcification presenting with chronic mesenteric ischemia. Often time, these patients may present with claudication that is relieved after this intervention provided there is no other hemodynamically significant disease burden downstream in the aorta, iliac, or femoral vessels. **A:** Arteriotomy line preserving the origin of the celiac and SMA. **B:** Endarterectomy. **C:** Postendarterectomy. **D:** Postclosure of the arteriotomy.

and ambulation is strongly encouraged in all extubated patients. Deep venous thrombosis prophylaxis is initiated in all patients. Postoperative ileus is managed expectantly, and plain abdominal x-ray films are obtained to follow progress. In the rare events of increasing leukocytosis, abdominal pain, and fevers, a CT angiography is obtained, and reexploration is performed only when there is a high index of suspicion. Large meals during the immediate postoperative period are generally avoided. Instead, the patient is recommended to have small, frequent meals. The patient should have a repeat ultrasound of the abdomen to evaluate velocities and repeat CT angiography if possible (Fig. 5).

TABLE 1. Mesenteric Revascularization

Key Technical Steps

- *Supraceliac aorta as inflow source:*
  1. Place an nasogastric tube
  2. Midline laparotomy with incision length and location depending on inflow source
  3. Divide the left triangular and gastrohepatic ligaments
  4. Incise the posterior peritoneum and divide the fibers of the diaphragm and the arcuate ligament to expose the supraceliac aorta
  5. Retract the esophagus and the left gastric leftward to expose the celiac artery and its major branches
  6. Mobilize the neck of the pancreas and gently retract it anteriorly to expose the SMA
  7. Tunnel the SMA limb under the pancreas, heparinize the patient, and complete the anastomosis

- *Iliac arteries as inflow source:*
  1. Steps 1 and 2 as above
  2. Expose the preferred common iliac artery
  3. Expose the SMA by dividing the ligament of Treitz
  4. Mobilize the fourth portion of the duodenum
  5. Retract the inferior border of the pancreas to enhance exposure
  6. Heparinize the patient and perform the anastomosis in the C-loop configuration
  7. Perform omentoplasty

Potential Pitfalls

- Inadvertent division of the replaced left hepatic artery while dividing the gastrohepatic ligament
- Injury to the vagus nerve and the esophagus
- Injury to the pancreaticoduodenal artery while exposing the SMA from above
- Injury to the pancreas while tunneling the graft
- Injury to the bowel
- Injury to the ureter while exposing the iliac artery
- Bleeding

Case Conclusion

This patient underwent successful ileo-SMA revascularization with a Dacron graft as described above. Postoperatively, the patient had a slow steady recovery and was discharged and was able to tolerate an oral diet. Six months later, she was eating without pain and had gained 10 pounds.

TAKE HOME POINTS

- Chronic mesenteric ischemia is a rare disease and presents a diagnosis dilemma.
- Early recognition and treatment is the best way to improve outcome and decrease excessive mortality associated with disease progression to acute mesenteric ischemia.
- Duplex ultrasound of the abdomen can reliably diagnose patients with chronic mesenteric ischemia, but CT angiography is crucial to delineate the anatomy for surgical planning and rule out other potential causes of abdominal pain.
- Endovascular repair is gaining steam as the primary modality for revascularization of patients with this condition.
- Open revascularization can be performed with excellent results in good-risk patients and should be considered for difficult lesions, failed percutaneous revascularization, or unusual etiologies.

SUGGESTED READINGS

Oderich GS, Bower TC, Sullivan TM, et al. Open versus endovascular revascularization for chronic mesenteric ischemia: risk-stratified outcomes. *J Vasc Surg*. 2009;49(6): 1472-1479.

Oderich GS, Gloviczki P, Bower TC. Open surgical treatment for chronic mesenteric ischemia in the endovascular era: when it is necessary and what is the preferred technique? *Semin Vasc Surg*. 2010;23(1):36-46.

Oderich GS, Malgor RD, Ricotta JJ II. Open and endovascular revascularization for chronic mesenteric ischemia: tubular review of the literature. *Ann Vasc Surg*. 2009;23(5):700-712.

Park VM, Cherry KJ Jr, Chua HS, et al. Current results of open revascularization for chronic mesenteric ischemia: a standard for comparison. *J Vasc Surg*. 2002;35(5):853-859.

Tallarita T, Oderich GS, Gloviczki P, et al. Patient survival after open and endovascular mesenteric revascularization for chronic mesenteric ischemia. *J Vasc Surg*. 2013;57(3): 747-755.

CLINICAL SCENARIO CASE QUESTIONS

1. Which of the following patients is a good candidate for open mesenteric artery revascularization?

   a. A 73-year-old male found to have heavy calcification at the origin of the SMA and celiac artery on a screening CT scan of the abdomen performed following a motor vehicle accident

   b. A 67-year-old female with history of hypertension, COPD, coronary artery disease, and postprandial abdominal pain found to have an occluded celiac artery and greater than 70% stenosis limited to the origin of the SMA

   c. A 70-year-old female current smoker with history of CAD, COPD on home oxygen, and postprandial abdominal pain with a high-grade, focal stenosis of the SMA

   d. A 62-year-old female ex-smoker with history of hypertension, hyperlipidemia, peripheral arterial disease, and postprandial abdominal pain with 20 pounds weight lost over 1 month found to have a high-grade stenosis of the celiac artery and flush, long-segment occlusion of the SMA

   e. A 50-year-old man with occluded SMA but patent celiac and IMA without weight loss and occasional abdominal pain of uncertain etiology

2. Optimal graft configuration in patient with chronic mesenteric ischemia:

   a. Is antegrade, aorto-SMA, and celiac bypass

   b. Depends on the patient's anatomy and cardiovascular risk factors

   c. Retrograde infrarenal aorta to SMA bypass

   d. Retrograde iliac to SMA bypass

   e. Thoracic aorta to SMA bypass

77 Endovascular Approach to Chronic Mesenteric Ischemia

AHSAN T. ALI and MATTHEW R. ABATE

Presentation

A 62-year-old man underwent an aortofemoral bypass graft (AFBG) for occlusive disease. In the immediate post-op period, he suffered mesenteric ischemia and underwent bowel resection (sigmoid and small bowel). Postoperatively, he developed aortic graft infection and nonhealing groin wounds in the setting of severe malnutrition and failure to thrive. Subsequent workup included computed tomography scan (CTA) demonstrating a stenosis of the superior mesenteric artery (SMA) and an occluded celiac artery. There was fluid around the graft indicating pan graft infection. Meanwhile, the patient had lost almost 35 pounds, and his prealbumin was 8.1 and albumin was 1.2.

Differential Diagnosis

There is usually little ambiguity about the diagnosis by the time the patient arrives in vascular clinic. Most patients have already undergone a cholecystectomy along with esophagogastroduodenoscopy (EGD) and colonoscopy, along with further imaging studies such as a CTA.

The hallmark of chronic mesenteric ischemia (CMI) is weight loss and postprandial pain. In certain clinical scenarios, the diagnosis can be in question if there is no weight loss. Occult malignancy can be associated with weight loss and "aversion from food" due to nausea. Thus, in patients with a history of smoking and unexplained weight loss, occult malignancy has to be ruled out before embarking on any mesenteric revascularization therapy. Other differential diagnoses to consider include nonocclusive mesenteric ischemia at watershed areas, median arcuate ligament syndrome, and aortic dissection.

Workup

In addition to history and physical examination, nutritional parameters and contrast imaging are essential in diagnosis and preoperative planning. CTA is most commonly utilized and will also demonstrate collateral pathways such as the arc of Riolan and marginal artery of Drummond. Other subtle findings are calcification of the origin of the SMA.

Case Continued

The patient had weight loss and postprandial pain. The preoperative CTA demonstrated severe stenosis of the SMA and occlusion of the celiac artery. The CTA also showed the presence of collaterals between the SMA and the inferior mesenteric artery; mainly the arc of Riolan and marginal artery of Drummond. The patient was scheduled for an arteriogram via the left brachial approach as an initial attempt to revascularize the SMA or the celiac artery.

Surgical Approach

Endovascular revascularization of the mesenteric vessels is indicated in acute or chronic clinical settings. A bypass to the celiac and/or the SMA from a supraceliac approach has the highest patency but comes with significant morbidity and mortality. However, if the patient is at a high risk, then an endovascular approach can be initially utilized as a bridge to an open and more durable procedure. The current trend is an endovascular approach first. Open mesenteric revascularizations are being performed less, and most vascular graduates have been exposed to only a handful of cases during their training. Hence, this trend may very well have to do with the comfort level of the vascular surgeon. However, the authors believe, an initial endovascular approach for CMI serves as a bridge to open surgical therapy especially if the patient is severely malnourished or very high medical risk.

For endovascular treatment of CMI, several things have to be considered: brachial versus femoral approach, type of catheter to engage the lumen, balloon expandable stent versus self-expanding, covered versus bare metal stent, and monorail versus coaxial systems.

Contraindications to Endovascular Approach

There are no absolute contraindications. Occlusions of the SMA with heavy calcifications can be a relative contraindication, especially if the occlusion is up to the middle colic artery.

Celiac vs. SMA or Both

The main objective is to treat the SMA. Celiac artery stenting can be attempted if SMA angioplasty is not possible or can not be done. In a comparative analysis of celiac versus SMA angioplasty and stenting, Ahanchi et al. found the primary patency of SMA interventions to be significantly higher bringing to question the clinical utility of celiac artery angioplasty and stenting. Unlike an open bypass, revascularization of both celiac and SMA is not the norm when attempting endovascular approach.

Angioplasty Versus Stenting

Stenting is recommended as the patency of angioplasty alone is dismal.

Brachial Versus Femoral

A femoral approach is preferred by some because it accommodates a larger sheath and a closure device can be used. For this particular approach, a curved catheter such as a Visceral Select (Cook Medical, Bloomington, IN) with a "Shepherd hook" is used with a hydrophilic wire. A Glide Cobra (Terumo Medical Corporation, Tokyo, Japan) can be used as well. However, a flush occlusion of the SMA usually precludes the femoral approach. The left brachial artery provides a straighter approach but has a higher complication rate. With access via the left brachial artery, the catheter does not need to be reversed;

a Vert or MPA 125 are popular choices (Cook Medical, Bloomington, IN). This approach can be performed with a cut down in high-risk patients (women, small caliber arteries). Lastly, it also depends on skill set and comfort level of the surgeon. The brachial approach clearly has advantages of torquability and pushability to facilitate crossing occlusions.

Balloon-expandable Versus Self-expanding

Most interventionalists prefer a balloon-expandable stent for accurate placement. However, if an abdominal procedure is planned in the future, a self-expanding stent can be used. It will keep its form and withstand retractor pressure during a subsequent open procedure, whereas the balloon-expandable stent may get crushed. Self-expanding nitinol stents are not as precise. Avoid the usage of more than one stent.

Covered Versus Bare Metal

With covered stents there are four options: Gore ViaBahn (Gore Medical, Flagstaff, AZ), Bard Fluency (Bard, Tempe, AZ), Wall Graft (Boston Scientific, Natick, MA), and iCast (Atrium, Hudson, NH). The first three require a large

---

TABLE 1. Key Technical Steps and Potential Pitfalls

Key Technical Steps

1. Approach via the left brachial artery. The authors recommend a cut down if the patient is at high risk for brachial complications (elderly, women, small caliber arteries). A femoral approach can be used, if the angle of the SMA is not very acute.
2. Place a 6-French 90-cm sheath if approaching via the brachial artery in the descending thoracic aorta at the level of the celiac artery (a 70-cm sheath is not long enough in most instances). Imaging can be obtained from a femoral sheath simultaneously through a separate catheter.
3. The image intensifier is placed at 80–90 degrees for a lateral view and initial angiogram obtained to identify the SMA and the celiac artery. The patients upper extremities have to be out of the way (above the head) for better imaging.
4. A slightly angled, moderately stiff catheter (e.g., MPA 125) is used with a hydrophilic stiff wire such as a Road Runner or Stiff Hydrophilic Glide (Cook Medical, Bloomington, IN) for crossing an occlusion. If there is a high-grade stenosis, a more pliable wire is preferred.
5. Once the wire has crossed the lesion, exchange it with a 0.35 or 0.18 working wire. Have adequate purchase of the exchange catheter into the target artery as it may get kicked out when introducing a stiffer wire, especially from the femoral approach.
6. Advance the sheath to cross the lesion, especially an occlusion.
7. Balloon angioplasty with a 20- to 40-mm length balloon can be used to assess the extent of area to be treated and visualize the waist seen during insufflation.
8. Once the stent is in the desired location, withdraw the sheath.
9. Deploy the stent hanging out 3–5 mm into the aorta as it is easy to miss disease at the origin. The angle of the SMA has to be factored in to have adequate coverage.

Potential Pitfalls

- The stent can sheer off the delivery catheter when going through a long heavily diseased segment. Hence, the sheath or guiding catheter should cross the lesion first if a balloon-expandable stent is used. Similarly, predilating with a balloon can make crossing the lesion with a stent less risky. This can be difficult if 0.18 or 0.14 wires are used, as they may not be able to provide enough support. Thus, the sheath has to cross the lesion on a 0.35 system.
- Plan on placing a single stent. Magnify the image during deployment for precision, as it can be difficult to visualize the extent of the diseased segment and the origin of the vessel.
- The lesion may require preangioplasty for the mounted stent to go through. During this, very judicious wire control cannot be over emphasized since there is not much purchase in the SMA and wire access can easily be lost. In addition, the location of the wire must be identified so it is not in one of the smaller SMA branches, which can lead to a perforation. Wire movement is inevitable during the procedure, and utmost caution has to be used to keep ensuring the position of the wire.
- Dissection of the SMA is a dreaded complication. It can be avoided by minimizing wire and sheath movement with catheter exchanges. Also, avoid advancing the sheath unprotected without a dilator.

caliber sheath (7 French or greater) and usually cannot be very precisely placed via the femoral approach. Hence, a cut down of the brachial artery may be necessary. The author prefers a balloon-expandable bare metal or covered (iCast, Atrium, Hudson, NH) stent. These can be deployed using a 6-French sheath. The longer the stent, the more difficult it is to deploy accurately. Anything longer than 40 mm is usually not needed.

Special Intraoperative Considerations

Abandon the procedure if:

1. The lesion is heavily calcified and there is a long segment occlusion in a small caliber vessel.
2. Flush occlusion of the SMA precludes femoral approach.

Case Conclusion

The cross table oblique arteriogram confirmed a high-grade proximal SMA stenosis and occluded celiac artery. A balloon-expandable bare metal stent (8 × 20 mm) was successfully placed in the SMA (Fig. 1).

He was then placed on nutritional supplements for the next 2 weeks. The patient gained weight while he was on supplemental nutrition and IV antibiotics. He then underwent replacement of the infected graft with femoral vein and has continued to do well postoperatively.

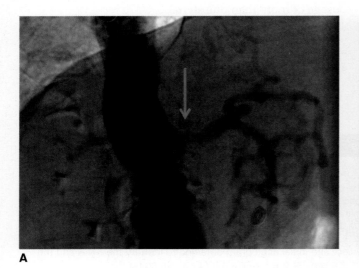

A

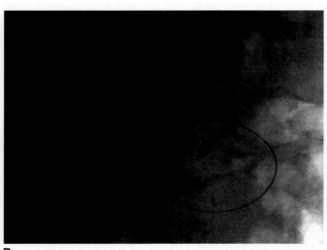

B

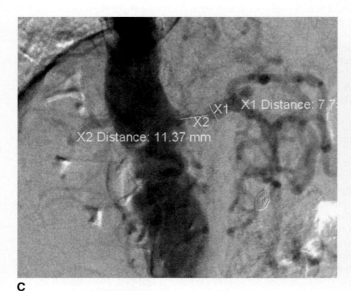

C

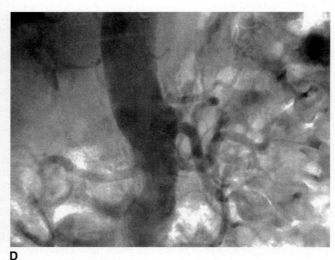

D

FIGURE 1 • **A:** Arteriogram from a steep oblique to show the origin of the SMA and high grade stenosis as indicated by arrow. **B:** After angiogram, measurements are made to size the PTA/stent with a 10-mm arterial size and 1.1-cm length. **C:** A confirmatory image with inflated balloon. **D:** A post-PTA/stenting arteriogram shows brisk flow without stenosis.

TAKE HOME POINTS

- Endovascular approach is usually a "bridge" to an open procedure in a severely malnourished patient where a combined mesenteric bypass and a major open procedure is a prohibitive risk.
- Use long sheaths and long catheters from the outset of the procedure. A stent will be needed for all ostial lesions. Avoid stenting long segments that extend to the middle colic artery and are heavily calcified.
- Balloon-expandable covered stents are available in 6 mm diameter through a 6-French sheath system. A brachial approach is preferred for a more anatomically aligned stent.

SUGGESTED READINGS

Ahanchi SS, Stout CL, Dahl TJ, et al. Comparative analysis of celiac vs mesenteric artery outcomes after angioplasty and stenting. *J Vasc Surg*. 2013;57(4):1062-1066.

Brown DJ, Schermerhorn ML, Powell RJ, et al. Mesenteric stenting for chronic mesenteric ischemia. *J Vasc Surg*. 2005;42(2):268-274.

Eidt JF, Mills J, Rhodes RS, et al. Comparison of surgical operative experience of trainees and practicing vascular surgeons: a report from the Vascular Surgery Board of the American Board of Surgery. *J Vasc Surg*. 2011;53(4):1130-1140.

Fioole B, van de Rest HJ, Meijer JR, et al. Percutaneous transluminal angioplasty and stenting as first-choice treatment in patients with chronic mesenteric ischemia. *J Vasc Surg*. 2010;51(2):386-391.

Kalapatapu VR, Murray BW, Palm-Cruz K, et al. Definitive test to diagnose median arcuate ligament syndrome: injection of vasodilator during angiography. *Vasc Endovascular Surg*. 2009;43(1):46-50.

CLINICAL SCENARIO CASE QUESTIONS

1. A 77-year-old woman presents with mild abdominal pain 3 weeks after colon resection for a left colon mass. She has a normal lactate but elevated WBC to 16K. Postoperatively, she has not been eating well and lost weight. After evaluation, mesenteric ischemia is suspected. She has an occlusion of the SMA 1.5 cm distal to the origin all the way to the middle colic on CTA. The celiac artery has a high-grade stenosis. What is the most appropriate approach:

   a. Systemic heparin and open embolectomy of the SMA
   b. Systemic heparin with systemic vasodilator
   c. Systemic TPA
   d. Angiogram via brachial approach and stent the celiac artery first
   e. Angiogram via the brachial artery approach and stent the SMA first past the middle colic

2. Decreasing the risk of mesenteric arterial dissection with an endovascular approach is best accomplished by:

   a. Using intravascular ultrasound
   b. Always approaching the artery orifice via a groin approach
   c. Preprocedural clopidogrel loading
   d. Care with advancing the catheter or sheath only after good wire access
   e. Using self-expanding stents only

78 Nonocclusive Mesenteric Ischemia

ELIZABETH A. JACKSON and ROBERT D. BROOK

Presentation

An 85-year-old female with a significant past medical history for coronary artery disease, cardiomyopathy with a reduced left ventricular ejection fraction of 20%, and chronic renal insufficiency (stage III) is admitted to the intensive care unit for increasing weight gain and dyspnea thought to be due to an exacerbation of heart failure. Workup for acute coronary syndrome was negative including no elevation in biomarkers (i.e., troponins) and no change in her electrocardiogram. She was treated with intravenous (IV) Lasix for heart failure. In addition, her angiotensin-converting enzyme (ACE) inhibitor dosage was increased, and spironolactone was added. Her clinical heart failure improved over the initial 24 hours; however, on transfer from the intensive care unit to the floor, she developed a low-grade fever and nausea. Vital signs revealed hypotension with a blood pressure of 78/40 mm Hg. IV fluids were initiated cautiously due to concern of her cardiomyopathy and worsening heart failure. Cardiac medications including her beta-blocker, ACE inhibitor, and diuretics were held. Several hours later, she complained of severe abdominal pain and her nausea increased.

On examination, blood pressure was 80/48 mm Hg, heart rate was 105 beats per minute, respirations were 26 per minute, and oxygen saturation was 92% with 3 L/min by nasal cannula. The patient appeared to be in acute distress with rapid respirations and complaints of severe abdominal pain. Neck veins were flat, and lungs were clear to auscultation. Heart sounds were regular with no gallops or murmurs. The patient's abdomen was painful to palpation diffusely with guarding but no rebound tenderness. Bowel sounds were absent. Stool was trace-positive for occult blood. Abdominal plain films and laboratories are ordered.

Test Reports

Abdominal plain films were ordered and read as normal without evidence of obstruction, ileus, mass, or lumen perforation. Laboratory studies included a complete blood cell (CBC) count notable for a mild leukocytosis (white blood cells [WBCs] = 11.9). Comprehensive metabolic panel was unchanged from the morning's labs and was within normal limits with the exception of serum bicarbonate of 19 mEq/L. Urinalysis was normal. Blood and urine cultures were drawn.

Differential Diagnosis

The differential diagnosis for acute periumbilical abdominal pain, fever, hypotension, and leukocytosis is broad. Peritonitis: lumen perforation (e.g., ulcer), ruptured diverticuli, or infections bacterial or nonbacterial organisms. Gastrointestinal: pancreatitis, early small bowel obstruction, diverticulitis, early appendicitis, inflammatory bowel disease, gastroenteritis, or *Clostridium difficile* colitis. Vascular: aortic dissection, aortic aneurysm leakage, and acute mesenteric ischemia. The latter includes splanchnic arterial thrombosis (usually in the setting of underlying atherosclerotic disease), arterial embolus or dissection, small vessel disease and vasculitis, venous thrombosis, watershed ischemia colitis, and small nonocclusive mesenteric ischemia (NOMI).

Discussion

In a patient with sudden (even relative) hypotension followed by severe abdominal pain greater than physical examination findings, NOMI should be immediately considered, particularly with a prior history of diminished left ventricular function and systemic atherosclerosis. In some cases, abdominal pain may be absent. Additional symptoms include abdominal bloating and nausea with vomiting. Mental status changes can also occur. The rectal examination being positive for occult blood and the concomitant metabolic acidosis are all nonspecific findings but are suggestive of mesenteric ischemia as well. Risk factors for NOMI include heart failure, vascular disease (cardiac or peripheral athero-sclerosis), chronic renal disease, aortic insufficiency, shock (septic or cardiogenic), cardiac arrhythmias, use of vasoconstrictive medications or cocaine, and dialysis. Hypotension and the use of digoxin increase the risk for NOMI by causing vasoconstriction of the splanchnic vessels. The use of diuretics may increase renal blood flow and further diminish mesenteric perfusion. Any concomitant infection, septicemia, and volume depletion will also further contribute to NOMI. Due to the high morbidity and mortality rates and emergent nature of this diagnosis, immediate testing should focus on excluding this diagnosis and differentiating between occlusive versus NOMI.

Diagnostic Tests

Abdominal computed tomography, magnetic resonance imaging, or ultrasonography cannot exclude NOMI. However, abdominal CT can demonstrate focal bowel wall thickening, or dilation. CT can also be used to exclude other causes of abdominal pain. Selective mesenteric angiography is the test of choice when mesenteric ischemia is suspected.

Mesenteric Angiography

An emergent mesenteric angiogram demonstrates NOMI. Four arteriographic criteria for NOMI have been presented: (1) narrowing at the origins of multiple superior mesenteric branches; (2) alternate arterial dilation and narrowing; (3) mesenteric arcade spasms; and (4) impaired perfusion of intramural vessels.

Discussion

Acute NOMI is caused by severe and diffuse superior mesenteric artery narrowing due to vasospasm that is triggered by malperfusion secondary to hypotension (heart failure), dehydration (aggressive diuresis with furosemide), and digoxin therapy.

Diagnosis and Recommendation

The diagnosis of acute NOMI is made. In contrast to acute occlusive mesenteric ischemic disease (e.g., emboli, thrombosis), surgery is not indicated for early NOMI without mucosal necrosis.

Approach

After angiography displays NOMI, IV fluid hydration and vasodilator therapy should immediately be initiated. Direct intra-arterial mesentery infusions of papaverine and prostaglandins have been used with success to relieve ischemia. Nitroglycerin can also be used. Vasospasm is known to persist even after correction or resolution of the inciting events. Correction of precipitating factors such as dehydration and/or hypotension and infection is recommended.

Surgical Approach

Control of NOMI with vasodilator therapy should be tried initially. Indications for initial or subsequent laparotomy are failure of intra-arterial vasodilators to restore splanchnic perfusion, an increase in serum markers suggesting bowel necrosis, peritonitis, and persistent symptoms of abdominal pain after 24 to 72 hours.

Case Conclusion

An initial 20-µg bolus of prostaglandin E1 was followed by an infusion of 2.5 to 5.0 µg/h. Symptoms of nausea with abdominal pain resolved within 24 hours. Lactate dehydrogenase enzymes and bicarbonate levels (acidosis) subsequently returned to normal. Repeat angiogram demonstrated a significant restoration of splanchnic perfusion (Fig. 1). IV glucagon may be used in this setting as a splanchnic vasodilator, though clinical experience is anecdotal.

Discussion

NOMI is a medical emergency associated with high mortality rates. It accounts for 20% to 30% of all syndromes of mesenteric ischemia. Conditions that predispose to the syndrome include previous heart disease and reduced cardiac function, older age, renal impairment, aortic insufficiency, and use of certain medications including diuretics and digoxin. Dehydration, hypotension, shock, and infection precipitate acute malperfusion of mesentery that triggers severe microvascular vasoconstriction and spasm. Immediate angiography and direct intra-arterial vasodilator therapy offer the best outcomes (Fig. 2).

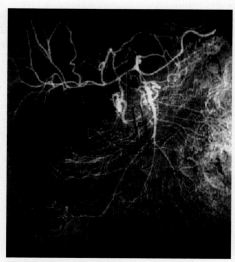

FIGURE 1 • Mesenteric angiography.

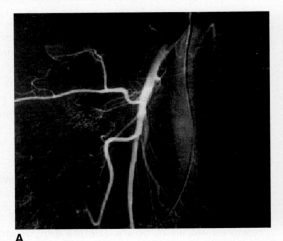
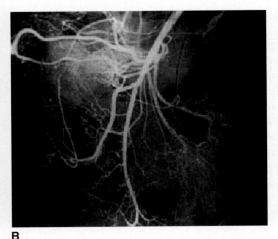

FIGURE 2 • **A:** Severe NOMI at baseline before vasodilator therapy. Extreme mesenteric vasoconstriction is evident. **B:** Posttreatment repeat angiogram demonstrates improved filling of vessels.

TAKE HOME POINTS

- Though rare, consideration of NOMI in clinical setting of abdominal pain, ileus, and septic parameters is important.
- Standard resuscitation for sepsis, including broad spectrum antibiotics, is indicated.
- Arteriography is the diagnostic method of choice.
- Direct arterial vasodilator therapy via arterial catheterization is typically the first-line therapy.
- Consider exploratory laparotomy for evidence of progression of bowel ischemia or perforation.

SUGGESTED READINGS

Bassiouny HS. Nonocclusive mesenteric ischemia. *Surg Clin North Am.* 1997;77:319-325.

Bobadilla JL. Mesenteric ischemia. *Surg Clin North Am.* 2013;93(4):925-940.

Kim AY, Ha HK. Evaluation of suspected mesenteric ischemia: efficacy of radiologic studies. *Radiol Clin North Am.* 2003;41:427-442.

Lock G. Acute mesenteric ischemia: classification, evaluation and therapy. *Acta Gastreoenterol Belg.* 2002;65:220-225.

Mansour MA. Management of acute mesenteric ischemia. *Arch Surg.* 1999;134:328-330.

Park WM, Gloviczki P, Cherry KJ. Contemporary management of acute mesenteric ischemia: factors associated with survival. *J Vasc Surg.* 2002;35:445-452.

Trompeter M, Brazda T, Remy CT, et al. Nonocclusive mesenteric ischemia: etiology, diagnosis, and interventional therapy. *Eur Radiol.* 2002;12:1179-1187.

CLINICAL SCENARIO CASE QUESTIONS

1. A 75-year-old woman with hear failure in the MICU develops severe abdominal pain, and a septic picture. No evidence of bowel perforation on CT scan is observed. After resuscitation, the most specific test to diagnose NOMI is:

   a. Duplex ultrasonography
   b. CTA
   c. MRA
   d. Angiography
   e. None—it is a clinical diagnosis

2. In a patient with angiographically confirmed NOMI, after resuscitation, the primary therapy is:

   a. Systemic calcium channel blocker therapy
   b. IV somatostatin
   c. IV glucagon
   d. Viagra
   e. IA prostaglandin E2

79 Mesenteric Venous Occlusive Disease

MICHELLE MUELLER

Presentation

A 48-year-old man with a past medical history of gastroesophageal reflux disease but no previous surgeries presents to the emergency department complaining of abdominal pain. He has had intermittent abdominal pain for years, but the symptoms have dramatically worsened over the last 2 weeks. The onset of pain occurs approximately 30 minutes after meals and lasts for hours, and is now associated with nausea and vomiting. The patient denies any weight loss, melena, or hematochezia. A recent upper endoscopy was unremarkable, and colonoscopy showed benign polyps.

On physical examination, the patient is noted to be afebrile and hemodynamically stable. The examination reveals the abdomen to be soft and mildly distended with moderate tenderness to palpation, but without peritoneal signs. There are no hernias. The white blood cell count is 7000, and hemoglobin is 40 mg/dL. The electrolyte levels, liver function tests, amylase, lipase, and lactate levels are normal. To further evaluate the abdominal pain, a computed tomography (CT) scan with oral and intravenous contrast is ordered.

Differential Diagnosis

The differential diagnosis for abdominal pain without peritonitis is extensive. Chronic abdominal pain narrows the differential, yet it remains lengthy. Possible diagnoses in this case include gastroesophageal reflux disease, inflammatory bowel disease, peptic ulcer disease, biliary colic, chronic cholecystitis, chronic pancreatitis, partial small bowel obstruction, tumor, chronic mesenteric ischemia, and mesenteric venous thrombosis (MVT).

Workup

CT scanning is an important part of the evaluation of abdominal pain. The addition of intravenous contrast to a CT scan of the abdomen and pelvis aids in the diagnosis of venous thrombosis, aneurysms, bowel ischemia, and bleeding. CT scan with venous phase contrast has greater than 90% accuracy in establishing the diagnosis of MVT. Important findings on the scan are thrombus, superior mesenteric vein dilation, target or "halo" sign, thickened bowel wall, and presence of collateral veins within the mesentery.

CT Scan
CT Scan Report

The CT scan reveals MVT (Fig. 1). There is mesenteric stranding and a filling defect in the superior mesenteric vein ringed with contrast, "halo" sign (*arrow*) (Fig. 2).

Diagnosis and Treatment

MVT is a broad term that includes thrombosis of the inferior mesenteric vein, superior mesenteric vein, splenic vein, or portal vein. MVT is responsible for approximately 2% to 15% of all cases of acute intestinal ischemia. MVT obstructs venous return, which can lead to edema of the bowel wall, distention, and eventual infarction. MVT is difficult to diagnose initially because of the typical insidious onset and subtle early clinical findings. Early symptoms are produced by congestion of the bowel and are visceral in character. Patients may present with signs and symptoms that are nonspecific and vague, including crampy abdominal pain, abdominal distention, nausea, anorexia, malaise, ascites, diarrhea, gastrointestinal bleeding, and pain out of proportion to examination. About half of patients will have leukocytosis; an elevated lactate is unusual. Delays in diagnosis are common and contribute to the reported high morbidity and 15% to 40% mortality.

The traditional separation of MVT into primary or secondary categories is arbitrary. *All patients with MVT should be regarded as harboring a hypercoagulable state.* The hypercoagulability may be endogenous and related to a defined abnormality in the coagulation system (e.g., protein C deficiency, protein S deficiency, antithrombin deficiency, antiphospholipid antibody syndrome, lupus anticoagulant, factor V Leiden, prothrombin

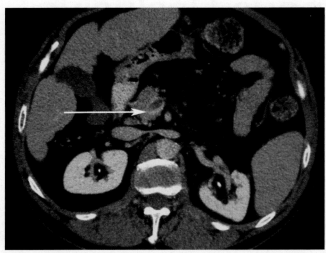

FIGURE 1 • CT scan with mesenteric vein thrombosis. *Arrow* highlights thrombus, with enhancing halo.

gene mutation). Alternatively, the hypercoagulable state producing MVT may result from other processes, such as intra-abdominal inflammation (pancreatitis, diverticular disease, peritonitis, appendicitis, inflammatory bowel disease), trauma, portal hypertension, intra-abdominal or hematologic malignancy, polycythemia vera, myelo-proliferative disorders, splenomegaly, oral contraceptives, cirrhosis, or even severe dehydration.

It is more relevant clinically to categorize MVT on the basis of duration of symptoms as well as whether portal or splenic vein thrombus is present. MVT can present acutely with a more fulminant course lasting only days or as a chronic condition (arbitrarily defined as lasting at least 4 weeks). Acute MVT more often results from small mesenteric vein branch involvement and is more difficult to diagnose with CT scanning or duplex ultrasound because the larger mesenteric veins may not contain thrombus. These patients have poor venous collateralization and are more

likely to have peritoneal signs on examination indicating bowel infarction. Acute MVT is often first recognized intraoperatively. A clear majority of patients with acute MVT will require an operation and probable bowel resection. Acute MVT has been more often associated with a thrombophilic complication than the chronic form.

Patients with chronic MVT often have symptoms lasting weeks, have involvement of larger vessels (focal thrombus at the portomesenteric confluence or splenic vein), and are usually diagnosed with a CT scan (MRI/MRA or possibly a duplex scan) identifying the large-vessel thrombosis as well as collateral circulation. When compared to acute MVT, these patients are more likely to have thrombosis related to a postoperative complication or cirrhosis. These patients rarely need an operation and almost never require a bowel resection. The Mayo Clinic experience suggests that patients with acute MVT fare worse than patients with chronic MVT. Mortality in acute MVT is higher at both 30 days (approximately 30% vs. 6%) and 3 years (64% vs. 17%).

Surgical Approach

Patients with suspected MVT and peritonitis should go to the operating room. Intra-operatively, the surgeon may find bloody ascites, and dusky, thick, and rubbery-appearing intestine. All patients should be anticoagulated as soon as possible once the diagnosis of MVT is made, preoperatively or even intraoperatively. If necrotic bowel is identified, resection should be performed. The surgeon should strongly consider a second-look laparotomy scheduled for 24 to 48 hours to reevaluate areas of questionable bowel viability. Additional bowel resections at second-look procedures are common (Table 1).

Very rarely, a large-vessel venous thrombectomy or local thrombolysis may be indicated. There are many reports in the literature using endovascular techniques. These can include mechanical thrombectomy, suction thrombectomy, and catheter-directed thrombolysis. These options should be reserved for patients who do not

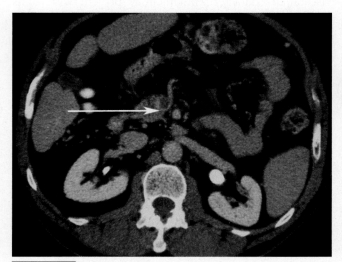

FIGURE 2 • CT scan showing thrombosed superior mesenteric vein. *Arrow* highlights thrombus with halo.

TABLE 1. Patients with Peritoneal Signs and Mesenteric Venous Thrombosis

Key Technical Steps

1. Midline laparotomy and full exploration
2. Full anticoagulation as soon as the diagnosis is made
3. Resect necrotic bowel
4. Consider surgical thrombectomy or other endovascular techniques
5. Second-look laparotomy

Potential Pitfalls

• Not recognizing MVT as the diagnosis
• Insufficient anticoagulation
• Forgetting to come back for a second look

respond to other therapies. It is not surprising that such treatment is often futile, because the patients most likely to need surgery are those with small vessel involvement.

Patients diagnosed with MVT, but without peritonitis, should be admitted to the hospital for fluid resuscitation and systemic anticoagulation. This is most often with intravenous heparin. These patients should be closely observed for the development of peritoneal signs, which should then prompt exploratory laparotomy. There is no benefit to surgery without signs of peritonitis. Again, there are some reports in the literature regarding the use of endovascular techniques in these patients as well. These small studies discuss possible quicker recovery and decreased length of stay; however, there is no long-term benefit proven at this time.

Complications associated with MVT include bowel necrosis, portal hypertension, variceal bleeding, and recurrent thrombosis. Indefinite (i.e., lifelong) anticoagulation is often recommended because patients so treated have a lower recurrence rate and better survival. However, if the cause of the MVT is clearly identified and temporary, it may be reasonable to discontinue the anticoagulation after 3 to 6 months. Individualized therapy is advised. The patient in this scenario was anticoagulated indefinitely because of the idiopathic nature of his MVT; it is presumed that he has a hypercoagulable state even though it is undefined.

Case Conclusion

At this point, the patient has no signs of bowel infarction and no indications for surgical exploration. The patient is admitted to the hospital for fluid resuscitation, immediate anticoagulation with full-dose intravenous heparin, and serial abdominal examinations. A hypercoagulability screen was sent prior to anticoagulation.

The patient remained NPO until the abdominal pain resolved. A diet was then resumed slowly, starting with clear liquid diet and advanced as tolerated. The patient's abdominal pain improves, and he tolerates oral intake. He is transitioned to subcutaneous low molecular weight heparin and then coumadin. Discharge occurs 2 days later. At follow-up approximately 2 weeks later, the patient is clinically well. His hypercoagulability screen revealed no abnormalities for protein C, protein S, or antithrombin III. Mutations in the factor V and prothrombin genes were absent. Lifelong anticoagulation is recommended.

TAKE HOME POINTS

- MVT is difficult to diagnose secondary to the vague presenting symptoms. *A high index of suspicion is essential*.
- The high morbidity and mortality is related to a delay in diagnosis. A high index of suspicion and liberal use of CT scanning in patients with abdominal pain may shorten this delay.
- It is useful to categorize patients based on duration of symptoms and isolated large mesenteric vein involvement.
- All patients with MVT should be anticoagulated as soon as possible after the diagnosis is made.
- Patients should be operated upon selectively, based on clinical findings that suggest bowel infarction.
- All patients with MVT should be regarded as hypercoagulable. Because of lower rates of recurrent MVT and better survival, indefinite anticoagulation is usually recommended.

SUGGESTED READINGS

Harnik IG, Brandt LJ. Mesenteric venous thrombosis. *Vasc Med.* 2010;15:407-418.

Kumar S, Kamath PS. Acute superior mesenteric venous thrombosis: one disease or two? *Am J Gastroenterol.* 2003;98:1299-1304.

Rhee RY, Gloviczki P, Mendonca CT, et al. Mesenteric venous thrombosis: still a lethal disease in the 1990s. *J Vasc Surg.* 1994;20:688-697.

Singal AK, Kamath PS, Tefferi A. Mesenteric venous thrombosis. *Mayo Clin Proc.* 2013;88:285-294.

CLINICAL SCENARIO CASE QUESTIONS

1. As soon as the diagnosis of MVT is made, which of the following is *most* essential (regardless of acuity or peritonitis)?

   a. Making the patient NPO
   b. Immediate exploratory laparotomy
   c. Immediate full anticoagulation
   d. Thrombolytic therapy
   e. Oral antiplatelet therapy

2. During surgery for acute MVT with peritonitis, which of the following principles is *not* recommended?

   a. Resection of nonviable bowel with immediate reanastomosis
   b. Full anticoagulation preoperatively or intraoperatively
   c. Consideration of mesenteric venous thrombectomy or thrombolysis
   d. Strongly considering a second-look laparotomy
   e. Aggressive intravenous hydration

80 Splenic Artery Aneurysm

TIMOTHY E. NEWHOOK, JOSHUA D. ADAMS, and GILBERT R. UPCHURCH Jr

Presentation

A 78-year-old grand multiparous woman with a past medical history significant for hypertension, aortic valve disease, Parkinson's disease, and sigmoid diverticulosis presented to the emergency department with a 5-month history of abdominal pain. She described the pain as being throughout her epigastrium and radiating to her left lower abdominal quadrant. Her abdominal pain is sharp in character and intermittent since onset. Furthermore, her pain does not change with eating and nothing makes it better or worse. She denies any changes in bowel habits, appetite, chest pain, cough, back pain, or shortness of breath. Her medications included clopidogrel. Her social history was negative for alcohol or tobacco use. Review of systems was negative for any other pathology. On physical examination, vital signs were normal other than moderate hypertension. She was appropriate on questioning. A parkinsonian tremor was observed. A systolic ejection murmur was noted on auscultation, and her heart rate and rhythm were regular. Her abdomen was obese, soft, and mildly distended; however, she reported tenderness to palpation over her epigastrium and left upper quadrant. Despite this, no rebound tenderness or guarding was detected. She had two-plus pitting edema in her lower extremities.

Differential Diagnosis

This patient presents with a complex and nebulous history of present illness. The differential diagnosis for chronic abdominal pain in an elderly patient with a history of hypertension, cardiovascular disease, and diverticulosis is broad. Despite this, a conservative differential diagnosis must include abdominal aortic aneurysm; acute, chronic, or acute-on-chronic mesenteric ischemia; diverticulitis; nephrolithiasis; urinary tract infection; malignancy; median arcuate ligament syndrome; and visceral artery aneurysms.

Case Continued

A chest and abdominal x-ray series are performed, which demonstrate no abnormalities. Due to her presentation and comorbidities, a surgical consultation is requested. A computed tomography arteriogram (CTA) is performed. Furthermore, a complete blood count with differential is indicated to rule out other diagnoses, such as infection or lymphoma. The exams and labs are within normal limits, except that a 2-cm splenic artery aneurysm (SAA), that is nonruptured, is noted (Figs. 1 and 2).

Discussion

Aneurysms of the splenic artery are the most common aneurysm of the splanchnic arterial circulation. Specifically, SAAs account for approximately 60% of all splanchnic arterial aneurysms and are the third most common intra-abdominal arterial aneurysm behind infrarenal aortic and arterial aneurysms. Despite this, SAAs are relatively rare and often insidious with an estimated incidence of 0.8% in retrospective reviews of nonselective arteriograms. SAAs occur in women four times more frequently than men and typically within the sixth decade of life. Moreover, SAAs are frequently multiple and most often occur in the distal segment of the splenic artery.

SAAs are most often asymptomatic; however, patients presenting with vague epigastric or left upper quadrant abdominal pain radiating to the left scapula may attribute their symptoms to this entity. Physical examination rarely yields any remarkable findings. Abdominal x-ray may reveal a curvilinear signet-ring calcification in the left upper quadrant; however, most SAAs are found incidentally during imaging studies, such as CT, CTA, or magnetic resonance imaging (MRI) for other pathologies. SAAs have been associated with three major risk factors: pregnancy, systemic arterial dysplasia, and portal hypertension. In regard to pregnancy, the majority of females diagnosed with SAA are multiparous with a mean number of pregnancies being between 4 and 5 in multiple series. It is believed that SAA formation in this population may be due to increased splenic arterial flow occurring during pregnancy, as well as hormonal effects on arterial elastic tissue. Furthermore, many patients with renal artery fibrodysplasia also harbor SAA. Finally, 1% to 20% of patients with portal hypertension have SAA for reasons that are incompletely understood. Increased

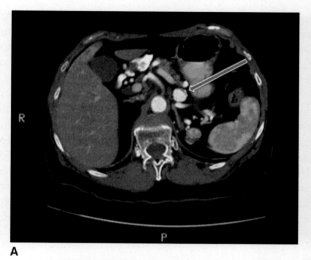
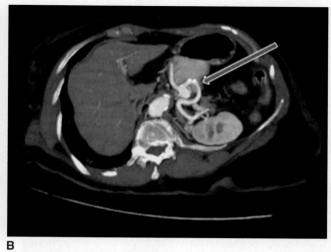

A   **B**

FIGURE 1 • **A,B:** CTA abdomen and pelvis demonstrating no evidence of aortic aneurysm. The celiac, superior mesenteric, and inferior mesenteric arteries are all widely patent. Aortic bifurcation, common, internal, and external iliac as well as common femoral arteries are widely patent without evidence of aneurysm disease. No evidence of mesenteric ischemia is observed. A 2-cm SAA arising 4 cm distal to the origin of the splenic artery is noted adjacent to the mid-pancreatic body (*arrows*). Multiple noninflamed diverticula arise from the sigmoid colon. No other abnormalities are present.

splenic arterial flow and hormonal imbalance increasing with end-stage cirrhosis may influence SAA formation in this population. Other factors that may contribute to SAA formation include pancreatitis, collagen vascular disease, atherosclerosis, and autoimmune disease (lupus).

SAAs have potential to rupture, which is often a lethal complication. Although rupture of SAA occurs in less than 2% of patients, it is imperative to recognize this as most SAA series report a high mortality after rupture. Patients believed to be at higher risk for SAA rupture include patients status post liver transplantation, women of childbearing age, pregnant women, and younger (less

than 60 years) patients. SAA in a pregnant patient is of particular concern as rupture has been reported in over 90% of cases, resulting in a reported maternal mortality of almost 75% and fetal mortality over 95% of cases. Finally, SAA diameter greater than 2 cm is associated with a higher risk of rupture. In order to prevent rupture, it is recommended that all symptomatic SAAs be repaired, as well as asymptomatic pregnant women and women of childbearing age because of the aforementioned risk of rupture and associated mortality. Moreover, patients with SAA over 2 cm should be offered elective repair.

Recommendations

Given the patient's presentation, risk factors, and subsequent radiologic studies, a diagnosis of symptomatic SAA is suspected. Therefore, a selective celiac arteriogram with consideration for endovascular repair is indicated.

Case Continued

After discussion of radiologic findings with the patient, consent was obtained to perform a selective celiac and splenic arteriogram with possible endovascular treatment of her SAA. The patient underwent intravenous conscious sedation and retrograde puncture of the right common femoral artery. First, the celiac artery was catheterized, and a selective celiac arteriogram was performed, after which a glidewire was utilized to catheterize the splenic artery. A selective splenic arteriogram was performed (Fig. 3A). A 2-cm saccular SAA was visualized arising from the inferior aspect of the mid-splenic artery, and the splenic artery was otherwise patent.

FIGURE 2 • A three-dimensional reconstruction of the CTA revealing a 2-cm SAA arising 4 cm distal to the splenic artery origin.

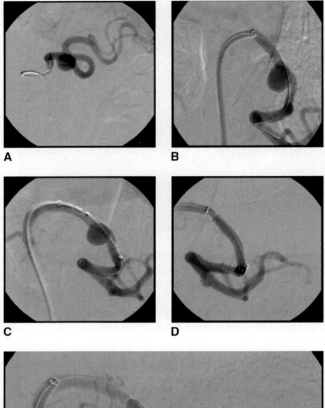

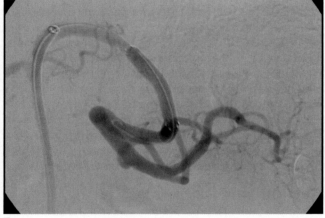

E

FIGURE 3 • **A:** A selective splenic arteriogram was performed. A 2-cm saccular SAA was visualized arising from the inferior aspect of the mid–splenic artery, and the splenic artery was otherwise patent. **B:** A Rosen wire was placed beyond the SAA, followed by the advancement of a 10-French long sheath into the proximal splenic artery. **C, D:** An 8 mm × 40 mm covered stent was placed beyond the SAA and deployed, which successfully excluded the SAA. **E:** A post–stent placement arteriogram revealed that the SAA was completely excluded, the splenic artery remained fully patent, and perfusion of the spleen was preserved.

Discussion

Repair of SAA has been traditionally performed by open or laparoscopic surgical aneurysmectomy or aneurysm exclusion; however, endovascular treatment of SAA has become the preferred mode of treatment. Due to the

amount of radiation involved with endovascular SAA treatment, open repair is preferred in pregnant patients. Otherwise, open repair should be reserved only for patients in whom endovascular treatment has failed or is inappropriate.

Endovascular therapy for SAA has distinct advantages as compared to open approaches including shorter length of stay, shorter recovery time, and no need for general anesthesia. Historically, poor operative candidates may be more amenable to percutaneous approaches for SAA treatment. Limitations include need for iodinated contrast, radiation exposure, and risk of splenic infarction. Also, postembolization syndrome, which consists of abdominal pain, fever, slowed gastric transit, pleural effusion, and pancreatitis, can occur.

Case Continued

The decision was made to perform an endovascular repair of the SAA at the time of initial angiogram. A Rosen wire was placed beyond the SAA, followed by the advancement of a 10-French long sheath into the proximal splenic artery (Fig. 3B). An 8 mm × 40 mm covered stent was placed beyond the SAA and deployed, which successfully excluded the SAA (Fig. 3C and D). A post–stent placement arteriogram revealed that the SAA was completely excluded, the splenic artery remained fully patent, and perfusion of the spleen was preserved (Fig. 3E). Following the procedure, the patient's right femoral arterial puncture site was closed in the usual fashion (Table 1).

TABLE 1. Splenic Artery Aneurysm

Key Technical Steps

1. Review of CTA with 3-D reconstructions to access potential for endovascular solution.
2. Access femoral artery under ultrasound guidance.
3. Selective catheterization of celiac and splenic artery.
4. Placement of stiff wire beyond the SAA, followed by the advancement of a sheath of adequate caliber to deliver stent graft.
5. Deployment of covered stent graft to exclude the SAA.
6. Consider leaving a microcatheter in the SAA to place coils if the SAA is not excluded following stent graft placement.
7. A poststent graft placement arteriogram should be performed to document complete exclusion of SAA.
8. Femoral arterial puncture site is closed.

Potential Pitfalls

• Inability to cannulate the splenic artery with standard catheter. Often requires use of microcatheters.
• Tortuous nature of splenic artery may make passage of large sheath and stent graft difficult. May need to consider coil embolization.
• Persistent flow in SAA after coiling/stenting. May require recurrent coiling. Need to be followed with CTA.

Discussion

Once an endovascular approach is selected, the decision must be made as to how to treat the SAA. The location of the SAA and the tortuosity of the artery are used to guide this decision. SAAs that are proximally located and without significant tortuosity may be treated by deployment of proximal and distal vascular occlusion plugs or by placing a covered stent across the aneurysm. The devices utilized to deploy these devices are stiff and therefore may limit their applicability in a tortuous artery. Coil embolization is typically best to treat distal SAAs in tortuous splenic arteries.

Although endovascular techniques are employed most often for SAA, more traditional surgical approaches should be considered. Laparoscopic SAA ligation is a viable alternative to open SAA repair. In regard to open procedures, various incisions may be made to access the SAA; however, the location of the SAA again guides the choice of procedure used to ultimately repair the aneurysm. Proximal SAAs typically require entering the lesser sac along the lesser curve of the stomach and ligating all entering and exiting vessels, followed by either excision or ligation of the aneurysm without arterial reconstruction. A retroperitoneal approach is typically employed to repair a mid–splenic artery aneurysm after a Kocher maneuver for pancreatic mobilization. The SAA is then ligated proximally. Finally, SAA of the distal artery or splenic hilum typically requires splenic mobilization for visualization, followed by either conventional splenectomy or simple suture obliteration.

Case Conclusion

The patient is admitted to the hospital overnight and remains pain free the next morning. She is discharged to home on her home medications which included Plavix. At 1 month, she is seen in follow-up. A CTA reveals the SAA to be excluded and the splenic artery to be widely patent. She remains pain free.

TAKE HOME POINTS

- The differential diagnosis for chronic abdominal pain in an elderly patient with a history of hypertension, cardiovascular disease, and diverticulosis is broad.
- Aneurysms of the splenic artery are the most common aneurysm of the splanchic arterial circulation.
- SAAs are most often asymptomatic, however patients presenting with vague epigastric or left upper quadrant abdominal pain radiating to the left scapula may attribute their symptoms to this entity.

- SAAs have been associated with three major risk factors: pregnancy, systemic arterial dysplasia, and portal hypertension.
- SAAs have potential to rupture, which is often a lethal complication.
- Although rupture of SAA occurs in less than 2% of patients, it is imperative to recognize this as most SAA series report a high mortality after rupture. Patients believed to be at higher risk for SAA rupture include patients status post liver transplantation, women of childbearing age, pregnancy, and younger (<60 years) patients.
- SAA in a pregnant patient is of particular concern as rupture has been reported in over 90% of cases, resulting in a reported maternal mortality of almost 75% and fetal mortality over 95% of cases.
- Repair of SAA has been traditionally performed by open or laparoscopic surgical aneurysmectomy or aneurysm exclusion; however, endovascular treatment of SAA has become the preferred mode of treatment.

SUGGESTED READINGS

Agrawal GA, Johnson PT, Fishman EK. Splenic artery aneurysms and pseudoaneurysms: clinical distinctions and CT appearances. *AJR Am J Roentgenol.* 2007;188(4):992-999.

Carr SC, Pearce WH, Vogelzang RL, et al. Current management of visceral artery aneurysms. *Surgery.* 1996;120:627-634.

Greene DR, Gorey TF, Tanner WA, et al. The diagnosis and management of splenic artery aneurysms. *J R Soc Med.* 1988;81:387-388.

Stanley JC, Fry WJ. Pathogenesis and clinical significance of splenic artery aneurysms. *Surgery.* 1974;76:898-908.

CLINICAL SCENARIO CASE QUESTIONS

1. Which of the following is *not* an indication for SAA repair?
   a. SAA diameter greater than 2 cm
   b. History of liver transplantation with a 2.3-cm SAA
   c. Female patient of childbearing age with a 2-cm SAA
   d. Symptomatic SAA
   e. Presence of incidental 7-mm SAA

2. Of the following, which is the most appropriate strategy for repair of a proximal, nontortuous 3-cm SAA in a healthy patient?
   a. Endovascular approach with deployment of a covered stent across the SAA
   b. Open surgical aneurysmectomy
   c. Laparoscopic SAA ligation
   d. Laparoscopic splenectomy
   e. Observation

81 Superior Mesenteric Artery Aneurysm

MATTHEW R. SMEDS and GUILLERMO A. ESCOBAR

Presentation

A 73-year-old man had a repair of a strangulated inguinal hernia and small bowel resection, complicated by a left ureteral injury and subsequent urinoma. A CT scan obtained 10 days after the index procedure revealed a 3-cm aneurysm of the mid–superior mesenteric artery (SMA) surrounded by loculated fluid collections (Fig. 1). The fluid collections are consistent with an infected urinoma, notable for septations, mesenteric stranding, and dilated bowel.

Differential Diagnosis and Epidemiology

Visceral artery aneurysms are rare clinical entities that are identified in less than 0.2% of autopsy studies. These aneurysms may be true aneurysms, mycotic, aneurysmal degeneration of dissections, or pseudoaneurysms. They are most commonly found in the splenic or hepatic distribution. However, aneurysms of the SMA and its branches are uncommon and represent only 6% to 7% of all visceral artery aneurysms. True, spontaneous SMA aneurysms are usually located in the proximal artery but can be located anywhere in the mesentery and sometimes appear as multiple aneurysms scattered in the mesentery.

Visceral artery aneurysms as a whole have the following etiologies: atherosclerotic (68%), mycotic (13%), traumatic (10%), collagen disorders (6%), and giant cell arteritis (3%). Meanwhile, SMA aneurysms are mycotic in almost two thirds of reported cases (usually endocarditis in younger patients or in concert with a severe intra-abdominal infection). Atherosclerotic degeneration accounts for the second most common cause of SMA aneurysms, while it is the most common etiology in older patients. SMA aneurysms can also follow primary dissections, or as a consequence of aortic dissections. Other causes include genetic disorders (Marfan's syndrome, Ehlers-Danlos syndrome, neurofibromatosis type I, Klippel-Trenaunay syndrome etc.), iatrogenic pseudoaneurysms, and inflammation from autoimmune disorders (giant cell arteritis).

Up to a third of visceral aneurysms may be associated with a nonsplanchnic aneurysm elsewhere in the body that usually is spontaneous, or they may be linked to arterial dissections. Historic reports of splanchnic artery aneurysm ruptures had high mortality rates between 20% and 70% (especially when related to pregnancy); however, recent reviews suggest that the modern mortality ranges between 15% and 20%.

Clinical Presentation of SMA Aneurysms

SMA aneurysms are usually asymptomatic and incidentally found on CT scans. Patients may experience vague abdominal pain, nausea, and vomiting—presumably secondary to distal embolization, perianeurysm inflammation, or compression. They may also present with various degrees of gastrointestinal hemorrhage secondary to fistulizing into bowel. Spontaneous intra-abdominal rupture of the aneurysm or acute SMA thrombosis can present with a more dramatic clinical presentation due to bleeding or acute mesenteric ischemia, respectively. Rupture rates are ill defined but estimated at approximately 10%. Bleeding may occur into the retroperitoneum or free rupture into the peritoneal cavity, the latter being linked to most fatalities. On physical exam, patients may have a palpable pulsatile mass or an audible bruit in the epigastrium. In patients presenting with abdominal pain alone, other causes of abdominal pain need to be ruled out first unless there is strong evidence of embolic injury to the bowel.

This case suggests the possibility of a mycotic etiology of the SMA aneurysm due to the associated infection and rather remote location from the origin of the artery. However, due to the patient's older age, it is possible to be from the more benign, spontaneous/atherosclerotic etiology. If so, then elective repair may be considered once his acute illness resolves. However, due to the real concern for a mycotic aneurysm, close surveillance with repeated short interval imaging should be obtained prior to dismissing the possibilities for urgent repair.

Case Continued

The patient was treated with intravenous antibiotics and underwent percutaneous drainage of the urinomas and had a percutaneous nephrostomy tube placed. Two weeks later, a CT angiography (CTA) demonstrated an increase

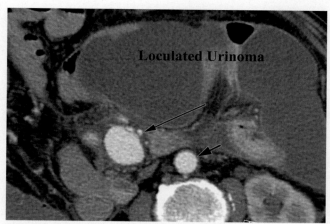

Loculated Urinoma

FIGURE 1 • Axial CTA images demonstrating a large, inflammatory rind surrounding an urinoma and SMA aneurysm. The *long arrow* indicates the SMA and a 3-cm SMA aneurysm. *Short arrow* indicates the aorta.

in size of the aneurysm to 4.5 cm (Fig. 2), and there is new stranding in the mesentery around the SMA without evidence of rupture. The celiac, superior mesenteric, and inferior mesenteric arteries are all grossly within normal limits. He denies abdominal or back pain, and there is no blood in his stool. On examination, his vital signs are normal. He has an open abdominal skin incision with good granulation tissue at the base, and the left nephrostomy tube has clear urine within. There are no pulsatile abdominal masses and has normal pulses in his extremities. Prior to this recent illness, he was in otherwise good health and was physically quite active for his age.

Discussion

The rapid interval growth and perimesenteric fat stranding are very concerning for a mycotic SMA aneurysm, as well as for impending rupture. Therefore, surgical

planning is to follow. Due to the infectious nature, either simple ligation or an autologous conduit (vein) should be chosen. Saphenous vein is the conduit of choice, and therefore, he should undergo preoperative vein mapping of the veins to select the ideal conduit.

Diagnosis, Natural History, and Treatment

Diagnosis of SMA aneurysms may be done via CT or MR angiography, conventional digital subtraction angiography, or duplex imaging in thin patients. Sonographic examination will demonstrate a hypoechoic pulsatile mass. Duplex is most helpful for screening or surveillance of known aneurysms, while angiography may be more useful for operative planning. High-resolution CT or MR angiography can determine the location of the aneurysm in relation to branch vessels, the degree of collateralization, and the presence of coexisting diseases. Three-dimensional reconstructions and straight line reconstruction software can be very helpful for endovascular case planning. Success at symptom management, aneurysm exclusion, and patency after open reconstructions is about 90% at 4 years, and there is a negligible mortality in elective procedures done in experienced centers, and about 15% overall.

Despite first being described in 1812, the natural history of SMA aneurysms remains unknown due to its scarcity and publication bias. Thus, the timing of SMA and visceral artery aneurysm repair is not well established, and their growth and rupture rates may be overestimated. As an example, while gastroduodenal artery aneurysms are associated with celiac artery occlusions and stenosis, they are reported to grow in only about 38% over 2 years, while the rest remain stable. Fear of rupture and embolization from aneurysms greater than 2 cm drive operative management. Patients with symptomatic aneurysms or

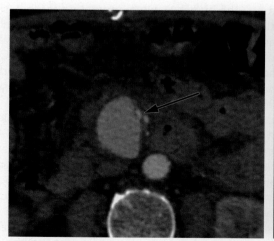
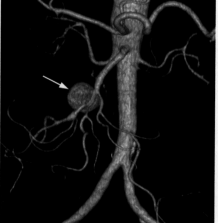

FIGURE 2 • **Left**-sided image demonstrates axial CTA images of the same patient, 2 weeks after draining the fluid collections. *Arrow* identifies the SMA aneurysm surrounded by inflammation, which has grown to 4.5 cm. **Right**-sided image is a 3-D reconstruction of the abdominal aorta and its branches. *Arrow* indicates the SMA aneurysm.

those larger than 2 cm should be considered for repair. Aneurysms found close to the wall of the intestine are managed with a limited segmental bowel resection including the affected mesentery. Multiple aneurysms scattered in the bowel cannot be managed in toto and therefore require watchful waiting and only intervening in symptomatic cases.

Smaller aneurysms, mesenteric dissections, and those felt to be too high risk for repair may be observed with serial ultrasound (when possible) or CT angiogram and generally have a rather slow growth rate. In patients with acute mesenteric dissections, anticoagulation for a few months, followed by antiplatelet agents, may be initially considered to decrease the risk of embolization and bowel ischemia, but these usually do not become aneurysmal after many years of observation.

Open Surgical Approach—Technical Tips and Outcomes

Surgical repair of SMA aneurysms can surprisingly be performed often via simple ligation (about 30% of reported cases), especially in cases of acute hemorrhage. The presence of collateral vessels will determine if simple ligation will suffice, and this can be further verified by temporary occlusion of the SMA segment to be ligated with assessment of bowel viability intraoperatively. Aneurysmorrhaphy is best done in primarily saccular aneurysms, where the top of the aneurysm can be removed and a linear repair can be done. If formal arterial reconstruction is needed, the greater saphenous vein is the conduit of choice in cases of infection or when a concomitant bowel resection is needed. In the absence of these conditions, a synthetic graft may be considered to replace or patch the artery.

Open surgical repair of SMA aneurysms is performed under general anesthesia in patients who are deemed acceptable surgical risk. A vertical midline abdominal incision is generally made (or transverse), and the omentum and transverse colon are retracted superiorly, with the small bowel and mesentery retracted caudally. If the aneurysm is in the proximal SMA, this will be retroperitoneal between the aorta and pancreas and posterior to the superior mesenteric vein and will require an approach via left-sided visceral rotation. Meanwhile, aneurysms that lie further out than the pancreas will require an anterior approach through the mesocolon-small bowel mesentery junction. Some aneurysms may require both types of exposures to obtain proximal vascular control (via the retroperitoneum) and then vascular reconstruction/repair from the anterior approach.

The SMA is located anteriorly within the mesentery, at the junction of the small bowel mesentery and transverse mesocolon where it crosses over the duodenum. Proximal and distal control is obtained while avoiding the superior mesenteric vein, which normally lays to the right of the artery. The further from the SMA origin,

greater care is needed to isolate and not injury branches that emerge from the lateral and posterior surfaces of the SMA. This is especially more challenging the more distal the aneurysm lies from the SMA origin where branches that are not seen are either avulsed during the dissection or will bleed continuously when entering the aneurysm sac during repair. Temporary occlusion of the SMA proximal and distal to the aneurysm, followed by an assessment of bowel viability, can allow for determination of the success of simple ligation. If aneurysmorrhaphy or bypass is planned, the patient is systemically heparinized, the vessels are clamped and the branches arising from the aneurysm sac are either temporarily occluded (for aneurysmorrhaphy or patching) or ligated (for SMA interposition grafting/bypass). The sac is opened and contents evacuated. Redundant wall is resected, and the SMA is reconstructed, or closed primarily (with or without a patch).

A more proximal aneurysm may require a retroperitoneal approach from the left side, with right medial reflection of the colon, pancreas, and spleen. Bypass arising from the aorta to a normal, distal SMA with ligation of the aneurysm is another option for very long or proximal aneurysms. After restoration of flow, the bowel should be investigated closely for viability. The mesentery is closed over the repair, heparin is reversed, and the abdomen is closed in the standard fashion.

Endovascular Approach—Technical Tips and Outcomes

Endovascular therapy provides an evolving option for patients in whom an open surgical approach may be suboptimal, but mostly limited to noninfectious etiologies. These alternatives include coil embolization of the aneurysm or feeding vessels and/or placement of a covered stent across the aneurysm and potentially the use of "flow-diverting" stents to theoretically allow flow into the branches, while promoting thrombosis of the aneurysm sac. As all these techniques can significantly impair intestinal blood flow, preprocedure evaluation of the small bowel branch vessels using 3-D CTA or a high-magnification angiogram is critical. Without adequate collateralization, bowel ischemia may result after endovascular exclusion of the blood flow.

Access is usually obtained via the left brachial or axial artery due to the acuity of the SMA angle off the aorta, and long or stiff stent grafts may not maneuver from the aorta into the SMA. Once the vessel is selected, a long sheath is advanced into the artery, and the covered stent or coils are delivered. Use of stent grafts requires adequate proximal and distal landing zones to ensure graft stability. There are no long-term data available to determine longevity of these repairs, but multiple case series describe their utility (mostly in emergent cases). "Flow-diversion" has been limited to about 28 cases reported using the Cardiatis Multilayer

Stent as a possible alternative to traditional open and endovascular approaches.

Operative Technique and Findings

After lysis of adhesions, the aneurysm is palpated at the base of the thickened mesentery. The lesser sac is entered, and the pancreas is elevated, allowing identification of the proximal SMA emerging beneath the uncinate process that is encircled with a vessel loop. The mesentery is pulled inferiorly, and the dissection is continued along the SMA until the aneurysm is encountered approximately 3 to 4 cm from the origin. The SMA distal to the aneurysm is identified and encircled with vessel loops. Five branches emanating from the aneurysm are also individually encircled with vessel loops. A length of greater saphenous vein is harvested from the left leg. The patient is systemically heparinized to a goal activated clotting time greater than 250 seconds, and the SMA is clamped proximally and distally. The aneurysm is opened and reveals that the back wall appears to have blown out. The five branches all have excellent back bleeding, and four are ligated. A segment of dilated bowel appears cyanotic, so the decision is made to reconstruct the artery. The saphenous vein is reversed and sewn as an interposition graft in an end-to-end fashion between the normal proximal and distal SMA. Flow is restored, and the bowel is inspected. There are good pulses and Doppler signals noted throughout the mesentery, and the bowel is now pink. The mesentery is closed over the vein graft, and the abdomen is irrigated with copious warmed saline. The abdominal incision is closed with the skin left open, and the leg incision is closed in multiple layers.

Postoperative Management

Postoperatively, the acuity of monitoring is dependent on the patient's preoperative clinical status and medical comorbidities. All patients should be monitored closely for bowel ischemia, which may be identified by progressive abdominal pain, bloody bowel movements, persistent nausea, vomiting or diarrhea, and hemodynamic instability. Laboratory studies associated to bowel ischemia are also obtained and may include liver function tests, as well as white blood cell counts and serum lactate levels. There should be a low threshold for return to the operating room for a second look if bowel ischemia is entertained.

Patients treated via an endovascular approach will typically have a lower perioperative morbidity and faster recovery. Access sites should be monitored for hematoma development, especially when the brachial artery was used. Endovascular techniques may result in "new" complications, including endoleak resulting from patent collateral vessels, and as such, long-term CTA monitoring of these patients may be necessary and conversion to open may be needed (Table 1).

TABLE 1. SMA Aneurysm Repair

Key Technical Steps

1. Meticulously review a high-resolution angiography study (CTA or conventional) to determine the location of the aneurysms and the mesenteric branches potentially involved in the repair.
2. Elevate the omentum and transverse colon superiorly to find most mesenteric aneurysms; however, some may require a concomitant left-sided approach for access or control.
3. Dissect the artery proximally and distally to aneurysm, taking care to control mesenteric side branches without injuring them.
4. Assess bowel viability for simple ligation with a clamp proximal and distal to the aneurysm. Preferred in cases of unstable rupture.
5. Reconstruction of the SMA is preferred and should be done with aneurysmorrhaphy (with or without patch), or by replacing with greater saphenous vein (or PTFE if no infection or bowel contents exposed).
6. Review the status of the bowel again prior to closure and have a high index of suspicion postoperatively.

Potential Pitfalls

- Failure to carefully dissect the mesenteric side and posterior branches leads to their injury and further damage to collateral flow.
- Inability to find aneurysms located far from the origin of the SMA, especially in a thick or bloody mesentery. You may need to dissect from below (via left or right visceral rotation) or use an intraoperative ultrasound.
- Injury to the duodenum or pancreas from retraction or careless dissection.
- Failure to examine the bowel after vascular intervention and miss intestinal or visceral ischemia.
- Not recognizing a replaced right hepatic artery originating in the proximal SMA. This can lead to potentially devastating liver ischemia when it is ligated or excluded endovascularly.
- Always consider infectious etiologies in patients with recent intra-abdominal infections (diverticulitis, appendicitis, etc.), endocarditis, or young patients and avoid repairs with prosthetic materials.

Case Conclusion

The patient's recovery is complicated by fascial dehiscence that is repaired with primary fascial closure. The patient is ultimately discharged home. Follow-up CT scan shows excellent flow through the bypass graft with no obvious defects or evidence of persistent infection. The patient reports no symptoms of abdominal pain or weight loss and does well through several years follow-up.

TAKE HOME POINTS

- Aneurysms of the SMA are uncommon, and half to two thirds of cases reported are of infectious etiologies.
- Repair should be performed in all symptomatic patients or those rapidly growing and should be considered in aneurysms greater than 2 cm in diameter.
- Nonoperative management may include observation with serial imaging (ultrasound if visible). Antiplatelet agents may be considered in smaller aneurysms, and cases of prohibitive surgical risk to theoretically reduce the risk of embolization and thrombosis.
- Surgical repair may be performed emergently via simple ligation and without mesenteric revascularization or aneurysmorrhaphy. However, reconstruction is preferred to minimize the risk of acute or chronic bowel ischemia.
- Saphenous vein grafts are the conduits of choice for mycotic aneurysms; however, prosthetic grafts have excellent patency when used for elective, noninfected fields.
- Endovascular therapy using covered stents, coil embolization, or "flow diversion" is becoming an increasingly popular option, especially those with prohibitive operative risk. Care must be taken to avoid the exclusion of critical mesenteric side branches and using stent grafts in cases of infection or in vessels with unfavorable anatomy for stenting.
- Bowel ischemia resulting from ligating/covering collateral vessels may result in significant morbidity and mortality, so a high index of suspicion must be kept after open or endovascular procedures.

SUGGESTED READINGS

Cochennec F, Riga CV, Allaire E, et al. Contemporary management of splanchnic and renal artery aneurysms: results of endovascular compared with open surgery from two European vascular centers. *Eur J Vasc Endovasc Surg.* 2011;42:340-346.

Grotemeyer D, Duran M, Park EJ, et al. Visceral artery aneurysms—follow-up of 23 patients with 31 aneurysms after surgical or interventional therapy. *Langenbecks Arch Surg.* 2009;394(6):1093-1100.

Jiang J, Diang X, Su Q, et al. Therapeutic management of superior mesenteric artery aneurysms. *J Vasc Surg.* 2011;53:1619-1624.

Pasha SF, Gloviczki P, Stanson AW, et al. Splanchnic artery aneurysms. *Mayo Clin Proc.* 2007;82(4):472-479.

Tulsyan N, Kashyap VS, Greenberg RK. The endovascular management of visceral artery aneurysms and pseudoaneurysms. *J Vasc Surg.* 2007;45:276-283.

CLINICAL SCENARIO CASE QUESTIONS

1. SMA aneurysms are most likely to have which of the following etiologies?

   a. Mycotic
   b. Atherosclerotic
   c. Connective tissue disease
   d. Pancreatitis
   e. Rheumatologic

2. Management of an unstable, ruptured 3-cm mycotic SMA aneurysm is best done with:

   a. Simple ligation of the involved segment of SMA
   b. Ligation and reconstruction with ilio-SMA bypass with PTFE
   c. Aneurysmorrhaphy by simply trimming the excess aneurysm sac and closing
   d. Saphenous vein interposition graft reconstruction and ligation
   e. Endovascular occlusion with a covered stent graft

82 Celiac Occlusion with Pancreaticoduodenal Aneurysm

AUDRA A. DUNCAN

Presentation

A 68-year-old woman with small bowel obstruction is incidentally found to have a 2.4-cm pancreatico-duodenal artery (PDA) aneurysm on a computed tomography (CT) scan performed for obstruction. Also identified on CT was an asymptomatic celiac artery occlusion due to median arcuate compression. She subsequently underwent abdominal exploration, lysis of adhesions, and bowel resection for the obstruction and remained asymptomatic regarding the PDA aneurysm.

Differential Diagnosis

PDA aneurysms and gastroduodenal aneurysms account for 1.5% to 2% of all splanchnic aneurysms and are frequently associated with pancreatic or biliary tract disease. Diagnosis must include a differentiation between true and false aneurysm because they have different etiologies and varying prognoses. For example, false aneurysm may occur in the setting of pancreatic necrosis, pseudocyst, septic emboli, or iatrogenic trauma from biliary or pancreatic interventions. Therefore, false aneurysms may require management of the primary problem first before or concomitant with aneurysm treatment. The mean age of PDA aneurysms is 50 years old with men:women ratio of 4:1, possibly because of the higher incidence of alcoholic pancreatitis in men. True PDA aneurysms, as in this patient, are less common and occur equally in men and women. It is hypothesized that these aneurysms occur in response to increased flow through pancreatic arcades in the setting of celiac stenosis or occlusion.

Workup

By history, patients with PDA aneurysms are typically asymptomatic or have vague epigastric or abdominal pain radiating to the back. If rupture occurs, as occurs in up to 75% of all PDA aneurysms, the pain can be sudden and severe. Because of the frequency of concomitant pancreatic or biliary tract disease, it is often difficult to differentiate the pain from the aneurysm compared to the pain from the underlying cause. Laboratory values of liver function studies, bilirubin, and pancreas enzymes may help differentiate underlying etiologies.

Diagnosis and Treatment

Although ultrasound may be an appropriate initial study in symptomatic patients, CT scan is often used to identify the anatomy of the biliary tract and visceral arterial anatomy. Many times, asymptomatic PDA aneurysms are identified incidentally, especially true aneurysms. CT angiography (CTA) can help delineate the presence of a celiac artery occlusion or stenosis and its cause (i.e., atherosclerotic vs. median arcuate compression) as well as identifying coexisting pancreatic or gastroduodenal disease (Fig. 1).

Digital subtraction angiography may be used as the first imaging modality in ruptured aneurysms in order to both diagnose and treat the aneurysm at the same time. Angiography may be superior to CT at identifying efferent and afferent arteries (Fig. 2). Inspiration and expiration views of the celiac artery origin with a CTA or angiogram may reinforce the diagnosis of median arcuate compression.

Surgical Approach

Regardless of size, PDA aneurysms should be treated due to the poor correlation between size and rupture risk. A ruptured PDA aneurysm can be treated solely with embolization or surgical ligation to facilitate hemodynamic stability. Open repair has been reported to include partial pancreatectomy or pancreaticoduodenectomy when necessary.

For PDA aneurysm in the setting of celiac stenosis or occlusion, treatment of celiac lesion should precede aneurysm treatment based on the theory that increased blood flow through collaterals is the primary cause (Fig. 3). In addition, the revascularization with bypass or

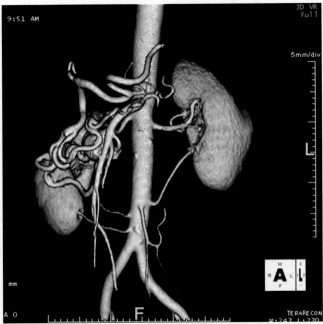

FIGURE 1 • CTA with 3D reconstruction demonstrates an occluded celiac artery origin and 2.4-cm pancreaticoduodenal artery aneurysm.

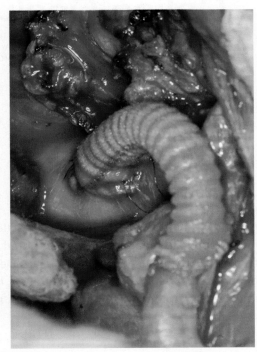

FIGURE 3 • Intraoperative photograph of aorta to common hepatic artery bypass with 7-mm prosthetic graft.

patch angioplasty of the celiac artery provides a pathway to place the endovascular sheath and catheters to treat the aneurysm. Once the celiac artery is reperfused, the PDA aneurysm can typically be coil embolized percutaneously (Fig. 4). Percutaneous and ultrasound-guided thrombin injection of PDA aneurysms may play a role in patients with acute pancreatitis.

Special Intraoperative Considerations

Because of the proximity of the pancreas to the aneurysm, open repair must be undertaken carefully to avoid aggravation of existing pancreatitis or cause de novo pancreatitis. Most authors advocate simple ligation in the

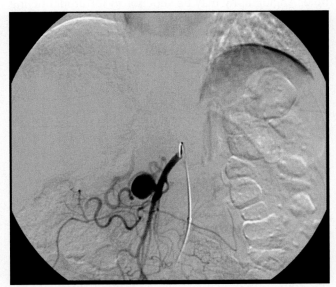

FIGURE 2 • Digital subtraction angiography identifies large PDA aneurysm.

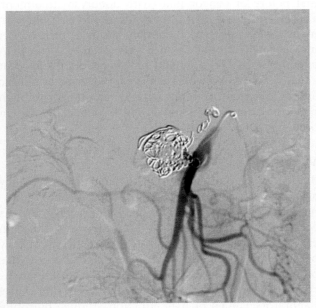

FIGURE 4 • Angiography 2 weeks after operative celiac revascularization, percutaneous coil embolization was successful at occluding flow into the aneurysm and afferent/efferent arteries.

TABLE 1. Key Technical Steps and Potential Pitfalls

Key Technical Steps

1. Percutaneous coil embolization may be facilitated by using a left brachial artery approach.
2. In ruptured PDA aneurysms, rapid control of bleeding can be secured with celiac artery balloon occlusion to stabilize the patient before embolization.
3. Afferent and efferent arteries should be embolized in addition to the aneurysm.
4. Coils are the preferred method of embolization, but liquid embolic material may be used as an adjunct.
5. If open ligation is attempted, involvement of the pancreas should be anticipated and care taken to avoid pancreatic injury.

Potential Pitfalls

- In percutaneous embolization—failure of embolization of inflow and outflow vessels may allow continuous filling of the aneurysm
- In open repair—bleeding, pancreatic leak, biliary tract, or liver injury

setting of rupture (Table 1). There is also some evidence that additional celiac trunk revascularization for true aneurysms may be unnecessary as small series do not demonstrate PDA aneurysm recurrence in the absence of celiac revascularization.

Postoperative Management

Serial imaging of the treated aneurysm and revascularization should be done, as coil-embolized aneurysms can become repressurized by increased flow through collateral arteries. Although ultrasound may identify the aneurysm well, CTA is often more definitive as a follow-up study (Fig. 5).

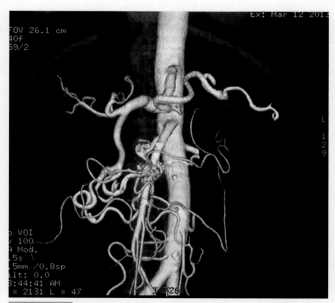

FIGURE 5 • Three months after treatment, CTA with 3D reconstruction demonstrates a patent prosthetic bypass and no flow into the PDA aneurysm.

Case Conclusion

After the patient recovered from her exploratory laparotomy and lysis of adhesions, she underwent a celiac artery revascularization with a supraceliac aorta to proximal common hepatic artery bypass with a 7-mm prosthetic graft. Two weeks later, she had coil embolization of the aneurysm and its outflow vessels, from a right femoral approach through the celiac graft. Completion angiography confirmed occlusion of aneurysm.

TAKE HOME POINTS

- All PDA aneurysms should be treated regardless of size because rupture risk does not correlate with size.
- The mortality of a ruptured PDA aneurysm is approximately 50%.
- Treatment is primarily with coil embolization or ligation, with or without celiac artery revascularization.

SUGGESTED READINGS

Boudghene F, L'Hermine C, Bigot JM, et al. Arterial complications of pancreatitis: diagnostic and therapeutic aspects in 104 cases. *J Vasc Interv Radiol.* 1993;4:551-558.

Gangahar DM, Carveth SW, Reese HE, et al. True aneurysm of the pancreaticoduodenal artery: a case report and review of the literature. *J Vasc Surg.* 1985;2:741-742.

Hildebrand P, Esnaashari H, Franke C, et al. Surgical management of pancreaticoduodenal artery aneurysms in association with celiac trunk occlusion or stenosis. *Ann Vasc Surg.* 2007;21:10-15.

Sutton D, Lawton G. Coeliac stenosis or occlusion with aneurysm of the collateral supply. *Clin Radiol.* 1973;24:49-53.

Teng W, Sarfati MR, Mueller MT, et al. A ruptured pancreaticoduodenal artery aneurysm repaired by combined endovascular and open techniques. *Ann Vasc Surg.* 2006;20: 792-795.

CLINICAL SCENARIO CASE QUESTIONS

1. A 54-year-old women experiences sudden-onset right upper quadrant pain and evidence of rupture of a previously known PDA with a stenotic but patent celiac artery. After stabilization, the most direct route to preventing further bleeding is:

   a. Open repair and supraceliac clamp occlusion
   b. Endoluminal approach with celiac artery balloon occlusion
   c. Endoluminal route with SMA catheterization and retrograde coil occlusion of the gastroduodenal artery

d. Endoluminal approach with covered stent grafting of the PDA

e. Transabdominal CT—guided glue occlusion of the PDA

2. The pathophysiology of PDA is thought to be due to:

a. Inherent genetic connective tissue disease

b. Smoking

c. Gender with women more commonly affected than men

d. High-flow state due to proximal celiac occlusion/stenosis

e. Portal hypertension

83 Hepatic Artery Aneurysm

WILLIAM M. STONE and THOMAS C. BOWER

Presentation

A 65-year-old man is referred for evaluation of celiac and hepatic artery aneurysms. His history dates back 1 year, at which time he underwent emergency operation for a ruptured splenic artery aneurysm. Operation included distal pancreatectomy, splenectomy, and ligation of the splenic artery. The patient currently has no symptoms from his aneurysms. He has not had fevers, weight loss, arthralgias, myalgias, hernia, joint swelling, laxity or dislocation, easy bruisability, visual changes, or lens dislocations, and has no family history of aneurysmal disease dissection, connective tissue disorders, or sudden death. He had a transient ischemic attack (TIA) 10 years ago presumably on the basis of hypertension. His only cardiovascular risk factor besides hypertension is hyperlipidemia. He has never had a myocardial infarction and has no pulmonary or renal problems.

CT imaging at the time of the splenic aneurysm rupture showed a celiac artery that measured approximately 20 mm in diameter. The common and proper hepatic arteries were normal. The left hepatic artery was diminutive. There was a focal dissection in the superior mesenteric artery.

On examination now, he is hypertensive with a blood pressure of 150/97 mm Hg. His heart rate is 69 beats per minute and regular. Examination of his neck, chest, heart, and abdomen is unremarkable. There are no abdominal masses or bruits. He has normal upper and lower extremity pulses, and there is no enlargement of the peripheral pulses.

Laboratory evaluation shows a normal blood count, electrolytes, liver function tests, sedimentation rate, and C-reactive protein. His serum creatinine is normal, as is his urinalysis.

Etiology, Incidence, and Clinical Presentation

The etiology of hepatic artery aneurysms has changed over the years. In the past, mycotic aneurysms were prevalent, whereas now, they are due to atherosclerosis, fibrodysplasia, vasculitis, polyarteritis nodosa, or systemic lupus erythematosus. Rarely, HAA has been seen in patients with Takayasu's arteritis, Kawasaki's disease, von Recklinghausen's neurofibromatosis, and Wegener's granulomatosis. HAA has been reported in patients with long-term oral amphetamine use and connective tissue disorders such as Marfan's and Ehlers-Danlos syndromes, Osler-Weber-Rendu, and hereditary hemorrhagic telangiectasia.

The true incidence of HAA is unknown, but they represent between 10% and 20% of all visceral artery aneurysms. More HAA are being discovered because of the rise in cross-sectional imaging studies. HAA are defined as true or false aneurysms, the latter increasing in frequency because of the growth of minimally invasive diagnostic and therapeutic hepatobiliary procedures. Men are more commonly affected, and time of presentation is in the sixth decade of life. Most patients have aneurysms in an extrahepatic location (75% to 80%). HAA can be solitary or multiple.

Approximately 10% of HAA present with symptoms in the absence of rupture. Most HAA currently detected are asymptomatic (75%). Patients with nonatherosclerotic aneurysms more often present with symptoms of rupture than do those with atherosclerotic HAA.

Assessment and Evaluation

The history does not support a diagnosis of vasculitis, so fibromuscular disease (FMD), segmental arterial mediolysis (SAM), or a connective tissue disorder are the most likely causes of the HAA. FMD and SAM can cause isolated spontaneous dissections of visceral, renal, or carotid arteries, which then can degenerate into aneurysms, sometimes rapidly. These dissections may involve more than one artery at the same presentation or occur at different time intervals.

Decisions for treatment should be based on the pathology of the splenic aneurysm, as it may provide clues as to the etiology of the HAAs; on whether the aneurysms are atherosclerotic or nonatherosclerotic; the size, location, growth rate, and rupture risk of the aneurysms; and the medical risk of the patient. The pathology report is sent, and the histologic analysis suggests medial dysplasia in the artery. The most likely etiology of these aneurysms based on this finding is FMD or SAM, the latter being on a continuum pathologically to FMD.

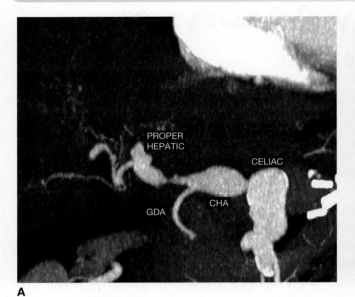
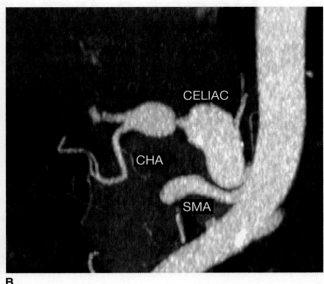

FIGURE 1 • Select CT angiographic images of the patient are shown in **(A** and **B)**. The proximal celiac artery was normal size, but the distal trunk was aneurysmal (23 mm). The common hepatic (CHA) and proper hepatic arteries had become aneurysmal in the past year (17 to 23 mm). The gastroduodenal (GDA) artery is patent, and the superior mesenteric artery (SMA) also is widely patent.

Imaging of the aneurysms has not been done for 1 year, so a new CT of the abdomen and pelvis is performed (Fig. 1). The celiac artery aneurysm has enlarged to 23 mm, and the common hepatic and proper hepatic arteries have become aneurysmal, measuring between 17 and 23 mm in diameter. The proper hepatic aneurysm is in the liver hilum. The right hepatic artery inside the hilar plate is 4 mm in diameter, but the remaining artery is of small caliber and irregular. The left hepatic artery is absent. There are two arteries near the base of the celiac that seem to supply the stomach. Other pertinent findings include a normal-size aorta, mildly dilated iliac arteries, mild dilatation of both renal arteries (8 to 9 mm in diameter), and a stable focal dissection of the superior mesenteric artery. There is no calcification within the walls of any of the aneurysms and no signs of periarterial inflammation, fluid, or air.

Rupture risk of HAA is poorly defined but seems to correlate with size and etiology. Although HAA is rare, and it is difficult to establish a relationship between rupture risk and size, most studies implicate a size greater than 20 mm in diameter as a predictor of rupture. In a large series from Mayo Clinic, the overall incidence of rupture was 14%, lower than other reports. However, of the nine patients who presented with rupture or symptomatic aneurysms, five had a nonatherosclerotic etiology, including fibromuscular dysplasia, polyarteritis nodosa, and infection. All five of these patients had aneurysm rupture, and some of the aneurysms were smaller than 2 cm. Importantly, mortality approaches 40% in patients with rupture. For these reasons, treatment is indicated for nonatherosclerotic or multiple HAA

in most circumstances, regardless of size. Atherosclerotic HAA over 2 cm in diameter in good risk patients should be treated. For older asymptomatic patients in marginal health, with atherosclerotic aneurysms between 2 and 5 cm, treatment remains controversial.

The patient is found to be good risk, with normal cardiac, pulmonary, and renal function. The remote history of TIA may not seem important now, but patients with FMD or SAM can have either intracerebral aneurysms or carotid dissection. An MRI/MRA of the head and neck is unremarkable. Medical genetics evaluation is completed and testing shows no specific connective tissue disorder.

Treatment

Since the etiology of the aneurysms is nonatherosclerotic, there has been new aneurysmal degeneration of the common and proper hepatic arteries since the previous CT, and the celiac and proximal hepatic artery aneurysm exceeds 20 mm, this patient requires treatment. Options for treatment are either open repair or endovascular therapy. Treatment by open repair in a good-risk patient can be done by ligation, resection, endoaneurysmorrhaphy, or reconstruction with a prosthetic or autogenous bypass or interposition graft. Arterial reconstruction with a graft requires an accessible and adequate-sized distal target artery, and a source of inflow. Figure 2 shows an example of such a reconstruction. Endovascular treatment can be done by coil occlusion, or placement of covered stents to exclude the aneurysm, provided the anatomy is appropriate. Durability of covered stents remains to be defined.

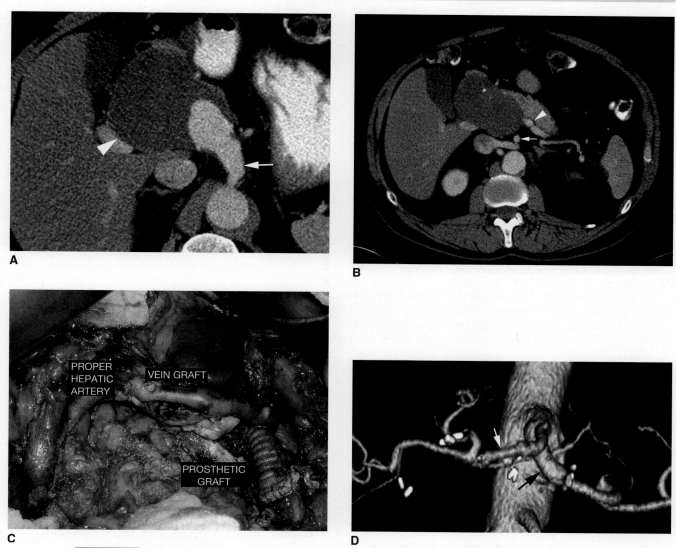

FIGURE 2 • A patient with a huge common hepatic artery aneurysm (9 cm) as shown in the CT images **(A,B)**. The proximal celiac artery is aneurysmal as shown by the *arrow* in **(A)**. The *arrow head* shows the caudal extent of the aneurysm, compressing the portal vein. In **(B)**, the splenic artery is normal sized (*arrowhead*), and the superior mesenteric artery is widely patent (*arrow*). The patient was reconstructed with a prosthetic graft from the supraceliac aorta to the splenic artery. A reverse vein graft was placed to the proper hepatic artery, with a distal anastomosis of that graft done with interrupted suture **(C)**. Postoperative CTA **(D)** shows a widely patent prosthetic graft to the splenic artery (*black arrow*) and vein graft to the proper hepatic artery (*white arrow*). The right and left hepatic arteries are seen.

Bypass in this patient will be difficult because the right hepatic artery would have to be accessed within the liver parenchyma, and outflow is poor. Similarly, the use of a covered stent is not possible in this patient. However, coil occlusion of the aneurysms is an option. Embolization plays an important role in the management of intrahepatic aneurysms, high-risk surgical candidates, and those in whom postprocedure liver dysfunction is felt to be low. The primary concerns with this intervention are hepatic ischemia, changes in liver function, and, in this patient, preservation of blood flow to the stomach. The latter is important because collateral blood supply to the stomach has been compromised by the splenic artery ligation and the distal pancreatectomy. Since the portal vein will be the primary supply of oxygen to the liver if the arteries are coiled, an ultrasound scan of the portal and hepatic veins is done. The study shows the portal vein blood flow to be antegrade toward the liver and the hepatic veins to be normal. Therefore, the potential for significant liver dysfunction with coil occlusion of the aneurysms ought to be low, especially because his liver function is normal despite poor intrahepatic arterial architecture.

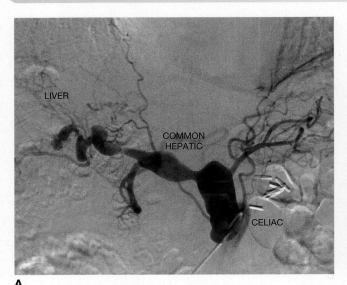

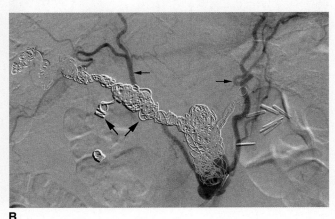

FIGURE 3 • Arteriographic images of the aneurysms before **(A)** and after **(B)** coil embolization. Note the poor intrahepatic arterial architecture. Image **(B)** shows the coils in the celiac, common hepatic, common proper hepatic, and gastroduodenal artery, illustrated in part by the *larger arrows*. Two proximal branches of the celiac artery that supply blood to the stomach were preserved (*small arrows*).

Case Conclusion

The patient undergoes successful coil occlusion of all the aneurysms as shown in Figure 3. Blood flow through the two proximal arteries originating from the celiac is preserved. The patient is monitored overnight in the hospital and has no postprocedure problems. The morning after the intervention, he has no fever, his abdomen is flat, soft and nontender, and liver function studies are normal. Follow-up 1 year later shows no recanalization of the aneurysms.

TABLE 1. Percutaneous Hepatic Aneurysm Treatment

Key Technical Steps

1. Percutaneous access and anticoagulation
2. Hepatic arterial cannulation
3. Diagnostic angiography
4. Confirm anatomy; coil embolization, possibly covered stent placement
5. Completion arteriogram

Potential Pitfalls

- Consider preprocedure imaging of both arterial and portal venous patency
- Avoid occluding important collateral flow
- Stent occlusion, severe liver ischemia

Whether a patient undergoes coil occlusion or open surgical treatment of an HAA, monitoring of liver function and/or an inflammatory response is important. The treated segment needs to be monitored for recanalization if the patient has been treated with coil occlusion of the aneurysm, or graft surveillance if reconstruction is done with a vein or prosthetic graft (Table 1).

TAKE HOME POINTS

- Hepatic artery aneurysms are rare but represent the second most common cause of visceral artery aneurysm.
- HAA can be true or false, with the latter increasing in frequency because of the higher number of hepatobiliary procedures being performed.
- The etiology of HAA has changed over the years, from mycotic to more atherosclerotic and nonatherosclerotic causes. Patients with multiple visceral aneurysms should be screened for a connective tissue disorder, active or burned out vasculitis, FMD, or SAM (SAM is a diagnosis by exclusion).
- Rupture risk seems to correlate with a size diameter greater than 2 cm or to nonatherosclerotic etiology. The latter group faces a high risk of rupture, so most patients with these aneurysms should be treated regardless of size.
- Treatment options include open or endovascular techniques. Open treatment includes ligation, excision, or reconstruction by a prosthetic or venous bypass graft, depending on the quality of the target artery. Embolization is preferred for intrahepatic aneurysms,

medically high-risk patients, or those with low risk of liver complications. Covered stent grafts may be used in select patients with appropriate anatomy.

SUGGESTED READINGS

Abbas MA, Fowl RJ, Stone WM, et al. Hepatic artery aneurysm: factors that predict complications. *J Vasc Surg.* 2003;38(1):41-45.

Christie AB, Christie DB, Nakayama DK, et al. Hepatic artery aneurysms: evolution from open to endovascular techniques. *Am Surg.* 2011;77:608-611.

Hulsberg P, De La Garza-Jordan J, Jordan R, et al. Hepatic artery aneurysm: a review. *Am Surg.* 2011;77:586-591.

Lal RB, Strohl JA, Piazza S, et al. Hepatic artery aneurysm. *J Cardiovasc Surg.* 1989;30(3):509-513.

Salcuni PF, Spaggiari L, Tecchio T, et al. Hepatic artery aneurysm: an ever present danger. *J Cardiovasc Surg.* 1995;36:595-599.

Saltzberg SS, Maldonado TS, Lamparello PJ, et al. Is endovascular therapy the preferred treatment for all visceral artery aneurysms? *Ann Vasc Surg.* 2005;19:507-515.

Tarazov PG, Ryzhkov VK, Polysalov VN, et al. Extraorganic hepatic artery aneurysm: failure of transcatheter embolization. *HPB Surg.* 1998;11(1):55-60.

Tessier DJ, Fowl RJ, Stone WM, et al. Iatrogenic hepatic artery pseudoaneurysms: an uncommon complication after hepatic, biliary, and pancreatic procedures. *Ann Vasc Surg.* 2003;17:663-669.

CLINICAL SCENARIO CASE QUESTIONS

1. An 80-year-old man is referred for evaluation of a 2.8-cm circumferentially calcified common hepatic artery. He is asymptomatic, has poor cardiac function, and has neither family history of aneurysms nor clinical evidence of aneurysms in other territories. A review of ultrasound and CT scans dating back 3 years shows no change in the size of the aneurysm.
Appropriate treatment is:

a. Surgical resection of the aneurysm and replacement with a prosthetic interposition graft
b. Surgical resection of the aneurysm and replacement with a vein interposition graft
c. Exclusion of the aneurysm with a covered stent
d. Continued observation

2. A 55-year-old is referred because of an enlarging but asymptomatic 5-cm common hepatic artery aneurysm. The aneurysm has grown in size by 2 cm over the past year. The aneurysm is noncalcified. CT imaging shows an aneurysm isolated to the common hepatic artery with a normal celiac artery trunk and normal intrahepatic vasculature. The gastroduodenal artery cannot be seen. The patient has no significant cardiopulmonary, renal, or liver abnormalities.
Which of the following is the best treatment option?

a. Resection of the hepatic artery aneurysm and reconstruction using a saphenous vein interposition graft between the celiac and proper hepatic arteries
b. Coil occlusion of the celiac, splenic, and hepatic arteries
c. Superior mesenteric to proper hepatic artery bypass graft
d. Placement of a covered stent from the celiac artery into the proper hepatic artery with coil occlusion of all other celiac artery branches

84 PVOD Medical Management

M. ASHRAF MANSOUR

Presentation

A 71-year-old man is sent to the vascular office by his Primary Care Physician because of absent pedal pulses and an abnormal CT of the chest that demonstrated a left subclavian stenosis. The patient is a former smoker (25 pack-years) with a history of hypertension and hyperlipidemia. He complains of bilateral calf cramping when walking, especially on an incline. He does not have any arm symptoms or dizziness with head turning. He denies angina with exertion. He denies rest pain or ulcers on the feet. He does have mild dyspnea with exertion.

Differential Diagnosis

Patients who complain of intermittent claudication, described as a cramp-like feeling in the calf that starts after walking and subsides with rest, should be suspected of having peripheral vascular occlusive disease (PVOD). It is important to ask if the symptoms are unilateral or bilateral. Patients with the classic risk factors for PVOD, including smoking, hypertension, and hyperlipidemia, will invariably have either aortoiliac or femoropopliteal occlusive disease. Other less common vascular conditions include thrombosed popliteal aneurysm, popliteal entrapment, or cystic adventitial disease of the popliteal artery. Nonvascular conditions mimicking claudication include neurogenic claudication (compression of lumbar nerves) and venous claudication (due to iliac vein stenosis or occlusion).

Workup

A good clinician can identify many clues about the location and extent of PVOD. For example, a diminished femoral pulse leads to a suspicion for iliac occlusive disease.

A complete physical examination should include palpation of all the peripheral pulses. An ankle-brachial index (ABI) should be obtained in the office, ideally with segmental arterial pressures and waveforms (Fig. 1). In some vascular laboratories, an arterial duplex mapping can be performed to image the lower extremity arterial tree. This is time consuming and requires a proficient vascular technologist performing the test.

More invasive imaging, such as computed tomography angiography (CTA) or magnetic resonance angiography (MRA), will require intravenous administration of contrast material (Isovue for CTA and gadolinium for MRA) both of which are contraindicated in patients with renal insufficiency. Digital subtraction angiography is also invasive since it involves intra-arterial injection of contrast and imaging in a Cath Lab or Endovascular Suite. In general, more invasive studies are obtained in cases where some intervention is being planned and not as screening tests.

Discussion

Claudication due to PVOD is a very common vascular problem. It is estimated that 10 to 12 million individuals in the United States suffer from claudication. There are many risk factors that contribute to PVOD, and they include tobacco use, hypertension, hyperlipidemia, and diabetes. The clinician who evaluates a patient with claudication must consider the patient as a whole, including the medical management of risk factors, and decide on the goals of therapy. It is unlikely that an elderly, obese patient with a sedentary life style will benefit significantly from an intervention aimed at improving the ABI.

Diagnosis and Treatment

The diagnosis of PVOD is established when the clinical findings on physical examination and noninvasive testing correlate with the patient's symptoms. With the widespread use of CTA, there are many patients who have evidence of PVOD but are not particularly symptomatic. Conversely, a patient may present with classic symptoms

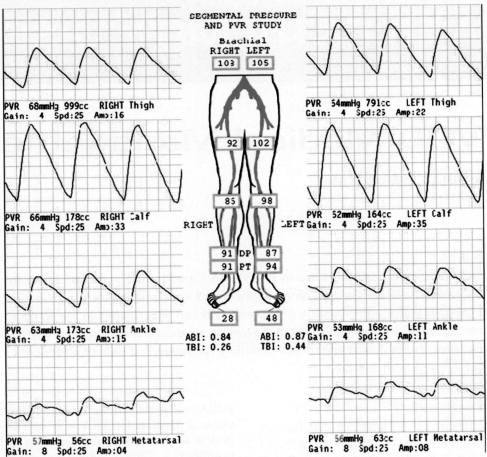

FIGURE 1 • Segmental arterial pressures and pulse volume recordings from a patient with mild claudication. Normal ABI is >0.94. This test suggests mild femoropopliteal occlusive disease.

of calf claudication, and yet palpable pedal pulses are present on exam. In the latter case, an exercise stress test is needed to confirm the diagnosis. If the ABIs are normal at rest, drop with treadmill walking, and return to baseline after a period of rest, the test is considered positive. Conversely, if the ABIs do not drop with walking, the test is considered negative.

The management of PVOD depends on the severity of symptoms and the disease. For example, a patient presenting with toe gangrene will require a more aggressive and urgent approach compared to a patient with three- to four-block calf claudication. In general, the management of PVOD will involve one or more of these three broad categories: medical, endovascular, and surgical management.

Medical Management

In most vascular patients, atherosclerotic changes are not confined to the peripheral vascular circulation. In fact, PVOD is a marker for cardiovascular complications (such as stroke and myocardial infarction) and death. Therefore, it is important to initiate medical management of all patients with PVOD (regardless of whether or not an intervention is planned). The cornerstone is primarily risk factor modification and counseling for a healthier lifestyle.

Risk factor modification includes smoking cessation, controlling hypertension, hyperlipidemia, and diabetes. Using an ACE inhibitor and lipid-lowering agents has been found to be beneficial to patients with PVOD. Similarly, aspirin (80 to 100 mg) daily is beneficial. The specific goals of medical management include maintaining a blood pressure of less than 140/90 mm Hg, LDL cholesterol level less than 100 mg/dL (although newer guidelines suggest not necessarily treating to a goal reduction), and hemoglobin A1c < 7.0%.

Cilostazol (Pletal) is a drug that has been approved for the treatment of intermittent claudication. It acts by a dual mechanism of platelet inhibition and peripheral vasodilation; it is a phosphodiesterase III inhibitor. However, this agent cannot be used in those with low ejection fractions (EF less than 30%) or with a history of Congestive Heart Failure.

In addition to prescribing medications, the physician should counsel patients to lose weight, adopt a Mediterranean diet, exercise regularly, and embrace a generally healthier lifestyle, although the evidence that these changes affect PVOD progression is lacking.

Long-Term Management

As previously mentioned, the long-term goals of treating patients with PVOD are to improve their symptoms and decrease the risk of cardiovascular complications, including myocardial infarction and stroke, and limb loss. It is paramount to convince patients that they need to adopt a healthy lifestyle and shun bad habits, such as smoking, excessive alcohol consumption, and a fatty diet. Indeed, smoking cessation is one of the most important changes a patient can make. Many studies have shown that regular supervised exercise, daily walking, can significantly improve the symptoms of PVOD. With a proper exercise regimen, patients are able to increase their walking distance and generally feel better.

Case Conclusion

The patient started a regular walking program with the help of his wife, with a goal to walk for 25 minutes at least five times a week. Cilostazol was started. At 3 months, the patient reported significant relief of his symptoms.

TAKE HOME POINTS

- The role of the treating physician is primarily to educate the patients and recommend a series of actions that are aimed at improving their symptoms and decreasing their risk of mortality and limb loss.
- Consider ASA, statins, and ACEI in all patients with PVOD.
- Consider cilostazol in patients for claudication symptoms.
- Smoking cessation is paramount.

SUGGESTED READINGS

Alonso-Coello P, Bellmunt S, McGorrian C, et al. Antithrombotic therapy in peripheral artery disease. *Chest.* 2013;141:669s-682s.

Ardati AK, Kaufman SR, Aronow HD, et al. The quality and impact of risk factor control in patients with stable claudication presenting for peripheral vascular interventions. *Circ Cardiovasc Interv.* 2013;5:850-855.

Dawson DL, Cutler BS, Meissner MH, et al. Cilostazol has beneficial effects in treatment of intermittent claudication. *Circulation.* 1998;98:678-686.

Gardner AW, Parker DE, Montgomery PS, et al. Efficacy of quantified home-based exercise and supervised exercise in patients with intermittent claudication: a randomized controlled trial. *Circulation.* 2011;123:491-498.

Murphy TP, Cutlip DE, Regensteiner JG, et al. Supervised exercise versus primary stenting for claudication resulting from aortoiliac peripheral artery disease: six months outcomes from the claudication: exercise versus endoluminal revascularization (CLEVER) study. *Circulation* 2012;125:130-139.

Norgren L, Hiatt WR, Dormandy JA, et al. Inter-society consensus for the management of peripheral arterial disease (TASC II). *J Vasc Surg.* 2007;45:S5A-S67A.

CLINICAL SCENARIO CASE QUESTIONS

1. A 70-year-old man presents with moderately limiting claudication. He has diabetes, hyperlipidemia, and hypertension and is a current smoker. He is on an aspirin and beta-blocker. The first most important step in his management is:

   a. Make sure his HbA1C is less than 7 mg/dL; refer to endocrinologist
   b. Begin a statin agent
   c. Begin an ACEI
   d. Counsel him to stop smoking immediately
   e. Begin Pletal

2. A new patient is referred to you for medical management of claudication. The agent with most evidence for specifically reducing claudication is:

   a. Trental
   b. Low-dose aspirin
   c. Ramipril
   d. Clopidogrel
   e. Cilostazol

PVOD with Claudication (SFA Stent)

GEORGE H. MEIER

Presentation

A 67-year-old male smoker presents to your office for evaluation of increasing pain in the right calf with walking. This was gradual in onset, beginning about 4 months ago, but has not resolved and continues to limit his daily activities. Initially, he thought that he had injured himself playing softball, but the pain has persisted. The "tightness" in his right calf is worse when he climbs stairs or when he is in a hurry. If he stops and stands in place, the discomfort resolves in a few minutes and he can resume walking. He has no other symptoms but does have a past history of hypertension and rare exertional chest pain. His examination demonstrates normal pulses in the left lower extremity with only a femoral pulse on the right side. He has no ulcerations or skin changes, and there is no dependent rubor.

Differential Diagnosis

Any symptom of exertional discomfort in the leg carries with it a differential diagnosis of not only peripheral arterial disease (PAD) but also musculoskeletal injury and lumbar radiculopathy. Smoking not only increases the risk of PAD but also increases the risk of lumbar disc disease. Neurogenic pseudoclaudication is a common diagnosis in this population and would be high in the differential diagnosis.

Generally, workup of the lumbar spine for causes of lower extremity pain is unwarranted unless lower back symptoms predominate. If necessary, plain x-rays of the lumbar spine, spinal CT, and spinal MRA all have some utility in this population. For most patients, plain x-rays of the lumbar spine are sufficient prior to any consideration of referral for evaluation for disc disease or bony impingement syndromes.

Rarer diagnoses are sometimes seen in younger patients due to muscular entrapment of the popliteal artery. In these settings, exertional pain in the calf may occur without atherosclerosis. If this is suspected, axial MRA can be performed and will demonstrate medial deviation of the popliteal artery around the muscles of the calf. Most commonly, the popliteal artery is medial to the medial head of the gastrocnemius muscle, leading to compression of the artery with tightening of the calf muscles.

Workup

The evaluation really begins with the physical examination. Most of the decisions concerning diagnostic testing start with an evaluation of the femoral pulses. If the femoral pulse to the symptomatic extremity is normal, then the occlusive arterial disease is likely confined to the infrainguinal vessels. If the femoral pulse is abnormal, then evaluation of the abdominal aorta and iliac vessels will also be needed.

Initial evaluation for exertional lower extremity symptoms, particularly with an abnormal pulse examination, should include baseline arterial noninvasive vascular testing. While most patients require only an ankle-brachial index to document the presence of significant vascular disease, a minority will require treadmill exercise testing with ankle-brachial index (ABI) measured before and after exercise. These patients may have normal circulation at rest but have a significant decrement in pulses and ABI under the stress of exercise.

With inflow disease, CTA is useful in the differential diagnosis of lower extremity claudication. Most commonly, this is in the setting of abnormal inflow to the lower extremity as represented by an abnormal femoral pulse. CTA provides anatomic information about the aorta and iliac vessels that can be used to then plan subsequent management. Alternatively, duplex ultrasound mapping of the aorta and iliac vessels can be performed to limit dye and radiation exposure.

Ultimately, the diagnostic test of choice will be an abdominal aortogram with bilateral runoff arteriography (Figs. 1 and 2). Whether this is done at the same time as an intervention, or at a separate setting, is up to the discretion of the interventionalist in conjunction with the patient's wishes.

Diagnosis and Treatment

With this history, the leading diagnosis is intermittent claudication due to arterial vascular insufficiency. Since the most common risk factor for claudication remains

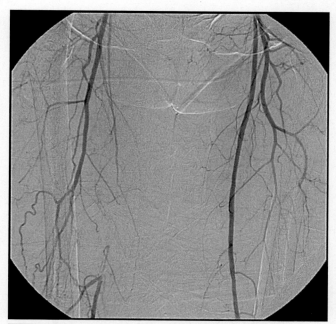

FIGURE 1 • Right superficial femoral artery occlusion.

cigarette smoking, initial management is smoking cessation, risk factor modification, and an exercise program of daily walking.

Risk factors for PAD include smoking, diabetes, hyperlipidemia, and a sedentary lifestyle. For this reason, the above initial management is generally appropriate. Goal for diabetic control is generally an HgbA1C

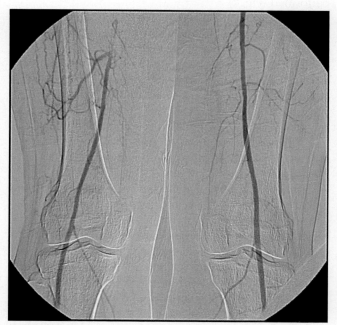

FIGURE 2 • Reconstitution of the above-knee popliteal artery in the same patient.

of less than 7%. Medically, all patients should be started on low-dose aspirin and a statin, both of which have a benefit relative to coronary events. While hypertension is a significant cardiac risk factor, hypertension is at most a minor risk factor for PAD. Control of hypertension is important nonetheless for lowering risk of a cardiac event.

Most atherosclerotic vascular disease is a systemic process, with coronary and cerebral involvement the norm. Since atherosclerosis is generally progressive over time, most treatment is initially focused on temporizing and controlling the symptoms. A daily walking program is effective at increasing exercise tolerance and decreasing leg symptoms. Generally, the disease remains stable for many years before progression may occur. In those patients with an ABI below 0.5, the risk of intervention is sufficiently high so that this should be discussed with the patient at that time in most cases.

While some medical therapies can alter the severity of PAD symptoms, it is unclear when these should be applied. Pentoxifylline has been used for many years but has only a modest benefit in patients with vasculogenic claudication. More appropriately, cilostazol seems to better improve walking ability but is generally contraindicated in patients with heart failure. Finally, ramipril, an ACE inhibitor, has been shown to improve walking distance in patients with PAD and may be an appropriate drug to consider in a PAD patient with hypertension.

Interventional Approach

The fundamental issue in the treatment of lower extremity claudication is the differentiation of inflow disease from outflow disease. Initial diagnostic arteriography including the abdominal aortic and iliac systems is essential to defining any abnormalities in the inflow arteries. If any aorta or iliac abnormalities are present, treatment of these issues should precede any treatment of outflow disease. Typically, open or endovascular treatment of iliac disease also tends to be more durable than treatment of lower extremity disease.

One of the challenges of performing diagnostic testing at the time of possible treatment is the need for immediate decision making during the procedure. If extensive inflow atherosclerosis is seen in the aorta, then this may necessitate open surgery. Iliac disease on the other hand usually requires endovascular treatment either prior to superficial femoral artery intervention or at the same time. In some cases, the presence of significant disease in the common femoral artery may require open intervention either at the time of the endovascular procedure (hybrid approach) or preceding endovascular treatment. If at any point the decision making is uncertain, delaying the intervention for further discussion or evaluation is warranted (Table 1).

TABLE 1. Endovascular SFA Treatment

Key Technical Steps

1. Complete angiography documenting the inflow and outflow from the diseased arterial segment
2. Wire traversal of the diseased segment, either within the lumen or subintimal, using a loop of wire as needed
3. Reentry into the normal outflow artery
4. Balloon angioplasty of the diseased segment of artery
5. Stent placement for arterial recoil with >30% residual stenosis

Potential Pitfalls

- Failed crossing of the diseased arterial segment
- Failed reentry into the true lumen after subintimal lesion transversal
- Significant extravasation of contrast from the artery
- Severe calcific residual stenosis limiting lumen of treated artery

Special Intraoperative Considerations

With complete occlusions of the superficial femoral artery, it is often impossible to cross the diseased arterial segment within the native arterial lumen. In this setting, subintimal wire dissection has been shown to be a viable alternative to intraluminal wire traversal. In this technique, the wire is intentionally passed into the subintimal space underneath the plaque (Fig. 3). In what is normally

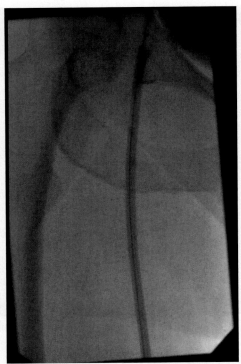

FIGURE 4 • Balloon angioplasty of right superficial femoral artery.

a traditional endarterectomy plane, the wire is allowed to traverse the diseased segment until it underlies a relatively normal lumen. Often a loop of wire is used to help keep the dissection within the main arterial tree. After the lesion is crossed, conventional balloon angioplasty is performed (Fig. 4).

Once adjacent to a relatively normal appearing arterial lumen, subintimal angioplasty requires reentry into the distal normal lumen to restore flow to the distal vascular tree. This reentry is often the major limitation associated with subintimal angioplasty. Technically, this is the most challenging portion of the intervention since reentry can be difficult if the atherosclerotic plaque remains thick or calcified. Fortunately, in the majority of cases, this reentry occurs at natural "feathering" points where the plaque thins as the arterial lumen begins to normalize.

If reentry cannot be achieved using guide wires and catheters, two options exist. First, reentry devices specifically for that purpose can be utilized to reenter the distal normal lumen. Devices such as the Outback catheter can be used to direct the needle back into the true lumen from the subintimal space. While these devices do add cost to the procedure, they can be invaluable in situations where true lumen reentry is otherwise challenging.

Second, distal arterial access from a pedal artery can be used as retrograde traversal can often be much easier

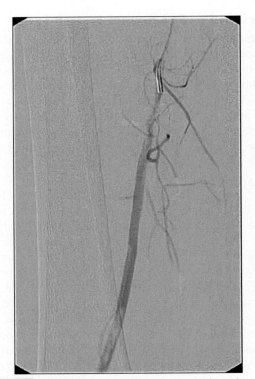

FIGURE 3 • Catheter traversal and reentry into the distal true lumen using a catheter.

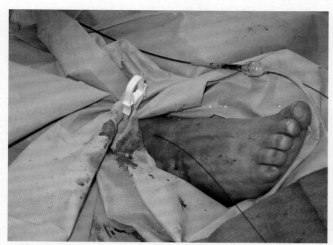

FIGURE 5 • Left femoral and right dorsalis pedis through-and-through arterial access to treat a right superficial femoral artery occlusion.

than antegrade (Fig. 5). While this ultrasound-guided retrograde entry can be tricky, with experience, this is often a relatively simple solution to a difficult reentry from the subintimal space.

Anticoagulation during the procedure is usually performed using unfractionated heparin but usually requires monitoring for adequacy during the procedure. Alternatively, bivalirudin can be used to provide a more rapidly reversible agent for these procedures.

During this portion of the procedure, extravasation from the artery can occur. When extravasation occurs, there are generally two issues. First, a risk of bleeding arises that must be limited. This is generally achieved by limiting the inflow to the segment, avoiding proximal angioplasty until an outflow channel is achieved. Only then is opening of the inflow channel completed. Second, the contrast extravasation can limit fluoroscopic visualization. Generally, half-strength contrast is used for the procedure, but if concerns for extravasation are present, this is further diluted to 1:4 contrast to saline. Generally, quarter-strength contrast is sufficiently dilute to allow fluoroscopic visualization through the area of extravasation.

Postoperative Management

The major issue in postprocedural management is the management of the puncture site into the artery. Like any angiogram, the size of the sheath used for access determines the risk of complications. In most cases, femoral access for interventional treatment requires the use of a 6-French sheath. The risk of complications with this access is minimal but increases with the use of anticoagulation.

Rarely, embolization of plaque or clot can occur, usually related to inadequate anticoagulation. During the procedure, routine anticoagulation is used to minimize the risk of clot formation, with a continuous infusion of agent or laboratory monitoring to ensure adequacy of anticoagulation.

Typically, no ultrasound or noninvasive surveillance is necessary after an angiogram other than a baseline ankle-brachial index measurement to document the postprocedure lower extremity arterial perfusion. If a significant hematoma is present at the access site, a duplex ultrasound to assess for the presence of a puncture site false aneurysm may be necessary.

Case Conclusion

The patient was felt to be a reasonable candidate for endovascular approach to treating his severe claudication. As shown in the figures above, he underwent successful recanalization and stenting of his right SFA. He was placed on periprocedural clopedigrel. At 6 months, he remained free of claudication symptoms and was in an exercise program.

TAKE HOME POINTS

- Vasculogenic claudication secondary to atherosclerosis is common in smokers.
- Initial management of claudication should consist of risk factor modification and an exercise program of daily walking.
- Treatment of vasculogenic claudication should be individualized based on the patient's symptoms and lifestyle.
- The endovascular treatment of a chronic SFA occlusion with claudication will generally require subintimal angioplasty and possible stent placement.
- Distal arterial access or a reentry device may be required to complete subintimal angioplasty in some patients.

SUGGESTED READINGS

Ahimastos AA, Pappas EP, Buttner PG, et al. A meta-analysis of the outcome of endovascular and noninvasive therapies in the treatment of intermittent claudication. *J Vasc Surg.* 2011;54(5):1511-1521.

Fakhry F, van de Luijtgaarden KM, Bax L, et al. Supervised walking therapy in patients with intermittent claudication. *J Vasc Surg.* 2012;56(4):1132-1142.

Fokkenrood HJ, Bendermacher BL, Lauret GJ, et al. Supervised exercise therapy versus non-supervised exercise therapy for intermittent claudication. *Cochrane Database Syst Rev.* 2013;(8):CD005263.

Frans FA, Bipat S, Reekers JA, et al. Systematic review of exercise training or percutaneous transluminal angioplasty for intermittent claudication. *Br J Surg.* 2012;99(1):16-28.

Jens S, Conijn AP, Koelemay MJ, et al. Randomized trials for endovascular treatment of infrainguinal arterial disease: systematic review and meta-analysis (Part 1: Above the knee). *Eur J Vasc Endovasc Surg.* 2014;47(5):524-535.

Lee C, Nelson PR. Effect of cilostazol prescribed in a pragmatic treatment program for intermittent claudication. *Vasc Endovascular Surg.* 2014;48(3):224-229.

Liu J, Wu Y, Li Z, et al. Endovascular treatment for intermittent claudication in patients with peripheral arterial disease: a systematic review. *Ann Vasc Surg.* 2013;14:pii: S0890-5096(13)00675-4.

Vodnala D, Rajagopalan S, Brook RD. Medical management of the patient with intermittent claudication. *Cardiol Clin.* 2011;29(3):363-379.

CLINICAL SCENARIO CLOSING QUESTIONS

1. Risk factors for lower extremity vasculogenic claudication include all of the following *except*:

   a. Hypertension
   b. Smoking
   c. Sedentary lifestyle
   d. Diabetes
   e. Obesity

2. Management of lower extremity vasculogenic claudication includes all of the following *except*:

   a. Exercise program
   b. Medical therapy such as cilostazol
   c. Anticoagulation
   d. Intervention, either surgery or endovascular
   e. Smoking cessation

86 Peripheral Vascular Disease with Claudication (Open Femoral Popliteal Bypass)

SUKGU M. HAN and CHRISTOPHER D. OWENS

Presentation

A 65-year-old male with a history of diabetes mellitus, hypertension, and a 30-pack-year history of smoking presents with pain in his left leg with walking. The patient describes the pain as dull aches, localized to the calf, and relieved with rest. He denies pain at rest or ulcers on his legs or feet. The pain started 8 months ago and has progressed in severity. During this time, walking distance at which the calf pain starts has progressively decreased to less than one block. On physical exam, he has normal bilateral femoral pulses, and faintly palpable right popliteal, dorsalis pedis, and posterior tibial pulses. On the left, pulses at the popliteal artery and below are absent. Only faint monophasic Doppler signals are detectable at his feet.

Differential Diagnosis

This patient presents with a classic description of lower extremity claudication from peripheral vascular disease (PVD): pain in the calf, reproducibly provoked by walking, and relieved with rest. Patients with claudication typically describe a sense of heaviness, weakness, or fatigue accompanying the pain. Occasionally, the exact cause of lower extremity pain becomes difficult to determine in patients with PVD, who also have neuropathy or radiculopathy from concomitant diabetes and spinal stenosis, respectively. Neuropathic pain is often described as a sharp, shooting, or burning sensation, while radiculopathy is worsened with prolonged sitting and is associated with particular position.

Workup

This patient's history and physical examination suggest arterial insufficiency as the most likely cause of his leg pain. Physical examination does not reveal lower back pain, or any maneuvers that elicit pain, which makes radiculopathy associated with spinal stenosis a less likely etiology.

The patient undergoes bilateral lower extremity arterial duplex ultrasound. His ankle-brachial indices (ABIs) are 0.9 and 0.75 on right and left, respectively. Noninvasive vascular laboratory studies allow dynamic quantitative assessment of lower extremity perfusion. Normal ABIs are greater than 1.0, while values less than 0.9 often correlate with claudication, and less than 0.7 with critical limb ischemia. In patients with long-standing diabetes mellitus or renal failure, where medial calcific sclerosis may be present in pedal arteries, their ABI values can be falsely elevated due to noncompressible vessels. In these instances, toe-brachial index (TBI) or percutaneous oxygen tension ($tcPO_2$) is used as a more reliable indicator of leg perfusion. In cases where claudication is strongly suspected with normal resting ABIs, exercise can induce a drop in ABIs by increasing flow across a given lesion. The abnormal ABIs in the setting of this patient's vascular examination suggest PVD as the most likely cause of pain. In addition to ABIs, duplex ultrasound can further characterize the stenosis by directly visualizing the plaque on gray-scale B-mode image and assessing the pulse wave form across the lesion on color-flow Doppler mode (Fig. 1). The degree of stenosis can be quantified by the elevation of peak systolic velocity (PSV) and broadening of the velocity waveforms across the lesion in the arterial segment. Typically, doubling of PSV compared to adjacent nondiseased arterial segment or PSV above 200 cm/s corresponds to greater than 50% luminal stenosis. Reconstituted arterial flow downstream to a complete occlusion shows blunted, monophasic waveforms with low PSV.

Anatomical evaluation of this patient's disease is traditionally done by angiography, with arterial access obtained typically at the contralateral groin. This patient's angiography (Fig. 2) shows chronic total occlusion of the superficial femoral artery with extensive collateral circulation arising from the profunda femoris reconstituting the popliteal artery below the knee. The popliteal artery gives branches to anterior and posterior tibial arteries. Some centers utilize CT angiogram (CTA) as the initial imaging study of choice. While CTA has the advantage of not requiring an arterial puncture, a detailed evaluation of infrapopliteal lesions is limited due to artifacts from calcification. In addition, formal angiography allows one to treat the lesion with balloon angioplasty or stenting in the same setting when appropriate.

Diagnosis and Treatment

Claudication due to superficial femoral artery lesion typically occurs at the calf and presents as tightness, fatigue, and pain with walking. Typically, one experiences claudication symptoms in the one muscle group below the level of disease. Natural course of the limb affected by claudication is relatively benign with low risk of progression to critical limb ischemia (less than 5%) and amputation

(1% at 5 years). However, claudication is a marker of the systemic atherosclerotic process and carries significantly increased risk of cardiovascular events by two to three times compared to age-matched controls. This cardiovascular disease burden poses a potential increased risk associated with intervention in these patients, when compared to general population without PVD. Therefore, the initial management of claudication consists of risk factor modification such as smoking cessation, diabetes control, and structured, supervised exercise walking program. Supervised exercise walking program, in particular, is thought to improve walking distance by inducing muscle cell adaptation to decreased oxygen delivery.

Given the relatively benign natural course of intermittent claudication, revascularization is reserved for

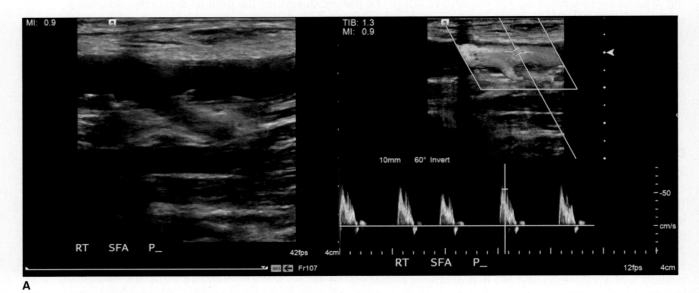

A

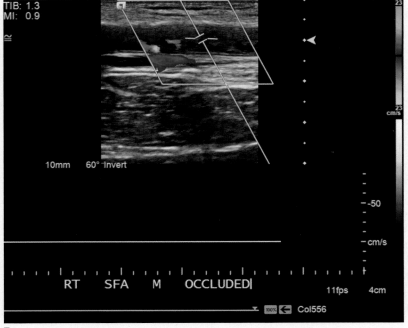

B

FIGURE 1 • **A:** Proximal superficial femoral artery with non–flow-limiting stenosis with normal pulse wave form. **B:** Complete occlusion of mid SFA.

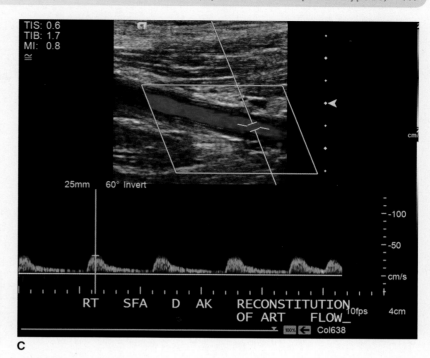

FIGURE 1 • (*Continued*) **C:** Monophasic flow seen in the distal SFA.

patients with debilitating symptoms, only after a trial of an optimized medical treatment. The cornerstone for treatment is cardiovascular risk factor reduction and smoking cessation. Optimal medical management should include a statin and aspirin. The perioperative risks as well as potential consequences of a failed revascularization on the claudicating limb would have to be considered against disability of claudication and the likelihood of symptom relief from the procedure. Namely, these consequences include neointimal hyperplasia at

the sites of intervention, and in the worst-case scenario, limb-threatening ischemia, caused by occlusion of stent or bypass graft itself.

In general, revascularization can be achieved by endovascular approach, open bypass, or a combination of both. While open bypass with autogenous vein conduit is thought to have the best long-term patency, the less invasive nature of endovascular therapy provides an attractive alternative in select cases. The decision-making process regarding the optimal approach for

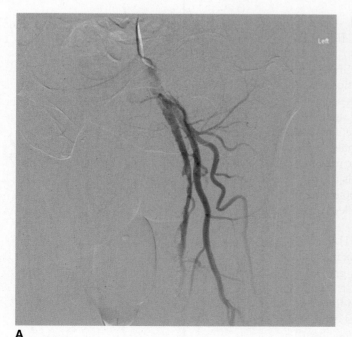

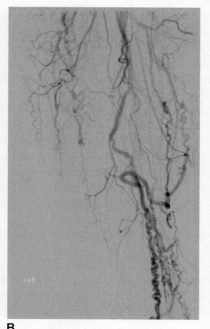

FIGURE 2 • **A:** Femoral angiography showing undiseased profunda femoris and heavily calcified superficial femoral artery with occlusion at the mid-thigh. **B:** Angiography of the left thigh showing extensive collateralization from branches of the profundafemoris.

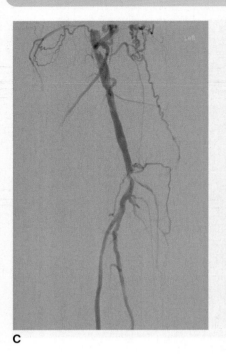
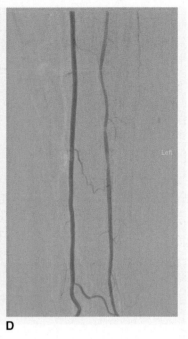

C   D

FIGURE 2 • (*Continued*) **C:** Angiography of the left knee, showing reconstitution of the above-knee popliteal artery. **D:** Angiography of the left calf showing patent anterior and posterior tibial arteries supplying the foot.

revascularization is complex. Lesion characteristics as specified by the Trans-Atlantic Inter-Society Consensus Document on Management of Peripheral Arterial Disease (TASC II) are only one of many factors to consider. The indications for revascularization, as well as the severity of various comorbid conditions, help weigh the benefits of the procedure against the associated risks for postoperative complications.

Surgical Approach

Open surgical bypass is accepted as the gold standard treatment for more extensive lesion types (TASC II type D, represented by total occlusions of the common femoral artery or greater than 20 cm occlusion of the SFA). The ideal bypass surgery would achieve revascularization based off a patent vessel with brisk flow, onto a target vessel with at least one continuous runoff to the foot, while using the shortest autogenous conduit. In this patient, the iliac and common femoral arteries appear undiseased, making the distal common femoral artery a suitable site for proximal anastomosis. A single piece of autogenous vein is the preferred conduit at all levels of bypass. An acceptable vein has characteristics of being compliant, thin walled, compressible, and at least 3 mm in diameter.

Key steps of any bypass surgery consist of (1) harvest and preparation of conduit, (2) exposure of proximal and distal vessels, and (3) tunneling of the bypass graft and anastomoses. Greater saphenous vein is most reliably found at the saphenofemoral junction 2 cm inferomedial to the pubic tubercle. Exposure of femoral artery is best achieved by a vertical groin incision. Femoral sheath is opened and common, superficial femoral, and profunda femoris arteries are dissected circumferentially

and controlled (Fig. 3). This often requires ligation of circumflex iliac vein in order to prevent avulsion of the vein and often marks the proximal extent of dissection. Exposure of the below-knee popliteal artery is achieved by a medial incision 1 cm below the tibia. As this incision lies directly over the great saphenous vein, care must be taken to avoid its injury. Investing fascia is entered, and popliteal space is entered between the gastrocnemius

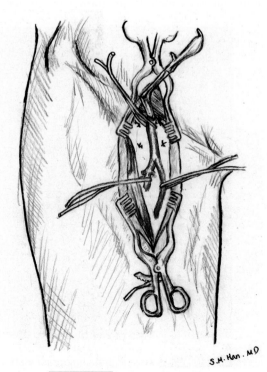

S.H.Han. MD

FIGURE 3 • Femoral exposure.

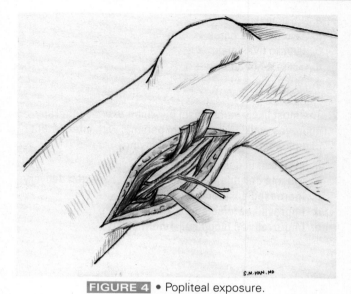

FIGURE 4 • Popliteal exposure.

and the soleus. The popliteal artery is found adherent to often coupled popliteal veins (Fig. 4). After administration of systemic heparin, an end-to-side proximal anastomosis is performed to the common femoral artery. If nonreversed configuration of the vein graft is chosen, lysis of valves is performed with valvulotome. Then, the vein is tunneled either superficially in the subcutaneous layer or anatomically through the adductor canal. Distal anastomosis is performed in similar fashion to the popliteal artery.

Special Intraoperative Considerations

Intraoperative evaluation of the bypass graft with duplex ultrasound and/or completion angiography may detect potential causes of early graft failures. Undetected defects in the graft, such as incompletely lysed valves, kinking, twisting, or compression during tunneling, and clamp injury to native vessels are some of the issues that should be considered.

Postoperative Management

Given the high prevalence of coronary artery disease, congestive heart failure, diabetes, and chronic obstructive pulmonary disease, management of these comorbidities is paramount in minimizing risk of perioperative complications. Particularly, continuation of beta-blockers, statins, and aspirin has been shown to decrease the rates of adverse cardiovascular events following bypass surgery. Perhaps equally important is the bypass graft surveillance. This is done to detect failing graft and to prevent complete thrombosis of the bypass graft. At our institution, this is typically done at intraoperatively at the conclusion of the case and then at 1, 3, 6 months, and then annually by duplex ultrasound.

Case Conclusion

This patient had adequate vein as conduit; all greater than 3 mm. He underwent a common femoral to AK popliteal bypass with reversed saphenous vein and had an unremarkable postoperative course. He was seen back at 3 months with a graft scan that showed no abnormalities. He reported no claudication symptoms since the surgery.

TAKE HOME POINTS

- Claudication due to PVD presents as reproducible, crampy pain in the calf provoked by walking and relieved by rest.
- Claudication carries a low risk of limb loss; however, it is a marker for increased risk of cardiovascular mortality.
- In addition to physical examination, diagnosis of PVD is most reliably established by resting or exercise ABI less than 0.9.
- Anatomical evaluation of PVD is performed by angiography or CTA and characterized according to TASC II classification.
- Medical management of claudication consists of risk factor modifications such as smoking cessation, diabetes control, and supervised exercise program.
- Endovascular procedures involving balloon angioplasty and/or stent have been successfully used to treat short-segment lesions.
- Open bypass with a single piece autogenous vein conduit of adequate size is the gold standard treatment for more extensive lesions (Table 1).

TABLE 1. Femoral Popliteal Bypass with Autogenous Vein

Key Technical Steps

1. Dissect the vein conduit without harvesting. The ipsilateral greater saphenous vein is the conduit of choice when available.
2. Unless in situ bypass is planned, create a tunnel either anatomically or superficially. Measure the length of the planned bypass using an umbilical tape or rubber tubing with the knee fully extended.
3. Harvest the vein of adequate length, and ensure adequate repair of all branches.
4. Tunnel the vein while making sure it is not twisted. Methylene blue marking may aid with this.
5. Perform tension-free proximal and distal anastomoses.

Potential Pitfalls

- Harvesting the vein before making sure the proximal and distal anastomotic sites are adequately free of disease.
- Creating the anastomosis without measuring the length with complete knee extension. This could lead to anastomosis under tension.
- Lack of confirmatory imaging may increase risk of early graft occlusion.

SUGGESTED READINGS

Devereaux PJ, Yang H, Yusuf S, et al. Effects of extended-release metoprolol succinate in patients undergoing non-cardiac surgery (POISE trial): a randomized controlled trial. *Lancet.* 2008;371(9627):1837-1847.

Dormandy J, Heeck L, Vig S. The natural history of claudication: risk to life and limb. *Semin Vasc Surg.* 1999;12(2):123-137.

Norgren L, Hiatt WR, Dormandy JA, et al. Inter-Society Consensus for the Management of Peripheral Arterial Disease (TASC II). *J Vasc Surg.* 2007;45S:S5-S67.

CLINICAL SCENARIO CASE QUESTIONS

1. The relative risk of a patient with intermittent claudication having a myocardial infarction or stroke compared with a nonclaudicant is increased by what factor?

   a. 1.5 times
   b. Two to three times
   c. Four to five times
   d. Six to eight times
   e. Ten times

2. The most likely mechanism by which exercise therapy improves walking distance in patients with intermittent claudication is which of the following?

   a. Increase in ankle-brachial index
   b. Muscle cell adaptation to decreased oxygen delivery
   c. Increased collateral formation
   d. Improved cardiac output
   e. Improved red blood cell deformability

87 Rest Pain and Nonhealing Ulcers

SUKGU M. HAN and MICHAEL S. CONTE

Presentation

An 81-year-old man with a history of hypertension, diabetes, and hyperlipidemia presents with a slowly enlarging ulcer on the left heel over a 5-month period. The ulcer was preceded by pain that localizes to the base of the toes, described as "burning pain." The pain is present at rest, worsens when lying in bed or with foot elevation, and is alleviated by dangling the foot in dependent position. In addition, he has a prior history of claudication symptoms, described as a dull achy pain in the left calf with walking two blocks, and relieved with rest. He is a former smoker with a 20 pack-year history, and denies history of stroke or known coronary artery disease. He has never had a deep venous thrombosis. Four months prior to presentation, the patient underwent stenting of the left superficial femoral artery (SFA) and balloon angioplasty of the peroneal artery. Following the procedure, the patient had a temporary relief of leg pain, but the ulcer failed to heal.

On examination, femoral pulses are easily palpable bilaterally. There are no other palpable pulses below this level in either leg. Doppler signals are insonated at both the dorsalis pedis (DP) and posterior tibial (PT) arteries bilaterally. There is an ulcer at the left medial aspect of the heel, measuring 3.5 cm in diameter, with necrotic tissue at the base (Fig. 1). There is no associated erythema or induration surrounding the ulcer. The left foot is cooler than the right, and demonstrates rubor when dependent and pallor on elevation. There is a marked absence of hair on the leg, and the skin appears atrophic, dry, and scaly. He has no carotid or abdominal bruits and no palpable abdominal masses.

Differential Diagnosis

The differential diagnosis of ischemic rest pain includes the pain and paresthesias of diabetic peripheral neuropathy, gout, rheumatologic disorders, osteoarthritis, and common foot conditions such as plantar fasciitis, bone spurs, and benign muscle cramps. The influence of dependency and elevation on this patient's foot pain and color are nearly pathognomonic of severe chronic limb ischemia and would not be typical of these other conditions. Ischemic rest pain is usually localized to the forefoot and is typically severe enough to require narcotics for symptomatic control. Benign nocturnal muscle cramps in the calf or thigh are a common condition not associated with circulatory disease. Trophic changes of the skin and loss of dermal appendages over the leg and foot are also characteristic of chronic ischemia. In this setting, it is important to examine both feet for additional ulcers that occur at points of pressure (heel) and friction (e.g., between the toes). A history of infection or poorly healing wound that leads to amputation following minor trauma is also suggestive of severe ischemia or poorly controlled diabetes. The reproducible calf pain provoked by ambulation and relieved with rest is characteristic of claudication secondary to arterial occlusive disease.

His prior history of leg claudication further supports peripheral arterial disease (PAD) as the etiology of his foot pain. However, it is important to note that many patients who present with signs or symptoms of critical limb ischemia (rest pain, tissue loss) do not relate an antecedent history of claudication, particularly those in whom disease is primarily at the infrapopliteal level.

Discussion

When evaluating a patient with PAD, one should keep in mind the systemic nature of atherosclerosis and assess by history other vascular beds (cerebral, coronary, mesenteric, renal, and aortoiliac) for ischemic symptoms. Recognized risk factors for PAD include age, tobacco use, diabetes, hyperlipidemia, and hypertension. Patients initially presenting with calf claudication are at a relative low risk for limb loss (1% per year). However, claudication, as a marker for overall cardiovascular disease, is associated with an increased risk for cardiovascular death (5% per year). In contrast to claudication, presence of rest pain or tissue loss signifies a more advanced stage of PAD, critical limb ischemia (CLI). Reported 5-year mortality rates for patients with CLI range from 30% to almost 90% in the literature. There is a wide spectrum of

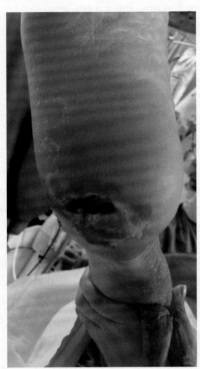

FIGURE 1 • Ischemic nonhealing heel ulcer with necrotic base.

CLI disease severity that relates to prognosis for both life and limb. Factors associated with higher mortality and amputation rates in CLI are diabetes, renal disease, tissue loss, and age.

The diagnosis of CLI is based on both the clinical symptoms (rest pain, tissue loss) and objective testing to document diminished lower limb perfusion. Noninvasive vascular laboratory studies such as ankle-brachial or toe-brachial systolic pressure index (ABI or TBI), segmental Doppler pressure (SDP) measurements, pulse volume recordings (PVRs), and duplex ultrasound (DUS) are helpful in distinguishing ischemic pain from other causes of limb pain. In addition, these studies aid in the assessment of the level (aortoiliac vs. femoropopliteal vs. infrapopliteal) and severity of the occlusive disease.

The ABI is a ratio of ankle systolic pressure to the higher brachial artery pressure and is easily performed in the clinic or at the bedside with the use of a hand-held Doppler. ABI values generally correlate with disease severity, and an ABI of less than 0.4 is often associated with CLI. ABI measurements can be significantly affected by the presence of tibial artery calcification, which is common in patients with diabetes and renal disease. Inability to achieve flow occlusion with the ankle cuff, absolute ankle pressure greater than 250 mm Hg, or an ABI > 1.4 all suggest false elevation of the ankle pressure due to noncompressible vessels. The toe-brachial index (TBI) is considered more accurate for diagnosing CLI in these settings. A digital cuff is used on the hallux, and a photoplethysmograph is placed on the pad of the digit.

TBI < 0.7 is abnormal, and <0.3 generally correlates with severe ischemia.

SDP measurements assess the drop-off in systolic blood pressure due to occlusive disease and can help to localize the level of obstruction. These are measured by inflating the blood pressure cuffs at several locations along the length of the leg. The systolic pressure at which a continuous wave Doppler signal insonated at the ankle returns is compared to the higher of the brachial artery pressures measured. The difference in the pressures measured is attributable to occlusive disease proximal to the blood pressure cuff. Pressure drops of greater than 20 mm Hg are generally considered physiologically significant. PVR are obtained with blood pressure cuffs inflated to 60 to 70 mm Hg placed along the leg in locations similar to SDP measurements. These partially inflated cuffs transmit changes in leg volume that occur with cardiac systole. The waveforms obtained indirectly correlate to the arterial pressure waves generated by the heart during systole. Damping (decrease) of the waveform is related to the presence and severity of occlusive disease proximal to the measuring cuff. PVRs are particularly useful in settings where cuff measurements of systolic pressure may be artificially elevated by noncompressible arteries with medial calcification (e.g., diabetes, renal failure). In patients with toe ulcers or other minor forefoot tissue loss, a PVR at the transmetatarsal level can be helpful to assess healing potential.

DUS is being used with increasing frequency to evaluate PAD. Through examining the velocity characteristics of arterial blood flow along the involved limb, one can localize a significant stenosis by looking for a peak systolic velocity (PSV) elevation as well as spectral broadening. Change of velocity waveform from multiphasic to monophasic across the lesion also signifies hemodynamic significance. The ratio of the PSV recorded across the lesion to that at the normal artery is used to quantify the degree of stenosis. The PSV ratio of 2.0 correlates to greater than 50% stenosis, while a ratio of 4.0 signifies greater than 75% stenosis.

Case Continued

The patient undergoes noninvasive vascular laboratory testing. ABIs are greater than 1.4 bilaterally due to noncompressible, calcified tibial arteries. However, the left TBI is significantly reduced at 0.1. DUS reveals normal velocity waveforms in the left external iliac and common femoral arteries. The previously placed stent in the SFA appears patent; however, there is an elevated PSV to 249 cm/min at the proximal SFA. The velocity waveforms in the popliteal artery show spectral broadening, and loss of multiphasicity. Distally, the DP artery appears patent, but with dampened monophasic waveforms and significant spectral broadening (Fig. 2). These findings are consistent with diffusely diseased left SFA, popliteal arteries, and total occlusion at the infrageniculate level with reconstitution of the DP artery.

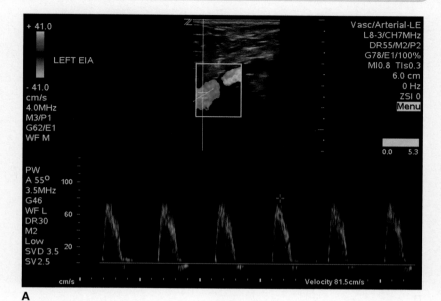

A

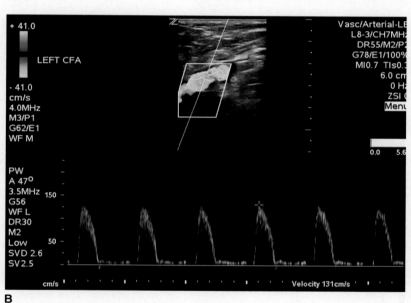

B

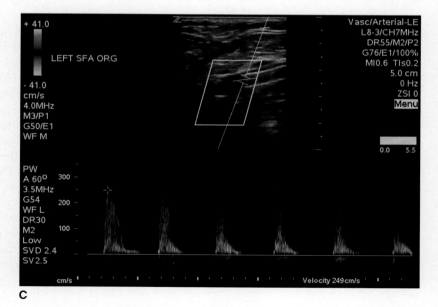

C

FIGURE 2 • Duplex ultrasound of left leg, showing (A) normal, triphasic velocity waveform in the external iliac artery, (B) normal PSV with biphasic waveform in the common femoral artery (C and D) elevated PSV to

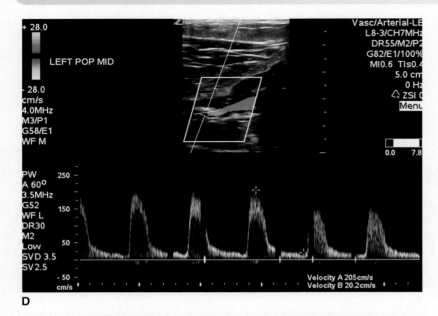

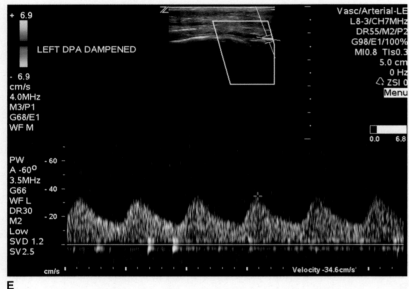

FIGURE 2 • (*Continued*) 249 cm/s and loss of multiphasicity in the proximal to the stented SFA, and the native popliteal artery **(E)** dampened monophasic signal with spectral broadening in the DP artery.

Discussion

The results of this patient's noninvasive vascular laboratory studies provide a functional confirmation of CLI in the left leg. Revascularization is indicated to salvage the left leg, and, at this point, a more detailed anatomical evaluation is required. An angiogram allows such evaluation, and an opportunity for an endovascular intervention. Vein mapping indicates that an adequate quality saphenous vein is present if bypass grafting is contemplated.

Case Continued

The patient undergoes an angiogram of the left leg from a contralateral femoral approach. The angiogram shows a widely patent CFA. The left profunda femoris appears patent proximally, but diffused diseased at multiple branches. The proximal SFA appears to have a high-grade stenosis at its origin. The stented portion of the SFA appears to be patent; however, the remainder of the SFA appears to be diffusely diseased. The proximal anterior tibial (AT) is patent for a very short distance, then occludes. The tibioperoneal trunk as well as the proximal PT, and the proximal peroneal arteries are occluded. The peroneal artery reconstitutes in the distal lower leg, then supplies a large collateral to the DP (Fig. 3).

Given the presence of CLI, and infrainguinal pattern of his PVD, this patient is offered bypass surgery for limb salvage. A bypass graft using an autogenous greater saphenous vein (GSV) from CFA to peroneal artery would provide flow to the dominant runoff to the affected foot. A preoperative cardiac assessment is initiated, focusing primarily on functional status. A history of significant coronary artery disease (prior MI, abnormal electrocardiogram,

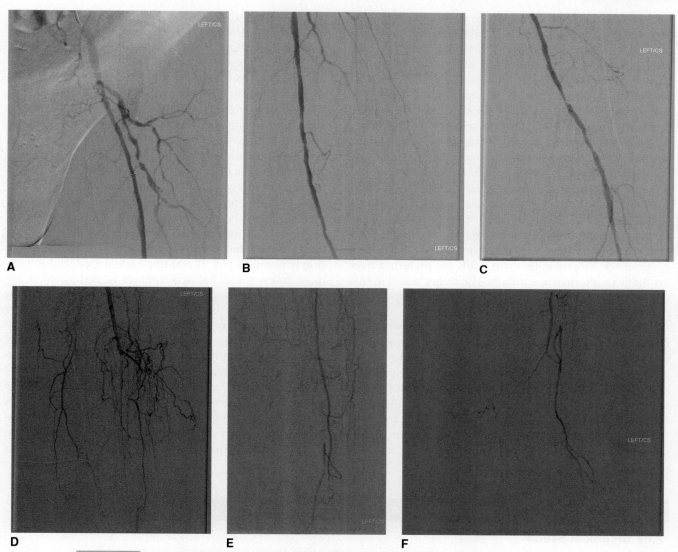

FIGURE 3 • Left leg angiogram showing **(A)** proximal SFA stenosis, and diffuse stenosis of profunda femoris; **(B)** diffuse moderate stenosis of mid-SFA; **(C)** severe stenosis of above-knee popliteal artery; **(D)** proximal AT occlusion. Chronic total occlusion of the tibioperoneal trunk, PT, and the peroneal arteries. **E and F:** The peroneal artery reconstitutes in the distal lower leg, and then supplies a large collateral to the DP.

or revascularizations), valvular heart disease, diabetes, and advanced age are important risk factors to identify. Because of his CLI and limited exercise capacity, cardiac stress testing (dobutamine echocardiography or persantine-thallium imaging) may be obtained if coronary revascularization with potential delay in treatment of PAD is an acceptable option. His preoperative echocardiogram showed normal ventricular function with 65% ejection fraction, and no significant valvular disease. Therefore, cardiac stress testing is not obtained. He is started on aspirin and a beta-blocker, and a statin preoperatively to reduce his perioperative cardiac morbidity and mortality. Based on his comorbid conditions, his risk of perioperative myocardial infarction is less than 5%, and the likelihood of early graft failure (30 days) is approximately 5%.

The patient is advised that between 50% and 70% of similarly constructed bypass grafts last 5 years without intervention, and patency approaches 80% with revisions. The limb salvage rate for patients having a successful bypass approaches 90% at 5 years. The potential complications of the procedure were discussed with the patient including wound infections, cardiac events, bleeding, graft failure, limb loss, renal failure, stroke, and death.

Discussion

The goals of revascularization in CLI are relief of pain, healing of wounds, and functional limb salvage. Open surgical bypass is accepted as the most durable, gold standard treatment for CLI with 5-year patency rate of

60% to 80% and limb salvage rate of 80% to 90%. The requirements for successful infrainguinal bypass surgery for CLI are unobstructed arterial inflow, a good quality autogenous vein conduit, and an outflow artery that provides direct in-line flow to the ankle and foot. Occasionally, hemodynamically significant stenosis in inflow vessels may need to be treated prior or concurrently to the bypass surgery. The selection of an appropriate conduit for the bypass is critical to its long-term success. Preoperative vein mapping is helpful to assess the availability and quality of conduit. An acceptable vein has characteristics of being compliant, thin-walled, compressible, and at least 3 mm in diameter. In general, a single segment of ipsilateral GSV is the conduit of choice, followed by contralateral GSV. Cephalic and basilic arm veins as well as the lesser saphenous vein, as either a single piece or as a composite graft, are preferred over synthetic or alternative conduits. The target vessel in this patient is the peroneal artery, which is the most proximal patent and dominant runoff vessel to the foot.

Key steps in infrainguinal bypass surgery consist of (1) harvest and preparation of conduit, (2) exposure of proximal and distal vessels, (3) tunneling of the bypass graft and anastomoses, and (4) completion imaging and assessment (Table 1). The GSV is first exposed at the saphenofemoral junction 2 cm inferomedial to the pubic tubercle. The vein is typically exposed over the required length using longitudinal incisions with intervening skin bridges. Exposure of the femoral artery is achieved by deepening the incision laterally and extending it proximally in the groin; in some patients with a large pannus, an oblique or transverse incision may be used. The femoral sheath is opened and common, superficial femoral, and profunda femoris arteries are dissected circumferentially and controlled (Fig. 4). Exposure of the peroneal artery is achieved by a medial calf incision 1 to 2 cm behind the posterior border of the tibia. As this incision lies directly over the great saphenous vein, care must be taken to avoid its injury. Investing fascia is entered, and the tibial attachment of the soleus is incised to enter the deep posterior compartment (Fig. 5). The PT is encountered first, and with continued dissection in this plane, the peroneal artery and vein is exposed deeper in the incision. An adequate length is exposed for the anastomosis, and the presence of any calcification is noted to pick the optimal site for arteriotomy. In most cases, the distal anastomosis is performed using tourniquet control; therefore, exposure and isolation of side branches is unnecessary. After administration of systemic heparin (70 to 100 U/kg intravenous), the vein is fully harvested from its bed and gently distended with a solution of heparin and vasodilator (e.g., papaverine) in a buffered, isotonic crystalloid solution (e.g., Plasmalyte). The vein graft may be oriented in either reversed or nonreversed orientation; the authors often prefer nonreversed for long GSV grafts to optimize the size match. However, graft orientation does not have a significant impact on outcomes in the literature. An

---

TABLE 1. Femoral Popliteal Bypass with Autogenous Vein

Key Technical Steps

1. Dissect the vein conduit without harvesting to minimize ischemia time. Handle the vein gently as excessive trauma may predispose to graft failure. The ipsilateral GSV is the conduit of choice when available. Carefully assess the caliber and quality of the vein; if areas of sclerosis or inadequate caliber are observed, a spliced vein or alternative conduit may be needed. While a good-quality vein is the optimal conduit for bypass, poor- or marginal-quality vein is a prescription for failure.
2. Obtain proximal and distal exposure for the bypass.
3. Unless in-situ bypass is planned, create a tunnel either anatomically or superficially. Measure the length of the planned bypass using an umbilical tape with the knee fully extended.
4. Following heparinization, harvest the vein of adequate length and ensure adequate repair of all branches.
5. Perform the proximal anastomosis. Insure normal inflow and absence of significant disease in the common and proximal deep femoral arteries.
6. Tunnel the vein after the proximal anastomosis with pressurization, while making sure it is not twisted or kinked.
7. Tourniquet control for the distal anastomosis facilitates exposure and minimizes target vessel dissection. Choose a minimally diseased area for the arteriotomy. After opening the artery, measure and trim the vein graft and perform the distal anastomosis in end-to-side fashion.
8. Obtain completion angiogram and/or duplex to insure patency without technical defect.

Potential Pitfalls

- Careful handling and assessment of the conduit is critical to success. It is better to excise a sclerotic or poor quality segment than to accept it. Know your options based on preoperative vein mapping.
- Harvesting the vein before making sure the proximal and distal anastomotic sites are adequately free of disease can result in inadequate length and need to splice segments.
- Creating the anastomosis without measuring the length with complete knee extension. This could lead to an anastomosis under tension.
- Choose the arteriotomy site in the distal artery carefully to avoid dealing with extensive calcification if this is possible.

is performed in similar fashion to the peroneal artery under tourniquet control (inflation to 250 to 300 mm Hg at the thigh level).

Intraoperative evaluation of the bypass graft with duplex ultrasound and/or completion angiography may detect potential causes of early graft failure. Undetected defects in the graft such as incompletely lysed valves, kinking, twisting, or compression during tunneling, and clamp injury to native vessels should be addressed prior to leaving the operating room. Angiography has the advantage of more easily imaging the native vessels and their collaterals that make up the runoff for the bypass. The authors typically employ both ultrasound and angiography at completion as the information is complementary.

Case Conclusion

The bypass is performed between the CFA and the peroneal artery using the ipsilateral GSV. Intraoperatively, the left CFA and proximal profunda femoris arteries were found to be diseased with dense posterior atherosclerotic plaque. In order to establish durable inflow, femoral endarterectomy is performed with patch angioplasty using bovine pericardium. The proximal anastomosis is performed in end-to-side fashion. The graft is oriented in nonreversed fashion, its valves lysed, and tunneled superficially. The distal anastomosis is fashioned to the peroneal artery in the distal 1/3 of the leg. A completion arteriogram is obtained, confirming a widely patent bypass graft to the peroneal artery (Fig. 6).

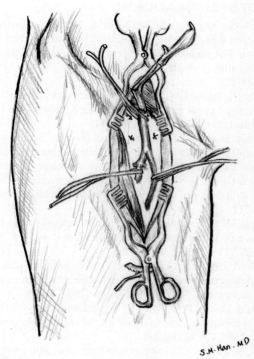

S.M.Han.MD

FIGURE 4 • Femoral artery exposure.

end-to-side proximal anastomosis is performed to the common femoral artery. If a nonreversed configuration of the vein graft is chosen, lysis of valves is performed with valvulotome. Then, the vein is tunneled either superficially in the subcutaneous layer or anatomically beneath the sartorius muscle and through the popliteal space to the distal target. The superficial graft tunnel has the advantage of being more readily accessible for surveillance and revision, if needed. The advantage of the deeper tunnel is that the graft is protected in the event of a wound infection or dehiscence. The distal anastomosis

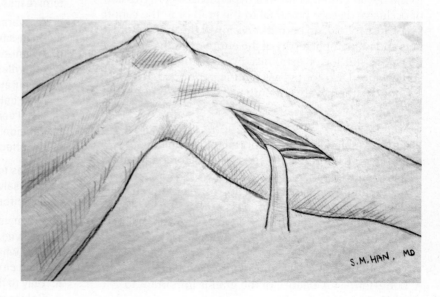

S.M.HAN, MD

FIGURE 5 • Peroneal exposure.

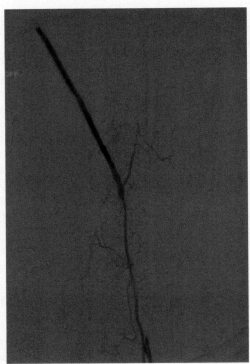

FIGURE 6 • Completion angiogram showing patent distal anastomosis to the peroneal artery.

The patient is discharged from the hospital on postoperative day 5. Follow-up is scheduled for a wound check in the office 1 week after discharge. His first graft surveillance duplex ultrasound performed 2 months after the operation shows patent bypass graft without velocity elevation along its entire length. The left TBI is improved to 0.58, and the heel ulcer has decreased in its size to 1.5 cm with clean base.

The patient should expect to have follow-up visits with a vascular surgeon for the remainder of his life. The goal of surveillance is to detect grafts that are failing due to the development of intimal hyperplasia or progression of occlusive disease proximal to the graft or in the runoff bed. Close follow-up permits revision of the graft before it fails and is an implicit part of the entire operative strategy for successful lower extremity bypass surgery. Typically, surveillance DUS for bypass graft is performed at 1, 3, 6, 12 months, then every 6 months.

TAKE HOME POINTS

- CLI has a high long-term mortality rate due to atherosclerotic burden and needs to be factored into any therapeutic plan.
- Arteriography is the best imaging for planning distal arterial bypasses.
- While inflow and outflow artery pressure and patency are critical, respectively, the conduit quality is most important.
- Vein orientation is less important than quality.
- Long-term surveillance of the graft is important to maximize patency.

SUGGESTED READINGS

Chew DKW, Conte MS, Belkin M, et al. Arterial reconstruction for lower limb ischemia. *Acta Chir Belg.* 2001;101:106-115.

De Frang RD, Edwards JM, Moneta GL, et al. Repeat leg bypass after multiple prior bypass failures. *J Vasc Surg.* 1994; 19:268-277.

Edwards JE, Taylor LM, Porter JM. Treatment of failed lower extremity bypass grafts with new autogenous vein bypass grafting. *J Vasc Surg.* 1990;11:136-145.

Effeney DJ, Stoney RJ. Femoropopliteal bypass. Disorders of the extremities. In: *Wylie's Atlas of Vascular Surgery;* 1993:56-91.

Grayburn PA, Hillis LD. Cardiac events in patients undergoing noncardiac surgery: shifting the paradigm from non-invasive risk stratification to therapy. *Ann Intern Med.* 2003;138: 506-511.

McDaniel MD, Cronenwett JL. Basic data related to the natural history of intermittent claudication. *Ann Vasc Surg.* 1989;3: 273-277.

Schanzer A, Hevelone N, Owens C, et al. Technical factors affecting autogenous vein graft failure: observations from a large multicenter trial. *J Vasc Surg.* 2007;46:1180-1190.

Taylor LM, Hamre D, Dalman RL, et al. Limb salvage vs amputation for critical ischemia: the role of vascular surgery. *Arch Surg.* 1991;126:1251-1258.

Tinder CN, Bandyk DF. Detection of imminent vein graft occlusion: what is the optimal surveillance program? *Semin Vasc Surg.* 2009;22(4):252-260.

Veith FJ, Gupta SK, Samson RH, et al. Progress in limb salvage by reconstructive arterial surgery combined with new or improved adjunctive procedures. *Ann Surg.* 1981;194:386-401.

CLINICAL SCENARIO CASE QUESTIONS

1. A 58-year-old female with diabetes mellitus presents with gangrene of the fourth toe. Contrast arteriography demonstrates occlusion of the superficial femoral and popliteal arteries with reconstitution of the posterior tibial artery in the mid-calf with continued patency to the foot. Her ipsilateral saphenous vein is intact. The configuration of the saphenous vein graft most likely to give her the best long-term results in terms of graft patency and limb salvage is:

    a. A reversed saphenous vein bypass
    b. An in-situ saphenous vein bypass
    c. A nonreversed translocated saphenous vein bypass regardless of the presence of any tapering
    d. A nonreversed translocated saphenous vein bypass if the caliber of the proximal vein is larger than the distal vein
    e. The configuration of the saphenous vein bypass does not affect graft patency or limb salvage

2. Bypasses to arteries below the knee may be considered for limb salvage with PTFE conduit in which of the following circumstances?

    a. When no acceptable autologous vein is present in the involved lower extremity
    b. Only when no suitable autologous vein is available
    c. In no circumstances
    d. Only to the posterior tibial artery
    e. Only to the peroneal artery

88 Peripheral Vascular Occlusive Disease—Rest Pain/Ulcers

HUITING CHEN and KATHERINE GALLAGHER

Adapted from a previous version by Leslie D. Cunningham and Michael S. Conte

Presentation

An 88-year-old man with a history of diabetes, congestive heart failure (CHF), hypertension, and hypercholesterolemia, status post three-vessel coronary artery bypass graft (CABG) × 10 years ago, presents to the clinic with 6 months of worsening left foot pain that localized to the forefoot. The pain is present at rest, improves with dependency, and worsens when lying in bed or with foot elevation. He has never had deep venous thrombosis. He lives alone and walks small distances around the house. On examination, he has no carotid or abdominal bruits and no palpable abdominal masses. His femoral pulses are easily palpable and equal. He has no other palpable pulses below this level on the left, but has a palpable right popliteal pulse. Biphasic Doppler signals are insonated in both the dorsalis pedis and posterior tibial arteries (DPA and PTA, respectively) on the right, and a monophasic signal is appreciated in the DPA and PTA on the left. His left foot demonstrates rubor when dependent and pallor on elevation. There is a marked absence of hair on the leg, and the skin appears atrophic, dry, and scaly. Of note, there are vein harvest incisions on the bilateral medial thighs.

Differential Diagnosis

The differential diagnosis of ischemic rest pain includes the pain and paresthesias of diabetic peripheral neuropathy, gout, rheumatologic disorders, osteoarthritis, and common foot conditions such as plantar fasciitis, bone spurs, and benign muscle cramps. The influence of dependency and elevation on this patient's foot pain and color are nearly pathognomonic of severe chronic ischemia and would not be typical of these other conditions. Ischemic rest pain is typically localized to the forefoot (toes, instep) and is usually severe enough to require narcotics for adequate management. Benign nocturnal muscle cramps in the calf or thigh are a common condition not associated with circulatory disease. Trophic changes of the skin and loss of dermal appendages over the leg and foot are characteristic of chronic ischemia. In this setting, it is important to examine the feet for ulcers that occur at points of friction. A history of poor healing or infection that leads to amputation following minor trauma is also suggestive of severe ischemia or poorly controlled diabetes.

Background and Workup

Background

Atherosclerosis is a systemic disease. This obligates one to assess other vascular beds (cerebral, coronary, mesenteric, renal, and aortoiliac) for ischemic symptoms when evaluating a patient for complaints of infrainguinal arterial insufficiency. Recognized risk factors for atherosclerosis include tobacco use, male gender, diabetes, hyperlipidemia, hypercholesterolemia, and hypertension. Patients initially presenting with calf claudication are at increased risk for cardiovascular death, but at relatively low risk for limb loss (approximately 5% and 1% per year, respectively). In contrast to patients with claudication, reported 5-year mortality rates for patients with critical limb ischemia (critical limb ischemia (CLI); rest pain or gangrene) range from 30% to almost 90%. Factors associated with higher mortality rates are diabetes, renal insufficiency, and renal failure. The goal of revascularization procedures in this patient population is limb salvage of inpatients with rest pain; approximately 75% will achieve relief from treatment of inflow disease alone. This is in contrast to patients with tissue loss who often require treatment of inflow and outflow disease.

Initial objective testing for lower limb ischemia is done in the noninvasive vascular laboratory. Studies performed include an ankle-brachial systolic pressure index (ABI), segmental Doppler pressure (SDP) measurements, and pulse volume recordings (PVRs). These are helpful in distinguishing ischemic pain from other causes of limb pain and aid in the assessment of the level (aortoiliac vs. femoropopliteal vs. tibial) and severity of the occlusive disease. The ABI is a ratio of ankle systolic pressure to the higher brachial artery pressure and is easily performed in the clinic or at the bedside with the use of a handheld Doppler. An index of less than 0.7 variably correlates with symptoms of calf claudication. An ABI of less than 0.4 is often associated with a history of rest pain or ulcer on physical examination. In diabetic or renal failure patients, TBI values should be performed as ABIs are often invalid due to severe calcification.

SDP measurements assess the drop-off in systolic blood pressure due to occlusive disease. These are measured by inflating blood pressure cuffs at several locations along the length of the leg. The systolic pressure at which a continuous wave Doppler signal insonated at the ankle returns is compared to the higher of the brachial artery pressures measured. The difference in the pressures measured is attributable to occlusive disease proximal to the blood pressure cuff. Pressure drops of greater than 20 mm Hg are generally considered physiologically significant. PVRs are obtained with blood pressure cuffs inflated to 60 to 70 mm Hg placed along the leg in locations similar to SDP measurements. These partially inflated cuffs transmit changes in leg volume that occur with cardiac systole. The waveforms obtained indirectly correlate to the arterial pressure waves generated by the heart during systole. Damping (decrease) of the waveform is related to the presence and severity of occlusive disease proximal to the measuring cuff. PVRs are particularly useful in settings where cuff measurements of systolic pressure may be artificially elevated by arterial calcification.

Workup

This patient will require noninvasive arterial testing and an angiogram to assess for outflow disease. Since this patient has palpable femoral pulses, we prefer angiogram over CTA to evaluate outflow disease.

Noninvasive Laboratory Workup

The patient has an ABI of 0.22 and a severely depressed waveform of the PVR at the metatarsal level on the left, consistent with critical ischemia of the left foot. On angiogram, there is significant arterial occlusive disease in the superficial femoral/popliteal artery and tibioperoneal system. Additionally, the superficial venous duplex confirms that the GSV bilaterally has been harvested and that the cephalic and small saphenous veins bilaterally are under 2 mm in diameter.

Arteriogram Report

There is no significant stenosis of the distal aorta, left common iliac artery, or external iliac artery (not shown). There is mild stenosis of the left common femoral artery (CFA). Arteriogram shows a patent CFA, occluded superficial femoral artery (SFA), and a patent profunda femoris artery (PFA) (Fig. 1). The left SFA is occluded at its origin

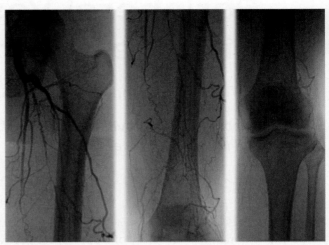

FIGURE 1 • Extremity angiograms demonstrating: left patent common femoral artery, occluded superficial femoray artery (SFA), and a patent profunda femoris. Multiple collaterals visualized along the length of the occluded SFA.

and reconstitutes at the level of the tibialis. The posterior tibial (PT) and peroneal (PE) artery are the major runoffs to the foot (Fig. 2).

Diagnosis and Treatment

This patient has severe CLI (rest pain) of the left leg. Ideally, this patient requires a bypass of the occluded SFA, popliteal, and diseased tibioperoneal trunk; however, given this patient's age, functional status, lack of autogenous conduit, and increased comorbid conditions, an endovascular approach may be preferred.

Using ultrasound guidance, a 4-French micropuncture needle is inserted into the contralateral common femoral artery. A 4-French sheath is placed in the CFA, and an omni catheter is placed in the terminal aorta. A soft tipped

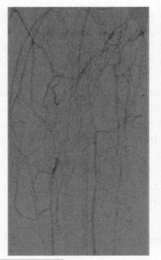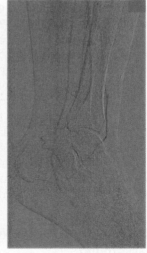

FIGURE 2 • Occluded SFA reconstitutes at the level of the tibialis, with the posterior tibial and peroneal arteries as the major runoffs to the foot. These runoffs are small and diseased.

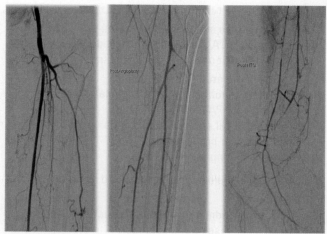

FIGURE 3 • Following PTA of the areas of stenosis/occlusion, the SFA, popliteal, PT and peroneal arteries were successfully treated with improved runoff to the foot.

glidewire is advanced up and over and into the ipsilateral CFA. Following this, a catheter/wire exchange is performed to allow for placement of a × 4S sheath up and over into the ipsilateral CFA. Following this, a glidewire is carefully manipulated through the area of occlusion/stenosis. The catheter is used to follow the wire across the lesions. If the subintimal plane is entered, care must be taken to reenter the true lumen in the area of reconstitution. In this case, the wire and catheter were used to cross the lesions, and then true lumen placement distally was confirmed prior to percutaneous transluminal angioplasty (PTA). The SFA, popliteal, PT, and peroneal were successfully opened with good runoff to the foot (Fig. 3).

Following completion of the procedure, complete run off studies should be obtained to ensure no distal embolization occurred. The sheath is then removed with manual pressure held for 30 minutes or a closure device can be used if the CFA is not calcified, and the sheath is in the CFA above the profunda and below the inguinal ligament.

With endovascular treatment, the patient should expect to have regular follow-up visits with a vascular surgeon. This follow-up includes routine surveillance by duplex ultrasonography, and ABI/TBI. The goal of surveillance is to identify areas of disease progression prior to occlusion, where intervention will be technically easier and successful outcomes more feasible. However, no prospective studies have been done to show it is efficacious to intervene prior to symptomatic progression.

The 5-year mortality rate for patients initially presenting with CLI is high. It is reiterated to the patient that atherosclerosis is a systemic disease and that control of blood pressure, hypercholesterolemia, blood sugar for diabetics, and smoking cessation are of paramount importance for both preservation of his limb as well as his life. Medical therapy is an important component in the treatment of PAD (peripheral artery disease). This patient has been

TABLE 1. Key Technical Steps/Potential Pitfalls

- Ultrasound-guided access with a 4-French micropuncture set should be used to allow for precise placement of access site 1 cm above profunda (PFA).
- A soft glidewire and catheter should be used as the initial approach to transverse the lesion.
- Heparinize the patient to an ACT of >250 prior to crossing the lesion.
- Start with a small sheath (4 French) and upsize as needed.
- Always confirm true lumen placement and distal to the lesion prior to performing PTA/stenting.
- Only place a stent for >30% residual stenosis or flow-limiting dissections.

taking aspirin and a statin. The potential complications of the endovascular procedure discussed with the patient include bleeding/hematoma, distal embolization, limb loss, renal failure, stroke, and death (Table 1).

Case Conclusion

The patient is discharged from the hospital on postoperative day 5. There is no groin hematoma. Follow-up is scheduled at 1 month after discharge with surveillance duplex ultrasound and ABI/TBI values.

TAKE HOME POINTS

- Ultrasound-guided access improves outcomes and decreases complication rates.
- Determine the site of occlusion/stenosis using physical exam and noninvasive imaging.
- Always start with the smallest sheath possible and upsize as needed.
- Always confirm true lumen placement distal to the lesion prior to performing any intervention.
- Full completion images should be obtained following treatment to assure no distal embolization.

SUGGESTED READINGS

Dippel E, Shammas N, Takes V, et al. Twelve-month results of percutaneous endovascular reconstruction for chronically occluded superficial femoral arteries: a quality-of-life assessment. *J Invasive Cardiol.* 2006;18(7):316-321.

Hirsch AT, et al. ACC/AHA 2005 Practice Guidelines for the management of patients with peripheral arterial disease (lower extremity, renal, mesenteric, and abdominal aortic): a collaborative report from the American Association for Vascular Surgery/Society for Vascular Surgery, Society for Cardiovascular Angiography and Interventions, Society for Vascular Medicine and Biology, Society of Interventional Radiology, and the ACC/AHA Task Force on Practice Guidelines (Writing Committee to Develop Guidelines for the Management of Patients With Peripheral Arterial Disease): endorsed by the American Association of Cardiovascular and Pulmonary Rehabilitation; National Heart, Lung, and Blood Institute; Society for Vascular Nursing; TransAtlantic Inter-Society Consensus; and Vascular Disease Foundation. *Circulation.* 2006;113(11): e463-e654.

Kalbaugh CA, et al. One-year prospective quality-of-life outcomes in patients treated with angioplasty for symptomatic peripheral arterial disease. *J Vasc Surg.* 2006;44(2):296-302; discussion 302-293.

Safley DM, et al. Quantifying improvement in symptoms, functioning, and quality of life after peripheral endovascular revascularization. *Circulation.* 2007;115(5):569-575.

Taylor LM, Hamre D, Dalman RL, et al. Limb salvage vs. amputation for critical ischemia: the role of vascular surgery. *Arch Surg.* 1991;126:1251-1258.

Wahlgren CM, Kalin B, Lund K, et al. Long-term outcome of infrainguinal percutaneous transluminal angioplasty. *J Endovasc Ther.* 2004;11(3):287-293.

CLINICAL SCENARIO CASE QUESTIONS

1. What maneuvers should be done at the end of an endovascular PTA/stent procedure to identify any distal embolization that occurred during the intervention?

   a. Image of the area of PTA/stenting
   b. Complete runoff images, including lateral foot
   c. Injection of TPA into tibial vessels
   d. Nothing; distal embolization is not a concern with endovascular procedures
   e. Duplex imaging of tibial vessels

2. CFA access should always be obtained using the following setup:

   a. Anatomic landmarks and hand palpation
   b. Blind stick based upon palpation
   c. Ultrasound guidance and micropuncture set
   d. Fluoroscopic guidance
   e. Groin crease

89 PVOD (Subintimal Recanalization—SAFARI)

NARASIMHAM L. DASIKA

Presentation

A 69-year-old man presented to the clinic with a 2-week history of progressively worsening right foot rest pain. He had multiple bilateral surgical bypass grafts and endovascular procedures in the past 11 years to treat peripheral arterial disease (PAD). Three weeks earlier, he had an unsuccessful thrombolysis of right external iliac artery (EIA) to posterior tibial artery (PTA) composite PTFE and vein graft and an attempted subintimal recanalization of right common femoral artery (CFA) and superficial femoral artery (SFA) from a contralateral left CFA access.

He was advised to have right above-the-knee amputation, but the patient is worried about the prospect of bilateral amputation from his advanced bilateral PAD. His past medical history includes CAD treated with stents, hyperlipidemia, obesity, and sleep apnea. He is a former smoker with a 50-pack-year smoking history. On physical examination, his vital signs are normal. Multiple well-healed groin and lower extremity surgical scars from prior surgeries are seen. He has no leg swelling and no ulcerations and has normal sensory and motor function, except for toe pain on touch. Vascular examination revealed absent palpable right femoral and popliteal pulses, but a dopplerable anterior tibial (AT) artery pulse is present. On the left, he has a feeble but palpable CFA pulse and dopplerable popliteal and pedal pulses.

Differential Diagnosis

Progressively worsening foot pain at rest that is worse in recumbent position with partial relief by standing suggests arterial insufficiency resulting in critical limb ischemia (CLI). Other causes of progressively worsening lower extremity pain include venous disease and peripheral neuropathy. The absence of swelling, relief of pain when the foot is in dependent position, and absence of edema are not in favor of venous disease. The protracted symptoms, rest pain, and examination findings exclude acute limb ischemia (ALI), pseudoclaudication, and neuropathy.

Workup

Workup of a patient with CLI should start with noninvasive vascular evaluation in the clinic. Patients with CLI typically have multilevel vascular lesions and ABI of less than 0.4. Resting segmental waveforms and pressures indicate the level of occlusion and multisegmental involvement. Additional noninvasive imaging with computed tomography angiography (CTA) or magnetic resonance angiography (MRA) is indicated to localize the level and morphology of occlusion, presence of calcium, reconstituted distal arterial anatomy, altered anatomy from prior surgeries, and patency of stents (Figs. 1 and 2). The imaging information allows appropriate treatment decisions to be made. In addition, CTA is very useful in preprocedure endovascular planning in terms of selection of access and devices and thereby reducing the procedure time and contrast load. The blood work should include evaluation of renal function and coagulation profile. Transthoracic echocardiography is recommended when there is history of concomitant ischemic heart disease. Vein mapping for surgical bypass grafts is performed to check for availability of suitable vein conduits for surgical treatment options. Admission and heparinization may have to be considered for patients with limb-threatening ischemia.

Diagnosis and Treatment

Surgical or endovascular revascularizations have to be considered in patients with CLI since medical management is unlikely to give relief from rest pain. When all the surgical options and endovascular options are expended over a period of time, amputation is inevitable. In the presence of advanced arterial disease of the contralateral lower extremity, the prognosis is very poor and the risk of bilateral amputation is high. Patients with CLI from long-segment femoropopliteal occlusions (greater than 15 cm) that are not suitable for surgical or transluminal endovascular options may benefit from PIER procedure (Percutaneous Intentional Extraluminal Recanalization), a technique that has been described by Bolia. PIER

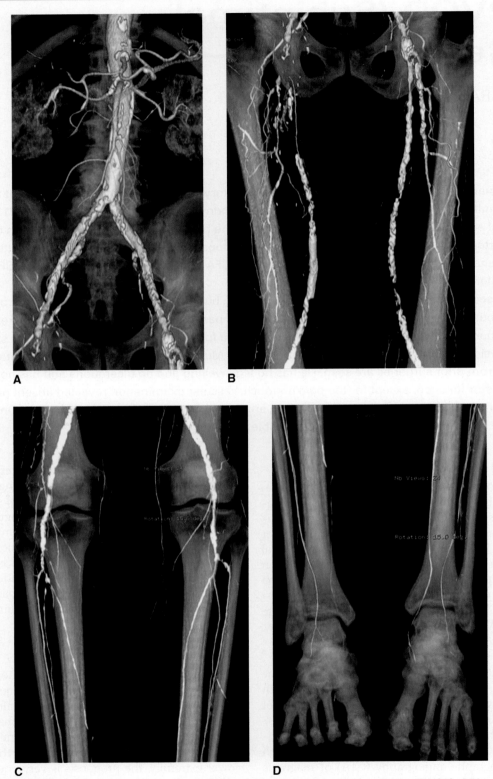

FIGURE 1 • CTA reformats showing heavily calcified arterial occlusion of right EIA **(A)**, CFA **(B)**, SFA **(C)**, and popliteal **(D)** arteries. The anterior tibial artery (D) is reconstituted in the leg. Note bilateral disease that is more severe on the right.

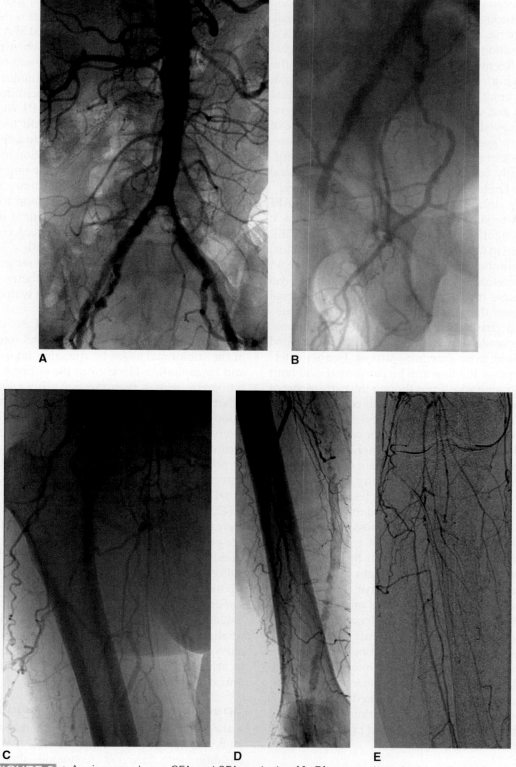

FIGURE 2 • Angiogram shows CFA and SFA occlusion **(A, B)**, reconstituted mid profunda femoris artery at mid-thigh **(C)** from internal iliac artery branches, providing poor collateral arterial supply **(D)** to AT and peroneal in the leg **(E)**.

procedure is recanalization of an occluded segment made subintimally through the medial layer of the arterial wall. This procedure has a reported success rate of 76% to 84% in revascularization of long-segment chronic total occlusions (CTO). Reentry into the distal patent lumen is the most challenging part of a PIER procedure, resulting in up to 25% technical failure, often due to heavily calcified distal arteries and vascular perforation. Successful reentry can be achieved in some of the failures by the use of reentry devices specifically developed for this purpose. These devices are often difficult to advance through long-segment heavily calcified occlusions from contralateral side and have limited role in reentry into tibial arteries.

A recently introduced technique called SAFARI (**S**ubintimal **A**rterial **F**lossing with **A**ntegrade-**R**etrograde **I**ntervention) significantly improved the success of PIER procedure even in CTOs that extend beyond the popliteal trifurcation into the tibial arteries. SAFARI technique, in principle, is a retrograde PIER procedure performed via retrograde access through a reconstituted distal arterial segment to enter the proximal patent lumen or the subintimal (PIER) channel created from antegrade access. The long retrograde recanalization wire is then grasped and externalized from antegrade access. Further intervention to improve the flow can be performed over both ends of this flossing wire. Even though the early report of this technique was performed through retrograde popliteal access in prone position, AT and PT arteries are most widely selected access arteries for retrograde distal access with the patient in supine position. SAFARI technique has been proven to be invaluable in minimizing the reentry failures and the need for reentry devices during the PIER procedure. The procedure is less invasive than surgery with high technical success and reported patency rates comparable to that of surgical bypass grafts. In addition, the SAFARI technique does not compromise the prospect of a future surgical bypass or the target artery for distal anastomosis. Other advantages of the SAFARI technique are the ability to (1) preserve the patency of large collateral arteries at the proximal and distal end of the CTO; (2) recanalize CTO of additional tibial arteries from antegrade access through the newly created subintimal channel; (3) treat the flow-limiting lesions of the pedal arteries; (4) perform secondary interventions such as plaque debulking if necessary; (5) successful revascularization following a failed PIER procedure in patients with heavily calcified lumen of the distal artery; and (6) recanalize through occluded stents and prior CFA endarterectomy (Figs. 3 and 4).

Endovascular Minimally Invasive Surgical Procedure

In preparation for the procedure, patients are loaded with Plavix and aspirin to minimize platelet aggregation and thrombosis during the procedure. Bilateral antegrade groin access sites (brachial access is uncommon) and the entire leg to be treated including the foot are prepped and draped. Contralateral CFA access is chosen for access when the CFA and the proximal SFA are occluded. Ipsilateral CFA access is preferable when proximal SFA is patent. Following access, antegrade subintimal recanalization is performed with PIER technique to the knee joint, and a wire is placed in the subintimal space. For distal retrograde access, the AT and PT with direct flow into the foot are preferred for SAFARI technique, even though any tibial or pedal artery including a metatarsal artery can be accessed. To avoid radiation to the operator, ultrasound (US)-guided access of the target tibial artery segment is performed under real-time imaging with intermittent color Doppler interrogation to avoid transgression of an adjacent vein. The patient is heparinized to keep the ACT between 250 and 300. A combination of 0.014 and 0.018 guidewires often with a 3-French support catheter are used for retrograde recanalization. The retrograde wire and the support catheter are gradually advanced to meet the antegrade wire within the subintimal space proximal to the knee joint.

Successful recanalization should be confirmed by mobility and contact of antegrade and retrograde wires in the subintimal space by changing fluoroscopy angles and by aspirating blood from the support catheter. The retrograde wire is then grasped with a loop snare and externalized through the antegrade access, providing a through-and-through body floss wire (SAFARI wire) for intervention with angioplasty. Following completion of recanalization and restoration, attempts should be made to provide 3-vessel outflows into the foot through the antegrade access. Angioplasty of the spiraling subintimal channel around the diseased rigid and calcified CTO lumen is performed at each level with appropriately sized balloons. Balloon angioplasty of channel may not provide uniformly smooth newly created lumen due to extrinsic compression by the densely calcified intima. Self-expanding bare metal nitinol or covered Viabahn stents may have to be deployed to provide uniform lumen in the SFA and suprageniculate popliteal artery. Exit angiography should be performed to document restoration of uninterrupted flow into the foot. At the conclusion of the procedure, hemostasis at the access sites is achieved by manual pressure following reversal of anticoagulation.

Special Intraoperative Considerations

If the popliteal artery occlusion extends below the knee joint into the proximal tibial arteries, retrograde recanalization with SAFARI technique should preferably started first. When US-guided distal access is not possible, fluoroscopy-guided access of calcified arteries or continuous contrast injection through the antegrade access to localize the artery for access is necessary. In patients with ischemic ulcers and tissue loss, angiosome concept-based retrograde access for recanalization of the

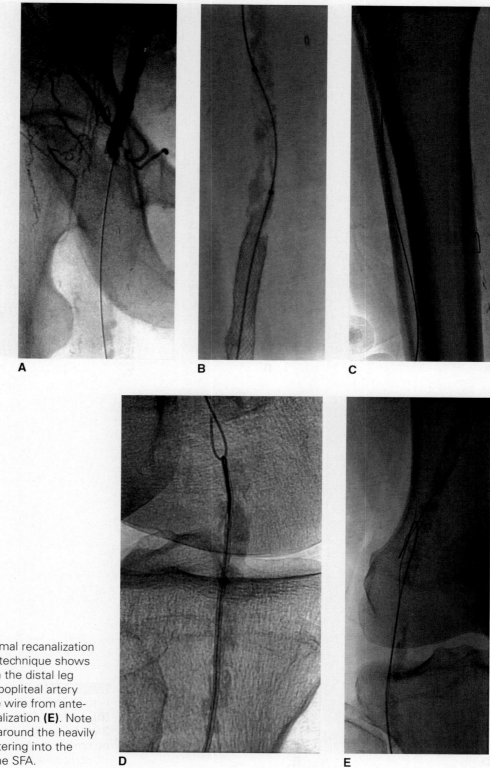

FIGURE 3 • Antegrade subintimal recanalization of CFA **(A)** and SFA **(B)**. SAFARI technique shows the retrograde access from AT in the distal leg **(C)**, retrograde recanalization of popliteal artery **(D)**, and snaring of the retrograde wire from antegrade access to complete recanalization **(E)**. Note the spiraling subintimal channel around the heavily calcified occluded lumen and entering into the fractured overlapping stents in the SFA.

tibial arteries is recommended. For recanalization of flush occlusions of the SFA, care should be taken to reenter anteromedially without compromising the ostium of the profunda femoris artery. Occasionally, the antegrade and retrograde channels may fail to communicate due to separation by a layer of arterial media. A double-balloon technique using simultaneous inflation of properly sized balloons from each access, with the tip of the balloons facing each other without overlap, allows communication between both channels by disrupting the separating layer

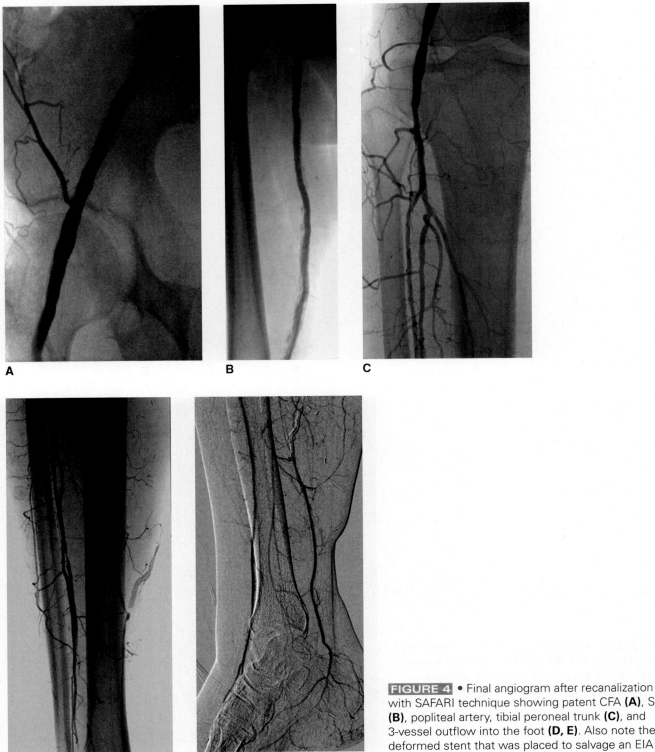

FIGURE 4 • Final angiogram after recanalization with SAFARI technique showing patent CFA **(A)**, SFA **(B)**, popliteal artery, tibial peroneal trunk **(C)**, and 3-vessel outflow into the foot **(D, E)**. Also note the deformed stent that was placed to salvage an EIA to PT composite vein graft at middle tibial level (D, E).

of arterial media. Complications from the recanalization steps are rare and most commonly include vessel perforation by guidewire or support catheter. If perforation or a major arterial venous communication is encountered, the wire is retracted by few centimeters and a new subintimal channel is created by changing the direction of the wire away from perforation. Similarly, when a reentry failure is encountered, changing the wire direction and creation of new channel at a slightly different plane often meets with success.

Atherectomy and debulking may improve the luminal diameter and eliminate the need for stenting. Prolonged

PTA at low pressure is recommended for PTA of tibial arteries. Angioplasty of the plantar arch and dorsalis pedis lesions should be considered to improve flow into the foot and wound healing. The new channel is often stented with self-expanding nitinol stents to achieve a larger smooth tubular lumen and to prevent focal narrowing by densely calcified plaques protruding into the lumen. Stents with open cell architecture may not fully expand due to focal extrinsic indentation by densely calcified plaques. Covered self-expanding stents are to be considered in the presence of extensive densely calcified CTO, focal intraprocedural perforations and arteriovenous fistula. Vasodilators such as intra-arterial nitroglycerin in multiple 100 to 200 µg boluses, papaverine, and verapamil should be considered to prevent arterial spasm from instrumentation. Distal embolization is not common with SAFARI procedure. However, when adjunct debulking and atherectomy devices are considered from antegrade access in patients with single tibial artery outflow, use of embolic protection devices may have a role. The retrograde pedal access sheath can also be used for aspiration of debris and clots. In the presence of occluded stents in the SFA, subintimal dissection outside of the stent may be difficult or may result in perforation. In this scenario, recanalization can be performed through the occluded stent and reenter the subintimal space after crossing the stent. During recanalization of long and multilevel CTO, the recanalization channel may be through a segment of native lumen. This may be unavoidable and does not alter the results of the procedure. Postprocedure hemostasis at distal access can also be obtained by inflation of a cuff over the site for 20 minutes at 30 mm Hg or by endoluminal inflation of an appropriately sized PTA balloon for 3 minutes from the antegrade access (Table 1).

TABLE 1. Key Technical Steps and Potential Pitfalls

Key Technical Steps

1. Gain US- or fluoroscopy-guided retrograde luminal access.
2. Recanalize with a straight or looped glidewire under real-time fluoroscopy.
3. Change the direction of wire when deviation of the wire from normal anatomic pathway is recognized.
4. Confirm successful recanalization before contrast injection.
5. Externalize retrograde wire through the antegrade sheath.
6. Perform antegrade or retrograde angioplasty over the SAFARI wire with properly sized balloons.
7. Perform adjunct procedures such as atherectomy, debulking, and stent placement for adequate luminal gain.

Potential Pitfalls

- Focal guidewire perforation or deviation into a branch artery
- Separation of antegrade and retrograde lumens due to different planes of subintimal dissection
- Occlusion of major branch artery origin by the subintimal dissection flap

Postoperative Management

Postoperatively, patients are admitted overnight for observation. Postprocedure lab evaluation includes, CBC, hematocrit, and renal function tests. Postprocedure ABIs are performed for baseline comparison prior to discharge. Two oral antiplatelet medications, aspirin 81 mg and Plavix 75 mg, are given for 6 weeks to 3 months following the procedure. Statins are administered for risk reduction. Oral anticoagulation is considered in patients that had extensive long-segment stenting.

Follow-up and surveillance is the key to the success of revascularization utilizing SAFARI technique. Every effort should be made to preserve the patency of revascularized arteries and the pedal arteries, since the procedure is most often performed when all other surgical and endovascular options are exhausted to treat the CTO. Arterial disease in the contralateral lower extremity is treated within 2 weeks, if necessary, to make the patient eligible for a supervised exercise program and postrevascularization rehabilitation. Patients are encouraged to increase activity level and initiate healthy diet for weight reduction and risk modification. Outpatient surveillance at 1, 3, 6, and 12 months, with noninvasive US imaging and Doppler evaluation in the clinic, is recommended for follow-up. Reintervention should be considered proactively in patients with evidence of focal recurrence of stenosis.

Case Conclusion

Postprocedure, the patient had significant improvement in ABI to 0.85 (PT) and 0.99 (AT), from a procedure 0.26 (PT) and 0.20 (AT). His rest pain resolved. At 3 years, following two secondary interventions for recurrence of disease in the popliteal artery on the right and one on the left for in-stent stenosis, he continued to be symptom free with an ABI bilaterally of 0.98 on the right and 1.10 on the left.

TAKE HOME POINTS

- SAFARI procedure preserves the collaterals at both ends of the occluded segment and the entire native reconstituted distal arteries.
- SAFARI technique can be attempted in all patients with a patent tibial artery with continuous flow into the foot.
- Following successful recanalization of proximal occlusion, distal tandem lesions should be treated to improve flow into the foot and for wound healing.
- Plantar loop technique performed through single access is not a SAFARI technique by definition but is a useful adjunct to recanalize additional crural arteries.
- SAFARI procedure does not compromise future surgical options, can be repeated, and is cost saving.

SUGGESTED READINGS

Bolia A, et al. Percutaneous transluminal angioplasty of occlusions of the femoral and popliteal arteries by subintimal dissection. *Cardiovasc Intervent Radiol.* 1990;13:357-363.

Gandini R, et al. The "Safari" technique to perform difficult subintimal infragenicular vessels. *Cardiovasc Intervent Radiol.* 2007;30:469-473.

Ikushima I, et al. Confluent two-balloon technique: an alternative method for subintimal recanalization of peripheral arterial occlusion. *J Vasc Interv Radiol.* 2011;22:1139-1143.

Nadal LL, Cynamon J, Lipsitz EC, et al. Subintimal angioplasty for chronic arterial occlusions. *Tech Vasc Interv Radiol.* 2004;7:16-22.

Schmidt A, et al. Retrograde recanalization technique for use after failed antegrade angioplasty in chronic femoral artery occlusions. *J Endovasc Ther.* 2012;19:23-29.

Spinosa DJ, et al. Subintimal arterial flossing with antegrade-retrograde intervention (SAFARI) for subintimal recanalization to treat chronic critical limb ischemia. *J Vasc Interv Radiol.* 2005;16:37-44.

CLINICAL SCENARIO CASE QUESTIONS

1. Distal embolization during SAFARI technique:
   a. Is the most common complication
   b. Should be prevented by using embolic protection devices
   c. Is more common than is transluminal recanalization procedure
   d. Is uncommon
   e. Often results in amputation

2. Limb salvage with SAFARI technique is least likely to be successful in a patient with:
   a. Atherosclerotic femoropopliteal occlusion and failed prior bypass grafts
   b. Flush occlusion of the SFA
   c. Diabetes, heel ulcer, and severe occlusive disease of plantar arch and dorsalis pedis arteries
   d. Contralateral below the knee amputation
   e. Occluded intra-arterial stents in the SFA

90 Failing Lower Extremity Bypass

NICHOLAS OSBORNE and PETER K. HENKE

Presentation

A 75-year-old man is seen for routine follow-up after undergoing reoperation on left femoral to below-knee popliteal bypass with reversed greater saphenous vein, which was done 6 months ago for rest pain. The patient had a prior femoral to above-knee popliteal bypass with prosthetic, and this had failed within 1 year. Past medical history includes diabetes, tobacco use times 30 years (and currently), hypertension, and hyperlipidemia. Medications include aspirin, a beta-blocker, an angiotensin-converting enzyme (ACE) inhibitor, and a multivitamin. The patient has no current symptoms and is ambulating more than half a mile without claudication. Physical examination shows a well-healed incision in his left groin and below-knee calf incision. The patient has a faintly palpable dorsalis pedis pulse with a biphasic Doppler signal. Ankle-brachial indices (ABIs) performed in the clinic prior to the visit demonstrate a decrease in his left (operative) leg of 0.61 from immediately post-op (0.86).

Differential Diagnosis

Although this patient is currently asymptomatic, they have an at-risk bypass graft. This early decrease in the ABIs suggests that there is a stenosis of the inflow, outflow, or bypass graft itself. The timing of the presentation correlates with the most common causes of graft failure. Within the first month following bypass, most bypass graft failures are due to technical problems or problems with conduit adequacy. These technical problems can range from anastomotic problems, persistent valve, or arteriovenous fistulae (especially in in situ grafts) and poor conduit. Between the period of 1 month and 2 years, failing bypasses are most likely due to intimal hyperplasia, but this may represent a technical problem such as an unrecognized sclerotic segment of vein, a frozen valve, or a stenosis of the inflow or outflow. Although long-segment stenoses are less likely, these can result from injury during vein harvest. After 1 to 2 years, the most common cause of bypass graft failure is progression of atherosclerotic disease of not only the inflow and outflow vessels but of the bypass graft itself.

Workup

All postoperative lower extremity bypass grafts should be followed with a standardized surveillance protocol; generally at first postoperative visit, then every 3 months for the first year, then biyearly, and then yearly. Recent studies of grafts followed with surveillance duplex have shown a primary assisted patency rate of 80% at 3 years. Although ABIs were not predictive of graft failure/revision, duplex ultrasonography (graft scans) has been correlated with improved patency rates. Graft stenoses may not manifest with dramatic changes in patient symptoms or changes in the ABI.

The patient's ABI is 0.61 on the left with biphasic Doppler waveforms. This suggests that there is a stenosis that will require reintervention to maintain graft patency.

Diagnosis and Treatment

Duplex graft surveillance is a well-established technique proven to significantly improve graft patency and limb salvage by 30% to 50% over 5 years and decrease early graft thrombosis by more than 50%. The concept is that a hemodynamically significant stenosis in the graft can be found and treated before the patient becomes symptomatic secondary to a thrombosed graft. Salvage techniques such as graft thrombolysis and revision are much less successful than if treated electively. Most graft stenoses occur within the first 2 postoperative years, and thus, more frequent early scanning is recommended (about every 3 to 6 months for the first year, every 6 months for the second year, and then yearly). Graft duplex velocities increase at the region of stenosis, and comparison between the highest velocity and just proximal to the stenosis velocity is essential. Table 1 shows an established classification of at-risk bypass grafts using duplex and ABI criteria. In general, as the velocity exceeds 300 cm/s, the graft is considered threatened. Highest-risk grafts have a loss of energy associated with a drop in the velocity following the stenosis to below 45 cm/s.

The patient underwent a duplex (graft scan), which showed a high-grade stenosis of the proximal

TABLE 1. Vein Graft Velocities and Risk of Graft Failure

Category	High-Velocity Criteria		Low-Velocity Criteria		Δ ABI
I. Highest risk	PSV > 300 cm/s or Vr > 3.5 or EDV > 100 cm/s	and	PSV < 45 cm/s	or	>0.15
II. High risk	PSV > 300 cm/s or Vr > 3.5	and	PSV > 45 cm/s	and	<0.15
III. Intermediate risk	300 cm/s > PSV > 200 cm/s or Vr > 2.0	and	PSV > 45 cm/s	and	<0.15
IV. Low risk	PSV < 200 cm/s or Vr < 2.0	and	PSV > 45 cm/s	and	<0.15

PSV, peak systolic velocity; EDV, end-diastolic velocity; Vr, velocity ratio.

anastomosis of 339 cm/s (Fig. 1). Early graft stenoses traditionally were treated with open surgical revision in the era prior to endovascular therapy. Currently, an endovascular approach can be attempted for a focal stenosis as first line.

Surgical Approach

Since this patient has an early graft stenosis that appears to involve the proximal anastomosis, an angiogram was performed to better delineate the nature of the stenosis. Since focal lesions may be amenable to treatment with balloon angioplasty, the patient was consented for an angiogram and possible intervention. Although a direct open repair may provide a long-term success, this would not interrogate the rest of the bypass graft.

Given the high-grade stenosis on duplex, the patient was admitted, and therapeutic intravenous heparin was administered to prevent graft occlusion. We treat these patients as urgencies given the high likelihood of occlusion that is unpredictable. The patient was taken the following day for an arteriogram from the contralateral femoral artery. The patient had a high-grade stenosis of the proximal graft on oblique views (Fig. 2). There was also an incidental stenosis of about 50% in the distal graft (not shown), which was balloon angioplastied with a 4-mm cutting balloon (on a 0.018 platform). The proximal lesion

was treated with a 5- and 6-mm cutting balloon with good results (Fig. 3). Pressure measurements before and after angioplasty demonstrated a gradient that decreased from 20 to 8 mm Hg across the lesion. Postoperatively, the patient did well. His ABIs improved to 0.87 on the left. At 1 month, he continued to have unchanged ABIs, but his graft duplex showed a residual stenosis proximally with a velocity of 266 cm/s. The patient was followed closely and returned to the clinic in 3 months with a repeat duplex and ABIs. Again, the ABIs remained unchanged (0.84), but his duplex again demonstrated an increased velocity of 365 cm/s in the proximal graft.

This patient now has a recurrent stenosis in the proximal graft, despite a successful endolumenal intervention. Although an endovascular approach could again be employed, given the quick recurrence of a flow-limiting lesion on duplex, an open revision with a vein patch may offer the best success and long-term patency. This patient was subsequently taken for an open revision of the proximal graft. In preparation, repeat vein mapping was performed, which demonstrated a usable segment of cephalic vein. He underwent a revision of the graft, and intraoperatively, he was found to have a stenotic segment of vein graft. This segment was patched with cephalic vein harvested from his left arm. Intraoperative duplex was used to

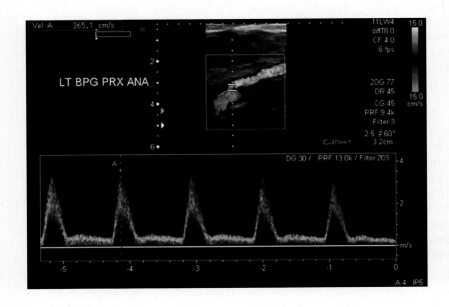

FIGURE 1 • Duplex ultrasound image showing high velocity in proximal vein graft. Note nice acoustic window, suggesting little turbulence.

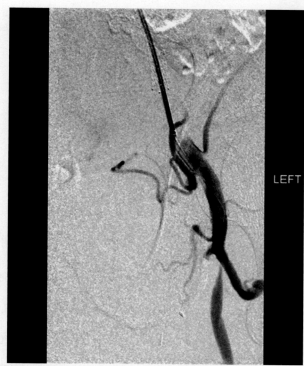

LEFT

FIGURE 2 • Contrast arteriogram showing high-grade proximal stenosis, likely due to neointimal hyperplasia.

demonstrate that the velocities were not elevated across the repair or distally (Table 2).

Special Intraoperative Considerations

Intraoperatively, it can help tremendously to have the stenosis marked using duplex prior to incision. This will help to guide the incision and avoid unnecessary dissection

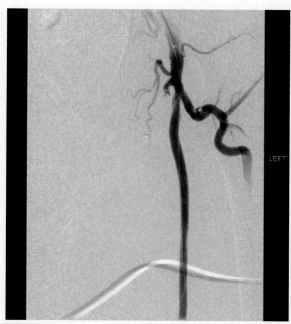

LEFT

FIGURE 3 • Post–cutting balloon angioplasty shows good result.

TABLE 2. Key Technical Steps and Potential Pitfalls

Key Technical Steps

1. Close follow-up of vein bypasses is essential, especially in the first 2 years.
2. Use of duplex ultrasonography is the standard method of following grafts.
3. If a high-grade stenosis identified, admission with heparinization is recommended, with early intervention.
4. Use of sequential cutting balloon angioplasty is recommended over noncutting balloon angioplasty.

Potential Pitfalls

- Ignoring duplex results suggesting high-grade stenosis
- Not treating critical stenosis in a timely fashion—that is, urgently
- Early (<30 d) graft stenosis is a problem as early graft angioplasty may cause rupture. Treating these patients with a 6-wk course of anticoagulation is recommended

and risk to the remaining bypass graft. The patient should have a usable segment of vein identified for patch angioplasty. Should the segment of vein be completely sclerotic, it may be interposed with a new vein graft, but this may lead to a higher risk of stenosis at the veno-veno anastomoses. Following repair, a completion duplex or angiogram is essential to judge the adequacy of the repair and rule out any other stenosis that could threaten the longevity of the bypass.

Case Conclusion

Postoperatively, he did well and was discharged home. His postoperative duplex showed a resolution of the stenosis with velocities in the 109 to 153 cm/s. Patient undergoing a reintervention for a threatened bypass should have the same routine follow-up schedule as a primary graft. He should remain on antiplatelet therapy, but in the absence of a high-risk graft (single vessel runoff, marginal conduit, spliced vein), he should not require anticoagulation with Coumadin postoperatively. Increased velocities on graft scan should again prompt repeat angiography.

TAKE HOME POINTS

- Recognition of a threatened bypass is crucial to prevent thrombosis/occlusion.
- Upon diagnosis of a threatened bypass, initiate anticoagulation immediately, and admit the patient for urgent intervention.
- An elevated velocity may be the only sign of a bypass graft stenosis.
- Perform an angiogram to investigate the possible stenosis and potentially treat the lesion.

- Recurrent stenosis is best treated with open repair (patch venoplasty or interposition).
- Use duplex to help guide the incision and exploration of a bypass stenosis.
- Routine surveillance of bypass grafts (especially in the first 2 years following surgery) will aid early recognition and treatment of these lesions.

SUGGESTED READINGS

Bergamini TM, George SM Jr, Massey HT, et al. Intensive surveillance of femoropopliteal-tibial autogenous vein bypass improves long-term graft patency and limb salvage. *Ann Surg.* 1995;221:507-516.

Mills JL, Bandyk DF, Gahtan V, et al. The origin of infrainguinal vein graft stenosis: a prospective study based on duplex surveillance. *J Vasc Surg.* 1995;21:16-25.

Mills JL Sr, Wixon CL, James DC, et al. The natural history of intermediate and critical vein graft stenosis: recommendations for continued surveillance or repair. *J Vasc Surg.* 2001;33:273-280.

Nehler MR, Moneta GL, Yeager RA, et al. Surgical treatment of threatened reversed infrainguinal vein grafts. *J Vasc Surg.* 1994;20:558-565.

Sanchez LA, Gupta SK, Veith FJ, et al. A ten-year experience with one hundred fifty failing or threatened vein and polytetrafluoroethylene arterial bypass grafts. *J Vasc Surg.* 1991;14(6):729-736.

Sullivan TR Jr, Welch HJ, Iafrati MD, et al. Clinical results of common strategies used to revise infrainguinal vein grafts. *J Vasc Surg.* 1996;24:909-919.

CLINICAL SCENARIO CASE QUESTIONS

1. A patient is seen for routine surveillance duplex of his bypass graft at 1 month post-op. What is the most common cause of a bypass graft failure at this time period?
   a. Anastomotic complication
   b. Vein graft atherosclerosis
   c. Progression of atherosclerosis in outflow vessels
   d. Inflow disease

2. A patient is seen in the clinic following a femoral to below-knee popliteal bypass with reversed saphenous vein graft. Which of the following is most consistent with a threatened bypass?
   a. CFA PSV 170, proximal anastomosis 186, mid graft 158, distal graft 230, outflow 156
   b. CFA PSV 170, proximal anastomosis 356, mid graft 38, distal graft 24, outflow 32
   c. CFA PSV 170, proximal anastomosis 356, mid graft 220, distal graft 180, outflow 186
   d. CFA PSV 170, proximal anastomosis 260, mid graft 158, distal graft 130, outflow 156

91 Acutely Thrombosed Bypass Graft (Including Lytics)

AMY B. REED

Presentation

A 57-year-old man arrives in the emergency department complaining of a 3-day history of a cool, painful left foot. He had previously undergone an aortobifemoral bypass graft at an outside institution. He is now 1 year out from a left femoral to posterior tibial artery bypass graft with greater saphenous vein, which you performed for rest pain after his prosthetic femoral above-knee popliteal artery bypass graft had occluded. On examination, the femoral pulses are palpable bilaterally. The left foot is cool and slightly mottled with a monophasic Doppler signal over the posterior tibial artery. The bypass graft is nonpalpable. His motorsensory examination is normal, except for slight numbness over the plantar arch.

Differential Diagnosis

The differential diagnosis for acute lower extremity ischemia typically includes arterial thrombosis secondary to underlying atherosclerotic arterial occlusive disease, atheromatous embolization from a more proximal unstable plaque, or thromboembolism from an aortic aneurysm or cardiac source. Early deep vein thrombosis can present in a similar manner; however, the leg will typically be swollen. Other less common causes of acute limb ischemia, such as thrombosed popliteal artery aneurysm, popliteal entrapment, and severe vasospasm, must also be kept in mind. In this patient with a previous history of peripheral bypass surgery, graft thrombosis must be considered the primary diagnosis.

Recommendation

After systemic heparinization, the initial diagnostic test in this patient is an aortogram with left lower extremity arteriogram. Acute limb ischemia is stratified into four categories based on severity and limb threat: class I—limb viable; class IIa—limb marginally threatened; class IIb—limb immediately threatened; and class III—irreversible limb changes. Patients with class I or IIa ischemia often have time for angiography and possible thrombolytic therapy in a semielective fashion, whereas patients with class IIb and early III typically require immediate revascularization. This patient has class IIa ischemia and would be best served by arteriography with possible thrombolysis of the suspected graft thrombosis.

Arteriography Report

Aortogram with left lower extremity runoff reveals a patent aortobifemoral bypass graft with occlusion of the superficial femoral, popliteal, and anterior tibial arteries. The stump of the bypass graft at the proximal anastomosis is visualized; however, the remainder of the graft is occluded. The posterior tibial artery is reconstituted in the proximal third of the calf.

Discussion

Catheter-directed thrombolysis for class I or IIa limb ischemia has several potential advantages, including more gentle clot lysis, the ability to clean out the involved segment as well as the distal vessels, and potentially revealing the underlying stenotic lesion. The decision to proceed with angiography and possible thrombolysis is dictated by the severity of the ischemia and perceived limb threat.

Approach

A Teflon-coated 0.035″ wire is used to select the stump of the proximal anastomosis and is able to be manipulated into the mid-portion of the occluded bypass graft. Percutaneous mechanical thrombectomy with a pulse spray of tissue plasminogen activator (TPA) 10 mg in 50 mL saline is laced throughout the extent of the thrombus. After 15 to 20 minutes of dwell time, percutaneous mechanical thrombectomy is performed. Repeat arteriography will typically show resolution of the thrombus and reveal the underlying culprit stenosis. If a significant amount of thrombus persists despite thrombectomy, an infusion catheter running TPA 1 mg/h along with systemic unfractionated heparin at 500 U/h may be run overnight. A repeat arteriogram is performed (Table 1 and Figure 1).

Arteriogram

Arteriogram Report

The bypass is able to be visualized after thrombolysis and reveals an area of narrowing just below the knee (Fig. 1).

TABLE 1. Key Steps and Potential Pitfalls of Thrombolysis

Key Technical Steps

1. Access with 6-French sheath to accommodate imaging and lysis catheter
2. TPA power pulse spray with 10 mg TPA in 50 mL heparinized saline with 15- to 20-min dwell time
3. Percutaneous mechanical thrombectomy and infusion catheter +/- infusion wire if residual thrombus
4. 500 U/hr IV heparin via sidearm of sheat

Potential Pitfalls

- Avoid full heparinization concomitantly with thrombolysis to reduce risk of remote bleed
- Follow fibrinogen levels, Hgb and PTT q 4-6hr to avoid potential complications from systemic thrombolysis

Approach

This area of narrowing will need to be addressed and revised in order to preserve long-term patency of the bypass graft. Ballon angioplasty with a cutting balloon is performed with less than 30% residual stenosis. A Duplex graft scan reveals proximal, mid-, and distal-portion graft velocities of 50 to 70 cm/s. Velocity at the distal anastomosis is 62 cm/s.

Diagnosis and Recommendation

Successful lysis of occluded femoral to posterior tibial artery bypass with underlying graft stenosis uncovered in the distal third of the bypass graft. The patient is offered graft revision using a short segment of distal greater saphenous vein from the ipsilateral extremity. It is explained to the patient that long-term graft patency is diminished, given the need for thrombolytics and graft revision, and that possible complications include graft failure as well as possible need for amputation, in addition to bleeding and infection.

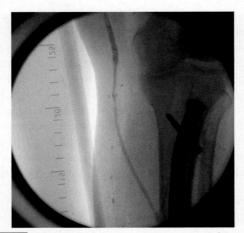

FIGURE 1 • Digital Subtraction Angiogram (DSA) image of distal graft showing narrowed area after successful thrombolysis.

Discussion

If thrombolytic therapy is successful, correction of the underlying graft lesion or distal runoff will be necessary. Intimal hyperplasia at valve sites and anastomoses are often the main culprits and may be amenable to balloon angioplasty if focal. Long areas of stenosis are best treated with open patch angioplasty or an interposition graft. Construction of a new distal anastomosis will often require a jump graft with vein to a more distal tibial arterial target.

Surgical Approach

The bypass graft is dissected free from surrounding soft tissue and scar via the previous medial incision. A segment of distal greater saphenous vein is harvested and is of excellent caliber. After systemic heparinization, proximal and distal control of the vein graft is achieved, followed by excision of the atretic segment of graft. End-to-end spatulated anastomoses are performed to interpose the harvested piece of greater saphenous vein. There is an excellent pulse in the vein graft with a palpable posterior tibial pulse at the ankle. Intraoperative duplex interrogation of the bypass graft shows complete resolution of the elevated velocities.

Discussion

Mature bypass grafts that have previously thrombosed are considered disadvantaged in terms of patency. Graft surveillance with duplex imaging should be employed on a regular basis to prevent this problem. Chronic warfarin anticoagulation may have a role in improving patency in these situations. Graft replacement versus salvage remains a controversial issue, particularly when autogenous conduit is limited.

Case Conclusion

This patient was heparinized and then he underwent arteriography and placement of thrombolytic catheter. After 24 hours, the graft was open and a distal stenosis was treated by cutting balloon angioplasty. He was anticoagulated for 6 months afterward and then transitioned to aspirin.

TAKE HOME POINTS

- Consider thrombolysis in cases where ischemia is nonembolic and grade level is IA or IIA.
- Contralateral remote arterial access with 6-French sheath.
- TPA power pulse spray with TPA, adequate dwell time, then percutanous thrombectomy.
- Treat underlying culprit lesion as able percutaneously or graft revision as needed.

- Anticoagulation and antiplatelet therapy with close graft surveillance.
- Consider new graft for those not successfully opened with thrombolysis.

SUGGESTED READINGS

Avino AJ, Bandyk DF, Gonsalves AJ, et al. Surgical and endovascular intervention for infrainguinal vein graft stenosis. *J Vasc Surg.* 1999;29:60-70.

Karthikeshwar K, Haskal ZJ, Ouriel K. The use of mechanical thrombectomy devices in the management of acute peripheral arterial occlusive disease. *J Vasc Interv Radiol.* 2001;12:405-411.

Nachman GB, Walsh DB, Fillinger MF, et al. Thrombolysis of occluded infrainguinal vein grafts: predictors of outcome. *J Vasc Surg.* 1997;25:512-521.

Sarac TP, Huber TS, Back MR, et al. Warfarin improves the outcome of infrainguinal vein bypass grafting at high risk for failure. *J Vasc Surg.* 1998;28:446-457.

CLINICAL SCENARIO CASE QUESTIONS

1. Percutaneous graft thrombolysis makes use of which thrombolytic agent?
   a. Urokinase
   b. Tissue plasminogen activator
   c. Snake viper venom
   d. Heparin
   e. Dabagatrin

2. _____ is a contraindication for thrombolytic therapy.
   a. Renal failure
   b. Age greater than 80
   c. Subarrachnoid hemorrhage 3 days prior
   d. Ventral hernia repair 3 weeks ago
   e. Factor V Leiden

92 Acute Limb Ischemia (Embolus)

NICHOLAS OSBORNE and PETER K. HENKE

Presentation

A 57-year-old man who had an acute myocardial infarction 6 weeks ago, treated with a percutaneous coronary intervention, presents to the emergency department with right lower extremity pain and numbness for 5 hours. The patient also feels light-headed and nauseated but is without chest pain. The patient notes having difficulty moving his right leg. No history of trauma is elicited. Past medical history includes tobacco use and hypertension, but no diabetes or hyperlipidemia. His discharge medications included an aspirin, a beta-blocker, an angiotensin-converting enzyme (ACE) inhibitor, and a diuretic.

On examination, his pulse is 140 beats per minute and irregular, and his blood pressure is 100/60 mm Hg. His abdomen is soft, and he has palpable femoral and pedal pulses in his left leg but no femoral or pedal pulses in his right leg. The right leg is cool and mottled, with decreased sensation and decreased motor function. Laboratory evaluation reveals creatinine, hematocrit, and leukocyte count and coagulation parameters within normal limits. His creatinine kinase is 290, and his lactate is 1.9.

Differential Diagnosis

A pulseless extremity warrants immediate attention. The patient presentation with pain, poikilothermia, pallor, paresthesias, and paralysis represent the classic five Ps of acute limb ischemia (ALI). ALI can be classified by the Society for Vascular Surgery (SVS) ALI grading system (Table 1). This patient represents grade IIB limb ischemia, which may be reversible with prompt intervention.

Workup

This patient has potential life- and limb-threatening problems with evidence of a new cardiac event (dysrhythmia), as well as ALI. It is common for patients with ALI to have multiple acute medical problems that must be treated appropriately, and saving life before limb is the overriding priority. First and foremost is evaluation and stabilization of his cardiac issues. An electrocardiogram suggests atrial fibrillation but no ST segment elevation or depression. The patient also denies any chest pain, and a rapid troponin I level is within normal limits. Thus, it is unlikely he has suffered a recurrent major myocardial infarction.

The most likely etiology of ALI in this case is a cardiac embolism and is the most common site of origin in general. Diagnostic tests, such as duplex and/or arteriography, may be considered, but minimizing delay in treatment for ALI is essential, because he has evidence of grade IIB limb ischemia. The patient needs revascularization within 1 to 2 hours (total ischemic time ≤6 hours), or he may suffer permanent muscle and nerve damage, rendering a nonsalvageable limb. A duplex or CT angiogram with runoff may be helpful to establish the level of thrombus/embolus, possibly identify a source (aortic thrombus), and demonstrate the presence of disease distal to the occlusion. Arteriography with thrombolysis is an option, but given the patient's classic history for an arterial thromboembolism (an antecedent cardiac event and normal vascular examination on his contralateral asymptomatic leg), this step may delay reperfusion that could be achieved more readily with surgery. The physical examination is very helpful to localize the site of occlusion in the setting of ALI. In this case, the patient has a diminished femoral pulse on the affected side, suggesting a more proximal lesion.

TABLE 1. Key Technical Steps/Potential Pitfalls

1. Circumferentially prep the extremity and contralateral groin to allow for catheter-directed interventions or below-knee/distal cut downs
2. Perform cut down of appropriate level vessels (femoral vs. popliteal)
3. If exposing the below-knee popliteal artery, control the tibioperoneal trunk and anterior tibial to allow for better control of the catheter direction in the tibialis
4. Make a transverse arteriotomy to avoid stenosis postoperatively
5. Start with a smaller embolectomy catheter and upsize as needed
6. Forcing the catheter can cause dissection—never force it
7. Always pass the embolectomy catheter one additional time following a clean passage
8. Confirm resolution of clot burden with back bleeding/forward bleeding and Doppler study following closure

Diagnosis and Treatment

This patient is suffering from both atrial fibrillation with rapid ventricular response and concomitant ALI. Upon establishing that this patient has ALI, the patient should be started on full-dose intravenous (IV) heparin (80 to 100 U/kg bolus and 18 U/kg/h). Intravenous heparin will not only improve outcomes from his ALI but will both decrease the risk of cardiac emboli from atrial fibrillation (which may also be the etiology of his lower extremity ischemia) and treat potential cardiac ischemia. An aspirin is given orally, as well. The patient's heart rate is controlled with an IV calcium channel blocker, and he converts to a sinus rhythm. The cardiac issues now seem to be stabilized. Cardiac enzymes are normal.

A CT angiogram of the abdomen pelvis and runoff demonstrates that the patient has an acute thrombus in the left external iliac and common femoral artery with distal reconstitution and three-vessel runoff to the foot. The contralateral side appears completely normal (Figs. 1 to 3).

Surgical Approach

In a patient with ALI with classic symptoms of an arterial atheroembolism (an antecedent cardiac event and normal vascular examination on his contralateral

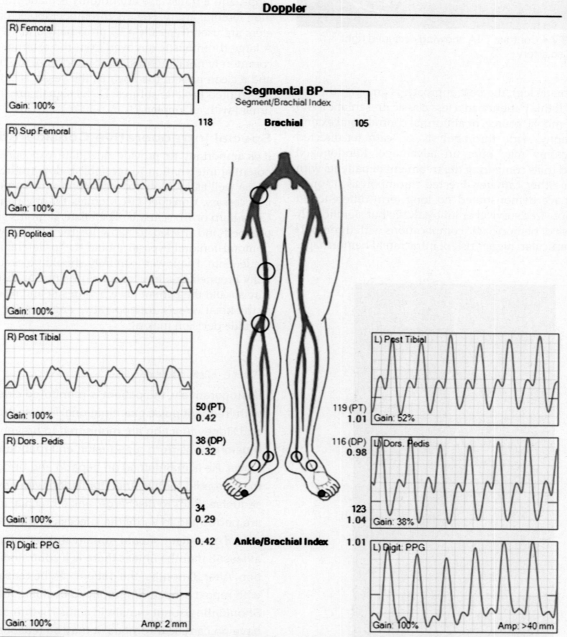

FIGURE 1 • Segmental doppler waveforms showing that his waveforms are monophasic from groin all the way to the foot, consistent with an occlusion above the inguinal ligament.

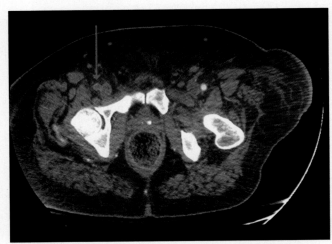

FIGURE 2 • Contrast CTA showing occluded right external iliac artery.

asymptomatic leg), the best approach is an open thrombectomy. If this patient had a less classic presentation (no obvious embolic source, or abnormal contralateral exam), arteriography with thrombolysis or catheter-directed thrombectomy may offer an advantage. Randomized controlled trials comparing the treatment of patients with ALI with either catheter-directed thrombolysis or open surgery have demonstrated no long-term difference in amputation-free survival or limb salvage but significantly higher risk of hemorrhagic complications with thrombolysis, in particular, higher risk of intracranial hemorrhage.

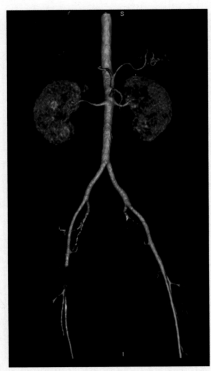

FIGURE 3 • Reformated CTA showing occluded right external iliac artery due to thromboembolism.

This patient is taken to the operating room. His abdomen and both lower extremities are prepped circumferentially and draped to allow an alternative arterial inflow vessel (e.g., contralateral femoral) if the ipsilateral iliac artery cannot be successfully embolectomized. Given the presentation, a femoral exposure is favored for removal of the thromboembolism. An open thromboembolectomy under local anesthesia with IV sedation is performed, given his recent myocardial infarction. A longitudinal incision is made from just below the inguinal ligament. The inguinal ligament is exposed, and the common femoral artery is dissected out along with its branches. Proximal and distal control is obtained with Pott's vessel loops, and a transverse arteriotomy is made in the common femoral artery. Fogarty thromboembolectomy catheters are used (typically a #5 proximally and #4 distally). A large thrombus is removed from the external iliac and common femoral arteries. After removal of the thrombus and a clean pass of the Fogarty, the vessel is closed with interrupted Prolene sutures. Distal signals are then confirmed with a Doppler.

Special Intraoperative Considerations

It is important to provide adequate exposure for any potential intervention to reestablish flow to the extremity, as well as to allow for fasciotomies to be performed if necessary. Consider fasciotomies for any patient with Class IIa/b or III ischemia. The bilateral groins should be prepped and draped to allow for the alternative inflow (femoral-femoral bypass) should the ipsilateral inflow be inadequate. The lower extremity should be circumferentially prepped to allow for a below-knee or distal exposure should the patient have poor result and residual clot in the tibial vessels. Intraoperative angiography can help to guide decision making.

Case Conclusion

Postoperatively, the patient is monitored closely with frequent pulse examinations. The electrolytes and kidney function are monitored to prevent any repercussions from reperfusion and rhabdomyolysis. He is maintained on heparin and bridged to Coumadin for his atrial fibrillation with embolic sequelae. Prior to discharge, ankle-brachial indices are performed to verify the success of the procedure. The patient should remain anticoagulated for at least 3 months unless there is a contraindication. After 3 months, the patient can be reassessed with repeat echocardiography to evaluate for clot. Should the patient remain in sinus rhythm and have no cardiac thrombus, it may be reasonable to stop anticoagulation.

TAKE HOME POINTS

- Prompt recognition of ALI is crucial.
- Determine the duration and reversibility of the ischemia (stage of ischemia).
- Early and therapeutic heparinization improves outcomes.
- Determine the site of occlusion using physical exam and noninvasive imaging.
- When performing an embolectomy, start with a smaller embolectomy catheter and then upsize the catheter.
- Consider the use of angiography and catheter-directed thrombolysis when the presentation and exam are not consistent with an embolic cause of ALI.
- Any embolectomy can be performed under local with sedation in the moribund patient.
- Consider fasciotomies in any patient with prolonged limb ischemia or advanced symptoms (Stage IIa or greater).

SUGGESTED READINGS

Berridge DC, Kessel DO, Robertson I. Surgery versus thrombolysis for initial management of acute limb ischaemia. *Cochrane Database Syst Rev.* 2013 PMID: 23744596.

Eliason JL, Wainess RM, Proctor MC, et al. A national and single institutional experience in the contemporary treatment of acute lower extremity ischemia. *Ann Surg.* 2003;238(3): 382-389; discussion 389-390.

Ouriel K, Veith FJ, Sasahara AA. A comparison of recombinant urokinase with vascular surgery as initial treatment for acute arterial occlusion of the legs. Thrombolysis or peripheral arterial surgery (TOPAS Investigators). *N Engl J Med.* 1998;338(16):1105-1111.

Rutherford RB, Baker JD, Ernst C, et al. Recommended standards for reports dealing with lower extremity ischemia: revised version. *J Vasc Surg.* 1997;26(3):517-538.

Weaver FA, Comerota AJ, Youngblood M, et al. Surgical revascularization versus thrombolysis for nonembolic lower extremity native artery occlusions: results of a prospective randomized trial The STILE Investigators Surgery versus thrombolysis for ischemia of the lower extremity. *J Vasc Surg.* 1996;24(4):513-521; discussion 521-523.

CLINICAL SCENARIO CASE QUESTIONS

1. A 75-year-old gentleman presents with a cold pulseless left leg. He has no Doppler signals in his DP or PT. He has mild sensory changes overlying the first web space. He has normal motor function. This represents:

   a. Class I ischemia
   b. Class IIa ischemia
   c. Class IIb ischemia
   d. Class III ischemia

2. As compared to open embolectomy, catheter-directed thrombolysis has been shown to have a(n):

   a. Inferior long-term amputation-free survival
   b. Higher degree of improvement in ABIs following therapy
   c. Higher rate of periprocedural hemorrhage
   d. Lower rate of intracranial hemorrhage

93 Paradoxical Embolism

BENJAMIN JACOBS, ANDREW KIMBALL, and THOMAS W. WAKEFIELD

Presentation

A 59-year-old woman presents to an outside institution with right-sided facial droop, right-sided hemiplegia, mild aphasia, and hypoxemia. She is resuscitated and put on oxygen with resolution of her hypoxemia. A computed tomography (CT) scan of the head was unremarkable, and a spiral chest CT scan revealed bilateral pulmonary emboli (PE). At this point, the patient is stabilized and transferred to your hospital.

On admission, the patient reports acute-onset shortness of breath and right-sided weakness roughly 12 hours ago. Without prompting, the patient recalls that 4 weeks ago she fell and dislocated her patella. She saw an orthopedic surgeon at that time—who recommended bed rest and non–weight bearing on that extremity. She continues to complain of pain in her left lower extremity. On exam, the patient is afebrile and in no respiratory distress. Vital signs reveal a regular pulse of 95 beats per minute, respiratory rate 22, and blood pressure 134/79; pulse oximetry is 91% on 4 L of oxygen and 100% on 100% oxygen by face mask. On physical examination, a systolic ejection murmur is appreciated; lungs are clear; there is ecchymosis of the left patella extending down to the shin without erythema or tenderness. Neurologic examination is significant for right-sided hemianopsia, facial droop, aphasia, and upper and lower extremity weakness.

Differential Diagnosis

The differential diagnosis in this case includes

1. Cerebral vascular accident (CVA—cardioembolic or thromboembolic)
2. Deep venous thrombosis with pulmonary embolism (DVT/PE)
3. CVA and DVT/PE
4. Paradoxical embolism—simultaneous DVT/PE and CVA from a venous embolus traversing a right-to-left shunt into the arterial system.

Initial Workup

In this case, a paradoxical embolism would account for all of the patient's symptoms and does not make the assumption that two conditions are happening simultaneously. Given concern for a paradoxical embolism, a transthoracic echocardiogram (TTE) with agitated saline injection ("bubble test") is ordered to look for a patent foramen ovale (PFO), and a lower extremity duplex scan is ordered to look for a DVT. Of note, transesophageal echocardiography (TEE) is considered more sensitive for the detection of a PFO—and should be ordered if the TTE is nondiagnostic.

Lower Extremity Duplex Scan

The lower extremity duplex scan reveals evidence of an acute DVT of the left leg involving the posterior tibial, peroneal, and anterior tibial veins.

Transthoracic Echocardiography with "Bubble Test"

The TTE with bubble test reveals no evidence of PFO—although the exam is limited by the patient's body habitus.

Transesophageal Echocardiography with "Bubble Test"

The TEE with bubble test reveals clear evidence of a PFO with right to left shunt. Of note, there is no valvular vegetations or intra-atrial thrombus.

Case Continued

The diagnosis of paradoxical embolism is made based on the clinical history and clear objective evidence of DVT/PE, a right-to-left shunt, and arterial embolism. The day after admission, a noncontrast head CT demonstrates mass effect consistent with a left cerebral nonhemorrhagic infarct. Given concern for hemorrhagic conversion of her stroke, she is not anticoagulated immediately and a Greenfield filter is placed. Three days after admission, the patient complains of increased right-sided weakness. She undergoes carotid duplex imaging.

Carotid Duplex Scan
Duplex Scan Report

A heterogeneous embolus (*arrow*) in the left common carotid artery creating a 60% to 80% diameter stenosis with instability is found (Fig. 1). The distal end of the embolus is imaged.

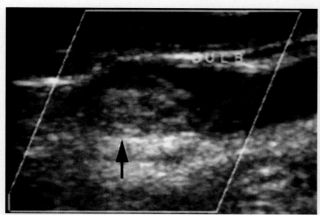

FIGURE 1 • Echogenic embolus (*arrow*) just below left carotid bulb. (Reproduced from Gada H, Jafer M, Graziano K, et al. Carotid embolectomy in the treatment of a paradoxical embolus. *Ann Vasc Surg.* 2003;17:457-461, with permission.)

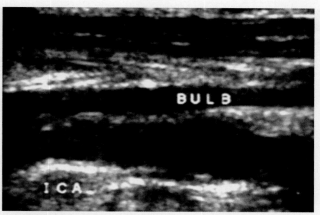

FIGURE 3 • Postprocedure duplex scan reveals no abnormalities. (Reproduced from Gada H, Jafer M, Graziano K, et al. Carotid embolectomy in the treatment of a paradoxical embolus. *Ann Vasc Surg.* 2003;17(4):457-461, with permission.)

Surgical Approach

The diagnosis of paradoxical embolus (PDE) to the left carotid artery is made. The patient is taken to the operating room for embolectomy, because the embolus appears to be unstable with the potential to cause further cerebrovascular injury. After systemic heparin administration, the left carotid artery is opened, revealing a large embolus at the carotid bifurcation. This embolus is removed, but because adequate retrograde flow is not obtained, a 3-French Fogarty catheter is carefully passed, extracting a tail of thrombus (6 cm long; Fig. 2). A number 12 shunt is rapidly placed, and flow is documented using Doppler. The arteriotomy is closed with a patch, and minimal atherosclerotic disease is found.

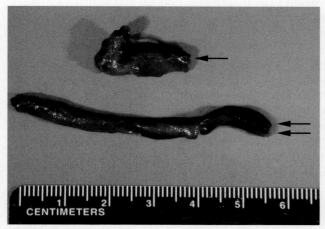

FIGURE 2 • Operative specimen revealing embolus. *Arrow* demonstrates echogenic embolus and correlates to the preoperative duplex image (see Fig. 55-1*A*). *Double arrows* point to thrombus tail. (Reproduced from Gada H, Jafer M, Graziano K, et al. Carotid embolectomy in the treatment of a paradoxical embolus. *Ann Vasc Surg.* 2003;17:457-461, with permission.)

A completion intraoperative duplex scan reveals excellent flow through the carotid and no debris (Fig. 3). The patient is awakened on the table and taken to the recovery room, where she remains stable. Her neurologic examination remains unchanged.

Case Continued

Six days following carotid embolectomy, the patient undergoes percutaneous closure of her PFO. The PFO is sized with a sizing balloon, and an Amplatzer atrial septal occluder device is delivered using fluoroscopic guidance.

After PFO closure, hemodynamic data indicates no significant shunt by oximetry. The patient is placed on long-term anticoagulation with warfarin for her lower extremity DVT. The patient is well at discharge with a stable neurologic exam. Six weeks later, a duplex scan of the left carotid artery is performed showing no abnormality. The patient was well at discharge from rehabilitation with a stable neurologic examination.

Discussion

PDE refers to venous embolism into the arterial circulation via a right-to-left shunt. A PFO is believed to be a major predisposing factor for PDE, especially in the presence of a large defect and concomitant atrial septal aneurysm. PFO is found in 25% to 30% of the population based on autopsy data. There is a reported fourfold increase in frequency of PFO in patients under 55 years old presenting with ischemic stroke. It is important to note, however, that the presence of a PFO is a sufficient but not necessary criterion for the diagnosis of paradoxical embolism, as intrapulmonary shunts are seen as well. *Indeed, these events are best characterized as belonging to the category known as cryptogenic stroke, or stroke that cannot be attributed to the common cardioembolic or atherosclerotic processes.*

TABLE 1. Carotid Embolectomy as Treatment of Paradoxical Embolus

Author	Age	Sex	Presentation	Location of Obstruction	Type of Surgery	Outcome	Follow-up Treatment
Turnbull et al. (1998)	54-year-old	M	Embolic stroke, pulmonary embolism, patent foramen ovale	Innominate artery	Combined carotid bifurcation and brachial embolectomy	Good	Long-term anticoagulation
McKinney et al. (2001)	67-year-old	M	Embolic stroke, patent foramen ovale, pulmonary hypertension	Right carotid bifurcation	Carotid embolectomy	Good	Long-term anticoagulation
Gada et al. (2003)	59-year-old	F	Embolic stroke, pulmonary embolism, patent foramen ovale	Left common carotid artery	Carotid embolectomy	Good	Long-term anticoagulation with percutaneous transcatheter closure of PFO

Modified from Gada H, Jafer M, Graziano K, et al. Carotid embolectomy in the treatment of a paradoxical embolus. *Ann Vasc Surg.* 2003;17:457-461.

The diagnosis of PDE requires

1. Confirmed presence of venous thromboembolism (VTE)
2. Evidence of abnormal communication between the systemic arterial and venous circulation
3. Evidence for arterial embolism
4. A gradient favoring right-to-left shunting

The present patient illustrates many of the classic features concerning for PDE. She presented with simultaneous symptoms of VTE and stroke. Her recent history of an orthopedic trauma and bed rest predispose her to the development of VTE and cross-sectional imaging from the outside institution confirmed the presence of a PE. A positive DVT scan and TEE with evidence of a PFO and right-to-left shunt help to solidify the diagnosis.

Current treatment of ischemic stroke of any type, including PDE, includes intravenous administration of Recombinant Tissue Plasminogen Activator (rt-PA). Fibrin-rich clots originating in the deep venous system, like those associated with PDE, are theoretically more amenable to thrombolysis with rt-PA. One study showed that patients with paradoxical embolic stroke had significantly better outcomes after rt-PA thrombolysis, though these data are best explained by age—younger in PDE patients—and admission NIH Stroke Scale, which was lower in PDE patients.

In PDE, anticoagulation should be started given the presence of VTE, but with concurrent acute stroke, the timing of initiation of anticoagulation is unclear. Per AHA and ACCP guidelines, early parenteral anticoagulation is not recommended in acute ischemic stroke due to the risk of hemorrhagic conversion. Early antithrombotic therapy with aspirin is recommended, however, within the first 48 hours. The use of Inferior Vena Cava (IVC) filter placement for the secondary prevention of early, recurrent, cryptogenic stroke has been described in the literature, but its effectiveness is unproven. IVC filters have been found to permit passage of emboli 3 mm in diameter. While these small emboli likely never cause significant

sequelae in the pulmonary circulation, they most certainly can have devastating sequelae in the cerebral circulation. While this continues to be studied, under present circumstances, there appears to be a general agreement among vascular surgeons that the potential benefits of IVC filter placement outweigh the potential risks.

Given the fact that most patients presenting with PDE have a PFO, it seems logical that closure of the PFO would be the preferable, definitive, treatment option. Over the past 10 years, this logic has been corroborated by numerous comparative, observational, and single-arm nonrandomized studies that have suggested decreased recurrence rates with PFO closure. In recent years, however, there have been many new randomized controlled trials with somewhat conflicted results. *While percutaneous PFO closure may seem like a logical solution, it is important to remember that it carries inherent risk and there is a significant amount of mounting data suggesting that it makes no difference in long term outcomes. Ultimately, the decision to proceed with PFO closure should be made on a case-by-case basis, guided by the surgeons clinical suspicion of PFO involvement and a meticulous analysis of the potential risks and benefits.*

Surgical treatment of carotid embolism caused by PDE is rare. Only three reported cases (including the present case) of surgical management have been described (Table 1). The major risk of carotid embolectomy is further ischemia caused by either distal embolization or reperfusion injury to the ischemic area.

Case Conclusion

In this case, the benefits of open embolectomy outweighed the risks of stroke extension because the patient still had movement in her right lower extremity, as well as improving aphasia. If she had evidence of a massive stroke or was unconscious, embolectomy would not have been recommended, as it would have exposed her to the risks of surgery without clear hopes of an improved outcome.

TAKE HOME POINTS

- PDE refers to venous embolism into the arterial circulation via a right-to-left shunt, for which PFO is believed to be the major predisposing factor.
- The diagnosis of paradoxical embolism is based on the clinical history and objective evidence of VTE, arterial embolism, and a right-to-left shunt.
- Initial treatment of PDE involves IV administration of rt-PA and initiation of antithrombotic therapy with aspirin within the first 48 hours.
- Data for percutaneous closure of PFO are equivocal, and this decision should be made after consideration of individual patient risk profiles.

SUGGESTED READINGS

Carroll JD, et al. Closure of patent foramen ovale versus medical therapy after cryptogenic stroke. *N Engl J Med.* 2013; 368(12):1092-1100.

Dalman R, Kohler TR. Cerebrovascular accident after Greenfield filter placement for paradoxical embolism. *J Vasc Surg.* 1989; 9(3):452-454.

Fazekas F. Management of right-to-left shunt in cryptogenic cerebrovascular disease: results from the observational Austrian paradoxical embolism trial (TACET) registry. *J Neurol.* 2013;260(1):260-267.

Fisher DC, Fisher EA, Budd JH, et al. The incidence of patent foramen ovale in 1000 consecutive patients: a contrast transesophageal echocardiography study. *Chest.* 1995;107:1504-1509.

Furlan AJ, et al.; for the CLOSURE I Investigators. PFO closure: closure. *Stroke.* 2013;44:S45-S47.

Gada HG, Jafer M, Graziano K, et al. Carotid embolectomy in the treatment of a paradoxical embolus. *Ann Vasc Surg.* 2003;17:457-461.

Hagen PT, Scholz DG, Edwards WD. Incidence and size of patent foramen ovale during the first 10 decades of life: an autopsy study of 965 normal hearts. *Mayo Clin Proc.* 1984;59(1):17.

Horner S, Niederkorn K, Gattringer T, et al. Paradoxical embolism. *Circulation.* 2010;122:1968-1972.

Martin F, Sanchez PL, Doherty E, et al. Percutaneous transcatheter closure of patent foramen ovale in patients with paradoxical embolism. *Circulation.* 2002;106:1121-1126.

McKinney WB, O'Hara W, Sreeram K, et al. The successful surgical treatment of a paradoxical embolus to the carotid bifurcation. *J Vasc Surg.* 2001;33:880-882.

Turnbull RG, Tsang VT, Teal PA, et al. Successful innominate thromboembolectomy of a paradoxic embolus. *J Vasc Surg.* 1998;28:742-745.

CLINICAL SCENARIO CASE QUESTIONS

1. Which of the following is not required for the diagnosis of PDE?

    a. Confirmed presence of venous thromboembolism (VTE)

    b. Echocardiographically proven atrial thrombus

    c. Evidence for arterial embolism

    d. A gradient favoring right-to-left shunting

2. The initial therapy of paradoxical embolism causing ischemic stroke includes:

    a. Early antithrombotic therapy with aspirin

    b. Carotid endarterectomy

    c. Oral anticoagulation with warfarin

    d. Caval interruption with Greenfield filter

94 Diabetic Foot Ulcer

JASON CROWNER and WILLIAM MARSTON

Presentation

A 26-year-old female with past medical history of end-stage renal disease requiring dialysis, hypertension, and type 2 diabetes presents to the wound care clinic for evaluation of a left great toe ulcer. Vital signs are grossly normal except for hypertension with systolic blood pressures in the 180s. Physical examination reveals an obese African American female with palpable left foot pedal pulses and an ulcer on the plantar aspect of the great toe (Fig. 1). A large callus surrounds the ulceration with necrotic tissue present within the base and apparent drainage. The patient states the wound has been present for several months and has been treated with Polysporin and oral antibiotics without significant improvement. She also reports a history of poorly controlled diabetes with a hemoglobin A1c of 9.9, persistent tobacco use, and continued ambulation on the foot.

Differential Diagnosis

Approximately 15% of diabetic patients will develop a full-thickness lower extremity ulcer, usually due to the combination of sensory neuropathy and motor neuropathy leading to toe and foot deformities. This is termed diabetic foot ulcer (DFU). In some cases, the condition is exacerbated by diabetes-induced peripheral arterial disease (PAD). Initial evaluation should consider the patient's diabetes and its complications to be the main causation of the ulcer until proven otherwise. Other common causes of lower extremity ulceration include nondiabetic arterial insufficiency, chronic venous insufficiency, trauma, and chronic pressure. Unusual causes include malignancy, lupus, Raynaud's syndrome, sickle cell disease, and gout.

In the evaluation of ulcerations present on the lower extremities, it is important to obtain a full and adequate history and physical examination. Diabetic ulcers frequently occur due to poor foot care in the setting of neuropathy, but the combined presence of PAD can exacerbate small wounds. Physical exam should include monofilament foot testing for neuropathy and noninvasive examination of the blood supply with an arterial duplex of the lower extremity. Routine laboratory evaluation should include hemoglobin A1c and plain x-rays of the foot to evaluate for osseous abnormalities or osteomyelitis.

Workup

Our patient's radiologic evaluation of the foot demonstrated soft tissue swelling and irregularity along the great toe distal phalanx consistent with possible infectious osteitis (Fig. 2). Laboratory values demonstrated an elevation of her hemoglobin A1c of 9.9, a white blood cell count within normal limits, and wound cultures demonstrating *Staphylococcus*. Arterial duplex of the right lower extremity demonstrated no evidence of PAD by presence of palpable pedal pulses.

Discussion

Diabetic foot ulceration is defined as a full-thickness wound penetrating through the dermis (the deep vascular and collagenous inner layer of the skin) located below the ankle in a diabetic patient according to the International Working Group on the Diabetic Foot. Multiple factors play into a DFU formation and inability to heal. The major factors in the formation of DFU are secondary to peripheral neuropathy and ischemia from PAD.

The DFU can thus be categorized into purely neuropathic, purely ischemic, or a combination of the two. A combination of the two, neuroischemia, makes up the majority, with a prevalence of approximately 50%, followed by neuropathic at 35%, and ischemic at 15%. The incidence of limb loss is highest in the neuroischemic group, estimated at 15% at 5 years. Early identification and treatment of PAD has been found to reduce the risk of limb loss.

Diagnosis and Treatment

A detailed evaluation of the wound is important to document the appearance, size, location, and the state of infection. This information should be available at follow-up visits to determine whether the wound is responding to the treatment. DFUs treated with a comprehensive management plan should demonstrate a significant reduction in size within 3 to 4 weeks of initiating treatment. If not, a full reevaluation of the wound and its potential underlying causes should be performed. The examination should

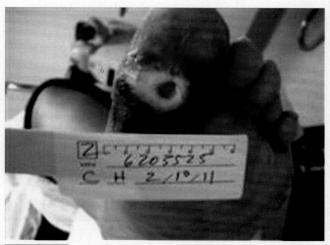

FIGURE 1 • Picture showing plantar base of great toe ulcer.

also include an investigation as to the specific cause of the ulceration: poor foot care, ill-fitting footwear, or bony changes causing pressure.

Operative management is warranted when there is nonviable tissue, infection, or need for improvement of blood flow. The need for wound cultures is controversial in the treatment of DFUs. In clearly infected wounds, tissue samples for culture are useful to identify the specific bacterial pathogens and guide antibiotic therapy. In wounds that do not appear to be clinically infected, it is unclear whether wound cultures are useful to identify and treat overgrowth of bacteria.

Several measures have been found to be useful in determining whether a lower extremity has adequate blood supply to heal with good wound care. Ankle-brachial

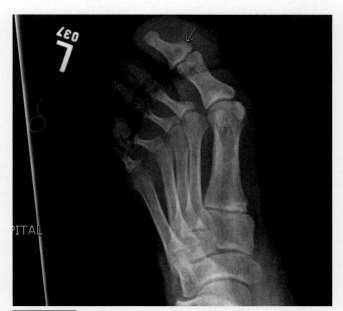

FIGURE 2 • Left foot x-ray—soft tissue swelling and irregularity along the great toe consistent with possible infectious osteitis at the base of the great toe phalanx.

indices (ABIs) are useful if the tibial blood vessels are not too calcified for compression. An ABI greater than 0.8 usually suggests that sufficient supply is available to support wound healing. An ABI between 0.5 and 0.8 is marginal, and an ABI below 0.5 is typically inadequate for an ankle or foot ulcer to heal. Patients with heavily calcified tibial vessels may yield falsely elevated ABIs. Toe pressures can be obtained with the use of a plethysmography cuff and are useful in situations where foot disease is present or ABIs are falsely elevated. An alternative to consider is to obtain transcutaneous oxygen measurement (TCOM) in the foot. A toe pressure greater than 50 mm Hg or a TCOM above 40 torr is typically associated with a favorable potential to heal, while lower numbers suggest that revascularization is likely to be necessary.

In regard to our case presentation, the patient's physical evaluation demonstrated the presence of infection and nonviable tissue. Arterial duplex examination of the limb resulted in an ABI of 0.95 and toe pressure of 140 consistent with normal arterial supply. The decision was made for operative debridement.

Ulcer Management

Nonsurgical

Conservative management involves aggressive wound care utilizing pressure offloading, topical wound agents, dressings, and adjuvant therapies. In a patient with adequate arterial supply, the primary underlying etiology relates to neuropathy-induced pressure. Thus, pressure offloading is critical to achieving reliable wound healing. A variety of options must be employed in individual patient cases to effectively relieve pressure including custom-molded orthotics, custom-designed shoes, full-length boots, and total contact casts (Fig. 3). The participation of a skilled podiatrist and/or orthotist is important to achieve optimal healing outcomes. Once healing of the wound has occurred, it is still important to counsel the patient on the importance of proper fitting footwear and daily monitoring.

A wide variety of topical wound agents and dressings are available for the treatment of DFUs and can assist with moisture, exudate, and bacterial control. In general, a moist wound environment is favored to support wound healing. Excess moisture in the wound bed is typically an inflammatory source and can become a nidus for infection. In this case, absorptive alginate or foam dressings are useful; however, many DFUs express little or no wound exudate and actually are susceptible to excess desiccation leading to poor healing. In these cases, the use of a moisture-donating hydrogel is useful to prevent tissue desiccation and support healing. Although there are a wide variety of dressings that claim to improve the healing of DFUs, there are no dressings that have been shown in robust randomized studies to significantly improve the rate of DFU closure.

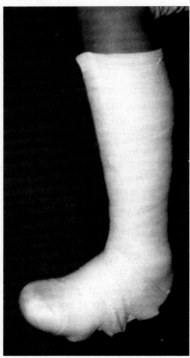

FIGURE 3 • Total contact cast.

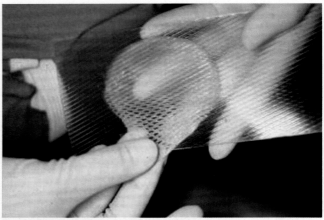

FIGURE 4 • Living cellular therapy.

Adjuvant Therapies

Negative Pressure Therapy

Application of negative pressure to the wound bed using a variety of devices has been found to improve the incidence of DFU healing. Two randomized studies using the Vacuum Assisted Closure (VAC) device (KCI—San Antonio, TX) have identified an increase in the incidence of DFU healing compared to standard wound dressings.

Living Cellular Therapies

Two living cellular therapies, Dermagraft and Apligraf, have been found in multicenter randomized studies to improve the incidence of wound closure of DFUs compared to standard treatment (Fig. 4). Other therapies that may be useful in selected cases to improve the incidence of wound healing include platelet-derived growth factor (Regranex) and hyperbaric oxygen (HBO) therapy.

Use of HBO therapy is an adjunct to wound care thought to increase cellular proliferation and angiogenesis. The patient is placed in a chamber at 2 to 3 atm of pressure while inhaling 100% oxygen; this dramatically increases oxygen partial pressure in the tissues resulting in increased oxygen carried by plasma. HBO therapy is thought to promote growth factors, increase collagen synthesis, help in the mobilization of stem/progenitor cells from bone and marrow, enhance antibacterial effects, and increase fibroblast activity. Evidence suggests that HBO may be useful in severe DFUs complicated by bone or tendon involvement after surgical debridement.

Surgical

The most compelling surgical indication is the presence of infection or gangrene. As mentioned previously, the initial workup of a DFU should include an x-ray, especially if signs of infection are present. Gas gangrene visualized on radiologic evaluation is an urgent surgical indication. The x-ray can also display bony changes such as osteomyelitis that can alter the surgical decision-making process.

Once the decision to operate is made (Table 1)—there are multiple tools to assist with the debridement itself along with wound healing. The operative debridement of devitalized or infected tissue can be performed with a scalpel, curette, or hydrosurgery using the Versajet. Once nonviable tissue is removed, wound care and healing once again become the main priorities.

In some cases, an amputation is necessary secondary to the disease process, location of ulcer, or infection involving a majority of the foot. In these instances, digit amputations may be necessary versus the use of a transmetatarsal or below-the-knee amputation. Most patients can fully function with loss of one or two digits, particularly if the

---

TABLE 1. Diabetic Ulcer Management

Key Technical Steps

1. Debridement of only nonviable tissue. Leave as much healthy tissue as possible.
2. Send proximal bone for culture to help with postoperative antibiotic management.
3. Tension-free closure of wound.
4. Ensure sufficient tissue for bone coverage and wound closure. Debride bone back to allow sufficient coverage.
5. End result of operation needs to leave the patient with a functional limb.

Potential Pitfalls

- Electing to perform operative management without evaluating blood flow
- Debridement of ulcer/limb in such a fashion that the limb will never be viable or usable for ambulation
- Leaving exposed bone with no soft tissue coverage

great toe is not involved, but once walking is not viable or operative debridement necessitates, it may be more beneficial to move forward with a midfoot or transmetatarsal amputation. The below-the-knee amputation should be reserved for circumstances in which the patient cannot heal distally or if the infection involves the entirety of the foot.

Postoperative Management

After adequate surgical debridement, an aggressive plan of pressure offloading, revascularization if needed, and wound management is initiated. If the postoperative wound is large, with a significant tissue defect, Negative Pressure Wound Therapy (NPWT) is commonly selected to accelerate granulation coverage of bone and tendon, reducing the incidence of recurrent infection. HBO may be selected in nonresponders to standard therapy, and living cellular preparations may be useful in the well-granulated wound bed to accelerate skin closure. The help of an occupational or physical therapist is also valuable to assist with proper ambulation after foot surgery, offloading, and other rehabilitation.

Case Conclusion

The patient underwent debridement of her left great toe—excisional debridement was performed for removal of nonviable skin and subcutaneous tissue. Surrounding callus was also trimmed away sharply. The wound extended down near the bone of the distal digit, but on palpation of the bone, there was no evidence of osteomyelitis. She tolerated the procedure well and continued conservative wound management with frequent trips to the wound care clinic for evaluation and maintenance of her ulcer. Along with wound care, she was evaluated and treated in the diabetes center by endocrinology and a diabetes nutritionist for better glycemic control. We also recommended the use of total contact casting to optimally eliminate pressure to the wound area. Unfortunately, the patient did not agree to this therapy that requires weekly clinic visits for care. Despite other therapies, her wound enlarged with further exposure of the bone and development of osteomyelitis. This required great toe amputation 4 months later after unsuccessful antibiotic therapy secondary to the presence of persistent osteomyelitis.

TAKE HOME POINTS

- DFUs can be neuropathic, ischemic, or a combination of both (neuroischemic). It is important to fully work up the patient with laboratory studies, radiologic evaluation, and noninvasive arterial blood flow studies.
- Aggressive wound care should be attempted initially along with use of pressure offloading and optimal footwear.
- Operative debridement is necessary if infection is present or large areas of nonviable tissue are present. Bony involvement can necessitate amputation.
- After control of infection, debridement, and revascularization, adjunctive therapies including NPWT, living cellular therapies, and HBO therapy should be considered to accelerate wound healing and reduce the risk of recurrent infection.
- Once wounds have healed, the patient should perform continued maintenance. This includes glycemic control, use of properly fitting footwear, and daily foot inspection.

SUGGESTED READINGS

Andros G, Lavery LA. *Rutherford's Vascular Surgery: Diabetic Foot Ulcers.* 7th ed. Philadelphia, PA: Saunders Elsevier; 2010:Chapter 112.

Armstrong DG, Cohen K, Courric S, et al. Diabetic foot ulcers and vascular insufficiency: our population has changed, but our methods have not. *J Diabetes Sci Technol.* 2011;5(6):1591-1596.

Moulik PK, Mtonga R, Gill GV. Amputation and mortality in new-onset diabetic foot ulcers stratified by etiology. *Diabetes Care.* 2003;26(2):491-494.

Singh N, Armstrong DG, Lipsky BA. Preventing foot ulcers in patients with diabetes. *JAMA.* 2005;293(2):217-228.

Sumpio BE, Armstrong DG, Lavery LA, et al. The role of interdisciplinary team approach in the management of the diabetic foot: a joint statement from the Society of Vascular Surgery and the American Podiatric Medical Association. *J Vasc Surg.* 2010;51(6):1504-1506.

Winkley K, Stahl D, Chalder T, et al. Risk factors associated with adverse outcomes in a population-based prospective cohort study of people with their first diabetic foot ulcer. *J Diabetes Complications.* 2007;6:341-349.

CLINICAL SCENARIO CASE QUESTIONS

1. If on physical exam one can probe to bone in a DFU on the great toe, the next step after ensuring the arterial supply is adequate is
   a. MRI
   b. Topical swab for culture
   c. Plain XR
   d. OR for toe amputation
   e. Hyperbaric oxygen therapy for 6 weeks

2. Use of hyperbaric oxygen for DFU is best in which scenario?
   a. Gas gangrene
   b. Nonhealing ulcer with TBI of 0.2
   c. After surgical debridement with slow healing in setting of well-vascularized limb
   d. Prior to major debridement in well-vascularized limb
   e. No evidence for its use in any cases

Chronic Gangrenous Foot, Nonvascularizable (Primary Amputation)

MARK NEHLER

Presentation

A 70-year-old man with diabetes, oxygen-dependent chronic obstructive pulmonary disease, hypertension, a 40-pack-year history of smoking, and end-stage renal disease presents with left heel gangrene. The patient has been minimally ambulatory after a recent hospitalization for a fall and fractured hip repair. On examination, the patient has femoral pulses and no pulses distally. There is a dry eschar on the left heel that encompasses most of the heel but no surrounding erythema and no odor (Fig. 1). He has a mild contracture at the left knee.

Differential Diagnosis

Heel lesions always involve some level of pressure and potentially neuropathy as components. Although they can occur in the setting of a fully ambulatory patient due to poorly fitting footwear, the current presentation is much more common. Patients with heel lesions often are at least briefly nonambulatory, frequently due to some acute event (in this case a hip fracture). In addition to the pressure issues, patients with heel lesions frequently have some level of peripheral vascular disease. Therefore, evaluation of the arterial circulation is important. Finally, there is no completely agreed-upon definition of an unsalvageable foot lesion. Heel lesions are notoriously difficult to manage due to poor local blood supply of the fat pad. Determination of the involvement of the

calcaneus is critical as most would consider that to be an indication of nonsalvageable.

Workup

Plain films demonstrate no soft tissue gas and no evidence of calcaneal osteomyelitis. Segmental pressures demonstrate suprasystolic pressures at multiple levels including the ankles. Toe pressures are 20 mm Hg bilaterally. Duplex shows both common femoral arteries are calcified but patent with biphasic waveforms and normal velocities. Both superficial femoral arteries show severe calcification and multiple stenoses with bilateral popliteal occlusions. After discussion with the patient and family, it is clear that his overall function has declined in the last 6 months. This has been markedly so since his fall and hip fracture where he has been minimally ambulatory since. He was living independently prior to the fall but now has required live-in assistance.

Discussion

The decision for a primary amputation is not an easy one for the surgeon or the patient. Most amputations done by vascular surgeons follow failed attempts at revascularization/limb salvage. However, a number of factors play into the decision for a primary amputation. The functional status of the patient is extremely important. Multiple series examining function in critical limb ischemia patients undergoing revascularization demonstrate that patients who are nonambulatory at baseline do not gain significant functional benefits and the patients who are ambulatory at baseline often take a functional hit in the first few weeks postoperatively that the majority will recover from over time (Fig. 2). Another issue that is critical is

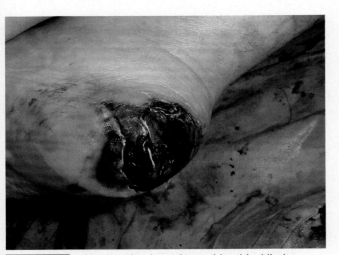

FIGURE 1 • Heel eschar in patient with critical limb ischemia and end-stage renal disease.

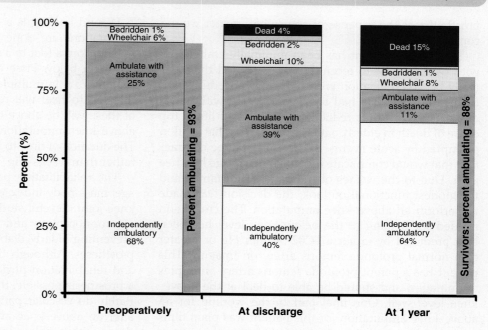

FIGURE 2 • Ambulation status preoperatively, at discharge, and at 1 year in patients undergoing bypass revascularization for critical limb ischemia. (From Goodney PP, et al. Predicting ambulation status one year after lower extremity bypass. *J Vasc Surg.* 2009;49:1431-1439, used with permission.)

the extent and nature of the foot lesion. Extensive necrosis theoretically can be managed with a variety of partial forefoot amputations and even free flap tissue coverage. In good-risk functional patients, this can be a useful strategy. However, the time for wound healing in these cases is usually measured in months not weeks, a substantial amount of downtime that often reduces function substantially due to deconditioning. A lack of revascularization option usually is an issue associated with secondary amputation after prior revascularization failure as the vast majority of patients with critical limb ischemia will have some revascularization option to attempt as a first-line therapy.

Patients with end-stage renal disease are especially problematic for limb salvage. The success rate for same is less than patients without end-stage renal disease. More importantly, the survival in patients with end-stage renal disease and critical limb ischemia is extremely limited. So decisions regarding heroic attempts for limb salvage in this population should be made with caution. The alternative of primary amputation also has high perioperative

morbidity and mortality and reduced survival over time but is often more of a palliative procedure (Fig. 3).

Diagnosis and Treatment

After discussion with the patient and family, it was decided to proceed with a primary amputation. This was primarily due to the patient's wish to have one procedure and not require repeat hospitalizations/procedures and also due to his declining functional status since his recent hip fracture. The next decision was above, through, or below the knee. The goal of saving the knee joint is to preserve ambulation with a prosthesis. However, a below-knee amputation often requires two procedures (if there is any question of pedal sepsis, a guillotine should be done first) and has a much greater wound failure rate than above-knee amputation. The trade-off is any potential ambulation in an elderly patient with critical limb ischemia is eliminated with loss of the knee joint. Through-knee amputations have gained popularity in select patients as the ambulation capability is much better than above-knee amputations with newer computerized

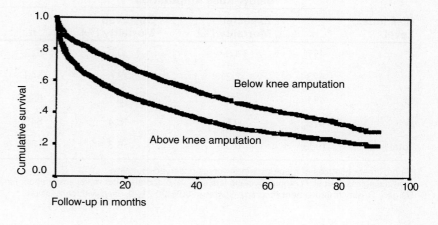

FIGURE 3 • Major amputee Kaplan-Meier survival. (From Feinglass J, et al. Postoperative and late survival outcomes after major amputation. Findings of the Department of Veterans Affairs National Surgery Quality Improvement Program. *Surgery.* 2001:130: 21-29, used with permission.)

prosthetics at the expense of somewhat greater wound complications.

The current patient has been minimally ambulatory with two legs due to recent hip fracture, and the focus really became palliation with reducing procedures and time in hospital. He had been considering withdrawal of dialysis due to his reduction in quality of life, a top cause of death in elderly patients on dialysis that is often prompted by acute events. He also has a knee contracture that would complicate his ability to salvage his knee joint. Due to the wishes of the patient and family and his modest functional outlook, the decision was made to perform an above-knee amputation. The circulation needed for healing at the below-knee level has been best predicted by either a TC02 35 mm Hg or greater or a normal profunda femoris artery on imaging. This patient has a patent profunda femoris artery on duplex examination and should be able to heal at the above-knee level well. One final part of the workup for an above-knee amputation for this patient was plain films to determine the length of the femoral portion of the recent hip reconstruction. The goal would be to transect the femur well below the existing hardware. Transecting the hardware would require special tools and risk hardware infection.

Postoperative Issues and Rehabilitation Potential

The morbidity and mortality of major limb amputation is not trivial. Multiple large databases state an operative mortality of 7% for below-knee amputations and roughly double that for above-knee amputations (Table 1). This mortality is primarily related to the comorbidities of the population undergoing amputation rather than the technical challenges of the procedure. Major postoperative morbidities are cardiac, thromboembolism, and also infection.

Wound healing is a major issue for amputees. Most amputations are done for necrosis, and transferring a wound from a foot to a stump is not ideal. Primary healing for a below-knee amputation varies widely but is roughly 75% in multiple series. Up to one third of those that fail to heal will require a reamputation, and half of these will be above the knee. Primary healing for an above-knee amputation is more uniform at 80% to 90%. The duration of time to heal is often measured in months rather than weeks (Fig. 4).

The rehabilitation potential of the patient relates to age, mass body index, comorbidities, and salvage of the knee joint. Several studies have demonstrated that lack of proprioception and thus balance is a key player in preventing elderly diabetics from ambulating well with prostheses. Although the majority of vascular patients and rehabilitation physicians consider ambulation with a prosthesis possible, the data are much more sobering. Rarely do vascular patients ambulate with a prosthesis after an above-knee amputation, and less than half of those with a below-knee amputation ambulate again. Despite these results, most nonambulatory amputees can remain in the community due to wheelchair access (Tables 2 and 3).

Case Conclusion

This patient underwent an above-knee amputation. He suffered a brief course of postoperative delirium that resolved. He was discharged to home with significant family support and a major goal of transfers and wheelchair use for ambulation. His wound healed without a complication. He ultimately died 6 months later from pneumonia but was able to remain in the community until that time.

TABLE 1. Thirty-day Postoperative Mortality in Various Risk Quartiles[a] for Above- and Below-Knee Amputation in the Veterans Affairs National Surgery Quality Improvement Program

Risk Index Level	Below-Knee Amputation			Above-Knee Amputation		
	n	Expected Mortality (%)	Observed Mortality (%)	n	Expected Mortality (%)	Observed Mortality (%)
I	477	1.0	0.8	522	3.5	2.3
II	473	2.2	2.8	543	6.2	7.2
III	481	4.2	3.1	538	10.9	11.8
IV	478	17.5	18.4	549	31.6	31.1
Total	1909	6.3	6.3	2152	13.3	13.3

[a]Approximate quartiles of mean expected versus observed mortality.
From Feinglass J, et al. Postoperative and late survival outcomes after major amputation. Findings of the Department of Veterans Affairs National Surgery Quality Improvement Program. *Surgery.* 2001:130:21-29, used with permission.

Time to heal

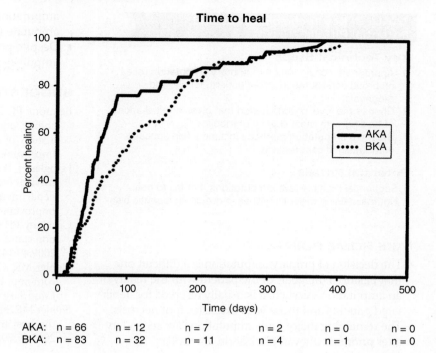

AKA: n = 66   n = 12   n = 7   n = 2   n = 0   n = 0
BKA: n = 83   n = 32   n = 11   n = 4   n = 1   n = 0

FIGURE 4 • Healing times in major lower extremity amputations. (From Nehler MR, et al. Functional outcome in a contemporary series of major lower extremity amputations. 2003;38:7-14, used with permission.)

TABLE 2. Functional Outcomes in Surviving Patients[a] after Major Lower Extremity Amputation

Parameter	Follow-up at 10.3 Months[b]		Follow-up at 17.5 Months[c]	
	n	%	n	%
All patients	(N = 90)		(N = 69)	
Ambulatory outdoors	19	21	20	29
Ambulatory indoors only	25	28	17	25
Nonambulatory	46	51	32	46
Prosthesis use	29	32	29	42
Community to care facility	15	17	6	8
Below-knee amputation group	(N = 60)		(N = 48)	
Ambulatory outdoors	17	28	18	38
Ambulatory indoors only	20	33	13	27
Nonambulatory	23	38	17	35
Prosthesis use	26	43	25	52
Community to care facility	9	15	3	6
Above-knee amputation group	(N = 30)		(N = 21)	
Ambulatory outdoors	2	7	2	10
Ambulatory indoors only	5	17	4	19
Nonambulatory	23	77	15	71
Prosthesis use	3	10	4	19
Community to care facility	6	20	3	14

[a]One hundred forty-three amputees who survived to discharge or >30 days.
[b]Mean follow-up for 6-month group.
[c]Mean follow-up for 12-month group.
From Nehler MR, et al. Functional outcome in a contemporary series of major lower extremity amputations. 2003;38:7-14, used with permission.

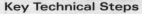

TABLE 3. Key Technical Steps and Potential Pitfalls

Key Technical Steps

1. Appropriate consideration of primary amputation relies on broad consideration of the patient, family, and prognosis.
2. Choose the level of amputation that gives most chance of healing with most chance of mobility.
3. Standard amputation methods include a flap apposed without significant tension.

Potential Pitfalls

- Sequential multiple level amputations that fail to heal
- Not maintaining patient's wishes in overall therapeutic plan

TAKE HOME POINTS

- The decision of primary amputation is a difficult one that balances the goals of the patient with the reality of an amputation. As such, it is usually reserved for debilitated patients and those with extensive foot necrosis. The remaining major limb amputations are secondary after prior failed revascularization attempts.
- The morbidity and mortality for major limb amputation is quite high. Much of this is related to the population of patients undergoing same. The rates are much higher for above- than below-knee amputation.
- The survival after major limb amputation is reduced as well. Five-year survival rates are much lower for populations following above- versus below-knee amputation. This is also significantly related to the comorbidities of the population.
- Wound healing is difficult for vascular amputees and is worse with amputations below the knee joint. Primary healing for a below-knee amputation is variable, but 75% is a common figure. Time to heal is often measured in months rather than weeks. Roughly one third of below-knee amputations that fail to heal are converted to an above-knee amputation.
- Ambulation after major limb amputation is poor in vascular patients. Rarely do vascular patients ambulate to any extent following an above-knee

amputation. Less than half of vascular patients will ambulate following a below-knee amputation.
- Despite poor rehabilitation, the majority of vascular amputees remain in the community.

SUGGESTED READINGS

Belmont PJ, Davey S, Orr JD, et al. Risk factors for 30 day complications and mortality after below-knee amputation: a study of 2911 patients from the National Surgery Quality Improvement Program. *J Am Coll Surg.* 2011;213:370-378.

Feinglass J, Pearce WH, Martin GJ, et al. Postoperative and late survival outcomes after major amputation. Findings of the department of Veterans Affairs National Surgery Quality Improvement Program. *Surgery.* 2001;130:21-29.

Goodney PP, Likosky DS, Cronenwett JL. Predicting ambulation status one year after lower extremity bypass. *J Vasc Surg.* 2009;49:1431-1439.

Nehler MR, Coll JR, Hiatt WR, et al. Functional outcome in a contemporary series of major lower extremity amputations. *J Vasc Surg.* 2003;38:7-14.

Nehler MR, Hiatt WR, Taylor LM Jr. Is Revascularization always the best treatment for critical limb ischemia? *J Vasc Surg.* 2003;37:704-708.

CLINICAL SCENARIO CASE QUESTIONS

1. Which patient finding most suggests that a patient may benefit from primary amputation rather than limb salvage interventions?

    a. An ABI of 0.1
    b. An occluded iliac and femoral system with intact three artery runoff
    c. Age greater than 80
    d. Significant overall debility
    e. Extensive toe gangrene

2. Factors that suggest an above-knee amputation may be better than a below-knee amputation include:

    a. Extensive heel necrosis with TBI = 0.5
    b. An occluded tibial arterial outflow
    c. A fixed knee contraction for greater than 6 months
    d. An occluded superficial femoral artery
    e. End-stage renal failure on hemodialysis

Wet Gangrene

SALVATORE DOCIMO Jr and ANIL HINGORANI

Presentation

A 68-year-old female presents with a chief complaint of pain located within the right foot. The pain is accompanied by a dark discoloration of toes two, three, and four, with an area of erythema that is migrating proximally. The first and fifth toes were amputated previously. The pain is constant, and the dark discoloration has worsened over the last 2 weeks. Her comorbidities include type II diabetes mellitus for 18 years, hypertension, hyperlipidemia, and a right femoropopliteal bypass with polytetrafluoroethylene graft 7 years ago. Her medications include hydrochlorothiazide, simvastatin, aspirin, and metformin. She uses alcohol socially and smokes half a pack of cigarettes daily for 25 years.

She is afebrile with vital signs within normal limits. Examination of the lower extremities demonstrates a left and right femoral pulse at 2+. No posterior tibial or dorsalis pedis pulses were palpable in either foot. No ulcerations of the left foot were noted.

Examination of the right lower leg reveals a lack of hair and rubor to the foot. A strong, foul odor emanating from her right lower extremity was noted. The first toe amputation site was noted to be dark and ischemic. The second and fourth toes were also noted to be dark and ischemic. The third and fourth toes were found to be swollen, cool, and cyanotic and noted to have capillary refill of 4 seconds. Figures 1 to 3 demonstrate the findings found on examination. The foot was found to be cool and erythematous, with blistering of the skin. Purulent material was expressed from the underside of the toes upon palpation.

Laboratory testing demonstrated a white blood cell (WBC) count of 8.0 K/UL, a normal hemoglobin and hematocrit, and a normal chemistry panel.

Differential Diagnosis

Dry Gangrene

Gangrene can be classified as dry or wet. Dry gangrene is often seen in patients with diabetes and atherosclerotic disease due to their diminished arterial flow. The decreased arterial flow creates ischemic, nonviable tissue, which becomes dry and at times dark. There is a lack of putrefaction. Another rare cause of dry gangrene is venous in origin. Venous gangrene occurs through the final phases of phlegmasia alba dolens and phlegmasia cerulea dolens.

Wet Gangrene

Wet gangrene involves putrefaction of tissue. Wet gangrene can progress from dry gangrene as the necrotic tissue becomes infected. Wet gangrene is accompanied by edematous, erythematous tissue surrounding the necrotic area. Infection itself can also directly lead to wet gangrene without the presence of prior ischemia. Mild erythema surrounding an area of dry gangrene does not constitute wet gangrene.

Necrotizing Fasciitis

Necrotizing fasciitis involves a rapidly spreading infection involving the subcutaneous tissue and deep fascia, which tends to spare the overlying skin initially. Edema and severe pain are often noted as the infection progresses and undermines the skin. Fluid-filled vesicles may appear, which is often followed by a brown to bluish skin discoloration and eventually gangrene. Numbness sets in due to destruction of the cutaneous nerves. The pathogens responsible include anaerobic organisms (*Bacteroides*, *Peptostreptococcus*), facultative organisms (streptococci, *E. coli*, *Klebsiella*, or *Streptococcus aureus*), or a single organism such as *S. pyogenes*.

Gas Gangrene

Gas gangrene is a form of wet gangrene most commonly caused by the exotoxin-producing Clostridium perfringens. Also known as "myonecrosis," the bacteria proliferate in the necrotic tissue and release exotoxin, known as alpha toxin, which further damages surrounding tissue, providing further nutrients for the anaerobic bacteria. The diagnosis is based upon the physical findings of infection with air in the soft tissues or crepitus. It is not based upon the finding of air on radiologic studies alone as this may not be associated with infection of the soft tissues. Treatment is urgent source control with surgical debridement and broad-spectrum antibiotic coverage.

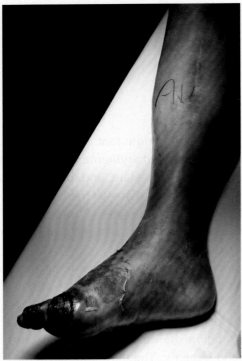

FIGURE 1 • Wet gangrene of the right lower extremity. Medial view. Note the edematous and erythematous tissue proximal to the necrotic tissue.

Diagnosis

Overall, the diagnosis of wet gangrene is clinical and based upon the physical examination. Wet gangrenous tissue will have a combination of characteristics that include edema, erythema, pungent smell, blisters, purulent discharge, and necrotic tissue. These findings are pathognomonic and confirmative for diagnosing wet gangrene. Prompt surgical and medical intervention should not be delayed in order to obtain radiographic studies.

In the setting of wet gangrene, analysis of the arterial system is not indicated prior to source control.

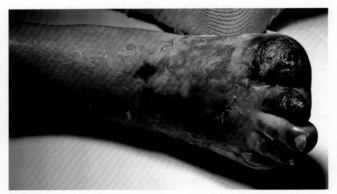

FIGURE 2 • Dorsal view of a right lower extremity with wet gangrene. Note the previous amputation of the hallux. Aspects of wet gangrene, such as edema, erythema, and necrotic tissue are present.

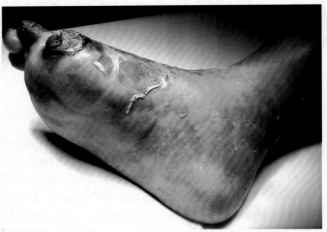

FIGURE 3 • Wet gangrene of the right lower extremity. Note the previous amputation of the hallux.

Noninvasive analysis, such as duplex scanning and the calculations of the ankle-brachial index (ABI) and toe-brachial index (TBI) are indicators of limb perfusion but do not play a vital role in the initial management of wet gangrene. More invasive studies, such as angiograms, can be also utilized to evaluate the arterial supply but only following source control.

Imaging, such as x-rays, may demonstrate changes associated with osteomyelitis such as soft tissue swelling, subperiosteal elevation, and sequestra or pieces of dead bone created during the process of necrosis leading to osteomyelitis. Magnetic resonance imaging (MRI) is the gold standard used to differentiate necrotizing soft tissue infections from nonnecrotizing cellulitis, with a sensitivity of nearly 100%. However, in the setting of wet gangrene, these studies are rarely indicated.

Approach to Management

Surgical Management

In the setting of wet gangrene, the only treatment option is source control with debridement and possible amputation. The timing of intervention will depend on the degree of pain, systemic toxicity, the presence of myoglobinuria, and extent of renal injury. Determination of amputation level is primarily based upon physical examination and also intraoperative findings. Intraoperatively, tissue will be removed until viable tissue is appreciated. Clinical judgment alone results in adequate healing of the stump in 80% of below-knee amputations and 90% of above-knee amputations. Repeated exams of the wound are necessary as repeat debridements may be needed.

In the setting of wet gangrene, broad-spectrum perioperative antibiotics should be administered. Anaerobic coverage in diabetic patients is recommended. A two-stage amputation involving a guillotine amputation followed by a definitive closure at a later stage may be an option.

Medical Management

Medical management often focuses on the prevention of ischemia leading to gangrene. Once gangrene has occurred, treatments often include pain relief, local ulcer care and pressure relief, treatment of infection, and modification of atherosclerotic risk factors, and also revascularization. Patients with peripheral artery disease should be receiving aspirin, beta-blockers, and statins—all shown to lower cardiovascular morbidity and mortality. Tight control of glucose levels to avoid hyperglycemia will also reduce the incidence of wet gangrene.

Wound care is based upon the tenets of adequate perfusion to the ischemic limb, adequate nutrition, and controlling infection. Surgical debridement of infected wounds or necrotic tissue is often required before healing can proceed. Hydrotherapy, vacuum-assisted closure, hyperbaric oxygen therapy, and wound dressing changes can also assist in wound healing after source control.

Discussion

Understanding the various types of gangrene and how to diagnose each are of vital importance.

Wet gangrene, a pathology requiring clinical diagnosis, is an ominous sign for amputation. Source control by way of debridement, with or without amputation, can prevent proximal progression and negate the risk of septic shock. Any other means of treatment, such as antibiotics, wound care, strict glucose control, or revascularization alone, will not prevent wet gangrene from advancing to sepsis and eventually septic shock (Table 1).

Case Conclusion

This patient received broad-spectrum antibiotics and IVF resuscitation. Then, the patient was taken for emergent guillotine amputation. Several days after this, with no physical exam evidence of ascending infection, the patient underwent a completion below-the-knee amputation.

TABLE 1. Key Technical Steps and Potential Pitfalls

Key Technical Steps
1. Wet gangrene is a clinical diagnosis based upon physical examination.
2. Antibiotics, wound care, glucose control, and revascularization will not prevent wet gangrene from advancing to sepsis and possibly septic shock.
3. Source control by prompt surgical debridement and amputation is the first line of treatment.

Potential Pitfalls
- Analysis of the arterial system by invasive studies, such as angiograms, is not necessary to diagnose wet gangrene.
- Noninvasive analysis of the extremity by duplex scanning, ABI, and TBI are not needed for diagnosis of wet gangrene.

TAKE HOME POINTS
- Limb wet gangrene represents a surgical emergency, and delay should not occur outside of resuscitation and initiation of broad-spectrum antibiotics prior to operating room.
- Consideration of forefoot amputation versus guillotine below-the-knee amputation can be made in the operating room, although consent of the patient for both is recommended.
- Determination of blood flow adequacy should be made after source control.

SUGGESTED READINGS

Dwars BJ, van den Broek TA, Rauwerda JA, et al. Criteria for reliable selection of the lowest level of amputation in peripheral vascular disease. *J Vasc Surg.* 1992;15(3):536.

Lille ST, Sato TT, Engrav LH, et al. Necrotizing soft tissue infections: obstacles in diagnosis. *J Am Coll Surg.* 1996;182(1):7-11.

McHenry CR, Piotrowski JJ, Teprinic JJ, et al. Determinants of mortality for necrotizing soft tissue infections. *Ann Surg.* 1995;221(5):558-565.

McIntyre KE Jr, Bailey SA, Malone JM, et al. Guillotine amputation in the treatment of nonsalvageable lower-extremity infections. *Arch Surg.* 1984;119(4):450-453.

Norgren L, Hiatt WR, Dormandy JA, et al. TASC II Working Group. Inter-society consensus for the management of peripheral arterial disease. *Int Angiol.* 2007;26(2):81-157.

CLINICAL SCENARIO CASE QUESTIONS

1. A 50-year-old man with long-standing diabetes, renal failure requiring hemodialysis, and peripheral artery disease presents to the ER with a foul-smelling R foot, elevated leukocytosis, and fever to 103°F. What imaging studies should be obtained prior to definitive surgical management?
   a. Plain foot x-ray
   b. MRI of foot to define extent of osteomyelitis
   c. Angiogram to determine healing of tissue
   d. None
   e. Duplex to determine waveform at ankle

2. All of these are essential therapies prior to definitive surgical management for wet gangrene except:
   a. Foot x-ray
   b. Broad-spectrum antibiotics
   c. IV fluid resuscitation
   d. Consent
   e. EKG

97 Transmetatarsal Amputation

ANNA ELIASSEN and DAWN M. COLEMAN

Presentation

A 70-year-old man with a history of hypertension, hyperlipidemia, insulin-dependent diabetes, and tobacco abuse presents with nonhealing, painful lower extremity tissue loss. He describes ulceration affecting the distal aspects of his left toes of approximately 4-month duration despite careful wound care. He denies history of antecedent trauma. He denies fever. Exam reveals palpable femoral and absent dorsalis pedis (DP) pulses bilaterally. There is a dry eschar affecting all toes on the left with demarcated tissue that appears healthy just proximal to his metatarsals (Fig. 1).

Differential Diagnosis

The differential diagnosis for nonhealing lower extremity ulcer and tissue loss includes ischemia (i.e., atherosclerosis and arteritis), venous insufficiency, diabetic neuropathy, pressure, and malignancy. Additionally, it is critical that any associated necrotizing soft tissue infection (i.e., wet gangrene) complicating a lower extremity ulcer is promptly recognized such that treatment with broad-spectrum parenteral antibiotics and surgical source control are not delayed.

Ulcer location and appearance will help identify wound etiology. Ischemic ulcers often accompany symptoms of rest pain. These ulcers are generally located over prominent bony areas that may result in pressure points for skin shear (i.e., toe tips, phalangeal heads, lateral malleolus, etc.) and typically appear even and sharply demarcated with punched-out wound margins. Tissue necrosis, cellulitis, and dry necrotic eschar may be present. Additionally, the surrounding skin is often blanched or purpuric, appearing at times shiny or "tight" with associated hair loss of the foot and ankle.

Ulcers of venous insufficiency typically spare the feet and toes, but rather occupy a location between the knee and ankle—most commonly these wounds affect the medial malleolus, but the lateral malleolus can also be affected. Surrounding skin will likely demonstrate additional findings consistent with advanced chronic venous insufficiency including eczematous changes, scaling, weeping, crusting, dermatitis, pruritus, hyperpigmentation, or lipodermatosclerosis. Diabetic neuropathic ulcers result from multiple factors that include neuropathy, autonomic dysfunction, and microvascular insufficiency. These ulcers are located at areas of repeated pressure-induced trauma (i.e., plantar metatarsal heads or dorsal interphalangeal joints) and are associated with an overgrowth of hyperkeratotic tissue (i.e., corn or callus) and signs of neuropathy on physical exam. These ulcers demonstrate undermined borders.

The patient in the above scenario presents with multiple risk factors for atherosclerotic occlusive disease. Additionally, the lesion location is highly suspicious for ischemic ulceration.

Workup

Additional clinical history should elicit symptoms of claudication or rest pain, lower extremity venous insufficiency (i.e., heaviness, aching, swelling), and diabetic neuropathy. Previous wounds and attempts at wound therapy should be documented. A complete lower extremity vascular exam that assesses for capillary refill, skin atrophy, hypertrophic nails, and hair loss in addition to pulses is necessary. Additionally, the wounds should be further qualified, specifically noting location, dimensions, presence of exposed tendon or bone, appearance of wound bed, and any associated cellulitis, drainage, and induration.

Noninvasive vascular lab studies including ankle-brachial index (ABI), duplex ultrasound, segmental blood pressures, and plethysmography will help confirm ischemic etiology and localize level of disease. In diabetics, the tibial vessels are often heavily calcified lending to noncompressibility and artificial elevation of the ABI. In these clinical situations, toe-brachial index (TBI) should be considered. Blood should be sent to assess for any leukocytosis; additionally, inflammatory markers (i.e., C-reactive protein) may be elevated in the setting of osteomyelitis. If there is any concern for bone infection, a bone scan or magnetic resonance imaging (MRI) may be considered for radiographic confirmation. Finally, computed tomography (CT) angiography and traditional angiogram are both adjuncts that will further identify arterial anatomy; angiography offers the benefit of simultaneous intervention if clinically appropriate.

On clinical exam, this patient has no sign of exposed bone, exposed tendon, or active cellulitis. While the toes have dry gangrene, the plantar surface is intact. There is hair loss about the ankle, palpable bilateral femoral

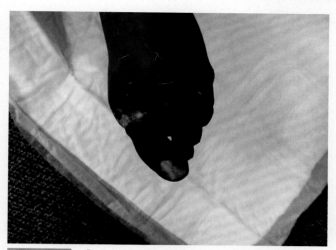

FIGURE 1 • Pedal photograph revealing dry eschar affecting all toes and demarcation of healthy proximal tissue.

pulses, and nonpalpable pedal pulses. Bilateral ABIs are 1.2, but tibial vessels are noted to be noncompressible. The right great toe has a TBI = 0.5, and the left DP and posterior tibial (PT) arterial waveforms are biphasic. MRI reveals osteomyelitis affecting the distal toes. Diagnostic arteriogram reveals preserved and regular inflow through the popliteal artery, peroneal occlusion at the midcalf, and preserved two-vessel outflow to the foot by way of diseased but patent anterior tibial and posterior tibial arteries.

Diagnosis and Treatment

This patient has nonhealing wounds of arterial insufficiency affecting multiple toes and associated with underlying osteomyelitis. Treatment options should consider the need for revascularization to ensure healing while identifying the indication for amputation and optimal level for such.

In situations of chronic critical limb ischemia, amputation is indicated for unreconstructable arterial disease, failed attempts at revascularization, patient comorbidities that prohibit candidacy for revascularization, and extensive tissue loss complicated by gangrene and/or infection (including pedal sepsis).

Given the dry gangrenous changes described and associated osteomyelitis, this patient requires amputation. While individual toe amputations may suffice, in clinical situations that require the removal of multiple toes, TMA offers a functional benefit; additionally, TMA is indicated for source control of extensive soft tissue infection of the forefoot.

While there is no definitive independent predictor of transmetatarsal healing when considering preoperative patient factors, skin temperature measurements, radioisotope scans, and skin perfusion pressure, a toe pressure of less than 38 mm Hg has been associated with failure of "minor amputations" in diabetic patients. This patient's biphasic waveform suggests the ability for TMA healing.

Surgical Approach

While it is likely that this patient will heal a TMA based on the above discussion, there are additional more proximal amputations that warrant discussion including the Lisfranc and Chopart amputations. Lisfranc's amputation results in a disarticulation of the first, third, fourth, and fifth tarsometatarsal joints, while the second metatarsal is divided up to two centimeters distal to the medial cuneiform. Chopart's amputation is performed through the talocalcaneonavicular joint and the calcaneocuboid joint. Both of these amputations result in a dramatic alteration in the biomechanics of the normal foot; additionally, comfortable and functional prosthetic fitting is challenging. Most authors suggest below-knee amputation (BKA) over the Lisfranc or Chopart amputations in clinical settings of tissue malperfusion that will not permit TMA healing in an effort to avoid altered ambulatory biomechanics and favor the more functional prosthetic limbs available to BKA patients.

The leg should be circumferentially prepped and draped; efforts at preserving a clean (albeit contaminated field in the setting of active tissue loss) should be maintained with occlusive dressings applied to any open wounds prior to skin preparation. A skin incision is made allowing for a plantar flap by constructing the transverse dorsal incision at the level of the midmetatarsal shafts from a point medial to the first metatarsal head to the opposing lateral side of the fifth metatarsal head. The incision is extended at right angles and along the metatarsophalangeal crease of the plantar aspect of the foot. The extensor tendons are divided proximal to the metatarsal heads, and each metatarsal shaft is divided using a power saw. It is important at this step to divide the bones approximately 1 cm proximal to the edge of the dorsal skin incision. The plantar tissues are then separated from the metatarsal shafts and dissected to excise exposed flexor tendons. The plantar flap is then extended over the dorsal aspect of the foot for closure. Ensure adequate hemostasis and consider pulse irrigation of the surgical bed prior to closure, especially in settings of active tissue loss. The flap should be closed in two layers with interrupted absorbable sutures reapproximating the fascia and a nonabsorbable suture by vertical mattress technique versus the use of staples reapproximating the skin to allow for minimal tension on the incision.

Potential pitfalls might result in a necessity for early reoperation, a delay in wound healing, or impaired prosthetic function and/or comfort. It is important to achieve adequate hemostasis prior to flap closure to avoid hematoma formation. Avoid unnecessary or overly restrictive compression bandages (i.e., ACE wrap) that may compromise skin flap viability. Ensure that the metatarsal shafts are divided 1cm proximal to the dorsal skin incision (as emphasized above) as this will prevent sharp bony protrusion into the incision and subsequent skin erosion in addition to minimizing the risk for potential future pressure points. Lastly, failure to excise all gangrenous or infected

TABLE 1. Transmetatarsal Amputation

Key Technical Steps

1. Make skin incision creating a plantar flap.
2. Divide extensor tendons.
3. Divide each metatarsal shaft with power saw.
4. Separate plantar tissues from metatarsal shafts.
5. Excise exposed flexor tendons.
6. Rotate plantar flap dorsally for closure.
7. Consider drain placement or wound vac prior to closure.

Potential Pitfalls

- Failure to achieve adequate hemostasis
- Failure to divide metatarsal shafts proximal to the dorsal skin incision
- Failure to excise all infected and gangrenous tissues

tissue will predictably result in worsening infection leading to nonhealing requiring subsequent reamputation, or possibly systemic spread and sepsis. In clinical scenarios of infected tissue loss, consider sending proximal bone samples for culture as this will guide postoperative antibiotic therapy selection and duration (Table 1).

Special Intraoperative Considerations

Pedal sepsis with and without ischemia constitutes a surgical emergency and is commonly identified in patients with diabetes and complicating neuropathy. In cases of suppurative infection (i.e., wet gangrene), it is prudent to consider guillotine TMA amputation for early source control. This can be followed at a later date by formal revision and flap creation for closure, or the wound may be left to heal by secondary intention with or without the assistance of a vacuum-assisted (negative pressure) dressing.

Postoperative Management

The common postoperative complications following TMA include wound infection (including persistent or recurrent osteomyelitis), nonhealing wound requiring reoperation, and phantom pain. While wound infection is more common following major lower extremity amputation, it frequently complicates patients with diabetes and those with preoperative infected tissue loss. Superficial surgical site infections typically respond to broad-spectrum antibiotic therapy, while deeper infections may necessitate more aggressive management including incision and drainage. In the latter situation, a vacuum-assisted (negative pressure) dressing should be applied to facilitate wound healing by secondary intention in an effort to reduce the increased risk of recurrent infection that would complicate primary closure. The level of reamputation for impaired wound healing should take into consideration tissue perfusion and the presence of underlying infection (including osteomyelitis). Diabetic patients are almost twice as likely to require reamputation as their nondiabetic counterparts, and the 5-year ipsilateral reamputation rate for diabetics after TMA approaches 45%.

Patients should be monitored regularly at short intervals (i.e., 2 weeks) postoperatively to gauge wound healing. Home nursing care is often required for those discharged with vacuum-assisted (negative pressure) dressings. Weight bearing should be avoided for approximately 4 to 6 weeks postoperatively; an off-loading prosthetic shoe or boot can accomplish this easily while permitting patient mobility and ambulation. Additionally, shoes with a steel shank in the sole or a curved sole will permit ambulation in a normal "toe-off" manner. With these prostheses, patients usually have minimal limb functional impairment and can ambulate well.

Case Conclusion

The patient underwent successful TMA with primary closure. He maintained compliance with an off-loading shoe for approximately 6 weeks and did not develop postoperative infectious complications. At last follow-up, his wound had healed, and he was ambulating without assistance.

TAKE HOME POINTS

- Tissue perfusion and underlying infection dictate the level of amputation.
- In patients with three or more affected toes, a TMA is functionally superior to amputation of the three toes alone.
- Suppurative infection identified pre- or intraoperatively negates wound closure—leave the wound open (i.e., guillotine amputation) and discuss with the patient surgical options that might include healing by secondary intention, TMA revision, or reamputation at a higher level (i.e., midfoot or below knee).
- All infected and nonviable tissue should be excised completely to decrease the patient's risk of residual infection, delayed wound healing, or reamputation.
- Patients should avoid weight bearing for 4 to 6 weeks postoperatively.

SUGGESTED READINGS

Armstrong DG, Lavery LA. Negative pressure wound therapy after partial diabetic foot amputation: a multicentre, randomised controlled trial. *Lancet.* 2005;366:1704-1710.

Eidt JF, Kalapatapu VR. Lower extremity amputation: techniques and results. In: Cronenwett J, et al. *Rutherford's Vascular Surgery.* Philadelphia, PA: Saunders Elsevier; 2010: 1772-1790.

Malone JM. Lower extremity amputation. In: Moore WS, ed. *Vascular and Endovascular Surgery: A Comprehensive Review.* 7th ed. Philadelphia, PA: Saunders; 2005:890-924.

Sideman MJ, Taubman KE, Beasley BD. Lower extremity amputation. In: Mulholland MM, Lillemoe KD, Doherty GM, et al., eds. *Greenfield's Surgery.* Philadelphia, PA: Lippincott Williams & Wilkins; 2011:1683-1696.

Thomas SRYW, Perkins JMT, Magee TR, et al. Transmetatarsal amputation: an 8-year experience. *Ann R Coll Surg Engl.* 2001; 83:164-166.

Vitti MJ, Robinson DV, Hauer-Jensen M, et al. Wound healing in forefoot amputations: the predictive value of toe pressure. *Ann Vasc Surg.* 1994;8:99.

Zhang WW, Abou-Zamzam AM. Lower extremity amputation: general considerations. In: Cronenwett J, Johnston KW, eds. *Rutherford's Vascular Surgery.* 7th ed. Philadelphia, PA: Saunders Elsevier; 2010:1761-1771.

CLINICAL SCENARIO CASE QUESTIONS

1. Which mid-foot amputation is performed through the talocalcaneonavicular joint and the calcaneocuboid joint?
   a. Lisfranc's
   b. Chopart's
   c. Transmetatarsal
   d. Syme's

2. Which of the following is the minimum toe-brachial index (TBI) thought necessary to heal a TMA?
   a. 0.75
   b. 0.6
   c. 0.5
   d. <0.3

98 Above-Knee Amputation— No Profunda Inflow

SCOTT A. BERCELI

Presentation

A 59-year-old male with a history of type II diabetes, hypertension, and a 40 pack-year smoking history presents with 2 months of increasing left forefoot pain and numbness. On further questioning, he provides a history of previous left external iliac and superficial femoral artery (SFA) stent placement, performed 10 years ago for symptoms of lifestyle-limiting claudication. Four years ago, he had return of his claudication, and workup revealed both stents to be occluded. Following a failed attempt at medical management, he underwent a right common femoral to left profunda femoral bypass using prosthetic graft. On examination today, his left foot demonstrates dependent rubor with no ulcerations. Pulse exam reveals a 3+ (out of 4) right femoral pulse and no left femoral, popliteal, or pedal pulses.

Differential Diagnosis

In a patient with a previous history of multilevel peripheral arterial occlusive disease, multiple previous interventions, and new onset of foot pain, critical limb ischemia should be entertained as the primary diagnosis. The presence of dependent rubor and an absent femoral pulse in the affected limb further supports this diagnosis. Alternate etiologies such as lumbar radiculopathy or diabetic neuropathy should be considered if the subsequent workup fails to support arterial occlusive disease as the underlying pathology.

The presence of a right femoral pulse and lack of left femoral pulse suggest thrombosis of the femorofemoral bypass graft as the initiating event for the left foot rest pain. Compromised right iliac inflow and left profunda femoral outflow are the most likely reasons for failure of the graft, but the normal right femoral pulse suggests a primary outflow problem. In this scenario, compromised outflow can result from intimal hyperplasia at the distal anastomosis or progressive atherosclerosis of the distal profunda branches, which in combination leads to reduced flow rates and graft thrombosis. Diabetes is frequently associated with diffuse, multifocal occlusive disease in the profunda femoral artery, and this may have contributed to the early graft failure observed in this patient.

Case Continued

Ankle-brachial indices (ABIs) were performed and show mild right and severe left leg ischemia, with an ABI of 0.78 on the right and 0.12 on the left. Segmental pressures demonstrate a greater than 25 mm Hg pressure drop in both the aortoiliac and femoropopliteal segments in the left leg, confirming multilevel occlusive disease.

Workup

Both conventional two-dimensional angiography and cross-sectional imaging (i.e., computed tomography [CT] or magnetic resonance [MR] angiography) are viable options as the next step in the evaluation. However, with the patient's severe occlusive disease, contrast delivery via an indwelling arterial catheter may be problematic, and cross-sectional imaging offers the best option for surveying the patient's complex anatomy following multiple failed revascularization attempts. While CT angiography (CTA) generally offers more consistent, less operator-dependent imaging and MRA offers the potential to avoid nephrotoxic agents, both studies provide similar information. Most commonly, local expertise has identified CT or MR imaging as the primary modality of choice, and this knowledge should be leveraged in these selections.

Return to Scenario

The current patient has normal renal function, and a CT angiogram is performed (Fig. 1). Notable findings include (1) a patent right and occluded left common and external iliac arteries; (2) occlusion of the femorofemoral bypass graft; (3) occlusion of the SFA in the midthigh, at the site of previous stent placement; (4) profunda femoral artery occlusion; (5) patent left popliteal artery; and (6) poor contrast delivery to the left tibial arteries that preclude accurate interpretation.

To further define the left profunda and tibial anatomy, the patient undergoes a digital subtraction arteriogram of the left leg, via a retrograde right femoral approach (Fig. 2). Contrast is injected at multiple locations along the thoracic and abdominal aorta to maximum opacification. Consistent with the CT scan, the left profunda femoral artery is occluded to the midthigh, where the primary profunda branch is noted to be diminutive. The popliteal

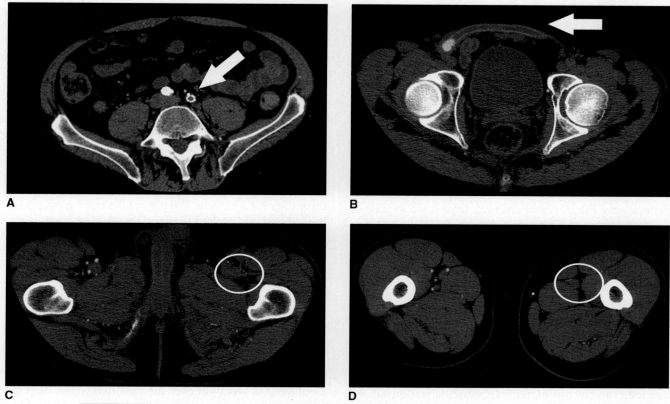

FIGURE 1 • CT angiogram performed upon initial presentation. **A:** Occlusion of a previously stented left common femoral artery (*arrow*). **B:** Occlusion of a femoral to femoral artery bypass graft (*arrow*). **C:** Occlusion of the left profunda femoral artery at the level of the femoral bifurcation. **D:** Occlusion of the left profunda femoral artery in the midthigh.

artery is patent, but all three tibial arteries occlude in the midcalf, with no evidence of pedal artery reconstitution.

Diagnosis and Treatment

The patient presents with acute or chronic left leg ischemia, resulting from thrombosis of the femorofemoral bypass graft. The severity of his ischemia is accentuated by occlusion of his profunda femoral artery and the corresponding loss of important collateral pathways between the common femoral and popliteal arteries. The patient's symptoms are almost exclusively unilateral, as failed endovascular and surgical revascularization procedures have significantly accelerated the natural history of occlusive disease. This coupled with severe tibial artery atherosclerosis, which is common to many diabetic patients, has resulted in a pattern of multilevel occlusive disease that presents multiple challenges for successful revascularization.

Surgical Approach

The primary goal for successful limb salvage in this patient is restoration of inflow into the left leg. With a long-segment SFA occlusion, the profunda femoral artery needs to serve as the primary outflow target. Both the CT scan and angiogram demonstrate left profunda occlusion, although the etiology remains unclear. The pathology

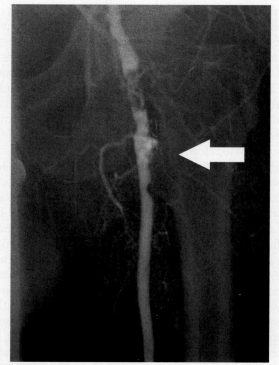

FIGURE 2 • Angiogram demonstrates occlusion of the proximal profunda femoral artery (*arrow*).

underlying this occlusion is the most important determinant of successful revascularization and dictates the potential for limb salvage. Intimal hyperplasia at the distal anastomosis of the femorofemoral graft and a corresponding low flow–induced thrombosis of the distal profunda would offer the best chance of success. Advanced atherosclerosis or chronic occlusive thromboemboli along the length of the profunda would significantly restrict the therapeutic options and portend a poor prognosis.

Given the extensive iliac and femoral occlusive disease, establishing inflow into the profunda is best accomplished via open surgical revascularization. An aortoprofunda bypass would offer the best durability, at the expense of increased perioperative risk. An extra-anatomic bypass, via revision of the femorofemoral bypass or a de novo left axilloprofunda bypass, would incur less perioperative risk with the trade-off of reduced long-term patency. Prosthetic grafts are traditionally the conduit of choice for inflow procedures, but large-diameter, autogenous conduit (such as femoropopliteal vein) may offer improved patency under extreme low-flow conditions. Placement of a sequential bypass from the profunda to a popliteal or tibial target may also be considered to improve outflow from a diseased or small caliber profunda.

Although a variety of surgical interventions could be reasonably defended, the patient's relatively young chronologic age and history of multiple revascularization failures would support the procedure that offers the best long-term durability. With left iliac occlusion, left SFA occlusion, and severe left profunda femoral disease, an aorto–left profunda bypass using contralateral femoral vein would be the most reasonable solution. Critical to this plan, however, is identification of a suitable profunda femoral target. Surgical exploration will be required to determine if a profunda thrombectomy can be performed to restore continuity with the rich collateral network that bridges the femoral and popliteal vasculature. Unfortunately, extensive atherosclerosis or chronic occlusion of the mid to distal profunda is highly probable and would essentially eliminate all reasonable options for revascularization. A preoperative discussion with the patient should be undertaken to inform him of this potential outcome.

With the success of the operation intimately connected to the status of the profunda, exploration of this artery should be the initial order of business. A longitudinal incision is made in the midportion of the thigh, along the lateral border of the sartorius muscle. The sartorius muscle is retracted medially, and a plane is developed between the adductor longus (medial) and vastus intermedius (lateral) muscles. The SFA is readily visible, and dissection is continued within the intramuscular plane until the profunda femoral artery and vein are identified. Palpation of the artery reveals a firm, diffusely calcified structure with no discernable pulse or Doppler signal. A longitudinal arteriotomy is performed, and subacute thrombus, consistent with the patient's 2-week history of rest pain, is encountered. A no. 3 embolectomy catheter is advanced proximally, but meets firm resistance at 10 cm. Withdrawal of the catheter produces thrombus but no back bleeding. Multiple attempts at proximal thrombectomy are performed with continued inability to pass the catheter beyond this occlusion. The catheter is then advanced into the distal profunda and meets firm resistance after a short distance. The arteriotomy is extended distally, and a fibrotic intraluminal cord is identified at the site of distal occlusion. Further extension of the arteriotomy fails to reveal a patent lumen. With an inability to identify a suitable distal target, the revascularization procedure is aborted. Postoperatively, the patient is informed of the operative findings and decides to delay major leg amputation at this time.

Case Continued

Over the next 3 months, the patient develops gangrene of the left first and second toes and presents for a semielective major leg amputation. Due to the relative ischemia of his calf musculature, the patient reluctantly agrees to a left above amputation. Although it is recognized that the arterial perfusion in his distal thigh is reduced, the overlying skin is warm, and the surgical team decides to proceed with an amputation at this level. At time of operation, the anterior and posterior thigh muscles are noted to be slightly pale, but viable. Although initial healing of the amputation site appears promising, the patient presents four weeks following the procedure with eschar along the incision. Continued observation over the next two weeks demonstrates progressive gangrene of the anterior flap (Fig. 3A).

Postoperative Management

Given the patient's severe inflow disease and profunda occlusion, he is at significant risk for primary nonhealing of a midthigh amputation. Although preemptive revascularization is a reasonable consideration in advancing this procedure, there is no definitive consensus regarding this issue. Primary amputation with close observation for early signs of ischemia and prompt intervention is also an appropriate strategy. Given the lack of distal targets in the left thigh, options for revascularization are focused primarily on improving pelvic perfusion, with the intent of increasing flow through the collateral networks that bridge the iliac and femoral vasculature. The ipsilateral internal iliac artery serves as the primary target, with revascularization accomplished via an aorta to internal iliac artery bypass. Extensive atherosclerosis of the internal iliac artery is not uncommon, especially in diabetic patients, and alternate targets such the middle sacral or inferior mesenteric artery may be considered in highly specialized situations (Table 1).

Case Conclusion

The patient has a suitable left internal iliac artery for placement of a bypass. Via a midline incision, he undergoes an infrarenal aorta to left internal iliac artery bypass using prosthetic graft. The amputation stump is debrided to viable tissue. With diligent wound care over the next 3 weeks, the above-knee

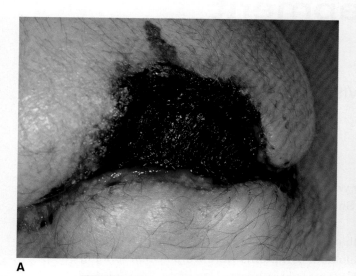
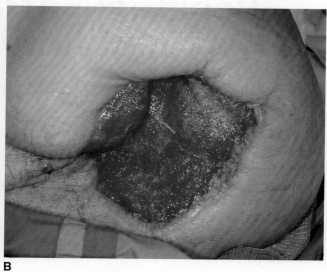

FIGURE 3 • **A:** Gangrene of an above-knee amputation stump secondary to local ischemia. **B:** Healing of the amputation stump following revascularization via an aorta to internal iliac artery bypass.

amputation stump demonstrates substantial healing (Fig. 3B). By 8 weeks postoperatively, the patient has healed his wound and is being evaluated for a prosthetic limb.

TAKE HOME POINTS

- Patients with multiple failed revascularization procedures can present with an atypical pattern of occlusive disease that places them at increased risk for limb loss.
- The profunda femoral artery is the critical target for inflow procedures into the leg, and an inability to revascularize this artery places the patient at high risk for a major leg amputation.
- Patients with diabetes have a characteristic pattern of occlusive disease that more frequently involves the profunda femoral and tibial arteries.
- In patients with inflow occlusive disease who require an above-knee amputation, early recognition and correction of wound ischemia is critical.

TABLE 1. Key Technical Steps and Potential Pitfalls

Key Technical Steps

1. Use all imaging necessary to assess for suitable pelvic or thigh arterial targets for revascularization.
2. Consideration of open, endovascular, or hybrid techniques is important.
3. Use of VAC primarily in a marginal AKA is often helpful.

Potential Pitfalls

- Failure to discuss severe and critical nature of disease process with the patient
- Failure to recognize long segment nonreconstructible profunda artery

- In patients with profunda femoral artery occlusion, the ipsilateral internal iliac artery serves as the most important source of collateral perfusion.

SUGGESTED READINGS

King TA, DePalma RG, Rhodes RS. Diabetes mellitus and atherosclerotic involvement of the profunda femoris artery. *Surg Gynecol Obstet.* 1984;159(6):553-556.

Natale A, Belcastro M, Palleschi A, et al. The mid-distal deep femoral artery: few important centimeters in vascular surgery. *Ann Vasc Surg.* 2007;21(1):111-116.

Okike N, Bernatz PE. The role of the deep femoral artery in revascularization of the lower extremity. *Mayo Clin Proc.* 1976;51(4):209-215.

Ouriel K, DeWeese JA, Ricotta JJ, et al. Revascularization of the distal profunda femoris artery in the reconstructive treatment of aortoiliac occlusive disease. *J Vasc Surg.* 1987;6(3):217-220.

CLINICAL SCENARIO CASE QUESTIONS

1. Which of the following arteries is *not* a potentially important source of midthigh perfusion to improve healing of an above-knee amputation site?

   a. Profunda femoral artery
   b. Superficial femoral artery
   c. Middle sacral artery
   d. Internal iliac artery
   e. Inferior mesenteric artery

2. Patients with diabetes have a higher frequency of atherosclerotic occlusive disease in which of the following arterial bed(s)?

   a. Superficial femoral artery
   b. Profunda femoral artery
   c. Tibial arteries
   d. Both A and B
   e. Both B and C

99 Popliteal Entrapment in Athletes

WILLIAM D. TURNIPSEED and TRAVIS L. ENGELBERT

Presentation

Scenario #1 A 19-year-old male collegiate soccer player with progressive right leg claudication over the competitive season was seen in the clinic. Symptoms: She had limited playing time but did not affect routine activity.

Scenario #2 A 15-year-old multisport female athlete with diffuse muscle cramping affecting the proximal and distal portion of the posterior calf muscles was evaluated. Symptoms were worse when running on inclines or going up stairs, infrequently associated with plantar paresthesia.

Evaluation

Claudication is an unusual complaint in healthy athletic adolescents and young adults particularly in the absence of musculoskeletal trauma. Screening tests are indicated in order to rule out uncommon causes for exercise-induced leg pain in these individuals. Noninvasive vascular studies including resting and postexercise ankle-brachial indices (ABIs) and stress positional plethysmography are helpful for detecting vascular occlusive or impingement syndromes. These conditions include premature atherosclerosis, medial cystic arterial disease, arterial dissections, and popliteal artery entrapment. Intramuscular compartment pressures are important to consider when isolated muscle group symptoms are present since chronic exertional compartment syndromes (CECSs) can occur in active individuals and frequently coexist with functional forms of popliteal artery entrapment. EMG and nerve conduction studies are occasionally indicated to rule out peripheral nerve impingement when exercise-induced footdrop or repetitive sensory changes occur on the plantar or dorsal aspect of the feet. Vascular imaging is essential when noninvasive circulatory screening tests are positive. Our preference is use of MRI/MRA with forced plantar and dorsiflexion if popliteal artery entrapment is suspected because this technique is less invasive and musculoskeletal anatomy can be visualized and good-quality vascular images obtained in these otherwise young and healthy individuals. Vascular imaging is the only accurate means of distinguishing anatomic from functional forms of popliteal entrapment.

Testing Results
Scenario #1

Vascular screening studies performed on the male soccer player suggested occlusive disease at rest and after exercise on the right (Figure 1 and Table 1). MR angiography demonstrated a segmental occlusion of the right popliteal artery and a normal-appearing left popliteal artery (Fig. 2). Stress positional testing with forced plantar and dorsiflexion demonstrated a static short-segment occlusion of the right popliteal artery and no impingement on the left (Fig. 3). T2-weighted coronal imaging demonstrated an anomalous musculotendinous band of gastrocnemius muscle crossing the popliteal vessels bilaterally (Fig. 4).

Scenario #2

Resting and postexercise vascular screening studies performed on the female athlete were normal (Fig. 5). However, stress positional plethysmography was markedly positive bilaterally (right > left) (Fig. 6). Neutral position MRA imaging demonstrated normal arterial positioning at rest (Fig. 7). Stress positional MRA demonstrated lateral displacement and long-segment vascular compression of the popliteal vessels bilaterally (Fig. 8A and B). Because of focal proximal muscle calf pain and cramping, compartment pressures were performed. Resting posterior superficial compartment pressures were markedly elevated at 40 mm in the posterior medial superficial and posterior lateral superficial compartments. Normal resting pressures are less than 15 mm. Although we do not routinely measure the distal deep posterior compartment pressures because of the risk of tibial neurovascular injury, distal retrotibial calf pain and plantar paresthesias can strongly suggest the presence of distal deep posterior compartment syndrome as well.

Treatment
Scenario #1

Adolescent males and young adults that present with ischemic claudication or atheroembolism of the feet should have vascular imaging. In this case, the preoperative noninvasive workup studies indicated the

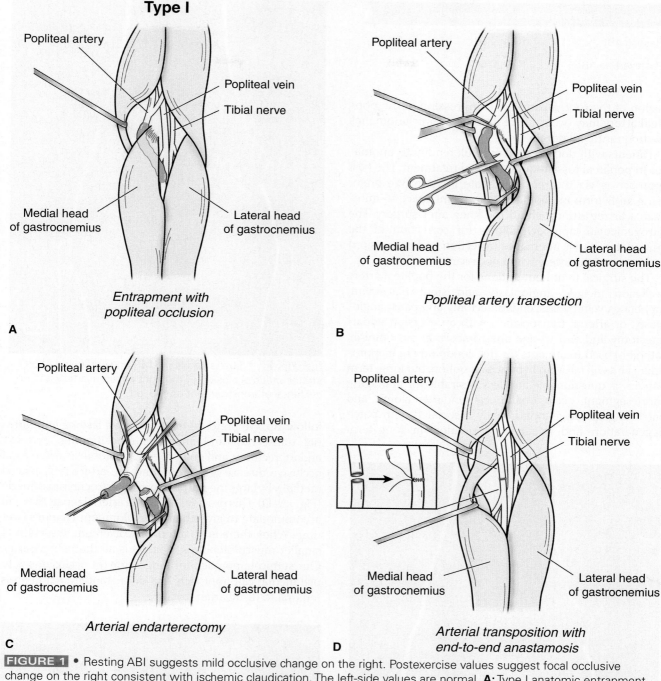

Type I

Entrapment with popliteal occlusion

A

Popliteal artery transection

B

Arterial endarterectomy

C

Arterial transposition with end-to-end anastamosis

D

FIGURE 1 • Resting ABI suggests mild occlusive change on the right. Postexercise values suggest focal occlusive change on the right consistent with ischemic claudication. The left-side values are normal. **A:** Type I anatomic entrapment with medial displacement and segmental occlusion of the popliteal artery is the cause for claudication in Scenario 1. **B:** The occluded popliteal artery is exposed through a posterior knee approach and transected. **C:** Eversion thromboendarterectomy is performed proximally and distally. **D:** The transected popliteal artery is transpositioned to its normal anatomic location and then approximated by end-to-end anastomosis.

presence of a symptomatic popliteal artery occlusion on the right. When a focal popliteal artery occlusion or aneurysmal change is detected in young adults, the anatomic form of popliteal entrapment should be suspected. Typically, angiograms of the symptomatic limb will demonstrate a short-segment occlusion of the popliteal artery with normal proximal superficial femoral

and distal tibial runoff vessels. If there is any doubt as to the cause for arterial occlusion, a stress positional MRA/MRI can confirm the presence of anomalous musculotendinous bands and the suspected diagnosis of anatomic PAES. Careful evaluation of the contralateral popliteal artery may demonstrate subtle medial deviation, and with forced plantar flexion or dorsal

TABLE 1. Exercise ABIs for scenario 1

Resting ABI	Right 0.86	Left 1.19
Postexercise ABI	Right 0.68	Left 1.25

flexion of the foot, a bandlike compression of the popliteal artery may occur, since these anatomic anomalies are frequently bilateral.

Patients with documented musculotendinous anomalies in popliteal fossa require surgical treatment. The best approach is via the retrogeniculate incision. We prefer using an S-form incision across the joint space to minimize scar retraction behind the knee after surgery. The retrogeniculate approach allows for correction of the musculotendinous anomalies (resection and/or excision) and repair of the artery when necessary.

The surgical treatment options for the popliteal artery occlusion include angioplasty and stent placement, saphenous vein bypass, endarterectomy and patch angioplasty, or arterial transposition with an eversion endarterectomy and end-to-end anastomosis. In our opinion, catheter-based treatments for this condition are inappropriate and will fail. Vein bypass is an option, but long-term patency is questionable and less desirable for managing short-segment occlusions. Local endarterectomy and patch angioplasty is occasionally associated with patch degeneration and aneurysm formation in long-term

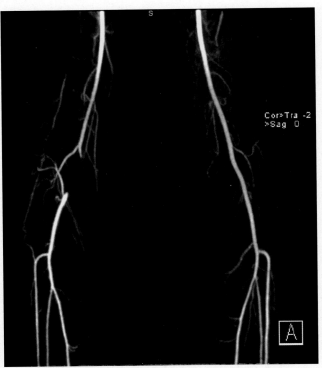

FIGURE 3 • Stress positional MR angiography demonstrates static occlusion of the right popliteal artery and no evidence of impingement on the left.

follow-up. We prefer to treat occlusive lesions with arterial transection and anatomic repositioning, eversion endarterectomy, and end-to-end anastomosis when focal occlusive disease is present, and the artery is displaced medially by large medial head of the gastrocnemius muscle (Fig. 1A–D). This provides a durable arterial repair that will accommodate to growth and development changes over time. When there is no arterial involvement, resection of smaller musculotendinous bands is all that is necessary. Our surgical approach for long-segment occlusions is to use medial calf approach and do a standard saphenous femoral to distal artery bypass.

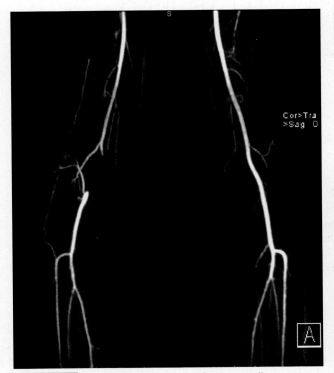

FIGURE 2 • MR angiography confirms a well-collateralized focal popliteal artery occlusion on the right and a normal left popliteal artery.

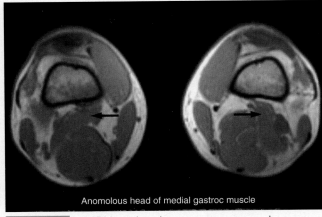

Anomolous head of medial gastroc muscle

FIGURE 4 • MRI imaging demonstrates anomalous gastrocnemius muscle bands bilaterally (*arrows*).

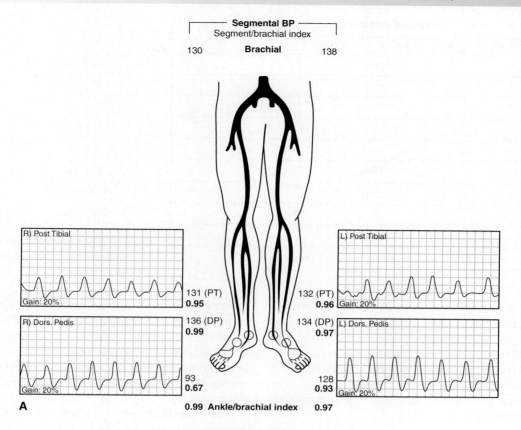

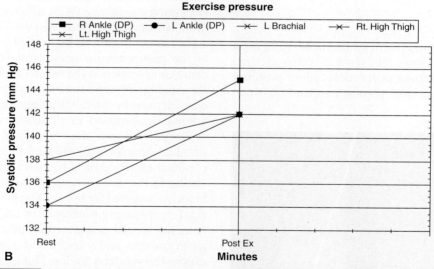

FIGURE 5 • **A:** Resting ABIs appear normal bilaterally. **B:** Postexercise ABIs appear normal bilaterally.

Take Home Points: Anatomic Popliteal Entrapment

- This condition is uncommon and most frequently occurs in males less than 40 years of age.
- Arterial complications are common in patients with anatomic politeal artery entrapment syndrome (PAES).

- Local resection of the musculotendinous band and/or direct arterial repair is preferred when occlusive or aneurysmal changes are present.
- Catheter-based treatment is contraindicated.
- Saphenous bypass maybe necessary when long-segment occlusions are present. Be careful in tunneling so as not to recreate entrapment.

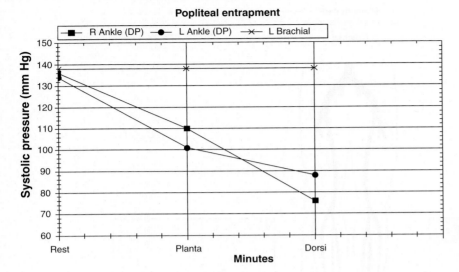

Popliteal entrapment

FIGURE 6 • Stress positional plethysmography demonstrates popliteal artery impingement bilaterally.

- Asymptomatic anatomic entrapment or musculotendinous anomalies should be surgically treated.
- We anticoagulate patients for 3 months following endarterectomy repair of occlusions and use 10 flat JP drains to minimize seroma accumulation in the popliteal fossa.
- Exertional compartment syndromes are uncommon in this patient group.

Treatment
Scenario #2

Functional popliteal entrapment syndrome (FPAES) most commonly occurs in female athletes and is characterized by tightness and cramping of the deep upper posterior calf muscles and occasional plantar paresthesias when running on inclines or with repetitive jumping. Vascular complications are very uncommon in FPAES patients and usually present as popliteal vein occlusions. At least 50% of all patients with FPAES have coexistent chronic exertional compartment syndrome (CECS). For optimal outcomes, both conditions should be identified and treated when present.

The second scenario patient had both problems. Surgical treatment for FPAES is technically quite different from the anatomic PAES. Clinical symptoms arise not from ischemia but from neuromuscular impingement associated with diffuse hypertrophy of the medial head of the gastrocnemius and plantaris muscles and from distal compression at the soleal canal by the soleus muscle. Angiographically functional popliteal entrapment is characterized by lateral displacement and long-segment arterial compression or occlusion with forced plantar or dorsiflexion on stress positional arteriography. Our standard approach for surgical treatment of functional popliteal entrapment is to use a medial calf approach, similar to that used to expose the distal popliteal artery branches targeted for bypass. The posterior medial superficial compartment is released by excising the fascia overlying the medial gastrocnemius and soleus muscles. The gastrocnemius and soleus muscles are then separated to expose the plantaris tendon. This is transected along with a distal third of the plantaris muscle (Fig. 9). Then the medial soleal attachments are taken down from the tibia using electrocautery from the level of the soleal canal to the midcalf. The fibrous band that forms the margin of the soleal canal is completely excised along with the fascia of the popliteus muscle. This widens the exit of the popliteal fossa (Fig. 10). Approximately 20% of our functional popliteal entrapment patients require additional resection of the proximal medial head of the gastrocnemius muscle using a posterior knee approach. Some surgeons prefer to use the posterior approach to resect the medial head of the gastrocnemius and plantaris muscle bellies as the primary operation. In our experience,

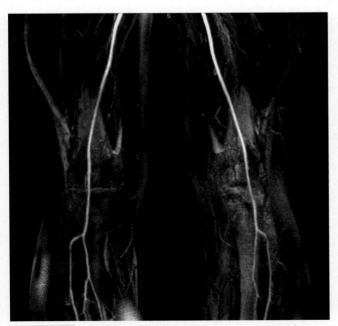

FIGURE 7 • MR imaging demonstrates normal resting arterial anatomy.

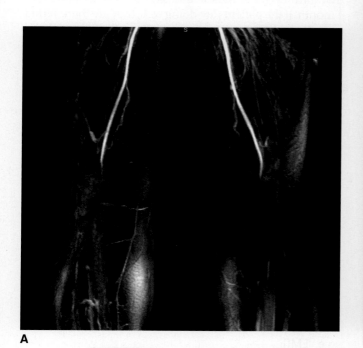

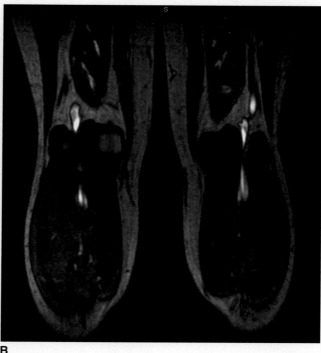

A

B

FIGURE 8 • **A:** Stress positional MR angiography demonstrates lateral arterial displacement with long-segment compression consistent with functional popliteal entrapment. **B:** Stress MR imaging demonstrates bilateral muscular impingement of vascular bundle with plantar flexion.

recovery is longer, wound management more problematic, and the likelihood of additional distal release surgery much higher when this approach is used as a primary treatment. Furthermore, the probability of a high-level

athletic rehabilitation appears to be lower when the posterior approach is used as sole treatment. We drain the popliteal space with a 10 flat JP drain that stays from 2 to 5 days. Based on preoperative compartment pres-

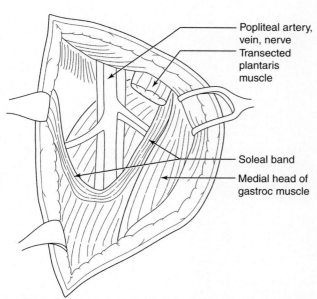

FIGURE 9 • This schematic demonstrates the superficial dissection via medial calf incision. The fascia overlying the gastrocnemius and soleus muscles has been excised and the plantaris muscle/tendon resected. This exposes the neurovascular bundle and the arcuate soleal band that forms the exit of the popliteal fossa.

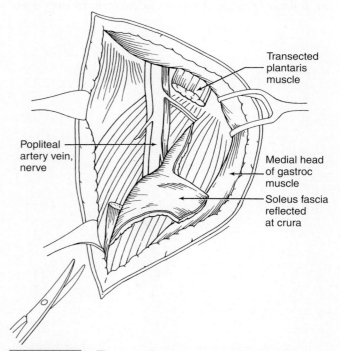

FIGURE 10 • The most important component of the functional entrapment release is resection of the crural fascia forming the soleal canal. This fascial band is the fulcrum against which the neurovascular bundle is compressed.

sures, fasciectomy is performed at the same time in appropriate compartments. We do not recommend fasciotomy for CECS treatment because recurrent rates are high (anterior compartment 15% to 25%, posterior compartments 48%). Recurrence rate for our fasciectomy technique is approximately 6% in either location.

Take Home Points: Functional Popliteal Entrapment

- FPAES is more common in females.
- Thirty percent of athletic individuals will have positive impingement studies, but less than 5% of these will have any associated symptoms.
- Functional impingement without symptoms should not be treated.
- Vascular complications with FPAES are rare and are manifest by popliteal occlusion (≤1%).
- Coexistent CECS should be treated at the same time when present.
- Additional proximal resection of the gastrocnemius may be required in up to 20% of patients treated.

Rehabilitation

Patients are in compression dressings until drains are removed. They are allowed to use crutches during this time. However, once the drains are out, the crutches are discarded. At 2 weeks, the nonimpact aerobic rehab program is started. This includes any activity in the pool, stationary biking, and the use of the elliptical trainer or stair master. The concept here is to maintain aerobic training and use of range of motion to break down early scars

that form between muscle and skin. This is continued for 1 month. If the patients are doing well, they are then started on a graduated running program. Once this is completed pain-free, they may return to unrestricted activity.

SUGGESTED READINGS

Pham TT, Kapur R, Harwood MI. Exertional leg pain: teasing out arterial entrapments. *Curr Sports Med Rep.* 2007;6:371-375.

Turnipseed WD. Popliteal entrapment syndrome. *J Vasc Surg.* 2002;35:910-915.

Turnipseed WD. Functional popliteal artery entrapment syndrome: a poorly understood and often missed diagnosis that is frequently mistreated. *J Vasc Surg* 2009;49:1189-1195.

CLINICAL SCENARIO CASE QUESTIONS

1. A young man has a history consistent with popliteal artery entrapment syndrome. The best imaging test to confirm this is:

   a. Stress position CTA
   b. Stress position MRA
   c. Stress position arteriogram
   d. Treadmill ABI test
   e. EMG

2. In a young person with suspected chronic exertional compartment syndrome, which compartment need not be measured?

   a. Superficial posterior
   b. Lateral
   c. Anterior
   d. Deep posterior
   e. medial deep

100 Persistent Sciatic Artery

AUDRA A. DUNCAN

Presentation

A 54-year-old woman with left calf claudication for 40 years has developed similar right-sided symptoms in the past year. Symptoms occur after walking four to five blocks. She has hypertension and hypercholesterolemia. On physical examination, she has 1+ (out of 4) femoral pulses and 3+ popliteal pulses bilaterally. Pedal pulses are 1 to 2+ bilaterally. She has no foot ulcers.

Differential Diagnosis

In a patient with risk factors for atherosclerosis, occlusive disease should be considered first as the etiology for claudication. However, the duration of this patient's symptoms suggests a potential congenital diagnosis, including aortic coarctation, embryologic arterial abnormalities, or cardiac lesions causing peripheral emboli. In a patient with a stronger pulse at the popliteal level compared to the femoral artery, persistent sciatic artery (PSA) should be suspected.

Workup

Although very rare with an incidence of 0.03% to 0.06%, PSA can result in limb loss if not identified and corrected in select cases, with aneurysms forming in 40% to 61% of PSA cases. The most common presentations are a painful, pulsatile gluteal mass; symptoms of sciatic nerve compression; and distal ischemia, although 40% to 50% are asymptomatic and identified incidentally on computed tomography (CT) scan. The mean age of PSA patients is 57 years with an equal distribution in men and women. PSAs are bilateral in 18% to 22%. Physical exam may identify a pulsatile mass in the buttocks or leg and diminished or absent femoral pulse with the presence of a palpable popliteal pulse (Cowie's sign). Concomitant findings of varicose veins, persistent sciatic veins, arteriovenous malformations, and abdominal wall capillary hemangiomas have been reported.

Diagnostic Tests and Results

Noninvasive vascular studies with exercise should be done to identify the degree of ischemia. This patient had ankle-brachial indices of 0.68 and 0.74 on the right and left, respectively, decreasing to 0.4 and 0.71 after 1 minute of exercise. She is able to exercise for 5 minutes, completing the 283-yard protocol with right calf weakness. Diagnostic imaging studies include ultrasound, CT angiogram (Fig. 1), and arteriography (Fig. 2A-D)

Magnetic resonance arteriography without contrast can be used in patients with renal insufficiency.

Diagnosis and Treatment
Surgical Approach

Management of PSA with or without aneurysmal changes depends on the degree of symptoms. No intervention is required if PSA is found incidentally or if the patient has stable mild ischemic symptoms, such as the described patient. PSA aneurysm rupture has not been reported, but aneurysm size should be followed serially with ultrasound or CT angiogram.

A PSA aneurysm alone, without significant distal ischemic disease, can be successfully managed with percutaneous embolization as well as exclusion with a stent graft. If catheter-based techniques are unsuccessful, open ligation with or without concomitant arterial revascularization has been described. Interposition grafting, with either prosthetic or vein conduit, from the normal femoral, external iliac, or hypogastric artery to the popliteal artery may be performed in

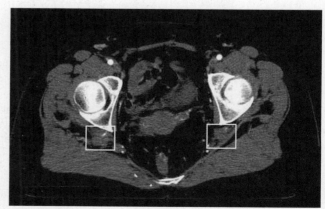

FIGURE 1 • CT scan of the abdomen and pelvis demonstrates bilateral thrombosed 2-cm PSA aneurysms (*white boxes*) from the pelvis to the popliteal arteries.

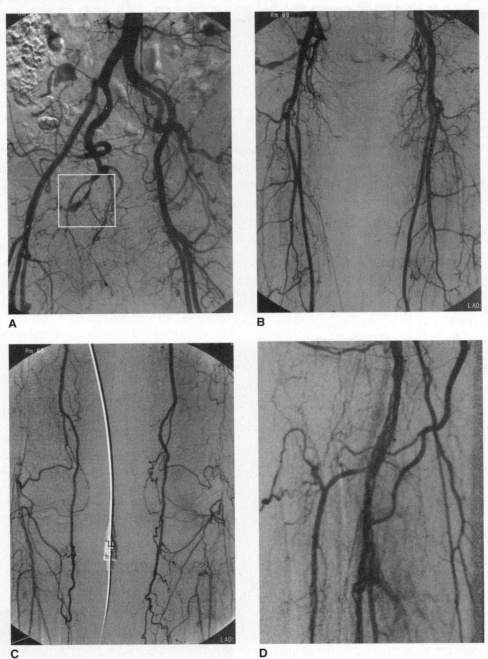

FIGURE 2 • Abdominal aortogram with bilateral lower extremity runoff shows a right remnant sciatic artery (*white box*) that is thrombosed as it exits the pelvis, refilling a tiny fragment at the lesser trochanter level **(A)**. No evidence of the left sciatic artery is noted on arteriogram. The distal bilateral superficial femoral arteries **(B)** end at the adductor hiatus, and the popliteal arteries refill via two collateral arteries **(C)**. There are luminal irregularities in both popliteal arteries indicative of partially recanalized thrombus **(D)**.

conjunction with aneurysm ligation or endoaneurysmorrhaphy via a retroperitoneal approach. The limb loss rate has been reported as high as 18%, but this includes many patients with primary amputations due to embolic events.

Special Intraoperative Considerations

Excision of the aneurysm should be avoided, as it is often adherent to the sciatic nerve, and foot-drop has been reported in open aneurysm repair. In addition, in comparing patients with aneurysm resection/endoaneurysmorrhaphy to those with exclusion/embolization, each had similar improvement in relief of compressive effects. Patients with PSA should also be treated carefully if undergoing hip operations due to the surgical proximity of the aberrant artery or if undergoing renal transplantation to the ipsilateral hypogastric artery.

Postoperative Management

Postoperative follow-up depends on the degree of revascularization or percutaneous treatment, with physical exam, noninvasive studies, and serial imaging (ultrasound or CTA). There is no data to support chronic anticoagulation, although antiplatelet agents would likely be used in patients with concomitant ischemia.

Case Conclusion

This 54-year-old woman has bilateral persistent sciatic arteries with aneurysmal degeneration and stable claudication. She has evidence of prior embolic events, but has little to no flow within the aneurysms on the present examination. Although femoropopliteal reconstruction could be considered, as she has adequate external iliac and common femoral arteries, the patient did not feel that her symptoms were lifestyle limiting and no operation was performed. Serial CT scans were recommended on a yearly basis to assess aneurysm size.

TAKE HOME POINTS

- Surgical treatment is necessary if lower limb ischemia is critical or if a PSA aneurysm is causing lower limb thromboembolism or severe buttock pain. (Table 1)
- Operative procedures, both open and endovascular, depend on the anatomy of the PSA and the indication (ischemia, compression or thromboembolism from aneurysm, or both).
- Endovascular procedures, either retrograde or antegrade, may become more common in treating PSA with or without aneurysms, but because of the rarity of the disease, comparison of open versus endovascular procedure outcomes will be impossible.

TABLE 1. Key Technical Steps and Potential Pitfalls

Key Technical Steps

1. Depending on the anatomy of the PSA, revascularization in addition to aneurysm ligation may be required.
2. Simple ligation may cause less sciatic nerve injury than attempted resection.
3. Percutaneous stent graft may allow treatment of PSA aneurysm without nerve injury.

Potential Pitfalls

- Consideration of the diagnosis is most important in those with palpable pedal pulses without femoral pulses and those with pulsatile buttock masses.
- The primary complications are nerve compression, embolism, and distal ischemia.
- Repair should be dictated on presentation, with endoluminal approaches reasonable as first option.
- Open repair with ligation is reasonable, but care of the surrounding sciatic nerve is critical.

SUGGESTED READINGS

Brantley SK, Rigdon EE, Raju S. Persistent sciatic artery: embryology, pathology, and treatment. *J Vasc Surg.* 1993;18:242-248.

Green PH. On a new variety of the femoral artery. *Lancet.* 1832;1:730-732.

Nuño-Escobar C, Pérez-Durán MA, Ramos-López R, et al. Persistent sciatic artery aneurysm. *Ann Vasc Surg.* 2013;27:1182.e13-1182.e16.

Parry DJ, Aldoori MI, Hammond RJ, et al. Persistent sciatic vessels, varicose veins, and lower limb hypertrophy: an unusual case or discrete clinical syndrome. *J Vasc Surg.* 2002;36:396-400.

Sultan SAH, Pacainowski JP, Madhavan P, et al. Endovascular management of rare sciatic artery aneurysm. *J Endovasc Ther.* 2000;7:415-422.

Yamamoto H, Yamamoto F, Ishibashi K, et al. Intermediate and long-term outcomes after treating symptomatic persistent sciatic artery using different techniques. *Ann Vasc Surg.* 2011;25:837.e9-837.e15.

Yang S, Ranum K, Malone M, et al. Bilateral persistent sciatic artery with aneurysm formation and review of the literature. *Ann Vasc Surg.* 2014;28:264.e1-264.e7.

CLINICAL SCENARIO CASE QUESTIONS

1. The origin of a persistent sciatic artery is:

   a. The common iliac artery
   b. The pudendal artery
   c. The internal iliac artery
   d. The external iliac artery
   e. The aortic bifurcation

2. A persistent sciatic artery is most commonly at risk of:

   a. No sequelae
   b. Acute occlusion with limb ischemia
   c. Aneurysmal degradation
   d. Source of distal arterial emboli
   e. Sciatic nerve ischemia

101 Popliteal Artery Aneurysm—Open Repair

PAUL D. DIMUSTO and PETER K. HENKE

Presentation

A 65-year-old man was referred to the vascular surgery clinic for evaluation of a large abdominal aortic aneurysm (AAA) discovered on screening ultrasound performed by his primary care physician given his 50-pack-year smoking history. The patient also has medical history significant for hypertension, hyperlipidemia, type 2 diabetes mellitus, and coronary artery disease with prior myocardial infarction, and he is morbidly obese. He has undergone coronary artery bypass grafting 10 years ago and coronary artery stent placement 3 years ago. He takes an aspirin, statin, and beta-blocker daily, among other medications. He has a family history of coronary artery disease, but no family history of aneurysms.

On examination in the clinic, he has a pulsatile abdominal mass and palpable femoral and pedal pulses bilaterally. As a part of his evaluation, he undergoes a duplex ultrasound scan of his bilateral femoral and popliteal arteries to survey for occult aneurysms, as well as ankle-brachial index (ABI). He is discovered to have bilateral popliteal aneurysms measuring 2.5 cm in diameter on the right (Fig. 1) and 2.2 cm on the left, with the right extending below the tibial plateau. His ABIs are 0.9 bilaterally with triphasic pedal waveforms.

Differential Diagnosis

Popliteal artery aneurysms (PAAs) are uncommon in the general population, with an incidence of less than 0.1%. However, in patients with AAAs, up to 14% will have femoral or popliteal aneurysms, with 10% having isolated PAA. They may present as a pulsatile mass in the popliteal fossa, but the majority are not detectable on physical exam, especially as the population becomes more obese. The differential diagnosis for a mass in the popliteal fossa includes a Baker's cyst, lipoma, hematoma, venous thrombosis, sarcoma, or lymphoma. These are all less likely in this patient.

Discussion

A PAA is defined as a dilation of the artery that is 1.5 to 2 times the diameter of the normal artery. Thus, a diameter of 1.5 to 2 cm is considered aneurysmal in most patients. PPAs occur almost exclusively in men with an approximately 30:1 male-to-female ratio in incidence. Ninety-six percent of PAAs were found in men in a large review of the literature. This is different than AAA, which typically has a 4:1 male-to-female ratio of incidence.

The pathophysiology of PAA is not entirely clear, but is thought to be more inflammatory in nature compared to the atherosclerotic degeneration seen in AAAs. In a study of patients with known AAAs, peripheral artery disease was more common in patients with PAA than in those AAAs and no peripheral aneurysms.

In this patient, his PAAs are asymptomatic and were discovered incidentally while undergoing workup for his AAA. However, 40% to 60% of patients will present with some form of symptoms. Most will present with ischemic symptoms, ranging from claudication (25%), to rest pain, to acute critical limb ischemia (25%). Patients may also present with evidence of repeated distal embolization, commonly referred to as "blue toe syndrome," and often have a slight decrease in perfusion and tibial occlusion. Finally, symptoms due to compression of the tibial nerve (neuropathy) or the popliteal vein (limb swelling or deep venous thrombosis) can also occur.

If a PAA is discovered de novo, the patient should undergo screening for AAA, as 38% to 62% of patients presenting with PAA will have a concomitant AAA and 15% will have a concomitant iliac aneurysm. Additionally, 35% to 48% of patients will have bilateral PAA as our patient does.

Imaging

Duplex ultrasonography, with both gray-scale imaging to detect the aneurysm size and any luminal thrombus present, as well as color Doppler flow to assess the flow above, through, and below the aneurysm, is the initial imaging study used in the workup. This is an excellent screening test as it is noninvasive and does not involve radiation or iodinated contrast. Duplex ultrasound can also be used to follow patients postrepair.

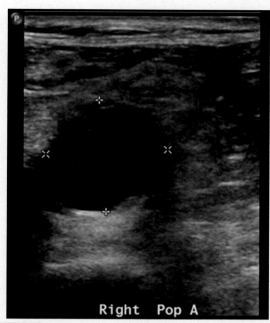

FIGURE 1 • Ultrasound image showing large right popliteal aneurysm.

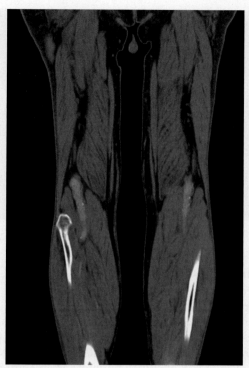

FIGURE 2 • Contrast CTA in sagital section showing right popliteal aneurysm.

Computed tomography angiography (CTA) or magnetic resonance angiography (MRA) can also be used to further evaluate a patient with a suspected or diagnosed popliteal aneurysm, particularly if the patient also has an AAA and is undergoing evaluation for repair. These can help define the inflow and outflow as well as the full extent of the aneurysm and surrounding anatomy (Table 1).

In patients who present with acute thrombosis of a PAA and acute limb ischemia, angiography with thrombolysis may be indicated as the initial imaging study. All patients being considered for PAA repair should undergo preoperative angiography, as this will help define the outflow vessels to the foot and a suitable distal target for bypass if the ABIs are abnormal. Up to 69% of patients will have 0 to 1 infrapopliteal arteries open due to embolization from the aneurysm. However, angiography should not be used as an initial evaluation of a suspected asymptomatic aneurysm, as

the aneurysm may not be detected due to thrombus in the aneurysm sac.

Case Continued

The patient underwent a CTA of the abdomen, pelvis, and lower extremities to further define the anatomy of his AAA as well as his PAA. This confirmed a 6.9-cm juxtarenal AAA as well as bilateral PAA greater than 2 cm in diameter (Figs. 2 and 3). The right extended to below the knee; the left was confined to behind the knee.

Recommendation

In patients presenting with both AAA and PAA, as in this patient, the more life-threatening problem should be repaired first. In our patient, as in most, his large AAA takes priority. Our patient underwent open juxtarenal AAA repair given his anatomy. Once he recovered from this, his bilateral PAA should be electively repaired in sequential fashion.

Vein mapping is performed that reveals suitable saphenous vein for a bypass on the right leg, but the left was previously harvested for his coronary bypass. He does have adequate cephalic vein bilaterally. Open bypass and aneurysm ligation via a medial approach is recommended. The right side is addressed first as it is slightly larger. A posterior approach is contraindicated in this case given the distal extent of the aneurysm. A posterior approach with bypass or interposition grafting can only be used for an aneurysm confined to behind the knee.

TABLE 1. Key Technical Steps and Potential Pitfalls

1. Once diagnosed, a good CTA or digital subtraction angiography (DSA) is appropriate for inflow and outflow target around the PAA.
2. A medial approach for above-knee to below-knee popliteal bypass is most common, but a posterior approach is reasonable in selected patients.
3. Do not forget to ligate the PAA proximally and distally.
4. Avoid conduit twisting by marking and passing the vein carefully.
5. Care with tissue is important as wound complications are frequent.

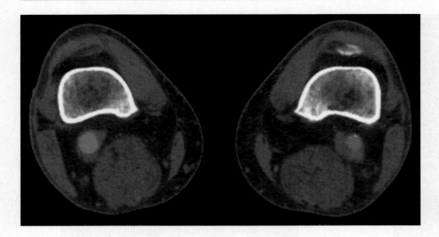

FIGURE 3 • Contrast CTA showing bilateral popliteal aneurysms.

Surgical Technique

The procedure is performed under general anesthesia in the supine position. The right leg is prepared and draped in sterile fashion, the knee is flexed slightly, and a bump is placed under the distal thigh. In this case, a bypass is performed from the distal superficial femoral artery (SFA) to the distal below the knee popliteal artery with ipsilateral reversed saphenous vein graft. In general, the shortest bypass possible to completely exclude the aneurysmal segment is preferred. Additionally, vein is strongly preferred over prosthetic as a conduit given better patency of a vein bypass below the knee.

The distal SFA and below the knee popliteal artery are exposed in standard fashion, and proximal and distal control is obtained. Care must be taken to not injure the saphenous vein during the arterial exposure. Preoperative marking of the vein with ultrasound can help avoid this complication. An anatomic tunnel is then created between the femoral condyles, and an adequate length of vein is then harvested. The patient is then heparinized, and an end-to-side anastomosis is performed proximally, then distally after distending the vein graft and taking care to not twist it while passing it through the tunnel. The native artery should be ligated both proximally and distally with a large silk tie and hemoclip to exclude the aneurysm from circulation. An intraoperative completion duplex is then performed to assess for any technical complications that need to be immediately addressed. Alternatively, a completion angiogram can be performed. Protamine is then given to reverse the heparin, the pedal Doppler signals are checked, and the wounds are closed in standard fashion.

Follow-Up

The patient has an uncomplicated postoperative course and is discharged home on postoperative day 4. He will follow up in the clinic at 1, 6, and 12 months postoperatively with a graft scan and ABI for graft surveillance. His

contralateral PAA will be excluded in a similar fashion using cephalic vein in approximately 8 weeks.

Overall, wound complications (4% to 5%), graft thrombosis (5%), and cardiac and respiratory complications (2%) are the most common following open exclusion of a popliteal aneurysm. Early mortality is approximately 2%, speaking to the extensive vascular comorbidities these patients have. In one large review, the early major amputation rate was 4% after open repair in all patients. The amputation rate in patients presenting with acute limb ischemia can be up to 25%, however. Long-term primary assisted patency rates are approximately 87% at 1 year, 86% at 3 years, and 64% to 75% at 5 years. The secondary patency is 90% at 1 year and 81% at 3 years. The 1-year amputation rate is about 7%.

In reasonable-risk patients, open exclusion of a popliteal aneurysm remains the gold standard of treatment.

Case Conclusion

This patient underwent staged repairs of his PAAs; first the right with ipsilateral reversed great saphenous vein as described above. He tolerated this well. Approximately 3 months later, he underwent a left PAA repair in a similar technical fashion. At 1 year out, his grafts remain patent.

TAKE HOME POINTS

- Recognition of PAA is a marker for AAA.
- PAA greater than 2 cm should be repaired in good-fit patients.
- PAAs in unfit patients can be followed with the patient on anticoagulation, but little evidence exists for this.
- Autologous bypass is the best strategy.

- Tibial artery embolization with occlusion, combined with sudden PAA thrombosis and occlusion, is associated with highest risk of limb loss.

SUGGESTED READINGS

Diwan A, Sarkar R, Stanley JC, et al. Incidence of femoral and popliteal artery aneurysms in patients with abdominal aortic aneurysms. *J Vasc Surg.* 2003;31:863-869.

Henke PK. Popliteal artery aneurysms: tried, true, and new approaches to therapy. *Semin Vasc Surg.* 2005;18:224-230.

Lovegrove RE, Javid M, Magee TR, et al. Endovascular and open approaches to non-thrombosed popliteal aneurysm repair: a meta-analysis. *Eur J Vasc Endovasc Surg.* 2008;36:96-100.

Pulli R, Dorigo W, Fargion A, et al. Comparison of early and midterm results of open and endovascular treatment of popliteal artery aneurysms. *Ann Vasc Surg.* 2012;26:809-818.

Tsilimparis N, Dayama A, Ricotta JJ II. Open and endovascular repair of popliteal artery aneurysms: tabular review of the literature. *Ann Vasc Surg.* 2013;27:259-265.

CLINICAL SCENARIO CASE QUESTIONS

1. A 70-year-old patient is found to have a 3-cm asymptomatic PAA, with thrombus, and has known 3v CAD, with mild angina. The next step is:

   a. CTA to better delineate anatomy
   b. Preoperative cardiology consultation
   c. Screening AAA duplex ultrasound
   d. DSA to better delineate anatomy
   e. Nothing, he is too high risk; treat medically

2. A patient with a 3-cm PAA is considered for repair. On duplex ultrasound vein exam, the right GSV is absent, the left GSV ranges from 1.5 to 2.5 mm, and the cephalic vein is greater than 2.5 mm. In this case, the best option would be:

   a. Use the contralateral vein.
   b. Use the cephalic vein.
   c. Use a prosthetic graft.
   d. Use a covered stent graft.
   e. Nothing; in a patient with marginal conduit, medical management is safer.

102 Endovascular Repair of a Popliteal Artery Aneurysm

ELIZABETH ANDRASKA, JOHN RECTENWALD, and PETER K. HENKE

Presentation

A 70-year-old man was referred to the clinic to evaluate a pulsatile mass felt in the left popliteal fossa by his primary care physician. His medical history is significant for hypertension, hyperlipidemia, and coronary artery disease with history of myocardial infarction. He has no family history of aneurysmal disease or coronary artery disease. A duplex ultrasound scan was performed on his femoral and popliteal arteries bilaterally. He was found to have bilateral popliteal artery aneurysms (PAAs) measuring 3 cm on the right and 3.4 cm on the left (Figs. 1 and 2). He was on a beta-blocker, aspirin, and a statin. In clinic, an ankle-brachial index (ABI) was measured to be 1.10 bilaterally, with triphasic pedal waveforms.

Differential Diagnosis

Any mass in the popliteal fossa should prompt a PAA workup. In this patient, the mass was pulsatile, and the ultrasound confirmed PAAs greater than 2 cm bilaterally. The differential diagnosis for a mass in this patient's popliteal fossa includes a Baker's cyst, venous thrombosis, hematoma, or neoplasm in addition to a PAA. An ultrasound should be performed to determine the presence of an aneurysm, size of the aneurysm, and presence or absence of intraluminal thrombus. While one third to one half of PAAs are asymptomatic, 20% to 40% present with some form of limb ischemia. Ischemic symptoms include claudication (25%), rest pain, foot ulceration, or acute limb ischemia. Patients may also present with "blue toe syndrome" (4% to 12%), which is caused by repeated thromboemboli from the PAA.

Workup

PAA disease is relatively uncommon in the general population, with an incidence of less than 0.1% in the general population. In patients with a diagnosed abdominal aortic aneurysm (AAA), the incidence of PAA is much higher (approximately 13% to 15%). Patients with PAAs are also at increased risk for other peripheral arterial aneurysms such as an iliac aneurysm (15%) or a femoral aneurysm. As with our patient, it is common for PAAs to occur bilaterally (35% to 48%). If a patient is found to have a PAA, abdominal and peripheral duplex ultrasound should be performed to rule out any synchronous aneurysms. Due to the morbidity of a ruptured AAA, prioritizing interventions in patients with both PAA and AAA is crucial. A large or rapidly growing AAA should be repaired prior to the PAA.

A computed tomography angiography (CTA) should be performed to better define the anatomy of the PAA and to establish inflow and outflow targets in case of surgical intervention. An ABI can be helpful in determining baseline limb perfusion, although it should not be considered a definitive test. If a patient has acute limb ischemia, urgent intervention is necessary due to high long-term amputation rates (9% to 36%). These patients should receive heparin anticoagulation and may be candidates for thrombolytic therapy before any other intervention is considered.

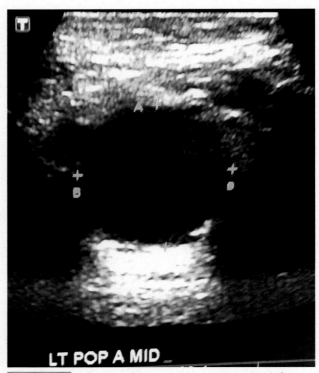

FIGURE 1 • Duplex ultrasound image showing left popliteal arterial dilation, consistent with an aneurysm.

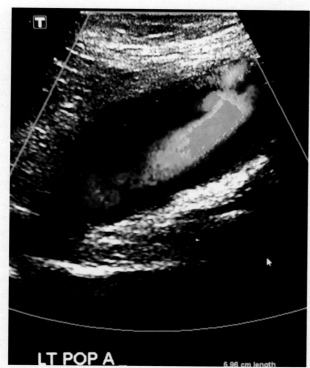

FIGURE 2 • Duplex ultrasound image with color flow showing blood flow and thrombus in popliteal aneurysm.

Diagnosis and Treatment

A PAA is defined as a popliteal artery that dilates to 1.5 to 2 times greater in diameter than the normal artery. The incidence of PAA in males as compared to females is extremely high (96%), and risk factors include coronary artery disease, hypertension, cerebrovascular disease, and a history of tobacco use.

Duplex ultrasonography should be used to screen and diagnose the PAA, as well as to evaluate for aneurysm size and presence of thrombus (Figs. 1 and 2). Duplex ultrasonography with power Doppler technique can be used to evaluate flow through the artery. These studies can also be done postoperatively to evaluate size and flow postrepair. Magnetic resonance angiography (MRA) or CTA can be used to further evaluate the inflow and outflow of a

patient's aneurysm and the surrounding anatomy (Fig. 3). Lower extremity angiography should be performed prior to a PAA repair to evaluate distal arterial runoff in cases where concomitant atherosclerosis exists (e.g., decreased ABI). Vein mapping should be done to determine presence of usable autologous conduit and, if none, may be a reason to repair the PAA via an endovascular technique.

Surgical or endovascular repair of the PAA is indicated in symptomatic patients and in asymptomatic patients with an aneurysm diameter of greater than 2 cm. However, some believe any PAA regardless of size should be repaired. Elective PAA repair for asymptomatic patients has been shown to provide better limb salvage than emergency revascularization due to a thrombosed PAA. While open surgical repair for a PAA remains the gold standard of treatment, endovascular repair has some advantages.

Endovascular repair avoids the morbidity associated with wound and possibly other major operative complications. If the patient is extremely high risk, anticoagulation therapy alone can be considered as an alternative to surgical intervention.

The patient underwent CTA of the abdomen, pelvis, and lower extremities. PAAs were confirmed bilaterally and were both focally confined to the popliteal fossa and with modest thrombus. Neither AAA nor other aneurysms were present. The anatomy of the aneurysm was not tortuous or extensive. Due to the relatively normal anatomy and the patient's preference, an endovascular repair of the left PAA was elected.

Surgical Approach

Anatomical parameters defined by the preoperative CTA or MRA should confirm that the PAA should not be extensive (e.g., long segment into below-knee popliteal artery) and that adequate landing zones (≥2 cm), both proximal and distal to the aneurysm, are present. The artery diameter between the two landing zones should be relatively similar and range usually 8 to 14 mm. Additionally, the patient must be able to tolerate antiplatelet therapy such as clopidogrel. Endovascular treatment is also a good alternative for patients that do not have adequate autologous

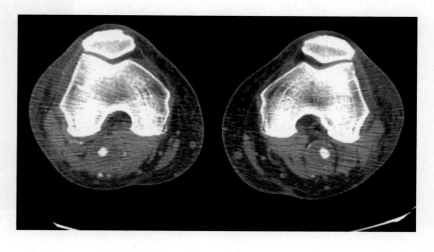

FIGURE 3 • Contrast CT scan showing bilateral popliteal aneurysms.

TABLE 1. Key Technical Steps and Potential Pitfalls

Key Technical Steps
1. Confirm that there is adequate normal artery both proximally and distally for the stent graft landing zones (>2 cm) and that the artery size is acceptable.
2. Avoid points of vessel flexion so stent does not kink.
3. Allow some oversizing of the covered stent to allow seal in the normal proximal and distal artery.

Potential Pitfalls
- Graft misdeployment.
- Avoid covering sites for potential surgical bypass and collaterals if possible.
- Ballooning outside of the covered stent can lead to dissection or rupture of the artery.

conduit for bypass repair. Success rate with endovascular treatment has not been extensively quantified, but a large review estimated the 5-year success rate to be 47% to 75%.

The procedure can be done under general, regional, or local anesthesia. The femoral artery is accessed by ultrasound-guided percutaneous or cutdown technique, per the surgeon's preference. A floppy followed by stiff guidewire is then threaded in an anterograde fashion, toward the popliteal artery. A nitinol stent lined with polytetrafluoroethylene such as the Viabahn (Gore, AZ) stent graft is slowly deployed along the guidewire, careful not to bend the graft into the aneurysm. Angiography of the aneurysm should be done prior to graft placement to aid in procedural planning and to confirm the proximal and distal landing zones and length of the graft. The diameter of stent graft should be chosen based on measurements taken by CTA and angiogram and should oversize the luminal diameter by 10% to 15%. The deployed graft should exclude the entire aneurysm and extend past the aneurysm endpoint to allow for shortening of the graft. The stent is then sealed both proximally and distally by ballooning within the stent. In this patient, no additional stents were needed. However, for more extensive PAAs, multiple stents may be indicated. In this case, stents should overlap to prevent endoleaks by 2 to 3 cm. The stent placement is then visualized with contrast angiography to check for presence of endoleak. The patient's knee is then flexed and observed under ultrasound guidance to ensure there is no occlusion due to stent bending. Intravenous heparin is given periprocedurally, based on the patient's weight, and any operative wounds are closed in the standard fashion (Table 1).

Special Intraoperative Considerations

Access may be direct via a superficial femoral artery (SFA) cutdown, percutaneously from the contralateral femoral artery, or antegrade from the ipsilateral CFA. Care must be taken to use a stiff wire (e.g., Amplatz) for which the device is navigated. Oftentimes, a preplaced arterial closure device can be used for a large-sheath placement with good results if done under ultrasound guidance. Care must be taken with cannulation past the PAA as

embolic material may be dislodged into the tibial arteries and then a suction thrombectomy or lysis may be needed.

Postoperative Management

The stent was properly placed in this patient, and he was able to be sent home the same day. He will follow up in the clinic at 1, 3, 6, and 12 months and then annually after that. His contralateral PAA will be repaired with endovascular treatment in about 6 weeks. An antiplatelet such as clopidogrel should be given postoperatively for a minimum of 6 weeks, although there is no direct evidence to support this.

While endovascular repair of PAA avoids the morbidity seen with open repair, there are many cases of repeat endovascular intervention and need for open bypass should the covered stent occlude. Additionally, graft occlusion and successive thrombus remain a significant complication with endovascular treatment (11%), often resulting in open surgical repair. Early endoleak is approximately 5%, 1-year amputation rate is 2%, and early mortality is 0.4%. Long-term primary assisted patency is 74% at 1 year and 87% at 3 years. Secondary patency is 87% at 1 year and 85% at 3 years in selected series. Due to the high incidence of graft occlusion and potential limb ischemia, endovascular repair of PAA should be reserved for patients that are otherwise unfit for open repair in the authors' opinion.

Case Conclusion

After bilateral PAA repair with endoprosthesis, this patient was monitored closely for a year and experienced no complications. Follow-up duplex (Fig. 4) and CTA (Fig. 5) showed a patent graft and an excluded PAA. He is now followed in clinic annually.

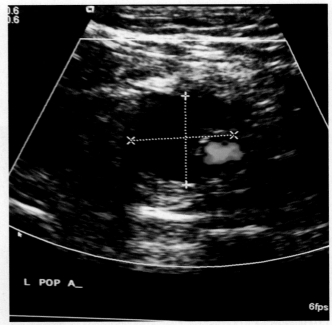

FIGURE 4 • Post–endovascular stent graft showing excluded PAA with flow in covered stent graft.

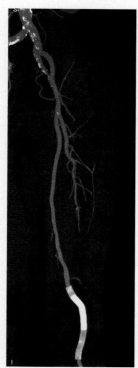

FIGURE 5 • Contrast CT scan showing in reformatted view the excluded PAA with a patent covered stent graft.

TAKE HOME POINTS

- Diagnosis of PAA is a marker for AAA.
- PAA greater than 2 cm should be repaired if the patient is a reasonable life expectancy.
- Open repair remains the gold standard for treatment of PAA, but endovascular repair of PAA is a reasonable alternative in selected patients.
- High rates of limb loss are associated with acute limb ischemia secondary to a thrombosed and occluded PAA.

SUGGESTED READINGS

Henke PK. Popliteal artery aneurysms: tried, true, and new approaches to therapy. *Semin Vasc Surg.* 2005;18: 224-230.

Lovegrove RE, Javid M, Magee TR, et al. Endovascular and open approaches to non-thrombosed popliteal aneurysm repair: a meta-analysis. *Eur J Vasc Endovasc Surg.* 2008;36: 96-100.

Pulli R, Dorigo W, Fargion A, et al. Comparison of early and midterm results of open and endovascular treatment of popliteal artery aneurysms. *Ann Vasc Surg.* 2012;26: 809-818.

Smialkowski AO, Huilgol RL. Outcome of endovascular repair of popliteal artery aneurysm using the Viabahn endoprosthesis. *J Vasc Surg.* 2012;55:1647-1653.

Tsilimparis N, Dayama A, Ricotta II JJ. Open and endovascular repair of popliteal artery aneurysms: tabular review of the literature. *Ann Vasc Surg.* 2013;27:259-265.

CLINICAL SCENARIO CASE QUESTIONS

1. A 65-year-old man has a recently diagnosed PAA of 3.0-cm size and no suitable venous conduit. The next step would be:

   a. Antiplatelet therapy only
   b. Anticoagulation therapy only
   c. Above-knee to below-knee ePTFE bypass
   d. An endovascular repair
   e. Duplex ultrasound of his abdomen

2. The best imaging modality to define the PAAs and arterial run off in patient with an ABI of 0.5 would be:

   a. Power duplex
   b. MRA
   c. CT
   d. Angiography
   e. None needed

103 Unilateral Leg Swelling Secondary to Venous Insufficiency

MARGARET CLARKE TRACCI and JULIE ARMATAS

Presentation

A 33-year-old woman with no past medical history presents with pain, swelling, and heaviness of her left leg. She first noticed these symptoms 4 years ago after giving birth to her second child. Her symptoms have progressed over time and are most pronounced at the end of the day or after prolonged standing. She has worn compression stockings for several months with persistence of her symptoms.

Physical examination reveals moderate edema of the left lower leg from midcalf to the ankle and a visible large varicosity traversing the medial thigh and proximal lower leg (Fig. 1). There are scattered telangiectasias and reticular veins around the ankles bilaterally; however, the right leg is without symptoms. The femoral and pedal pulses are palpable, and there are no skin changes noted.

Differential Diagnosis

While up to one third of the population is affected by venous disease, there are a variety of pathophyiologic processes that may underlie leg edema. Bilateral lower extremity edema may be systemic in nature, associated with underlying renal, cardiac, or hepatic disease, malnutrition, or inciting medications. Careful review of the patient's history is necessary to distinguish these.

Lymphedema may cause unilateral or bilateral edema, which is generally nonpitting in nature and involves the toes and dorsum of the foot. The skin often assumes a thickened, peau d'orange appearance. A positive Stemmer's test, indicated by the inability to pinch and lift a skinfold at the base of the second toe, is typical of lymphedema. Lymphedema may occur in association with venous insufficiency and is, in this setting, called phlebolymphedema.

Venous disease may be unilateral or bilateral and may involve physiologic elements of both obstruction and insufficiency. Symptoms include aching, throbbing, a sensation of heaviness or fatigue of the affected limb, or burning, itching, or "pins and needles" sensation in the skin. These will tend to be more prominent toward the end of the day and after periods of prolonged standing. Elements of patient history, such as female gender, parity, the presence of obesity, and family history of varicose veins, may support the diagnosis. The identification of occlusive disease is essential.

The most common etiology of venous occlusive disease is deep vein thrombosis, which may be provoked or associated with various thrombophilias. External compressive syndromes may result from pelvic or other tumors or from iliac vein compression by the right iliac artery or distal aorta, known commonly as May-Thurner syndrome. Patients may or may not present with the visible varicosities, reticular veins, or telangiectasias commonly associated with venous insufficiency.

Physical examination may demonstrate palpable varicosities or the cords or tenderness of chronic phlebitis. Skin changes associated with venous disease range from hemosiderin deposition to severe lipodermatosclerosis

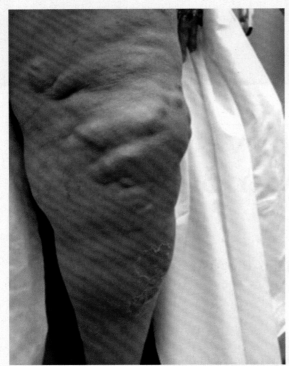

FIGURE 1 • Visible large varicosity traversing the medial thigh and proximal lower leg.

and even skin ulceration, typically in a gaiter distribution. The presence of unsightly veins leads some patients to seek treatment for cosmesis in the absence of significant symptoms. It is important to note that visible telangiectasias, reticular veins, and varicosities may occur in the absence of other symptoms or axial reflux.

Workup

A thorough history and physical exam can typically distinguish systemic, lymphatic, or venous causes of lower extremity edema. When venous insufficiency is suspected, duplex ultrasound (DU) is the inexpensive, noninvasive, and safe workhorse of diagnosis and is useful not only to establish the diagnosis but also to guide treatment and assess outcomes.

Duplex Ultrasound

A thorough venous duplex examination should comprise visualization of both deep and superficial systems as well as assessments of vessel compressibility, flow (including the presence and duration of reflux), and augmentation. The reflux examination is ideally obtained in a standing position, using patient Valsalva to elicit reflux at the common femoral vein, saphenofemoral junction, and more central portion of the greater saphenous vein (GSV) and manual or cuff compression and release to do the same

in veins of the distal leg. Pathologic reflux is defined as retrograde flow that lasts greater than 1000 ms in the common femoral, femoral, and popliteal veins (deep system) and greater than 500 ms for the greater and small saphenous veins, the deep femoral vein, tibial veins, and perforating veins.

Plethysmography

Plethysmography provides a physiologic measurement of venous volume or pressure and is used to detect and characterize venous disease. Volume changes, amount of reflux, degree of venous outflow obstruction, and the efficiency of the calf muscle pump can be estimated. The availability of plethysmography has also limited its use in recent years, although it is still felt to be useful in the setting of advanced disease for the clarification of pathophysiology.

Advanced Imaging (CT and MR Venography)

These modalities are used selectively primarily in the evaluation of congenital malformations (primarily gadolinium-enhanced magnetic resonance [MR]) or central pathologies such as thrombotic or nonthrombotic iliocaval obstruction or compressive syndromes such as May-Thurner, pelvic congestion, or nutcracker syndromes (MR or computed tomography [CT]).

Contrast Venography and Intravascular Ultrasound

For patients with complex obstructive or mixed disease, ascending and descending venography may play a critical role in diagnosis and management. It provides physiologic as well as anatomic information regarding both reflux and obstruction as well as the opportunity to treat obstructive disease, particularly in central locations. Intravascular ultrasound can serve as an important adjunct to a catheter-based study or intervention, as it provides excellent data regarding the cross-sectional area of the vein and may be more sensitive in the detection and characterization of compressive or obstructive lesions than contrast venography alone.

Medical Evaluation

In the event of recurrent or unprovoked venous thrombosis, thorough review of patient and family history as well as laboratory investigation for thrombophilia is appropriate.

Results

DU on this patient revealed reflux in the left GSV, greater than 5 seconds. The left GSV measured 5.3 mm, and there was no reflux in the small saphenous vein. These findings led to a diagnosis of left GSV reflux (Fig. 2).

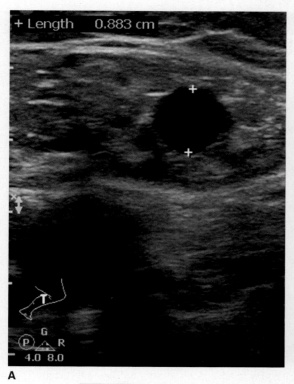
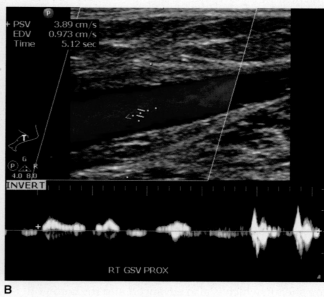

FIGURE 2 • Axial view (**A**) of GSV in sheath and longitudinal view (**B**) demonstrating reflux.

Diagnosis and Treatment

Typically, the first-line therapy for symptomatic varicose veins is moderate (20 to 30 mm Hg) compression therapy. Its effectiveness may be augmented by lifestyle modifications such as weight loss, exercise, and periodic leg elevation. Patients with saphenous reflux and symptoms that persist despite a trial of compression are generally excellent candidates for ablative therapy.

Vein stripping and ambulatory phlebectomy, once the mainstay of treatment for venous reflux, are performed less frequently since the advent of catheter-based treatments. The limitations of open surgical treatment for saphenous reflux, high ligation, and inversion stripping include the use of general anesthesia, increased morbidity, and deep vein thrombosis (DVT) rates approaching 5%. Some argue that conventional high ligation and stripping are preferable for patients with a very large saphenous vein at the saphenofemoral junction (higher risk of thrombus extension into the common femoral vein) or for very superficial, partially obstructed, or extremely tortuous saphenous veins.

For symptomatic patients with superficial reflux, radiofrequency (RF) ablation and endovenous laser ablation (EVLA) have been found to be safe and effective, with results comparable to high ligation and stripping. The anatomic features listed above should be viewed as relative, rather than absolute, contraindications, and surgeons who perform endovenous ablation frequently are adept at addressing such challenges. Hydrophilic wires may be used to traverse very tortuous veins with success, and, where needed, multiple access sites may be used to address occlusive segments through which the sheath cannot be advanced. Endovenous ablative therapy may be applied to greater and short saphenous veins, large accessory veins, and many perforating veins. Foam sclerotherapy of axial veins is also used and recently has an FDA approval for this indication.

Based on the patient's duplex findings of severe reflux in the left GSV from the saphenofemoral junction to the distal thigh, as well as the complaints of aching and burning despite compliance with compression therapy, this patient was deemed an appropriate candidate for EVLA, with planned treatment from just peripheral to the saphenofemoral junction to the level of the knee or proximal calf. This would be followed by sclerotherapy or ambulatory phlebectomy of any remaining symptomatic varicosities.

Surgical Decision Making

The decision to proceed with surgical intervention for varicose veins is in large part dependent on the patient's symptoms. If the patient can be compliant with compression and lifestyle changes and symptoms are adequately relieved, conservative management may be suitable. For those with persistent symptoms or more severe presentations such as ulceration, outcomes with regard to ulcer recurrence are improved when superficial reflux is addressed.

Surgical Approach: Endovenous Ablation

The etiology of the patient's symptoms is venous insufficiency (incompetent venous valves) of the left GSV. Treatment with endovenous ablation, in this case EVLA, is preferred.

EVLA may be performed in the office, often with the adjunct of oral or IV sedation. If oral sedation is to be used, the patient may be premedicated prior to preparation. The left GSV is examined under ultrasound to evaluate anatomy from the saphenofemoral junction to proposed access site, typically at or just distal to the knee. The patient's entire leg is prepped and draped to afford access to the course of the saphenous vein from ankle to saphenofemoral junction. Using ultrasound guidance, the distal left GSV is visualized and access is obtained using a 21-gauge micropuncture needle. A 0.018-inch wire is advanced into the vein and used to exchange the needle for a 4-French introducer. The inner dilator and wire are then removed, and a 0.035-inch wire may then be advanced beyond the saphenofemoral junction into the common femoral vein. The 4-French introducer sheath is then exchanged for a 5-French procedure sheath, which is also advanced into the common femoral vein. The wire and introducer of the long sheath are then removed and the laser catheter advanced and locked in place. Laser fiber and introducer may then be carefully withdrawn under ultrasound guidance until a longitudinal view demonstrates laser tip placement approximately 1.5 to 2 cm peripheral to the saphenofemoral junction.

Tumescent (buffered 0.1% lidocaine without epinephrine) is then used either with hand injection or utilizing a continuous pump controlled by a pedal to infiltrate circumferentially around the saphenous vein, providing analgesia, a thermal shield to protect skin and saphenous nerve, and to ensure thorough treatment of the vein by compressing it closely around the laser fiber. Ultrasound is then once again used to confirm the location of the catheter tip position. Appropriate eye protection for operator and patient is donned, and the laser is activated and withdrawn slowly through the length of the saphenous vein to be treated. The rate of catheter movement is targeted to deliver energy in the range of 30 to 50 joules/cm at a setting of 5 to 7 W. A premarked sheath and auditory cues aid the operator in maintaining the appropriate delivery of energy. The catheter and sheath are then removed and hemostasis obtained with direct pressure. Ultrasound is used to visualize the saphenofemoral junction and to confirm patency of the common femoral vein. A sterile dressing is placed on the entry site and gentle compression held. Thirty- to forty-mm Hg compression hose are donned, and the patient is discharged home following an appropriate period of observation (Table 1).

TABLE 1. Endovenous Laser Ablation

Key Technical Steps

1. Identify appropriate candidate for EVLA.
2. Access vein using ultrasound guidance and a micropuncture kit.
3. A guidewire and sheath are advanced through the saphenous vein to the junction.
4. A laser fiber is then advanced and fiber and sheath withdrawn until the fiber tip is 1–2 cm peripheral to the saphenofemoral or saphenopopliteal junction.
5. Tumescent (0.1% buffered lidocaine) is injected along the length of the vein to externally compress the vein and protect the surrounding tissue from thermal injury.
6. The activated laser is withdrawn slowly to deliver 30–50 joules/cm to the treated segment of the vein.
7. The catheter and sheath are removed, and a dressing is applied.
8. Completion imaging is performed to confirm patency of the common femoral vein at the saphenofemoral junction.
9. 30–40 mm Hg compression hose are donned.
10. Follow-up venous imaging is performed (time range from 24 h to 7–10 days reported).

Potential Pitfalls

- Inability to obtain access in the vein due to venospasm
- Inability to advansce the catheter due to tortuosity
- Inadvertent treatment of deep vein and EHIT
- Thermal injury (skin or saphenous nerve)

Postoperative Management

Patients are permitted to opt for daytime wear only following an initial 36-hour period of continuous wear if compliance is difficult. Patients are asked to walk hourly the day of the procedure to lessen the risk of DVT and to stay well hydrated and active throughout the week. Acetaminophen or NSAIDs generally provide sufficient postprocedure pain control.

Follow-up is arranged at one week (reported range 24 hours to 7 to 10 days) with ultrasound to assess for DVT (endothermal heat–induced thrombosis [EHIT]) and again at 6 weeks to assess resolution of symptoms and need for further therapy, as for residual symptomatic varicosities. If DVT is detected extending into the common femoral vein, patients are treated with low molecular weight heparin and followed with serial ultrasound until thrombus retraction is observed. Other potential issues include thermal injury to the saphenous nerve in the lower leg; however, this is generally avoided by accessing the saphenous vein several inches proximal to the gaiter region. Thermal injury to the skin may also occur, although careful tumescent technique maintaining at least 1 cm of buffer between catheter and skin and improved performance of the latest generation of catheters have rendered this quite rare. Lack of vein closure or late recanalization may occur. The most commonly encountered issue is local phlebitis, which typically responds to conservative therapy.

Case Conclusion

The patient underwent successful EVLA of the left GSV and is seen in follow-up 1 week later. Ultrasound at one week confirmed closure of the vein and no evidence of DVT. The symptoms of aching, heaviness, and swelling have greatly subsided.

TAKE HOME POINTS

- Patients with measured venous reflux may or may not be symptomatic, and those with visible varicosities or telangiectasias may or may not demonstrate abnormal axial vein reflux.
- Duplex ultrasonography is the mainstay of diagnosis of venous insufficiency.
- Abnormal reflux is considered to be greater than 1 second of reversed flow in the femoral or popliteal veins or greater than 0.5 seconds of reversed flow in saphenous, tibial, deep femoral, and perforating veins.
- Treatment options for saphenous reflux include high ligation and stripping of the greater or small saphenous veins or catheter-based therapies such as EVLA and RFA.
- RFA and EVLA are safe and effective treatments for venous insufficiency, and the outcomes are comparable to each other and to open surgical stripping. As they are less morbid than open surgical therapy, they are typically considered first-line therapy.

- Potential complications of catheter-based therapy include DVT, thermal injury to the nerve or skin, phlebitis, and recanalization.
- Surveillance for DVT should be routinely performed following treatment of saphenous veins.

SUGGESTED READINGS

Eklof B, Rutherford RB, Bergan JJ, et al. Revision of the CEAP classification for chronic venous disorders: consensus statement. *J Vasc Surg.* 2004;40(6):1248-1252.

Gloviczki P, Comerota AJ, Dalsing MC, et al. The care of patients with varicose veins and associated chronic venous diseases: clinical practice guidelines of the Society for Vascular Surgery and the American Venous Forum. *J Vasc Surg.* 2011;53(5 suppl):2S-48S.

Murad MH, Coto-Yglesias F, Zumaeta-Garcia M, et al. A systematic review and meta-analysis of the treatments of varicose veins. *J Vasc Surg.* 2011;53(5 suppl):49S-65S.

CLINICAL SCENARIO CASE QUESTIONS

1. Which of the following is the favored diagnostic modality for identification of venous insufficiency?

   a. Duplex ultrasound with provocative maneuvers
   b. Catheter venography
   c. Magnetic resonance venography
   d. Ambulatory venous pressures
   e. Plethysmography

2. When evaluating a patient presenting with a history of left leg swelling and heaviness and a normal exam on the right, what condition should be considered?

   a. Paget-Schroetter syndrome
   b. Venous malformation
   c. May-Thurner syndrome
   d. Femoral vein compression following a poorly healed femoral fracture
   e. Lymphedema

Varicose Veins

ANDREA T. OBI and THOMAS W. WAKEFIELD

Presentation

A 47-year-old man with no significant past medical history presents to your office complaining of right leg pain and swelling with prolonged standing. Results of the physical examination are normal, except for large, bulging varicose veins (Fig. 1) and edema of the right lower extremity.

Differential Diagnosis

Leg edema can be caused by a pathophysiologic process limited to the leg or by a systemic process. Systemic processes responsible for lower extremity edema, which is generally bilateral, include organ failure (heart, liver, kidney), certain medications, and paralysis and muscle atrophy resulting in prolonged periods of extremity dependency. Lymphedema can cause unilateral or bilateral leg swelling.

Swelling may be the result of varicose veins alone or may be attributable to deep venous pathology that can coexist with varicose veins. Thrombosis and congenital anomalies can cause deep venous obstruction and deep venous insufficiency; both of these latter conditions can be associated with unilateral or bilateral edema, with or without varicose veins. The symptoms of deep venous pathology are similar to those associated with varicose veins caused by superficial venous insufficiency, but the treatment of these entities is different.

Discussion

The edema that results from organ failure, paralysis, muscle atrophy, prolonged extremity dependency, or medications can generally be ruled out by a thorough history and physical examination. Unlike the "pitting" edema associated with venous insufficiency, which begins in the ankles and calves, the "nonpitting" edema of lymphedema begins in the dorsum of the foot, usually involves the toes, and progresses proximally with time. The skin of a lymphedematous limb is characterized by a peau d'orange appearance and papillomas. The skin associated with superficial venous insufficiency and varicose veins can show no changes at all or can display lipodermatosclerosis and stasis pigmentation changes in the gaiter region.

The etiology of varicose veins is the result of three pathophysiologic states: valvular insufficiency, obstruction, or calf pump malfunction. Valvular insufficiency occurs most frequently in the superficial system and is associated with development of varicose veins. The most commonly affected veins include the great saphenous (70% to 80%) followed by small saphenous (15% to 20%) and nonsaphenous (10%). Increasing severity of symptoms occurs with involvement of more than one venous system. Chronic reflux results in transmission of high venous pressures to the lower leg while standing. Valvular insufficiency occurs as the valve becomes elongated and floppy or by dilation of the valvular ring. Deep venous thrombosis accounts for half of the cases of deep vein valvular dysfunction due to vein wall fibrosis and valve scarring. Other causes of reflux include high levels of estrogen during pregnancy and prolonged standing, which both cause vein dilation.

Venous hypertension can also be the result of an obstruction to blood exiting the lower extremity. Obstruction can be due to a vascular occlusive lesion from a deep venous thrombosis or from nonthrombotic occlusion, such as compression of the left common iliac vein by the right common iliac artery (May-Thurner syndrome).

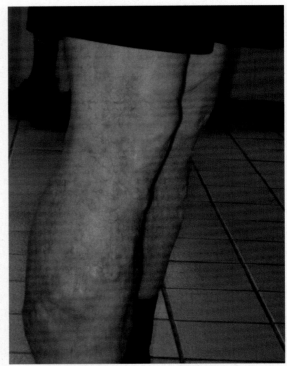

FIGURE 1 • Symptomatic varicosities.

TABLE 1. CEAP

Clinical Classification

C0	No visible or palpable signs of venous disease
C1	Telangiectasies or reticular veins
C2	Varicose veins
C3	Edema
C4	Pigmentation or eczema
C5	Healed venous ulcer
C6	○Active venous ulcer
S	Symptomatic: ache, pain, tightness, skin irritation, heaviness, muscle cramps

Anatomic Classification

As	Superficial veins
Ap	Perforator veins
Ad	Deep veins
An	No venous location identified

Etiologic Classification

Ec	Congenital
Ep	Primary
Es	Secondary (postthrombotic)
En	No venous cause identified

Pathophysiologic Classification

Pr	Reflux
Po	Obstruction
Pr, o	Reflux, obstruction
Pn	No venous pathophysiology identifiable

Adapted from Eklöf B, Rutherford RB, Bergan JJ, et al. American Venous Forum International Ad Hoc Committee for Revision of the CEAP Classification. Revision of the CEAP classification for chronic venous disorders: consensus statement. *J Vasc Surg.* 2004;40(6):1248-1252.

The diagnosis of chronic venous disease begins with a thorough history and physical exam. Severity of illness is categorized by the Clinical, Etiology, Anatomy, Pathophysiology (CEAP) (Table 1) and Venous Clinical Severity Scoring System (VCSS) (Table 2). Venous duplex ultrasonography is capable of detecting both deep and superficial venous thrombosis or insufficiency. In our practice, duplex imaging is performed on all patients presenting with venous disease. The patient is positioned standing with weight on the contralateral limb. The standing position allows for filling of the deep venous system and accentuates the hydrostatic effects of venous insufficiency. The deep venous system is assessed for acute and chronic disease. If acute deep venous thrombosis (DVT) is discovered, the investigation is ended. If there is not a DVT, the pulse wave Doppler is performed during Valsalva and during distal compression if possible, and time of reflux is measured. Duration of valve closure greater than 500 ms (0.5 seconds) in the superficial or perforator veins is considered pathologic (Fig. 2). Retrograde flow in the deep veins of up to 1000 ms (or 1.0 seconds) is considered normal. Importantly, reflux should be determined in all the veins including the great saphenous, small saphenous, accessory saphenous, common femoral, popliteal, and perforating veins. Such a practice will prevent missed pathologic refluxing veins and will provide the surgeon with a "road map" of disease. In a review of 1091 patients, we discovered 30% to have reflux in locations other than the saphenofemoral junction. Oftentimes,

TABLE 2. Revised VCSS

Clinical Descriptor	Absent (0)	Mild (1)	Moderate (2)	Severe (3)
Pain	None	Occasional	Daily not limiting	Daily limiting
Varicose veins	None	Few	Calf or thigh	Calf and thigh
Venous edema	None	Foot and ankle	Below knee	Knee and above
Skin pigmentation	None	Limited perimalleolar	Diffuse lower 1/3 calf	Wider above lower 1/3 calf
Inflammation	None	Limited perimalleolar	Diffuse lower 1/3 calf	Wider above lower 1/3 calf
Induration	None	Limited perimalleolar	Diffuse lower 1/3 calf	Wider above lower 1/3 calf
No. active ulcers	None	1	2	3 or more
Ulcer duration	None	<3 mo	3–12 mo	>1 y
Active ulcer size	None	<2 cm	2–6 cm	>6 cm
Compression therapy	None	Intermittent	Most days	Fully comply

Reprinted with permission from Vasquez MA, Rabe E, McLafferty RB, et al., American Venous Forum Ad Hoc Outcomes Working Group. Revision of the venous clinical severity score: venous outcomes consensus statement: special communication of the American Venous Forum Ad Hoc Outcomes Working Group. *J Vasc Surg.* 2010;52(5):1387-1396.

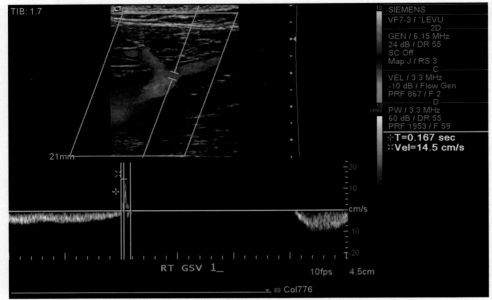

A

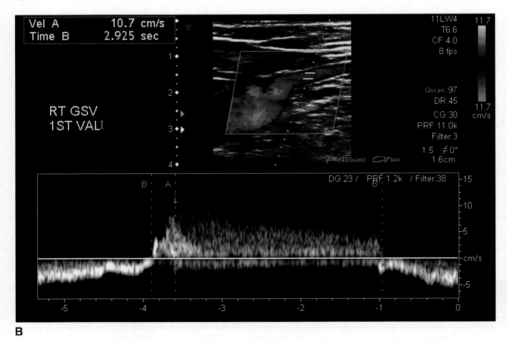

B

FIGURE 2 • Duplex ultrasonography demonstrating competent (**A**) great saphenous vein and refluxing (**B**) great saphenous vein.

venous duplex represents the only imaging study necessary to determine appropriate treatment.

Recommendation

Venous Duplex Ultrasound

Venous Duplex Ultrasound Report

The right great saphenous vein displays saphenofemoral reflux (duration longer than 0.5 second). No significant reflux is noted in the left lower extremity. No reflux or obstruction is noted in the deep venous system.

Diagnosis and Recommendation

The venous duplex ultrasound shows the etiology of the patient's varicose veins to be saphenofemoral reflux in the right lower extremity. The first line of treatment is compression therapy; intermittent leg elevation; exercise such as walking, cycling, and swimming; and protection of the skin barrier. Had the ultrasound shown significant deep venous insufficiency alone or in conjunction with superficial venous insufficiency, the nonoperative management noted above would be the recommended first treatment. In this patient, who has superficial venous insufficiency alone, surgical intervention is indicated if he remains symptomatic, develops a complication, or is unable to wear and tolerate compression therapy.

Surgical Approach

Treatment of Reflux

The widespread adoption of duplex ultrasound and development of endovenous therapies have significantly altered the treatment of varicose veins. The majority of patients presenting with varicosities will have concomitant venous reflux identified on duplex ultrasound. All patients with superficial reflux with a valve closure time of greater than 500 ms should be considered for an antireflux procedure if conservative therapy has not alleviated the symptoms. Currently, the use of endovenous thermal ablation, encompassing radiofrequency ablation (RFA) and endovenous laser therapy (EVLT), is the recommended therapy of choice over traditional open surgery (high ligation and stripping) with a grade 1B by the Society for Vascular Surgery (SVS) and American Venous Forum (AVF) varicose vein guidelines (Table 3). Foam sclerotherapy, while safe, is not as efficacious as is RFA, EVLT, or open surgery and thus is not recommended as first-line treatment for saphenous reflux.

Endovenous ablation may be performed in an office-based setting or in the operating room. The patient is positioned supine in reverse Trendelenburg with knee externally rotated (Fig. 3B). The great saphenous vein is accessed at or below the knee with a micro guidewire, and a 4-French sheath is placed. This is replaced using Seldinger technique with a 5-French venous catheter. The device (RF or EVL catheter) is passed through the sheath to the saphenofemoral junction. Use of ultrasound is critical to position the tip of the catheter prior to starting the ablation procedure (Fig. 3C). Ensuring a distance of 2.5 cm from the saphenofemoral junction decreases the risk of endovenous heat-induced thrombosis (EHIT). The perivenous tissue is then infiltrated with tumescent anesthesia to act as a heat sink, provide local analgesia, and produce venoconstriction for closer contact of the catheter and the vein wall. The catheter is slowly withdrawn as the vein is ablated in a retrograde fashion. If RFA catheter is utilized, the catheter is heated to 120°C for 20-second intervals. The vein is heated sequentially, most commonly in 7-cm segments (according to the length of the selected catheter), with the first segment of vein treated twice. The Endovenous Laser Ablation (EVLA) technique allows for continuous withdrawal of the catheter at 1 to 2 mm/s for the first 10 seconds, followed by 2 to 3 mm/s for the remainder. At the end of the procedure, the length of the vein is reimaged to ensure occlusion. Although uncommon with modern devices, incomplete occlusion warrants immediate re-treatment.

Treatment of Varicosities

Some patients will experience regression of varicosities with treatment of reflux alone, although at the current time, there is no clinical prediction rule that can reliably select these patients. Treatment of symptomatic varicosities can be undertaken either through traditional stab phlebectomy or via a minimally invasive approach via transilluminated powered phlebectomy (TIPP). Reported data thus far on the TIPP procedure are promising, but are not robust enough to determine whether one approach should be favored over the other.

Regardless of technique chosen, the patients must be met in the preoperative holding area and the areas of varicosities marked in the standing position, as they may regress significantly in the supine position (Fig. 3A and B). If stab phlebectomy is to be performed, the veins are marked directly over their course. If TIPP is chosen, the area of the veins is encircled but not marked directly as this would interfere with the transillumination of the technique. The subcutaneous tissue is then infiltrated with tumescent anesthesia. If ambulatory phlebectomy is the

TABLE 3. Methods of Endovenous Ablation

Method	Recommended Use	Advantages/Disadvantages
Endovenous laser ablation	• Current standard of care	• Safe, efficacious, few contraindications, low risk for complications • *Requires use of tumescent anesthesia*
Radiofrequency ablation	• Current standard of care	• Safe, efficacious, few contraindications, low risk for complications • *Requires use of tumescent anesthesia*
Foam sclerotherapy	• Second-line therapy	• Least invasive method, safe, low risk of complications • *Less efficacious than EVLA or RFA*
Superheated steam	• Experimental	• No need for a guidewire • *Limited data on efficacy and safety* • *Not widely available*
Mechanicochemical ablation	• FDA approved; not enough data for guideline recommendation	• No risk of thermal injury, no need for tumescent anesthesia • *Limited data on efficacy and safety*

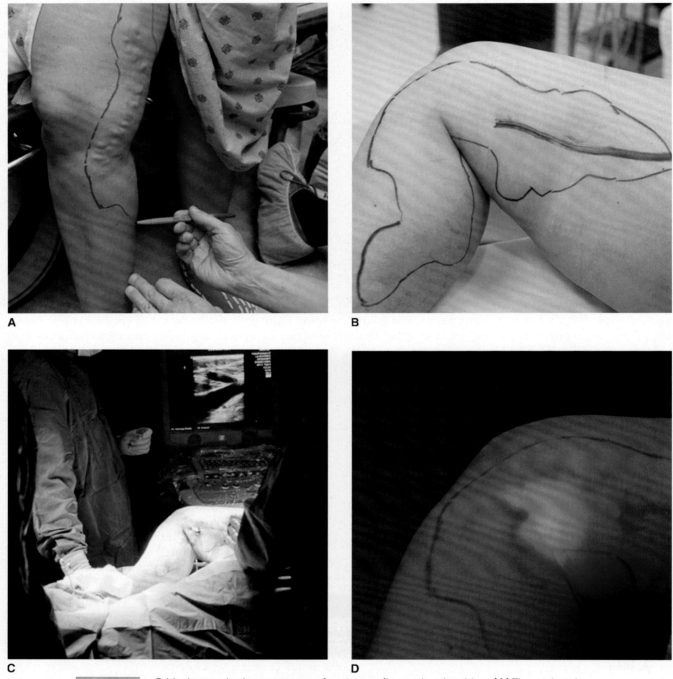

FIGURE 3 • Critical steps in the treatment of venous reflux and varicosities. **(A)** The patient is marked in standing position as clusters of varicosities will often regress in supine **(B)** position. Note that the trajectory of the saphenous vein is marked in a different color **(B)** to allow for easy identification. The saphenofemoral junction is visualized with ultrasound **(C)** during ablation to ensure sufficient distance to protect against EHIT. Transillumination **(D)** of varicosities expedites visualization and removal of veins during TIPP procedure.

method chosen, the skin just adjacent to the varicosities is incised with a no. 11 Beaver blade, a 15 ophthalmologic blade, or a 19-gauge needle. The veins are avulsed with hooks or forceps. If TIPP is utilized, the instruments are passed through tiny incisions adjacent to the area of varicosities. An illuminator cannula delivers tumescent anesthesia and provides transillumination of the veins (Fig. 3D). A resector handpiece mobilizes and suctions varicosities. Tiny "punch" incisions allow flushing of blood from the subcutaneous tissue with the tumescent solution.

TABLE 4. Key Technical Steps and Potential Pitfalls

Key Technical Steps
1. Mark all varicosities in standing position.
2. Place the patient in reverse Trendelenburg and access the vein at or below the knee. Infiltrate perivenous space with tumescent anesthesia solution.
3. Ablate the vein under live ultrasound 2 to 2.5 cm from the saphenofemoral junction in a retrograde fashion.
4. Insert a lighted cannula subdermally for transilluminated powered phlebectomy. Remove varicosities via a hand-held resector. Many tiny "punches" to drain tumescent anesthesia and blood.
5. Wrap the leg in compression bandage and elevate.

Potential Pitfalls
- Marking the patient in the supine position may lead to inadequate identification and removal of varicosities.
- Ablation <2 cm to the saphenofemoral junction may lead to development of EHIT.
- Inadequate postoperative compression may lead to hematoma.

The main advantage of TIPP appears to be much more complete and faster removal of large clusters of varicosities with fewer incisions compared to traditional stab phlebectomy (Table 4).

Postoperative Care

The limb is wrapped in a compression dressing, and patients are discharged to home following the procedure. Ambulation is encouraged. In our practice, patients have a routine follow-up ultrasound in 1 to 2 weeks postoperative. Postoperative complications identified by routine duplex screening include deep venous thrombosis and endovenous thrombosis. Paresthesias are common but seldom significantly impact quality of life. Hematoma, superficial venous thrombosis, and surgical site infections occur infrequently. When postoperative edema has subsided, the patient is fitted for compression stockings (20 to 30 mm Hg) and the stockings are used for a short period of time during healing, typically approximately 2 weeks (longer if concomitant phlebectomies are performed). They are used long term (30 to 40 mm Hg) if there is underlying deep vein insufficiency.

Discussion

There currently exists clinical equipoise with regard to the best treatment strategy for these individuals: is it better to treat the varicose veins at the same time or allow regression of the veins following treatment of the reflux? Performing both the antireflux procedure and the varicose vein procedure at the same time eliminates the need for additional anesthesia and cost. However, this may result in overtreatment and unnecessary anesthesia and operative risk. Delayed treatment has the benefit of minimizing

intervention; however, not all patients will have regression of varicosities and will require additional intervention. The current recommendation from the Society for Vascular Surgery (SVS) and American Venous Forum (AVF) varicose vein guidelines is to perform the phlebectomy with saphenous vein ablation, either during the same procedure or at a later stage. However, if general anesthesia is required for the phlebectomy, the suggestion is to perform the procedures at the same time (Grade IB). It is currently our practice to selectively perform concurrent antireflux and varicose vein removal, with simultaneous procedures preferred in approximately 70% to 80% of cases.

Case Conclusion

This patient underwent right great saphenous vein RFA, along with right leg phlebectomies using TIPP. He was wrapped for 48 hours postoperatively, followed by his first dressing change. He was encouraged to ambulate immediately after surgery. After 48 hours, he wrapped his leg daily and then used compression for approximately 2 weeks following his procedure. He did very well.

TAKE HOME POINTS
- Patients presenting with suspected chronic venous insufficiency should undergo evaluation with duplex ultrasound of the great saphenous, small saphenous, accessory saphenous, common femoral, popliteal, and perforating veins. About 30% of patients will have accessory reflux, and thus, complete evaluation will ensure treatment of pathologic refluxing veins.
- Criteria for surgical treatment of superficial reflux must include failure of compression therapy or inability to use compression therapy and valve closure time of greater than 500 ms. Ablation of reflux should be avoided in cases of deep venous obstruction without adequate venous flow, as the superficial system may represent the majority outflow of the lower limb.
- Current evidence favors ablation of reflux via RFA or EVLT over open ligation or sclerotherapy.
- Varicosities should be marked in the standing position to avoid undertreatment. The use of TIPP may offer the advantageous of more complete and expedient removal of large clusters of varicosities with fewer incisions.

SUGGESTED READINGS
Bergan JJ. Varicose veins: hooks, clamps, and suction. Application of new techniques to enhance varicose vein surgery. *Semin Vasc Surg.* 2002;15(1):21-26.

Bergan JJ, Schmidt-Schonbein GW, Coleridge Smith PD, et al. Chronic venous disease. *N Engl J Med.* 2006;355:488-498.

Gloviczki P, Comerota AJ, Dalsing MC, et al. The care of patients with varicose veins and associated chronic venous diseases: clinical practice guidelines of the Society for Vascular Surgery and the American Venous Forum. *J Vasc Surg.* 2001; 53(5 suppl):2S-48S.

Lurie F, Creton D, Eklof B, et al. Prospective randomized study of endovenous radiofrequency obliteration (closure procedure) versus ligation and stripping in a selected patient population (EVOLVeS Study). *J Vasc Surg.* 2003;38(2):207-214.

Scurr JH, Tibbs DJ. Clinical patterns of venous disorder: incompetence in superficial veins: simple or primary varicose veins. In: *Varicose Veins, Venous Disorders, and Lymphatic Problems in the Lower Limbs.* Oxford: Oxford University Press; 1997:47-101.

Weiss RA, Feied CF, Weiss MA. Venous physiology and pathophysiology. In: *Vein Diagnosis and Treatment: A Comprehensive Approach.* New York, NY: McGraw-Hill; 2001:23-30.

CLINICAL SCENARIO CASE QUESTIONS

1. What valve closure times define pathologic refluxing veins?

   a. Superficial (greater than 500 ms), perforator (greater than 500 ms), deep (greater than 500 ms)

   b. Superficial (greater than 1000 ms), perforator (greater than 500 ms), deep (greater than 500 ms)

   c. Superficial (greater than 500 ms), perforator (greater than 1000 ms), deep (greater than 1000 ms)

   d. Superficial (greater than 500 ms), perforator (greater than 500 ms), deep (greater than 1000 ms)

2. In a patient with pathologic refluxing superficial veins, what is the current treatment of choice?

   a. High ligation and division of saphenous vein

   b. RFA or EVLT

   c. Sclerotherapy

   d. Hook phlebectomy

105 Acute Iliofemoral Deep Vein Thrombosis

AMIR AZARBAL, GIYE CHOE, and GREG MONETA

Presentation

A 68-year-old woman presents with a 2-day history of a painful, swollen left lower extremity. She is otherwise healthy and has been in her usual state of health until the sudden onset of left leg pain and swelling. She does not smoke or take medications. On exam, her left lower extremity is swollen from her ankle to her thigh and tender to palpation. Her motor and sensory exam is intact, her calf compartments are soft, and she has palpable pedal pulses.

Differential Diagnosis

Sudden onset of painful, unilateral lower extremity swelling represents a lower extremity deep vein thrombosis (LE DVT) until proven otherwise. Provoked DVTs occur in the setting of trauma, surgery, or immobilization. Unprovoked DVTs require investigation of environmental, genetic, and anatomic reasons risk factors for DVT.

Workup

The preferred imaging modality for diagnosis of LE DVT is a duplex ultrasound. D-Dimer blood tests are useful in excluding DVT in cases with low pretest probability of DVT and do not have a role in cases where the clinical presentation is suggestive of DVT. Initiation of anticoagulation should not be delayed until completion of confirmatory testing. Detection of DVT in the iliac veins may be possible using duplex ultrasound, but computed tomography and magnetic resonance venography may be needed to determine the proximal extent of the thrombosis (Fig. 1).

Discussion

Iliofemoral deep vein thrombosis (IFDVT) is a subset of LE DVT that involves the common femoral and/or iliac veins. Immediate pain, swelling, paradoxical stroke, respiratory compromise, and full cardiopulmonary collapse after a pulmonary embolism (PE) can all arise without warning. Venous insufficiency, venous claudication, postthrombotic syndrome (PTS), and chronic thromboembolic pulmonary hypertension (CTPH) can plague patients for the rest of their life. IFDVTs occur more commonly on the left side, and many series also report a higher incidence of IFDVT in women as compared to men.

Virchow's triad of venous stasis, endothelial injury, and hypercoagulability are commonly named risk factors of LE DVT. IFDVTs have a fourth potential precipitating factor, anatomy. In the absence of precipitating factors causing IFDVT, a hypercoagulable disorder workup and investigation of anatomic causes of IFDVT are warranted. The most common cause of iliac vein compression is May-Thurner syndrome (MTS). MTS describes the mechanical compression of the left common iliac vein by the overlying right common iliac artery. The chronic compression may result in reactive intimal changes that can cause typical intimal "spurs" or webs, which can lead to IFDVT. Other anatomic derangements that fit in the category with MTS include pelvic radiation changes, postsurgical changes, tumor compression, and postthrombotic iliac vein occlusion (Fig. 2).

Treatment

Anticoagulation

Systemic anticoagulation remains the cornerstone of treatment for IFDVT. Treatment with anticoagulation is based on a single randomized trial published in 1960, showing that 1.5 days of heparin and just 14 days of oral vitamin K antagonism markedly reduced recurrent PE and mortality. Current recommendations for the treatment of DVT are provided by the American College of Chest Physicians and rigorously reviewed and updated every few years. Treatment of iliofemoral DVT falls under the recommendations for proximal DVT and includes the following:

- Initiation of parenteral anticoagulation such as low molecular weight heparin (LMWH) or fondaparinux and oral vitamin K antagonist without delay and continuation of parenteral agent for at least 5 days and until INR > 2.0 on two separate reads (1B)
- Three months of therapy for provoked DVT with transient risk factor
- Continued therapy past 3 months for unprovoked DVT and acceptable bleeding risk (2B)

While prolonged anticoagulation can decrease the incidence of PTS and recurrent DVT, the benefit of prolonged

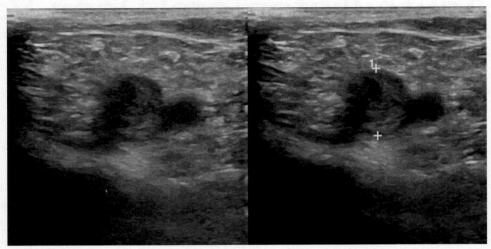

FIGURE 1 • Venous duplex ultrasound demonstrating acute deep vein thrombosis of the common femoral vein.

anticoagulation must be weighed against the increased risk of bleeding. It is important to maintain therapeutic anticoagulation levels as subtherapeutic anticoagulation is associated with risk of recurrence and subsequently PTS.

The use of LMWH for 3 months followed by oral vitamin K antagonism is also reasonable and has some data supporting this regimen is associated with reduced PTS.

Newer oral anticoagulants are now available and emerging as viable alternatives to warfarin for treatment of acute DVTs. Rivaroxaban, dabigatran, and apixaban have been demonstrated in randomized control trials and a systematic review to be as effective as warfarin in preventing overall death, death from PE, and recurrent DVT and PE. Rivaroxaban, edoxaban, and apixaban are direct factor Xa inhibitors. Rivaroxaban and edoxaban are dosed once daily, while apixaban is dosed twice daily. Dabigatran is a direct thrombin inhibitor that is dosed twice daily.

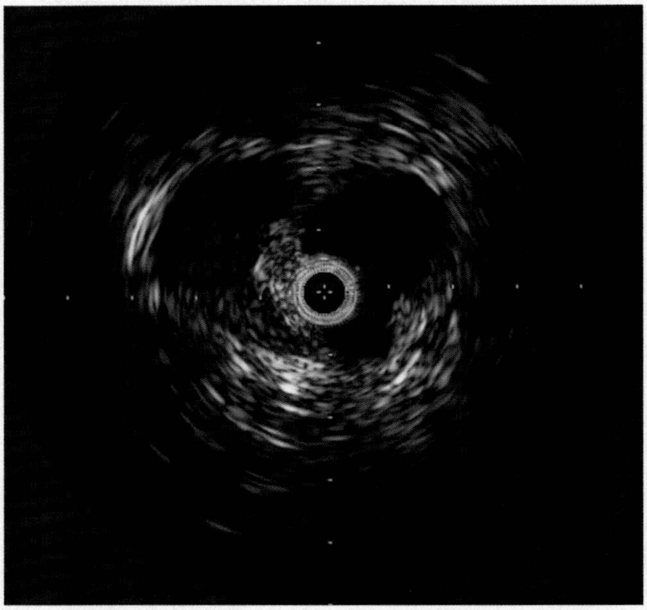

While anticoagulation is quite effective at preventing PE and death, long-term venous function is quite poor. IFDVTs treated with anticoagulation have recanalization rates of about 30% and even worse functional outcomes, with greater than 80% of patients demonstrating abnormal venous function after treatment.

Ambulation

Evidence shows that early ambulation is safe and likely beneficial for patients with LE DVT. According to CHEST guidelines, early ambulation is recommended over bed rest (2C). A number of randomized trials have examined this issue and are summarized in two meta-analyses, both of which demonstrated no increased risk of PE or adverse event. None of the studies that composed the meta-analyses were specific to IFDVT, and rates of IFDVT were not specifically reported in the studies; however, it is unlikely that a study focusing on IFDVT would change these recommendations for early ambulation.

Compression

The first randomized trial of compression stockings showed a 50% reduction in PTS as judged by a nonvalidated scale. A second randomized trial and two meta-analyses have also shown similar decreases in PTS. However, the most recent and largest randomized trial of compression stockings, the SOX trial, did not show any benefit in cumulative incidence or severity of PTS with the use of compression stockings for 2 years after an episode of first proximal DVT. One criticism of this study is that compliance was poor, with only 56% of patients using compression stockings more than 3 days a week. Even before the results of the SOX trial were published, the most recent ACCP guidelines downgraded its recommendation for compression stockings to a 2B level. While the data for compression

FIGURE 2 • Intravascular ultrasound demonstrating an intimal web within the left common iliac vein.

stockings preventing PTS are not very robust, compression stockings are generally included in the standard of care for patients with DVT due to their low cost and high safety profile and that they often reduce pain.

Endovascular Therapy

Evidence continues to emerge to support an aggressive approach to clearance of IFDVT such as catheter-directed thrombolysis (CDT) and percutaneous mechanical thrombectomy (PMT). A large randomized trial and a meta-analysis have shown better outcomes in terms of PTS occurrence, venous patency, and venous reflux for CDT compared to conventional therapy. The precise technical aspects of this have yet to be standardized, which is part of the reason the ACCP guidelines continue to formally recommend anticoagulation alone over CDT (grade 2C). In cases of IFDVT secondary to iliac vein compression by the overlying iliac artery, consideration should be given to stenting of the compressed iliac vein. There are no randomized data to support the use of venous stents to decrease the incidence of PTS or prevent DVT recurrence; however, the generally poor prognosis of IFDVTs and the good initial results seen with iliac vein stents have made this treatment approach popular.

Case Conclusion

The patient was started on therapeutic LMWH. Duplex US confirmed a left-sided IFDVT. A discussion regarding the risks and benefits of CDT was held, and the decision was made not to proceed with endovascular therapy. The patient was maintained on LMWH, started on warfarin, and discharged home. LMWH was continued until her INR was therapeutic on two separate readings. She was also prescribed 30 to 40 mm Hg compression stockings and given instruction on early ambulation and leg elevation. A complete review of systems and review of health maintenance was not concerning for underlying malignancy. After 3 months of anticoagulation, the risks and benefits of continued anticoagulation were discussed with the patient. Given her low bleeding risk and the fact that she had an unprovoked proximal DVT, she was continued on warfarin therapy indefinitely.

TAKE HOME POINTS

- Iliofemoral DVTs represent a subset of proximal lower extremity DVTs associated with worse outcomes including acute PE, recurrent DVTs, and PTS.
- Prompt anticoagulation and maintenance in the therapeutic range is necessary to prevent PE and recurrent DVT.
- Consider early and consistent ambulation.
- Consider 30 to 40 mm Hg compression for symptom relief.
- CDT and PMT may improve long-term venous function and prevent PTS, but should be determined on a case by case basis.

SUGGESTED READINGS

Guyatt GH, et al. Antithrombotic therapy and prevention of thrombosis, 9th ed. American College of Chest Physicians Evidence-Based Clinical Practice Guidelines. *Chest.* 2012;141:e351S-418S.

Eden T, et al. Long-term outcome after additional catheter-directed thrombolysis versus standard treatment of acute iliofemoral deep vein thrombosis: a randomized control trial. *Lancet.* 2012;379(9810):31-38.

CLINICAL SCENARIO CASE QUESTIONS

1. What are the features of iliofemoral DVT that are different compared to other lower extremity DVTs?
   a. They are more common in younger patients.
   b. There is no difference in laterality.
   c. They have a higher rate of progression to postthrombotic syndrome.
   d. Catheter-based mechanical thrombectomy is the mainstay of treatment.
   e. They are more commonly associated with fatal PE.

2. Acute iliofemoral DVT:
   a. Should all receive intravenous thrombolytic therapy
   b. Can be prevented by early high-grade compression therapy
   c. Are associated with anatomical abnormalities in most cases
   d. Should be treated with rapid and full therapeutic anticoagulation regardless of other adjunctive therapies
   e. Should be treated with at least 48 hours of bed rest

106 Endovascular Treatment of Acute Iliofemoral DVT

RAFAEL D. MALGOR and ANTONIOS P. GASPARIS

Presentation

A 35-year-old female, otherwise healthy, with a 17-pack-year history of smoking presents to the emergency department complaining of left lower extremity pain and swelling over the past 2 days. She states that 3 days ago, she returned home from her summer vacation in the New England region and had to drive herself back home for about 6 hours. She also informs you that she has been taking oral contraceptives for about 15 years, but no other medications. She denies any chest pain, history of similar episodes of lower extremity edema, any trauma, or long bone fractures in the past. Her vital signs are within normal limits except for an elevated respiratory rate. She appears to be uncomfortable holding her left thigh and calf that is notably more swollen compared to the right. Her left distal thigh, calf, and foot are cyanotic, and multiple engorged, nonvaricose veins are noticeable. Due to significant edema, pedal pulses are difficult to palpate, but are present. She denies any foot numbness, and she is able to flex and extend her ankle and toes that elicits calf pain. Noteworthy, her mother and one of her aunts had vein stripping in the past and her paternal uncle had an episode of cardiorespiratory collapse that was related to leg swelling.

Differential Diagnosis

Lower extremity pain associated or not with edema can be caused by several entities. One must always investigate if the patient had any recent trauma that could have caused a muscle tear, soft tissue hematoma, or bone fractures. A ruptured Baker's cyst should be considered regardless of the evidence of fall or body collision. Traumatic injuries are often suggested by localized tenderness and edema of a specific affected portion of the lower extremity. Patients with history of travel to mountains or forest or those who practice hiking must also be asked about any insect bite or skin tear that can be related to infectious process. It is not rare to have a patient with signs of initial necrotizing fasciitis caused by a bug bite or skin excoriation. A warm, hyperemic leg coupled with some signs of sepsis, such as fever and chills, is not always present but definitely helps to differentiate an infected leg from other causes.

The most important differential diagnosis to be excluded in any patient with acute onset of leg pain is acute limb ischemia that has to be addressed in a timely manner in order to ultimately avoid devastating consequences, such as limb loss. This particular patient has some findings that aid to a diagnosis other than acute arterial occlusion. On the physical exam, the patient has palpable pulses. Further, when evaluating the motor and sensory status of the limb, the physician also noted a completely intact neurologic exam that is often present only in very initial stages of acute arterial occlusion. A quick review of symptoms of acute arterial occlusion and deep venous thrombosis is provided in Table 1.

The presence of risk factors such as a long car ride, use of oral contraceptives, tobacco use in a female patient coupled with positive findings of asymmetric limb edema, pain, enlarged nonvaricose veins, palpable pedal pulses, and intact neurologic function makes the diagnosis of deep vein thrombosis (DVT) very appealing.

TABLE 1. Typical Clinical Presentation of Acute Arterial Occlusion and DVT

Physical Examination	Acute Arterial Occlusion	DVT
Lower extremity pain	Often severe	Often tolerable
Limb edema	Often absent	Likely present
Sensorial deficit (i.e., numbness, no sensation)	Likely present	Often absent or mild
Motor deficit (loss of flexion/extension toes, ankle)	Likely present	Very rare
Calf tenderness to palpation	Yes	Yes
Distal pulses in the affected extremity	Absent	Palpable
Coolness to touch (thermal skin gradient sensation)	Likely present	Very likely absent

However, DVT diagnosis is difficult to be made based only on physical exam findings that have low sensitivity and specificity as many conditions can mimic the signs and symptoms of DVT. Thus, an imaging study must be obtained in order to confirm the DVT diagnosis.

Workup

In the emergency department, a quick assessment using a clinical DVT probability score (Wells' criteria) plus measurement of D-Dimer levels can potentially rule out DVT before any imaging study or vascular specialist consultation is requested. The Wells' criteria, their interpretation, and decision-making algorithm are summarized in Figure 1. It is important to note that in many patients, D-Dimer is falsely positive, and therefore, such patients should not be tested. Also, those patients with high probability for DVT should not have D-Dimer test but an imaging test.

The first and most important step in the workup for lower extremity venous thromboembolism is the duplex ultrasound (DU). DU has many advantages over other imaging studies because it is a low-cost, portable, safe to use, easy to repeat, and noninvasive tool. Evaluation of the suprainguinal veins is at times necessary such as when thrombus extends to the level of the common femoral vein or when there is suspicion of pathology above the inguinal ligament. This can be achieved with DU, but when the suprainguinal veins cannot be clearly evaluated, computed tomographic venography (CTV) or magnetic resonance venography (MRV) can be obtained to further delineate the extent of DVT and patency of inferior vena cava (IVC).

In this particular scenario, iliac vein compression must be considered. May-Turner syndrome occurs when the left common iliac vein (CIV) is compressed by the right common iliac artery (RCIA) and often affects female patients. Other iliac vein compression syndromes have been described including right common iliac and external iliac vein (EIV) compression.

Imagining Workup (DU/CTV)

Intraluminal echolucent material is seen in the left popliteal and femoral veins extending into the EIV. The veins are dilated and noncompressible and have no flow augmentation. Additionally, a reduced diameter is noted in the proximal CIV with thrombosis of CIV and external and internal iliac veins (Fig. 2A–D). A CTV is obtained confirming that the IVC is widely patent, and the left CIV is compressed by the RCIA (Fig. 2E).

Diagnosis and Treatment

The diagnosis is acute iliofemoral DVT, which was confirmed by DU. Treatment options for this patient include anticoagulation, thrombolysis, and surgical thrombectomy. The latter is only indicated in patients with impending venous gangrene or contraindication to thrombolytic therapy. Thrombolysis is appealing due to early thrombus resolution, preservation of valve function, and possibly lower incidence of postthrombotic syndrome. Thrombus lysis can be accomplished locally, directed through a catheter (catheter-directed thrombolysis, CDT) or combined with a device that performs mechanical thrombectomy (pharmacomechanical

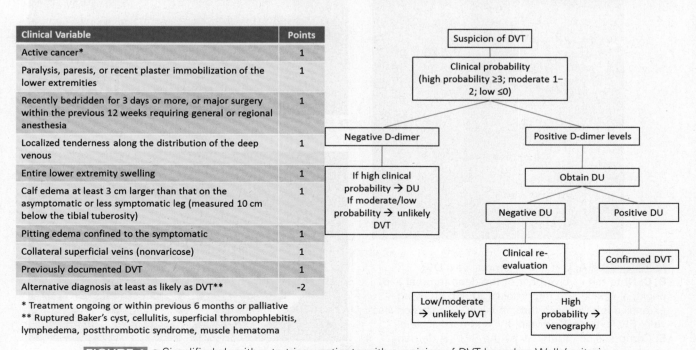

Clinical Variable	Points
Active cancer*	1
Paralysis, paresis, or recent plaster immobilization of the lower extremities	1
Recently bedridden for 3 days or more, or major surgery within the previous 12 weeks requiring general or regional anesthesia	1
Localized tenderness along the distribution of the deep venous	1
Entire lower extremity swelling	1
Calf edema at least 3 cm larger than that on the asymptomatic or less symptomatic leg (measured 10 cm below the tibial tuberosity)	1
Pitting edema confined to the symptomatic	1
Collateral superficial veins (nonvaricose)	1
Previously documented DVT	1
Alternative diagnosis at least as likely as DVT**	-2

* Treatment ongoing or within previous 6 months or palliative
** Ruptured Baker's cyst, cellulitis, superficial thrombophlebitis, lymphedema, postthrombotic syndrome, muscle hematoma

FIGURE 1 • Simplified algorithm to triage patients with suspicion of DVT based on Wells' criteria.

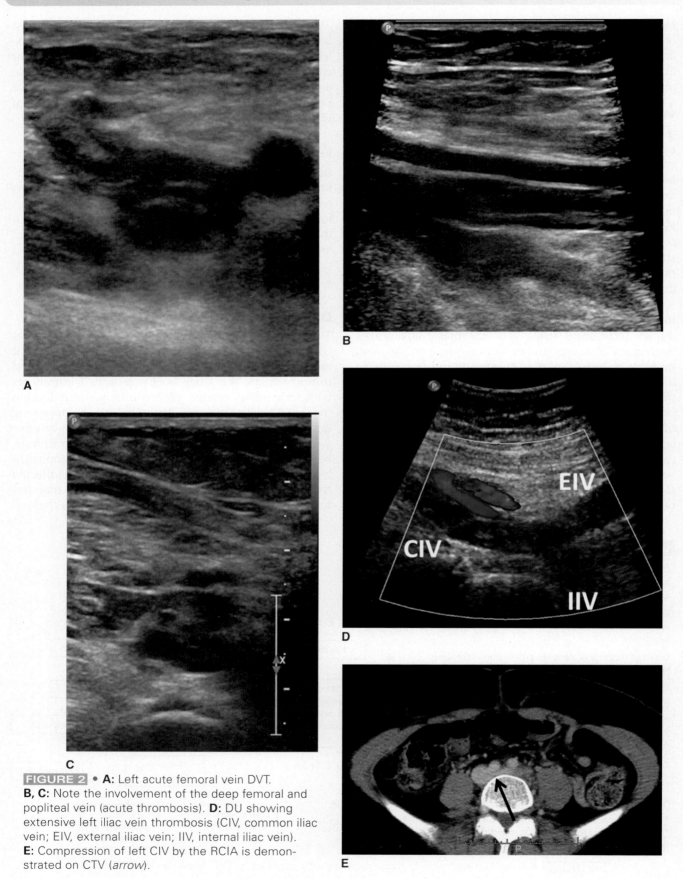

FIGURE 2 • **A:** Left acute femoral vein DVT.
B, C: Note the involvement of the deep femoral and popliteal vein (acute thrombosis). **D:** DU showing extensive left iliac vein thrombosis (CIV, common iliac vein; EIV, external iliac vein; IIV, internal iliac vein). **E:** Compression of left CIV by the RCIA is demonstrated on CTV (*arrow*).

thrombectomy, PMT). Systemic thrombolysis has been abandoned due to its significant risk of bleeding complications and inconsistent efficacy.

Several studies comparing anticoagulation versus CDT have demonstrated superior recanalization rates in patients who underwent CDT. The ongoing experience and excellent results of PMT have also been reported with lower dosage of thrombolytic, less duration of treatment, and lower bleeding complications.

Patient selection for thrombolysis is very important and includes presence of contraindications, patient comorbidities, and age of thrombus. Absolute contraindications to thrombolysis include history of previous intracranial hemorrhage (ICH), arterial puncture at a noncompressible site, intracranial neoplasm, cerebral arteriovenous malformation or aneurysm, recent intracranial or spinal surgery, uncontrolled blood pressure (systolic greater than 185 mm Hg or diastolic blood pressure greater than 110 mm Hg), active internal bleeding, or any acute bleeding diathesis (i.e., platelet count less than 100,000/mm^3). The 9th edition of the *Chest Guidelines* indicates that venous thrombolysis is most likely to be beneficial in patients with iliofemoral DVT with symptoms for less than 14 days, good functional status, life expectancy of greater than 1 year, and a low risk of bleeding. It remains to be further investigated whether or not thrombolysis in patients with femoropopliteal DVT, thrombus greater than 14 days, and the use of PMT in patients with higher risk of bleeding

(i.e., isolated segment thrombolysis with Trellis device) can improve clinical outcomes.

Case Continued

An informed consent including the potential risks, such as major bleeding, pulmonary embolism, and death, and the benefits of resolving or diminishing the clot burden is obtained. A blood sample is drawn to determine the baseline of fibrinogen levels, platelet count, hematocrit and hemoglobin levels, activated partial thromboplastin, and prothrombin time.

The patient is taken to the interventional suite or operating room, prepped, and draped in the prone position. A direct popliteal vein ultrasound-guided puncture is then performed using a micropuncture needle, wire, and catheter, which is subsequently exchanged by a 4-Fr sheath over a hydrophilic wire. An initial venogram is obtained, which in this patient shows filling defects in the entire femoral vein extending into left iliac veins (Fig. 3A and B). Then, an angled glide wire and glide catheter are advanced into the IVC. Venogram of the IVC demonstrates that it is patent. A 30-cm long Trellis catheter (Trellis-8 Peripheral Infusion System, Covidien, Mansfield, MA) is chosen and parked in the entire length of the thrombosed left iliac veins. The proximal balloon is inflated in the IVC and pulled back to the origin of the left CIV (Fig. 3C). The distal balloon is inflated in the femoral vein, isolating the treatment segment (Fig. 3D). Infusion of r-tPA through the Trellis catheter allows lysing the thrombus during the

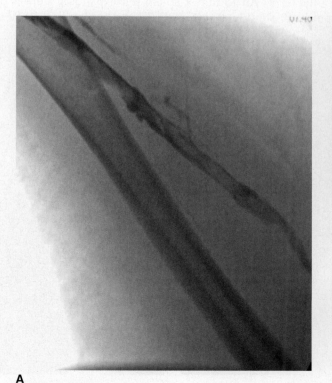
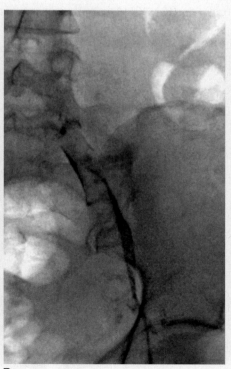

A   **B**

FIGURE 3 • **A:** An initial venogram showed thrombosis of the left femoral vein. **B:** Extensive involvement of left iliac veins is also noted.

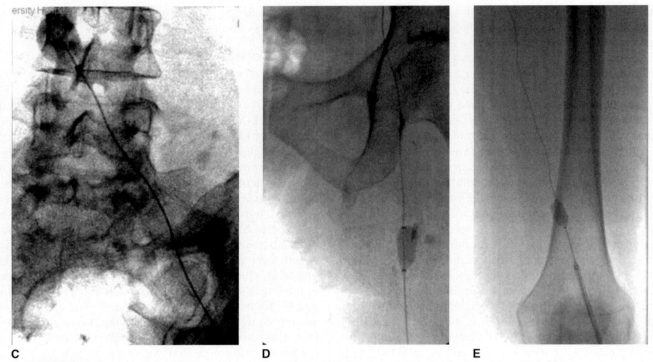

C **D** **E**

FIGURE 3 • (*Continued*) **C:** PMT is initiated using a 30-cm-long Trellis catheter (Trellis-8 Peripheral Infusion System, Covidien, Mansfield, MA). Note that the proximal balloon is inflated in the IVC and then back off to engage the proximal CIV. **D:** The distal balloon is initially parked in the femoral vein isolating the treatment segment. **E:** After treating the iliofemoral segment, the distal balloon is parked in the transition between the femoral and the popliteal vein to complete the treatment.

treatment cycles. Following treatment of the iliofemoral segment, the femoropopliteal segment is treated in a similar fashion with distal balloon now inflated in the distal femoral vein (Fig. 3E). A completion venogram is obtained showing patent proximal iliac veins with compression at the level of left CIV (Fig. 4A).

An 18 mm × 90 cm self-expanding stent is deployed starting at proximal CIV and ending in the EIV vein due

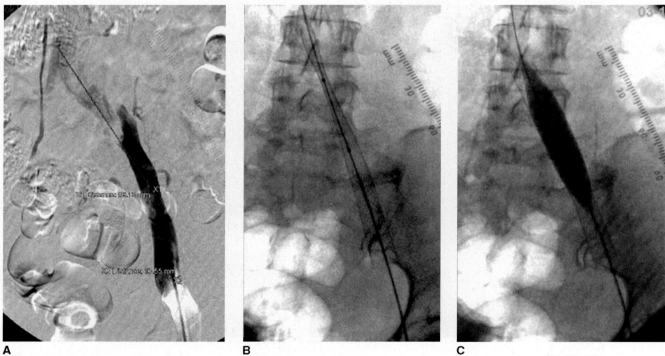

A **B** **C**

FIGURE 4 • **A:** Completion venogram showed a high-grade stenosis of the common iliac vein due to extrinsic compression by the right common iliac artery. **B:** A 18 mm × 90 cm self-expanding stent is deployed proximally and distally the stenotic area. **C:** Balloon angioplasty is performed using a 16-mm noncompliant balloon to ensure good stent apposition to the vein wall.

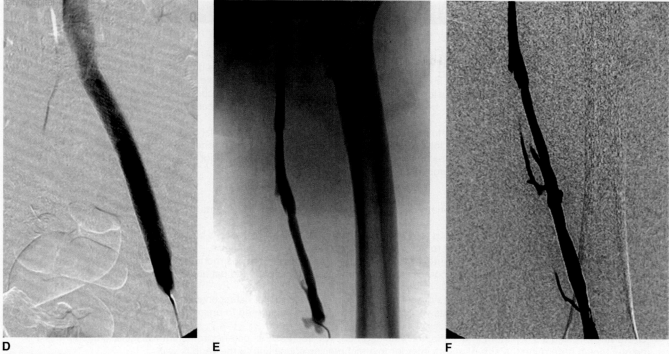

D   **E**   **F**

FIGURE 4 • (*Continued*) **D:** Completion venogram demonstrated an excellent result with brisk inflow and outflow. **E and F:** Patency of the left femoral vein is also confirmed at the end of the procedure.

to persistent stenosis caused by left CIV compression (Fig. 4B). The stent is dilated using a 16-mm noncompliant balloon. No recoiling is noted on completion venography after the dilation (Fig. 4C). Completion lower extremity venography confirms widely patent left iliofemoral and femoropopliteal segments (Fig. 4D–F).

Surgical Approach: Key Technical Points and Pitfalls to Avoid

Initial contrast venography is obtained to evaluate the extent and chronicity of the DVT, the presence of tributaries (collateral pathways), and the patency of the IVC. It can be carried out either through a popliteal (in the prone position), ipsilateral femoral, contralateral femoral, or jugular vein (in the supine position) approach. The most common access site used for thrombolysis is the popliteal approach. CDT is commonly chosen as either an initial treatment strategy or to clean up residual thrombus following PMT. The advantages of PMT include overall shorter treatment time, lower bleeding complications, and the ability to treat in a single session in selected patients.

There are several PMT devices, none of which have been shown to be superior but each having its own advantages and disadvantages. The goal with PMT is to mechanically macerate the thrombus and therefore increase the surface area for the thrombolytic to bind. The ability for the devices to achieve this depends on the diameter of the vein treated and the chronicity of the thrombus. If single session treatment is not obtained, short adjunctive treatment with CDT will often clean up residual thrombus.

Some questions remain unanswered at this point, such as the role of prophylactic temporary filter placement, role of posterior tibial vein access, and device selection regardless of method employed. There is no evidence that routine placement of an IVC filter has a role during thrombolysis, but there may be selected patients that may benefit. A retrievable filter may be considered in patients with extensive iliocaval clot burden, those with associated pulmonary embolism, or those with marginal cardiorespiratory reserve. In patients with involvement of the entire popliteal and tibial vein, posterior tibial vein access can be performed along with popliteal vein puncture to increase the amount of lytics delivered in the infrapopliteal segment and maximize inflow from below. Regarding PMT device selection, as mentioned above, none have been shown to have clear advantages and selection is often made based on personal preference and experience.

Venous outflow obstruction of the iliac veins is often present in patients with iliofemoral thrombosis. Following thrombolysis, the underlying lesion is revealed and should be addressed in order to prevent rethrombosis. Venous angioplasty alone has technically very poor results because of recoiling or inability to overcome persistent extrinsic compression. Therefore, stenting is necessary to resolve the obstruction and achieve good outflow.

Currently, we do not have a dedicated venous stent and the most common used stent is the Wallstent, given that this is the only stent that comes in large sizes. The stent diameter for the common iliac should be 14 to 18 mm, for the external iliac 12 to 16 mm, and the common femoral vein 10 to 14 mm. The main goals of

TABLE 2. Key Technical Steps and Potential Pitfalls

Key Technical Steps

1. Position the patient properly on the table (supine vs. prone); obtain access guided by DU.
2. Perform an initial venogram to assess the extent of thrombosis including IVC thrombus burden.
3. Choose preferably a pharmacomechanical device over multihole lysis catheter if possible to expedite thrombus removal.
4. Proceed with continuous lytic agent infusion if significant residual thrombus found on completion venogram.
5. Monitor fibrinogen levels, platelet count, hematocrit and hemoglobin levels, activated partial thromboplastin, and prothrombin time in between lytics checks.
6. Obtain follow-up venography within 12 h to redefine thrombolysis goals based on residual thrombus and iliac vein compression.
7. Evaluate for iliac vein compression with intravascular ultrasound if available; perform venous stenting if indicated.
8. Ensure there is acceptable flow and no residual thrombus on completion venogram prior to ending the procedure.
9. Discontinue sheath and continue anticoagulation for 3–6 mo.

Potential Pitfalls

- Acute vein thrombosis has to be differentiated from acute arterial occlusion in all patients with acute lower extremity pain not related to trauma.
- Selecting the right patient for early thrombus removal is key to avoid complications, such as bleeding, neurologic deficits and death.
- Ultrasound-guided angioaccess is critical to ensure venous rather than arterial puncture.
- Admission to high level of care, such as intensive care unit or a unit with continuous monitoring and dedicated nursing staff is critical to detect access site bleeding complications and to assess constantly the patient's cardiorespiratory and overall neurovascular status.
- Periodic blood drawn to assess the patient's coagulation status in order to avoid or detect ongoing bleeding is highly recommended.
- After thrombus removal, all vein segments with residual disease must be stented to ensure good inflow and outflow. Failing to do so will decrease patency rates.
- Oversizing or using a small stent in the affected vein segment will decrease its patency rates. Intravascular ultrasound is a helpful tool to determine the size of stents in order to attain precise apposition to the venous wall.
- If the stents are deployed below the inguinal ligament, patency of the femoral or deep femoral veins must be always ensured to avoid thrombosis later on.

venous stenting are to cover all diseased segments and obtain good inflow and outflow. In some circumstances, the stent can be safely extended into the IVC or below the inguinal ligament in order to ensure brisk inflow and outflow. Balloon angioplasty after stenting is required to fully expand the stent.

The presence of residual stenosis can be evaluated with venography or intravascular ultrasound (IVUS). Indirect signs of residual stenosis on venography include presence of collaterals, intraluminal filling defects, or poor venous outflow. If available, IVUS has been shown to be superior in detecting obstruction and evaluating extent of disease when compared to venography. Precise evaluation of the length to be treated and selection of stent size can be easily attained using IVUS.

Following thrombolysis and venous stenting, completion venogram or IVUS must be performed to evaluate flow and look for significant filling defects or residual stenosis that may lead to technical failure. A quick review of technical steps and pitfalls to avoid can be found in Table 2.

Special Intraoperative Considerations

When performing the initial diagnostic venogram, a few anatomic variations may be noted. Inferior vena cava and iliac veins hypoplasia or agenesis is rare, but it may be present. While these findings are often detected in a preoperative CTV or MRV, care must be exercised to detect these anatomic variations that can drastically impact the outcomes. Some anecdotal reports of thrombolysis in cases of IVC/iliac veins hypoplasia have demonstrated success on decreasing the clot burden and reestablishing flow through collaterals, such as lumbar veins or paraspinal vein plexus.

The presence of caval thrombosis in the presence of IVC filter is not unusual. Successful thrombus removal can be achieved while working around the filter. We have not experienced any issues, such as filter migration or IVC wall perforation during PMT or CDT. In addition, stents can be safely deployed into the IVC covering a previously placed filter without complications if necessary.

Postoperative Management

Minor bleeding may occur from oozing and ecchymosis at the venous puncture site. Often, it does not require any treatment. Major bleeding that requires blood transfusion, such as into the retroperitoneum, gastrointestinal, or genitourinary tract, is rare, but ominous. The most threatening bleeding complication is ICH. Complaints of headache, nausea, vomiting, altered mental status, and uncontrolled hypertension may be an early sign of ICH with increasing intracranial pressure. Thrombolytics and heparin infusion should be immediately discontinued, CT of the head obtained, and neurology consultation requested. Pulmonary embolism must be considered in patients with respiratory distress especially in the immediate postoperative course.

Imagining surveillance is warranted after thrombolysis and stenting to ensure long-term venous patency. The patient must remain on anticoagulation for at least 6 months. Our imaging surveillance protocol includes DU prior to discharge, 1 month, 6 months, and yearly DU thereafter.

Case Conclusion

This case scenario exemplifies an episode of acute iliofemoral DVT secondary to left iliac vein compression that was successfully treated by endovascular means. Catheter-based therapy must always be pursued in similar cases of DVT provided there are no contraindications to administration of thrombolytic agents and treatment criteria are met, such as onset of symptoms less than 14 days and life expectancy of greater than 1 year with good functional status. It has been suggested that early thrombus removal reduces the risk of future post-thrombotic complications in the affected limb.

TAKE HOME POINTS

- Venous DU must be the first imaging study obtained not only to confirm but also to determine DVT extent in order to aid patient's selection for thrombolysis.
- CT or MRV can be utilized to further investigate the IVC and iliac vein involvement. The presence and patency of the iliac veins and IVC must always be confirmed prior to thrombolysis. Presence of iliac vein compression and intra-abdominal pathology can be evaluated.
- Good candidates for thrombolysis are those with acute iliofemoral DVT, symptoms less than 14 days, good performance status, life expectancy greater than 1 year, and low risk of bleeding.
- Close hemodynamic monitoring and attention to laboratory results are required while the patient remains on thrombolytics.
- CDT and PMT are both efficacious techniques to treat acute iliofemoral DVT. PMT may expedite the treatment and reduce number of venograms and amount of thrombolytic drug infused.
- The indications of prophylactic IVC filter prior to CDT or PMT have to be individualized based on IVC and iliac clot burden and respiratory status in presence/extent of PE.

SUGGESTED READINGS

Enden T, Haig Y, Kløw NE, et al. Long-term outcome after additional catheter-directed thrombolysis versus standard treatment for acute iliofemoral deep vein thrombosis (the CaVenT study): a randomised controlled trial. *Lancet.* 2012;379(9810):31-38.

Kearon C, Akl EA, Comerota AJ, et al. Antithrombotic therapy for VTE disease: antithrombotic therapy and prevention of thrombosis, 9th edition: American College of Chest Physicians Evidence-Based Clinical Practice Guidelines. *Chest.* 2012;141(2 suppl):e419S-e494S.

Klein SJ, Gasparis AP, Virvilis D, et al. Prospective determination of candidates for thrombolysis in patients with acute proximal deep vein thrombosis. *J Vasc Surg.* 2010;51(4):908-912.

Malgor RD, Gasparis AP. Pharmaco-mechanical thrombectomy for early thrombus removal. *Phlebology.* 2012;27(suppl 1):155-162.

Meissner MH, Gloviczki P, Comerota AJ, et al. Society for Vascular Surgery; American Venous Forum. Early thrombus removal strategies for acute deep venous thrombosis: clinical practice guidelines of the Society for Vascular Surgery and the American Venous Forum. *J Vasc Surg.* 2012;55(5):1449-1462.

Patterson BO, Hinchliffe R, Loftus IM, et al. Indications for catheter-directed thrombolysis in the management of acute proximal deep venous thrombosis. *Arterioscler Thromb Vasc Biol.* 2010;30(4):669-674.

CLINICAL SCENARIO CASE QUESTIONS

1. Based on the current recommendations for endovenous treatment of acute iliofemoral DVT, which patient is most likely to benefit?

   a. A 55-year-old female, 10 weeks' pregnant with history of left acute DVT affecting her left popliteal and distal femoral vein

   b. A 48-year-old man, bedbound, recently diagnosed with stage 4 glioblastoma multiforme with bilateral moderate lower extremity edema and a positive DU for bilateral acute femoral and distal iliac vein thrombosis

   c. A 10-year-old female with acute onset of bilateral lower extremity edema with positive DU for bilateral femoropopliteal DVT; the IVC and iliac veins could not be visualized

   d. A 67-year-old active male with previous left posterior tibial vein DVT, now presenting with acute right iliofemoral lower extremity DVT after a 12-hour flight

   e. An 85-year-old female with previous left iliofemoral DVT who complains of left lower extremity edema and pain for the past 3 weeks; her DU is positive for chronic iliac vein DVT and acute or chronic femoral vein DVT

2. A 56-year-female, otherwise healthy, complaining of moderate right lower extremity pain and edema for 3 days is diagnosed with right acute iliofemoral DVT. She has been very active working in an office and has no family history of thrombophilia. She has smoked 1 pack of cigarettes a day for the past 20 years. Her past surgical history is significant for a right lumpectomy for breast cancer 3 years ago. She was also diagnosed with a solitary brain metastasis that is scheduled to be excised within 2 weeks. She has been on tamoxifen for the past 3 years. At this point, the best treatment for this patient with acute iliofemoral DVT is:

   a. Catheter-directed thrombolysis followed by 6 months of anticoagulation

   b. Pharmacomechanical thrombectomy along with anticoagulation

   c. Anticoagulation with low molecular weight heparin for at least 6 months and compression therapy

   d. Inferior vena cava filter placement, thrombolysis, and lifelong anticoagulation

   e. Lifelong anticoagulation with a direct thrombin inhibitor

107 Calf Vein Thrombosis (or Tibial DVT)

ELNA MASUDA

Presentation

Case 1 A 76-year-old male patient with active colon cancer presents with severe left leg calf pain and swelling for 5 days. He has no shortness of breath, chest pain, or hemoptysis. No prior history of deep vein thrombosis (DVT) or pulmonary emboli (PE).

Case 2 A 50-year-old female with mild right calf pain and swelling 1 week after undergoing right knee arthroscopy. She has no chest symptoms, and her past history is negative for prior DVT/PE. She has chronic active hematuria from nephrolithiasis and required blood transfusions 1 week ago. She has been compliant with all her doctor appointments and remains ambulatory and active.

Differential Diagnosis

Leg pain and swelling during the postoperative period should prompt early investigation of DVT which could involve the inferior vena cava (IVC), iliac, femoral, popliteal, and/or calf veins. For isolated calf DVT, which is a likely cause, treatment with anticoagulation versus duplex surveillance depends on clinical risk factors, including the severity of symptoms and contributing risk factors for clot propagation. It is imperative that the physician recognizes and treats the blood clot sufficiently to avoid potential propagation, recurrence, and serious consequences of PE. The differential diagnosis should also include other less serious but common diagnoses below the knee including hematoma, ruptured Baker's cyst, and cellulitis.

With calf vein thrombosis, the clot may involve either one or both paired "axial veins": posterior tibial, peroneal, and anterior tibial veins. Other calf vein thrombi that qualify as deep vein thrombosis are clots involving the "muscular veins," which include soleal and gastrocnemius veins as they drain the calf muscles.

Notably, when isolated calf DVT (CDVT) is reported, they usually involve the posterior tibial and/or peroneal and rarely if ever involve the anterior tibial vein alone. Therefore, many vascular laboratories elect not to include the anterior tibial in the initial test for DVT below the knee, and the Accreditation Laboratories do not require initial scanning of the anterior tibial vein.

The diagnosis of hematoma is usually associated with a history of trauma. Ruptured Baker's cyst can mimic DVT and is frequently identified by duplex ultrasound scanning, MRI, or CT.

Workup

Clinical suspicion should always be high in any postoperative patient with leg pain and/or swelling. A thorough history and physical exam should include a past history of previous DVT or PE, which would represent a significant risk for recurrence. A complete history should include examining for risk factors listed in Table 1.

If the clinical suspicion for DVT is moderate to high, there should be a low threshold to proceed directly to ultrasound testing by either compression ultrasound or color flow duplex scanning. Although compression

TABLE 1. Stratifying Treatment Based on Clinical Risks Factors for DVT

	Low Risk	High Risk
	Transient risk	Active malignancy
	Postsurgical (uncomplicated)	Unprovoked
		Permanent risk
	Pregnancy	Antiphospholipid antibody syndrome
	Air travel	
Risk for recurrence after stopping anticoagulation for 3 mo	3% per year first 2 y, 15% over 5 y	7%–10% per year first 2 y (for unprovoked)
		>10% per year first year for active cancer
Treatment options	Anticoagulation OR serial duplex surveillance and repeat clinical f/u[a]	Anticoagulation

[a]Duplex surveillance reserved for those reliable for follow-up and minimal symptoms.

ultrasound with gray scale alone is sufficient in most cases particularly in proximal or femoral popliteal DVT, the addition of color to the duplex scanning improves resolution of calf veins. If DVT is identified, then the opposite leg from the index DVT limb should be scanned because of approximately 20% chance of finding a DVT in the opposite limb.

D-Dimer levels can be useful in the outpatient setting and if the clinical suspicion for DVT is low. Positive D-Dimer has limited value since it lacks specificity and can be elevated by inflammatory states, cancers, advanced age, infection, and pregnancy. A negative D-Dimer is very useful for excluding an acute DVT, particularly in a low-risk clinical scenario. In the current scenario presented, D-Dimer would be of little value given the high clinical risk for DVT.

Diagnosis and Treatment

All patients with calf DVT must be clinically examined for symptoms and signs of PE such as dyspnea, pleuritic chest pain, hemoptysis, and tachycardia that should lead to proper workup with CT angiogram of the chest. If PE is identified, all must undergo standard anticoagulation for at least 3 to 6 months.

Once PE have been clinically excluded, treatment choices for calf DVT include standard anticoagulation for 3 to 6 months or serial duplex ultrasound surveillance with repeat clinic follow-up. Several factors should be considered in determining best treatment strategy for the patient. This includes clinical risk category (Table 1), degree of symptoms, logistics of treatment, dependability of follow-up, and patient preference.

Patients should be stratified into low or high risk for propagation based on presenting clinical risk factors.

High-risk patients for clot propagation and recurrence should be treated with anticoagulation and not duplex surveillance. These include those with active malignancy, unprovoked DVT, antiphospholipid syndrome, large clot burden such as bilateral calf vein DVT, those with prior history of DVT, and/or severe symptoms of pain and swelling. Patients with severe pain or swelling may benefit from heparin therapy in addition to its anticoagulant effect, by its anti-inflammatory effects, and symptomatic relief (Table 2).

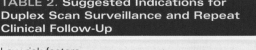

TABLE 2. Suggested Indications for Duplex Scan Surveillance and Repeat Clinical Follow-Up

Low risk factors
Asymptomatic or mildly symptomatic
Reliable for follow-up
Resources of US duplex scanning available
Anticoagulation contraindicated, bleeding risks too high
If anticoagulation contraindicated, suggest duplex surveillance over inferior vena cava (IVC) filter particularly in low-risk group.

Anticoagulation

Typical anticoagulation regimen consists of heparin (unfractionated or low molecular weight heparin [LMWH] or fondaparinux) followed by vitamin K antagonist (VKA). The initial bridging with either unfractionated heparin or LMWH is necessary for at least 5 to 7 days to provide rapid coverage while VKA take effect and to avoid a transient hypercoagulable period produced by VKA.

LMWH possesses a predictable pharmacologic response and therefore allows this class of drugs to be given weight-adjusted subcutaneous injections without the need for laboratory monitoring. For enoxaparin, the usual dosing is 1.0 mg/kg every 12 hours or 1.5 mg/kg daily for at least 5 days while awaiting the INR goal of 2.0 to 3.0. High dosing of VKA initially (10 to 20 mg daily) is discouraged as this can potentiate the hypercoagulable response. Lower doses of VKA such as 5 mg daily are generally recommended.

Optimal duration of anticoagulation is dependent on ongoing risk factors for recurrent venous thromboembolism (VTE). In cases of low risk, 6 weeks of anticoagulation is probably adequate based on two randomized controlled trials (RCTs). In high-risk groups, a minimum of 3 to 6 months is recommended and if risk factors such as ongoing active malignancy and unprovoked calf DVT (CDVT) are encountered, extended anticoagulation beyond 3 to 6 months should be considered and weighed against the risk of bleeding.

Serial Duplex Ultrasound Surveillance

For patients with *low* clinical risk, anticoagulation or serial duplex scanning and repeat clinical follow-up can be offered for treatment. Serial repeat duplex scanning and clinical follow-up should be reserved for select patients who have mild symptoms, are reliable to return for follow-up for serial exams, and are able to return earlier than scheduled if symptoms were to worsen or change. Surveillance would not be a good option for those who live remotely from the clinician's office or have logistical or cognitive restrictions limiting follow-up. Surveillance ultrasound and clinic follow-up every 5 to 7 days for at least 2 weeks are recommended and with mild symptoms controlled with stockings, leg elevation, and avoidance of prolonged sitting and standing.

Novel Oral Anticoagulants

The burden of treatment with LMWH injections and bridging to VKA is now simplified by new oral anticoagulant agents that do not require parenteral bridging or laboratory monitoring. If an oral agent such as factor Xa inhibitor or thrombin inhibitor is selected, disclosure should be made that a direct antidote is not yet available (at the time of this review); however, RCTs have shown equivalent if not lower risks of major bleeding with some novel oral agents over standard VKA.

Compression Stockings

All patients regardless of treatment with anticoagulation or duplex surveillance should be properly fitted with elastic support stockings 30 to 40 mm Hg, instructed to ambulate and avoid prolonged sitting with the leg in dependent position, avoid prolonged standing, and exercise regularly once symptoms have abated to prevent early recurrence.

Special Considerations

What if the patient had an active malignancy with CDVT?

Anticoagulation is recommended over duplex surveillance. Cancer induces a hypercoagulable state when tumor cells produce procoagulant factors such as tissue factor leading to higher recurrence rates. Depending on costs and burden of treatment, extended treatment beyond 3 to 6 months should be considered if active malignancy persists. With active malignancy and DVT in general (including proximal leg DVT and PE), LMWH as primary treatment over LMWH plus VKA has been shown to reduce recurrent VTE events. However, due to costs and burden of treatment, LMWH as primary treatment for several months may not be a practical option for CDVT, and standard treatment with VKA may be preferred.

What is the risk for pulmonary emboli or propagation of calf vein DVT into the popliteal vein or higher during duplex surveillance?

Risk for PE is about 3% based on prospective studies with serial duplex surveillance and repeat clinical exams. The risk for clot propagation with duplex surveillance is in the range of 8% to 15%; therefore, patients need to be counseled regarding the risks prior to embarking on duplex surveillance as option.

What if the patient had a contraindication to anticoagulation such as recurrent gross hematuria?

If the patient has low clinical risk factors, mild symptoms, and a contraindication to anticoagulation, monitoring of the clot by serial duplex surveillance and repeat clinical exams is a feasible option. An IVC filter would not be needed in a low risk clinical scenario. However, if the patient has high risk factors for recurrence, has severe symptoms, and has a contraindication to anticoagulation, an IVC filter may be considered.

What are current recommendations for thrombophilia screening?

Currently, there is no role for routine screening for thrombophilia in first episode of CDVT. In fact, the role for screening is unusual for any VTE including PE and proximal DVT. If PE or proximal DVT is encountered, thrombophilia testing should be limited to young females with history of miscarriages or suspected of having the antiphospholipid syndrome. If the patient already has an established diagnosis of thrombophilia, they should be considered high risk and treated as such.

Case conclusion

Case 1 This patient had a calf vein thrombus associated with a major risk factor for recurrence due to active malignancy. Optimal treatment was anticoagulation, with either the standard LMWH and VKA or oral anti Xa or thrombin inhibitors.
Case 2 This patient had a posterior tibial and peroneal DVT diagnosed by duplex ultrasonography (Fig. 1). Given this was associated with a transient risk, and mild symptoms she was given the

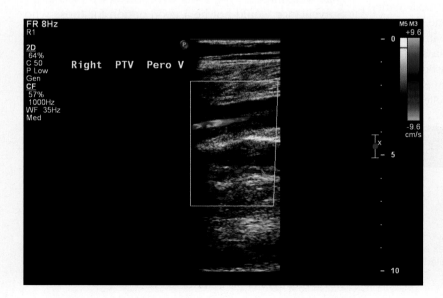

FIGURE 1 • Pic of calf DVT involving the right peroneal and posterior tibial veins. Note the typical appearance of veins with no color flow, dilated, and noncompressible found adjacent to the associated arteries seen with color flow.

option of duplex surveillance. Furthermore, she had hematuria, and a relative contraindication to anticoagulation. She remained active and reliable and returned for repeat duplex scans every 5 to 7 days for at least 2 to 3 weeks with follow up clinical visits.

TAKE HOME POINTS

- CDVT is associated with *pulmonary emboli at presentation* in up to 30% of most prospective series. A thorough exam for pulmonary symptoms or signs of PE should always be part of the *initial* and ongoing follow-up.
- If treatment consists of serial duplex scanning without initial anticoagulation, and CDVT propagates to the popliteal vein or higher, or shows signs of extension to adjacent veins or opposite leg, anticoagulation should be initiated immediately.
- If serial duplex scanning is selected, treatment should include repeat studies and clinical follow-up every 5 to 7 days for 2 to 3 weeks.
- If close follow-up with scans is not feasible, the best treatment option is anticoagulation.

SUGGESTED READINGS

East AT, Wakefield TW. What is the optimal duration of treatment for DVT? An update on evidence-based medicine of treatment for DVT. *Semin Vasc Surg.* 2010;23:182-191.

Kearon C, Akl EA, Comerota AJ, et al. Antithrombotic therapy for VTE disease: Antithrombotic Therapy and Prevention of Thrombosis, 9th ed.: American College of Chest Physicians Evidence-Based Clinical Practice Guidelines. *Chest.* 2012;141:e419S-94S.

Masuda EM, Kistner RL, Musikasinthorn C, et al. The controversy of managing calf vein thrombosis. *J Vasc Surg.* 2012;55: 550-561.

Philbrick JT, Becker DM. Calf deep venous thrombosis. A wolf in sheep's clothing? *Arch Intern Med.* 1988;148:2131-2138.

CLINICAL SCENARIO CASE QUESTIONS

1. Which of the following is the best imaging method for diagnosis and surveillance of tibial DVT?

   a. Venography of the lower extremity
   b. Two-point serial duplex scanning of femoral and popliteal veins
   c. Duplex scanning including color flow and gray-scale imaging
   d. CT venography of the calf

2. A patient has a small 4-cm-length clot in the peroneal vein near the ankle, has mild pain and swelling, and recently had an arthroscopic procedure on his knee 5 days previously. Which of the following is *not* an appropriate treatment option?

   a. Anticoagulation
   b. Duplex scan surveillance every 5 to 7 days for at least 2 weeks with close clinical follow-up
   c. Stockings alone
   d. Anticoagulation with a Xa inhibitor without heparin bridging

108 Acute Superficial Thrombophlebitis of the Great Saphenous Vein

FEDOR LURIE

Presentation

A 58-year-old man with no history of varicose veins presents with pitting edema in his left distal calf and ankle. Measurements of his contralateral leg show a 1-cm difference in circumference at the ankle and 1.5 cm at midcalf. He reports that he had recently developed redness and pain in his left medial calf, with the redness extending to his middle thigh 2 days later. His calf is tender upon palpation, and a hard painful cord is palpable under the skin in the distal and medial thigh. He is afebrile and has no chest pain, shortness of breath, or cough.

Differential Diagnosis

The diagnosis of superficial thrombophlebitis is primarily based on the clinical presentation. The combination of pain, erythema, and tenderness in the medial thigh with a palpable tender cord in the anatomical position of the greater saphenous vein (GSV), often accompanied by a mild edema of the leg, is sufficient for establishing a clinical diagnosis.

Superficial thrombophlebitis is relatively easy to differentiate from other inflammatory conditions in the lower extremities, especially when the patient has pre-existing varicose veins. It is important to exclude cellulitis that may be accompanied by lymphangitis in the medial thigh. The appearance in such cases resembles superficial phlebitis, but the patients usually have fever and general symptoms of inflammation at the onset of the disease.

When superficial phlebitis occurs in extremities without varicose veins, as in the case of this patient, an underlying condition should be suspected, with the most frequent being malignancy, thrombophilia, or vasculitis (Buerger's, Behçet's, and others).

Workup

A duplex ultrasound examination is performed to determine the proximal extension of the thrombus and to rule out deep vein thrombosis (DVT). The scan also confirms the diagnosis of superficial thrombophlebitis as demonstrated by an enlarged vein with endoluminal echogenic filling, absence of flow, and noncompressibility (Fig. 1).

Superficial thrombophlebitis in extremities without varicose veins is associated with malignancy in 5% to 12% and with thrombophilia in 50% of cases. Screening for malignancy may be necessary if suggestive symptoms are present. Testing for thrombophilia is not indicated unless the patient is pregnant or has a history of venous thromboembolism (VTE).

More than half of patients with Behçet's disease are affected by superficial thrombophlebitis. The presence of erythema nodosum or inflammatory bowel disease can assist in the diagnosis of Behçet's. When phlebitis occurs in several separate veins (thrombophlebitis saltans), or affects several segments of the same vein (thrombophlebitis migrans), a workup for Buerger's disease is necessary.

In our patient, a duplex ultrasound scan confirmed acute thrombosis of his left GSV, with proximal extension to 10 cm from the saphenofemoral junction. He showed no evidence of DVT. Because he had a family history of venous thromboembolic disease, including a sister who had suffered multiple miscarriages, a coagulation panel was ordered, and he was positive for anti-β_2-glycoprotein antibodies and factor V Leiden.

Diagnosis and Treatment

Compression therapy with bandages or graduated stockings can relieve symptoms and facilitate resolution of the thrombus. Compression therapy and ambulation alone can be sufficient treatment in as many as 80% of patients. Adding nonsteroidal anti-inflammatory drugs provides better pain relief and faster resolution of inflammation. Anticoagulation may also be beneficial. The CALISTO trial demonstrated that the risk of VTE was reduced by 85% in patients receiving 2.5 mg/d of fondaparinux compared with those receiving a placebo. However, a cost analysis has suggested that anticoagulation may not be a cost-effective option.

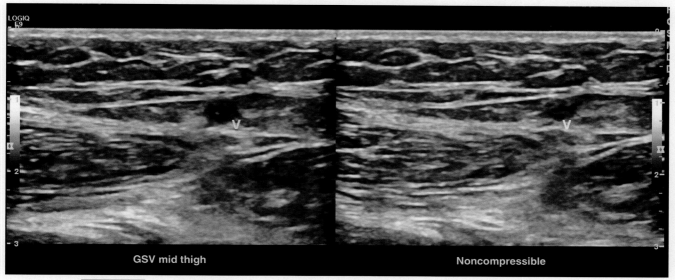

GSV mid thigh   Noncompressible

FIGURE 1 • Gray scale ultrasound image of GSV. Left panel shows GSV, that in the right panel shows noncompression. This is confirmatory for a thrombosed segment.

The American Venous Forum Guidelines recommend surgical treatment of the proximal extension of the thrombus within 1 cm from the saphenofemoral junction and conservative treatment for more distal thrombi. Surgical treatment consists of high ligation of the GSV. Stripping may be done simultaneously or delayed depending on the severity of inflammation. Revision of the saphenofemoral junction should be performed, and if thrombus extends into the common femoral vein, surgical thrombectomy may be performed.

Although there are no level 1 data comparing surgical treatment to medical management, a systematic review of six studies suggests that medical management is at least as effective as surgery. The 9th edition of the American College of Chest Physicians guidelines suggests the use of a prophylactic dose of low molecular weight heparin (LMWH) or fondaparinux for 45 days versus no anticoagulation if thrombus is at least 5 cm in length. These guideline committee also recommends medical rather that surgical treatment.

If medical management is selected for patients with proximal GSV thrombosis, a follow-up duplex scan may be necessary, especially if symptoms persist or new symptoms and signs, such as swelling or heaviness, develop. Although pulmonary embolism (PE) is a rare complication of superficial thrombophlebitis, patients should be informed of the risk and manifestations of PE.

Case Conclusion

The patient was treated with enoxaparin (Lovenox) at 1 mg/kg twice daily for 5 days and warfarin. Once his international normalized ratio (INR) was within the therapeutic range for two consecutive tests, he was managed on 5 mg of warfarin daily.

TAKE HOME POINTS

- Patients with superficial thrombophlebitis without varicose veins should be evaluated for coexisting malignancy, thrombophilia, and vasculitis.
- Duplex ultrasound should be performed to identify proximal extension of the thrombus and rule out DVT.
- Medical treatment should include compression therapy, ambulation, and anti-inflammatory drugs, with possible anticoagulation.
- Surgical treatment or anticoagulation with duplex ultrasound follow-up should be considered if the proximal extension of the thrombus is within 1 cm from saphenofemoral junction.

SUGGESTED READINGS

Decousus H, Prandoni P, Mismetti P, et al. The CALISTO Study Group. Fondaparinux for the treatment of superficial-vein thrombosis in the legs. *N Engl J Med.* 2010;363:1222-1232.

Decousus H, Quéré I, Presles E, et al. POST (Prospective Observational Superficial Thrombophlebitis) Study Group. Superficial venous thrombosis and venous thromboembolism: a large, prospective epidemiologic study. *Ann Intern Med.* 2010;152:218-224.

Gloviczki P. *Handbook of Venous Disorders. Guidelines of the American Venous Forum.* 3rd ed. London, UK: Hodder Arnold; 2009.

Goldman L, Ginsberg J. Superficial phlebitis and phase 3.5 trials. *N Engl J Med.* 2010;363:1278-1280.

Kalodiki E, Stvrtinova V, Allegra C, et al. Superficial vein thrombosis: a consensus statement. *Int Angiol.* 2012;31:203-216.

Mouton WG, Kienle Y, Muggli B, et al. Tumors associated with superficial thrombophlebitis. *Vasa.* 2009;38:167-170.

Sullivan V, Denk PM, Sonnad SS, et al. Ligation versus anticoagulation: treatment of above-knee superficial thrombophlebitis not involving the deep venous system. *J Am Coll Surg.* 2001;193:556-562.

CLINICAL SCENARIO CASE QUESTIONS

1. Primary diagnostic goals of duplex ultrasound scan in patients with superficial thrombophlebitis include:

   a. Identification of reflux in deep veins
   b. Ruling out arterial disease
   c. Identification of proximal extension of the thrombus and ruling out DVT
   d. Evaluation of the age of the thrombus

2. Conservative therapy of the superficial thrombophlebitis should include:

   a. Thrombolysis with tPA
   b. Compression therapy with bandages or stockings
   c. Unfractionated heparin
   d. Antibiotics

Chronic Venous Insufficiency— Postthrombotic Syndrome

JOSEPH D. RAFFETTO

Presentation

A 45-year-old male presents with a 5-year history of left lower extremity swelling, which is progressive over the course of the day. The swelling involves his leg and knee and extends into the thigh. The patient wears 30 to 40 mm Hg thigh-high compression stockings. His past history is significant for traumatic injury of the back at age 35, which required an anterior open fusion of his L4-L5 spine. The surgery was complicated by a hematoma requiring an exploratory laparotomy. One week later, the patient developed a venous thromboembolism (VTE) requiring an inferior vena cava (IVC) filter. Given his progressive edema, he underwent left iliac angioplasty 3 year ago with minimal relief. His pulse exam is normal, there are no skin changes or ulcers, and he has no other medical issues.

Differential Diagnosis

Both the clinical history and presentation are suggestive of a chronic venous insufficiency and postthrombotic syndrome. In addition, his history of iliac vein angioplasty is suggestive that he has a central venous problem in the iliac vein. Because of his history of VTE, one needs to consider recurrent deep venous thrombosis. Other possibilities of unilateral edema are infection, lymphedema, trauma, and tumors.

Workup

Color flow duplex ultrasound was performed and demonstrated recanalized left femoral vein with chronic thrombus that was not occlusive and flow in the vein (Fig. 1).

Further evaluation determined that the left popliteal vein had chronic recanalized thrombus with venous flow (Fig. 2A), but significant reflux (4.84 seconds) in the popliteal vein (Fig. 2B). The common femoral vein (CFV), deep femoral vein (DFV), tibial veins, and great/small saphenous veins were all normal. The suggestion of central vein obstruction and significant swelling that involved both the leg and thigh warranted further evaluation of the iliac venous system. A computerized axial tomographic venography (CTV) demonstrated a patent IVC (Fig. 3A), a severely compressed left common iliac vein (CIV, Fig. 3B), a patent left external iliac vein (EIV) but with postthrombotic changes (Fig. 3C), and patent left

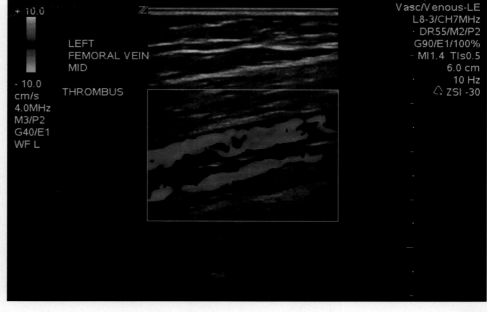

FIGURE 1 • Color flow duplex ultrasound (CFDUS) demonstrating the femoral vein (blue on CFDUS, the red color is the femoral artery). Note the irregularity on the vein wall.

525

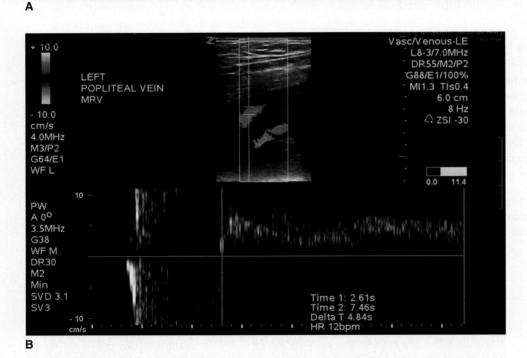

FIGURE 2 • **A:** Color flow duplex ultrasound (CFDUS) demonstrating the popliteal vein (*arrow*) with chronic thrombus (hyperechoic). **B:** Spectral Doppler waveform demonstrating reflux in the popliteal vein of 4.84 seconds.

femoral vein but with chronic postthrombotic changes (Fig. 3D). Both the ultrasound and CTV favor a diagnosis of chronic venous insufficiency with postthrombotic syndrome and CIV obstruction. In fact, there is no suggestion of pelvic tumors in the pelvis and no evidence of infection or clinical presentation of lymphedema.

Diagnosis and Treatment

The patient's symptoms are related to several problems. He has postthrombotic syndrome secondary to recanalized chronic DVT with severe reflux in the popliteal vein, which explains the leg edema; however, the edema of the lower extremity extends into the thigh, suggesting

that the CIV obstruction and EIV with a postthrombotic recanalized vein are also contributing to the problem. The primary treatment of postthrombotic syndrome is compression therapy. Vein valve transplantation is reserved for patients with recalcitrant venous ulcers and skin changes, which the patient does not exhibit. There is no indication or studies to support endovascular angioplasty and stent treatment of the femoral-popliteal recanalized vein segments. Importantly, given the central venous obstruction, both surgical and endovascular approaches need to be considered to relieve the venous hypertension in the limb. Endovenous treatment of iliofemoral or iliocaval obstruction is the primary treatment modality,

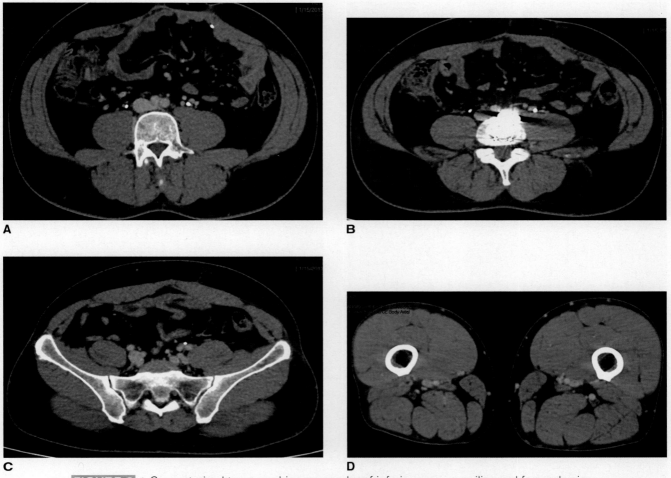

FIGURE 3 • Computerized tomographic venography of inferior vena cava, iliac and femoral veins. **A:** Normal inferior vena cava. **B:** Compressed left iliac vein, note metallic prosthesis in the lumbar spine. **C:** Left external iliac vein patent with minimal post-thrombotic changes (right external iliac vein patent and normal). **D:** Left femoral vein patent with post-thrombotic changes (right femoral vein patent and normal).

and open surgical venous reconstruction techniques are reserved for failed endovenous procedures.

Surgical Approach

Endovenous procedures involving the iliac vein and IVC can be approached from either the femoral vein or popliteal vein. Procedures should be performed in a fixed imaging suite for optimal imaging, reduction in radiation exposure, and safety. Approaching from the popliteal vein provides further options to treat the entire iliac vein, including stenting into the CFV if needed, but this is usually reserved for acute DVT of the iliofemoral region. In addition, if there is segmental occlusion of the femoral vein, a popliteal approach would not be favorable. In chronic postthrombotic iliocaval and iliofemoral vein obstruction, the common femoral vein or femoral vein is the optimal access site. All venous access sites should be performed under ultrasound guidance to avoid the artery, especially in the femoral region, and by micropuncture technique. In this patient, the CFV approach was performed with ultrasound-guided micropuncture

with a 0.018-inch wire and 5-French sheath, since the most significant problem was in the left CIV and proximal EIV. The patient is administered intravenous heparin. Venography is performed via the side port of the sheath and in multiple views including anterior-posterior (AP), right anterior oblique (RAO), and left anterior oblique (LAO) in order to provide the required information of the venous anatomy (Fig. 4A–C). The venogram demonstrated a compressed left CIV in the area of the lumbar spine hardware and postthrombotic trabeculations within the EIV. It is important to note that venography can be normal in appearance, but it does not exclude the possibility of iliac vein obstruction, hence the importance of using intravascular ultrasound (IVUS).

A 0.035-inch glidewire and Kumpe catheter were used to cross the venous lesions and passed into the IVC. Once the lesion is crossed, a wire exchange is performed with a 0.035-inch Amplatz wire. A sheath exchange was performed and a 10-French sheath placed. Further delineation of the venous pathology and anatomical detail is obtained with IVUS. IVUS demonstrated

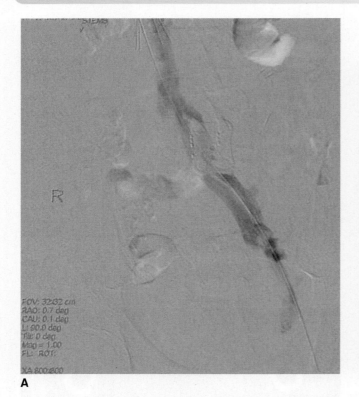

A

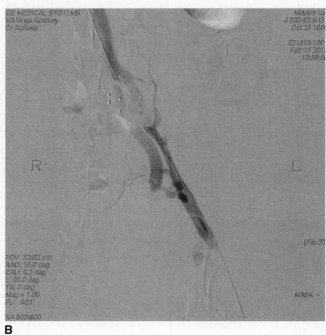

B

C

FIGURE 4 • Venography of the left iliofemoral veins.
A: Anterior-posterior view, note compression of the left common iliac vein, but contrast is lightly opacifying the vein.
B: Right anterior oblique view, persistent compression of the left common iliac vein, with visualization of left internal iliac vein, and narrowed but patent left external iliac vein.
C: Left anterior oblique view, with compression of the left common iliac vein.

a compressed postthrombotic left CIV (Fig. 5A), post-thrombotic trabeculations in the left EIV (Fig. 5B), and a normal distal left EIV (Fig. 5C). IVUS is essential in venous work to confirm and define the obstruction, to determine proper sizing of the stents and delineate the area of vein pathology requiring treatment, to confirm positioning of the stent, and to visualize and confirm resolution of the obstruction. The CIV and EIV were pre-dilated with a 6 mm × 100 mm balloon (Fig. 6A). The

left CIV severe stenosis was treated with a 14 mm × 90 mm self-expanding Wallstent starting from the distal IVC to the proximal EIV and was postdilated to profile with a 9 × 40 balloon (Fig. 6B). Repeat venography and IVUS defined a narrowed segment of the EIV and normal CFV (Figs. 5C and 6C). Next, predilation of the EIV with the 9 mm × 40 mm balloon was performed, and a second Wallstent (16 mm × 90 mm) with 2-cm overlap with the first stent was used to treat

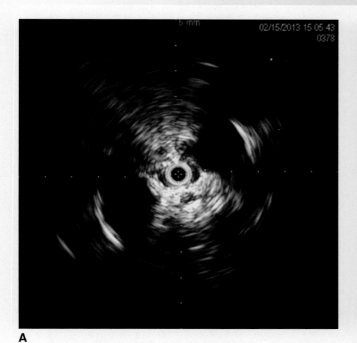

A

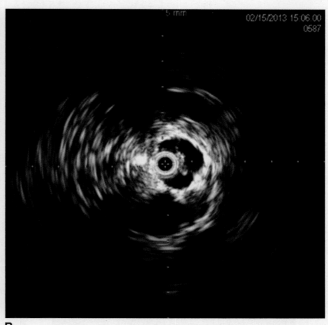

B

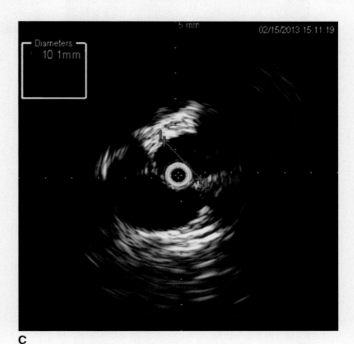

C

FIGURE 5 • Intravascular ultrasound (IVUS) of left iliofemoral venous system before endovascular intervention. **A:** Severely compressed postthrombotic left common iliac vein. **B:** Postthrombotic trabeculae in the left external iliac vein. **C:** Normal distal left external iliac vein.

the entire EIV (Fig. 7A). One should avoid untreated vein segments that are less than 5 cm between stents due to increased risk of secondary stenosis. Postdilation of the left CIV and proximal EIV vein with a 12 mm × 4 mm balloon was performed and postdilation of the distal aspect of the stents and the proximal CFV with a 10 mm × 4 mm balloon. Repeat venography demonstrated rapid contrast and patent iliac vein system (Fig. 7B). However, imaging was not well defined because of artifact caused by the metal hardware near the CIV. IVUS demonstrated a well-positioned CIV stent that protrudes into the IVC (Fig. 8A, which is the correct positioning of the stent to

prevent restenosis in the untreated CIV); the areas of previous near obstruction were significantly improved with good stent wall apposition. However, the stenosis was not completely resolved, indicating significant fibrosis of the CIV wall as seen on IVUS by the hyperechoic spectra (Fig. 8B) and well-expanded stent in the EIV, with resolution of the postthrombotic trabecular changes (Fig. 8C). Once the procedure is complete, the sheath is removed and pressure held over the entry site for 15 to 20 minutes. A completion ultrasound of the access site is not mandatory but recommended to document patency and flow and the presence or absence of any hematoma.

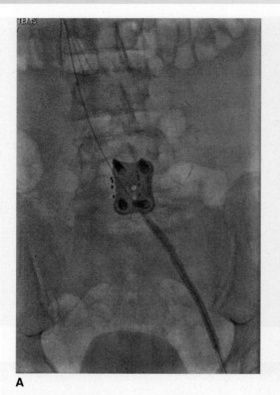

A

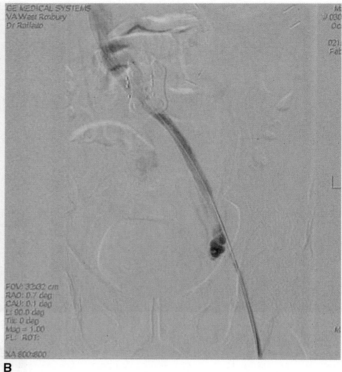

B

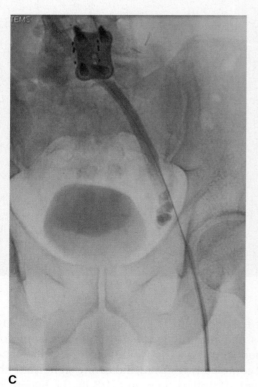

C

FIGURE 6 • Venography demonstrating balloon angioplasty and stent placement in left iliac venous system. **A:** Predilation of the left common iliac and external iliac veins. **B:** Placement of 14 × 90 mm Wallstent in left common iliac vein and post-dilated with 9 × 40 mm balloon. **C:** Left external iliac vein with stenosis that was pre-dilated with 9 × 40 mm balloon.

Special Intraoperative Considerations

It is absolutely imperative that IVUS rather than venography be utilized to clearly demonstrate the area of pathologic obstruction and define the treatment strategy. If occlusive disease is determined to extend into the CFV,

it is acceptable to place the self-expanding stents across the inguinal ligament and into the CFV. This approach requires that the access be obtained at the femoral vein. However, caution is advised as to ensure adequate outflow from the DFV and not to "jail" the DFV and

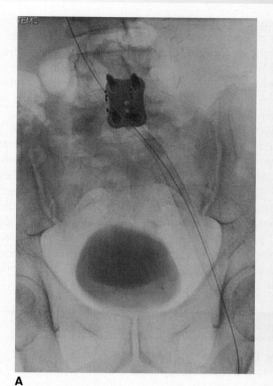
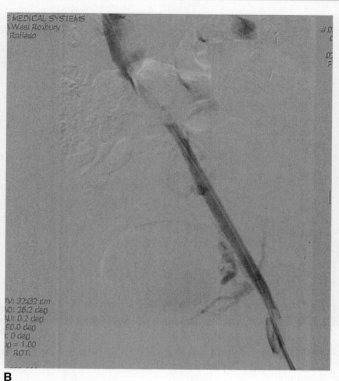

A   **B**

FIGURE 7 • Venography demonstrating balloon angioplasty and stent placement in left external iliac venous system. **A:** A 16 × 90 mm Wallstent in the left external iliac vein with 2 cm overlap with stent placed in common iliac vein, and post-dilated the common and external iliac veins with a 12 × 40 mm balloon. **B:** Final venography of iliac vein system. Note that it is difficult to appreciate the presence of residual luminal disease of the common iliac vein due to metal hardware.

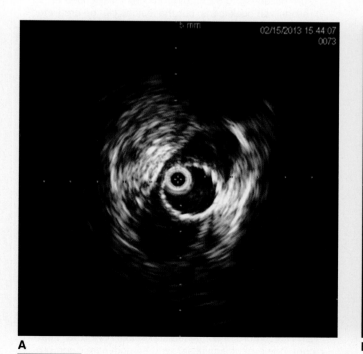
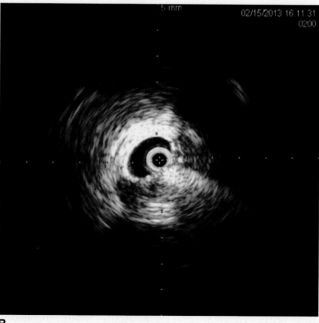

A   **B**

FIGURE 8 • Intravascular ultrasound (IVUS) of left iliofemoral venous system after endovascular intervention. **A:** Stent 14 × 90 mm in the IVC and entering the left common iliac vein. **B:** The 14 × 90 mm stent in the left common iliac vein at the area of original compression with excellent apposed stent, the severe obstruction is significantly improved but not completely relieved.

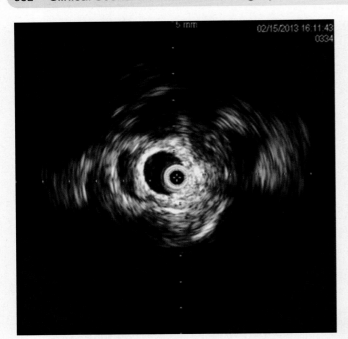

C

FIGURE 8 • (Continued) **C:** The 16 × 90 mm stent in left external iliac vein with excellent resolution of trabeculae and well apposed stent.

compromise the outflow. If at the time of iliac vein intervention there is significant CFV postthrombotic disease, one should consider performing a hybrid procedure with endophlebectomy of the CFV to ensure adequate inflow from the DFV and simultaneous treatment of the iliac venous obstruction. In patients with chronic obstruction of the iliocaval and iliofemoral venous system, the pelvic collateral veins may drain into the ascending lumbar veins and be mistaken for the iliac veins or the IVC; therefore, appropriate anatomic knowledge during venography is important to avoid injuring or stenting these structures inadvertently.

Postoperative Management

Following interventions of the iliac venous system, patients are usually monitored in hospital for 24 hours. Anticoagulation is not necessary, unless the patient was on anticoagulation prior to the procedure for DVT, has acute or chronic iliac venous obstruction with suspicion of new thrombus, or has a known hypercoagulable disorder. Most patients are placed on aspirin 81 mg. If a patient had a recanalization and stent of the iliac venous system, 4 to 6 weeks of anticoagulation is recommended. Patients should be maintained with knee high compression stockings. Potential complications that can occur are hematoma and retroperitoneal bleeding. Acute stent thrombosis may require reintervention, while contrast-induced nephropathy is usually self-limiting. Transient back pain is relieved with analgesics. Outpatient follow-up,

although not standardized, should encompass clinical visits at 6 weeks to 3 months and at 6 and 12 months, since the majority of stent-related thrombosis and restenosis occur in the first year. However, iliac veins that are recanalized secondary to postthrombotic occlusions may be seen more frequently, as their risk for early stent thrombosis is higher.

Color flow duplex ultrasound imaging can be performed both to assess stent patency in the iliac venous system and to evaluate the CFV to assess for phasic flow. After the first year, patients can be monitored every 6 to 12 months. Patients presenting with worsening symptoms of edema, pain, and skin changes should be evaluated with venous ultrasound of the deep and superficial veins, including evaluation of the stent-treated iliac venous outflow. If too deep to image, other modalities such as CTV, venography, or IVUS are reasonable (Table 1).

TABLE 1. Endovascular Iliac Vein Angioplasty and Stent

Key Technical Steps

1. Appropriate imaging studies with CTV to delineate venous anatomy and area of pathology.
2. Ultrasound-guided micropuncture venous access in the femoral or popliteal vein.
3. Administer intravenous heparin.
4. Intravascular ultrasound (IVUS) to define anatomic detail and area to be treated.
5. Predilate iliac vein obstruction with small high pressure balloon (4 to 6 mm balloons are initially used for recanalized occlusions, but the lesions can be predilated with 12 to 16 mm balloons without an increased risk of rupture).
6. Deploy self-expanding stents (Wallstent) of at least 14 to 16 mm diameter in the iliac venous system. When treating, CIV obstructions need to place the proximal portion of the stent in the IVC at the confluence of the right and left CIV. If multiple stents are required, at least several centimeters of overlap is required.
7. Long-term anticoagulation is with aspirin 81 mg, unless the patient was already on anticoagulation for DVT and/ or has a hypercoagulable disorder which then would require prolonged therapy.

Potential Pitfalls

- Unable to cross obstruction, especially in chronic postthrombotic iliac veins. This may require advanced endovenous techniques with specialized wires and catheters to cross the obstruction.
- Undersizing of the stent with inadequate radial force to alleviate obstruction or stent migration.
- Oversizing of the stent with stent elongation and overtreating the iliac vein pathology.
- Severe vein wall fibrosis with incomplete resolution of the obstruction requiring additional balloon-expandable stents.
- Vein wall rupture, if contained and stable no further treatment; however, if significant with hemodynamic compromise, then will need treatment with endovenous covered stent.

Case Conclusion

The patient's edema significantly improved and his symptoms also resolved. He underwent repeat color flow duplex ultrasound at 1 month, demonstrating a patent stent system in EIV and normal phasic flow in the CFV. At 6 months, he had worsening leg swelling to his knee, and a repeat ultrasound demonstrated patent stent in the EIV, and a CTV demonstrated a widely patent stents in the left iliac venous system. The edema in the leg was attributed to his postthrombotic disease affecting the femoral-popliteal vein, and knee high compression therapy with 30 to 40 mm was maintained.

TAKE HOME POINTS

- Unilateral leg swelling in the presence of postthrombotic syndrome can indicate iliofemoral venous obstruction.
- Patients with a history of VTE are at increased risk for recurrent deep venous thrombosis and worsening symptoms of edema, pain, or skin changes, including venous ulcers.
- IVUS is essential in defining venous obstruction, morphology, sizing for venous stent, and pre- and postplacement of the venous stent as venography may appear "normal" or with minimal venous pathology.
- Stents are always required to treat the venous system obstruction, as balloon angioplasty alone is not sufficient. In the iliac and femoral venous segments, a 14- to 18-mm-diameter self-expanding stents should be employed.
- Compression stockings of at least 30 to 40 mm Hg should be continued in patients with postthrombotic changes in the lower extremity deep veins.

SUGGESTED READINGS

de Wolf MA, Arnoldussen CW, Wittens CH. Indications for endophlebectomy and/or arteriovenous fistula after stenting. *Phlebology.* 2013;28(suppl 1):123-128.

Labropoulos N, Gasparis AP, Tassiopoulos AK. Prospective evaluation of the clinical deterioration in post-thrombotic limbs. *J Vasc Surg.* 2009;50:826-830.

Neglen P, Berry MA, Raju S. Endovascular surgery in the treatment of chronic primary and post-thrombotic iliac vein obstruction. *Eur J Vasc Endovasc Surg.* 2000;20:560-571.

Neglen P, Hollis KC, Olivier J, et al. Stenting of the venous outflow in chronic venous disease: long-term stent-related outcome, clinical, and hemodynamic results. *J Vasc Surg.* 2007;46:979-990.

Neglén P, Tackett TP Jr, Raju S. Venous stenting across the inguinal ligament. *J Vasc Surg.* 2008;48:1255-1261.

Raju S. Best management options for chronic iliac vein stenosis and occlusion. *J Vasc Surg.* 2013;57:1163-1169.

Raju S, Neglén P. Percutaneous recanalization of total occlusions of the iliac vein. *J Vasc Surg.* 2009;50:360-368.

CLINICAL SCENARIO CASE QUESTIONS

1. Currently, the best method to define a venous stenosis is:
   a. Venous pressure gradient
   b. Venography
   c. IVUS
   d. CTV
   e. Venous duplex ultrasound

2. All of the following are acceptable stent placement strategies except:
   a. Extending into the IVC
   b. Avoid un-stented regions between stents to prevent restenosis
   c. Placement of a stent across the inguinal ligament to treat proximal common femoral vein disease
   d. Placement of stents in recanalized femoral veins
   e. Placement of 14- to 18-mm stents in the iliac veins

110 Incompetent Venous Perforators

RANDOLPH TODD C. JONES and LOWELL S. KABNICK

Presentation

A 68-year-old man presents to the office with recurrent edema, pain, and ulceration of the right lower extremity. The patient is well known and has a long history of venous disease: Deep Venous Thrombosis (DVT), superficial venous insufficiency, and venous ulcers. He has had several endovenous thermal ablations involving his superficial axial veins, including the right small and great saphenous veins. In addition, he underwent intravascular ultrasound (IVUS) with percutaneous transluminal angioplasty (PTA) and stenting of the right common and external iliac veins for significant stenosis (77% area reduction) and Intraluminal scarring. Until his presentation today, his ulcer had been healed.

On physical exam, he is afebrile and his vital signs are within normal limits.

The patient has bilateral lower extremity pitting edema, which is significantly worse on the right. Most notably, there is an area of ulceration just superior to the medial malleolus measuring 3.5 cm × 6 cm in diameter (Fig. 1). The ulcer bed is moist, clean, and with no overt signs of infection. There is mild epidermal erythema, hyperpigmentation, and induration. His dorsalis pedis and posterior tibial pulses are 2+, equal, and bilateral.

Differential Diagnosis

Lower extremity ulcer etiologies are numerous. Patients presenting with lower extremity ulceration require workup for both venous and arterial insufficiencies. Before proceeding with any ulcer therapy, malignancy and arterial ulcer etiologies must be excluded. Biopsy may be necessary to identify the root cause.

In the above patient, consideration for recurrent DVT, in-stent restenosis, and/or stent occlusion should be ascertained before proceeding with further evaluation and treatment.

Workup

The evaluation of all patients with lower extremity ulceration includes identifying the causal factor(s) of the ulceration and excluding other more morbid and potentially life-threatening etiologies. After arterial, traumatic, or infectious etiologies are excluded, the exact nature and extent of peripheral venous insufficiency is determined.

Understanding venous anatomy of the lower extremities is paramount to accurate diagnosis and optimal treatment of superficial venous reflux. This is further emphasized by the fact that the perforating veins are numerous, occur at relatively regular anatomic locales in the lower extremities (Fig. 2), and can often be missed, even by the most experienced ultrasonographers. Of note,

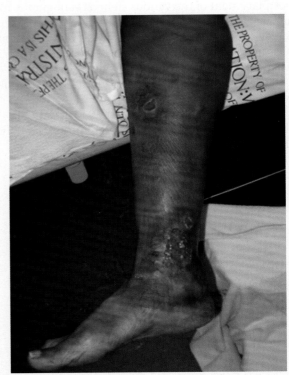

FIGURE 1 • Typical appearing venous stasis ulcer of the lower extremity. Note the hyperpigmentation surrounding the ulcer, and its location on the medial malleolus.

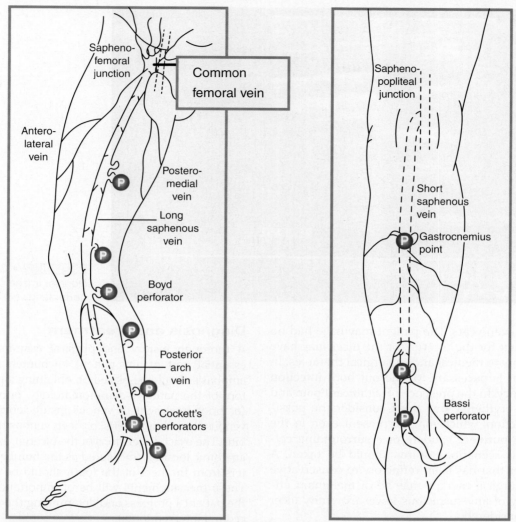

Saphenofemoral junction

Common femoral vein

Anterolateral vein

Posteromedial vein

Long saphenous vein

Boyd perforator

Posterior arch vein

Cockett's perforators

Saphenopopliteal junction

Short saphenous vein

Gastrocnemius point

Bassi perforator

FIGURE 2 • This diagram of the various perforating and axial veins of the thigh and leg uses older nomenclature.

the short and long saphenous veins have since been renamed the "small saphenous" and "great saphenous" veins, respectively. In addition, the named perforating veins have fallen out of favor for more descriptive anatomic nomenclatures such as the medial thigh, popliteal, and posterior tibial perforators. The importance of knowing the locations of the various perforators and understanding that incompetent perforating veins (IPVs) can be a major source of recurrent varicose veins and venous ulcers cannot be overemphasized.

Duplex ultrasound has a high degree of diagnostic accuracy, low cost, and widespread availability. Presently, ultrasound is considered by most as the gold standard for diagnosis of peripheral venous insufficiency and DVT. Using duplex ultrasound for perforator investigation, we can document the location, diameter, degree of reflux, and its connection to any superficial tributaries that might be contributing to varicosities, advanced skin changes, or ulceration (Figs. 3 and 4).

Typically, when using duplex imaging for perforator size determination, the diameter is measured horizontally at the level where the perforator exits the fascia (Fig. 4). Some venous interventionalists prefer to measure the size where the perforator is largest, which is usually just superficial to where it exits the muscular fascia. Refluxing perforators need to be a minimum of 3.5 mm in diameter with duration of reflux lasting greater than 0.5 seconds to be considered of hemodynamic significance.

CEAP and Venous Clinical Severity Scores (VCSS) should be documented on all patients with symptomatic superficial or deep venous insufficiency. Additionally, the clinical score of the CEAP classification is of particular importance, as it is a key component of the American Venous Forum (AVF) and Society for Vascular Surgery (SVS) guidelines for perforator treatment.

The duration of a nonhealing ulcer is very important in determining treatment options. In some cases, lower extremity ulcers may have been present for several

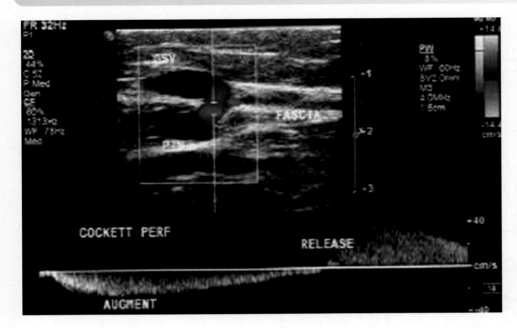

months and even years. The patient may have had no prior treatment for the ulcer(s), or the ulcer may have been refractory to medical and/or surgical therapies. In either case, it is necessary to rule out both infection and malignancy. In the presence of significant pain and surrounding erythema, one must consider the possibility of infection, which may be present even in the absence of a purulent exudate or a surrounding cellulitis. In this scenario, cultures should be taken. A painless ulcer that has been refractory to conservative medical or surgical therapy may be of malignant etiology. Biopsy of any suspicious lower extremity ulcer should be considered.

Diagnosis and Treatment

A thorough history and physical examination are an essential part of any patient encounter. In particular, emphasis should be placed on obtaining a pertinent history of the patient's symptomatology, prior procedures (or prior treatment of venous insufficiency), superficial venous thrombophlebitis, or deep venous thrombophlebitis. The exact dimensions of the ulcer(s), as well as their anatomic location (measured as the number of centimeters from the heel of the foot), should be documented. These measurements will be of importance in tracking the patient's progress and determining the need for procedural intervention(s).

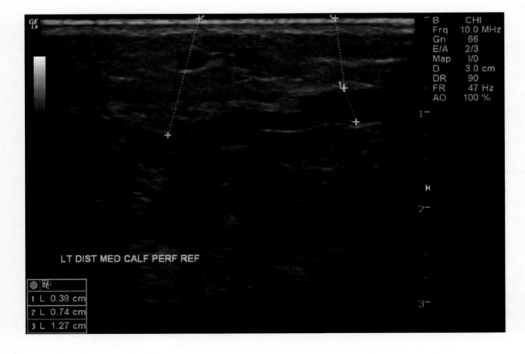

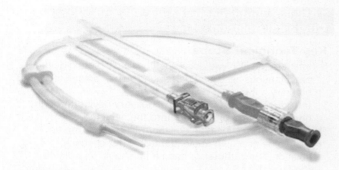

FIGURE 5 • An 0.018″ microintroducer set, which includes a 21-g needle, 0.018″ guidewire, and a 4-French introducer sheath.

Duplex ultrasound is of vital importance in the diagnosis and treatment of incompetent venous perforators. The contribution of IPVs to ambulatory venous hypertension is significant. Up to 70% of IPVs are of hemodynamic significance, and nearly half (45%) of IPVs are not abolished with saphenous ablation. Surgical therapy for superficial venous reflux has not been shown to improve the rate of ulcer healing, but it has been shown to decrease the incidence of recurrence.

Perforator Treatment Guidelines

The current indications for incompetent perforator interruption according to the AVF and SVS are as follows: (1) The patient must have C5 or C6 disease (either an active venous ulcer or a healed ulcer); (2) the perforator must have demonstrable reflux of 0.5 seconds or greater; (3) the perforator must be greater than 3.5 mm in diameter, measured where it exits the muscular fascia; and (4) the perforator must be anatomically related to the area of the ulcer or healed ulcer.

Surgical Approach

There are several efficient ways of interrupting IPVs. Each technique has its individual advantages and disadvantages. Proper technique selection is essential to clinical success.

Open perforator ligation using ultrasound guidance to hook the perforator or a communicating tributary is a technique that can be quite useful in some patients with C3 or C4a disease. This procedure can be done in combination with ambulatory phlebectomy of any associated varicosities; however, it may be of limited utility in a patient with more advanced disease such as lipodermatosclerosis (C4b) or an active or healed ulcer. Healing of wounds around a previous or active ulcer bed is unpredictable at best, and making an incision (however small) into this area is not recommended.

Endovenous techniques include ultrasound-guided chemical, laser, and radiofrequency ablation. Common steps to all three techniques include the use of duplex ultrasound to gain needle access to the perforator (Fig. 5) or a communicating tributary in close proximity, after which the chosen ablative device is introduced into the vein via a catheter or directly through the needle access.

Ultrasound-guided chemical ablation can be needle or catheter directed. The initial steps are essentially the same; however, catheter-directed sclerotherapy involves the use of a guidewire and the modified Seldinger technique to introduce it into the perforator and/or its communicating tributaries. Once access is confirmed via aspiration, and on duplex (Fig. 6), a sclerosing agent is then injected into its epifascial tributary and stopped when it reaches the perforator. Currently approved sclerosants are sodium tetradecyl sulfate (Sotradecol) and polidocanol (Asclera). The use of a proprietary foam sclerosant just approved by the FDA (November 2013, BTG, Philadelphia, PA) is unknown; however, injection of physician-made foam has been well documented in the literature. If the sclerosant is foamed, the patient should be placed in the Trendelenburg position during the injection process and proximal pressure should be applied to minimize the amount of foam that enters the central venous system.

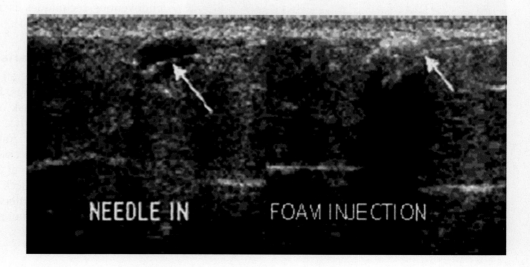

FIGURE 6 • Duplex ultrasound showing needle access of a perforating vein.

NEEDLE IN   FOAM INJECTION

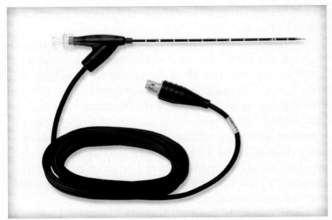

FIGURE 7 • An RFA perforator ablation device (Image courtesy of Covidien). This device is seldom used by the authors, as we feel that the use of laser is substantially easier and quicker than radiofrequency for perforator ablation.

Endovenous thermal ablation with the radiofrequency device (Fig. 7) is performed with direct introduction of the device through the skin. For laser ablation, once percutaneous access is obtained via ultrasound guidance, the modified Seldinger technique may be used to introduce a sheath (or if a 400-μm laser fiber is used, it may be introduced directly through the needle) (Fig. 8). The device is advanced under ultrasound guidance into the perforator at the level of the fascia, and tumescent anesthesia is injected around the vein and catheter. Care should be taken not to advance the tip of the device beyond the fascia, as this may result in DVT or nerve injury. The patient should be placed in the Trendelenburg position to facilitate vein wall contact around the device. The specifics regarding optimal treatment energy levels are beyond the scope of this chapter, as the recommended energy levels vary greatly with the type of device used.

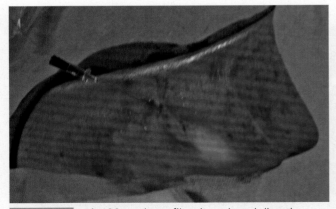

FIGURE 8 • A 400-μm laser fiber introduced directly through the needle into an incompetent perforator.

TABLE 1. Endovenous Laser, RF, and Chemical Ablation

Key Technical Steps

1. Infiltrate the skin with local anesthesia ultrasound-guided percutaneous access of perforating vein or connected tributary.
2. Introduce thermal or chemical delivery device through needle, sheath, or catheter into the selected IPV.
3. Confirm device location (for thermal devices, the tip should be at or just above the fascia; for chemical ablation, the catheter or needle tip should be outside the fascia).
4. Infiltrate with tumescent anesthesia around vein and device (skip step if using chemical ablation).
5. Place patient in the Trendelenburg position.
6. Deliver energy according to specific device recommendations.
7. Confirm lack of flow in treated vein and patency of deep vessels.

Potential Intraoperative Pitfalls

- Loss of access
- Improper device position, resulting in injury to the deep system, paresthesia, or the accompanying perforating artery
- Injection of accompanying perforator artery
- Distal embolization of sclerosant

Immediately following ablation, duplex ultrasound is used to confirm a lack of flow in the target vein and to assess the patency of the underlying deep vessels.

Potential pitfalls of any perforator ablation include inability to obtain access for the device or accessing the accompanying perforating artery instead of the vein. If the perforating artery is damaged by thermal ablation, usually there will be no significant sequelae. However, if the artery is injected, the fluid or foam will embolize to the dermal branches and can cause tissue necrosis. Regardless of the modality chosen, recanalization is not an infrequent occurrence, and we have demonstrated occlusion rates of 100% at 4 months and 86% at 12 months. Fortunately, perforator management by endovenous techniques is not technically challenging and is repeatable (Table 1).

Postoperative Management

Postoperatively, we place all patients into 30- to 40-mm Hg compression stockings. In addition to the compression garment, we also ask our patients to ambulate for several minutes in the office before leaving.

Patients are seen for routine follow-up and duplex ultrasound at 1 week to assess the patency of the deep veins. Routine follow-up at 3 months is performed with duplex ultrasound to check the efficacy of the closure, although a shorter time interval would be reasonable if the clinician is concerned about recurrent or active ulceration.

Case Conclusion

The patient was managed nonoperatively with appropriate medical therapy (Unna boot and, subsequently, compression hose). His ulcer was reepithelialized within 6 weeks. After ulcer healing, the patient underwent endovenous laser ablation of two separate incompetent medial distal calf posterior tibial perforators along with catheter-directed foam sclerotherapy of the superficial tributaries beneath the healed ulcer bed.

Fortunately, for the past 15 months, the patient has been free of ulcer recurrence. He has enjoyed complete resolution of his lower extremity pain accompanied by a decrease in ankle circumference of 1.5 cm. According to duplex ultrasound reports, the patient's stent is patent without evidence of recurrent stenosis. Finally, he continues to wear graduated compression hose and returns to our office at regular intervals.

TAKE HOME POINTS

- Endovenous access should be established using ultrasound guidance.
- Access may be obtained directly by needle into the offending perforating vein or via a connected tributary and subsequently passing a catheter or sheath into the perforator.
- Venous blood should be aspirated through the needle and confirmed with ultrasound to ensure proper access when performing endochemical ablation.
- Laser is preferred over RF by us due to its ease of use and shorter procedure time.

SUGGESTED READINGS

Almeida J. *Atlas of Endovascular Venous Surgery*. Philadelphia, PA: Saunders, an imprint of Elsevier; 2012.

Coleridge-Smith P, Labropoulos N, Partsch H, et al. Duplex ultrasound investigation of the veins in chronic venous disease of the lower limbs—UIP consensus document. Part I. Basic principles. *Eur J Vasc Endovasc Surg.* 2006;31:83-92.

Delis KT, Ibeguna V, Nicolaides AN, et al. Prevalence and distribution of incompetent perforating veins in chronic venous insufficiency. *J Vasc Surg.* 1998;28(5):815-825.

Gloviczki P, Comerota AJ, Dalsing MC, et al. Society for Vascular Surgery; American Venous Forum. The care of patients with varicose veins and associated chronic venous diseases: clinical practice guidelines of the Society for Vascular Surgery and the American Venous Forum. *J Vasc Surg.* 2011;53(5 suppl): 2S-48S.

Gloviczki P. *Handbook of Venous Disorders*. 3rd ed. Guidelines of the American Venous Forum. London, UK: Hodder Arnold Publishers; 2009.

CLINICAL SCENARIO CASE QUESTIONS

1. According to the AVF/SVS consensus, the following conditions are all indications for perforator interruption except:

    a. C5 or higher disease
    b. Anatomic relation to the site of the active or previous ulcer bed
    c. Diameter of 3.5 mm or greater
    d. Reflux of duration 0.5 seconds or longer
    e. Pitting edema

2. Which of the following is the most common potential complication of endovenous ablation of a perforating vein?

    a. Tissue necrosis
    b. DVT
    c. Treatment failure
    d. Paresthesia
    e. Infection

111 IVC Filter Placement

ELIZABETH ANDRASKA, PETER K. HENKE, and JOHN RECTENWALD

Presentation

A 65-year-old woman presents to the ED with pain and swelling in her left leg. This patient has a medical history significant for left femur fracture, which was repaired 2 months ago. She also has a history of left leg tibial vein deep vein thrombosis (DVT) and had been taking chronic warfarin. However, she suffered a recent 4U gastrointestinal bleed and now cannot take anticoagulation for at least 6 weeks. She has no family history of DVT.

On physical exam, the left leg is noted to be warm and swollen. The patient reports acute pain and tenderness when asked to walk across the examination room. She undergoes a duplex ultrasound scan of each lower extremity. She is discovered to have a new acute, occluding DVT in her left external iliac vein.

Differential Diagnosis

In a patient with such a classic presentation, a DVT workup and immediate ultrasonography is imperative. In addition to DVT, a possible pulmonary embolism (PE) must be considered in the differential diagnosis. However, most patients who present with such symptoms will not have a DVT. A differential diagnosis for lower extremity pain and swelling includes a muscle or orthopedic injury, lymphatic obstruction, venous insufficiency, cellulitis, or Baker's cyst. Patients who present with bilateral leg swelling may need to be evaluated for potential systemic causes of leg swelling such as cirrhosis, congestive heart failure, or nephrotic syndrome.

Workup

DVT and PE, collectively referred to as venous thromboembolism (VTE), is a common clinical problem. Timely diagnosis and therapy is necessary to avoid embolism and potentially death. Many tests can be done to assess VTE risk; however, a D-Dimer test in conjunction with a Well's score can reliably determine pretest probability of VTE. Additionally, duplex ultrasonography with grayscale imaging to detect luminal thrombus and Doppler flow to assess the flow within the vessel should be performed on each extremity to assess the presence and extent of possible DVT. If suspicion for PE remains high, computed tomography angiography has replaced pulmonary angiogram and is now the gold standard for diagnosis of PE.

This patient was found to have an elevated D-Dimer of 4.5 (normal 0.4 to 2.5) and a Well's score criteria of 3 due to recent trauma and medical history significant for DVT. As stated, the duplex ultrasound study showed a DVT in the left external iliac vein.

Diagnosis and Treatment

The gold standard for treatment of VTE is anticoagulation therapy. However, in certain patient populations, anticoagulation therapy is contraindicated. Contraindications to anticoagulation include patients who cannot be safely anticoagulated such as those with brain metastasis, severe thrombocytopenia, or active bleeding at the time of diagnosis. Patients who have failed or have poorly controlled anticoagulation therapy or those who develop a complication due to anticoagulation therapy are also candidates for placement of an IVC filter. Less strong indications include those at high risk for bleeding or falls while on anticoagulants. In these patients, an inferior vena cava filter should be considered to prevent a fatal PE. Patients who are at high risk for bleeding may also be contraindicated for anticoagulation therapy. Risk factors for bleeding include age greater than 65, previous bleeding, thrombocytopenia, antiplatelet therapy, recent surgery, previous stroke, diabetes, anemia, cancer, renal failure, and liver failure. Both permanent and retrievable optional filters are available. In patients with acute, short-term contraindication for anticoagulation, a retrievable filter is a reasonable choice.

Although controversial, IVC filters are used as prophylaxis in high-risk individuals. In one large review, IVC filters were indicated both as prophylaxis in high-risk individuals (58%) and therapeutically in patients with a diagnosed acute proximal venous thrombus or VTE and contraindicated for anticoagulation therapy (42%). Individuals that may benefit from IVC filter prophylaxis include high-risk trauma patients, orthopedic and neurosurgical patients, and cancer patients. However, strong evidence for prophylactic filters is lacking.

This patient's indication for a filter is an anticoagulation complication as well as need for PE protection for at least 1 to 3 more months. Given the limited time frame required for an IVC filter, a retrievable IVC filter would be indicated for this patient.

Surgical Approach

There are many types of IVC filters. When deciding on which one to place, one should consider its ability to trap clot without compromising venous return within the cava and the ease of placement and removal. With this patient, a Denali vena cava filter (Bard, Tempe, AZ) was chosen due to a reasonable efficacy and safety profile. This particular filter should only be used in IVCs less than 30 mm.

A venogram is performed first. The IVC can be accessed from either femoral vein or jugular vein. The right femoral vein is most often used to access the site because it provides direct access to the IVC and a straighter lie for filter, minimizing filter tilting. In patients that are hypercoagulable, have iliac vein thrombi, or are obese, the right internal jugular vein may be a less complicated access site. The procedure should be done under fluoroscopic guidance. To access the femoral vein, puncture the vein using the Seldinger technique. Next, a guidewire is advanced into the vein. The coaxial introducer sheath is introduced over the guidewire. Once in the common iliac vein, a vena cavagram is performed. It is important to assess for the presence of a duplicated cava, patency of the vessels, and any caval thrombus near the planned filter site as well as the landmarks for the renal veins (Fig. 1).

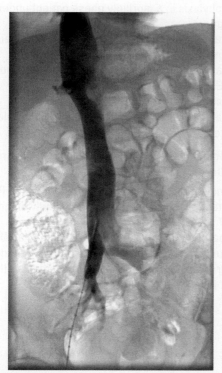

FIGURE 1 • Contrast venocavagram showing the iliac bifurcation and the renal veins; important landmarks for filter placement.

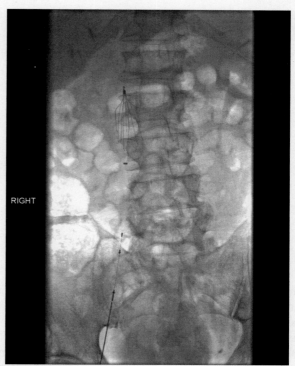

FIGURE 2 • Removable IVC filter is in good position by single-shot x-ray.

The filter should be placed just below the inflow of the renal veins. Once this site is visualized by venogram, the filter is deployed (Fig. 2). If the renal veins cannot be visualized on venogram, then each renal vein can be selectively catheterized to confirm their location. Each device has slightly different deployment mechanisms, and the surgeon placing the filter should be familiar with the instructions for use for the filter being placed.

Special Intraoperative Considerations

A large vena cava may require bilateral common iliac vein filters, a suprarenal IVC filter, or a permanent IVC filter such as the Bird's nest. Misdeployment of retrievable filters can usually be corrected by snaring and capturing the filter and redeploying the filter or, in the case of permanent IVC filters, placing a new filter in the correct location. Placement of a suprarenal filter is indicated for woman who may be pregnant and in those with perirenal vein DVT (Table 1).

Postoperative Management

Insertion site and general health status should be evaluated 24 hours after placement. The filter should be removed once the risks of anticoagulation have resolved. This is usually within 6 to 12 weeks. Filter mortality compared to anticoagulation therapy is not well defined due to study design limitations. Because filters are recommended only when anticoagulation is contraindicated, it is difficult to compare the groups.

Procedural complications include hematoma near the insertion site, DVT at the vein site of insertion, and IVC

TABLE 1. Key Technical Steps and Potential Pitfalls

Key Technical Steps

1. Choose access site wisely—jugular vs. femoral
2. Confirm the following with the venogram:
    a. Lowest renal vein
    b. Caval diameter
    c. Presence of thrombus near renal veins
    d. Contralateral iliac vein—need to see it
3. Deploy infrarenal in most cases

Potential Pitfalls

- Be careful to apply appropriate tension during filter deployment, to avoid tilting of the filter.
- Misplacement into azygos or above the renal veins inadvertently
- Cava diameter large and potential filter embolism

thrombosis. There are also a number of complications related to the filter device itself such as filter migration, fracture, embolism, or filter erosion into the IVC wall to the retroperitoneum or duodenum. The rate of DVT after placement of IVC filters is 5% to 21% after 2 years, compared to 10% to 12% in individuals treated with anticoagulation therapy. The incidence of PE is low at 1 year (1% to 3.6%). While short-term data on filter complications are well researched, the long-term complication rates are relatively unknown. Long-term complications include IVC perforation, occlusion, rupture, thrombosis, or migration of the device.

Thus, the indications for filter placement should be monitored closely, and the filter should be removed as soon as the risks subside.

Case Conclusion

This patient underwent an uneventful removable IVC filter placement as shown in Figure 2. She remained without symptoms or signs of pulmonary embolism, as well as no further GI bleeding. Given this was a provoked DVT related to an orthopedic injury, at 3 months post-DVT, she was deemed low risk after a D-dimer was checked and was normal. The filter was removed via a jugular approach without incident.

TAKE HOME POINTS

- An IVC filter placement is indicated in patients that have a known DVT or PE and are contraindicated for, developed a complication of, or have failed anticoagulation therapy.
- To avoid long-term complications, the filter should be removed as soon as it is no longer indicated. This is well documented by a warning letter issues by the FDA in August of 2010.
- Removable filters should be retrieved whenever possible. Retrieval rates of removable filters are extremely low. If the patient has reasons for a persistent risk, consider a permanent filter.

SUGGESTED READINGS

Angel LF, Tapson V, Galgon RE, et al. Systematic review of the use of retrievable inferior vena cava filters. *J Vasc Interv Radiol.* 2011;22:1522-1530.

Kaufman JA. Retrievable vena cava filters. *Tech Vasc Interven Radiol.* 2004;7:96-104.

Kaufman JA. Optional vena cava filters: what, why, and when. *Vascular.* 2007;15:304-313.

Rectenwald JE. Vena cava filters: uses and abuses. *Semin Vasc Surg.* 2005;18;166-175.

Streiff MB. Vena caval filters: a comprehensive review. *Blood.* 2000;95(12):3669-3677.

CLINICAL SCENARIO CASE QUESTIONS

1. The accepted indications for an IVC filter include:
    a. Prophylaxis in a morbidly obese patient undergoing a surgery
    b. A trauma patient without bleeding and no neurologic injury
    c. A patient on therapeutic anticoagulation who suffers a PE
    d. A patient with an iliocaval DVT
    e. A patient with two documented hypercoagulable states

2. An indication for permanent as compared with retrievable filter is:
    a. Transient risk of bleeding in a patient with a PE
    b. Metastatic career in patient with newly diagnosed DVT
    c. Hypercoagulable disorder in setting of iliac DVT
    d. Trauma patient with DVT and subdural hematoma
    e. Untreated pancreatic cancer in a patient with DVT and failed anticoagulation

112 Lymphedema

JAMES LAREDO and BYUNG BOONG LEE

Presentation

A 56-year-old man with a history of recurrent lower extremity cellulitis is referred by his primary medical doctor for chronic bilateral lower extremity swelling. He reports a 5-year history of progressive swelling of his lower extremities involving his feet, toes, ankles, and calves. He notes hardening of the skin of his legs below the knees and development of wartlike lesions. He was initially treated with compression stockings, but has been noncompliant over the past 5 years. He denied any history of deep vein thrombosis or history of varicose veins. There was no family history of leg swelling.

Differential Diagnosis

Leg edema is a common condition that is seen by all practicing clinicians. The differential diagnosis of lower extremity edema is extensive and includes systemic causes such as congestive heart failure, renal insufficiency, hepatic insufficiency, hypoalbuminemia, medications, and local causes such as deep vein thrombosis, venous insufficiency, lymphedema, lipedema, and cellulitis.

Workup

On physical examination, the patient is an obese man with normal arterial pulses in both lower extremities. There is no groin adenopathy. He has nonpitting edema of the bilateral lower extremities below the knees, with warty projections, lichenification, cobble stoning of the skin, and a malodorous fungal infection. There was no ulceration or drainage. Both feet had the presence of the Stemmer sign (inability to pinch a fold of skin at the base of the second toe) and puffiness of the forefoot (buffalo hump) (Fig. 1).

Venous duplex exam of the bilateral lower extremities was negative for deep vein thrombosis and venous insufficiency. Based on the presentation and past history of recurrent bilateral lower extremity cellulitis, a diagnosis of secondary lymphedema is made.

To confirm the diagnosis, bilateral lower extremity lymphoscintigraphy was performed.

Lymphoscintigraphy

Subcutaneous injection of radiolabeled sulfur colloid is administered in the first and second web space of the toes of both feet, followed by radionuclide scanning.

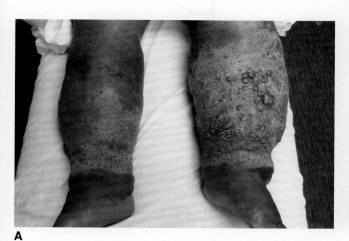
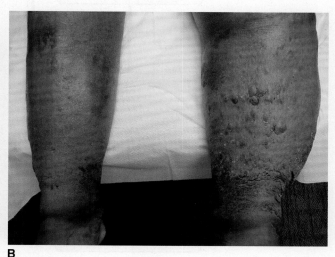

A   **B**

FIGURE 1 • Bilateral lower extremity lymphedema in a 56-year-old man before and after complex decongestive therapy. **A:** Before treatment. Note the significant limb swelling and chronic skin changes (lichenification, warty projections, and cobblestone appearance) associated with lymphedema. **B:** After treatment. Note the significant improvement in limb swelling and chronic skin changes.

Delayed isotope egress from the injection site, with decreased uptake and dermal back flow, was seen consistent with lymphedema.

Diagnosis and Treatment
Secondary lymphedema: Stage III

The patient was treated with a combination of compression wrapping, manual lymphatic drainage (MLD), and pneumatic compression therapy. Meticulous skin care including topical antifungal cream and skin moisturizers and skin cleansers was also part of his treatment regimen. Because of his history of recurrent lower extremity cellulitis, the patient was started on prophylactic antibiotic treatment with daily oral penicillin.

Lymphedema

Lymphedema is characterized by a progressive and usually painless swelling of tissues, most commonly involving the lower extremities in 80% of cases. It can also occur in the arms, face, trunk, and external genitalia. Lymphedema is the result of decreased transport capacity of the lymphatic system. Lymphedema can be primary or secondary (Fig. 2). Primary lymphedema is due to a defect in the lymph-conducting pathways. Secondary lymphedema is due to an acquired cause

that results in injury and impairment of the lymphatic system.

Primary lymphedemas have been classified into three groups depending on the age of onset: congenital (before age 2), praecox (onset between age 2 and 25), and tarda (after age 35). Lymphedema praecox is the most common form of primary lymphedema with a female-to-male ratio of 10:1. It is usually unilateral and often limited to the foot and calf in most patients.

Secondary lymphedema is far more common than primary lymphedema and represents 90% of cases of lymphedema. The most common causes of lower extremity lymphedema are tumor (e.g., lymphoma, prostate cancer, ovarian cancer), surgery involving the lymphatics, radiation therapy, trauma, and infection.

Stages of Lymphedema
Treatment of Lymphedema
General Considerations

The importance of patient education and compliance cannot be overemphasized when treating patients with lymphedema. The patient must first understand that lymphedema is a chronic condition and will never be completely cured. In addition, they must also understand that there is no "quick fix" operation, medication, or

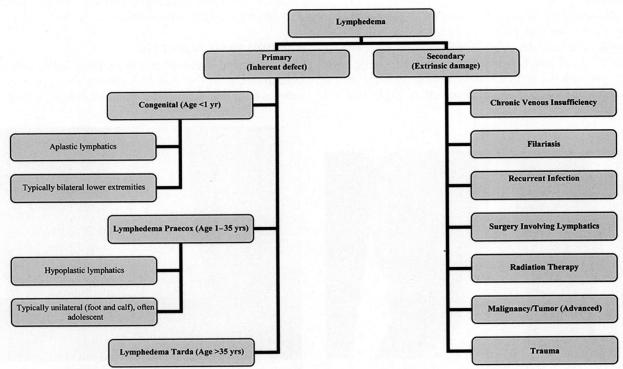

FIGURE 2 • Primary and secondary lymphedema. Lymphedema is the result of decreased transport capacity of the lymphatic system. Lymphedema can be primary or secondary. Primary lymphedema is due to a defect in the lymph conducting pathways. Secondary lymphedema is due to an acquired cause. (From Kerchner K, Fleischer A, Yosipovitch G. Lower extremity lymphedema update: pathophysiology, diagnosis, and treatment guidelines. *J Am Acad Dermatol.* 2008;59(2):324-331.)

TABLE 1. Stages of Lymphedema

Latency	Risk for lymphedema present. No clinical change evident
Stage I	Pitting, reduces overnight with simple measures (elevation). No fibrosis
Stage II	No longer pitting, no full reduction with elevation, evident fibrosis
Stage III	Nonreversible, hardened fibrosis and sclerosis of cutaneous and subcutaneous tissues

From International Society of Lymphology. The diagnosis and treatment of peripheral lymphedema. 2009 Consensus Document of the International Society of Lymphology. *Lymphology.* 2009;42(2):51-60.

TABLE 2. Physical Treatments for Lymphedema

Treatment	Effect
Exercise	Dynamic muscle contractions encourage movement of lymph along tissue planes and noncontractile, initial lymph vessels (passive drainage) and increased contractility of collecting lymph vessels (active drainage).
Compression garments	Opposes capillary filtration Acts as a counterforce to muscle contractions generating greater interstitial pressure changes
Manual lymphatic drainage	Form of massage therapy that stimulates lymph flow in more proximal, normally draining lymphatics to "siphon" lymph from congested areas
Compression bandaging	Used as an intensive treatment in combination with exercise to reduce large, misshapen lower limbs and permit subsequent maintenance treatment with compression stockings
Pneumatic compression	Softens and reduces limb volume but can forcibly displace fluid into trunk and genitalia. Compression garments must be worn after treatment.
Elevation	Does not stimulate lymph drainage, but lowers venous pressure and therefore capillary filtration, allowing lymph drainage to catch up

From Mortimer PS. ABC of arterial and venous disease swollen lower limb—2: lymphoedema. *BMJ.* 2000;320:1527-1529.

therapy that will completely reverse the clinical condition. Treatment of lymphedema is essentially management of the medical condition and prevention of progression of the disease process. Lymphedema can be successfully managed (Table 1).

The goals of lymphedema therapy are to arrest progression, reduce swelling, maintain that reduction, prevent infection, restore mobility and range of motion, and train patients for self-management.

Physical Treatments

Physical treatment to reduce swelling is aimed at controlling lymph formation and improving lymph drainage through existing lymphatic vessels and collateral routes by applying normal physical processes that stimulate lymph flow (Table 2).

Manual therapies in multiple forms remain the most widely used interventions for the therapeutic management of lymphedema, regardless of etiology. MLD is a highly specialized form of massage therapy that employs very light and gentle cutaneous distension to enhance lymph transport. MLD is believed to stimulate and increase the intrinsic contractility of lymph collecting vessels and encourage increased protein molecule sequestration and subsequent transport.

Complex decongestive therapy (CDT) is a combined approach to lymphedema therapy that has been standardized by multiple international lymphatic treatment organizations and specialized lymphedema treatment programs. The treatment regimen is composed of two phases, intensive reduction therapy followed by maintenance therapy (Table 3). This treatment regimen utilizes MLD, compression wrapping, exercise therapy, and skin care. This highly successful treatment regimen has become the standard of care for lymphedema management. Significant improvement and reduction of swelling is often readily apparent after treatment (Fig. 1).

Compression wrapping in various forms has been a long-standing treatment of both venous and lymphatic edemas. Lymphatic wrapping techniques are complex and utilize low-stretch bandages instead of the more traditional high-stretch elastic bandages. High-stretch wrapping produces high pressures at rest that decrease with limb muscle contraction and movement. This decreases the ability of the wrap to raise the tissue

TABLE 3. Complex Decongestive Therapy

Phase I: Intensive reduction therapy
  Manual lymphatic drainage massage
  Multilayered low-stretch wrapping techniques
  Specific exercise regimen
  Skin care education and techniques

Phase II: Maintenance therapy
  Daily wear of pressure garment
  Continued nightly multilayered wrapping
  Self-manual lymphatic drainage massage
  Exercise
  Continued meticulous skin management

From Gamble GL, Cheville A, Strick D. Lymphedema: medical and physical therapy. In: Gloviczki P, ed. *Handbook of Venous Disorders.* 3rd ed. London, UK: Hodder Arnold, 2009:649-657.

pressure during exercise, reducing the hydrostatic pressure gradient and resulting in a reduction in stimulation of lymphatic flow.

In contrast, low-stretch wrapping provides resistance during muscle pump action that results in an increase in pressure gradient and stimulates increased fluid flow. Patients with significant obesity, pain problems, or advanced disease may not be able to comply with the complexities of wrapping. For these patients, static gradient compression devices are available.

The use of elastic compression garments is the mainstay of the maintenance portion of any lymphedema management program. Compliance with daily use of compression stockings is critical for maintenance of limb size and volume. Compression garments should have graduated compression where pressure is highest distally and decreases proximally where the pressure is lowest at the highest level. For a lower extremity graduated compression stocking, pressure is highest at the ankle and is lowest at the knee, thigh, or waist, depending on the length of the stocking. Recommended graduated compression is 30 to 40 mm Hg for the lower extremity.

Prevention of Infection

Prevention of acute episodes of cellulitis or lymphangitis is critical because they cause severe deterioration in swelling and result in further injury to the lymphatic system. Care of the skin, good hygiene, control of skin diseases such as tinea pedis, and careful antiseptic dressing application after minor wounds are all important. Antibiotics must be administered promptly when an acute inflammatory episode occurs. There are no definitive studies addressing antibiotic prophylaxis for patients at risk for lymphedema, but evidence has shown the relationship between chronic fungal infection and the development of cellulitis, which is known to increase the potential for lymphatic failure.

Surgical Therapy

In situations where CDT fails to improve the size and weight of a lymphedematous limb that is so large, it inhibits its use and interferes with mobility and function, surgery may be of value. Surgery is aimed at either removing excessive tissue (excisional procedures) or bypassing local lymphatic defects (lymphatic reconstruction procedures). CDT is still required after surgical excision and reconstruction.

Excisional procedures usually involve staged removal of the lymphedematous subcutaneous tissue of the leg. The most radical excisional operation, the Charles procedure, involves total skin and subcutaneous tissue excision of the lower extremity from the tibial tuberosity to the malleoli, followed by skin grafting. The main complication associated with this procedure and other excisional procedures is infection and necrosis of the skin graft.

Chronic lymphedematous tissue transforms with time into adipose tissue, which cannot be reduced by massage or compression treatment. Liposuction aimed at removing this adipose tissue has been reported to be beneficial in treating lymphedematous limbs. This procedure is not routinely performed for treatment of lymphedema.

Developments in microvascular techniques have allowed surgical attempts at direct lymphatic reconstructions, performance of lymphatic-venous anastomoses, or lymphatic grafting. These reconstructions are usually indicated in only a small subset of patients who have proximal obstruction with preserved lymphatic vessels distally.

The best outcomes are seen in patients with secondary lymphedema, with well-defined trauma to the lymphatics, seen on lymphatic imaging, who underwent lymphatic to venous anastomoses.

Lymphatic bypass procedures are only performed in a few selected cases and in only a few specialized medical centers. This is reflected in the literature by small patient numbers in most series reported.

Case Conclusion

This patient likely has lymphedema tarda. He was treated intensively with manual lymphatic drainage and, once the swelling was reduced, was fitted with compression garments. He was also instructed on a weight reduction program as well as exercise. With this, his lower extremities remain stable, and he has not had further cellulitis episodes.

TAKE HOME POINTS

- Lymphedema is the result of decreased transport capacity of the lymphatic system.
- Primary lymphedema is due to a congenital defect in the lymph conducting pathways.
- Secondary lymphedema is due to an acquired cause that results in injury and impairment of the lymphatic system.
- Secondary lymphedema represents over 90% of all cases of lymphedema.
- Manual therapies in multiple forms remain the most widely used interventions for the therapeutic management of lymphedema, regardless of etiology.
- Compression therapy remains the mainstay of treatment for lymphedema.
- Surgical therapy is seldom required for the treatment of lymphedema.

SUGGESTED READINGS

Badger C, Preston N, Seers K, et al. Physical therapies for reducing and controlling lymphoedema of the limbs. *Cochrane Database Syst Rev.* 2004;18(4):CD003141.

Gamble GL, Cheville A, Strick D. Lymphedema: medical and physical therapy. In: Gloviczki P, ed. *Handbook of Venous Disorders*. 3rd ed. London, UK: Hodder Arnold; 2009: 649-657.

Gloviczki P. Principles of surgical treatment of chronic lymphedema. In: Gloviczki P, ed. *Handbook of Venous Disorders*. 3rd ed. London, UK: Hodder Arnold; 2009:658-664.

International Society of Lymphology. The diagnosis and treatment of peripheral lymphedema. 2009 Consensus Document of the International Society of Lymphology. *Lymphology*. 2009;42(2):51-60.

Lee B, Andrade M, Bergan J, et al. Diagnosis and treatment of primary lymphedema. Consensus document of the International Union of Phlebology (IUP)-2009. *Int Angiol*. 2010;29(5): 454-470.

Mayrovitz HN. The standard of care for lymphedema: current concepts and physiological considerations. *Lymphat Res Biol*. 2009;7(2):101-108.

Mortimer PS. ABC of arterial and venous disease swollen lower limb—2: lymphoedema. *BMJ*. 2000;320:1527-1529.

Rooke TW, Felty C. Lymphedema: pathophysiology, classification, and clinical evaluation. In: Gloviczki P, ed. *Handbook of Venous Disorders*. 3rd ed. London, UK: Hodder Arnold; 2009:629-634.

Thanaporn PK, Rockson SG. Disease of the lymphatic vasculature. In: Dieter RS, Dieter RA Jr, Dieter RA, eds. *Venous and Lymphatic Diseases*. New York, NY: McGraw Hill; 2011: 569-594.

Tiwari A, Cheng KS, Button M, et al. Differential diagnosis, investigation, and current treatment of lower limb lymphedema. *Arch Surg*. 2003;138(2):152-161.

CLINICAL SCENARIO CASE QUESTIONS

1. A 24-year-old patient presents with new-onset left lower extremity swelling. A DVT duplex scan is negative, and the swelling involves the forefoot. What is the most likely diagnosis?

   a. Congenital lymphedema
   b. Lymphedema praecox
   c. Lymphedema tarda
   d. Secondary lymphedema
   e. Filariasis

2. Primary therapy for lymphedema includes:

   a. Intravenous antibiotics
   b. Manual lymphatic drainage
   c. Surgical removal of excess tissue with skin grafting
   d. Surgical lymphovenous anastomotic construction
   e. Anticoagulation

113 Brachial Artery Injury Following Humerus Fracture

ANDREW S. KAUFMAN and TODD E. RASMUSSEN

Presentation

Case 1 A 21-year-old male presents to the emergency department complaining of right arm pain 2 hours after falling from a ladder onto his outstretched arm. The patient has no relevant past medical or surgical history, and on physical exam, he is in significant pain holding his right arm. There is obvious swelling in the right upper extremity surrounding the elbow, which is tender to palpation. Examination of arm strength and range of motion is limited because of pain in the extremity. Examination of the distal arm reveals a normal-appearing hand with slightly delayed (greater than 3 seconds) capillary refill. Neither the radial nor the ulnar pulse is able to be palpated although there are Doppler signals audible at the distal aspect of both of the arteries at the wrist. On radiographic assessment, the patient is found to have a Gartland type III displaced supracondylar humerus fracture (Fig. 1A and B). A manual blood pressure cuff is used on the forearm in combination with the continuous wave Doppler to calculate the injured extremity index (IEI), which is 0.70.

Case 2 A 22-year-old Marine presents to the resuscitation room 40 minutes following an improvised explosive injury during which he sustained multiple penetrating injuries including a significant soft tissue wound to the right upper extremity. There is a tourniquet tightly secured in place over the proximal portion of the arm, and although there is no active bleeding, there is a significant amount of blood on the bandages covering the arm and hand. Following primary survey and initiation of resuscitation, the patient is found to have a pulseless and pale right hand and with no Doppler signals over the radial or ulnar arteries at the wrist. Radiographic imagining of the extremity demonstrates a complex fracture of the midportion of the humerus.

Differential Diagnosis

A fractured humerus should always lead to a clinical suspicion of a brachial artery injury. Although the artery is injured in a minority of these types of fractures, the proximity of the vessel to the humerus and the harmful consequences of a missed vascular injury call for an astute clinical evaluation. One may encounter two categories of humerus fracture, open and closed. In both of these categories of fracture, the likelihood of brachial artery injury is proportional to the severity of the fracture including the degree of displacement or malalignment. Closed fractures are most common after a fall such as in the first case vignette or other forms of blunt trauma. In contrast, open fractures result from penetrating mechanisms such as gunshot or explosive events. In the most severe of injuries, a blunt humerus fracture may result in the bone penetrating through the skin, which is also considered an open fracture. The differential diagnosis of patients with an injured upper extremity with arm and hand symptoms includes brachial artery injury with varying degrees of ischemia, compression or entrapment of the main peripheral nerves coursing distally through the extremity (radial, ulnar, or median), and/or pain from the fracture.

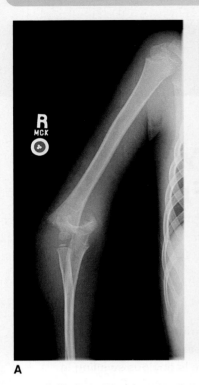
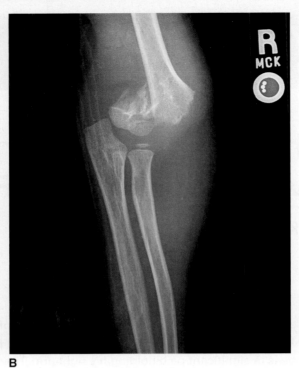

A   **B**

FIGURE 1 • **A, B:** Radiographic images of a Gartland type III fracture of the right supracondylar humerus (Case vignette 1).

Workup

Physical Examination

As one examines the patient with an injured upper extremity, it is useful to consider the differential diagnosis, which, in addition to fracture pain fracture, includes brachial artery spasm, peripheral nerve (i.e., median, radial and ulnar) entrapment, or brachial artery injury with varying degrees of ischemia. In the presence of a humerus fracture, spasm of the brachial artery may result in an initially abnormal-appearing arm and hand with reduced or absent pulses or Doppler signals. This phenomenon is especially common in younger patients, and the secondary vasospasm will often resolve with return of pulses and Doppler signals after reduction and alignment of the fracture. Similarly, after fracture reduction, any artery or nerve entrapment will often resolve with improvement of more distal signs and symptoms.

The physical examination of patients with a suspected or obvious humerus fracture includes assessing the extremity for deformity and a careful evaluation of perfusion to the hand and fingers. Depending on the setting, the physical exam can be performed simultaneous with plain radiographs (multiple views of the humerus, the shoulder, and the elbow) to diagnose and assess the severity of the fracture (Fig. 1A and B). A general guide is that a posterior or lateral fracture dislocation of the humerus is more commonly associated with a brachial artery injury, whereas a medial or anterior dislocation is more commonly associated with radial nerve injury.

The vascular exam of the upper extremity begins with observing for hard signs of vascular injury such as arterial bleeding from open wound(s), an expanding or tense hematoma, or obvious ischemia of the hand and fingers. Palpation for the brachial pulse just above and medial to the antecubital fossa and the radial and ulnar pulses at the wrist should be performed, and capillary refill should be estimated on the distal aspect of the fingers.

Continuous wave Doppler is an extension of the physical exam in patients with a humerus fracture. Doppler signals should be assessed in the same locations at which pulses were palpated (antecubital fossa, radial and ulnar arteries at the wrist). Strong, biphasic signals audible at these locations argues against a brachial artery injury, while weak, monophasic, or absent arterial signals signify a flow-limiting arterial defect. To more objectively assess perfusion of the arm and hand, one can measure the IEI.

The IEI is a ratio of the occlusion pressure of the distal arterial Doppler signal in the injured compared to the noninjured upper extremity. To accomplish this, a manual blood pressure cuff is placed over the forearm of the injured upper extremity and inflated while the Doppler signal is being listened to at the radial and then the ulnar artery. The cuff pressure at which the arterial signal occludes at each of the arteries should be recorded and then these steps repeated on the uninjured upper extremity. The IEI is calculated by dividing the highest occlusion pressure on the injured extremity by the occlusion pressure of the uninjured extremity with a normal index being 0.9 or greater. The IEI provides an objective and repeatable measure by which to assess for arterial injury and is especially useful in scenarios where perfusion distal to the humerus fracture may not be obvious.

Additional Imaging versus Operation

Patients with hard signs of brachial artery injury (i.e., external hemorrhage, profound or obvious ischemia, arteriovenous fistula, and expanding hematoma) typically do not need additional imaging or workup prior to being taken to the operating room for exploration and treatment. One exception to this is the case in which the patient has additional injuries that require further imaging. For example, the patient in the second case vignette had the hard sign of hemorrhage requiring tourniquet application and requires little additional imaging of the arm before the operation. However, this patient may very well require imaging of other injuries (i.e., head, chest, and abdomen) prior to initiating treatment of the arm.

Patients who have a humerus fracture and soft or less clear signs of vascular injury (i.e., modestly reduce IEI, audible but abnormal sounding Doppler signals, equivocal capillary refill) pose a more challenging diagnostic scenario. In the first clinical vignette, additional imaging with arteriography, contrast tomography (CT), or duplex ultrasonography may be useful in making the decision as to whether or not to operate on the brachial artery. Because of the relatively superficial nature of the brachial artery, duplex ultrasound is often the imaging modality of choice as it is quick, inexpensive, and noninvasive. However, standard catheter-based arteriography or CT angiography may also be used to discern the presence of flow-limiting defects or injuries in the brachial artery following humerus fracture.

It is important to restate that in all cases of humerus fracture that the initial step of management, often even before additional imaging, is fracture reduction and stabilization of the extremity. This can often be performed outside of the operating room following hemorrhage control, initiation of resuscitation, and pain control measures. In nearly all cases of significant fracture with dislocation or misalignment, this management step should be pursued regardless of initial signs of vascular injury. Depending on the severity of and the time since the injury, reducing and stabilizing the fracture may favorably change perfusion to the arm and the associated vascular exam. In most cases of mild to moderate humerus fracture, the decision as to whether or not to operate on or further image a brachial artery is made after the fracture is reduced and the vascular exam is repeated. If signs of vascular injury persist after fracture reduction and stabilization, then additional imaging with one of the previously noted modalities is indicated. In cases of extreme open humerus fracture (i.e., the mangled extremity) such as the second case vignette, fracture reduction and stabilization and exploration of the brachial artery should occur simultaneously in the operating room.

Treatment Decision

If physical signs of malperfusion persist or evidence of brachial artery injury are evident after fracture reduction, efforts to restore normal perfusion to the arm and hand should be undertaken in most cases. In rare instances of damage control surgery or those cases in which the ischemia is incomplete (i.e., injury distal to the profunda brachii) and felt to be tolerable, brachial artery injuries can be observed. However, like lower extremity ischemia, chronic malperfusion to the arm and hand can lead to debilitating neuromuscular atrophy and dysfunction and even tissue loss.

Surgical Approach

Brachial artery injury should be approached with an open surgical incision in nearly all cases. While isolated reports of catheter-based treatment of this injury pattern exist, the brachial artery's superficial and accessible position in the upper extremity and its relatively small size make it most amenable to open repair. To expose and operate on the brachial artery, the patient should be placed supine on the operating table with the arm extended out onto an arm table. To facilitate concurrent management of the humerus fracture, it is often useful to have a radiolucent arm board and mobile fluoroscopy.

The axilla should be shaved and the hand and fingers included in the surgical scrub so that they are accessible to examine during and after revascularization. The brachial artery should be approached through a median incision in the upper arm in the crease between the biceps and triceps muscle groups. The incision should be positioned proximal enough to allow exposure and control of the brachial artery, which can include extending the exposure proximal into the axilla through an S-shaped incision if needed.

The brachial artery rests in the groove between the biceps and triceps muscle groups and is adjacent and often crossed by one or more brachial veins. From its proximal segment, the brachial artery gives rise to a deep arterial branch referred to as the profunda brachii. Depending on its size, this artery can provide a significant amount of perfusion to the distal upper extremity assuming it or its collateral branches have not been injured with the fracture. In some instances in which the extent of the profunda brachii is preserved, ligation of the main brachial artery distal to the profunda origin is well tolerated. If this approach is considered, it will be necessary to monitor distal perfusion in the intra- and perioperative period to assure that the deep brachial artery is sufficient to avoid adverse effects of ischemia.

The median nerve courses adjacent to the brachial artery and veins through most of the upper arm, and some have referred to this relatively fixed compartment as the axillary and brachial sheath. Once the area of brachial artery injury is exposed, proximal and control of the vessel with loops or small vascular clamps should be obtained. The zone of brachial artery injury should be dissected free of surrounding structures and the extent of injury determined. Depending on the severity of injury, vascular repair will require primary closure, patch angioplasty, or interposition grafting. Because of its relatively small and elastic nature, most significant brachial artery repairs will require removal of the injured segment and restoration of flow using an interposition graft.

Prior to repairing the brachial artery, removal of thrombus proximal and distal to the injury should be accomplished using a small (2 or 3 French) Fogarty thromboembolectomy catheter. Once this has been accomplished, one should assure that there is ample fore and back bleeding and then instill heparinized saline solution proximal and distal to the injured segment. The edges of the injured vessel should be debrided to assure that the suture repair is performed through normal or nontraumatized, full-thickness vascular wall. Regardless of the type of reconstruction (primary, patch, or interposition), repair should be completed using fine (6-0 or 7-0), monofilament, permanent suture such as polypropylene (Prolene). In most cases, autologous saphenous vein should be used for the patch or the interposition graft. If vein is not available, synthetic path or conduit such as ePTFE (expanded polytetrafluoroethylene) may be used. Assessment of perfusion following completion of the vascular repair can be made using intraoperative Doppler or duplex and occasionally contrast arteriography. The vascular repair should be covered with viable muscle and soft tissue to reduce the likelihood of anastomotic infection or desiccation and disruption.

Special Considerations for Operative Repair

Temporary Vascular Shunt

The use of temporary vascular shunts as a quicker and simpler way to restore perfusion to the arm and hand in instances of severe brachial artery injury is an accepted damage control maneuver. This adjunct may be especially useful to reduce ischemic times in cases in which the operating team has limited experience with formal vascular reconstruction or in cases where the patient has higher priority, life-threatening injuries. Shunts have also been shown to be effective at quickly restoring perfusion to the arm and hand prior to formal fixation of the humerus fracture. In these cases, the injury is explored, the shunt placed, the fracture reduced and fixated, and then the shunt removed for formal vascular repair.

Use of a temporary vascular shunt for a brachial artery injury should be preceded by the previously described steps including exploration of the injury, proximal and distal control, removal of thrombus, and assurance of proximal inflow and distal back bleeding. At this juncture, the temporary vascular shunt is gently inserted and secured either with the vessel loops or with a silk free tie. Patency of the shunt can be confirmed using continuous wave Doppler. The most commonly used shunts are the smaller (8 or 10 French) Argyl or the shorter (15 cm) Sundt shunt.

Anticoagulation

Heparin sulfate as an anticoagulant should be used when possible in the setting of brachial artery injury and repair. In cases where the injury is isolated and not associated with a significant soft tissue wound, normal or full doses (50 to 75 U/kg) of systemic heparin can be given at the time that the arterial injury is being explored. If the patient has other injuries or a large open, soft tissue wound, which preclude the use of systemic anticoagulation, "regional" heparin can be administered in the form of heparinized saline solution. Typically, heparinized saline contains anywhere between 1000 and 10,000 U of heparin per liter of sterile saline, and this can be flushed proximal and distal to the vascular reconstruction as well as used to irrigate the vessel during the time of the repair. Unless there are untoward events that accompany the vascular repair such as large amounts of distal thrombus or a repair that thromboses and requires revision, the use of heparin in the postoperative period is not required.

Fasciotomy

Fasciotomy is not usually required in the case of brachial artery injury repair because of the relative small mass of muscle in the forearm and hand and the less constrained compartments of the forearm. However, in cases in which the ischemic time has been greater than 6 hours or in which there has been significant blast or crush injury, it is recommended that a fasciotomy be performed. The forearm has three compartments that should be opened at the time of fasciotomy: dorsal or extensor, volar or flexor, and mobile wad. If the volar compartment is tight upon opening, it is recommended that the carpal tunnel be released in order to avoid entrapment or compression of the median nerve.

Postoperative Care and Management

The upper extremity must be closely monitored in the postoperative setting including repeat assessment for adequate perfusion. In most instances, this is performed with a continuous wave Doppler machine and pen although a duplex ultrasound machine is also useful in the mid- and longer-term period. Unless unusual complications accompanied the brachial artery repair, systemic anticoagulation is not required in the postoperative period. In most cases, the heparin from the operating room is allowed to dissipate, and then patients receive low-dose, low molecular weight heparin or antiplatelet therapy or both. If a vascular reconstruction has been performed (primary, patch, or interposition repair), duplex surveillance of this should be performed at 6 and 12 months after the operation. Annual duplex ultrasounds of the repair are desired thereafter although these can be difficult to continue in younger trauma patients.

Case Conclusion

In the first case vignette after initiation of monitored sedation and pain control, the patient has the right supracondylar fracture reduced and aligned. After this maneuver, pulses were able to be palpated in the radial and ulnar arteries. The IEI was repeated and found to be 0.90. The patient underwent duplex ultrasound of the brachial artery at the time of open reduction and internal fixation (ORIF) of the humerus demonstrating no flow-limiting defects. The patient was closely monitored after repair of the fracture including repeat duplex of the brachial artery at 7 and 30 days both of which showed normal flow through the brachial artery.

The patient in the second case vignette was initially treated at a forward surgical team (FST) facility where the tourniquet was removed in the operating room when the penetrating wound was explored. In addition to the open humerus fracture, the brachial artery and median nerve were found to be severed by the penetrating fragment. As a matter of damage control or abbreviated operating, the patient had a shunt placed in the right brachial artery reperfusing the right arm and hand prior to forearm fasciotomy and external fixation of the humerus fracture. At the conclusion of this 60-minute operation, the patient's arm was stabilized and there were palpable pulses in the radial and ulnar arteries.

The patient was evacuated to a higher echelon of care (level III surgical hospital) where he arrived with a well-perfused hand. A radiograph was taken of his right arm upon arrival demonstrating an aligned humerus fracture and an indwelling temporary vascular shunt (Fig. 2). The patient was taken to the operating room where the right upper extremity wounds were explored and the Javid shunt found to be patent by Doppler exam. The median nerve was identified as severed and tagged with monofilament suture (Fig. 3). The patient was positioned and prepped such that distal great saphenous vein could be harvested and used as conduit for the interposition graft following shunt removal (Figs. 4 and 5). Following removal of the shunt and placement of a reversed great saphenous vein interposition graft, the patient's wounds were debrided and irrigated and viable tissue used to close over the vascular reconstruction and severed median nerve. A closed, negative pressure wound therapy device was used to cover the wounds (Fig. 6), and the patient was evacuated out of the theater of war 18 hours later (Table 1).

TAKE HOME POINTS

- Complete neurovascular exam should be documented with any humerus fracture.
- Triage injuries; life over limb and a limb tourniquet use can be lifesaving.

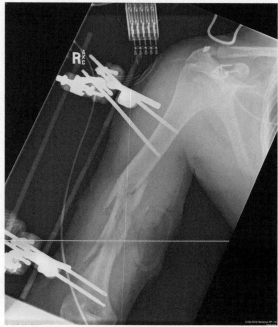

FIGURE 2 • Radiograph of right upper extremity showing open humerus fracture and a temporary vascular shunt, which was placed as a damage control adjunct to restore perfusion prior placement of the external fixator and patient evacuation to a high echelon of care (Case vignette 2).

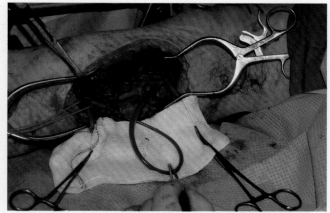

FIGURE 3 • Operative photograph showing a Javid temporary vascular shunt in the right brachial artery (Case vignette 2). The Javid shunt was confirmed to be patent with a continuous wave Doppler machine. Note that the severed median nerve has been identified and tagged with fine polypropylene suture.

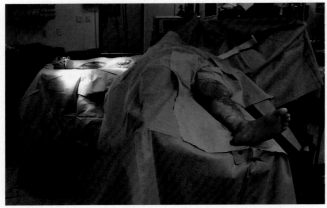

FIGURE 4 • The patient in vignette 2 is shown in the higher echelon operating room at the time of shunt removal and formal vascular repair. The patient's distal left leg has been prepped for harvest of the distal great saphenous vein to be used as conduit.

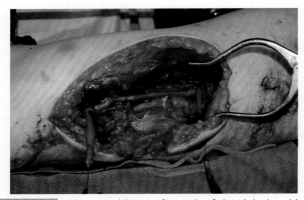

FIGURE 5 • Interposition graft repair of the right brachial artery after shunt removal. The interposition graft is a reverse greater saphenous vein taken from the patient's left ankle. Note that the severed median nerve has been tagged with polypropylene sutures for repair at a later time (Case vignette 2).

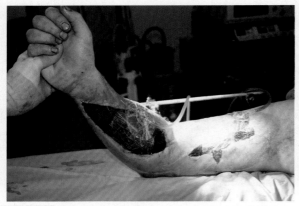

FIGURE 6 • Following soft tissue coverage over the interposition graft and the tagged median nerve, a closed negative pressure wound therapy device (VAC) has been applied to the wounds of the right upper extremity including the fasciotomy wound on the right forearm (Case vignette 2).

TABLE 1. Key Technical Steps and Potential Pitfalls

Key Technical Steps

1. Proper and complete neurovascular exam is essential with a humerus fracture.
2. Use IEI for quantifying blood flow between injured and noninjured arm.
3. Can use local heparinization if systemic heparinization is contraindicated.
4. In severe injury, use of a temporary shunt is indicated.
5. Use autologous tissue for definitive repair.

Potential Pitfalls

- Always reduce the fracture first.
- Soft tissue coverage over arterial repair is essential—don't place VAC (vacuum assisted dressing device) over artery directly.
- Consider fasciotomy of distal arm if tight—particularly in pediatric patients.

- Reduce fracture first—often, impaired blood flow will improve to normal.
- Use temporary arterial shunt if a prolonged time is needed for other injuries to be treated.
- Definitive revascularization should be with autologous tissue, usually greater saphenous vein.

SUGGESTED READINGS

Choi PD, Melikian R, Skaggs DL. Risk factors for vascular repair and compartment syndrome in the pulseless supracondylar humerus fracture in children. *J Pediatr Orthop.* 2010;30:50-56.

Clouse WD, Rasmussen TE, Perlstein J, et al. Upper extremity vascular injury: a current in-theater wartime report from operation Iraqi Freedom. *Ann Vasc Surg.* 2006;20:429-434.

Franz RW, Goodwin RB, Hartman JF, et al. Management of upper extremity arterial injuries at an urban levels I trauma center. *Ann Vasc Surg.* 2009;23:8-16.

Stranes BW, Beekley AC, Sebesta JA, et al. Extremity vascular injuries on the battlefield: tips for surgeons deploying to war. *J Trauma.* 2006;60(2):432-442.

Zellweger R, Hess F, Nicol A, et al. An analysis of 124 surgically managed brachial artery injuries. *Am J Surg.* 2004;188:240-245.

CLINICAL SCENARIO CASE QUESTIONS

1. The IEI is defined as:

    a. Intraosseous blood flow by duplex
    b. Similar to traumatic brain injury (TBI) in number ranges
    c. Allows comparison of injured to noninjured arm
    d. It is the occlusion pressure of the proximal brachial artery
    e. It is most useful in dealing with a mangled extremity

2. In a patient with a multi-injury trauma and right upper extremity (RUE) open humerus fracture with nonpalpable radial and ulnar pulses, after stabilization and resuscitation, the next first step is:

    a. Administer systemic heparin to prevent further thrombosis.
    b. Reduce the fracture.
    c. At bedside, place arterial shunt.
    d. Fixate the fracture externally.
    e. Perform nerve assessment and repair if transected.

114 Endovascular Repair of Acute Aortic Transection

STEPHANIE M. CARVALHO and MARK F. CONRAD

Presentation

A 54-year-old man with no past medical history presents to the emergency department after he struck the handlebars of his dirt bike while attempting to jump 75 feet. He was wearing a helmet and had no loss of consciousness. He was ambulating at the scene but complained of difficulty breathing. First responders noted subcutaneous emphysema and decreased breath sounds. They attempted bilateral needle decompression of his lungs in the field with no relief of symptoms. He continued to decompensate in the field and was intubated and transported to the emergency department. His vitals upon presentation are blood pressure (BP) 90/50, heart rate (HR) 110 beats per minute, oxygen saturation (O_2 Sat) 90%, and Glasgow Coma Scale 4T (patient is intubated and withdraws to pain). He has bruising on his sternum and substantial subcutaneous emphysema that extends from the shoulders to the diaphragm. The normal trauma protocol is followed, during which he receives two large-bore IVs, undergoes a negative FAST exam, and has bilateral 36-F chest tubes placed with return of 500 mL of blood from the left chest and no blood from the right. He responds to the fluid and chest decompression, and his vitals improve to BP 120/60 and HR 80, and pulse oximetry is 100%. The following x-ray is obtained (Fig. 1).

Differential Diagnosis

The main pathologic causes of a widened mediastinum on chest x-ray are chest masses and enlargement of the great vessels. Common masses include lymphoma, thyroid enlargement, teratoma, and thymus tumors. An aneurysm of the aortic arch or descending thoracic aorta will also lead to a widened mediastinum. However, in a patient with a significant mechanism of blunt injury to the chest, the most likely cause is a traumatic aortic tear, and this must be diagnosed expediently.

Workup

A high-velocity head-on motor vehicle crash or blunt force to the chest leads to rapid deceleration of the body and can cause the aorta to tear along its attachment at the ligamentum arteriosum. A history of this mechanism of injury should increase the index of suspicion for a traumatic aortic tear. Other major injuries to the chest such as multiple rib fractures, flail chest, or pulmonary contusion should also make one think of an acute aortic tear, as should a widened mediastinum on chest x-ray. In the setting of blunt chest trauma, if there is a suspicion of traumatic aortic tear, the next test to obtain is a CT angiogram of the chest. These patients usually present with multiple injuries, and most trauma protocols involve scanning the chest, abdomen, and pelvis at the same time to identify occult solid organ injuries. It is important to stabilize the patient using the ABCs of trauma resuscitation prior to traveling from the trauma bay to radiology for further imaging studies.

Chest CTA

In the region of the aortic isthmus distal to the origin of the left subclavian artery, there is intimal injury with elevation of an intimal flap and pseudoaneurysm of the descending aorta at the level of the ligamentum arteriosum (Fig. 2). There is also accompanying intraluminal thrombus. The pseudoaneurysm is located approximately 2.2 cm distal to the origin of the left subclavian artery. There is an intermediate density hematoma surrounding the descending aorta to the level of the renal arteries with no evidence of active extravasation.

Diagnosis

Grade 3 traumatic aortic tear.

Discussion

Although rare, injury to the thoracic aorta is the second leading cause of death (head injury is most common) after blunt force trauma. This is usually a lethal condition with a greater than 80% mortality rate at the scene of the accident, and contemporary autopsy studies of patients after blunt trauma have reported the incidence of aortic rupture to be approximately 30%. The most common mechanism for this injury remains motor vehicle crashes,

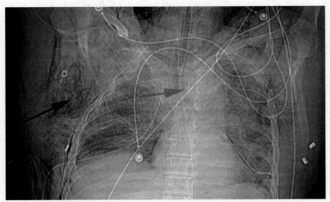

FIGURE 1 • The patient's initial supine chest x-ray. It shows that the patient has an endotracheal tube and bilateral chest tubes in place. The *red arrow* points to the widened mediastinum. The *black arrow* points to the extensive subcutaneous emphysema seen throughout the x-ray.

especially head on collisions because of the transfer of energy between the two vehicles and the rapid deceleration that is experienced by their occupants.

Traumatic aortic injuries occur across a spectrum of lesions, and a grading system has been developed to help guide management. A grade 1 injury amounts to an intimal tear with no violation of the media or adventitia of the aorta. These are usually treated conservatively with medical management. Grade 2 injuries involve the intima and media of the aorta and present as in intramural hematoma. These represent a gray zone of management as many can be treated medically with serial CTA follow-up, but some will progress to rupture and need treatment. Although the general recommendation is

to treat grade 2 injuries, it is important to consider the patient's overall condition when addressing these lesions. A grade 3 injury involves all three layers of the aorta with pseudoaneurysm formation, and a grade 4 injury is a frank rupture. Both of these injuries require early intervention.

Medical management consists of strict BP control with beta blockade and afterload reduction in order to decrease aortic wall stress. It is common for these patients to have other injuries and repair of a grade 2 to 3 tear may have to be deferred for more pressing injuries such as an actively bleeding pelvic fracture or solid organ injury. The current Society for Vascular Surgery (SVS) guidelines recommend that all patients with grade 2 to 4 injuries undergo repair. In the absence of other injuries, repair should be performed within 24 hours of the initial presentation if possible.

Preoperative Planning

The CTA should be used to develop an operative plan. It is important to have 2 cm of normal aorta proximal to the tear in order to obtain an adequate seal. Due to the location of the aortic tear, it is common to have to cover the left subclavian artery but the graft rarely needs to extend beyond the origin of the left common carotid artery. In the emergent setting, we have not routinely revascularized the left subclavian artery with a carotid to subclavian bypass as this will delay therapy and is unnecessary in most patients. The diameter of the aorta is measured in the proximal seal zone and then 10 cm distally. It is best to obtain these measurements in the centerline fashion using three-dimensional image planning software. If this is not available or an accurate diameter cannot be obtained, intravascular ultrasound (IVUS) can be used to obtain an accurate centerline measurement during the procedure. Finally, the access vessels

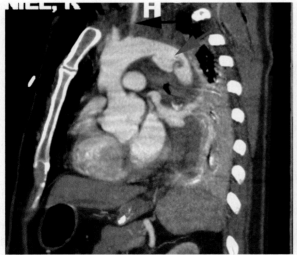

A

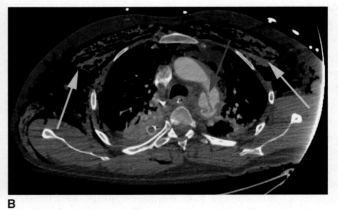

B

FIGURE 2 • **A:** This is an oblique view of the aorta showing the aortic tear (*red arrow*) with intima floating free within the aorta and surrounding hematoma of the pseudoaneurysm. The left subclavian artery (*black arrow*) is proximal to the tear. **B:** Axial view of the chest showing the extensive subcutaneous emphysema (*yellow arrows*). The aortic tear has led to a complex infolding of the intima with surrounding hematoma (*red arrow*).

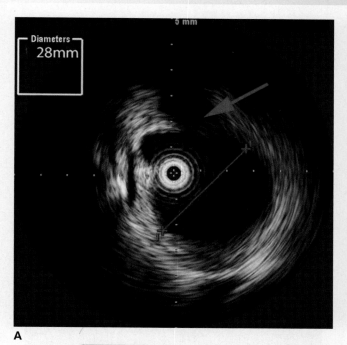
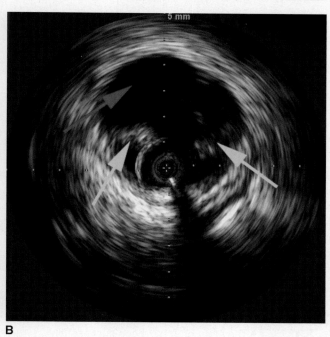

A

B

FIGURE 3 • **A:** Static IVUS image of the aorta proximal to the traumatic tear. The *purple line* gives a true centerline measurement of 28 mm at the level of the origin of the left subclavian artery (*red arrow*). **B:** Static IVUS image of the aortic tear. The intimal flaps are free flowing in the aorta (*yellow arrows*), and there is a contained pseudoaneurysm outside the aortic wall (*red arrow*).

need to be assessed for adequate size to deliver a 20- to 24-F sheath (needs to be at least 7 mm in diameter without calcium). This can be an issue in young females, and a conduit may be needed to safely deliver the device.

There are currently two commercially available stent grafts in the United States with an indication for traumatic tear. They are the Conformable GORE TAG Thoracic Endoprosthesis (W.L. Gore and Associates Inc., Flagstaff, AZ) and the Valiant Captivia Stent Graft (Medtronic, Santa Rosa, CA). Grafts are chosen based upon the sizing recommendations of the manufacturer. Ultimately, the oversizing may be determined by what is stocked on the OR shelves such that centers with a high volume of blunt thoracic injuries should have a good selection of grafts available.

Case Continued

The patient was placed in the supine position with a roll under the left chest to improve visualization of the aortic arch. The abdomen and groins were prepped and draped in a sterile fashion. The left common femoral artery was exposed through a small transverse incision. The patient was given 5000 U of heparin. A Kumpe catheter was used to drive a glidewire beyond the lesion and into the arch. A stiff wire was then placed. The IVUS catheter was advanced over the wire through a 9-F sheath and was used to identify the pseudoaneurysm and the proximal and distal seal zones (Fig. 3). The proximal seal zone was measured to be 28 mm by IVUS, and the distal was 24 mm. A tapered stent graft (32 to 28 mm) with a 120-mm length was chosen. A pigtail catheter was advanced into the aorta from a 5-F sheath placed in the opposite groin. An angiogram

was performed prior to graft deployment (Fig. 4), and the graft was deployed so that it partially covered the left subclavian artery (Fig. 5). There were no endoleaks so the graft was not ballooned. The hardware was removed and the artery was repaired with a 5-0 Prolene stitch.

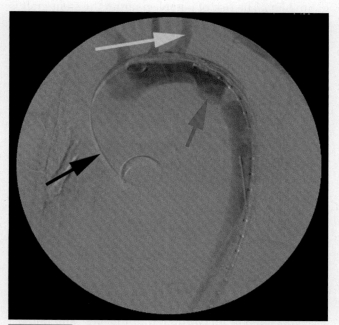

FIGURE 4 • Predeployment angiogram with a stiff wire in the ascending aorta (*black arrow*). The stent graft has been advanced to the level of the pseudoaneurysm (*red arrow*). The landing zone will be at the level of the left subclavian artery (*yellow arrow*).

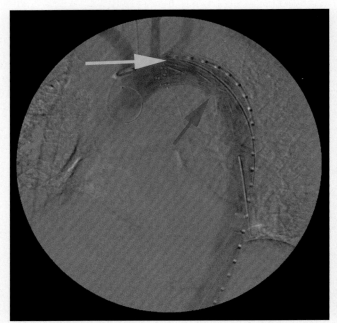

FIGURE 5 • The stent graft has been successfully deployed with partial coverage of the left subclavian artery (*yellow arrow*) and complete exclusion of the pseudoaneurysm (*red arrow*). There is no evidence of endoleak.

Postoperative Management

The patient is kept in the ICU for at least 24 hours. However, most have long recovery times secondary to the concomitant injuries that often accompany acute aortic transection. The BP parameters can be liberalized as necessary for optimal treatment of things like traumatic brain injury. The risk of paraplegia from the stent graft is low due to the short lengths of coverage. If paraplegia/paraparesis does occur, the patient can be treated with a spinal drain and increased systolic BP. If the subclavian artery was covered, a carotid subclavian bypass can also be performed. Assessing the status of the vertebral arterial bed is important, and if compromised with coverage of the left subclavian, this suggests that a carotid subclavian should be performed.

Patients should be followed with serial CTA. It is recommended that a scan is obtained at 4 to 6 weeks to establish a baseline followed by a scan at 1 year. If the lesion has completely healed around the graft, patients can be surveyed with a noncontrast scan.

Case Conclusion

The patient recovered slowly from his chest injuries and was discharged to a rehabilitation center. He was seen in follow-up 6 months later and had a CTA (Fig. 6). He had returned to his normal life and was still jumping dirt bikes.

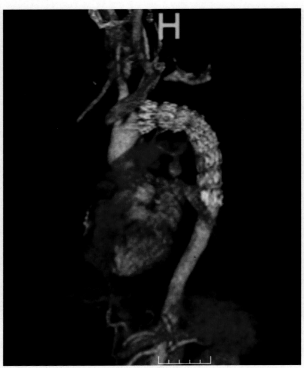

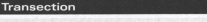

FIGURE 6 • Three-dimensional reconstruction of the descending thoracic aorta at 6-month follow-up visit. The pseudoaneurysm has completely healed around the stent graft, and the aorta is now normal.

TABLE 1. TEVAR for Acute Aortic Transection

Key Technical Steps

1. Accurately plan the procedure by measuring the proximal and distal seal zones and selecting an appropriate stent graft.
2. Ensure that the patient has adequately sized iliac vessels to deliver the device.
3. Routine heparin administration—can be lower dose than standard TEVAR.
4. IVUS can be used to identify landmarks and accurately measure the diameter of the proximal and distal landing zone.
5. Often need to cover the left subclavian artery—rarely revascularize
6. Deploy the graft under fluoroscopic guidance.
7. Ensure adequate treatment with a completion aortogram.
8. Only balloon the graft if an endoleak persists.
9. Repair artery and close the groin.

Potential Pitfalls

- These are usually acute cases, and you will need to make the stent grafts in stock work for the patient's anatomy.
- Young patients have steep aortic arches, and the graft can form a "bird's beak" at the proximal seal zone that can lead to collapse of the graft.
- Access vessels can be too small to deliver the device, especially in the young.
- Aggressive oversizing can lead to pleating of the graft or collapse.

Discussion

The use of TEVAR for treatment of traumatic aortic tear has rapidly increased among surgeons in the United States. A review of the Medicare database showed that the percentage of patients with blunt aortic injuries treated with TEVAR increased from 11% in 2004 to 76% in 2007 and the number is likely higher now. This is in part due to the fact that the short-term mortality rate of patients undergoing TEVAR is half that of those for open repair (10% to 14% for TEVAR vs. 25% to 35% for open repair). There are several additional advantages of TEVAR over open repair of acute aortic injuries including a shorter hospital stay, lower transfusion requirement, and almost no reported cases of paraplegia after TEVAR. Long-term survival also appears to favor TEVAR (Table 1).

TAKE HOME POINTS

- Mechanism of injury should increase your suspicion for acute aortic transection.
- CTA is the best imaging modality to diagnose and plan treatment.
- Grade 2 to 4 injuries should be repaired.
- TEVAR requires advanced endovascular skill to perform expeditiously.
- Plan the case using grafts you have in stock and stock your shelves accordingly.
- Make sure the access vessels are adequate and that you have a good proximal seal zone.
- Limit heparin if the patient has other injuries (especially head trauma).
- Early mortality is better with TEVAR than with open repair.

SUGGESTED READINGS

Akowuah E, Angelini G, Bryan AJ. Open versus endovascular repair of traumatic aortic rupture: a systemic review. *J Thorac Cardiovasc Surg.* 2009;138(3):768-769.

Cambria RP, Crawford RS, Cho JS, et al. A multicenter clinical trial of endovascular stent graft repair of acute catastrophes of the descending thoracic aorta. *J Vasc Surg.* 2009;50: 1255-1264.

Conrad MF, Ergul EA, Patel VI, et al. Management of diseases of the descending thoracic aorta in the endovascular era: a Medicare population study. *Ann Surg.* 2010;252: 603-610.

Lee WA, Matsumura JS, Mitchell RS, et al. Endovascular repair of traumatic thoracic aortic injury: clinical practice guidelines of the Society for Vascular Surgery. *J Vasc Surg.* 2011;53(1): 187-192.

Xenos ES, Abedi NN, Davenport DL, et al. Meta-analysis of endovascular vs open repair for traumatic descending thoracic aortic rupture. *J Vasc Surg.* 2008;48:1343-1351.

CLINICAL SCENARIO CASE QUESTIONS

1. A patient who presents with a full-thickness aortic tear (across the intima, media, and adventitia) that is contained by a pseudoaneurysm would be graded as:

   a. Grade 1
   b. Grade 2
   c. Grade 3
   d. Grade 4
   e. Grade 5

2. Is there a way to accurately size the proximal landing zone if you do not have access to a program that allows you to make a centerline measurement?

   a. No, but this is a trauma so just put in a 25-mm graft and hope for the best.
   b. Yes, IVUS can be used to accurately measure the diameter of the proximal seal zone.
   c. Yes, the candy cane view of the aorta will give an accurate diameter.
   d. Yes, you can serially inflate balloons in the aortic arch until you find the correct size.
   e. Assess with reconstructed MRA.

115 Intra-abdominal Vascular Trauma

NAM T. TRAN and AMELIA J. SIMPSON

Presentation

A 23-year-old patient is brought to the emergency department after a snowmobile crash where he was ejected and landed 100 feet from the vehicle. At the scene, the patient was unconscious and was intubated for airway protection. En route, the patient's vital signs were BP of 80/45 and HR 130s. Initial trauma evaluation was remarkable for normal chest x-ray and lateral C-spine film. His pelvic AP film demonstrated a left pelvic ring fracture. Focused Assessment with Sonography in Trauma (FAST) exam was equivocal for intra-abdominal fluid. Given concern for pelvic bleeding, the patient was taken to the angiography suite. Pelvic angiogram did not show evidence of extravasation.

Differential Diagnosis

Abdominal vascular injuries are among the most lethal injuries in the trauma patient and are also some of the most difficult to deal with by the trauma surgeon. Typically, blunt injury to the abdomen results in injury to the solid organs such as spleen or liver. On the other hand, major vascular injury is seen in only 5% to 25% of patients admitted to the hospital with abdominal trauma. However, this is the most common cause of death in these patients. The high mortality associated with abdominal vascular trauma is multifactorial with the main reasons being massive acute blood loss, associated injuries, and difficulty with gaining rapid control of the injured bleeding vessel.

In our case presentation, the most likely diagnosis should be intra-abdominal hemorrhage. While this is most likely due to solid organ disruption, the possibility of vascular injury should not be excluded. Imaging modality such as multidetector CT can be especially helpful in blunt abdominal trauma. With the use of multiphasic image acquisition, one can not only differentiate arterial versus venous hemorrhage but also characterize areas of "contrast blush" as either contained or active hemorrhage. In recent years, advances in endovascular techniques have transition arteriography from just a diagnostic exam into a therapeutic treatment modality as well.

Case Continued

While in the angiography suite, the patient also underwent abdominal arteriography with the thought that one can embolize solid organ bleed if a contrast blush was present. Instead, the abdominal aortogram demonstrated extravasation from the perivisceral abdominal aorta (Fig. 1).

The patient was then taken urgently to the operating room for definitive treatment.

Operative Approach

The retroperitoneal space along with its vascular structures has been traditionally divided into three zones: zone I (midline), zone II (para median), and zone III (pelvic) (Fig. 2). From an anatomic surgical approach, these zones can be further divided into segments based on the retroperitoneal attachment of the mesentery. This facilitates the exposure and surgical management of vascular structures within each specific zone.

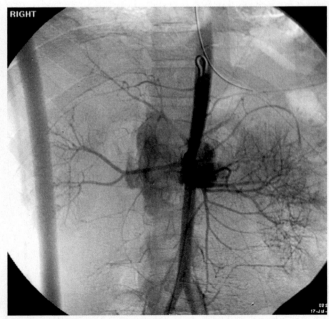

FIGURE 1 • Abdominal aortogram demonstrating contrast blush from the para visceral aorta.

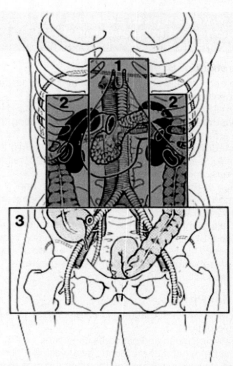

Zone I Supramesocolic

This space contains the suprarenal abdominal aorta, celiac trunk, superior mesenteric artery (SMA) and vein, and the origin of the renal vessels. Exposure of vascular structures in this zone is best accomplished via a left medial visceral rotation. In cases where rapid vascular control is required due to expanding hematoma or active hemorrhage, proximal control of the aorta should be obtained at the supraceliac aorta.

The left medial visceral rotation is best accomplished by initially dividing the retroperitoneal attachments along the line of Toldt and then reflecting the left colon, spleen, left kidney, tail of the pancreas, and gastric fundus to the midline (Fig. 3). With this exposure, the surgeon can visualize the entire abdominal aorta from the diaphragm to the aortic bifurcation. This maneuver, however, does take time and can potentially injure the spleen, left kidney, or left renal artery. Lastly, a critical step to gain proximal control of the aorta with the left medial visceral rotation is adequate division of the left crus so that a vascular clamp can be applied to the supra celiac aorta. Failure to fully mobilize the crus can lead to suboptimal proximal aortic control and ongoing hemorrhage.

Alternative approach to zone I supramesocolic vascular structure is an extended Kocher maneuver (Fig. 4). In this instance, the "C" loop of the duodenum and the head

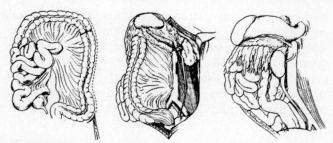

of the pancreas are elevated toward the midline. This approach will allow the surgeon to visualize the suprarenal aorta between the celiac axis and the SMA. However, one will not be able to gain control of the supra celiac aorta from this approach.

Traditionally, one can gain access to the supra celiac aorta via the lesser sac. This is accomplished by dividing the gastrohepatic ligament, pushing the stomach to the left, and using one's fingers to bluntly dissect around the crura of the supra celiac aorta. Placement of a nasogastric tube (NGT) can facilitate identification of the aorta especially in the severely hypotensive patient as the aorta may be flaccid; the aorta will be medial to the esophagus and the NGT as one tries to bluntly dissect in the region of the diaphragmatic hiatus. Lastly, the use of an aortic occlusion device or manual compression with one's hand is an effective method of rapid aortic control at the diaphragm by direct application of pressure to compress the aorta against the spine.

Celiac Trunk

Dense neural and lymphatic tissues surround the celiac artery origin, thus making exposure of this area difficult especially in an actively bleeding patient. Typically, ligation is well tolerated for the left gastric artery, proximal splenic artery, or the common hepatic artery proximal

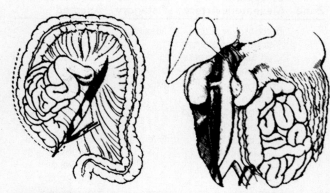

to the origin of the gastroduodenal due to rich collateral networks in this area. Repair to the proper hepatic artery, due to its larger size, can be accomplished via lateral arteriorrhaphy, primary end-to-end anastomosis, or end-to-end bypass graft. Due to the high likelihood of associated hollow viscus injury and spillage, the use of prosthetic conduit is discouraged if arterial bypass is needed.

Superior Mesenteric Artery

Injury to the SMA is thankfully rare as mortality can be high with approximately one third of patients dying within 24 hours of presentation. Outcomes are related to the presence of hypotension, location of injury, presence of bowel infarction, and associated injuries. In 1972, Fullen and colleagues classified SMA injury into four zones with management of either ligation or repair dependent on the zone of injury (Table 1).

In Fullen's zone I, the SMA can be easily visualize and repair via left medial visceral rotation. Alternatively, many surgeons have described directly transecting the pancreas when approaching this area from an anterior approach. As the SMA has not divided into branches, repair of SMA injury in this location is critical, as ligation would lead to necrosis of the entire small bowel and the right colon.

In Fullen's zone II, the SMA gives off branches to the pancreaticoduodenal and the middle colic. In this area, one typically encounters exsanguinating hemorrhage from branch vessel avulsion or complete SMA transection. In the coagulopathic and hypotensive patient, the use of a temporizing vascular shunt at the first damage control laparotomy is much better than either SMA ligation or taking the time needed

TABLE 1. Fullen's Anatomic Classification of SMA Injury

Zone	Segment of Superior Mesenteric Artery	Ischemic Category	Bowel Segments Affected
I	Trunk proximal to first major branch (inferior pancreaticoduodenal)	Maximal	Jejunum, ileum, right colon
II	Trunk between inferior pancreaticoduodenal and middle colic	Moderate	Major segment of small bowel, right colon
III	Trunk distal to middle colic	Minimal	Minor segment of small bowel or right colon
IV	Segmental branches, jejunal, ileal, colic	None	No ischemic bowel

TABLE 2. Key Steps to Exposure and Management of Intra-abdominal Vascular Trauma

Key Technical Steps

1. Exploration should only be done for active hemorrhage or expanding hematoma.
2. Proximal control of the aorta is accomplished by dividing the gastrohepatic ligament and bluntly dissecting the crura around the diaphragmatic hiatus.
3. Left medial visceral rotation involves taking down the line of Toldt and rotating the left colon, spleen, tail of pancreas, and gastric fundus medially.
4. Ligation of the proximal left gastric, splenic, and common hepatic proximal to the gastroduodenal artery origin is well tolerated.
5. SMA injury in Fullen's zones I, II, and III should be revascularized. SMA injury in Fullen's zone IV can be ligated.
6. Prosthetics bypass can be used if there is no spillage. Otherwise, autologous conduit such as greater saphenous vein (GSV) is best.

Potential Pitfalls

- Left medial visceral rotation can take precious time in an unstable patient.
- Injury to the spleen and pancreas can occur.
- Need to be mindful of profound "acid wash out" and irreversible bowel ischemia with prolonged proximal aortic cross clamp.

to perform vascular reconstruction. Once the patient has stabilized, one has time to perform adequate debridement of devitalized tissue as injury to this area often involved the pancreas. Simple lateral arteriorrhaphy is best as long as it does not narrow the lumen of the artery. In cases of extensive injury, the SMA origin can be ligated and the inflow to the SMA can be based on the infrarenal aorta well away from the area of injury to protect the suture lines from potential pancreatic enzyme breakdown.

Injuries to the more distal SMA beyond the transverse colon, Fullen's zone III, should be repaired to maintain perfusion to the distal jejunum and ileum. As the vessel caliber in this region is smaller, interposition bypass will be better than simple arteriorrhaphy repair with choice of conduit such as autologous or prosthetic materials dictated by associated injury and whether or not there is spillage of abdominal contents. Fullen's zone IV injury, or injury to the segmental braches, is best treated with ligation (Table 2).

Renal Artery

Proximal injury to the renal vessels necessitates gaining proximal aortic control at the diaphragmatic hiatus prior to exploration of the hematoma. Once vascular control has been accomplished, a direct anterior approach should be used. This is accomplished by lifting the transverse colon superiorly with the small bowel packed to the right upper quadrant. The ligament of Treitz is divided, and the inferior mesenteric vein is pushed to the left or ligated. With the retroperitoneum overlying the aorta divided, the crossing left renal vein can be visualized. With mobilizing of the left renal vein either superiorly or inferiorly, one can gain access to the origin of both the right and left renal arteries. Repair such as simple arteriorrhaphy or proximal ligation and bypass from the aorta can then be performed to control hemorrhage and restore perfusion to the kidney.

Endovascular Treatment

Within the last 10 years, the application of endovascular surgery has found its way into the management of vascular trauma. A recent report by de Mestral and colleagues examined the National Trauma Data Bank of those patients admitted with the diagnosis of blunt abdominal aortic injury. In a cohort of over 262,000 patients, they identified 436 patients with blunt abdominal vascular injuries. Of these, 42 patients underwent repair with over half (69%) done using endovascular techniques.

A key component of gaining control of the aorta is via prelaparotomy thoracotomy with cross clamping of the thoracic aorta in those patients with abdominal vascular injuries and shock. A report from Detroit Receiving Hospital showed that those patients who respond to aortic cross clamping have a significant higher survival than those that did not. In this regard, the use of endovascular aortic occlusion balloon is an attractive technique to gain control of the aorta in those patients with abdominal vascular injuries. Proximal exposure of the aorta at the diaphragmatic hiatus can be difficult, especially in those patients with expanding supramesocolic hematoma or active hemorrhage. An exploratory laparotomy can decompress the hematoma and send the patient into irreversible hypovolemic shock. By placing an aortic occlusion balloon via transfemoral approach, the trauma surgeon can gain control of the aorta prior to entering the abdomen.

Case Continued

In the operating room, the patient was hemodynamically unstable and became severely hypotensive with general anesthetic induction. Thus, rapid percutaneous entry into his right femoral artery was accomplished, and a Coda balloon was placed above the area of injury and inflated to profile (Fig. 5). The patient had immediate improvement in his hemodynamics. Exploratory laparotomy was carried out with left medial visceral rotation. Proximal aortic control at the hiatus was not required as this was already done with the aortic occlusion balloon. Operative findings include avulsion of the SMA at its origin, or Fullen's zone I. There was no other associated injury. The patient underwent retrograde SMA bypass from the left common

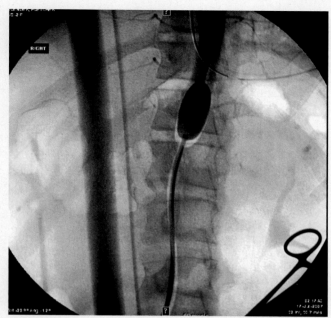

FIGURE 5 • Aortic occlusion balloon for proximal aortic control.

iliac artery with a 6-mm polytetrafluoroethylene (PTFE) graft. Total aortic cross clamp and ischemic time was 35 minutes.

Case Conclusion

The patient's abdomen was left open, and he returned to the operation room 36 hours later for relook laparotomy. At that time, no further injury was identified, and his abdomen was closed. He had an uneventful postoperative course subsequently and was discharged to a rehabilitation unit on hospital day 20. Annual abdominal duplex follow-up of his mesenteric bypass showed it to be widely opened without flow abnormality. At last clinical follow-up, the patient has returned to full activities without any residual effects from his traumatic injury.

TAKE HOME POINTS

- Abdominal vascular injuries are uncommon, but mortality is high (33% to 67%), due to their location as well as associated intra-abdominal trauma pathologies.
- Rapid proximal aortic control at the diaphragm should be done definitively and expediently. Recent advances allow the surgeon to gain proximal aortic control via endovascular aortic balloon occlusion.

- Surgical exposure of the region is best accomplished via extended Kocher maneuver or left medial visceral rotation.
- The use of Fullen's anatomic classification can facilitate intra-operative decision to perform either revascularization or ligation of SMA injury.

SUGGESTED READINGS

Asensio JA, Britt LD, Borzotta A, et al. Multiinstitutional experience with the management of superior mesenteric artery injuries. *J Am Coll Surg.* 2001;193(4):354-365; discussion 365-366.

Asensio JA, Chahwan S, Hanpeter D, et al. Operative management and outcome of 302 abdominal vascular injuries. *Am J Surg.* 2000;180(6):528-533; discussion 533-5334.

Berthet JP, Marty-Ané CH, Veerapen R, et al. Dissection of the abdominal aorta in blunt trauma: endovascular or conventional surgical management? *J Vasc Surg.* 2003;38(5):997-1003.

Castelli P, Caronno R, Piffaretti G, et al. Emergency endovascular repair for traumatic injury of the inferior vena cava. *Eur J Cardiothorac Surg.* 2005;28(6):906-908.

de Mestral C, Dueck AD, Gomez D, et al. Associated injuries, management, and outcomes of blunt abdominal aortic injury. *J Vasc Surg.* 2012;56(3):656-660.

Fox CJ, Gillespie DL, O'Donnell SD, et al. Contemporary management of wartime vascular trauma. *J Vasc Surg.* 2005;41(4):638-644.

Genovese EA, Fonio P, Floridi C, et al. Abdominal vascular emergencies: US and CT assessment. *Crit Ultrasound J.* 2013;5(suppl 1):S10. doi:10.1186/2036-7902-5-S1-S10

Martinelli T, Thony F, Decléty P, et al. Intra-aortic balloon occlusion to salvage patients with life-threatening hemorrhagic shocks from pelvic fractures. *J Trauma.* 2010;68(4):942-948. doi:10.1097/TA.0b013e3181c40579

Mosquera VX, Marini M, Cao I, et al. Traumatic aortic injuries associated with major visceral vascular injuries in major blunt trauma patients. *World J Surg.* 2012;36(7):1571-1580. doi:10.1007/s00268-012-1536-x

Shalhub S, Starnes BW, Tran NT, et al. Blunt abdominal aortic injury. *J Vasc Surg.* 2012;55(5):1277-1285. doi:10.1016/j.jvs.2011.10.132

CLINICAL SCENARIO CASE QUESTIONS

1. With regard to injury to the celiac trunk, which of these vessels should *not* be ligated?
   a. Splenic artery
   b. Left gastric artery
   c. Common hepatic artery proximal to the gastroduodenal origin
   d. Common hepatic artery distal to the gastroduodenal origin

2. Which of the following vascular structures is not located in zone I supramesocolic region?
   a. Superior mesenteric artery
   b. Celiac trunk
   c. Renal artery
   d. Superior mesenteric vein
   e. Left renal vein

116 Upper Extremity Trauma

DAVID L. GILLESPIE and MARLENE O'BRIEN

Presentation

A 31-year-old male presents as a level 2 trauma alert for multiple gunshot wounds to the extremities. Upon arrival in the trauma bay, he is agitated and writhing in pain, although protecting his airway with an oxygen saturation of 98%. He is hemodynamically stable with HR 85, RR 24, and BP 125/98 mm Hg. On careful examination, he has lacerations over his right shoulder, two penetrating injuries over his bilateral buttocks, and a through-and-through penetrating injury of his left forearm. He has 2+ bilateral radial pulses and no associated pulsatile bleeding.

Left Upper Extremity X-Ray

Two paper clips overlie the proximal to mid forearm. Tiny metallic opacities are noted in this region amidst marked soft tissue swelling and some subcutaneous emphysema. No acute fracture is seen (Fig. 1).

Approach

As with any acute trauma, the treatment algorithm starts with Advanced Trauma Life Support (ATLS): airway, breathing, circulation, disability, and exposure. The patient has palpable bilateral radial pulses, but has a penetrating through-and-through injury of his left forearm that raises concern for potential vascular injury. Only a minority of patients actually present with hard signs of traumatic vascular injury, including observed pulsatile bleeding, palpable thrill, audible bruit on auscultation, absent distal pulse, or a visible expanding hematoma (Table 1). A pulse deficit may not initially be present due to extensive collaterals in the arm; therefore, soft signs of traumatic vascular injury warrant further diagnostic workup: significant hemorrhage by history, neurologic abnormality, diminished pulse compared with contralateral extremity and proximity of bony injury, or penetrating wound (Table 1). A through-and-through penetrating injury of the left forearm, despite a palpable radial pulse, necessitates further investigation.

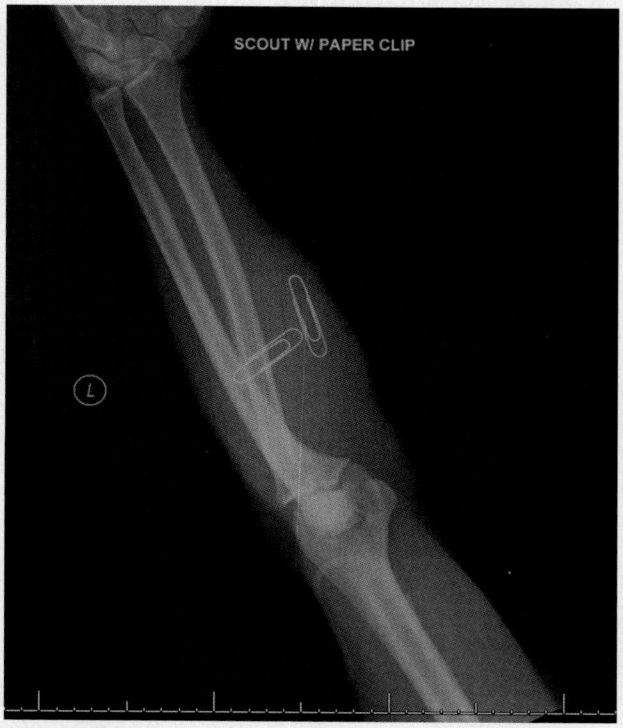

Case Continued

The patient's left upper extremity is tender to palpation without crepitus. Sensory and motor function of both upper extremities is intact, although the left hand is markedly cooler than the right. Because he is hemodynamically stable and has multiple penetrating injuries, the decision is made to send him to the CT scanner for further imaging, including CT angiography of his left upper extremity.

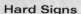

SCOUT W/ PAPER CLIP

FIGURE 1 • Left upper extremity x-ray demonstrating tiny metallic opacities and soft tissue swelling by an area of penetrating trauma (*paper clips*).

TABLE 1. Signs of Traumatic Vascular Injury

Hard Signs
- Pulsatile bleeding
- Arterial thrill on palpation
- Bruit auscultated over arterial injury
- Absent distal pulse
- Visible expanding hematoma

Soft Signs
- Close proximity of bony injury or soft tissue destruction
- Diminished pulses
- Neurologic abnormality
- Significant hemorrhage by history

Workup and Diagnosis

The patient has no hard signs of vascular trauma and is hemodynamically stable. At this time, the diagnostic test of choice is CT angiography. The main indications for CTA of upper extremity arterial injuries are as follows: (1) exclusion of vascular injury in the absence of clinical hard signs and (2) determination of injury location, nature, and extent of vascular injury when not clearly evident on physical examination. CTA has acceptable sensitivity and specificity for diagnosing vascular injury and has increasingly replaced both Doppler ultrasound and conventional angiography in the diagnosis of upper extremity vascular injury, except when a comminuted fracture may decrease its sensitivity.

Left Upper Extremity CT Angiogram

Abrupt cut off of the radial artery suspicious for arterial injury. No active extravasation. Irregularity of the ulnar artery. There is an associated large hematoma. No active extravasation. This may represent an arm compartment syndrome due to hematoma (Fig. 2).

Recommendations

The patient should be taken to the operating room for a left upper extremity exploration and potential vascular repair. In cases of nonocclusive vascular injury, such as pseudoaneurysms or intimal flaps that do not threaten limb viability, conservative therapy with the initiation of antiplatelet therapy and repeat delayed imaging may be acceptable. In this case, however, the injury appears occlusive despite a reassuring physical exam.

In situations where bony injury coexists with vascular trauma, vascular repair is usually undertaken prior to orthopedic repair because ischemic time is critical to overall outcome. Exceptions to this are in cases of unstable fractures, where external fixation is required immediately to stabilize the limb to prevent further injury to surrounding structures. Fortunately, this patient does not have coexisting fractures in the left upper extremity and his forearm exploration and repair can be initiated without delay.

Surgical Approach

Preoperative antibiotics with strong gram-positive coverage should be instituted before making a skin incision, and, in cases with known bony injuries, coverage for gram-negative organisms should be used as well. The entire extremity should be prepared and draped to make multiple options for revascularization readily available. In addition, an uninjured extremity should be included in the operative field in the event that autogenous vein grafting is warranted.

In most cases, extremity incisions are placed longitudinally, directly over the injured vessel, and extended proximally or distally as necessary. The first goal is proximal control of the injury to abate hemorrhage. When proximal control is challenging, the option of endoluminal balloon occlusion with fluoroscopic guidance from a remote site should be considered.

Once the injury has been identified, there are several options for arterial repair, including patch angioplasty, end-to-end anastomosis, interposition graft, or

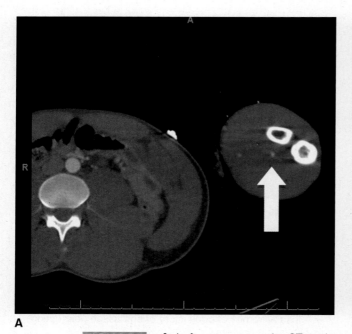

A

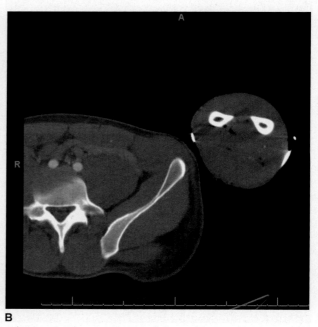

B

FIGURE 2 • **A:** Left upper extremity CT angiogram demonstrating a patent radial artery proximally. **B:** Occluded radial artery with multiple surrounding flecks of air.

TABLE 2. Upper Extremity Vascular Repair

Key Steps

1. CTA to determine vessel injury/occlusion
2. Open exploration with longitudinal incision
3. Proximal control with arterial clamp or occlusion balloon
4. Single-vessel injury in the upper extremity may be treated with ligation.
5. Primary repair for injuries <2 cm in length
6. Reverse greater saphenous vein bypass graft for injuries >2 cm
7. Proximal and distal ends flushed with heparinized saline
8. Completion angiogram and/or intraoperative Doppler

Potential Pitfalls

- Reperfusion injury
- Unintentional nerve injury
- Missed arterial injury
- Distal embolization
- Fogarty catheter endothelial injury

autogenous vein bypass graft. In cases where soft tissue damage is extensive and the segment of injured vessel is greater than 2 cm, bypass grafting is indicated. In general, autogenous vein is preferred to Polytetrafluoroethylene (PTFE), except in cases where autogenous vein is inadequate or unavailable, when the patient is unstable and quick repair of the artery is critical, or when a large size discrepancy between the vein graft and native artery exists. In both blunt and penetrating trauma, the degree of intimal injury and/or occlusion can extend beyond the area of obvious injury, so care should be taken to pass a Fogarty catheter proximal and distal to the arterial injury to remove intraluminal thrombus. Both the proximal and distal ends should be flushed with heparinized saline solution.

Single-vessel injury in the forearm may not need to be repaired, but sometimes can be ligated or embolized because of collateralization provided by the superficial palmar arches. Incomplete arches, however, do exist in 3.6% to 21.5 % of patients. When both radial and ulnar arteries are injured, repair of the ulnar should be undertaken preferentially, because it is the dominant blood supply to the hand (Table 2).

Case Continued

Upon exploration of the left forearm, significant hematoma is encountered. A short-segment (approximately 1 cm) penetrating injury to the left radial artery is identified. The ulnar artery appears intact, although in the field of injury. Ligation of the radial artery is considered, but due to the possibility of ulnar artery involvement, the decision is made to primarily repair the radial artery. The left radial artery is repaired primarily with 6-0 Prolene suture. Upon restoration of arterial flow, the forearm

is noticeably tense and the surrounding soft tissue is highly edematous.

Diagnosis and Recommendations

Because there is an obvious short-segment injury to the radial artery and the ulnar artery appeared irregular on CT angio and is in the field of blast injury, primary repair of the radial artery is undertaken. Compartment syndrome is a frequent manifestation of reperfusion injury following restoration of arterial flow in a traumatic setting. Risk factors for developing compartment syndrome include ischemic time greater than 6 hours and the presence of extensive orthopedic, soft tissue, or venous injuries. Because this patient's vascular injury is associated with considerable hematoma and moderate ischemic time (approximately 4 hours), fasciotomy for compartment syndrome should be considered to prevent further neurovascular injury. The forearm is comprised of three compartments: dorsal, volar, and mobile wad. The dorsal compartment contains extensors of the fingers and wrist, while the volar compartment contains flexors and pronators of the forearm as well as the radial and ulnar arteries. The dorsal is the most susceptible to compartment syndrome. Because the mobile wad compartment is closely associated with the dorsal component, it frequently does not require separate decompression.

Surgical Approach

A "lazy S"-shaped incision is typically used over the volar compartment to prevent future skin contracture and to allow freeing of superficial and deep flexor wads and decompression of the median nerve by carpal tunnel release. The incision begins at the antecubital fossa with release of the lacerates fibrosis (biceps aponeurosis) to decompress the median nerve and is carried no farther radially than the midaxis of ring finger to avoid injury to the superficial palmar branch of the median nerve. Care is taken distally to release the carpal tunnel. Once the volar compartment is decompressed, the dorsal compartment may not require further decompression. In situations that it does, a linear, longitudinal forearm incision is made between mobile extensor wad and extensor digitorum communis muscle bellies.

Case Continued

The volar compartment of the forearm is opened with extensive bulging of the muscle, which appears viable. A Vacuum Assisted Closure (VAC) sponge dressing is placed over the fasciotomy site, and Doppler signals are obtained intraoperatively to confirm an intact palmar arch with flow through the radial and ulnar arteries. The patient then undergoes diagnostic laparoscopy to rule out visceral injury. His flank wounds are debrided and irrigated. He is left intubated and transported to the ICU for fluid resuscitation and q1h Doppler pulse checks.

Discussion

Upper extremity vascular trauma is less common than lower extremity vascular trauma, with injury to the brachial artery being the most common and injury to the radial artery being the least common. Long-term follow-up for open surgical repair of upper extremity vascular injury demonstrates a primary patency of greater than 90%, with limb salvage rates ranging from 92% to 100%. A multidisciplinary approach to care at a level 1 trauma center expedites care for patients with vascular trauma, ensuring superior outcomes. An intraoperative completion angiogram should be considered when intraoperative Doppler is inconclusive or troubling. Intra-arterial vasodilators such as papaverine can be used to reverse severe spasm in the distal arterial tree. In the case of axillary and/or subclavian artery injury, an endovascular approach is increasingly being utilized to circumvent the difficulty in obtaining proximal with an open approach due to anatomical considerations.

Case Conclusion

The patient is extubated and continues to recover. His VAC dressing is changed at the bedside, and the fasciotomy excision is examined at the bedside (Fig. 3). The plastic and reconstructive surgery team is consulted. They make the decision that the volar compartment is viable and provides adequate coverage of the radial artery. The wound is covered with wet-to-dry dressings that are changed twice daily, and plans are made for delayed split-thickness skin grafting.

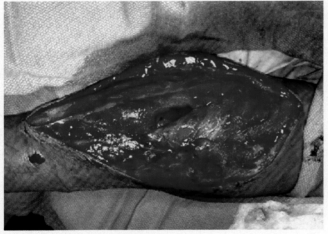

FIGURE 3 • Left forearm fasciotomy site on postoperative day 3.

Postoperative Management

In cases of large soft tissue defects of the upper extremity, it is prudent to enlist the assistance of plastic or orthopedic reconstructive surgeons to ensure adequate soft tissue coverage. For upper extremity trauma, the latissimus dorsi muscle makes an ideal pedicled flap because of its long neurovascular pedicle, large size, ease of mobilization, and expendability. For this patient, the fasciotomy incision can be reconstructed with a split-thickness skin graft once the edema has decreased. Diligent wound care during the postoperative period is crucial to prevent infection and encourage granulation tissue formation. Patients with a recent vascular anastomosis or bypass graft should have q1h or q2h Doppler checks of the reconstructed artery for the first 48 hours and then can be liberalized to q4h. While therapeutic anticoagulation is not typically necessary, initiation of an antiplatelet drug is usually recommended. A multidisciplinary approach in upper extremity vascular injury and trauma is paramount to ensuring expeditious care and successful outcomes.

TAKE HOME POINTS

- Hard signs of vascular injury warrant immediate exploration.
- Vascular injury may be present despite a reassuring physical examination.
- Limitation of ischemic time is critical for successful outcomes.
- Computed tomographic angiography is the first-line diagnostic imaging tool for upper extremity vascular injury.
- Nonocclusive vascular injuries can be managed conservatively.
- Single-vessel injuries can be treated with ligation.
- Primary repair is indicated for injured arterial segments less than 2 cm.
- Autogenous vein is preferred over PTFE for bypass grafting for injured segments greater than 2 cm.
- Patients with upper extremity vascular injury may require forearm fasciotomy with delayed reconstruction following restoration of arterial flow.

SUGGESTED READINGS

DuBose J, Rajani R, Gilani R, et al. Endovascular management of axillo-subclavian arterial injury: a review of published experience. *Injury.* 2012;43:1785-1792.

Franz R, Skytta C, Shah K, et al. A five-year review of management of upper-extremity arterial injuries at an urban level I trauma center. *Ann Vasc Surg.* 2012;26:655-664.

Klocker J, Falkensammer J, Pellegrini L, et al. Repair of arterial injury after blunt trauma in the upper extremity—immediate and long-term outcome. *Eur J Vasc Endovasc Surg.* 2010;39:160-164.

Patterson B, Holt P, Cleanthis M, et al. *Br J Surg.* 2012;99: 494-505.

CLINICAL SCENARIO CASE QUESTIONS

1. A 25-year-old man presents with a stab wound to the right arm. There is no pulsatile bleeding, hematoma, thrill, or bruit. His right radial pulse is diminished compared to the left. The most appropriate diagnostic study to order at this time is:

   a. Duplex ultrasound
   b. Upper extremity angiography
   c. Noncontrast CT scan
   d. CT angiography of the upper extremity
   e. MRI of the upper extremity

2. A 55-year-old female sustains multiple injuries in a motor vehicle accident, including crush injury of her left arm. In the operating room, approximately 4 cm of the brachial artery is injured. The preferred method of revascularization is:

   a. Primary repair
   b. Ligation with forearm fasciotomy
   c. Autogenous repair using greater saphenous vein from the lower extremity
   d. Repair with PTFE interposition graft

117 Inferior Vena Cava Filter Removal

OLUFUNMI ONAOPEMIPO AWONUGA and MARC A. PASSMAN

Presentation

A 28-year-old woman with a history of morbid obesity, 10-pack-year history of smoking, and hypertension presents for a follow-up regarding her inferior vena cava (IVC) filter. An optional IVC filter was placed during admission to the trauma intensive care unit following a motor vehicle accident 2 months ago. Her injuries consisted of intraparenchymal hemorrhage, subdural hemorrhage, grade IV liver laceration, multiple rib fractures, and right hemopneumothorax, which precluded pharmacologic thromboprophylaxis with anticoagulation at that time. She was in the intensive care unit and was on a ventilator for 10 days, during which time a deep vein thrombosis (DVT) was identified on ultrasound without evidence of pulmonary embolism (PE) on additional imaging. An optional IVC filter was placed due to relative contraindications to therapeutic anticoagulation due to her injuries. It has been 30 days since IVC filter placement, and she has been home for 2 weeks, ambulating without difficulty. She presents for IVC filter removal consideration.

Discussion

Systemic anticoagulation is primary standard therapy for DVT and PE based on evidence-based guidelines from the American College of Chest Physicians (ACCP), with IVC filter placement reserved for patients with documented DVT or PE and a contraindication to anticoagulation, complication of anticoagulation, or recurrent venous thromboembolism (VTE) despite therapeutic anticoagulation. The recommendations are controversial for IVC filter use as prophylaxis in patients without documented DVT but at high risk due to medical conditions, such as trauma or critically illness, when primary pharmacologic thromboprophylaxis is not feasible secondary to bleeding risk. While ACCP recommends against prophylactic IVC filter use, the Eastern Association for the Surgery of Trauma (EAST) and the Society for Interventional Radiology (SIR) guidelines support selected use of IVC filter placement for VTE prophylaxis.

There are multiple different FDA-approved and commercially available filter designs (Table 1). When an IVC filter is placed, decision should be made regarding permanent versus optional filter placement based on perceived duration of filter need. Although all optional filters also carry an FDA indication for permanent use, if a permanent need is determined at time of placement, a filter specific to permanent use is preferred, while optional filters should be considered if a temporary need is determined. Patients chronically at high risk of clinically significant PE irrespective of management with primary therapy, short life expectancy, or noncompliance with primary therapy or follow-up appointments should have a permanent filter placed.

Known long-term risks associated with IVC filters include, but are not limited to, access site thrombosis, filter fracture, filter migration, filter embolization, and IVC perforation. Between 2005 and 2010, the FDA received 921 device adverse event reports involving IVC filters, of which 328 involved device migration, 146 involved embolizations (detachment of device components), 70 involved perforation of the IVC, and 56 involved filter fracture. Some of these events led to adverse clinical outcomes in patients. The FDA recommends retrievable IVC filters be removed as soon as protection from PE is no longer needed.

Several studies have indicated that a variable percentage of optional IVC filters are actually removed, ranging between 20% and 80%, with higher follow-up reported with actively managed protocols. If an optional filter is used, it should be placed with intention of retrieval, with a retrieval timeline determined at the time of placement. The time frame within which a filter should be retrieved is recommended for each device based on FDA indications for use (IFUs), but in practice is poorly defined. Recommended retrieval time frames for each filter vary significantly, and understanding of optimal retrieval times is important prior to placement. In general, an earlier time frame is associated with higher retrieval success rates and planned retrieval should be as soon as clinically indicated. Using standard timelines and retrieval techniques, 80% to 100% of filter retrieval attempts will be successful.

Workup

The patient undergoes a focused history and physical examination. She is fully ambulatory with no residual disabilities from her trauma. She did not have any planned procedures upcoming in the future. She has been wearing compression stockings and had no lower extremity swelling or evidence of venous congestion in her lower extremities. A lower extremity venous duplex ultrasound was performed that showed no evidence of residual DVT. Abdominal x-ray showed that a conical filter was upright in anatomic position within the IVC, right side of vertebral bodies with apical hook tip at L2-3 level, full expansion of base of filter, without tilt or filter leg distortion. Serum laboratory studies reveal a hemoglobin of 13 g/dL, a platelet count of 200,000, and a creatinine of 0.6 mg/dL.

Discussion

According to the SIR, IVC filters may be removed when the indication for the IVC filter is no longer present and/or when anticoagulation either therapeutic or prophylactic can be used based on decreasing potential for bleeding risk. Filters should be removed when the risk of clinically significant PE is acceptably low as a result of improved clinical status with decreased VTE risk, or achievement of sustained appropriate primary VTE treatment with anticoagulation and no further indication for filter need. Appropriate primary VTE treatment will vary depending on the VTE risk status of the patient. Patients should demonstrate the ability to tolerate sustained primary VTE treatment before removal of the filter. The period of time required will vary based on the patient's clinical and functional status and ability to resume evidence-based standard therapy for VTE. Prior to discontinuation of the IVC filter, one should assure that the patient is not anticipated to return to a high-risk state for VTE because of interruption of primary treatment, change in clinical management, or change in clinical condition. The life expectancy of the patient should be long enough that the presumed benefits of discontinuation of filtration can be realized. Limited evidence suggests that some complications of filters may take years to manifest. Patients not anticipated to survive more than 6 months are unlikely to derive any discernible benefit from filter retrieval.

Prior to IVC filter retrieval, workup should include a physical examination to assess for signs of DVT. Lower extremity venous duplex ultrasound is performed prior to filter removal to confirm the presence or absence of DVT. A finding of a DVT on lower extremity venous duplex ultrasound requires initiation of anticoagulation therapy prior to filter removal. If patients are already on therapeutic anticoagulation for documented DVT, there should be consideration of conversion to a low molecular weight heparin bridge prior to filter retrieval with resumption of longer-acting oral anticoagulation postretrieval. Patients who require laboratory monitoring for anticoagulation should have stable measurements with no evidence of bleeding for at least 7 days before the discontinuation procedure. Patients with established VTE should not have clinical or objective evidence of failure or a complication of primary therapy before filter retrieval. Otherwise, continued IVC filter, possibly permanently, may be warranted.

Diagnosis and Treatment

Prior to IVC retrieval, the integrity of the IVC filter should be radiographically confirmed to make sure that there are no filter-related problems that would render retrieval technically challenging or impossible with endovascular techniques. Filter positioning and anatomic characteristics that are commonly cited as predictors of failure are filter tilt, caval penetration, and caval angulation. The most powerful predictors of failure in multiple studies have been hook apposition to the caval wall and increased filter dwell time.

Venography of the vena cava and implanted filter is performed at the time of the retrieval procedure. Position of the filter retrieval hook relative to the IVC wall and potential angulation issues are determined. Substantial filling defects present within the filter indicating clot preclude successful filter retrieval, and the procedure should be discontinued.

Case Continued

The patient was brought to the Endo Suite. She was placed supine on the operating room table. Intravenous sedation was provided. The right neck was prepped and draped in usual sterile fashion. With ultrasound guidance, the patency of the right internal jugular vein was confirmed, and with real-time imaging, a single puncture needle access was obtained using micropuncture needle, wire, and sheath. Sheath was then upsized to a 5-French sheath. A 0.035-inch glide wire was advanced down into the infrarenal IVC, followed by a flush catheter. Digital subtraction venography was performed with findings of an IVC filter in straight alignment to the IVC wall, apical hook at the level of the renal veins, and no evidence of filling defects within the filter device.

Surgical Approach

Depending on the type of optional IVC filter used, different approaches and techniques are required for filter removal and providers should be familiar with specific filter retrieval techniques and kits as per each device's IFUs. Most filters require percutaneous access from either jugular approach or femoral approach, with need to engage the filter retrieval hook with a snare. Once the filter hook is engaged, the snared filter is retracted into an appropriately sized sheath (Fig. 1). Independent of filter type, during the retrieval process, difficulty releasing the filter from the IVC attachment may occur, and retrieval should be aborted if the filter does not release with modest tension. Retrieved filters should be inspected for integrity, directly and with postretrieval imaging to make sure there are no retained filter components (Table 1).

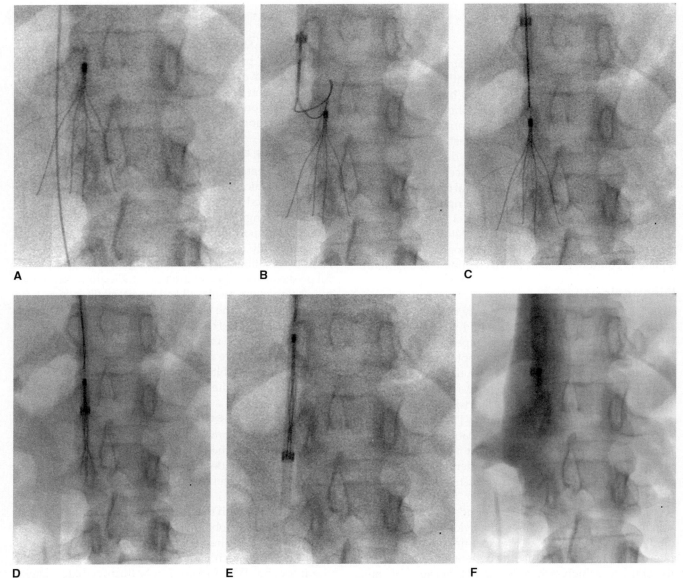

FIGURE 1 • **A:** IVC filter in place with guidewire in the vena cava. **B:** Snare capture of the IVC filter apical hook. **C:** Advance the sheath over the filter. **D, E:** Retracting filter into sheath. **F:** Completion venogram.

TABLE 1. Key Technical Steps and Potential Pitfalls

Key Technical Steps

1. Puncture the right jugular vein (for filters with apical hook) or femoral vein (for filters with caudal hook) using ultrasound guidance; Seldinger access technique preferred.
2. Advance guidewire and flush catheter to the level of infrarenal IVC below filter.
3. Perform diagnostic venography of IVC to exclude clot (Fig. 1A).
4. Dilate the puncture site with the dilator over the guidewire.
5. Insert the retrieval sheath over the guidewire to level followed by snare system.
6. Snare the filter hook (Fig. 1B).
7. Advance the sheath over the filter as a gentle pull is placed on snared filter to retrieve filter into sheath (Fig. 1C–E).
8. Inspect the removed filter to make sure there are no missing components.
9. Completion venography of IVC to confirm patency and no extravasation (Fig. 1F)
10. Remove the sheath and hold pressure over the puncture site.

Potential Pitfalls

- Injury to the IVC
- Acute PE
- Extravasation of contrast material at the time of completion venography
- Hematoma at retrieval vascular access site
- Inability to retrieve filter

Special Intraoperative Considerations

Multiple endovascular techniques have been used to aid in difficult filter retrieval. A simple technique is to use a snare with a different configuration. Additional use of a 10- to 14-mm angioplasty balloon from either jugular or femoral vein access positioned between the filter apical hook and the caval wall or within the filter struts can release intimal attachments and/or reorient the filter into a straighter alignment to facilitate retrieval. Another realignment technique involves using a wire looped through the apical struts of the filter and snared to provide traction on the filter while a second snare catheter from the same direction is used to secure the hook.

Case Conclusion

Under imaging guidance, the apical hook of the filter was engaged with a snare catheter and successfully removed via the sheath from the jugular vein access. Completion venogram showed a patent IVC with no extravasation or retained filter elements in the abdomen or chest. After postoperative observation, the patient was discharged home later that day.

Postoperative Management

For elective IVC filter removal, outpatients usually do not require admission. All patients should be evaluated for a few hours postprocedure to monitor for access site bleeding, pain management, and observations of major problems such as IVC rupture and PE. Admission to the hospital should be reserved only for complications that may have occurred during filter removal.

TAKE HOME POINTS

- Systemic anticoagulation is the standard of care for DVT and PE.
- Removal of retrievable IVC filters should be performed as soon as possible based on risk profile for DVT/PE and decreased bleeding risk that allows for anticoagulation if needed.
- Patients should be evaluated prior to filter retrieval to ensure that the risk of clinically significant PE is acceptably low and that the retrieval procedure can be performed safely.
- Venography should be performed to determine whether thrombus is present within the filter, in which case the filter should be left in place as a permanent filter.

- Depending on the type of filter used, different approaches and techniques are required for filter removal. Most filters require percutaneous access and engagement of a hook attached to the filter with a snare for successful retrieval.

SUGGESTED READINGS

Avgerinos ED, Bath J, Stevens J, et al. Technical and patient-related characteristics associated with challenging retrieval of inferior vena cava filters. *Eur J Vasc Endovasc Surg.* 2013;46(3):353-359.

Decousus H, Leizorovicz A, Parent F, et al. A clinical trial of vena caval filters in the prevention of pulmonary embolism in patients with proximal deep-vein thrombosis. *N Engl J Med.* 1998;338(7):409-416.

Gyang E, Zayed M, Harris EJ, et al. Factors impacting follow-up care after placement of temporary inferior vena cava filters. *J Vasc Surg.* 2013;58(2):440-445.

Kaufman JA, Kinney TB, Streiff MB, et al. Guidelines for the use of retrievable and convertible vena cava filters: report from the society of interventional radiology multidisciplinary consensus conference. *J Vasc Interv Radiol.* 2006;17(3):449-459.

Ni H, Win LL. Retrievable inferior vena cava filters for venous thromboembolism. *ISRN Radiology.* 2013;2013:8; Article ID 959452, *http://dx.doi.org/10.5402/2013/959452*

Rogers FB, Cipolle MD, Velmahos G, et al. Practice management guidelines for the prevention of venous thromboembolism in trauma patients: the EAST practice management guidelines work group. *J Trauma.* 2002;53(1):142-164.

Zakhary EM, Elmore JR, Galt SW, et al. Optional filters in trauma patients: Can retrieval rates be improved? *Ann Vasc Surg.* 2008;22(5):627-634.

CLINICAL SCENARIO CASE QUESTIONS

1. IVC filters should be removed when:

   a. An indication for a permanent filter is present
   b. The patient has short life expectancy
   c. Patients are noncompliant with primary therapy or follow-up appointments
   d. The risk of clinically significant PE is acceptably low as a result of achievement of sustained appropriate primary anticoagulation treatment or improved clinical status with decreased venous thromboembolism risk

2. Prior to retrieval of an IVC filter, one should:

   a. Perform lysis of any DVT that is present at the time of IVC filter removal
   b. Obtain ankle-brachial indices
   c. Therapeutically anticoagulate all patients for 1 year
   d. Assure that the patient is not anticipated to return to a high-risk state because of interruption of primary treatment, change in clinical management, or change in clinical condition

118 Removal of IVC Filter Adherent to IVC Wall

DAVID M. WILLIAMS

Presentation

A 41-year-old woman presented in the clinic with chronic left iliac vein occlusion with left leg pain, heaviness, and swelling. She had acute left leg deep venous thrombosis (DVT) 2 months before, which was unprovoked except for the presence of May-Thurner anatomy (Fig. 1). She had a failed attempt at thrombolysis. After suspension of anticoagulation due to gastrointestinal bleeding, a Celect inferior vena cava (IVC) filter (Cook, Inc., Bloomington, IN) was placed in the infrarenal IVC. One month after her clinic visit (3 months after her DVT), she underwent successful recanalization and stenting of her left iliac common and external iliac veins. She was discharged on clopidogrel 75 mg/d, aspirin 81 mg/d, and enoxaparin 100 mg twice per day. The patient tolerated anticoagulation. Clopidogrel was discontinued after 2 months, and the patient was successfully transitioned to Coumadin. Her INR was successfully maintained between 2.2 and 3.2. Nearly 6 months after recanalization, she presented for follow-up venography to evaluate the venous stent, and requested that her filter be removed at the same time.

Assessment

In judging whether to remove a filter, we review the current indications for the filter (Table 1) as well as the anticipated difficulties in removing a filter (Table 2). According to the manufacturer's instructions for use, the Kaplan-Meier curve of attempted retrieval of the Celect filter shows a 90% probability of successful retrieval at 1 year. At the time of venographic follow-up of her iliac vein stents, the filter would have been implanted for 8 months, and she was currently tolerating Coumadin, with an INR of 2.6. Consequently, she no longer needed the filter, and the odds of successful retrieval were considered good.

Initial Filter Retrieval Attempt

Filter retrieval was anticipated to be straightforward, so anticoagulation was maintained. From the right internal jugular (IJ) vein approach, a Cook retrieval loop snare was advanced into the IVC. Inferior venacavogram showed the filter retrieval hook (Fig. 1) abutting the wall of the IVC and no thrombus within the filter itself. The loop snare could not be made to engage the retrieval hook. Because the patient was anticoagulated, no aggressive attempt to secure the filter was made.

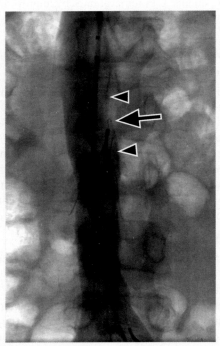

FIGURE 1 • Inferior venacavogram prior to first attempt at filter retrieval, following treatment of left common iliac vein compression syndrome. The filter apex (*arrow*) abuts the medial wall of the IVC (*arrowheads*). It was not technically possible to engage the apical hook, which was embedded in the IVC wall.

TABLE 1. When to Remove the Filter

Prophylactic filter is no longer needed
   Risk of venous thromboembolism has passed
   Anticoagulation can be resumed
   No additional elective surgical procedure is planned
Filter contains no significant thrombus burden
Anticoagulation
   Do not interrupt if retrieval is uncomplicated
   Suspend (transition to heparin) if retrieval is complicated

TABLE 2. Technical Difficulty of Filter Retrieval

Uncomplicated
  Within approved window of filter removal (Cook Gunther-
    Tulip, Cordis OptEase) according to Instructions for Use
  Window not so critical (Cook Celect, Bard G1 and G2)
Intermediate
  G-T or OptEase outside window, normal coagulation
    parameters
Complicated
  G-T or OptEase outside window, anticoagulated
  Forceful extraction
  Laser extraction
Other considerations
  Vascular access (patent IJ vein)
  Anatomic position of filter
    Apex tilted against IVC wall
    Apex tilted into and tenting roof of renal or hepatic vein wall

Case Continued and Advanced IVC Filter Removal Techniques

The patient returned 3 months later. At this time, she had discontinued Coumadin. Her advanced D-Dimer value was 1.5 (normal 0.4 to 2.5).

From the right IJ approach, an 8 French × 45 cm sheath was placed into the IVC. Through the sheath, a recurved catheter was used to direct a wire below the hook and medial to the converging apex of the filter legs (Fig. 2),

allowing the free end of the wire to be captured by a loop snare and retracted from the IJ sheath. Using firm but reasonable traction on both ends of the catheter from the jugular access, we were unable to advance the sheath over the filter hook and unable to retract the loop free of the upper body of the filter. The wire was then removed. From the right common femoral vein, an 8 × 40 balloon was directed medial to the filter and inflated, displacing the upper body of the filter laterally, in an effort to position the filter hook more centrally in the IVC lumen (Fig. 3). However, a transjugular loop snare continued to slide over the filter apex, without passing medial to the hook, suggesting that the filter hook was embedded in the IVC wall. Biopsy forceps (7 French × 55 cm Bioptome, Cordis, Bridgewater, NJ) were advanced from the 8-Fr transjugular sheath, and, after verifying proper position using rotational fluoroscopy, the opened jaws were directed onto the hook and closed (Fig. 4). Several bits of tissue were retrieved by the jaws until, after 4 passes, the hook itself was engaged. The hook was tightly grasped to allow countertraction on the filter as the sheath was advanced, closing and capturing the filter, which was then removed. Inferior venacavogram after filter retrieval showed no filling defect at the filter site, no IVC stenosis, and no contrast extravasation (Fig. 5).

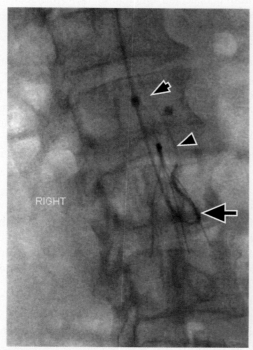

FIGURE 2 • Through a recurved catheter (*arrow*) passed below the filter apex, a guidewire (*arrowheads*) has been passed medial to the converging filter legs. The wire tip was captured by a loop snare and withdrawn from the jugular sheath, creating a loop encircling the embedded filter apex. Despite traction on the loop, the sheath could not be advanced over the filter apex, and the tissue entrapping the filter apex could not be disrupted.

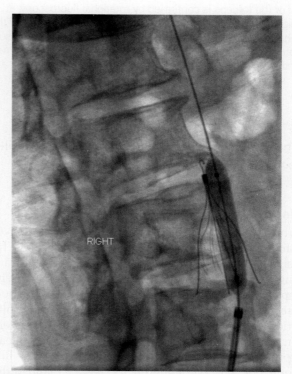

FIGURE 3 • Through a sheath in the right common femoral vein, an 8 × 40 balloon has been passed anteromedial to the upper body of the filter. After balloon inflation, the filter apex was deflected closer to the central axis of the IVC. Note that if the apex is embedded in IVC wall, the apical hook is still not accessible to the retrieval snare. In this case, maneuvers to ensnare the retrieval hook were fruitless.

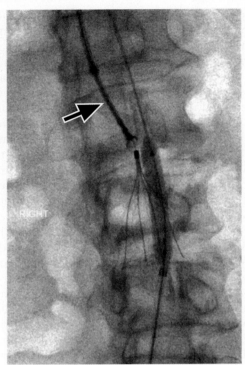

FIGURE 4 • Failure to engage the filter hook has been attributed to tissue engulfing the filter apex. Since the patient is not anticoagulated, the biopsy forceps (*arrow*) are being used to debride the tissue surrounding the hook. Proper position of the forceps is confirmed by rotational fluoroscopy, at which time the jaws are closed. After several repetitions of this maneuver, the filter hook has been uncovered, and jaw closure captures the hook. The sheath is then advanced while countertraction on the filter is maintained by the biopsy forceps.

Case Conclusion

The patient did well with no complication from filter extraction and required no further follow-up.

Discussion

Fortunately, this IVC filter was removed with relatively straightforward and uncomplicated maneuvers. The design of the Celect filter with relatively straight radiating legs and alignment arms and without crossing loops makes it relatively easy to remove, once the hook is secured. At a certain point during complicated filter retrievals, the question arises whether further escalation of the procedure is, on balance, preferable to leaving the filter in place. For example, the Gunther-Tulip filter (Cook, Inc., Bloomington, IN) has a garland of thin wire looping from leg to leg, and both the hook and the wire loops can become embedded in tissue. Failure to advance the sheath over these wire loops is the usual

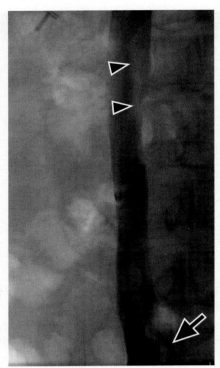

FIGURE 5 • Inferior venacavogram after filter removal, with contrast injection in the transfemoral flush catheter. The left common iliac vein stent is visible (*arrow*). No IVC stenosis, filling defect, or extravasation is present. Flow defect from unopacified left renal vein inflow is seen in the suprarenal IVC (*arrowheads*).

cause of unsuccessful retrieval of this filter. In patients with this filter who have been insistent about filter removal, we have used laser-assisted extraction, which does expose the patient to risk of IVC laceration. In cases such as this, decision to escalate the procedure must be based on the indication for removal, the risks of more aggressive retrieval techniques, and operator experience (Table 3).

TAKE HOME POINTS

- Verify absence of need for filter, including no imminent elective surgical procedure.
- Be familiar with recommended window of filter removal.
- Be familiar with the manufacturer's recommended retrieval technique.
- For the difficult filter, chose your target level of intervention:
  - Tilted apex: deflect upper body of filter with angioplasty balloon
  - Tilted apex embedded in IVC mural tissue: free apex with transjugular wire loop or forceps
  - Wire loops resist sheath advancement: laser extraction

TABLE 3. Key Technical Steps and Potential Pitfalls

- Verify minimal or no thrombus in filter (intravascular ultrasound or inferior venacavogram).
- Attempt filter capture by recommended snare device or grasper, and then advance sheath over filter.
- If filter tents are next to the aortic wall, precluding simple capture of the filter hook or apex, attempt to deflect filter apex more centrally into the IVC lumen, using an angioplasty balloon inflated between the IVC wall and the filter apex.
- If filter apex is embedded in IVC mural tissue, attempt breaking tissue adhesion by passing a transjugular wire underneath the adhesion and between filter and IVC wall, constructing a loop, then retracting the loop from the IJ sheath. Alternatively, debride adherent tissue from the filter hook using biopsy forceps.
- If wire loops (e.g., found with Gunther-Tulip or Simon-Nitinol filter) in the filter structure adhere to IVC wall and resist sheath advancement, reconsider indications for removal. If, after balancing indications for removal, preferences of patient, risks of retrieval, and operator experience, aggressive filter extraction is warranted, consider laser extraction.
- Pitfalls of filter removal include pulmonary embolism (if filter contains unrecognized thrombus burden), damage to filter with fracture or bending of filter legs with altered filter orientation and competence.
- Care must be taken to not be so aggressive as to cause damage to IVC, renal, or hepatic veins.

SUGGESTED READINGS

Iliescu B, Haskal ZJ. Advanced techniques for removal of retrievable inferior vena cava filters. *Cardiovasc Intervent Radiol.* 2012;35:774-750.

Imberti D, Ageno W, Carpenedo M. Retrievable vena cava filters: a review. *Curr Opin Hematol.* 2006;13:351-356.

Kaufman JA. Optional vena cava filters: what, why, and when. *Vascular.* 2007;15:304-313.

Kaufman JA. Retrievable vena cava filters. *Tech Vasc Interv Radiol.* 2004;7:96-104.

Kuo WT, Cupp JS, Louie JD, et al. Complex retrieval of embedded IVC filters: alternative techniques and histologic tissue analysis. *Cardiovasc Intervent Radiol.* 2012;35:588-597.

CLINICAL SCENARIO CASE QUESTIONS

1. A patient with quiescent ulcerative colitis had a Gunther-Tulip filter placed prophylactically 6 months ago, before elective knee surgery. He has heard of filter complications including fracture and migration and would now like the filter removed. Your first step is to:

   a. Get a contrast CT to observe the orientation of the filter in the IVC
   b. Review indications for continued filter prophylaxis in the patient
   c. Schedule the patient for filter retrieval, after explaining that filter position like excessive tilting may be encountered, which would prevent straightforward retrieval
   d. Review the specific complications worrying the patient in the context of the actual record of the Gunther-Tulip in long-term implantation

2. In a patient with a difficult-to-remove IVC filter, a primary reason for failure of retrieval is:

   a. Filter tilt
   b. A malpositioned filter from the initial placement
   c. Organ compression
   d. Filter ingrowth to the IVC wall
   e. Thrombosed filter

119 Retroperitoneal Hematoma after Angiogram

KATHERINE GALLAGHER

Presentation

A 77-year-old female presented to the post anesthesia care unit (PACU) following treatment of her left lower extremity for claudication. Per the operative report, the patient had an unremarkable procedure. An 18-gauge needle was used to cannulate the left common femoral artery, and her right superficial femoral artery (SFA) was treated with percutaneous angioplasty via an up-and-over approach. On the operative note, it was noted that the wire passed without resistance. She did receive a loading dose of 300 mg of clopidogrel.

Her medical history is significant for a coronary artery disease status plus coronary stenting, hypertension, and a 50-pack-year history for smoking. The patient has been recovering reasonably well in the PACU and has no obvious evidence of groin hematoma; however, she has had several episodes of hypotension, and she has responded to 500-mL boluses of IV fluid. She reports that she is feeling somewhat lightheaded and nauseated but is without any chest pain. On examination, her pulse is 130 beats per minute and her blood pressure is 90/50. She is reporting some pain in her iliac fossa region on the left, which has been requiring analgesics. Her abdomen is soft. She has palpable bilateral femoral pulses and no evidence of hematoma in the left groin. Laboratory evaluation reveals normal creatinine, leukocyte count, and coagulation parameters; however, her hematocrit is noted to be 10 points lower than her baseline.

Differential Diagnosis

Differential diagnosis for this scenario includes complications related to the procedure (percutaneous access, perforation at the site of endovascular treatment) as well as cardiac issues (e.g., MI). The leading diagnosis is retroperitoneal hematoma as the retroperitoneum can hold a significant volume of blood without any obvious signs on physical exam. Often by the time hemodynamic compromise occurs, the patient has already lost a significant volume of blood, which can result in devastating complications in many of the vascular patients with significant heart disease and little volume reserve.

Background and Workup

Background

This patient has a potential life-threatening problem, with suspicion of retroperitoneal hematoma. First and foremost is evaluation and stabilization of the patient. Diagnostic evaluation can include abdominal CTA in order to evaluate for retroperitoneal hematoma; however, prompt volume resuscitation preferably with blood/colloid is warranted. Although most retroperitoneal hematomas can be treated conservatively, extravasation may require surgical treatment or endovascular management. Patients who continue to have persistent hypotension despite adequate resuscitation may require operative intervention. Additionally, those who fail to respond appropriately following transfusion may warrant imaging in the endovascular suite.

Patients who develop femoral neuropathy require hematoma evacuation and exploration. Endovascular embolization or stent graft placement for active extravasation is occasionally necessary. What is most important in management of the retroperitoneal hematoma is prompt recognition of the complication. Delays in recognition add to increase morbidity and mortality. Mortality rates approach 0.5% to 2% in patients who develop this complication. The most common symptoms of retroperitoneal hematoma include back pain and groin discomfort, which occur in approximately 75% to 80% of patients. Profound hypotension is also present in a significant number of patients, ranging anywhere from 40% to 65%. This complication may be more common with difficult access or wire and sheath maneuvers in the iliac arteries, as well as if the patient is on potent antiplatelet or anticoagulant therapies.

Approximately 10% to 15% of patients will require intervention for ongoing blood loss. The use of the micropuncture technique along with ultrasound guidance to assure proper needle placement can significantly reduce the risk of retroperitoneal hematoma. Arterial sticks that occur above the inguinal ligament are often the inciting event for development of a retroperitoneal hematoma. This is often due to difficulty in achieving adequate compression of the vessel at this level. Retroperitoneal hematomas, however, can occur with lower sticks in areas of scarring where the blood can spread along fascial planes. Visualization of the femoral head on fluoroscopy as well as the use of ultrasound guidance and micropuncture set can reduce the risk of retroperitoneal hematomas.

Workup

The first step for a hypotensive patient in the PACU is to assess the airway, breathing, and circulation, the "ABCs." Fluid/volume and resuscitation efforts should be initiated promptly. The patient should undergo a workup including full labs, EKG, and cardiac enzymes. Particular attention should be paid to the patient's volume status. Making sure the patient's coagulation parameters are normal is also essential. For example, not reversing the heparin after the procedure may increase the postprocedure bleeding rate.

Preoperative/baseline hematocrit values should be considered as well as intraoperative details reviewed regarding fluid management. If the patient is stable, a CT scan of the abdomen and pelvic imaging should be considered. If the patient is unstable, aggressive resuscitation is warranted. If the patient fails to stabilize with initial resuscitation, prompt return to the OR for exploration is likely necessary.

Diagnosis and Treatment

This patient has a large retroperitoneal hematoma, and given her advanced age and low cardiac reserve, this has resulted in a significant blood loss with the inability to fully compensate for these volume losses.

In this patient, she was responsive to resuscitation and quickly ruled out for an MI/cardiac event. Since she had stabilized, a CT was obtained (Fig. 1). This CT

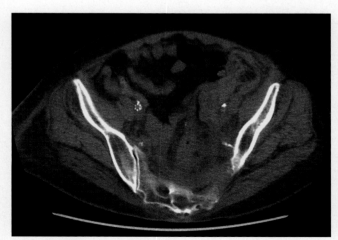

FIGURE 1 • Pelvic CT.

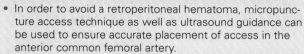

TABLE 1. Key Technical Steps and Potential Pitfalls

- In order to avoid a retroperitoneal hematoma, micropuncture access technique as well as ultrasound guidance can be used to ensure accurate placement of access in the anterior common femoral artery.
- Vigilant postoperative monitoring is important to allow for early detection of a retroperitoneal hematoma.
- There should be a high index of suspicion for retroperitoneal hematoma in anyone experiencing intermittent hypotension within several hours postoperatively following endovascular access.
- The lack of a hematoma at the site of puncture is not an indication of whether retroperitoneal hematoma may be present. If any question exists regarding the presence of retroperitoneal hematoma, a prompt evaluation should be performed if the patient is stable using abdominal CT.
- In most cases, treatment involves aggressive resuscitation and stabilization with conservative management. Evacuation of the hematoma would be warranted in cases where significant femoral neuropathy is present or in cases of active extravasation, where either endovascular or surgical repair is needed.

demonstrates a large left-sided retroperitoneal hematoma. Serial hematocrits were trended, and the patient required 2 units of packed red blood cells (PRBCs) for a hematocrit drop from a baseline 32 to 18. She responded to conservative therapy and did not require operative intervention/exploration. Her antiplatelet therapy was held (Table 1).

Case Conclusion

The patient was discharged from the hospital on postoperative day 5. Follow-up was scheduled for 1 month. Antiplatelet therapy was restarted on discharge.

TAKE HOME POINTS

- Using ultrasound guidance and a micropuncture technique can decrease the incidence of retroperitoneal hematoma.
- If the access site is above the inguinal ligament, and a smaller (≤6-French) sheath was used, direct pressure and careful postoperative monitoring is warranted for retroperitoneal hematoma.
- Hypotension is often the first sign of a retroperitoneal hematoma in the PACU.
- In cases where larger sheaths (greater than 9 French) were placed above the inguinal ligament. In cases of large retroperitoneal hematomas, either open or endovascular repair may be needed.

- The majority of retroperitoneal hematomas can be managed conservatively with aggressive resuscitation and careful monitoring and is more common in those with potent antiplatelet therapy or anticoagulant therapy.

SUGGESTED READINGS

Farouque HM, Tremmel JA, Raissi Shabari F, et al. Risk factors for the development of retroperitoneal hematoma after percutaneous coronary intervention in the era of glycoprotein IIb/IIIa inhibitors and vascular closure devices. *J Am Coll Cardiol.* 2005;45(3):363-368.

Kent KC, Moscucci M, Mansour KA, et al. Retroperitoneal hematoma after cardiac catheterization: prevalence, risk factors, and optimal management. *J Vasc Surg.* 1994;20(6):905-910.

Kinnaird TD, Stabile E, Mintz GS, et al. Incidence, predictors, and prognostic implications of bleeding and blood transfusion following percutaneous coronary interventions. *Am J Cardiol.* 2003;92(8):930-935.

Popma JJ, Satler LF, Pichard AD, et al. Vascular complications after balloon and new device angioplasty. *Circulation.* 1993;88(4 Pt 1):1569-1578.

Sreeram S, Lumsden AB, Miller JS, et al. Retroperitoneal hematoma following femoral arterial catheterization: a serious and often fatal complication. *Am Surg.* 1993;59(2):94-98.

CLINICAL SCENARIO CASE QUESTIONS

1. An 84-year-old man develops hypotension 2 hours following an endovascular procedure. Exam is completely normal. What management strategy should you employ?

   a. Immediate return to the OR for open exploration
   b. Five-hundred milliliter bolus of crystalloid and reevaluate in 4 hours
   c. Fluid resuscitation, aggressive monitoring, CT scan, EKG, serial hematocrits if the patient is stable
   d. Nothing; he is old and this is due to the 20-mL intraoperative blood loss
   e. Return to OR and angiography

2. Factors that may increase the risk of a retroperitoneal bleed include:

   a. Obesity
   b. Diabetes
   c. Aspirin therapy
   d. Nonreversal of heparin after completion of the procedure
   e. Male gender

120 | Iatrogenic Femoral Arteriovenous Fistulas

JASON P. JUNDT and TIMOTHY K. LIEM

Presentation

A 71-year-old female with hypertension, hyperlipidemia, atrial fibrillation on warfarin therapy, and a 50-pack-year smoking history presents for follow-up 2 weeks after an aortogram with bilateral lower extremity runoff. The procedure was performed for right lower extremity claudication symptoms. Noninvasive studies demonstrated ankle-brachial indices (ABIs) of 0.68 on the right and 0.81 on the left. The procedure was performed via left femoral access with anticoagulation managed by low molecular weight heparin bridge. The patient's vital signs are normal, but she complains of worsening left leg claudication symptoms since the procedure. There are no groin hematomas but mild swelling in the location of the left femoral puncture. Distal signals are present but biphasic. Auscultation demonstrates a bruit over the left common femoral artery.

Differential Diagnosis

Complications from femoral artery access are common, occurring in 1% to 14% of procedures. The complications are diverse and include hematoma (10%), pseudoaneurysm (2% to 8%), active bleeding (2.5%), arteriovenous fistula (AVF) (0.1%), thrombosis (less than 0.1%), embolism (less than 0.1%), and retroperitoneal hematoma (less than 0.1%). While the majority of these complications are minor and do not require intervention, some are severe and insidious and occasionally require urgent operative intervention (e.g., hemorrhage into the retroperitoneum).

A history and physical examination consistent with worsening claudication in conjunction with swelling and bruit are suspicious for an iatrogenic AVF. Furthermore, this patient has risk factors for AVF formation following percutaneous intervention, such as female gender (OR = 1.84), arterial hypertension (OR = 1.86), warfarin therapy (OR = 2.34), and left-sided puncture (OR = 2.21). An additional risk factor, not present in our patient, includes intraprocedural heparin dosage of greater than 12,500 units.

Workup

The patient undergoes further evaluation with an arterial duplex examination. Using an 8- to 12-MHz probe and color flow pulsed Doppler duplex ultrasound, an iatrogenic AVF is diagnosed (Fig. 1) between the profunda femoris artery and the femoral vein. A less than 0.2-cm communicating channel is visualized, and no pseudoaneurysm is seen. Laboratory findings are unremarkable.

Diagnosis and Treatment

Arteriovenous fistulas and pseudoaneurysms of the lower extremity arteries are most commonly iatrogenic or secondary to traumatic injury. Over the past 20 years, percutaneous interventions have exponentially increased, making iatrogenic AVFs a more frequently encountered clinical entity. A history of prior intervention in the setting of worsening claudication, nonhealing ulcers, and symptoms of congestive heart failure are suspicious for an iatrogenic AVF. Physical examination can demonstrate stigmata of previous groin access, swelling, bruising, erythema, and a palpable thrill. Auscultation over the previous access point will demonstrate a continuous machinery type bruit, and occasionally, temporary occlusion of large AVFs will cause a reflexive slowing of the heart rate (Nicoladoni-Branham sign).

Imaging studies including duplex ultrasound with pulsed Doppler and color flow imaging (DUS), computerized tomography angiogram (CTA), and conventional angiogram (CA) all can confirm the diagnosis and define the anatomy. Specific findings associated with AVFs on DUS include the presence of flow jets, and conversion of the typical high-resistance arterial waveform to a lower-resistance pattern with persistent diastolic flow (Fig. 2). In addition, some AVFs demonstrate a "visual bruit" (color mixing outside of the vessel wall), caused by turbulence-associated soft tissue vibration (Fig. 3). Computerized tomography typically will demonstrate early opacification of the vena cava during the arterial phase, with asymmetric enhancement and distention of venous structures due to venous hypertension ipsilateral and distal to the AVF. Conventional angiography will demonstrate the location,

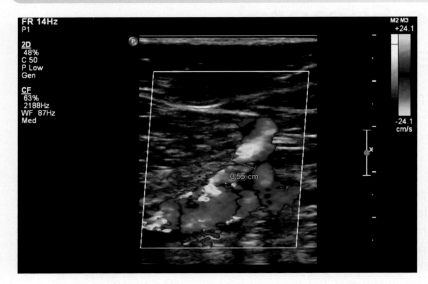

FIGURE 1 • Iatrogenic arteriovenous fistula between the deep femoral artery and the femoral vein.

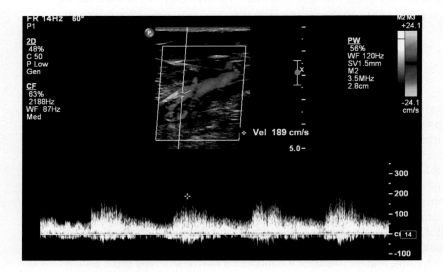

FIGURE 2 • Doppler-derived waveforms in a femoral artery, demonstrating low-resistance flow caused by an arteriovenous fistula.

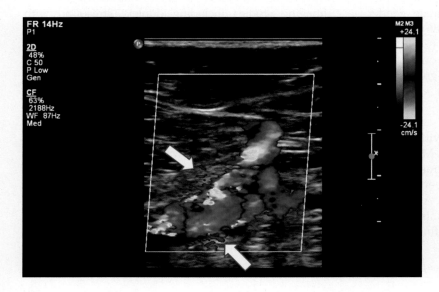

FIGURE 3 • Soft tissue vibration caused by an arteriovenous fistula may cause a "visual bruit" or flow artifacts outside of the vessel wall.

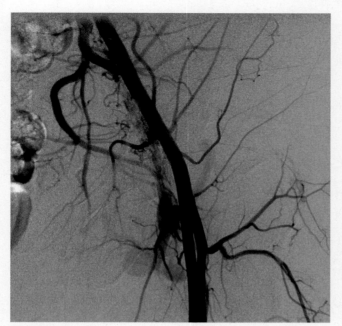

FIGURE 4 • Conventional angiography demonstrating early venous filling associated with an iatrogenic arteriovenous fistula.

neck if present, and flow jet with characteristic rapid venous filling through the AVF. It can be useful both for diagnosis and concurrent treatment (Fig. 4).

Surgical treatment for iatrogenic AVFs seldom is necessary, since the spontaneous closure rate at 1-year follow-up is greater than 80% with nonoperative management. Of the iatrogenic AVFs that close at 1 year, nearly 70% will close within the first 4 months, with the remainder closing within 12 months. Surgical or catheter-based treatment should be considered in patients with symptoms such as severe pain and edema, and in the unusual patient with worsening congestive heart failure.

There are three treatment options for iatrogenic AVFs: ultrasound-guided compression repair (UGCR), endovascular exclusion (either with a covered stent graft or vascular plug in the communicating channel), or open repair. Although UGCR is the least invasive option, it is typically poorly tolerated, and given the nature of iatrogenic AVFs (short necks and high flow), it has the lowest rate of treatment success. Endovascular therapy, consisting of covered stent placement or embolization with a vascular plug, is becoming utilized more commonly with numerous case reports and series demonstrating both safety and efficacy. Open surgical repair has a very high technical success rate, but adverse event rates as high as 20% have been reported, mostly in relation to groin wounds complications.

Endovascular and Surgical Approach

If noninvasive attempts to close symptomatic iatrogenic AVFs are not successful, either endovascular or open intervention is indicated. Patients with a hostile groin

(due to multiple prior surgeries), those who are deemed to be at high risk for infection or wound complications (large pannus), and unstable patients (recall that many of these patients underwent coronary angiogram and stenting due to myocardial infarction) may benefit from a minimally invasive approach, either with embolization or placement of a covered stent. Embolization is more suitable for chronic AVFs that have well-developed tortuous fistulous tracts and for distal or deep femoral fistulas that may be the result of blunt or penetrating trauma. Stent graft coverage is more suitable for patients with large artery fistulas (common femoral or superficial femoral), especially when the fistulous tract may be short.

Endovascular repair of a femoral AVF often is approached with a retrograde crossover technique from the contralateral groin, since antegrade femoral puncture results in inadequate working lengths. Access is obtained using DUS or fluoroscopic guidance as needed and a 4-French or 5-French micropuncture set. A Benson wire is advanced into the distal aorta. A 4-French or 5-French pigtail catheter is then placed in the distal aorta, with aortography perform to delineate the iliofemoral anatomy as well as the iatrogenic AVF. At this point, measurements are obtained to plan for stent or Amplatzer selection as well as sheath size for delivery. The aortic bifurcation is navigated using a RIM catheter, Sos Omni, or other appropriate catheter. A J-wire or glidewire can then be advanced down the contralateral common iliac, external iliac, and common femoral arteries.

In anticipation of sheath placement, the patient is anticoagulated with 80 U/kg of heparin sulfate. A long precurved sheath, with a diameter appropriate for deployment of the selected stent, is advanced over the guidewire and stationed proximal to the AVF. An angiogram is performed through the sheath, and SmartMask or roadmap setting is used to precisely place a covered stent across the abnormal communication. Completion angiogram is performed to confirm sealing of the fistula. The patient receives a follow-up duplex evaluation and typically is discharged home on the same day. Postoperative medications include 3 months of dual antiplatelet therapy followed by indefinite aspirin.

Patients who are a good operative risk, those with unsuitable endovascular anatomy, and those who have failed endovascular repair may undergo open surgical correction. Open surgical repair usually is performed under general anesthesia. A longitudinal or oblique incision is made directly over the arterial segment of the iatrogenic AVF. The skin and subcutaneous tissue are divided using electrocautery with proximal and distal control of both venous and arterial structures. Longer fistulous tracts usually can be divided without clamping the adjacent femoral artery or vein. If the artery is injured or if the fistula closure results in significant arterial or venous stenosis, then heparin should be administered and patch angioplasty performed. Continuous wave Doppler should then been used to confirm venous patency and conversion of the arterial waveform into a typical higher-resistance signal (Table 1).

TABLE 1. Key Technical Steps and Potential Pitfalls

Key Technical Steps

Endovascular Repair of Iatrogenic Arteriovenous Fistula

1. Safe arterial access
2. Identification of the iatrogenic AVF and availability of appropriate stent graft
3. Placement of a guidewire beyond iatrogenic AVF
4. Imaging to size graft and approximate location
5. Administration of heparin and placement of sheath
6. Successful deployment of the graft with subsequent imaging to confirm exclusion of the fistula
7. Hold pressure to ensure no groin complications at the access site
8. Check distal pulses
9. Clopidogrel for 3 months following the procedure, and indefinite aspirin

Open Repair of Iatrogenic Arteriovenous Fistula

1. Longitudinal or oblique incision over the iatrogenic AVF
2. Proximal and distal control of artery and vein
3. Administration of heparin and clamping of vessels for short/wide AVFs
4. Ligation of fistula with or without repair of the artery
5. Continuous Doppler signal evaluation after repair to confirm fistula ligation and high-resistance arterial signal

Potential Pitfalls

- Access complications
- Inability to access the iatrogenic AVF due to preexisting severe peripheral vascular disease
- Persistent leak after stent deployment
- Embolism, thrombosis, ischemia

Special Intraoperative Considerations to Endovascular and Open Repair

While there is no evidence that preexisting peripheral artery disease increases the risk of iatrogenic AVF, there is evidence that peripheral artery disease (PAD) may increase the risk of other femoral artery complications such as pseudoaneurysm (PSA) and embolization. Furthermore, severe PAD may complicate the ability to repair an iatrogenic AVF using endovascular techniques. Endovascular techniques also carry the risk for iatrogenic dissection, thrombosis, and embolization, most of which are treatable, if recognized at the time of the procedure. Open repair with proximal and distal control prior to dissecting the AVF or a PSA can be difficult due to exposure limitations and the presence of previous hematoma. In such situations, balloon occlusion techniques with an appropriately sized Fogarty balloon, three-way stopcock, and small Luer-Lock syringe can provide hemostasis during repair. Severe PAD may compromise the success of a simple repair, and more extensive operations such as femoral endarterectomy, profundaplasty, and possibly arterial replacement with graft may be warranted. The unanticipated finding of infection at the site of PSA or iatrogenic AVF can complicate the issue, further requiring resection of the infected arteries and veins followed by arterial reconstruction with autogenous graft conduits or extra-anatomic bypass and ligation.

Postoperative Management

Case series regarding endovascular repair of iatrogenic AVFs have documented technical success rates of greater than 90%. However, several complications associated with this technique may occur in the early and late postoperative period. Early complications include contralateral access site issues (PSA, iatrogenic AVF, bleeding, hematoma, etc.), embolization, thrombosis, and exclusion (jailing) of collateral vessels with resultant ischemia. Late complications include intimal hyperplasia, in-stent restenosis, and thrombosis. The majority of patients in these series (83%) had resolution of the iatrogenic PSA or AVF without short- or long-term complications.

The optimal medical management for patients who receive a covered stent graft has not been studied in a prospective fashion. Extrapolating from clinical trials involving patients who undergo percutaneous coronary intervention using bare metal stents, most interventional physicians and surgeons treat with dual antiplatelet therapy for a defined period. Currently, the Journal of the American Heart Association recommends indefinite aspirin therapy and 3 months of an additional antiplatelet agent, most commonly clopidogrel. Patients who undergo open surgical repair for an AVF do not require any additional antiplatelet therapy beyond that which is indicated for their underlying medical comorbidities. Postoperative surveillance should include arterial and venous duplex ultrasound prior to discharge from the hospital and at 2 months, 6 months, and 1 year.

Case Conclusion

The patient underwent successful treatment via an endovascular approach as a day procedure, using a 5 mm × 4 cm covered stent graft placed from the contralateral femoral artery. Postprocedure ultrasound demonstrated no areas of stenosis and resolution of the fistula. At a 2-month follow-up appointment, duplex ultrasound demonstrated a peak systolic velocity (PSV) of 353 cm/s in the middle of the stent, while just proximal to the stent, the external iliac artery PSV measures 82 cm/s. The patient complained of recurring claudication after walking two blocks. The patient returned to the endovascular suite, and in-stent stenosis was identified. Using a 4 mm × 4 cm cutting balloon, the area of intimal hyperplasia was scored, and the covered stent was re-treated with a 5 mm × 4 cm angioplasty balloon. The lesion responded well to the treatment with improvement of symptoms. At the subsequent follow-up appointment, the patent was doing well with no claudication symptoms and no identifiable velocity elevation on duplex ultrasound imaging.

TAKE HOME POINTS

- Iatrogenic AVF occurs in 0.1% of femoral access procedures.
- Most iatrogenic AVF (81%) will close spontaneously within 12 months.
- Symptomatic or iatrogenic AVFs that do not close within 12 months can be treated effectively with both endovascular and open techniques.
- Endovascular repair exposes the patient to contralateral access complications, such as embolization and thrombosis. However, there is less postoperative pain, fewer wound complications, and a shorter hospital stay. The open approach has a higher technical success rate and a higher risk of wound complications.
- Dual antiplatelet therapy is recommended after covered stent placement.
- Patients need follow-up with duplex imaging prior to discharge and at 2 months, 6 months, and 1 year.
- Late complications of repair such as intimal hyperplasia can be readily identified by duplex ultrasound and treated appropriately with either endovascular or open technique.

SUGGESTED READINGS

Castillo-Sang M, Tsang AW, Almaroof B, et al. Femoral artery complications after cardiac catheterization: a study of patient profile. *Ann Vasc Surg.* 2010;24(3):328-335.

Kelm M, Perings SM, Jax T, et al. Incidence and clinical outcome of iatrogenic femoral arteriovenous fistulas: implications for risk stratification and treatment. *J Am Coll Cardiol.* 2002;40(2):291-297.

Perings SM, Kelm M, Jax T, et al. A prospective study on incidence and risk factors of arteriovenous fistulae following transfemoral cardiac catheterization. *Int J Cardiol.* 2003;88(2-3):223-228.

Seay T, Soares G, Dawson D. Postcatheterization arteriovenous fistula: CT, ultrasound, and arteriographic findings. *Emerg Radiol.* 2002;9(5):296-299.

Thalhammer C, Kirchherr AS, Uhlich F, et al. Postcatheterization pseudoaneurysms and arteriovenous fistulas: repair with percutaneous implantation of endovascular covered stents. *Radiology.* 2000;214(1):127-131.

Toursarkissian B, Allen BT, Petrinec D, et al. Spontaneous closure of selected iatrogenic pseudoaneurysms and arteriovenous fistulae. *J Vasc Surg.* 1997;25(5):803-809.

CLINICAL SCENARIO CASE QUESTIONS

1. The most common complication associated with femoral artery access is:
   a. Femoral artery pseudoaneurysm
   b. Profunda femoris—femoral vein fistula
   c. Hematoma
   d. Bleeding

2. Arteriovenous fistula associated with femoral artery access will spontaneously close in what percentage of patients?
   a. 10%
   b. 40%
   c. 50%
   d. 80%
   e. 100%

121 Posterior Knee Dislocation

ANDREW G. GEORGIADIS and ALEXANDER D. SHEPARD

Presentation

A 37-year-old morbidly obese female (BMI 46) is brought to the emergency department after slipping on a carpet at home and presenting with left knee pain. She is triaged to a low-acuity bed. She has swelling and pain in her left lower extremity but no discernible deformity or open wounds. After examination, this is determined to be an isolated injury. At the time of orthopedic and vascular surgical consultation, dorsalis pedis and posterior tibial pulses are absent in the injured left lower extremity but are present in the uninjured right. Femoral pulses are palpable bilaterally. Sensation is grossly intact but altered on the dorsal and plantar left foot. The patient cannot tolerate any passive motion of her left knee.

Differential Diagnosis

Based on the physical exam, there is an arterial occlusion in the left lower extremity below the level of the femoral artery. Despite the lack of physical deformity in the injured extremity, the main differential diagnosis is a periarticular fracture or knee dislocation. The popliteal artery is relatively fixed proximally and distally at the adductor hiatus and fascial arch of the soleus and is therefore susceptible to injury with any traumatic knee deformity. Injury to the popliteal artery results from direct avulsion, transection, or most commonly a stretch injury leading to intimal disruption and thrombosis.

In the setting of dislocation, closed reduction must be performed immediately under appropriate pharmacologic muscle relaxation, usually administered by the emergency department physician. Reassessment of distal pulses is made thereafter.

Case Continued

Radiographs reveal a knee dislocation with the patient's tibia posterior to her femur (Fig. 1). Closed reduction was unsuccessfully attempted in the emergency department. Warm ischemia time at the time of attempted reduction was 4 hours. The patient was immediately taken to the operating room for closed reduction of the knee under general anesthesia with intraoperative arteriography.

Workup

A focused history and physical are essential in determining the mechanism and chronicity of extremity ischemia. Radiographs of the knee should be obtained immediately in any patient with knee pain and an asymmetric pulse exam (Fig. 1). Hard signs of vascular injury include active hemorrhage, expanding hematoma, distal ischemia, or bruit at the injury site. Asymmetric pulses or return of a palpable pulse after reduction mandates further evaluation with Doppler-derived ankle-brachial indices (ABIs). An ABI less than 0.9 constitutes an indication for arterial imaging. Palpable pulses do not exclude vascular injury as pulse waves can propagate through developing thrombus and an undetected intimal injury can lead to later thrombotic complications. An ABI greater than 0.9 reliably excludes a significant arterial injury.

Angiography remains the gold standard for extremity arterial imaging but is increasingly being supplanted by computed tomographic angiography (CTA) particularly for injuries at or above the level of the knee. In the setting of potential knee dislocation, CTA can also provide information about the vein as well as fractures that could change management. Duplex scanning is another imaging modality that is particularly useful when trying to rule out an intimal injury in a patient with palpable pulses and reduced ABIs. In the absence of palpable pulses following reduction, further evaluation should be undertaken in the operating room.

Case Continued

After closed reduction in the operating room, the patient's knee was grossly unstable and recurrent posterior dislocation occurred with any manipulation of the extremity. Postreduction pulses and signals were absent. Warm ischemia time at this juncture was 5 hours.

Diagnosis and Treatment

Radiographic evaluation confirms the direction of dislocation and any associated fractures. The direction of a dislocation is termed by the distal portion of the articulation, here the tibia, and anterior dislocations are more common. Early studies suggested that the popliteal artery failed by intimal tearing, stretch, and thrombosis in anterior dislocation versus frank transection in posterior dislocation. It is now known that any direction of dislocation can result in any morphology of vessel compromise.

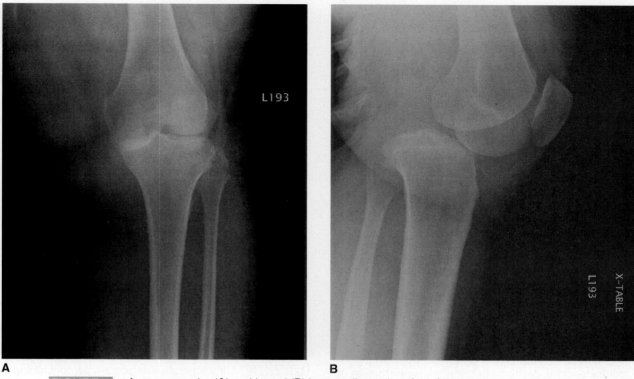

FIGURE 1 • Anteroposterior (**A**) and lateral (**B**) knee radiographs of a left knee posterior dislocation.

Ultimately, the direction of dislocation is irrelevant for the purposes of acute treatment. Emergent closed reduction should be performed followed by immediate reassessment of distal pulses and ABIs. In the setting of acute ischemia, patients should be immediately heparinized. If distal pulses are restored, ABIs should be performed. If the ABI is greater than 0.9, the patient can be safely observed with serial exams. If the ABI is less than 0.9, further arterial imaging is required as outlined above. Institutions with protocols for ABI-based selective arterial imaging have reported very low false-negative rates. For nonobese patients with minor changes in their ABI, we prefer duplex scanning of the popliteal artery/vein and distal vasculature. For more profound ABI changes (less than 0.8), we prefer catheter angiography or CTA. Most detected popliteal artery injuries should be repaired unless minor in nature. Intimal injuries involving less than 30% of the vessel circumference can be safely observed with serial duplex ultrasounds and ABIs. We usually treat these patients with a short course of anticoagulation and discharge on clopidogrel. Patients without restoration of pulses following knee reduction should go directly to the operating room for exploration with or without intraoperative angiography based on surgeon preference. Full-dose heparin anticoagulation should be continued.

Traditionally, knee dislocation after high-energy trauma has been associated with the highest rates of popliteal vascular injury, with a reported incidence of 7%

to 40%. There are now increasing reports of low-energy knee dislocation in obese patients (often following a slip or fall from level ground) resulting in even higher rates of associated vascular and nerve injury. Obese patients with seemingly innocuous trauma may be overlooked and triaged inappropriately, leading to delay to diagnosis of limb-threatening ischemia. In the setting of delayed diagnosis (greater than 6 hours) or if the surgeon has high suspicion for severe muscle necrosis intraoperatively, consent for primary amputation should be obtained preoperatively. Although tibial nerve injury is more common in obese patients with knee dislocation than in nonobese patients, nerve disruption is rare (Table 1).

Surgical Approach

The patient should be placed supine on a radiolucent table and after the induction of general anesthesia, both lower extremities prepped from groin to toes in anticipation of contralateral saphenous vein harvest. The knee should be closed reduced, if this could not be accomplished preoperatively, in conjunction with the orthopedic surgery team. Assessment of knee stability is important after reduction, as gross instability is common after dislocation and usually necessitates placement of spanning external fixation. Placement of an external fixator prior to definitive vascular repair, however, delays revascularization and prevents knee flexion, which is critical to exposure and repair of the injured segment. If pulses return following operative reduction, intraoperative angiography can be

TABLE 1. Popliteal Artery Repair Associated with Knee Dislocation

Key Technical Steps

1. Avoid definitive skeletal stabilization with external fixator until vascular repair completed. The unstable knee can be supported with rolled packs during vascular reconstruction.
2. Expose the popliteal artery through a medial distal thigh proximal calf incision, dividing the medial attachments of the knee.
3. Excise all injured vessel wall, and remove any occluding or partially occluding thrombus in inflow and runoff vessels.
4. Even for short defects, interposition grafting with reverse GSV, harvested from the contralateral extremity, is recommended to ensure a tension-free repair.
5. Repair an injured popliteal vein whenever possible.
6. Have a low threshold for performing fasciotomies.

Potential Pitfalls

- In any situation with lower extremity orthopedic and/ or vascular trauma, ensure the patient is placed on a radiolucent table.
- Fasciotomy should be performed in patients with prolonged (4–6 hours) ischemia and should usually precede vascular reconstruction.
- Avoid injury to ipsilateral GSV during popliteal artery exposure and fasciotomies.
- Ensure complete clearance of distal clot by performing an intraoperative, postthrombectomy, prereconstruction angiogram if there is any doubt.

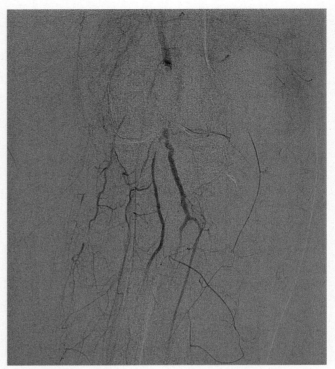

FIGURE 2 • Intraoperative angiogram demonstrating popliteal artery occlusion with an aberrant (high) origin of the posterior tibial artery.

performed to rule out a popliteal injury (Fig. 2). Patients with persistent ischemia or an angiographically defined major injury after reduction require popliteal exploration. If warm ischemia time is greater than 5 to 6 hours, we recommend four compartment fasciotomies of the leg through liberal medial and lateral incisions and notation of muscular contractility.

The injured segment of popliteal artery is invariably directly behind the knee joint at the level of the tibial plateau. Direct visualization of this segment requires knee flexion, which can be problematic with a grossly unstable knee; usually, the knee can be safely supported with appropriately placed rolled packs. A medial incision beginning just above the knee anterior to the sartorius is carried distally on to the calf 1 to 2 cm posterior to the medial edge of the tibia. Exposure of the injury site usually requires division of all the medial knee structures (gracilis, semimembranosus, semitendinosus, and medial head of the gastrocnemius), which can have further adverse effects on knee stability. The divided ends should be tagged and an attempt made at reapproximation at the time of closure. Occasionally, a posterior approach can be used when there is a documented short-segment thrombosis without distal propagation of clot, but this approach severely limits additional operative options (i.e., vein harvest, concomitant fasciotomy, distal thrombectomy). A posterior approach, however, avoids further knee destabilization and is ideal in an obese patient. Some authorities advocate bypass of the injured segment through standard above-knee and below-knee popliteal

exposures. This approach avoids division of the medial knee structures but precludes direct exposure of the injured arterial segment and vein.

Exposure of the popliteal vessels can be challenging as normal anatomy is frequently disturbed by edema, hematoma, or deformity. The injured segment is connoted by a dusky, purplish hue to the external vessel wall. Once the extent of the injury has been determined, preparations are made for repair. Excision of the injured segment and creation of an end-to-end tension-free anastomosis is virtually never possible without extensive mobilization and division of geniculate branches. Interposition grafting with a segment of reversed greater saphenous vein (GSV) harvested from the contralateral extremity is the standard treatment for most of these injuries. With this in mind, a longitudinal arteriotomy is performed at the injury site to identify the junction between normal and abnormal artery. Occasionally, a limited dissection is noted, which can be repaired locally after thrombectomy followed by arterial closure with a vein patch. More significant injuries are the rule and require excision of the injured segment. Normal popliteal artery is transected distally and clot removed from the distal vascular bed with a # 3-French balloon thrombectomy catheter. Complete clearance of the distal vascular bed can be documented with an angiogram. The proximal artery is prepared in a similar fashion with restoration of pulsatile inflow sufficing to document the clearance of proximal thrombus. In cases of profound limb ischemia, a small intraluminal shunt can be placed to restore flow while vein is harvested. We have found this maneuver much more useful in penetrating trauma where bone and/or patient stabilization is necessary prior to definitive vascular repair. In addition, further arterial length is sacrificed as the ends of the artery where the shunt is placed almost invariably require further resection.

An appropriate length of GSV is harvested from the contralateral groin. The proximal anastomosis is performed first in end-to-end fashion after spatulating the two ends. Great care is taken to ensure an appropriate length of graft to avoid being either too short or redundant when the knee is in appropriate extension. The distal anastomosis is then performed in end-to-end fashion to the distal popliteal artery. Following stabilization of the knee with or without an external fixator, a postreconstruction angiogram is obtained to assess the adequacy of repair and (if not done prior to repair) the status of the runoff vessels. Popliteal vein injuries are much less frequent than arterial injuries with knee dislocations (10% to 15% in our experience), but when detected should be repaired whenever possible to enhance limb salvage. Venous repair should usually precede arterial repair. Necrotic/nonviable muscle and soft tissue should be debrided prior to closure and every attempt made to reapproximate the medial knee structures with coverage of the interposition graft with loosely coapted, healthy tissue. If fasciotomies have not been previously performed, careful consideration should be paid to proceeding with them now. Fasciotomy sites, if performed, are treated with negative pressure, vacuum-assisted sponge dressings.

Special Intraoperative Considerations

In situations with prolonged ischemia (4 to 6 hours), always consider four compartment fasciotomies, which in most cases should precede arterial reconstruction. In cases of low-velocity dislocation in morbidly obese patients, it may be helpful to place two operating tables adjacent to one another, gather multiple assistants, and procure large retractors. Significant technical intraoperative difficulty has been noted in the bypass grafting of such patients. Mannitol can be helpful in managing reperfusion injuries in patients with prolonged ischemia. With nonviable muscle in all four compartments or a disrupted tibial nerve (very rare), consider primary amputation.

Case Continued

The patient was placed supine on two adjacent radiolucent tables. After orthopedic reduction, four compartment fasciotomies were the first step performed because of the length of time elapsed since injury. The popliteal artery was exposed and proximal and distal control obtained. A long area of injury was identified and a 6-cm segment of artery resected. Following proximal and distal thrombectomy, an angiogram was obtained to confirm clearance of the distal vasculature. An interposition graft of reversed saphenous

vein, harvested from the contralateral thigh, was placed with immediate return of posterior tibialis and dorsalis pedis Doppler signals. External fixation was placed anterolaterally and a completion angiogram performed to reveal a technically satisfactory result.

Postoperative Management

Hourly pulse monitoring is necessary for 24 hours, the most common window for graft thrombosis or bleeding. If fasciotomies have not been performed, compartment surveillance should be performed concomitantly. Aspirin antiplatelet therapy (325 mg/day) and prophylactic doses of low molecular weight heparin should be administered to all with consideration for full-dose anticoagulation in patients with concomitant venous injuries. Limb elevation and selective use of intermittent pneumatic compression sleeves should be instituted in all patients. Any early change in pulse or signal exam, whether sudden or gradual, should be considered graft occlusion until proven otherwise. Nearly all patients should have regained palpable pedal pulses within the 12 hours of surgery with failure to do so suggesting a problem that warrants further investigation. Patients with knee dislocation have high rates of tibial and peroneal nerve injury, which should be managed expectantly. If fasciotomy was not performed, then particular attention should be paid to the development of compartment syndrome, which can be particularly difficult to diagnose in obese patients with concomitant nerve injuries. We have not found compartmental pressures to be of any help. Even without a compartment syndrome, there can be significant muscle damage leading to rhabdomyolysis and possible myoglobinuria. For this reason, we check serial (q8 hour) creatine phosphokinase levels for the first 24 hours and institute aggressive dieresis as necessary. If the patient has an insensate foot secondary to tibial neuropraxia, attention to providing pressure relief is necessary to avoid skin breakdown as is an ankle-foot orthosis to prevent a plantar flexion deformity. Multiligamentous knee reconstruction should not be performed during the initial hospital stay.

Case Conclusion

Hourly pulse and signal surveillance was continued for 48 hours. The fasciotomy sites were closed on postoperative day 4 using a Dermaclose device. The patient developed a superficial wound infection and was treated with parenteral antibiotics with a transition to oral antibiotics and supportive local wound care. Paresthesias persisted in the superficial and deep peroneal nerve distributions without motor deficit. The patient was discharged from the hospital on postoperative day 8.

TAKE HOME POINTS

- Have a high index of suspicion for knee dislocation in obese patients with seemingly innocuous trauma.
- An evidence-based protocol for the evaluation of vascular injury associated with knee dislocation results in faster diagnosis and improved outcomes.
- Selective arterial imaging avoids unnecessary testing.
- Irreversible tissue damage may occur after 6 hours of trauma-induced ischemia, and revascularization should be accompanied by fasciotomy.
- Restoration of arterial continuity after blunt popliteal injury is best accomplished by interposition vein grafting.

SUGGESTED READINGS

Georgiadis AG, Mohammed FH, Mizerik KT, et al. Changing presentation of knee dislocation and vascular injury from high energy trauma to low energy falls in the morbidly obese. *J Vasc Surg.* 2013;57(5):1196-1203.

Nicandri GT, Dunbar RP, Wahl CJ. Are evidence-based protocols which identify vascular injury associated with knee dislocation underutilized? *Knee Surg Sports Traumatol Arthrosc.* 2010;18:1005-1012.

Stannard JP, Sheils TM, Lopez-Ben RR, et al. Vascular injuries in knee dislocations: the role of physical examination in determining the need for arteriography. *J Bone Joint Surg Am.* 2004;86-A:910-915.

Wagner WH, Calkins ER, Weaver FA, et al. Blunt popliteal artery trauma: one hundred consecutive injuries. *J Vasc Surg.* 1988;7(5):736-743.

CLINICAL SCENARIO CASE QUESTIONS

1. Which of the following is an indication for arteriography in the setting of knee dislocation?
   a. Posterior knee dislocation
   b. Anterior knee dislocation
   c. Postreduction ABI of 0.85
   d. Symmetric postreduction dorsalis pedis pulses
   e. Patient history of peripheral vascular disease

2. A 25-year-old is evaluated in the trauma bay after a motor vehicle collision. He has an obvious left knee deformity and absent distal pulses, and all other workup is negative. Radiographs reveal an isolated anterior knee dislocation. After reduction, pulses return and are symmetric bilaterally. ABIs in the affected extremity are 0.95. What is the next most appropriate treatment?
   a. Arteriography
   b. Discharge with close follow-up
   c. External fixation
   d. Serial pulse exam for 24 to 48 hours
   e. Exploration of the popliteal artery

122 Penetrating Injury to the Lower Extremity

KIRA N. LONG and TODD E. RASMUSSEN

Presentation

A 24-year-old male is transferred to the resuscitation room from an outlying facility by emergency medical system (EMS) paramedics after having been shot in his left thigh just above the knee. The patient had initially been treated in the operating room of a smaller outlying facility. At the time of the initial operation, the field tourniquet had been removed and the wound explored revealing a transected above-knee popliteal artery and vein. Because of limited resources and experience at the facility, flow across the arterial and venous injuries was restored by placing temporary vascular shunts after the vessels had been controlled and thrombus removed. A left lower extremity fasciotomy was performed at the outlying facility, and the leg was dressed and wrapped for transfer including positioning but not tightening tourniquets above and below the wound in case the shunts became dislodged during transport (Fig. 1). The patient arrives in the resuscitation room with normal vital signs and a well-perfused left foot including a palpable dorsalis pedis pulse.

Diagnosis

Signs of Vascular Injury

Penetrating wounds to the lower extremities should always raise suspicion for injury to one of the main arteries or veins in the limb. The diagnosis of vascular injury in this setting is fairly straightforward if the patient has hard signs, which include bleeding from the penetrating wound or wounds, an expanding hematoma around the wound, the presence of an audible bruit, a palpable thrill, or obvious ischemia of the leg. The diagnosis of lower extremity vascular injury is more challenging in the absence of hard signs, and in these cases, a high index of suspicion and additional testing (Doppler or radiographic imaging) is required. Soft signs of vascular injury include the presence of a penetrating fragment or munition near a major vessel, a nonexpanding hematoma, or the report of significant blood loss at the scene of the injury. Neurologic deficit in the extremity is often considered a soft sign of vascular injury as are certain fracture patterns including displaced femur fractures and a displaced fracture of the tibial plateau. Even in the absence of clear ischemia, the examiner's index of suspicion should be raised if one or more of these soft signs of lower extremity vascular injury are present.

Workup

As one examines the patient with penetrating wounds to the lower extremity, it is useful to consider the differential diagnosis, which , in addition to vascular injury, includes pain from fracture, peripheral nerve injury, or entrapment of a nerve from an adjacent fracture. Pain from the penetrating soft tissue wound itself is often significant and in some cases may be the only significant finding. In the presence of a fracture, the axial vessels of the thigh (femoral or popliteal) and/or leg (tibial vessels) may be misaligned, thus causing reduced or absent pulses or Doppler signals in the foot. In these instances, if the wall of the vessel is uninjured, reduction and alignment of the lower extremity fracture will often result in restoration of perfusion. Similarly, nerve entrapment will also frequently resolve with improvement of distal signs and symptoms after reduction and alignment of the extremity fracture.

Physical examination of patients with penetrating wounds to the lower extremity, gunshot, or other includes assessing the extremity for deformity and evaluation of perfusion to the foot and toes. Depending on the setting, the physical exam can be performed simultaneously with plain radiographs (views of the femur, knee, tibia, and fibula) to diagnose and assess the severity of any fracture. Palpation for the femoral pulse at the inguinal ligament, the popliteal pulse behind the knee, and the posterior tibial and dorsalis pedis pulses in the foot should be performed and capillary refill estimated in the toes.

Continuous wave Doppler is an extension of the physical exam in patients with penetrating wounds to the lower extremity and Doppler signals should be assessed at the same locations at which pulses were palpated. Strong, biphasic signals audible at these locations argue against a significant artery injury, while weak, monophasic or

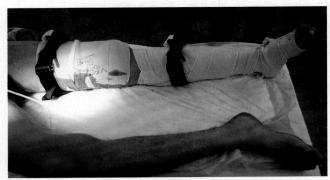

FIGURE 1 • Left lower extremity gunshot wound resulting in transected above-knee popliteal artery and vein. The injury was explored at a smaller outlying facility at which time the artery and vein were managed with vascular shunts, a left lower extremity fasciotomy was performed, and the extremity was dressed as shown in the image. The loosely applied Combat Application Tourniquets were positioned at the time of transport in case the shunts became dislodged. Note also the *writing* on the ace bandage indicating that vascular shunts are in place.

TABLE 1. Management Considerations

Key Technical Steps

1. Proper and complete neurovascular exam is essential with a penetrating injury.
2. Confirm whether hard signs of vascular injury are present or soft signs.
3. Use IEI for quantifying blood flow between injured and noninjured extremity.
4. Can use local heparinization if systemic heparinization is contraindicated.
5. In severe injury, use of a temporary shunt is indicated.
6. Use autologous tissue for definitive repair.

Potential Pitfalls

- Always reduce the fracture first if present with penetrating injury.
- Soft tissue coverage over arterial repair is essential—do not place VAC over artery directly.
- Consider four-compartment fasciotomy in most cases after reperfusion.
- If the patient is stable, consider venous repair—neglect may lead to severe swelling if a proximal vein is injured.

---

absent arterial signals indicate a flow-limiting arterial defect. To more objectively assess perfusion of the leg and foot, one should measure the injured extremity index (IEI). Also referred to as the ankle-brachial index (ABI), the IEI is a ratio of the occlusion pressure of the distal arterial Doppler signal in the injured compared to the noninjured lower extremity. To accomplish this, a manual blood pressure cuff is placed over the leg of the injured extremity and inflated while the Doppler signal is assessed at the posterior tibial and then the dorsalis pedis artery. The cuff pressure at which the arterial signal occludes or is no longer audible at each of the arterial locations should be recorded and these steps repeated on an uninjured upper extremity (i.e., the brachial artery). The IEI or ABI is calculated by dividing the highest occlusion pressure on the injured lower extremity by the occlusion pressure of the upper extremity with a normal index being 0.9 or greater. The IEI or ABI provides a more objective and repeatable measure by which to assess for lower extremity arterial injury and is especially useful in scenarios where perfusion distal to a femur or tibial fracture may not be obvious (Table 1).

Additional Imaging versus Operation

Patients with hard signs of lower extremity arterial injury (i.e., external hemorrhage, profound or obvious ischemia, arteriovenous fistula, and expanding hematoma) such as those in the case scenario provided at the beginning of the chapter typically do not need additional imaging or workup prior to being taken to the operating room. One exception to this is the case in which the patient has additional injuries that require further imaging. For example, if a patient has hard signs of lower extremity hemorrhage requiring tourniquet application, little additional imaging

of the leg may be necessary before exploring the wound in the operating room. However, if this same patient has other penetrating or blunt injuries, he or she may very well require imaging (i.e., head, chest, and abdomen) prior to commencing treatment of the penetrating lower extremity wounds.

Patients who have femur and/or a tibial fracture and less clear signs of vascular injury (i.e., modestly reduce ABI, audible but abnormal sounding Doppler signals, equivocal capillary refill) pose a more challenging diagnostic scenario. In these cases, additional imaging with arteriography, contrast tomography (CT), or duplex ultrasonography may be useful in making the decision as to whether or not to operate on the artery. However, unlike blunt or closed trauma, patients with gunshot or fragmentation injury to the lower extremity require operative debridement and washout of the soft tissue wound(s) regardless of concern for vascular injury.

Because of the relatively superficial nature of the arteries of the lower extremity, duplex ultrasound is often the imaging modality of choice as it is quick, inexpensive, noninvasive, and able to be repeated. However, traditional catheter-based arteriography or CT angiography may also be used to discern the presence of flow-limiting defects or injuries in the femoral, popliteal, or tibial vessels with CT providing particularly detailed information when there is concern for fracture.

It is important to note that in all cases of penetrating lower extremity with fracture, the initial step in management, often even before additional imaging, is fracture reduction and stabilization of the extremity. This can often be performed outside of the operating room following hemorrhage control, initiation of resuscitation, and pain control measures. In nearly all cases of significant fracture with dislocation or misalignment, this management step should be pursued regardless of initial signs of vascular injury. Depending on the severity of and the time since the injury, reducing and stabilizing a femur or tibial fracture may favorably change perfusion to the leg and foot and improve the vascular exam. In most cases of mild to moderate fracture, the decision as to whether or not to operate on or further image the lower extremity vessels is made after the fracture is reduced and the vascular exam is repeated. If signs of vascular injury persist after fracture reduction and stabilization, then additional imaging with one of the previously noted modalities is indicated. In cases of extreme open femur or tibial fracture (i.e., the mangled extremity), fracture reduction and stabilization and exploration of the vessels should occur simultaneously in the operating room.

Treatment Decision

If physical signs of ischemia are present or persist after fracture reduction, efforts to restore normal perfusion to the leg and foot should be undertaken in most cases. In the lower extremity, the decision to operate on an arterial injury is highly dependent on the anatomic location of the injury. Proximal injuries to the common femoral artery require repair in nearly all cases as the degree of collateral circulation around this large inflow vessel is not sufficient to maintain viability to the leg and foot. Although injuries distal to the profunda femoris artery are somewhat better tolerated, the superficial femoral and popliteal arteries should also be repaired in the majority of cases. This is especially true in the setting of penetrating injury in which collaterals from the proximal common, profunda, and superficial femoral arteries will have been interrupted by the soft tissue wound(s).

In contrast to the femoral and popliteal arteries, a selective approach to tibial artery repair is recommended (i.e., repair some but not all). Because of the redundant nature of the tibial vessels (anterior tibial, posterior tibial, and peroneal), it is common that one or even two of these arteries may be injured without rendering the leg or foot critically ischemic. The selective approach to tibial artery repair is made while balancing the severity of extremity ischemia with the patient's overall injury and physiologic condition. The complexity of a tibial vessel reconstruction in the setting of penetrating trauma will require seasoned vascular surgery experience and several hours of operating. In some cases in which the degree of ischemia to the leg and foot is in question or incomplete, the tibial artery may be ligated or restored with a temporary vascular shunt while the patient is resuscitated and an experienced vascular team assembled.

The practice of damage control surgery or abbreviated operating refers to limiting the physiologic stress or compromise from the initial operation, which should focus only on controlling hemorrhage and contamination and restoring critical ischemia. Within the bounds of damage control surgery, it is also recognized that extremity vascular ligation with or without immediate amputation may be the necessary operation. This maneuver typically applies to the significantly mangled extremity in which repair would be futile or judged to put the patient's physiologic condition or life at risk.

Surgical Approach

Lower extremity vascular injury should be approached with an open surgical incision in nearly all cases. While isolated reports of catheter-based (i.e., endovascular) treatment of this injury pattern exist, the superficial and accessible nature of the lower extremity vasculature makes it most amenable to open repair. To expose and operate on any lower extremity vascular injury from a penetrating mechanism, the patient should be placed supine on the operating table and the lower abdomen and groins shaved and included in the surgical scrub. Including these proximal aspects in the surgical field allows one access to the external iliac and common femoral arteries should inflow control be needed or access for arteriography. The surgical scrub and prep should also include both lower extremities from the groin to and including the feet and toes. Access to the distal aspect of the extremity allows one to fully position the limb and assess perfusion following exploration and management of the injury—repair, ligation, or shunting. To facilitate concurrent management of any extremity fracture(s) and/or performance of angiography, it is useful to have the patient positioned on a radiolucent table and to have mobile fluoroscopy available in the room.

The common, profunda, and proximal superficial femoral arteries should be approached through a longitudinal incision at and just distal to the inguinal ligament. The incision should be positioned proximal enough to allow exposure and control of the femoral artery, which can include extending the exposure proximal onto the lower abdomen and retroperitoneum. In the inguinal space and just distal to this, the femoral artery rests between the femoral vein and nerve.

The superficial femoral artery extends distally in the thigh exiting through the adductor magnus (i.e., adductor or Hunter's canal) above the knee where it transitions to the popliteal artery (Fig. 2). The femoral vessels in the thigh should be approached through a medial incision reflecting the sartorius muscle either up (superior or lateral) or down (inferior) depending on whether the incision is proximal or distal, respectively. Throughout its course in the thigh, the superficial femoral and then popliteal artery is adjacent and often adherent to its sister femoral vein. There are three notable anatomic features of the adductor canal: (1) the superficial femoral artery becomes the above-knee popliteal artery, (2) the saphenous nerve becomes a superficial structure, and (3) the supreme geniculate artery or arteries arise from the axial femoral artery.

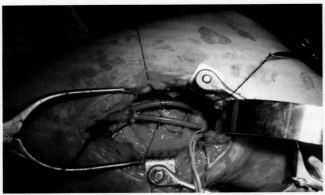

FIGURE 2 • At the time of exploration of the injury in the case, vascular shunts were found in the proximal popliteal artery and vein. The shunts had been secured with silk suture ties, and both were patent with Doppler flow several hours after the injury. Note also the operative approach that includes a Wietlaner retractor proximally, a Henly popliteal retractor, and a short handheld Wylie renal vein retractor to expose the behind the knee segment.

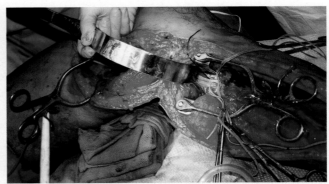

FIGURE 3 • Exposure of the below-knee popliteal space of the left lower extremity in a case other than the provided scenario. Note that the lift or "bump" is placed behind the thigh and the leg is slightly flexed to allow the gastrocnemius muscle to hang down and open the below-knee operative space. In this image, the Henly popliteal retractor with adjustable depth blades is used to open the below-knee popliteal space and a short, narrow handheld Wylie renal vein retractor is used to expose the behind the knee segment. The popliteal artery, which has a patent shunt in it, has been encircled by a blue vessel loop as has the uninjured popliteal vein.

To expose the distal superficial femoral and above-knee popliteal artery and vein, the knee should be slightly flexed (i.e., "frog-leg" position) with a small bump or elevation placed below the knee. This maneuver enlists the help of gravity in opening up the above-knee popliteal space by slightly suspending the thigh musculature such that it "hangs down" and is not compressed up against the vessels to be exposed. To expose above and behind the knee, the medial incision should be extended distally to the level of the knee with care taken not to injure the ipsilateral saphenous vein. A deep Wietlaner or Henly popliteal self-retaining retractor with adjustable depth blades is often a necessity for this exposure as is a handheld narrow (1″) Wylie renal vein retractor (5″ length or depth) (Fig. 2). Using this approach, one should be able to expose the above- and behind-knee popliteal vessels without dividing the medial attachments of the pes anserinus (sartorius, gracilis, and semitendinosus).

The operative exposure of the below-knee popliteal artery requires much of the same equipment, although the elevator or "bump" should be placed underneath the thigh allowing gravity to pull the musculature of the leg down away from the popliteal space (Fig. 3). The below-knee popliteal vessels should also be approached through a medial incision with division of the gastrocnemius fascia allowing opening of the space. Care should be taken not to divide the saphenous vein with this incision, and one should recognize that the popliteal artery often rests between the popliteal vein and the tibial nerve from this medial approach (Fig. 4). The origin of the anterior tibial artery marks the distal extent of the popliteal artery, which then transitions to become the tibial-peroneal trunk behind the proximal most fibers of the soleus muscle or fascia (entering the posterior deep compartment).

The operative approach to the posterior tibial and peroneal arteries, both of which rest in the posterior deep compartment, is through a medial approach in the leg. The fascia of the gastrocnemius muscle is first

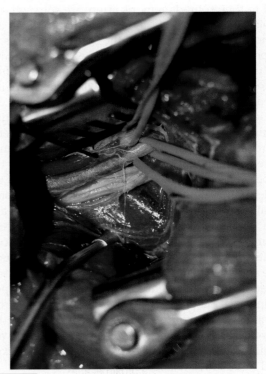

FIGURE 4 • A close view of the structures of the below-knee popliteal space including the popliteal artery with a patent vascular shunt in place, the popliteal vein, and the tibial nerve. In this case, the popliteal vein was uninjured and has been dissected free from the medial portion of the artery and encircled with a blue vessel loop to allow retraction away from the artery.

incised, facilitating entry into the posterior superficial compartment. With this muscle retracted inferiorly, the attachment of the soleus muscle to the edge of the tibia must be divided over a distance in order to enter the desired compartment and expose the posterior tibial and peroneal vessels. When entering the posterior deep compartment from the medial approach, the first artery to be encountered is the posterior tibial artery. The peroneal artery, which resides in this same compartment, is deeper or more lateral than the posterior tibial. Because the anterior tibial artery takes a lateral course from below the knee and rests in the anterior compartment of the leg, it must be approached through a lateral incision.

The zone of injury should be dissected free of surrounding structures and the extent of injury determined. Depending on the severity, vascular repair will require one of three categories of approach: primary closure, patch angioplasty, or interposition grafting. Because of their relatively small and elastic nature, most significant lower extremity arterial injuries from penetrating mechanisms will require removal of the injured segment and restoration of flow using an interposition graft (Figs. 5 and 6).

Prior to repairing the artery, removal of thrombus proximal and distal to the injury should be accomplished using a small (2- or 4-French) Fogarty thromboembolectomy catheter. Once this has been accomplished, one should assure that there is ample fore and back bleeding and then instill heparinized saline solution proximal and distal to the injured segment. The edges of the injured vessel should be debrided to assure that the suture repair is performed through normal or nontraumatized, full-thickness vascular wall. Regardless of the type of recon-

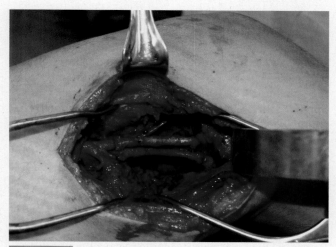

FIGURE 6 • Operative photograph showing interposition vein graft repair of the proximal popliteal artery and vein. The interposition grafts consisted of reversed greater saphenous vein from the right (contralateral) lower extremity.

struction (primary, patch, or interposition), repair should be completed using fine (6-0 or 7-0), monofilament, permanent suture such as polypropylene (Prolene) or polytetrafluoroethylene (ePTFE). In most cases, autologous saphenous vein from the contralateral extremity should be used for the patch or the interposition graft (Figs. 5 and 6). If vein is not available, synthetic path or conduit such as ePFTE may be used. Assessment of perfusion following completion of the vascular repair can be made using intraoperative Doppler or duplex and occasionally contrast arteriography. The vascular repair should be covered with viable muscle and soft tissue to reduce the likelihood of anastomotic infection or desiccation and disruption. This final point is particularly important in the setting of significant soft tissue injury from penetrating mechanisms. Depending on the extent of soft tissue injury, one may need to plan on repeat operations to assess the viability of evolving muscle and soft tissue assuring adequate debridement. Occasionally, a local, rotational, vascularized muscle flap is necessary to provide coverage of the vascular reconstruction.

Special Considerations for Operative Repair

Temporary Vascular Shunt

The use of temporary vascular shunts as in the case scenario (Fig. 2) is a quicker and simpler way to restore perfusion to lower extremity in the setting of some extremity vascular injuries. This damage control adjunct may be especially useful to reduce ischemic time in cases in which the operating team has limited experience with formal vascular reconstruction (e.g., the case vignette) or in cases where the patient has higher priority, life-threatening injuries. Shunts have also been shown to be effective at quickly restoring perfusion to the leg and foot prior to formal fixation of a femur or tibial fracture. In these cases, the lower extremity vascular injury is explored and the shunt placed following

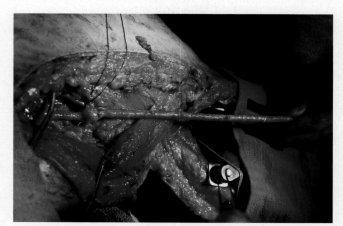

FIGURE 5 • Formation of an interposition reversed greater saphenous vein graft for a left lower extremity popliteal artery injury. In this case, the proximal anastamosis has been completed and the vein graft is distended with blood from excellent inflow. Note that the medial attachments (pes anserinus) to the medial tibial tuberosity have been preserved in this case. The next step in this sequence was reapplying proximal control, decompressing the interposition graft, and tunneling it behind the knee (anatomic location) to the below-knee position for the distal anastamosis.

thrombectomy and infusion of local-regional heparin. The fracture is then reduced and fixated, and then, the shunt is removed and formal vascular repair performed.

Patency of the shunt can be confirmed using continuous wave Doppler. The most commonly used shunts are the smaller (8- or 10-French) Argyl, the shorter (15 cm) Sundt, or the Javid (Fig. 2). Experience has shown that shunts placed in larger proximal arteries and veins such as those in the case description are quite effective and remain patent without anticoagulation for a period of hours in most cases. In contrast, shunts are less likely to remain patent over longer periods of time when placed in the smaller tibial vessels of the leg.

Vein Repair

Repair of lower extremity vein injuries resulting from penetrating injuries should be considered and performed on a selective basis (i.e., repair some but not all). Foremost, there is no role for repair of small tibial level veins, which should be ligated if they are bleeding. In most cases, more proximal (popliteal and femoral) extremity vein repair is not indicated as the collateral venous drainage compensates for ligation of the injury. However, in cases of extensive penetrating soft tissue injury in which the collateral network has been disrupted or in cases of larger proximal, watershed veins, repair is often necessary to avoid the sequelae of venous hypertension. Specifically, the author has pursued repair of the proximal superficial and common femoral veins as a matter of routine if there is evidence of interruption of collaterals and significant venous hypertension (i.e., significant pressure gradient). Experience from this and the Vietnam War has also showed a benefit to limb salvage associated with selective popliteal vein repair (Fig. 5). If lower extremity vein repair has been accomplished, the authors prefer to place an intermittent pneumatic compression device around the slightly elevated leg to augment flow through the repair in the immediate and early postoperative period. Importantly, vein repair must also be considered in context of the patient's overall injury constellation and physiologic status. In cases in which the patient has had prolonged operating for other life- or limb-threatening injuries or in which the flow of casualties does not permit additional operating time, proximal lower extremity vein injuries should be ligated (or shunted) as a matter of damage control.

Anticoagulation

Heparin sulfate as an anticoagulant should be used when possible in the setting of lower extremity vascular injury and repair. In cases where the injury is isolated and not associated with a large soft tissue wound, normal or full doses (50 to 75 U/kg) of systemic heparin can be given at the time that the arterial injury is being explored. If the patient has other injuries or a large soft tissue wound that precludes the use of systemic anticoagulation, "regional" heparin can be administered in the form of heparinized saline solution. Typically, heparinize saline contains anywhere between 1000 and 10,000 U of heparin per liter of sterile saline, and this can be flushed proximal and distal to the vascular reconstruction as well as used to irrigate the vessel during the time of repair. Unless there are untoward events that accompany the vascular repair such as large amounts of distal thrombus or a repair that thromboses and requires revision, the use of heparin in the postoperative period is not required.

The two scenarios in which low-dose systemic heparin may be necessary in the postoperative period are the uncommon tibial artery revascularization and the more proximal popliteal or femoral vein repair (Fig. 5). Because of the tenuous nature and a lower flow rates associated with these reconstructions, it is the author's preference to use systemic anticoagulation in these cases.

Fasciotomy

Prophylactic lower extremity fasciotomy is recommended in cases of prolonged ischemic time (4 to 6 hours), significant blast or crush injury, and large volume resuscitation. Prophylactic fasciotomy is also recommended in cases in which the patient will not be able to be examined by the treating surgeon (i.e., cases of continued evacuation) and in cases in which the patient will not be able to participate the postoperative physical examination (i.e., continued sedation and ventilation).

Fasciotomy of the leg requires opening of four compartments through two (medial and lateral) generous incisions. The posterior superficial and deep compartments are released through a medial incision beginning just distal to the medial tibial tuberosity, extending to within 4 to 5 cm of the medial malleolus. Importantly, the posterior deep compartment can only be released by dividing the fibrous attachment of the soleus muscle from the inferior aspect of the tibia along its length. A common mistake involves opening only the posterior superficial compartment of the leg, which contains no significant neurovascular structures, while neglecting the deep compartment, which houses the posterior tibial and peroneal vessels and the tibial nerve. The anterior and lateral compartments of the leg are opened using a lateral incision positioned 2 to 3 cm inferior to the lateral edge of the tibia and nearly the same extent as the medial approach. During this aspect of the procedure, one must be sure to generously open of the anterior compartment, which houses the anterior tibial artery and the deep peroneal nerve. Fasciotomy wounds can be covered with a moist dressing and loose wrap or with variations of the closed, negative pressure wound therapy devices.

Postoperative Care and Management

The lower extremity must be closely monitored in the postoperative setting including repeat assessment for adequate perfusion. In most instances, this is performed with a continuous wave Doppler machine and pen, although a duplex ultrasound is also useful in the mid- and longer-term period.

If vascular reconstruction has been performed (primary, patch, or interposition repair), duplex surveillance of the repair should be performed at 6 and 12 months after the operation. Annual duplex ultrasounds of the reconstruction are desired thereafter, although these can be difficult to continue in younger trauma patients. Other considerations in the postoperative period include managing any complex open wounds and the mid- and long-term management of the lower extremity fracture(s), both of which are beyond the scope of this chapter.

Case Conclusion

In the case vignette, the patient was taken to the operating room where the above-knee penetrating wound was explored revealing patent popliteal artery and vein shunts (Fig. 2). Following administration of systemic heparin and control of the vessels, the shunts were removed and the transected vessels repaired with greater saphenous vein interposition grafts from the contralateral extremity. In this case, the venous shunt was removed first with interposition repair of the venous injury (nonreversed greater saphenous vein) followed by a similar repair of the popliteal artery (reversed greater saphenous vein). After vascular repair, patency was confirmed with continuous wave Doppler and the wound closed over a closed suction (Jackson-Pratt) drain. The fasciotomy incisions were covered with a closed, negative pressure wound therapy dressing or device. Because of the venous repair, the patient had an intermittent pneumatic compression on the leg and the leg slightly elevated in the immediate and early postoperative period.

TAKE HOME POINTS

- Complete neurovascular exam should be documented with any penetrating trauma—determine hard signs and soft signs.
- Hard signs of injury mandate operative exploration and repair; soft signs may allow observation or later therapy.
- Triage injuries: life over limb and a limb tourniquet use can be lifesaving.
- Damage control operative approach is indicated in multiply injured patients, and the use of a temporary

arterial shunt is indicated if transport to another center or stabilization is required.
- Reduce fracture first—often, impaired blood flow will improve to normal.
- Definitive revascularization should be with autologous tissue, usually greater saphenous vein.

SUGGESTED READINGS

Burkhardt GE, Cox M, Clouse WD, et al. Outcomes of selective tibial artery repair following combat-related extremity injury. *J Vasc Surg.* 2010;52(1):91-96.

Clouse WD, Rasmussen TE, Peck MA, et al. In theater management of wartime vascular injury: a report from Operation Iraqi Freedom. *J Am Coll Surg.* 2007;204(4):625-632.

Gifford SM, Aidinian G, Clouse WD, et al. Effect of temporary vascular shunting on extremity vascular injury: an outcome analysis from the GWOT vascular initiative. *J Vasc Surg.* 2009;50(3):549-555.

Rasmussen TE, Clouse WD, Jenkins DH, et al. The use of temporary vascular shunts as a damage control adjunct in the management of wartime vascular injury. *J Trauma.* 2006;61(1):15-21.

White JM, Stannard A, Burkhardt GE, et al. The epidemiology of vascular injury in the wars in Iraq and Afghanistan. *Ann Surg.* 2011;253(6):1184-1189.

Woodward EB, Clouse WD, Eliason JE, et al. Penetrating Femoropopliteal injury during modern warfare: experience of the Balad Vascular Registry. *J Vasc Surg.* 2008;47:1259-1265.

CLINICAL SCENARIO CASE QUESTIONS

1. A 47-year-old man sustains gunshot wounds to his abdomen and left leg. He is hemodynamically stable, but has obvious ischemia of his leg without pedal pulses. The next steps in triage of care for this patient would be:
   a. Duplex exam of LLE, if arterial occlusion documented, place temporary shunt
   b. Arteriogram with possible recanalization and stent; then explore abdomen for definitive therapy
   c. Heparinization and exploration of his abdominal injury
   d. Tourniquet application without inflation, exploration and placement of arterial shunt, explore abdomen for definitive therapy
   e. Tourniquet application, heparinization, explore abdomen for definitive therapy, placement of arterial shunt

2. Which compartment in the lower leg is most likely to be missed when doing a four-compartment fasciotomy?
   a. Anterior
   b. Superficial posterior
   c. Deep posterior
   d. Lateral
   e. Both lateral and superficial posterior

123 Compartment Syndrome

MARK R. HEMMILA

Presentation

A 31-year-old man with no significant past medical history presents to the emergency department 3 hours following an altercation. He has multiple gunshot wounds in his left anterior thigh from a handgun, and a small amount of blood is emanating from these wounds. On physical examination, he has an obvious left femur deformity with swelling in the region of the wound and associated long bone instability. Examination of bilateral lower extremities reveals a cool, mottled left lower extremity with numbness and weakness in the foot. The right femoral, popliteal, dorsalis pedis, and posterior tibial pulses are all easily palpable and normal. The left femoral pulse is 2+, and the left popliteal, dorsalis pedis, and posterior tibial pulses are absent on both palpation and Doppler interrogation.

Differential Diagnosis

Potential injured neurovascular structures in this patient include the superficial femoral artery, popliteal artery, superficial femoral vein, popliteal vein, and sciatic nerve. The neurologic changes can be associated with direct trauma to the peripheral nerves or secondary injury from ischemia. Concern for compartment syndrome should be entertained secondary to potential vascular injury with ischemia and the presence of long bone fractures with associated swelling.

Compartment syndrome develops when tissue expansion in a rigidly confined space generates pressure that exceeds the capillary perfusion pressure of the tissue residing in the closed space.

Noncompliance of the fascial envelope leads to a rapid increase in the compartmental pressure, which may exceed the capillary perfusion pressure. This causes further ischemia, added tissue injury, more edema, and increased pressure—a cycle that eventually results in severe and permanent tissue damage. Traditionally, compartment syndrome has been considered a disease of the fascial compartments that enclose muscle and neurovascular structures within the extremities. However, compartment syndrome can occur in other fascial compartments of the body, such as the abdomen. The development of compartment syndrome is usually an unavoidable process associated with trauma or acute vascular occlusion and ischemia. However, permanent damage to the compartmental contents is preventable and in most circumstances represents a delay in diagnosis or inadequate treatment.

Compartment syndrome should be considered in every patient with an injured extremity or acute vascular compromise. Conditions that are associated with a high incidence of compartment syndrome include fractures, crush injuries, large volume resuscitation, acute arterial compromise, and acute venous occlusion. Less common potential causes of compartment syndrome are a tight dressing or cast, eschar from a circumferential burn, soft tissue swelling from envenomation, and application of military antishock trousers.

The five Ps (pain, paresthesias, paralysis, pulselessness, and pallor) are a common mnemonic for signs and symptoms consistent with compartment syndrome. Pain out of proportion to the severity of injury is a sensitive symptom in an awake patient. Stretching of the muscle group involved often exacerbates the pain caused by excessive pressure in the compartment. The appearance of paresthesias can be early, and sensory abnormalities are indicators of nerve compression and ischemia. Paralysis is typically a late finding due to prolonged nerve compression or irreversible muscle damage. Pulselessness from compartment syndrome alone is a late event and indicates a delay in diagnosis. Often, pulselessness results from acute occlusion of the artery from emboli, thrombus, or trauma and initiates the tissue ischemia leading to compartment syndrome. Early discovery of pulselessness and paralysis, which are typically late findings in the setting of compartment syndrome, should raise the possibility of neurovascular injury. As pressure builds in the compartment, it causes compression of the capillaries, leading to decreased skin perfusion and localized pallor. Physical examination revealing a tense, firm extremity during palpation of the tissue is worrisome and can be easily compared to the contralateral fascial compartment.

Open long bone fractures with extensive soft tissue injury is an unusual setting in which compartment syndrome can occur. A common pitfall is to assume that the open nature of injury provides complete decompression. This rationale is false and can lead to catastrophic results.

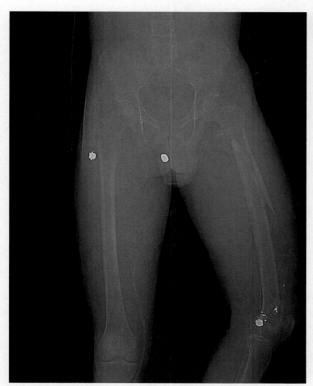

FIGURE 1 • Computed tomography scan scout film.

Initial treatment should be triggered when suspicion arises for compartment syndrome based on clinical findings. Orthopedic casts or tight dressings are removed; escharotomies are performed in burn patients. If the patient's symptoms do not improve, a decompressive fasciotomy is indicated. In equivocal cases, measurement of the compartment pressure may be helpful. No established benefit has been proven in humans from the administration of pharmacologic agents such as antioxidants or mannitol.

Workup

The patient undergoes performance of a pelvic x-ray and plane film examination. To evaluate for vascular injury, a computed tomography angiogram is obtained of the left lower extremity. Findings are a severely comminuted fracture of left proximal femur diaphysis and left medial femoral condyle extending into the distal femoral metadiaphysis with possible extension to the articular surface. Soft tissue changes with adjacent foreign bodies consistent with history of gunshot wound (Fig. 1). There is a high-grade laceration of the left superficial femoral artery with associated pseudoaneurysm and thrombosis (Fig. 2).

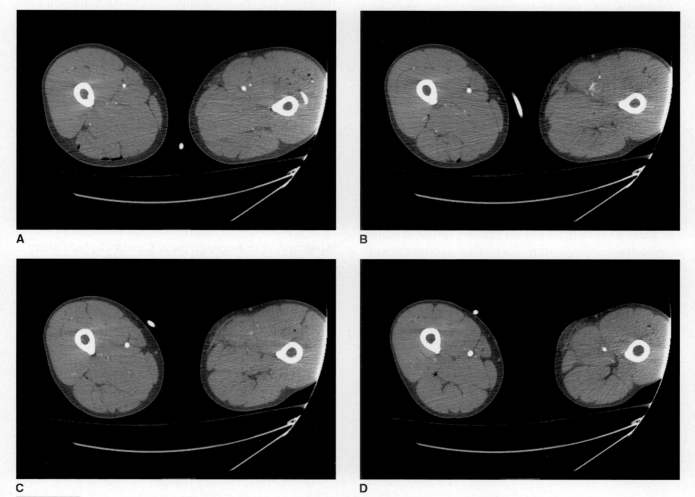

FIGURE 2 • Selected cuts of CT angiogram through bilateral thighs (**A**, proximal; **B and C**, mid; **D**, distal).

Diagnosis and Treatment

The patient is taken emergently to the operating room where he undergoes rigid sigmoidoscopy to rule out rectal injury. This is followed by left medial thigh exposure of the superficial femoral and popliteal artery, debridement of the damaged arterial tissue, thromboembolectomy of the popliteal and both tibial arteries, and placement of a temporary arterial shunt. Orthopedic surgery stabilizes his femur fracture by placing a spanning external fixator and performs arthroscopic irrigation and debridement of the left knee. Definitive vascular repair is performed by placing a 6-cm segment of saphenous vein graft to replace the damaged artery. It is now 7 hours since his injury and 1 hour since his left lower extremity was revascularized.

This extremity has been ischemic for 6 hours. Arterial circulation has been reestablished, and the patient is currently in the reperfusion period. Concern for compartment syndrome of the left lower leg should be extremely high based on the injury sustained, duration of ischemia, and the preoperative neurologic examination. Three options exist: (1) assume presence of compartment syndrome based on the history of the case and immediately perform four-compartment fasciotomies, (2) measure compartment pressures and proceed with fasciotomy if values greater than 25 to 30 mm Hg are obtained, and (3) observe the patient postoperatively for signs and symptoms of compartment syndrome and return to the operating room for fasciotomy if clinically indicated. You choose option 1 as the safest approach for the patient in this case. Option 3 requires an awake, cooperative patient, with the ability to perform hourly neurovascular examinations. To safely pursue option 3, the patient must have no neurologic deficits preoperatively or postoperatively and must have the ability to return promptly to the operating room should the need for fasciotomy arise.

Surgical Approach

Release of pressure in the compartment is performed by longitudinally incising the fascia in one location per compartment in the affected extremity. In general, all compartments of the involved portion of the extremity should undergo fasciotomy. The calf has 4 compartments, the thigh 2, the foot 10, the arm 3, and the forearm 2. Following release of the compartment, the exposed muscle should be assessed clinically for tissue damage and viability. Does it bulge through the fascial incision? Is it beefy red or dusky, purple, gray, black, or brown? Does the muscle contract when stimulated with the electrocautery? All clearly nonviable tissue should be debrided. Equivocal tissue should be reassessed for viability with serial examinations, and the patient returned to the operating room for debridement if marginal tissue progresses to nonviability.

The standard incisions for a four-compartment lower leg fasciotomy are lateral and medial through the skin of the calf (Table 1). The lateral incision is placed slightly

TABLE 1. Key Technical Steps and Potential Pitfalls

Key Technical Steps

1. Identification of need for fasciotomy.
2. Placement of medial and lateral incision.
3. Finding of intermuscular septum and opening of both compartments (lateral: anterior and posterior, medial: superficial and deep).
4. Elevate fascia off of muscle with blunt, closed, upturned tip of Metzenbaum scissors.
5. Use push technique to divide fascia in cephalad and caudad direction with slightly opened tips (0.5 cm) of sharp Metzenbaum scissors.

Potential Pitfalls

- Inadequate fasciotomy length
- Failure to open all four compartments
- Peroneal nerve injury

anterior to the fibula and lateral to the anterior tibial crest. This provides access to the anterior and lateral compartments of the lower leg. Creating a short transverse incision through the leg fascia can aid in locating the intramuscular septum between the two compartments. The superficial peroneal nerve lies posterior to this membrane in the lateral compartment. When longitudinally dividing the fascia of the lateral compartment, care must be taken to avoid dividing or injuring this nerve. The medial incision is created 2 cm posterior to the posterior crest of the tibia, which is midway between the anterior and posterior calf borders. The surgeon should avoid injuring the saphenous nerve and vein. Another transverse incision is made to identify the intramuscular septum between the superficial and deep posterior compartments. Using Metzenbaum scissors, longitudinal fasciotomies are performed to open the two posterior compartments. Generous skin incisions should be made and usually run at least 15 to 20 cm in length. If any doubt is present about the adequacy of fasciotomy, the incisions in the skin and fascia should be extended until this uncertainty is eliminated.

Special Intraoperative Considerations: Measurement of Compartment Pressures

Intracompartmental tissue pressure in the extremities can be measured directly using a sterile needle connected to a pressure transducer. A commercial device manufactured by Stryker Instruments (Stryker Corporation, Kalamazoo, MI) is commonly used for this purpose (Fig. 3) and has a needle with a side hole to avoid incorrect readings from tissue occlusion of the needle lumen. To perform a pressure measurement, the skin over the central region of the compartment is swabbed with aseptic solution and anesthetized with local anesthetic. A tiny incision is made in the skin with a No. 11 scalpel blade, and the needle of the pressure transducer is inserted through the opening

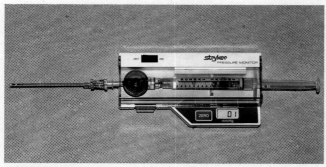

FIGURE 3 • Stryker intracompartmental pressure monitor.

and advanced until it penetrates the fascia surrounding the compartment to be measured. A small amount (0.5 mL) of saline is injected and the equilibrated pressure measured. It is important to measure all of the individual compartments in the region of interest because the different compartments can have elevated pressures independent of each other. A pressure of less than 10 mm Hg is considered normal. Pressures of 10 to 20 mm Hg are considered mildly elevated, but present a low risk for permanent tissue injury. The capillary hemostatic pressure in a normal patient is 35 mm Hg. Thus, a pressure greater than 30 mm Hg with clinical signs is indicative of compartment syndrome and requires immediate fasciotomy. Pressures between 20 and 30 mm Hg represent a "gray zone" where the concern for compartment syndrome must be entertained, but the choice to perform a fasciotomy is usually correlated with the clinical course and whether or not continued tissue swelling is expected. It must be emphasized that pressure measurements are not a substitute for sound clinical judgment and prudent operative management when compartment syndrome is suspected.

Postoperative Management

Many different techniques exist for managing the open wound following a lower extremity fasciotomy. The "Roman sandal"technique involves placement of surgical stables parallel to the wound edges and lacing the staples with a crisscrossing elastic vessel loop that can be tightened gradually over time. Sterile dressings can be placed over this setup. Alternatively, a wound vacuum can be utilized. Bridging the two wounds with a piece of sponge allows for a single vacuum line to be used per extremity. Dressings should be nonrestrictive and allow for continued examination of the tissue to assess viability and swelling. Returning the patient to the operating room every few days for examination, debridement, and gradual wound closure is recommended. Most wounds can eventually be closed with dermal and skin sutures. No attempts should be made to reclose the fascia. Wounds that cannot achieve skin closure are treated with placement of a meshed split-thickness skin graft.

Case Conclusion

A four-compartment, two-incision left lower extremity fasciotomy is performed. Extensive bulging of the muscle bellies through the fasciotomy and skin openings occurs. The open skin wound is approximated using staples, elastic vessel loops, and the shoelace technique. Two days later, the patient is taken to the operating room by orthopedic surgery for removal of his external fixator and open reduction and internal fixation of his left supracondylar femur fracture. The skin incisions of his fasciotomy wounds are closed with a combination of delayed primary closure and split-thickness skin grafting on postinjury day 10.

TAKE HOME POINTS

- Most of the negative sequelae from compartment syndrome can be avoided by early diagnosis if the clinician has a high index of suspicion.
- Implement appropriate monitoring in patients who are at risk for elevated compartmental pressures as well as correcting the underlying cause (e.g., acute limb ischemia).
- Pain out of proportion to the injury sustained is an important finding in the setting of potential compartment syndrome and should not be ignored.
- Correlation of the history, physical findings, and pressure measurements will yield the best results when ruling in or out the diagnosis of compartment syndrome.
- Be wary of overlying dressings, tight casts, and splints in the newly injured patient, and be vigilant in examining these patients for signs and symptoms of compartment syndrome.
- When performing a fasciotomy and caring for patients with fasciotomies, use sterile technique because infection of the muscle tissue can lead to further tissue loss and morbidity.

SUGGESTED READINGS

Bergstein JM. Extremity compartment syndrome. In: Cameron JL, ed. *Current Surgical Therapy.* 7th ed. St. Louis, MO: Mosby; 2001:1140-1144.

Blaisdell FW. The pathophysiology of skeletal muscle ischemia and the reperfusion syndrome: a review. *Cardiovasc Surg.* 2002;10:620-630.

Farber A, Tan TW, Hamburg NM, et al. Early fasciotomy in patients with extremity vascular injury is associated with decreased risk of adverse limb outcomes: a review of the National Trauma Data Bank. *Injury.* 2012;43:1486-1491.

Kragh JF Jr, San Antonio J, Simmons JW, et al. Compartment syndrome performance improvement project is associated with increased combat casualty survival. *J Trauma Acute Care Surg.* 2013;74:259-263.

Nypaver T. Fasciotomy in vascular trauma and compartment syndrome. In: Ernst CB, Stanley JC, eds. *Current Therapy in Vascular Surgery.* 4th ed. St. Louis, MO: Mosby; 2001:624-628.

Ulmer T. The clinical diagnosis of compartment syndrome of the lower leg: are clinical findings predictive of the disorder? *J Orthop Trauma.* 2002;16:572-577.

Velmahos GC, Toutouzas KG. Vascular trauma and compartment syndromes. *Surg Clin North Am.* 2002;82:125-141.

CLINICAL SCENARIO CASE QUESTIONS

1. What is the normal capillary hydrostatic pressure in the lower leg?
   a. 10 mm Hg
   b. 20 mm Hg
   c. 35 mm Hg
   d. 50 mm Hg

2. Which are risk factors for compartment syndrome?
   a. Vascular injury
   b. Long bone injury
   c. Tight cast
   d. Soft tissue injury with swelling
   e. All of the above

124 Intravenous Drug Injection into Femoral Artery

JEFFREY R. RUBIN and YEVGENIY RITS

Presentation

A 63-year-old man underwent noninvasive vascular studies for a pulsatile ulcerated mass in the right groin. The patient had been admitted to the medicine service with complaints of fever and chills with a history of intravenous drug use since the age of 14. The patient admits to a recent injection of heroin into the right groin vessels.

While being held in the waiting area of the inpatient vascular laboratory, the patient complained of a warm sensation in the right groin spreading over the right leg. He was found to have active pulsatile bleeding originating from right groin area. A medical code was called, and the ultrasound technician applied direct pressure to the groin. Upon the evaluation by the on-call physicians, vascular surgery was called and the patient was taken directly to the operating room for resuscitation and emergent groin exploration.

Differential Diagnosis

The differential diagnosis of a pulsatile mass in the groin, in a patient with a history of intravenous drug use, includes a mycotic aneurysm, or an infected pseudoaneurysm of the femoral artery. With local signs of infection, skin changes, mass expansion, and/or bleeding, no further evaluation is necessary and surgical exploration is required.

Laboratory Data and Imaging

Groin abscesses in patients with a history of drug use should never be drained without thorough investigation. Radiographic studies should be focused on confirming the diagnosis, mapping of the involved vessels, identifying the associated pathology, and the planning of surgery.

With a history of a pulsatile mass and intravenous drug abuse (IVDA), without local symptoms or signs of impeding rupture (skin changes, erythema, drainage, and local expansion), several additional tests could be helpful. Vascular duplex ultrasound is the least invasive, least expensive, and the easiest to obtain for evaluating the nature of the mass, that is, pseudoaneurysm versus true mycotic aneurysm, or abscess, as well as the size and extent of the arterial involvement. Vein mapping of both legs may also be helpful for surgical planning. CT scan is more expensive and not as accessible as ultrasound, but is more accurate and sensitive for determining anatomical location, tissue planes, and extent of the arterial involvement.

Laboratory information should include type and cross-match, coagulation studies, sedimentation rate, and blood cultures.

Case Continued

The patient was brought to the operating room, with pressure being applied to the groin. Both groins, abdomen, and legs were prepped, and patient was intubated. A "hockey stick" incision was made in the right lower abdomen 3 to 5 cm above the inguinal ligament. A standard retroperitoneal exposure of the external iliac artery was performed, and proximal control was achieved. The patient was heparinized, and distal control of the femoral artery was achieved distal to the area of rupture, obtaining control of the superficial and profunda femoral arteries (Fig. 1). Two sets of instruments were separately used for clean and contaminated portions of the procedure to minimize cross-contamination. Contralateral saphenous vein was harvested for the reconstruction. The infected common femoral, proximal superficial, and profunda femoral arteries were resected, and the area was widely debrided and curetted. Stat Gram stains were taken of the remaining margins and were debrided until they were negative for presence of bacteria. A distal external iliac artery to profunda femoris bypass was performed with reversed saphenous vein, and a jump graft was performed to the superficial femoral artery (SFA) (Fig. 2). Anastomoses were covered with a sartorius muscle flap. A vacuum-assisted dressing was applied. The patient was initially placed on broad-spectrum antibiotics, and these

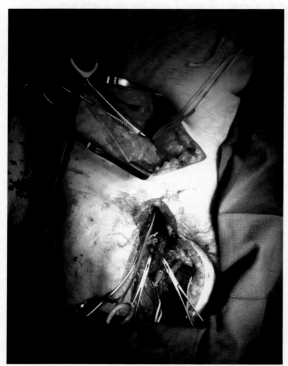

FIGURE 1 • Retroperitoneal exposure for proximal control (*arrow*). Standard femoral exposure for the distal control (*double arrow*). **A:** Clamp on eternal iliac artery. **B:** Profunda femoris artery. **C:** Superficial femoral artery.

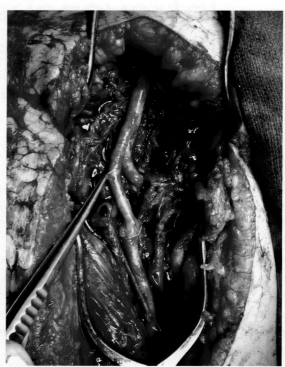

FIGURE 2 • External iliac to profunda and superficial femoral arteries bypass with the reversed greater saphenous vein.

were adjusted to organism-specific antibiotics, which were given intravenously for 6 weeks.

Discussion

The groin is the most common area of septic complications in the intravenous drug abuser. The incidence of mycotic pseudoaneurysm is unknown; however, a study by Tsao et al., that reviewed 7795 hospital visits related to IVDA, resulted in 11 pseudoaneurysms with an annual prevalence of 0.14%. The right groin and upper thigh are the most often used areas for the intravenous drug user. Infected femoral pseudoaneurysms are usually the result of repetitive needlestick injuries; however, septic emboli to the arterial wall have also been reported.

Most patients present with painful swelling and erythema. Seventy percent of pseudoaneurysms are associated with a pulsatile mass. A rapidly expanding mass and free rupture with skin erosion present less commonly. Vascular compromise with extremity ischemia is uncommon.

Broad-spectrum antibiotics should be started immediately to cover polymicrobial flora. The most common organism found in the mycotic pseudoaneurysm is *Staphylococcus aureus*, which may be methicillin resistant. Mixed cultures with pseudomonas species, yeast, and genitourinary flora are also frequently reported. Patients are often immunosuppressed due to malnourishment

and/or from concomitant infection with human immunodeficiency virus and hepatitis C.

Endovascular therapy for mycotic pseudoaneurysm is limited to emergent isolation techniques for proximal and distal control and has no true long-term therapeutic value. Endovascular therapy has been reported for the ruptured anastomotic pseudoaneurysm. Standard therapy is surgical exploration with wide local debridement of the infected tissues. There have been many proponents of ligation without immediate revascularization since the rate of reinfection is high. Simple ligation of the SFA results in a high rate of amputation as high as 85%. This is based on the military wound experience. Reddy et al. reported a 33% incidence of amputation in patients that underwent common femoral artery (CFA) ligation, without revascularization. To the contrary, if after ligation of the femoral vessels, the patient has Doppler signals, several studies reported 100% limb salvage. Delayed vascular reconstruction with extra-anatomic bypass, if the patient develops severe ischemia, is also possible. Muscle coverage, especially with sartorius muscle flap, decreases chances of anastomotic breakdown.

Intravenous broad-spectrum antibiotics should be started immediately upon presentation and modified once sensitivity results are available. We recommend 6 weeks of intravenous antibiotics followed by oral antibiotics for 6 months if a bypass was inserted or if contamination is severe (Table 1).

TABLE 1. Key Technical Steps and Potential Pitfalls

Key Technical Steps

1. Always admit.
2. If actively bleeding, go directly to the OR.
3. If not actively bleeding, obtain duplex ultrasound or CTA.
4. Resect all infected artery.
5. Reconstruct with autologous tissue.
6. Continue IV antibiotics for at least 6 weeks.

Potential Pitfalls

- Nonrecognition and not obtaining history of IVDA.
- Do not use prosthetic material in infected bed.
- Not covering autologous repair with soft tissue, preferably muscle.

Case Conclusion

The patient was followed at home by a visiting nurse who changed the negative pressure dressing per routine and administered IV antibiotic therapy. Two weeks later, the patient was seen in clinic and was doing well. At 6 weeks, the patient's wound was completely granulated and was ready for skin graft (Fig. 3). After the wound was completely healed, a duplex ultrasound examination was performed for baseline and scanning is performed every 6 months for the first year and annually thereafter if test results are unremarkable.

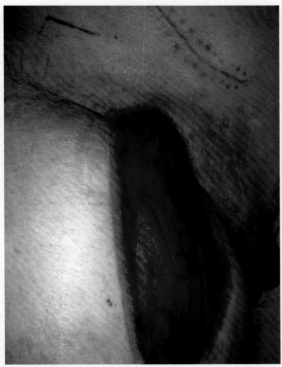

FIGURE 3 • Wound prior to the split-thickness skin graft.

TAKE HOME POINTS

- Admit all patients with pulsatile femoral masses in clinical setting consistent with infection given potential for rupture and exsanguination, start empirical antibiotics and type, and cross for blood.
- Duplex ultrasonography is the first-line diagnostic modality for suspected femoral mycotic aneurysms.
- Autologous tissue reconstruction is suggested given the acuity and virulence of the likely bacterial infection.
- Consider extra-anatomical routes when necessary.
- Soft tissue well-vascularized muscle flaps in conjunction with VAC wound therapy are effective.

SUGGESTED READINGS

Arora S, et al. Common femoral artery ligation and local debridement: a safe treatment for infected femoral artery pseudoaneurysms. *J Vasc Surg.* 2001;33(5):990-993.

Chan YC, Burnand KG. Management of septic groin complications and infected femoral false aneurysms in intravenous drug abusers. *Br J Surg.* 2006;93(7):781-782.

De BM, Simeone FA. Battle injuries of the arteries in World War II; an analysis of 2,471 cases. *Ann Surg.* 1946;123:534-579.

Jayaraman S, et al. Mycotic pseudoaneurysms due to injection drug use: a ten-year experience. *Ann Vasc Surg.* 2012;26(6):819-824.

Klonaris C, et al. Emergency stenting of a ruptured infected anastomotic femoral pseudoaneurysm. *Cardiovasc Intervent Radiol.* 2007;30(6):1238-1241.

Peirce C, et al. The management of mycotic femoral pseudoaneurysms in intravenous drug abusers. *Ann Vasc Surg.* 2009;23(3):345-349.

Reddy DJ, et al. Infected femoral artery false aneurysms in drug addicts: evolution of selective vascular reconstruction. *J Vasc Surg.* 1986;3(5):718-724.

Tsao JW, et al. Presentation, diagnosis, and management of arterial mycotic pseudoaneurysms in injection drug users. *Ann Vasc Surg.* 2002;16(5):652-662.

CLINICAL SCENARIO CASE QUESTIONS

1. A 30-year-old man with IVDA history presents to the ER with a 24-hour history of fever, pain, swelling, and redness in the left groin. On exam, a tender pulsatile mass is noted with overlying cellulitis. The first choice in diagnostic testing includes:

   a. Nothing; admit and take to OR for incision and drainage
   b. Duplex ultrasound
   c. CTA
   d. MRA
   e. Angiography with possible intervention

2. In a patient with a mycotic femoral aneurysm, the least good choice for arterial reconstruction is:

   a. Autologous saphenous vein with muscle flap coverage
   b. Obturator bypass with autologous vein
   c. Dacron interposition grafting with coverage and closed suction drainage
   d. Arterial homograft with muscle flap coverage
   e. Femoral vein reconstruction with closed suction drainage

Answer Key

Chapter 1: E, E

Chapter 2: D, C

Chapter 3: E, A

Chapter 4: B, C

Chapter 5: D, C

Chapter 6: C, D

Chapter 7: D, D

Chapter 8: C, D

Chapter 9: D, D

Chapter 10: D, C

Chapter 11: C, A

Chapter 12: C, B

Chapter 13: D, A

Chapter 14: A, B

Chapter 15: B, D

Chapter 16: C, B

Chapter 17: A, D

Chapter 18: B, E

Chapter 19: D, C

Chapter 20: C, D

Chapter 21: C, D

Chapter 22: C, C

Chapter 23: A, B

Chapter 24: B, A-E

Chapter 25: D, C

Chapter 26: D, B

Chapter 27: E, A

Chapter 28: B, D

Chapter 29: B, C

Chapter 30: D, D

Chapter 31: A, C

Chapter 32: B, C

Chapter 33: C, B

Chapter 34: B, D

Chapter 35: C, E

Chapter 36: B, C

Chapter 37: B, C

Chapter 38: C, D

Chapter 39: E, A

Chapter 40: C, D

Chapter 41: D, D

Chapter 42: C, B

Chapter 43: E, B

Chapter 44: B, C

Chapter 45: E, E

Chapter 46: A, B

Chapter 47: C, C

Chapter 48: C, B

Chapter 49: C, B

Chapter 50: E, D

Chapter 51: C, B

Chapter 52: C, B

Chapter 53: D, A

Chapter 54: D, E

Chapter 55: C, B

Chapter 56: D, D

Chapter 57: B, C

Chapter 58: B, D

Chapter 59: B, D

Chapter 60: B, B, C

Chapter 61: A, A

Chapter 62: B, C

Chapter 63: B, C

Chapter 64: C, D

Chapter 65: C, A

Chapter 66: D, E

Chapter 67: B, E

Chapter 68: C, D

Chapter 69: D, B

Chapter 70: B, C

Chapter 71: E, C

Chapter 72: A, C

Chapter 73: D, C

Chapter 74: D, B

Chapter 75: B, E

Chapter 76: D, B

Chapter 77: D, D

Chapter 78: D, E

Chapter 79: C, A

Chapter 80: E, A

Chapter 81: A, A

Chapter 82: B, D

Chapter 83: D, A

Chapter 84: D, E

Chapter 85: E, C

Chapter 86: B, B

Chapter 87: E, B

Chapter 88: B, C

Chapter 89: D, C

Chapter 90: A, B

Chapter 91: B, C

Chapter 92: C, C

Chapter 93: B, A

Chapter 94: D, C

Chapter 95: D, C

Chapter 96: D, A

Chapter 97: B, C

Chapter 98: B, E

Chapter 99: B, D

Chapter 100: C, C

Chapter 101: C, B

Chapter 102: E, D

Chapter 103: A, C

Chapter 104: D, B

Chapter 105: C, D

Chapter 106: D, C

Chapter 107: C, C

Chapter 108: C, B

Chapter 109: C, D

Chapter 110: E, C

Chapter 111: C, E

Chapter 112: D, B

Chapter 113: C, B

Chapter 114: C, B

Chapter 115: D, E

Chapter 116: D, C

Chapter 117: D, D

Chapter 118: B, D

Chapter 119: C, D

Chapter 120: C, D

Chapter 121: C, D

Chapter 122: D, C

Chapter 123: A, E

Chapter 124: B, C

Index

Notes: Page numbers followed by f denote figures; those followed by a t denote tables.